NETTER'S
CARDIOLOGY

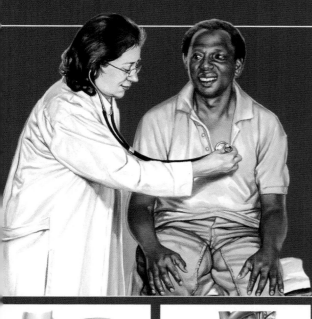

NETTER'S CARDIOLOGY

3rd EDITION

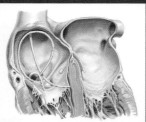 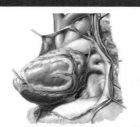 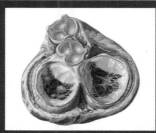 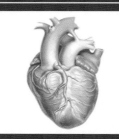 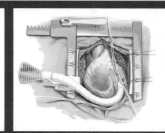

EDITED BY

George A. Stouffer, MD
Ernest and Hazel Craige Distinguished Professor of Medicine
Chief, Division of Cardiology
Physician in Chief, UNC Heart and Vascular Service Line
University of North Carolina at Chapel Hill
Chapel Hill, North Carolina

Marschall S. Runge, MD, PhD
Professor of Internal Medicine
Dean, University of Michigan Medical School
Executive Vice President for Medical Affairs
Chief Executive Officer, Michigan Medicine
Ann Arbor, Michigan

Cam Patterson, MD, MBA
Chancellor
University of Arkansas for Medical Sciences
Little Rock, Arkansas

Joseph S. Rossi, MD
Associate Professor of Medicine
Director, Cardiac Catheterization Laboratory
University of North Carolina at Chapel Hill
Chapel Hill, North Carolina

ILLUSTRATIONS BY

Frank H. Netter, MD

CONTRIBUTING ILLUSTRATORS

Carlos A. G. Machado, MD

John A. Craig, MD

David J. Mascaro, MS

Enid Hatton

Steven Moon, MA

Kip Carter, MS, CMI

Tiffany S. DaVanzo, MA, CMI

ELSEVIER

ELSEVIER

1600 John F. Kennedy Blvd.
Ste 1600
Philadelphia, PA 19103-2899

NETTER'S CARDIOLOGY, THIRD EDITION

ISBN: 978-0-323-54726-0

Notices

Knowledge and best practice in this field are constantly changing. As new research and experience broaden our understanding, changes in research methods, professional practices, or medical treatment may become necessary.

Practitioners and researchers must always rely on their own experience and knowledge in evaluating and using any information, methods, compounds, or experiments described herein. In using such information or methods they should be mindful of their own safety and the safety of others, including parties for whom they have a professional responsibility.

With respect to any drug or pharmaceutical products identified, readers are advised to check the most current information provided (i) on procedures featured or (ii) by the manufacturer of each product to be administered, to verify the recommended dose or formula, the method and duration of administration, and contraindications. It is the responsibility of practitioners, relying on their own experience and knowledge of their patients, to make diagnoses, to determine dosages and the best treatment for each individual patient, and to take all appropriate safety precautions.

To the fullest extent of the law, neither the Publisher nor the authors, contributors, or editors, assume any liability for any injury and/or damage to persons or property as a matter of products liability, negligence or otherwise, or from any use or operation of any methods, products, instructions, or ideas contained in the material herein.

Previous editions copyrighted 2010 and 2004.

Library of Congress Cataloging-in-Publication Data
Names: Stouffer, George A., editor. | Runge, Marschall Stevens, 1954- editor. | Patterson, Cam, editor. |
    Rossi, Joseph S., editor. | Netter, Frank H. (Frank Henry), 1906-1991, illustrator.
Title: Netter's cardiology / edited by George A. Stouffer, Marschall S. Runge, Cam Patterson, Joseph S. Rossi ;
    illustrations by Frank H. Netter ; contributing illustrations, Carlos A. G. Machado [and 6 others].
Other titles: Cardiology
Description: 3rd edition. | Philadelphia, PA : Elsevier, [2019] | Includes bibliographical references and index.
Identifiers: LCCN 2018013552 | ISBN 9780323547260 (hardcover : alk. paper)
Subjects: | MESH: Cardiovascular Diseases | Diagnostic Techniques, Cardiovascular
Classification: LCC RC667 | NLM WG 120 | DDC 616.1/2—dc23 LC record available at https://lccn.loc.
    gov/2018013552

Content Strategist: Marybeth Thiel
Publishing Services Manager: Catherine Albright Jackson
Senior Project Manager: Claire Kramer
Design Direction: Patrick Ferguson

Working together
to grow libraries in
developing countries

www.elsevier.com • www.bookaid.org

Printed in China
Last digit is the print number: 9 8 7 6 5 4 3 2 1

ABOUT THE EDITORS

George A. Stouffer, MD, was born in Indiana, Pennsylvania, and was graduated from Bucknell University and the University of Maryland, School of Medicine. He completed his internal medicine residency, cardiology fellowship, and interventional cardiology fellowship at the University of Virginia. During his cardiology fellowship, he completed a 2-year National Institutes of Health research fellowship in the laboratory of Gary Owens at the University of Virginia. He was on the faculty at the University of Texas Medical Branch from 1995 to 2000, where he became an associate professor and served as Co-Director of Clinical Trials in the Cardiology Division and as Associate Director of the Cardiac Catheterization Laboratory. He joined the faculty at the University of North Carolina in 2000 and currently serves as the Henry A. Foscue Distinguished Professor of Medicine and Chief of Cardiology. Dr. Stouffer's main focus is clinical cardiology with an emphasis on interventional cardiology, but he is also involved in clinical and basic science research. His basic science research is in the areas of regulation of smooth muscle cell growth, the role of the smooth muscle cytoskeleton in regulating signaling pathways, thrombin generation, and renal artery stenosis.

Marschall S. Runge, MD, PhD, was born in Austin, Texas, and was graduated from Vanderbilt University with a BA in general biology and a PhD in molecular biology. He received his medical degree from the Johns Hopkins School of Medicine and trained in internal medicine at Johns Hopkins Hospital. He was a cardiology fellow and junior faculty member at Massachusetts General Hospital. Dr. Runge's next position was at Emory University, where he directed the Cardiology Fellowship Training Program. He then moved to the University of Texas Medical Branch in Galveston, where he was Chief of Cardiology and Director of the Sealy Center for Molecular Cardiology. He was at the University of North Carolina from 2000 to 2015, where he served as Charles Addison and Elizabeth Ann Sanders Distinguished Professor of Medicine, Chair of the Department of Medicine, President of UNC Physicians, and Vice Dean for Clinical Affairs. He is currently Dean of the Medical School at the University of Michigan, Executive Vice President for Medical Affairs, and Chief Executive Officer of Michigan Medicine. Dr. Runge is board-certified in internal medicine and cardiovascular diseases and has spoken and published widely on topics in clinical cardiology and vascular medicine.

Cam Patterson, MD, MBA, was born in Mobile, Alabama. He was a Harold Sterling Vanderbilt Scholar and studied psychology and English at Vanderbilt University, graduating summa cum laude. Dr. Patterson attended Emory University School of Medicine, graduating with induction in the Alpha Omega Alpha Honor Society, and completed a residency in Internal Medicine at Emory University Hospitals and Chief Residency at Grady Memorial Hospital. He completed 3 years of research fellowship under the guidance of Edgar Haber at the Harvard School of Public Health, developing an independent research program in vascular biology and angiogenesis that was supported by a National Institutes of Health fellowship. He did a cardiology fellowship and was on the faculty at the University of Texas Medical Branch from 1996 to 2000. Dr. Patterson was at the University of North Carolina at Chapel Hill from 2000 to 2014 where he served as founding director of the UNC McAllister Heart Institute, Chief of Cardiology, and the Ernest and Hazel Craige Distinguished Professor of Cardiovascular Medicine. He received his MBA from the UNC Kenan-Flagler School of Business in 2008. He is an elected member of the American Society of Clinical Investigation and the Association of University Cardiologists. Until recently he was Senior Vice President and Chief Operating Officer at New York Presbyterian–Weill Cornell Medical Center and currently serves as Chancellor of the University of Arkansas for Medical Sciences.

Joseph S. Rossi, MD, was born in Hopedale, Illinois. He completed his undergraduate studies at the University of Illinois and then completed his medical education at the University of Illinois–Chicago, graduating with induction into the Alpha Omega Alpha Honor Society. He completed residency and fellowships in internal medicine, cardiovascular disease, and interventional cardiology at Northwestern University, where he also obtained a master's degree in clinical investigation. Dr. Rossi is currently the Director of the Cardiac Catheterization Lab at the University of North Carolina. He is actively involved in multiple clinical trials and has received research grants to support his interest in the pharmacogenomics of dual antiplatelet therapy and complex coronary artery revascularization among Medicare beneficiaries. Dr. Rossi is particularly interested in pairing clinical and administrative data to enhance our knowledge of trends and resource utilization for patients with advanced vascular disease.

PREFACE

Our goal for the third edition of *Netter's Cardiology* was to provide a concise and practical overview of cardiovascular medicine that has been updated to include new information and important clinical areas that were not well covered in the previous editions or in other cardiology texts. To accomplish this expansion while maintaining a focused text that could be used as a ready reference, we again avoided exhaustive treatment of topics. We also have made every effort to present the essential information in a reader-friendly format that increases the reader's ability to learn the key facts without getting lost in details that can obfuscate the learning process.

The first two editions of *Netter's Cardiology* were an effort to present in a concise and highly visual format the ever-increasing amount of medical information on cardiovascular disease. The challenge that clinicians face in "keeping up" with the medical literature has continued to grow in the 14 years since the first edition of *Netter's Cardiology*. This need to process the ever-expanding medical information base and apply new findings to the optimal care of patients is acute in all areas of medicine, but perhaps it is most challenging in disciplines that require practitioners to understand a broad spectrum of evidence-based medicine, such as the field of cardiovascular diseases. The explosion of medical knowledge is also a real educational challenge for learners at all levels—students, residents, and practicing physicians—who must rapidly determine what is and is not important, organize the key information, and then apply these principles effectively in clinical settings.

The third edition includes substantial changes. All the chapters have been updated, there is a new section on Structural Heart Disease, and new chapters have been added on Basic Anatomy and Embryology of the Heart, Stem Cell Therapies for Cardiovascular Disease, Diabetes and Cardiovascular Events, Coronary Hemodynamics and Fractional Flow Reserve, Epidemiology of Heart Failure: Heart Failure with Preserved Ejection Fraction and Heart Failure with Reduced Ejection Fraction, Management of Acute Heart Failure, Cardiac Transplantation and Mechanical Circulatory Support Devices, Cardiovascular Manifestations of Rheumatic Fever, Clinical Presentation of Adults with Congenital Heart Disease, Transcatheter Aortic Valve Replacement, Transcatheter Mitral Valve Repair, Tricuspid and Pulmonic Valve Disease, Deep Vein Thrombosis and Pulmonary Embolism, Cardiac Tumors and Cardio-oncology, and Cardiovascular Disease in the Elderly.

As in the first two editions, the contributing authors have taken advantage of the genius of Frank Netter by carefully selecting the best of his artwork to illustrate the most important clinical concepts covered in each chapter. When Netter artwork was unavailable or difficult to apply to illustrate modern clinical concepts, we again used the great artistic talents of Carlos A. G. Machado, MD, to create new artwork or to skillfully edit and update some of Frank Netter's drawings. The combination of Dr. Machado's outstanding skills as a medical artist and his knowledge of the medical concepts being illustrated was an invaluable asset.

As in the first two editions, we chose to use authors from the University of North Carolina School of Medicine at Chapel Hill or those with close ties to the university. This allowed us to select authors who are clinical authorities, many of whom are also well known for their national and international contributions. All have active clinical practices that require daily use of the information covered in their chapters, and all are well aware of the approach to patient management used by their peers at other institutions and in other practice settings. Many of the contributing authors for this edition also contributed to prior editions of this textbook. Each author, whether a previous contributor or not, was given clearly defined guidelines that emphasized the need to distill the large amount of complex information in his or her field and to present it concisely in a carefully prescribed format maintained across all chapters. The result is a text that is truly clinically useful and less of a compendium than is commonly the case in many medical texts.

We believe that the changes we have made in the third edition substantially improve *Netter's Cardiology* and ensure that it will continue to be a highly useful resource for all physicians, both generalists and subspecialists, who need to remain current in cardiology—from trainees to experienced practitioners. Whether we have succeeded will obviously be determined by our readers. We welcome the comments, suggestions, and criticisms of readers that will help us improve future editions of this work.

George A. Stouffer, MD
Ernest and Hazel Craige Distinguished Professor of Medicine
Chief, Division of Cardiology
Physician in Chief, UNC Heart and Vascular Service Line
University of North Carolina at Chapel Hill
Chapel Hill, North Carolina

Marschall S. Runge, MD, PhD
Professor of Internal Medicine
Dean, University of Michigan Medical School
Executive Vice President for Medical Affairs
Chief Executive Officer, Michigan Medicine
Ann Arbor, Michigan

Cam Patterson, MD, MBA
Chancellor
University of Arkansas for Medical Sciences
Little Rock, Arkansas

Joseph S. Rossi, MD
Associate Professor of Medicine
Director, Cardiac Catheterization Laboratory
University of North Carolina at Chapel Hill
Chapel Hill, North Carolina

Algorithms have been color coded for quick reference.

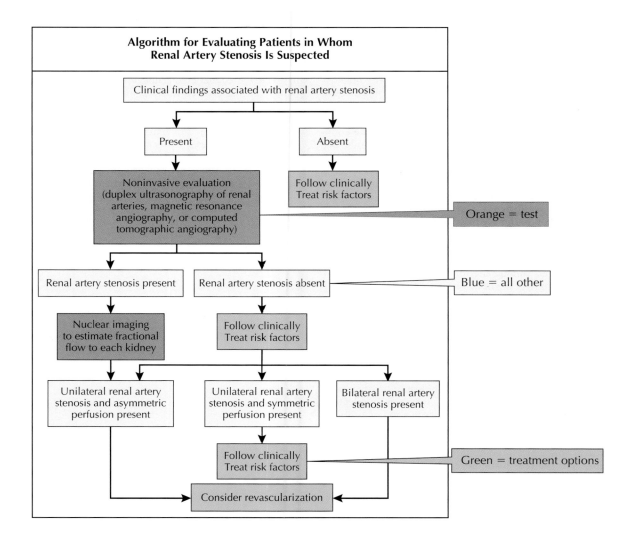

**Algorithm for Evaluating Patients in Whom
Renal Artery Stenosis Is Suspected**

Clinical findings associated with renal artery stenosis

Present

Absent

Noninvasive evaluation
(duplex ultrasonography of renal
arteries, magnetic resonance
angiography, or computed
tomographic angiography)

Follow clinically
Treat risk factors

Orange = test

Renal artery stenosis present

Renal artery stenosis absent

Blue = all other

Nuclear imaging
to estimate fractional
flow to each kidney

Follow clinically
Treat risk factors

Unilateral renal artery
stenosis and asymmetric
perfusion present

Unilateral renal artery
stenosis and symmetric
perfusion present

Bilateral renal artery
stenosis present

Follow clinically
Treat risk factors

Green = treatment options

Consider revascularization

ABOUT THE ARTISTS

Frank H. Netter, MD

Frank H. Netter was born in 1906 in New York City. He studied art at the Art Student's League and the National Academy of Design before entering medical school at New York University, where he received his medical degree in 1931. During his student years, Dr. Netter's notebook sketches attracted the attention of the medical faculty and other physicians, allowing him to augment his income by illustrating articles and textbooks. He continued illustrating as a sideline after establishing a surgical practice in 1933, but he ultimately opted to give up his practice in favor of a full-time commitment to art. After service in the United States Army during World War II, Dr. Netter began his long collaboration with the CIBA Pharmaceutical Company (now Novartis Pharmaceuticals). This 45-year partnership resulted in the production of the extraordinary collection of medical art so familiar to physicians and other medical professionals worldwide.

In 2005, Elsevier, Inc., purchased the Netter Collection and all publications from Icon Learning Systems. There are now more than 50 publications featuring the art of Dr. Netter available through Elsevier, Inc. (www.elsevierhealth.com).

Dr. Netter's works are among the finest examples of the use of illustration in the teaching of medical concepts. The 13-book *Netter Collection of Medical Illustrations*, which includes the greater part of the more than 20,000 paintings created by Dr. Netter, became and remains one of the most famous medical works ever published. The Netter *Atlas of Human Anatomy*, first published in 1989, presents the anatomic paintings from the Netter Collection. Now translated into 16 languages, it is the anatomy atlas of choice among medical and health professions students the world over.

The Netter illustrations are appreciated not only for their aesthetic qualities, but also, more important, for their intellectual content. As Dr. Netter wrote in 1949, ". . . clarification of a subject is the aim and goal of illustration. No matter how beautifully painted, how delicately and subtly rendered a subject may be, it is of little value as a *medical illustration* if it does not serve to make clear some medical point." Dr. Netter's planning, conception, point of view, and approach are what inform his paintings and what makes them so intellectually valuable.

Frank H. Netter, MD, physician and artist, died in 1991.

Learn more about the physician-artist whose work has inspired the Netter Reference collection at https://www.netterimages.com/artist-frank-h-netter.html.

Carlos A. G. Machado, MD

Carlos Machado was chosen by Novartis to be Dr. Netter's successor. He continues to be the main artist who contributes to the Netter collection of medical illustrations.

Self-taught in medical illustration, cardiologist Carlos Machado has contributed meticulous updates to some of Dr. Netter's original plates and has created many paintings of his own in the style of Netter as an extension of the Netter collection. Dr. Machado's photorealistic expertise and his keen insight into the physician/patient relationship inform his vivid and unforgettable visual style. His dedication to researching each topic and subject he paints places him among the premier medical illustrators at work today.

Learn more about his background and see more of his art at https://www.netterimages.com/artist-carlos-a-g-machado.html.

ACKNOWLEDGMENTS

This third edition of *Netter's Cardiology* benefited enormously from the hard work and talent of many dedicated individuals.

First, we thank the contributing authors. All are current or former faculty members at the University of North Carolina School of Medicine, Chapel Hill, or have close ties to the institution. Without their intellect, dedication, and drive for excellence, *Netter's Cardiology*, third edition, could not have been published. We had a solid foundation on which to build the third edition, thanks to the hard work of the contributing authors of the second edition, many of whom we were fortunate to have continue on to this edition. We are also grateful for the invaluable editorial contribution that Dr. E. Magnus Ohman made to the first edition.

Special recognition goes to John A. Craig, MD, and Carlos A. G. Machado, MD. They are uniquely talented physician-artists who, through their work, brought to life important concepts in medicine in the new and updated figures included in this text. Marybeth Thiel at Elsevier was invaluable in bringing the third edition to fruition.

We would especially like to acknowledge our families: our wives—Susan Runge, Meg Stouffer, Emma Rossi, and Kristine Patterson—whose constant support, encouragement, and understanding made completion of this text possible; our children—Thomas, Elizabeth, William, John, and Mason Runge; Mark, Jeanie, Joy, and Anna Stouffer; Paul, Samuel, and James Rossi; and Celia, Anna Alyse, and Graham Patterson—who inspire us and remind us that there is life beyond the computer; and, finally, our parents—whose persistence, commitment, and work ethic got us started on this road many, many years ago.

CONTRIBUTORS

EDITORS

Cam Patterson, MD, MBA
Chancellor
University of Arkansas for Medical Sciences
Little Rock, Arkansas

Joseph S. Rossi, MD
Associate Professor of Medicine
Director, Cardiac Catheterization Laboratory
University of North Carolina at Chapel Hill
Chapel Hill, North Carolina

Marschall S. Runge, MD, PhD
Professor of Internal Medicine
Dean, University of Michigan Medical School
Executive Vice President for Medical Affairs
Chief Executive Officer, Michigan Medicine
Ann Arbor, Michigan

George A. Stouffer, MD
Ernest and Hazel Craige Distinguished Professor of Medicine
Chief, Division of Cardiology
Physician in Chief, UNC Heart and Vascular Service Line
University of North Carolina at Chapel Hill
Chapel Hill, North Carolina

AUTHORS

Basil Abu-el-Haija, MD
Clinical Cardiac Electrophysiology
Staff Physician, Kaweah Delta Hospital
Visalia, California

Tiffanie Aiken, BS
MD Candidate 2019
University of South Carolina School of Medicine Greenville
Greenville, South Carolina

Sameer Arora, MD
Cardiovascular Disease Fellow
University of North Carolina at Chapel Hill
Chapel Hill, North Carolina

Matthew S. Baker, MD
Assistant Professor of Medicine
Division of Cardiology
University of North Carolina School of Medicine
Chapel Hill, North Carolina

Charles Baggett, MD
Cardiologist
The Harbin Clinic
Rome, Georgia

Thomas M. Bashore, MD
Professor of Medicine
Senior Vice Chief, Division of Cardiology
Duke University Medical Center
Durham, North Carolina

Sharon Ben-Or, MD
Assistant Professor
Department of Surgery
University of South Carolina at Greenville
Greenville, South Carolina

Hannah Bensimhon, MD
Cardiology Fellow
Department of Medicine
University of North Carolina at Chapel Hill
School of Medicine
Chapel Hill, North Carolina

Christoph Bode, MD, PhD
Chairman of Internal Medicine
Medical Director, Department of Cardiology and Angiology
Albert-Ludwigs-Universität Freiburg
Freiburg, Germany

Michael Bode, MD
Cardiovascular Disease Fellow
Department of Medicine
Division of Cardiology
University of North Carolina at Chapel Hill
Chapel Hill, North Carolina

Weeranun D. Bode, MD
Assistant Professor
Department of Medicine
Division of Cardiology
University of North Carolina at Chapel Hill
Chapel Hill, North Carolina

Mark E. Boulware, MD
Interventional Cardiologist
University of Colorado Health Heart and Vascular Center
Colorado Springs, Colorado

Michael E. Bowdish, MD
Director, Mechanical Circulatory Support
Assistant Professor of Surgery
Keck School of Medicine of University of Southern California
Los Angeles, California

Timothy Brand, MD
Cardiothoraic Surgery Resident
University of North Carolina Hospitals
Chapel Hill, North Carolina

Bruce R. Brodie, MD, FACC
Past President, LeBauer Cardiovascular Research Foundation
Cone Health Heart and Vascular Center
Greensboro, North Carolina

Adam W. Caldwell, MD
Cardiovascular Disease Fellow
Division of Cardiology
University of North Carolina School of Medicine
Chapel Hill, North Carolina

Eric P. Cantey, MD
Department of Medicine
Feinberg School of Medicine at Northwestern University
Chicago, Illinois

Thomas G. Caranasos, MD
Assistant Professor
Department of Surgery
University of North Carolina at Chapel Hill
Chapel Hill, North Carolina

Wayne E. Cascio, MD
Director
Environmental Public Health Division
National Health and Environmental Effects Research Laboratory
Office of Research and Development
U.S. Environmental Protection Agency
Chapel Hill, North Carolina

Matthew A. Cavender, MD, MPH
Assistant Professor of Medicine
Department of Medicine
Division of Cardiology
University of North Carolina at Chapel Hill
Chapel Hill, North Carolina

Patricia P. Chang, MD, MHS
Associate Professor of Medicine
Director of Heart Failure and Transplant Program
Division of Cardiology
University of North Carolina at Chapel Hill
Chapel Hill, North Carolina

Christopher Chien, MD FACC
Clinical Assistant Professor
Division of Cardiology
University of North Carolina
Chapel Hill, North Carolina
Medical Director, Heart Failure Clinic
UNC-Rex Hospital
Raleigh, North Carolina

Christopher D. Chiles, MD
Clinical Assistant Professor of Medicine
Texas A&M Health Science Center
Program Director, Cardiovascular Disease Fellowship
Baylor Scott & White Health/Texas A&M
Temple, Texas

Eugene H. Chung, MD
Associate Professor
Cardiac Electrophysiology Service
Department of Internal Medicine
Michigan Medicine
University of Michigan
Ann Arbor, Michigan

David R. Clemmons, MD
Kenan Professor of Medicine
Division of Internal Medicine
University of North Carolina School of Medicine
Chapel Hill, North Carolina

Romulo E. Colindres, MD, MSPH, FACP
Clinical Professor of Medicine
Division of Nephrology and Hypertension
Department of Medicine
University of North Carolina at Chapel Hill
Chapel Hill, North Carolina

Frank L. Conlon, PhD
Professor
Departments of Biology and Genetics
University of North Carolina at Chapel Hill
Chapel Hill, North Carolina

Jason Crowner, MD
Assistant Professor of Surgery
Division of Vascular Surgery
University of North Carolina School of Medicine
Chapel Hill, North Carolina

Xuming Dai, MD, PhD
Assistant Professor of Medicine
Division of Cardiology
University of North Carolina at Chapel Hill
Chapel Hill, North Carolina

Arjun Deb, MD
Associate Professor
Department of Medicine (Cardiology) and Molecular, Cell, and Developmental Biology
Broad Stem Cell Research Center
University of California, Los Angeles
Los Angeles, California

Cody S. Deen, MD
Assistant Professor of Medicine
Division of Internal Medicine/Cardiology
University of North Carolina at Chapel Hill
Chapel Hill, North Carolina

Gregory J. Dehmer, MD, MACC, MSCAI
Vice President, Medical Director Cardiovascular Services
Baylor Scott & White Health
Central Texas Division
Temple, Texas
Professor of Medicine
Department of Internal Medicine
Division of Cardiology
Texas A&M College of Medicine
Bryan, Texas

John S. Douglas, Jr., MD
Professor of Medicine
Director of Interventional Cardiology Fellowship Program
Emory University School of Medicine
Atlanta, Georgia

Allison G. Dupont, MD
Interventional Cardiologist
The Heart Center of Northeast George Medical Center
Gainesville, Georgia

Fredy H. El Sakr, MD
Fellow in Cardiovascular Medicine
University of Michigan Hospital
Ann Arbor, Michigan

Joseph J. Eron, MD
Professor of Medicine
Director, Clinical Core
University of North Carolina Center for AIDS Research
Division of Infectious Disease
University of North Carolina School of Medicine
Chapel Hill, North Carolina

Mark A. Farber, MD, FACS
Professor of Radiology and Surgery
Division of Vascular Surgery
Director, Aortic Center
University of North Carolina School of Medicine
Chapel Hill, North Carolina

Sunita Juliana Ferns, MD, MRCPCH(UK), FHRS
Assistant Professor of Pediatrics
Director, Pediatric Invasive Electrophysiology
University of North Carolina at Chapel Hill
Chapel Hill, North Carolina

Michelle A. Floris-Moore, MD, MS
Associate Professor
Department of Medicine
Division of Infectious Diseases
University of North Carolina School of Medicine
Chapel Hill, North Carolina

H. James Ford, MD
University of North Carolina
Division of Pulmonary and Critical Care
Chapel Hill, North Carolina

Elizabeth Boger Foreman, MD, FAASM
Sleep Medicine Specialist
Sentara Martha Jefferson Medical and Surgical Associates
Charlottesville, Virginia

Elman G. Frantz, MD
Professor of Pediatrics
Division of Cardiology
University of North Carolina School of Medicine
Director, Pediatric Cardiac Catheterization Laboratory
North Carolina Children's Hospital
Co-Director, Adult Congenital Heart Disease Program
University of North Carolina Heart and Vascular Center
Chapel Hill, North Carolina

Anil K. Gehi, MD
Associate Professor of Medicine
Director, Clinical Cardiac Electrophysiology Service
Division of Cardiology
University of North Carolina School of Medicine
Chapel Hill, North Carolina

Leonard S. Gettes, MD
Professor Emeritus
Department of Medicine
Division of Cardiology
University of North Carolina at Chapel Hill
Chapel Hill, North Carolina

Olivia N. Gilbert, MD
Advanced Heart Failure and Transplant Cardiologist
Novant Health Forsyth Heart and Wellness
Winston-Salem, North Carolina

Allie E. Goins, MD
Department of Medicine
Emory University
Atlanta, Georgia

Anna Griffith, MD
Clinical Fellow
Division of Hematology and Oncology
Department of Internal Medicine
University of North Carolina Hospitals
Chapel Hill, North Carolina

Thomas R. Griggs, MD
Professor Emeritus
Medicine, Pathology, and Laboratory Medicine
University of North Carolina School of Medicine
Chapel Hill, North Carolina

Benjamin Haithcock, MD
Associate Professor of Surgery and Anesthesiology
University of North Carolina Hospitals
Chapel Hill, North Carolina

Eileen M. Handberg, PhD
Professor of Medicine
Department of Medicine
University of Florida
Gainesville, Florida

Alan L. Hinderliter, MD
Associate Professor of Medicine
Division of Cardiology
University of North Carolina at Chapel Hill
Chapel Hill, North Carolina

Lucius Howell, MD
Asheville Cardiology Associates/Mission Health
Asheville, North Carolina

James P. Hummel, MD
Visiting Associate Professor of Medicine
Division of Cardiovascular Medicine
University of Wisconsin School of Medicine and Public Health
Madison, Wisconsin

Thomas S. Ivester, MD, MPH
Professor of Maternal Fetal Medicine
Department of Obstetrics and Gynecology
University of North Carolina School of Medicine
Chief Medical Officer and Vice President for Medical Affairs
UNC Health Care
Chapel Hill, North Carolina

Brian C. Jensen, MD
Associate Professor of Medicine and Pharmacology
Department of Medicine
Division of Cardiology
University of North Carolina School of Medicine
UNC McAllister Heart Institute
Chapel Hill, North Carolina

Beth L. Jonas, MD
Reeves Foundation Distinguished Professor of Medicine
Division of Rheumatology, Allergy, and Immunology
University of North Carolina at Chapel Hill
Chapel Hill, North Carolina

Golsa Joodi, MD, MPH
Post-Doctoral Research Fellow
Department of Medicine
Division of Cardiology
University of North Carolina at Chapel Hill
Chapel Hill, North Carolina

Jason N. Katz, MD, MHS
Associate Professor of Medicine
Department of Internal Medicine
University of North Carolina
Chapel Hill, North Carolina

Audrey Khoury, BS, AB
Medical Student
University of North Carolina School of Medicine
Chapel Hill, North Carolina

J. Larry Klein, MD
Professor of Medicine and Radiology
Department of Cardiology and Radiology
University of North Carolina at Chapel Hill
Chapel Hill, North Carolina

Martyn Knowles, MD, FACS
Adjunct Assistant Professor of Surgery
Division of Vascular Surgery
University of North Carolina at Chapel Hill
Chapel Hill, North Carolina

David W. Lee, MD
Chief Cardiology Fellow
Division of Cardiology
University of North Carolina School of Medicine
Chapel Hill, North Carolina

Daniel J. Lenihan, MD, FACC
Professor of Medicine
Director, Cardio-Oncology Center of Excellence
Advanced Heart Failure
Clinical Research
Cardiovascular Division
Washington University
St. Louis, Missouri

Fong T. Leong, MBChB, PhD, FRCP, FHRS
Consultant, Cardiac Electrophysiologist
University Hospital of Wales
Cardiff, United Kingdom

Gentian Lluri, MD, PhD
Assistant Professor
Department of Medicine
Division of Cardiology
University of California, Los Angeles
Los Angeles, California

Robert Mendes, MD, FACS
Adjunct Assistant Professor
Division of Vascular of Surgery
University of North Carolina School of Medicine
Chapel Hill, North Carolina

Phil Mendys, PharmD
Co-Director, Lipid and Prevention Clinic
Department of Medicine
Division of Cardiology
University of North Carolina Healthcare
Chapel Hill, North Carolina

Venu Menon, MD, FACC, FAHA
Director, Cardiac Intensive Care Unit
Director, Cardiovascular Fellowship
Associate Director, C5 Research
Professor of Medicine
Cleveland Clinic Lerner College of Medicine
Case Western Reserve University
Cleveland, Ohio

Michael R. Mill, MD
Professor of Surgery and Pediatrics
University of North Carolina at Chapel Hill
Chapel Hill, North Carolina

Paula Miller, MD
Clinical Associate Professor of Medicine and Cardiology
Department of Medicine
Division of Cardiology
University of North Carolina School of Medicine
Chapel Hill, North Carolina

Timothy A. Mixon, MD, FACC, FSCAI
Interventional Cardiologist
Baylor Scott & White Health
Temple, Texas
Associate Professor of Medicine
Department of Internal Medicine
Division of Cardiology
Texas A&M College of Medicine
Bryan, Texas

J. Paul Mounsey, PhD, BSc, BM, BCh
Chief of Electrophysiology, East Carolina Heart Institute
Professor of Medicine
Brody School of Medicine
East Carolina University
Greenville, North Carolina

E. Magnus Ohman, MD, FRCPI
Professor of Medicine
Associate Director, Duke Heart Center—Cardiology Clinics
Director, Program for Advanced Coronary Disease
Duke Clinical Research Institute
Duke University Medical Center
Durham, North Carolina

Rikin Patel, DO
Cardiovascular Disease Fellow
Baylor Scott & White Health/Texas A&M
Temple, Texas

Kristine B. Patterson, MD
Associate Professor of Medicine
Division of Infectious Disease
Columbia University Medical Center
New York, New York

Eric D. Pauley, MD
Cardiovascular Disease Fellow
University of North Carolina Hospitals
Chapel Hill, North Carolina

Pamela S. Ro, MD
Associate Professor
Department of Pediatrics
University of North Carolina at Chapel Hill
Chapel Hill, North Carolina

Rachel D. Romero, MD
Fellow
Division of Rheumatology, Allergy, and Immunology
University of North Carolina at Chapel Hill
Chapel Hill, North Carolina

Lisa J. Rose-Jones, MD
Assistant Professor of Medicine
Division of Cardiology
University of North Carolina at Chapel Hill
UNC Center for Heart and Vascular Care
Chapel Hill, North Carolina

Richard S. Schofield, MD
Professor of Medicine
Division of Cardiovascular Medicine
University of Florida College of Medicine
Department of Veterans Affairs Medical Center
Gainesville, Florida

Kristen A. Sell-Dottin, MD
Assistant Professor
University of Louisville
Louisville, Kentucky

Jay D. Sengupta, MD
Clinical Cardiac Electrophysiologist
Minneapolis Heart Institute at Abbott Northwestern Hospital
Minneapolis, Minnesota

Faiq Shaikh, MD
Molecular Imaging Physician Consultant
Cellsight Technologies, Inc.
San Francisco, California

Arif Sheikh, MD
Associate Professor
Department of Radiology
Columbia University
New York, New York

David S. Sheps, MD, MSPH
Professor
Department of Epidemiology
University of Florida
Gainesville, Florida

Brett C. Sheridan, MD
San Francisco Cardiology
San Francisco, California

Ross J. Simpson, Jr., MD, PhD
Director of the Lipid and Prevention Clinic at University of
    North Carolina
Professor of Medicine and Adjuvant Professor of Epidemiology
University of North Carolina at Chapel Hill
Chapel Hill, North Carolina

Christopher E. Slagle, PhD
Postdoctoral Fellow
Departments of Biology and Genetics
University of North Carolina at Chapel Hill
Chapel Hill, North Carolina

Sidney C. Smith, Jr., MD, FAHA, FESC, FACP, MACC
Professor of Medicine
Department of Medicine/Division of Cardiology
University of North Carolina at Chapel Hill
Chapel Hill, North Carolina

Mark A. Socinski, MD
Professor of Medicine
Division of Hematology and Oncology
Multidisciplinary Thoracic Oncology Program
Lineberger Comprehensive Cancer Center
University of North Carolina School of Medicine
Chapel Hill, North Carolina

Robert D. Stewart, MD, MPH
Staff, Pediatric and Congenital Heart Surgery
Heart and Vascular Institute
Cleveland Clinic
Cleveland, Ohio

Thomas D. Stuckey, MD, FACC
Medical Director, LeBauer Cardiovascular Research and
    Education
Cone Health Heart and Vascular Center
Greensboro, North Carolina

Carla A. Sueta, MD, PhD
Professor of Medicine Emerita
Division of Cardiology
University of North Carolina School of Medicine
Chapel Hill, North Carolina

Khola S. Tahir, MD
Cardiovascular Disease Fellow
University of North Carolina at Chapel Hill
Chapel Hill, North Carolina

Walter A. Tan, MD, MS
Associate Professor of Medicine
Director, Cardiac Catheterization Laboratories
Wake Forest—Baptist Health
Winston-Salem, North Carolina

David A. Tate, MD
Associate Professor of Medicine Emeritus
Division of Cardiology
University of North Carolina School of Medicine
Chapel Hill, North Carolina

Rebecca E. Traub, MD
Assistant Professor
Department of Neurology
University of North Carolina at Chapel Hill
Chapel Hill, North Carolina

Bradley V. Vaughn, MD
Professor of Neurology
University of North Carolina School of Medicine
Chapel Hill, North Carolina

John P. Vavalle, MD, MHS, FACC
Assistant Professor of Medicine
Director of Structural Heart Disease
University of North Carolina at Chapel Hill
Chapel Hill, North Carolina

Anirudh Vinnakota, MS
Case Western Reserve University School of Medicine
Department of Thoracic and Cardiovascular Surgery
Cleveland, Ohio

Raven A. Voora, MD
Assistant Professor of Medicine
Division of Nephrology
University of North Carolina at Chapel Hill
Chapel Hill, North Carolina

Thelsa Thomas Weickert, MD
Assistant Professor
Department of Medicine
Division of Cardiology
University of North Carolina at Chapel Hill
Chapel Hill, North Carolina

Andy Wessels, PhD
Professor and Vice-Chair, Department of Regenerative Medicine
and Cell Biology
Co-Director, Cardiovascular Developmental Biology Center
Medical University of South Carolina
Charleston, South Carolina

John T. Wilkins, MD, MS
Assistant Professor of Medicine (Cardiology) and Preventive
Medicine
Northwestern University Feinberg School of Medicine
Chicago, Illinois

Park W. Willis IV, MD
Sarah Graham Kenan Distinguished Professor of Medicine and
Pediatrics Emeritus
Director, Cardiac Ultrasound Laboratories
Division of Cardiology
University of North Carolina School of Medicine
Chapel Hill, North Carolina

Eric H. Yang, MD, MBA
Director of Interventional Cardiology and Cardiac
Catheterization Laboratories
Department of Cardiovascular Disease
Mayo Clinic Arizona
Phoenix, Arizona

Michael Yeung, MD
Assistant Professor of Medicine
University of North Carolina School of Medicine
Chapel Hill, North Carolina

Andrew O. Zurick III, MD, MSEd, FACC, FASE
Director of Advanced Cardiovascular Imaging
Cardiovascular Medicine
St. Thomas Heart
Nashville, Tennessee
Affiliated Assistant Professor
Division of Internal Medicine in the Department of Clinical
Medical Education
University of Tennessee Health Science Center, College of
Medicine
Knoxville, Tennessee

ONLINE CONTENTS

Visit **www.ExpertConsult.com** for the following:

VIDEOS

SECTION VIII: STRUCTURAL HEART DISEASE

Chapter 52 Catheter-Based Therapies for Adult Congenital Heart Disease

Video 52-1 Bedside echo-guided balloon atrial septostomy

Video 52-2 Free pulmonary regurgitation after tetralogy of Fallot repair, stepwise Melody valve implantation after prestenting, and competent Melody valve postimplantation

Video 52-3 Stepwise transcatheter closure of a patent ductus arteriosus with the Amplatzer Duct Occluder

Video 52-4 Stepwise transcatheter closure of a secundum atrial septal defect with the Amplatzer Septal Occluder

Video 52-5 Stepwise transcatheter closure of a patent foramen ovale with an Amplatzer Occluder

PRINTABLE PATIENT EDUCATION BROCHURES FROM
FERRI'S NETTER PATIENT ADVISOR, 3RD EDITION

1. STRESS TEST USED TO PREDICT HEART ATTACK RISK
2. MANAGING YOUR DIAGNOSTIC HEART CATHETERIZATION
3. MANAGING YOUR PERCUTANEOUS CORONARY INTERVENTION
4. MANAGING YOUR CORONARY ARTERY BYPASS SURGERY
5. MANAGING YOUR HYPERTROPHIC CARDIOMYOPATHY
6. MANAGING YOUR SUPRAVENTRICULAR TACHYCARDIA
7. MANAGING YOUR CARDIAC PACEMAKER AND DEFIBRILLATOR
8. MANAGING YOUR AORTIC VALVE DISEASE
9. MANAGING YOUR MITRAL VALVE DISEASE
10. MANAGING YOUR PULMONARY HYPERTENSION AND THROMBOEMBOLIC DISEASE
11. MANAGING YOUR SLEEP DISORDER AND HEART DISEASE
12. MANAGING YOUR EXERCISES AND CARDIOVASCULAR HEALTH
13. MANAGING YOUR ATRIAL FIBRILLATION
14. MANAGING YOUR ATRIAL SEPTAL DEFECT
15. MANAGING YOUR CONGESTIVE HEART FAILURE (CHF)
16. MANAGING YOUR CORONARY ARTERY DISEASE
17. MANAGING YOUR DEEP VEIN THROMBOSIS
18. MANAGING YOUR HEART ATTACK
19. MANAGING YOUR HIGH CHOLESTEROL
20. MANAGING YOUR HIGH BLOOD PRESSURE (HYPERTENSION)
21. MANAGING YOUR MYOCARDITIS
22. MANAGING YOUR RENAL ARTERY STENOSIS
23. MANAGING YOUR VENTRICULAR SEPTAL DEFECT
24. MANAGING YOUR HEART ATTACK: FOR WOMEN

CONTENTS

SECTION I

Introduction

Basic Anatomy and Embryology of the Heart

Frank L. Conlon, Christopher E. Slagle, Andy Wessels

ORIGINS OF CARDIAC PRECURSOR POPULATIONS

Heart development begins as the primary germ layers—ectoderm, mesoderm, and endoderm—are induced and progressively changed to various cell types during the morphogenetic process of gastrulation. Combinatorial networks of intercellular signaling events cooperate with massive tissue migrations and internalizations to lay out the basic body plan of the vertebrate embryo. Mesoderm-derived cardiac precursors are among the first cell populations to internalize, coalescing into 2 bilateral populations toward the anterior end of the embryo between 13 and 15 days of human development. The identity of these progenitor pools as cardiac precursors is defined and maintained by expression of a core cohort of developmental gene regulators or transcription factors. These cardiac transcription factors function cooperatively and hierarchically to induce expression of appropriate structural proteins, including components of the specialized cardiomyocyte contractile apparatus and ion channels. Many cardiac transcription factors function not only in the initial specification of cardiac precursors, but also in later aspects of heart morphogenesis, such as establishing chamber identity, chamber-vessel alignment, and conduction system development. Therefore proper spatial and temporal functions of cardiac transcription factors dictate development of a healthy and functional heart. This requirement of correct genetic regulation is exemplified by the numerous congenital heart defects associated with or caused by mutations in cardiac transcription factors.

Even at such early stages of embryonic development, the cardiac precursor pools have been subdivided into two distinct sources of progenitors according to expression of different subsets of cardiac transcription factors. The first, designated as the first heart field, will form the primitive linear heart tube, which will give rise to the left ventricle and most of the atrial tissues. The second heart field, incorporated into the primitive embryonic heart at various stages of development, contributes to the right ventricle and outflow tract. The developing heart receives further contributions from the cardiac neural crest and the mesothelium. The cardiac neural crest is made of ectodermal cells arising outside the heart fields at the lateral borders of the neural plate and because of neural induction from the midline ectoderm. The cardiac neural crest migrates to the heart-forming region, where it contributes to septation of the outflow tract into the arterial and pulmonary vessels. The mesothelium is the embryonic cell source that gives rise to the epicardium, an epithelium that covers the surface of the heart and that plays a role in a number of processes, such as the development of the coronary system and the formation of the annulus fibrosis.

FORMATION OF THE PRIMITIVE LINEAR HEART TUBE

Even before gastrulation has completed, the internalized bilateral cardiac precursor pools continue to migrate in response to signaling cues from neighboring tissues. Remaining as cohesive epithelia, the heart fields move anteriorly and ventrally between 15 and 20 days of development, fusing at the embryonic midline to form the transient cardiac crescent (Fig. 1.1). Proper midline fusion of the bilateral cardiac primordia is essential for development of the heart. Several cardiac transcription factors are required for this process, and loss of function of any one of them causes extensive defects in further morphogenesis, including cardia bifida in severe cases.

Newly united as the cardiac crescent, the multipotent cardiac progenitors coalesce further to form a linear tube by 3 weeks of development, segregating into the future endocardial lining and myocardial walls (Fig. 1.2). The linear heart tube consists exclusively of differentiated first heart field cells; the second heart field persists as a mesenchymal population, which is a loose association of rapidly dividing precursor cells adjacent to the heart tube. Although no specialized electrical conduction system has yet arisen, the myocardium of the linear heart tube already exhibits autonomous contractions. Compared with those of a mature heart, these contractions are slow and weak, driven only by the intrinsic depolarizing activity and conductivity of the still-maturing cardiomyocytes. Once the conduction system develops and connects to the mature working myocardium, it will serve as an extrinsic regulator of the electrical impulses within the myocardium. Sufficient contractile force will, in turn, allow the heart to beat at the strength required to circulate blood throughout the body.

LOOPING OF THE LINEAR HEART TUBE

As a consequence of its formation, differentiation, and rudimentary functionality, the linear heart tube is mostly postmitotic. During the fourth week of human gestation, growth and elongation of the linear heart tube occur by means of contribution and division of second heart field cells at both the sinus venosus and truncus arteriosus (posterior and anterior poles, respectively). Concurrently, an embryo-wide genetic program breaks the final axis of symmetry—the left-right axis. Asymmetrical intercellular signaling on the left side of the embryo governs the migration and division of second heart field cells in the lengthening heart tube, leading to two major morphological cardiac asymmetries. First, the entire linear heart tube displaces to the right and rotates 90 degrees about its anterior-posterior axis, so that the original ventral surface of the linear tube is now the left side of a C-shaped tube (Fig. 1.3). Second, asymmetrical mitotic expansion of the second heart field contributions leads to localized "ballooning" of the primitive atrial and ventricular regions of the heart tube, transforming the C-shaped tube into an S-shaped heart (Fig. 1.3).

Further gross morphogenetic movements of the embryo bring the two poles in close apposition, anterior to the primitive chambers. This repositioning prepares the inflow and outflow tracts for appropriate connections to the developing vasculature, thereby contributing to proper segregation of oxygenated and deoxygenated blood flow among the heart, lungs, and body. By 30 days of gestation, the prospective atria

Approximately 20 days postconception

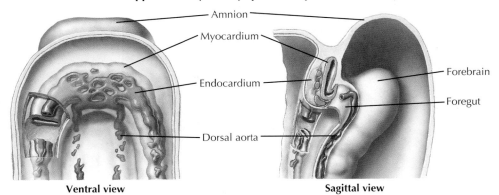

Amnion
Myocardium
Endocardium
Forebrain
Foregut
Dorsal aorta

Ventral view　　　　　　**Sagittal view**

Approximately 21 days postconception

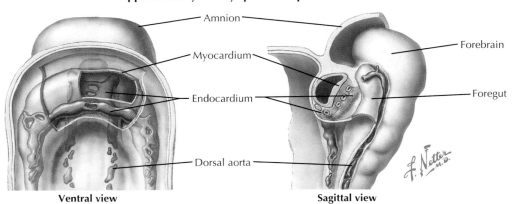

Amnion
Myocardium
Endocardium
Forebrain
Foregut
Dorsal aorta

Ventral view　　　　　　**Sagittal view**

FIG 1.1 Formation of the heart tube.

Approximately 22 days postconception

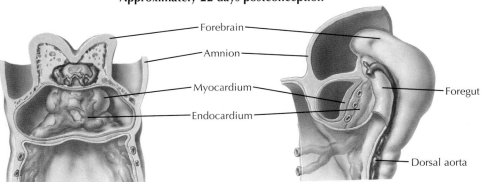

Forebrain
Amnion
Myocardium
Endocardium
Foregut
Dorsal aorta

Ventral view　　　　　　**Sagittal view**

Approximately 23 days postconception

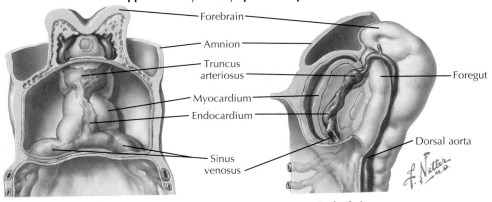

Forebrain
Amnion
Truncus arteriosus
Myocardium
Endocardium
Sinus venosus
Foregut
Dorsal aorta

Ventral view　　　　　　**Sagittal view**

FIG 1.2 Formation of the heart tube (*continued*).

Approximately 23 days postconception

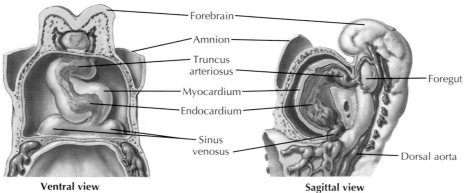

Forebrain

Amnion

Truncus arteriosus

Myocardium

Endocardium

Sinus venosus

Foregut

Dorsal aorta

Ventral view

Sagittal view

Approximately 24 days postconception

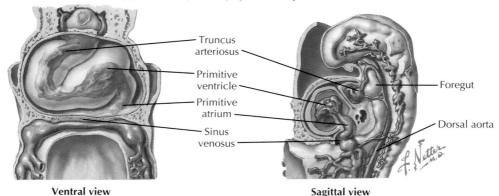

Truncus arteriosus

Primitive ventricle

Primitive atrium

Sinus venosus

Foregut

Dorsal aorta

Ventral view

Sagittal view

FIG 1.3 Formation of the heart loop.

are repositioned anterior to the ventricular region, marking the first resemblance of the embryonic heart to its future adult structure.

Formation of the S-looped heart overlaps with the beginnings of ventricular and outflow tract septation and valve development as endocardial cushions emerge within the atrioventricular junction and the outflow tract.

CHAMBER FORMATION

During the time of cardiac looping, at approximately 3 weeks of development, the arterial and venous poles of the heart decrease or cease cell division. At the same time, cardiomyocytes at two distinct locations within the intervening tissue reinitiate cell proliferation. This localized expansion of cardiomyocytes gives rise anteriorly to the atria and posteriorly to the left ventricle, with the area separating the two regions giving rise to the atrioventricular canal. Studies in chickens and mice demonstrated that the atria grow not only through proliferation but also by the recruitment of cells to the venous pole of the heart. The left ventricle and the atria are largely derived from a common pool of progenitors termed the first heart field (Fig. 1.4). In contrast, the second heart field gives rise to the dorsal mesenchymal protrusion and primary atrial septum, which are tissues that are critically important for atrioventricular septation, the outflow tract, and the right ventricle. A conserved role for the second heart field is supported by the observations that abnormalities that affect the expansion of the second heart field are associated with congenital heart disease in mouse models and humans, including atrial and atrioventricular defects, as well as outflow tract abnormalities.

Contribution of cells from the second heart field to the heart is complete by the fifth week of human development. At this stage, chamber identity can be established by inspecting anatomic features and/or by the expression of left or right ventricular chamber-specific genes. As the cardiovascular system develops to support postnatal systemic and pulmonary circulations, the heart goes through a series of complex remodeling events. Critical steps in this process are the formation of the septa between individual components of the heart, with the purpose of separating the respective blood flows within the heart, and the formation of valves facilitating unidirectional flow among the respective components. Together, these two events are commonly referred to as valvuloseptal morphogenesis.

SEPTATION

Atrial septation is initiated when the second heart field–derived dorsal mesenchymal protrusion and the myocardial primary atrial septum (or septum primum) extend ventrally into the, yet undivided, common atrium. In the mouse, this process takes place between embryonic day (ED) 9.5 to 10.5; in humans the process occurs around day 30. The space between the leading edge of the atrial septum and the fusing atrioventricular cushions in the atrioventricular canal is the primary atrial foramen. As the primary atrial septum grows toward the mesenchymal atrioventricular cushions, thereby closing the primary interatrial foramen, perforations appear in the upper part of the primary atrial septum. These perforations will eventually coalesce and form the secondary interatrial foramen. As this part of atrial septation process nears completion, the secondary atrial septum (or septum secundum) appears

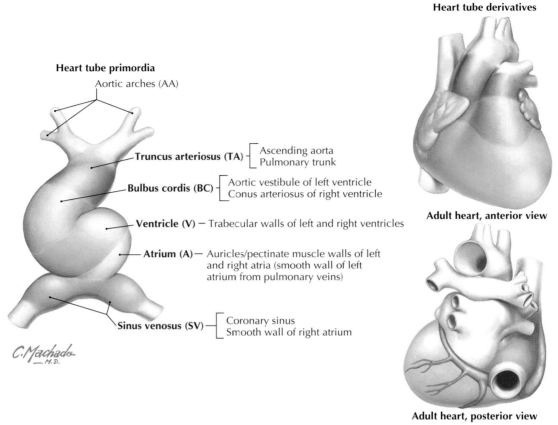

Heart tube primordia

Aortic arches (AA)

Truncus arteriosus (TA) — Ascending aorta / Pulmonary trunk

Bulbus cordis (BC) — Aortic vestibule of left ventricle / Conus arteriosus of right ventricle

Ventricle (V) — Trabecular walls of left and right ventricles

Atrium (A) — Auricles/pectinate muscle walls of left and right atria (smooth wall of left atrium from pulmonary veins)

Sinus venosus (SV) — Coronary sinus / Smooth wall of right atrium

Heart tube derivatives

Adult heart, anterior view

Adult heart, posterior view

FIG 1.4 Summary of heart tube derivatives.

in the space between the primary atrial septum and the left venous valve in the roof of the right atrium. Eventually, the upper part of the primary atrial septum will fuse with the secondary atrial septum, thereby closing off the secondary atrial foramen and completing the atrial septation process. Failure of fusion of the two atrial septa will lead to the congenital defect patent foramen ovale.

Compared with atrial septation, the creation of the ventricular septum is a rather straightforward process. As the tubular heart expands, undergoes looping, and remodels, distinctive left and right ventricular components appear. During this process, a myocardial ridge, the interventricular septum, emerges between the left and right ventricle. Subsequent outward expansion of the ventricles, a process sometimes referred to as "ballooning," in combination with upward growth of the interventricular septum and eventual fusion of crest of the septum with the atrioventricular cushions, completes the process of ventricular septation. Cell lineage tracing experiments in the mouse demonstrated that, like the right ventricle, the interventricular septum is largely derived from the second heart field.

The third septal structure that is required for separating the respective blood flows in the heart is found in the outflow tract. After completion of cardiac looping, a single outflow tract can be found connected to the right ventricular component of the yet unseptated heart. Septation of this outflow tract is required for the formation of an aorta, which eventually connects to the left ventricle, and a pulmonary trunk that comes from the right ventricle. Two sets of endocardial ridges are located within the outflow tract, and as a result of their fusion, these will separate the common outflow tract into an aorta and a pulmonary trunk. Failure of fusion can lead to congenital defects, including a double outlet right

ventricle. The cardiac neural crest is also important in the septation process that separates aorta and pulmonary trunk. Abnormal development of the cardiac neural crest specifically affects the formation of the aorticopulmonary septum downstream of the semilunar valves (Fig. 1.5). This can result in the congenital defect common arterial trunk (or truncus arteriosus) or in aorticopulmonary window.

FORMATION OF THE CARDIAC VALVES

The fully formed heart contains two sets of one-way valves. In the atrioventricular junction, the atrioventricular valves facilitate unidirectional flow through the left and right atrioventricular orifices, whereas at the ventriculoarterial junction, the semilunar valves serve the same function at the junction of the left ventricle and the aorta, and at the junction of the right ventricle and the pulmonary trunk.

Atrioventricular valve formation is initiated at the atrioventricular junction of the looping heart (see previous description); two atrioventricular cushions appear as a result of local accumulation of extracellular matrix between the atrioventricular endocardium and myocardium. A process of endothelial-to-mesenchymal transformation leads to the generation of a population of mesenchymal cells that colonize the cushions. As the heart grows, and these major atrioventricular cushions become bigger, they eventually fuse, thereby separating the common atrioventricular junction into the left and right atrioventricular orifices. As this process takes place, on the lateral walls of these respective orifices, two additional atrioventricular cushions form. These are known as the left and right lateral atrioventricular cushions. These lateral cushions also become populated with endocardially derived mesenchyme. Recent

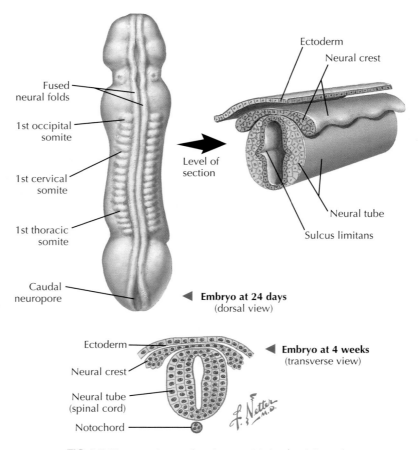

Fused
neural folds

1st occipital
somite

1st cervical
somite

1st thoracic
somite

Caudal
neuropore

Level of
section

Ectoderm

Neural crest

Neural tube

Sulcus limitans

◀ **Embryo at 24 days**
(dorsal view)

Ectoderm

Neural crest

Neural tube
(spinal cord)

Notochord

◀ **Embryo at 4 weeks**
(transverse view)

FIG 1.5 Nervous tissue of embryo at 24 days and 4 weeks.

cell fate studies in mice showed that epicardially derived cells migrate into these lateral cushions. Epicardially derived cells do not populate the major cushions. Further remodeling of the cushion-derived tissues eventually leads to the formation of the mitral valve leaflets in the left atrioventricular orifice and the tricuspid valve leaflets in the right atrioventricular orifice.

In many respects, the development of the semilunar valves is similar to that of the atrioventricular valves. It involves the fusion of two mesenchymal tissues, the parietal and septal endocardial ridges, which result in the separation of the left and right ventricular outflows. The emergence of a set of smaller endocardial ridges, the intercalated ridges at the opposite sides of the formed septum, resembles the process of formation of the lateral cushions in the atrioventricular junction. The remodeling of these two sets of mesenchymal ridges will eventually lead to the formation of the semilunar valves.

CARDIAC NEURAL CREST

The neural crest is a transient population of cells that form from the dorsal ectoderm at the time of neural tube closure (Fig. 1.5). The neural crest population arises through a series of inductive interactions with surrounding tissues around the fourth week of development. Once formed, the cells undergo an epithelial-to-mesenchymal transition, migrating ventrally and laterally to contribute to a wide array of tissue types, including the epinephrine-producing cells of the adrenal gland, the parasympathetic neurons, cartilage, bone, connective tissue, and pigment cells. The neural crests themselves are multipotential at the

time of their formation; their ultimate fate is a reflection of their relative position along the anterior-to-posterior axis of the embryo. In the cranial portions of the embryo, classic fate mapping studies showed that a subpopulation of neural crest cells enter the arterial pole or the venous pole of the heart to give rise to all of the parasympathetic innervation of the heart, the smooth muscle layer of the great vessels, and portions of the outflow tract. This population is termed the cardiac neural crest. Ablation studies in chicks and genetic studies in mammals demonstrated not only that the cardiac neural crest cells contribute to these regions of the heart but also that they are also essential for the proper formation of each of these structures.

EPICARDIUM AND EPICARDIALLY DERIVED CELLS

The walls of the developed heart essentially consist of three cell layers: the endocardium, the myocardium, and the epicardium. The endocardium and myocardium are generated early in development during the formation of the primitive linear heart tube (see previous description). However, the epicardium, a layer of epithelial cells covering the heart, is like the cardiac neural crest, a late addition to the developing heart. The source of the epicardium is the proepicardium, a local proliferation of the mesothelium found in association with the sinus venosus at the venous pole. In the mouse, the proepicardium can be seen around ED 9.5; in humans, this happens around day 30. Shortly after its generation, the proepicardium attaches to the myocardial surface in the atrioventricular junction. From there, the cells spread out as an epicardial sheet and eventually cover nearly the entire heart. Cell fate studies in animal models indicated that the epicardial-like cells covering the distal part of the outflow tract are not derived from the proepicardium proper but instead come from the pericardial mesothelium associated with the aortic sac.

After formation of the epicardium, epithelial-to-mesenchymal transformation of a subpopulation of epicardial cells leads to the formation of epicardially derived cells that migrate into the space between the epicardium and the myocardium. This process is most pronounced at the junction between the atria and ventricles, where it leads to the formation of the atrioventricular sulcus. Furthermore, cell fate studies in animal model systems demonstrated that epicardially derived cells also migrate into the ventricular myocardial walls where they differentiate into interstitial fibroblasts and coronary smooth muscle cells. In addition, these animal studies also revealed that epicardially derived cells contribute significantly to the leaflets of the atrioventricular valves that are derived from the lateral atrioventricular cushions.

ADDITIONAL RESOURCES

Bruneau BG. Signaling and transcriptional networks in heart development and regeneration. *Cold Spring Harb Perspect Biol.* 2013;5:a008292.

A comprehensive review of primary literature on the genetic and molecular underpinnings of cardiac morphogenesis.

De la Cruz M, Markwald RR, eds. *Living Morphogenesis of the Heart.* Birkhauser.

An excellent detailed summary of the original studies in cardiac development.

Kirby ML. *Cardiac Development.* Oxford University Press; 2007.

An outstanding comprehensive text on vertebrate heart development.

Männer J. Cardiac looping in the chick embryo: a morphological review with special reference to terminological and biomechanical aspects of the looping process. *Anat Record.* 2000;259:248–262.

An in-depth review of primary literature documenting looping of the linear heart tube, illustrated with electron micrographs of the morphological process in chicken embryos.

Rana MS, Christoffels VM, Moorman AFM. A molecular and genetic outline of cardiac morphogenesis. *Acta Physiol.* 2013;207:588–615.

A synthesis of literature detailing contributions of various cardiac progenitor sources to development of the mature vertebrate heart.

2

The History and Physical Examination

Marschall S. Runge, Fredy H. El Sakr, E. Magnus Ohman, George A. Stouffer

The ability to determine whether disease is present or absent—and how that patient should be treated—is the ultimate goal for clinicians who evaluate patients with suspected heart disease. Despite the number of diagnostic tests available, the importance of a careful history and physical examination has never been greater. Opportunities for errors in judgment are abundant, and screening patients for coronary risk using a broad and unfocused panel of laboratory and noninvasive tests can lead to incorrect diagnoses and unnecessary testing. Selection of the most appropriate test and therapeutic approach for each patient is based on a skillfully performed history and physical examination. Furthermore, interpretation of any test results is based on the previous probability of disease, which again is based on the history and physical. Although entire texts have been written on cardiac history and physical examination, this chapter specifically focuses on features of the cardiac history and the cardiovascular physical examination that help discern the presence or absence of heart disease.

THE CONCEPT OF PREVIOUS PROBABILITY

The history and physical examination should allow the clinician to establish the previous probability of heart disease, that is, the likelihood that the symptoms reported by the patient result from heart disease. A reasonable goal is to establish the risk of heart disease in a patient as "low," "intermediate," or "high." One demonstration of this principle in clinical medicine is the assessment of patients with chest pain, in which exercise stress testing to accurately diagnose coronary heart disease (CHD) depends on the previous probability of disease. In patients with a low risk of CHD based on clinical findings, exercise stress testing results in a large number of false-positive test results. Because up to 15% of exercise stress tests produce positive results in individuals without CHD, use of this test in a low-risk population can result in an adverse ratio of false-positive to true-positive test results and unnecessary cardiac catheterizations. Conversely, in patients with a high risk of CHD based on clinical findings, exercise stress testing can result in false-negative test results, which is an equally undesirable outcome, because patients with significant coronary artery disease (CAD) and their physicians may be falsely reassured that no further evaluation or treatment is necessary.

Emphasis is increasing on quantifying previous probability to an even greater degree with various mathematical models. This is a useful approach in teaching and may be clinically feasible in some diseases. However, for most patients with suspected heart disease, categorizing risk as low, intermediate, and high is appropriate, reproducible, and feasible in a busy clinical practice. Therefore obtaining the history and physical examination represents a key step before any testing, to minimize use of inappropriate diagnostic procedures.

THE HISTORY

A wealth of information is available to clinicians who carefully assess the history of the patient. Key components are assessment of the chief complaint; careful questioning for related, often subtle symptoms that may further define the chief complaint; and determination of other factors that help categorize the likelihood of disease. Major symptoms of heart patients include chest discomfort, dyspnea, palpitations, and syncope or presyncope.

Chest Discomfort

Determining whether chest discomfort results from a cardiac cause is often a challenge. The most common cause of chest discomfort is myocardial ischemia, which produces angina pectoris. Many causes of angina exist, and the differential diagnosis for chest discomfort is extensive (Box 2.1). Angina that is reproducible and constant in frequency and severity is often referred to as stable angina. For the purposes of this chapter, stable angina is a condition that occurs when CAD is present, and coronary blood flow cannot be increased to accommodate for increased myocardial demand. However, as discussed in Chapters 12 through 14, there are many causes of myocardial ischemia, including fixed coronary artery stenoses and endothelial dysfunction, which lead to reduced vasodilatory capacity.

A description of chest discomfort can help establish whether the pain is angina or of another origin. First, characterization of the quality and location of the discomfort is essential (Fig. 2.1). Chest discomfort because of myocardial ischemia may be described as pain, a tightness, a heaviness, or simply an uncomfortable and difficult-to-describe feeling. The discomfort can be localized to the mid-chest or epigastric area, or may be characterized as pain in related areas, including the left arm, both arms, the jaw, or the back. The radiation of chest discomfort to any of these areas increases the likelihood of the discomfort being angina. Second, the duration of discomfort is important because chest discomfort due to cardiac causes generally lasts minutes. Therefore pain of short duration ("seconds" or "moments"), regardless of how typical it may be of angina, is less likely to be of cardiac origin. Likewise, pain that lasts for hours, on many occasions, in the absence of objective evidence of myocardial infarction (MI), is not likely to be of coronary origin. Third, the presence of accompanying symptoms should be considered. Chest discomfort may be accompanied by other symptoms (including dyspnea, diaphoresis, or nausea), any of which increase the likelihood that the pain is cardiac in origin. However, the presence of accompanying symptoms is not needed to define the discomfort as angina. Fourth, factors that precipitate or relieve the discomfort should be evaluated. Angina typically occurs during physical exertion, during emotional stress, or in other circumstances of increased myocardial

BOX 2.1   Differential Diagnosis of Chest Discomfort

Cardiovascular
Ischemic
- Hyperthyroidism
- Tachycardia (e.g., atrial fibrillation)
- Coronary spasm
- Coronary atherosclerosis (angina pectoris)
- Acute coronary syndrome
- Aortic stenosis
- Hypertrophic cardiomyopathy
- Aortic regurgitation
- Mitral regurgitation
- Severe systemic hypertension
- Severe right ventricular/pulmonary hypertension
- Severe anemia/hypoxia

Nonischemic
- Aortic dissection
- Pericarditis
- Mitral valve prolapse syndrome: autonomic dysfunction

Gastrointestinal
- Gastroesophageal reflux disease
- Esophageal spasm
- Esophageal rupture
- Hiatal hernia
- Cholecystitis

Pulmonary
- Pulmonary embolus
- Pneumothorax
- Pneumonia
- Chronic obstructive pulmonary disease
- Pleurisy

Neuromusculoskeletal
- Thoracic outlet syndrome
- Degenerative joint disease of the cervical or thoracic spine
- Costochondritis
- Herpes zoster

Psychogenic
- Anxiety
- Depression
- Cardiac psychosis
- Self-gain

BOX 2.2   Conditions That Cause Increased Myocardial Oxygen Demand

- Hyperthyroidism
- Tachycardia of various etiologies
- Hypertension
- Pulmonary embolism
- Pregnancy
- Psychogenic
- Central nervous system stimulants
- Exercise
- Psychological stress
- Fever

increased myocardial oxygen demand due to anemia, hyperthyroidism, or similar conditions (Box 2.2). Angina occurring at rest, or with minimal exertion, may denote a different pathophysiology, one that involves platelet aggregation, which is clinically termed "unstable angina" or "acute coronary syndrome" (see Chapters 20 and 21).

Patients with heart disease need not present with chest pain at all. Anginal equivalents include dyspnea during exertion, abdominal discomfort, fatigue, or decreased exercise tolerance. Clinicians must be alert to and specifically ask about these symptoms. Often, a patient's family member or spouse notices subtle changes in the endurance of the patient or that the individual no longer performs functions that require substantial physical effort. Sometimes, patients may be unable to exert themselves due to comorbidities. For instance, the symptoms of myocardial ischemia may be absent in patients with severe peripheral vascular disease who have limiting claudication. One should also be attuned to subtle or absent symptoms in individuals with diabetes mellitus (including type 1 and type 2 diabetes), which is a coronary risk equivalent as defined by the Framingham Risk Calculator.

When the likelihood that CHD accounts for a patient presenting with chest discomfort or any of the aforementioned variants is considered, assessment of the cardiac risk factor profile is important. The Framingham Study first codified the concept of cardiac risk factors, and over time, quantification of risk using these factors has become an increasingly useful tool in clinical medicine. Cardiac risk factors determined by the Framingham Study include a history of cigarette smoking, diabetes mellitus, hypertension, or hypercholesterolemia; a family history of CHD (including MI, sudden cardiac death, and first-degree relatives having undergone coronary revascularization); age; and sex (male). Although an attempt has been made to rank these risk factors, all are important, with a history of diabetes mellitus being perhaps the single most important factor. Subsequently, a much longer list of potential predictors of cardiac risk has been made (Box 2.3). Multiple risk calculators have since been created, such as the atherosclerotic cardiovascular disease algorithm used by the American College of Cardiology, the American Heart Association cholesterol guidelines, and the Multi-Ethnic Study of Atherosclerosis (MESA), which uses classic risk factors with the addition of a coronary artery calcium score to predict a 10-year risk of CHD.

Symptoms suggestive of vascular disease require special attention. Peripheral vascular disease may mask CHD because the individual may not be able to exercise sufficiently to provoke angina. A history of stroke, transient ischemic attack, or atheroembolism in any vascular distribution is usually evidence of significant vascular disease. Sexual dysfunction in men is not an uncommon presentation of peripheral vascular disease. The presence of Raynaud-type symptoms should also be elicited because such symptoms suggest abnormal vascular tone and function, and increase the risk that CHD is present.

oxygen demand. When exercise precipitates chest discomfort, relief after cessation of exercise substantiates the diagnosis of angina. Sublingual nitroglycerin also relieves angina, generally over a period of minutes. Instant relief or relief after longer periods lessens the likelihood that the chest discomfort was angina.

Although the presence of symptoms during exertion is important in assessing CHD risk, individuals, especially sedentary ones, may have angina-like symptoms that are not related to exertion. These include postprandial and nocturnal angina, or angina that occurs while the individual is at rest. As described herein, "rest-induced angina," or the new onset of angina, connotes a pathophysiology different from effort-induced angina. Angina can also occur in persons with fixed CAD and

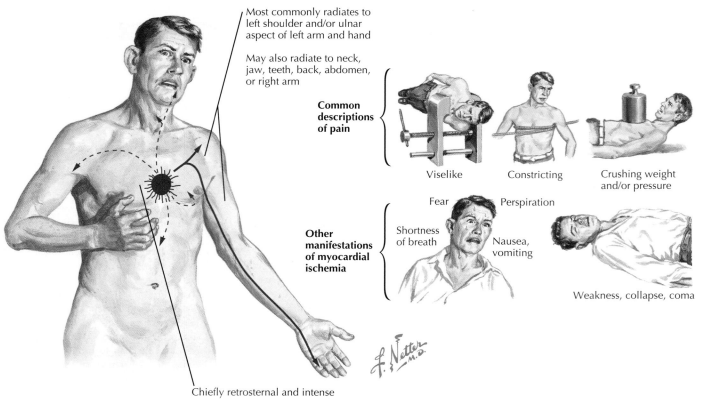

Most commonly radiates to left shoulder and/or ulnar aspect of left arm and hand

May also radiate to neck, jaw, teeth, back, abdomen, or right arm

Common descriptions of pain

Viselike   Constricting   Crushing weight and/or pressure

Other manifestations of myocardial ischemia

Fear   Perspiration

Shortness of breath   Nausea, vomiting

Weakness, collapse, coma

Chiefly retrosternal and intense

FIG 2.1 Pain of myocardial ischemia.

BOX 2.3 Cardiac Risk Factors

- Diabetes
- Smoking
- Hypertension
- High cholesterol
- Hyperlipidemia
- Sedentary lifestyle
- High-fat diet
- Stress
- Metabolic syndrome
- Family history of CHD (including history of MI, sudden cardiac death, and first-degree relatives who underwent coronary revascularization)
- Age
- Male sex
- Obesity

CHD, Coronary heart disease; *MI,* myocardial infarction.

Determining whether the patient has stable or unstable angina is as important as making the diagnosis of angina. Stable angina is important to evaluate and treat but does not necessitate emergent intervention. However, unstable angina or acute coronary syndrome carries a significant risk of MI or death in the immediate future. The types of symptoms reported by patients with stable and unstable angina differ little, and the risk factors for both are identical. The severity of symptoms is not necessarily greater in patients with unstable angina, just as a lack of chest discomfort does not rule out significant CHD. The important distinction between stable and unstable coronary syndromes is whether the onset is new or recent, and/or progressive (e.g., occurring

more frequently or with less exertion). The initial presentation of angina is, by definition, unstable angina, although for a high percentage of individuals this may merely represent the first recognizable episode of angina. For those with unstable angina, the risk of MI in the near future is markedly increased. Likewise, when the patient experiences angina in response to decreased levels of exertion or when exertional angina has begun to occur at rest, these urgent circumstances require immediate therapy. The treatment of stable angina and acute coronary syndrome is discussed in Chapters 19 to 21.

The Canadian Cardiovascular Society Functional Classification of Angina Pectoris is a useful guide for everyday patient assessment (Box 2.4). Categorizing patients according to their class of symptoms is rapid and precise and can be used in follow-up. Class IV describes the typical patient with acute coronary syndrome.

Finally, it is important to distinguish those patients who have noncoronary causes of chest discomfort from those with CHD. Patients with gastroesophageal reflux disease (GERD) often present with symptoms that are impossible to distinguish from angina. In numerous studies, GERD was the most common diagnosis in patients who underwent diagnostic testing for angina and were found not to have CHD. The characteristics of the pain can be identical. Because exercise can increase intraabdominal pressure, GERD may be exacerbated with exercise, especially after meals. Symptoms from GERD can also be relieved with use of sublingual nitroglycerin. GERD can also result in early morning awakening (as can unstable angina) but tends to awaken individuals 2 to 4 hours after going to sleep, rather than 1 to 2 hours before arising, as is the case with unstable angina. Other causes (see Box 2.1) of angina-like pain can be benign or suggestive of other high-risk syndromes, such as aortic dissection or pulmonary embolus. Many of these "coronary mimics" can be ruled out by patient history, but others, such as valvular aortic stenosis, can be confirmed or excluded by physical examination.

BOX 2.4 Canadian Cardiovascular Society Classification of Angina Pectoris

I. Ordinary physical activity, for example, walking or climbing stairs, does not cause angina; angina occurs with strenuous, rapid, or prolonged exertion at work or recreation.

II. Slight limitation of ordinary activity; for example, angina occurs when walking or stair climbing after meals, in cold, in wind, under emotional stress, or only during the few hours after awakening, when walking more than two blocks on the level, or when climbing more than one flight of ordinary stairs at a normal pace and during normal conditions.

III. Marked limitation of ordinary activity; for example, angina occurs when walking one or two blocks on the level or when climbing one flight of stairs during normal conditions and at a normal pace.

IV. Inability to carry on any physical activity without discomfort; angina syndrome may be present at rest.

From Campeau L. Grading of angina pectoris [letter]. *Circulation.* 1976;54:522–523.

The goal of taking the history is to alert the clinician to entities that can be confirmed or excluded by physical examination or that necessitate further diagnostic testing.

Dyspnea, Edema, and Ascites

Dyspnea can accompany angina pectoris or it can be an anginal equivalent. Dyspnea can also reflect congestive heart failure (CHF) or occur because of noncardiac causes. The key to understanding the etiology of dyspnea is a clear patient history, which is then confirmed by a targeted physical examination.

Dyspnea during exertion that quickly resolves at rest or with use of nitroglycerin may be a result of myocardial ischemia. It is important to establish the amount of activity necessary to provoke dyspnea, the reproducibility of these symptoms, and the duration of recovery. As with angina, dyspnea, as an anginal equivalent or an accompanying symptom, tends to occur at a given workload or stress level; dyspnea that occurs one day at low levels of exertion but not prompted by vigorous exertion on another day is less likely to be an anginal equivalent.

In patients with CHF, dyspnea generally reflects increased left ventricular (LV) filling pressures (Fig. 2.2). Although LV systolic dysfunction is the most common cause of the dyspnea, dyspnea also occurs in individuals with preserved LV systolic function and severe diastolic dysfunction. However, these two entities present differently, and physical examination can distinguish them. With LV systolic dysfunction, dyspnea tends to gradually worsen, and its exacerbation is more variable than that of exertional dyspnea resulting from myocardial ischemia, although both are due to fluctuations in pulmonary arterial volume and left atrial filling pressures. Typically, patients with LV systolic dysfunction do not recover immediately after exercise cessation or use of sublingual nitroglycerin, and the dyspnea may linger for longer periods. Orthopnea, the occurrence of dyspnea when recumbent, or paroxysmal nocturnal edema provides further support for a presumptive diagnosis of LV systolic dysfunction. Patients with LV diastolic dysfunction tend to present abruptly with severe dyspnea that resolves more rapidly in response to diuretic therapy than does dyspnea caused by LV systolic dysfunction. The New York Heart Association (NYHA) functional classification for CHF (Table 2.1) is extremely useful in following patients with CHF and provides a simple and rapid means for longitudinal assessment. The NYHA functional classification also correlates well with prognosis. Patients who are in NYHA functional class I have a low

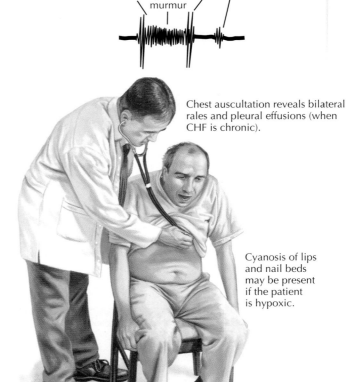

Left-Sided Cardiac Heart Failure

Cardiac auscultation for third heart sounds (S_3) and murmurs should be performed in standard positions, including that with the patient sitting forward.

S_1 Systolic murmur S_2 S_3

Chest auscultation reveals bilateral rales and pleural effusions (when CHF is chronic).

Cyanosis of lips and nail beds may be present if the patient is hypoxic.

C. Machado —M.D.

Patients with left-sided CHF may be uncomfortable lying down.

FIG 2.2 Physical examination. *CHF,* Congestive heart failure.

risk of death or hospital admission within the following year. In contrast, the annual mortality rate of those with NYHA functional class IV symptoms exceeds 30%.

As with chest discomfort, the differential diagnosis of dyspnea is broad, encompassing many cardiac and noncardiac causes (Box 2.5). Congenital heart disease, with or without pulmonary hypertension, can cause exertional dyspnea. Patients with significant intracardiac or extracardiac shunts and irreversible pulmonary hypertension (Eisenmenger syndrome) are dyspneic during minimal exertion and often at rest. It is also possible to have dyspnea because of acquired valvular heart disease, usually from aortic or mitral valve stenosis or regurgitation. All of these causes should be easily distinguished from CHD or CHF by physical examination. Primary pulmonary causes of dyspnea must be considered, with chronic obstructive pulmonary disease and reactive airways disease (asthma) being the most common causes. Again, a careful history for risk factors (e.g., cigarette smoking, industrial exposure, allergens) associated with these entities and an accurate physical examination should distinguish primary pulmonary causes from dyspnea due to CHD or CHF.

TABLE 2.1   Comparison of the ACC/AHA and the NYHA Classifications of Heart Failure

ACC/AHA STAGE		NYHA FUNCTIONAL CLASS	
Stage	**Description**	**Class**	**Description**
A	At high risk for HF but without structural heart disease or symptoms of heart failure	None	
B	Structural heart disease but without signs or symptoms of heart failure	I (mild)	No limitation of physical activity. Ordinary physical activity does not cause undue fatigue, palpitation, or dyspnea.
C	Structural heart disease with previous or current symptoms of heart failure	1 (mild)	No limitation of physical activity. Ordinary physical activity does not cause undue fatigue, palpitation, or dyspnea.
		2 (mild)	Slight limitation of physical activity. Comfortable at rest, but ordinary physical activity results in fatigue, palpitation, or dyspnea.
		III (moderate)	Marked limitation of physical activity. Comfortable at rest, but less than ordinary activity causes fatigue, palpitation, or dyspnea.
D	Refractory heart failure requiring specialized interventions	IV (severe)	Unable to carry out any physical activity without discomfort. Symptoms of cardiac insufficiency at rest. If any physical activity is undertaken, discomfort is increased.

ACC/AHA, American College of Cardiology/American Heart Association; *HF,* heart failure; *NYHA,* New York Heart Association.
NYHA data from the Criteria Committee of the New York Heart Association. *Diseases of the Heart and Blood Vessels: Nomenclature and Criteria for Diagnosis.* Boston: Brown; 1964.
ACC/AHA data from Yancy CW, Jessup M, Bozkurt B, et al. 2013 ACCF/AHA guideline for the management of heart failure: a report of the American College of Cardiology Foundation/American Heart Association Task Force on Practice Guidelines. *J Am Coll Cardiol.* 2013;62:e147–e239.

BOX 2.5   Differential Diagnosis of Dyspnea

Pulmonary
- Reactive airways disease (asthma)
- Chronic obstructive pulmonary disease
- Emphysema
- Pulmonary edema
- Pulmonary hypertension
- Lung transplant rejection
- Infection
- Interstitial lung disease
- Pleural disease
- Pulmonary embolism
- Respiratory muscle failure
- Exercise intolerance

Cardiac
- Ischemic heart disease/angina pectoris
- Right-sided heart failure
- Aortic stenosis or regurgitation
- Arrhythmias
- Dilated cardiomyopathy
- Hypertrophic cardiomyopathy
- Congestive heart failure
- Mitral regurgitation or stenosis
- Mediastinal abnormalities
- Pericardial tuberculosis
- Transposition of the great arteries

Other
- Blood transfusion reaction
- Measles

Peripheral edema and ascites are physical examination findings consistent with pulmonary hypertension and/or right ventricular (RV) failure. These findings are included in the history because they may be part of the presentation. Although patients often comment on peripheral edema, with careful questioning, they may also identify increasing abdominal girth consistent with ascites. Important questions on lower extremity edema include determination of whether the edema is symmetrical (unilateral edema suggests alternate diagnoses) and whether the edema improves or resolves with elevation of the lower extremities. The finding of "no resolution overnight" argues against RV failure as an etiology. In addition, for peripheral edema and ascites, it is important to ask questions directed toward determining the presence of anemia, hypoproteinemia, or other causes. The differential diagnosis of edema is broad and beyond the scope of this chapter.

Palpitations and Syncope

It is normal to be aware of the sensation of the heart beating, particularly during or immediately after exertion or emotional stress. Palpitations refer to an increased awareness of the heart beating. Patients use many different descriptions, including a "pounding or racing of the heart," the feeling that their heart is "jumping" or "thumping" in their chest, the feeling that the heart "skips beats" or "races," or countless other descriptions. A history that shows that palpitations began to occur during or immediately after exertion, and not at other times, raises the concern that these sensations reflect ventricular ectopy associated with myocardial ischemia. It is more difficult to assess the significance of palpitations occurring at other times. Supraventricular and ventricular ectopy may occur at any time and may be benign or morbid. As discussed in Chapters 41 and 42, ventricular ectopy is worrisome in patients with a history of MI or cardiomyopathy. Lacking this information, clinicians should be most concerned if lightheadedness or presyncope accompanies palpitations.

Syncope generally indicates an increased risk for sudden cardiac death and is usually a result of cardiovascular disease and arrhythmias.

BOX 2.6 Differential Diagnosis for Syncope

Cardiogenic
- Mechanical
  Outflow tract obstruction
  Pulmonary hypertension
  Congenital heart disease
  Myocardial disease: low-output states
- Electrical
  Bradyarrhythmias
  Tachyarrhythmias
- Neurocardiogenic
  Vasovagal (vasodepression)
  Orthostatic hypotension

Other
- Peripheral neuropathy
  Medications
  Primary autonomic insufficiency
  Intravascular volume depletion
  Reflex
  Cough
  Micturition
  Acute pain states
  Carotid sinus hypersensitivity

If a syncopal episode is a presenting complaint, the patient should be admitted for further assessment. In approximately 85% of patients, the cause of syncope is cardiovascular. In patients with syncope, assessment for CHD, cardiomyopathy, and congenital or valvular heart disease should be performed. In addition, neurocardiogenic causes represent a relatively common and important possible etiology for syncope. Box 2.6 shows the differential diagnosis for syncope. It is critical to determine whether syncope really occurred. A witness to the episode and documentation of an intervening period are helpful. In addition, with true syncope, injuries related to the sudden loss of consciousness are common. However, individuals who report recurrent syncope (witnessed or unwitnessed) but has never injured themselves may not be experiencing syncope. This is not to lessen the concern that a serious underlying medical condition exists but, instead, to reaffirm that the symptoms fall short of syncope, with its need for immediate evaluation.

THE PHYSICAL EXAMINATION

There are several advantages to obtaining the history of the patient before the physical examination. First, the information gained in the history directs the clinician to pay special attention to aspects of the physical examination. For instance, a history consistent with CHD necessitates careful inspection for signs of vascular disease; a history suggestive of CHF should make the clinician pay particular attention to the presence of a third heart sound. Second, the history allows the clinician to establish a rapport with patients and to assure patients that the clinician is interested in their well-being; clinicians are then allowed to perform a complete physical examination, which is imperative in a complete evaluation. In this light, the therapeutic value of the physical examination to the patient should not be underestimated. Despite the emphasis on technology today, even the most sophisticated patients expect to be examined, to have their hearts listened to, and to be told whether worrisome findings exist or whether the examination results were normal.

General Inspection and Vital Signs

Much useful information can be gained by an initial "head-to-toe" inspection and assessment of vital signs. For instance, truncal obesity may signal the presence of type 2 diabetes or metabolic syndrome. Cyanosis of the lips and nail beds may indicate underlying cyanotic heart disease. Hairless, dry-skinned lower extremities or distal ulceration may indicate peripheral vascular disease. Other findings are more specific (Fig. 2.3). Abnormalities of the digits are found in atrial septal defect; typical findings of Down syndrome indicate an increased incidence of ventricular septal defect or more complex congenital heart disease; hyperextensible skin and lax joints are suggestive of Ehlers-Danlos syndrome; and tall individuals with arachnodactyly, lax joints, pectus excavatum, and an increased arm length-to-height ratio may have Marfan syndrome. These represent some of the more common morphological phenotypes in individuals with heart disease. Vital signs can also be helpful. Although normal vital signs do not rule out CHD, marked hypertension may signal cardiac risk, whereas tachycardia, tachypnea, and/or hypotension at rest suggest CHF.

Important Components of the Cardiovascular Examination

The clinician should focus efforts on those sites that offer a window into the heart and vasculature. Palpation and careful inspection of the skin for secondary changes because of vascular disease or diabetes is important. Lips, nail beds, and fingertips should be examined for cyanosis (including clubbing of the fingernails) and, when indicated, for signs of embolism. Examination of the retina using an ophthalmoscope can reveal evidence of long-standing hypertension, diabetes, or atheroembolism, denoting underlying vascular disease. Careful examination of the chest, including auscultation, can help to differentiate causes of dyspnea. The presence of dependent rales is consistent with left-sided heart failure. Pleural effusions can result from long-standing LV dysfunction or noncardiac causes and can be present with predominantly right-sided heart failure, representing transudation of ascites into the pleural space. Hyperexpansion with or without wheezing suggests a primary pulmonary cause of dyspnea, such as chronic obstructive pulmonary disease or reactive airways disease. The presence of wheezing rather than rales does not rule out left-sided heart failure. It is not uncommon to hear wheezing with left-sided CHF. Wheezing from left-sided CHF is most commonly primarily expiratory. Inspiratory and expiratory wheezing, particularly with a prolonged inspiratory-to-expiratory ratio, is more likely to be caused by intrinsic lung disease.

The vascular examination is an important component of a complete evaluation. The quality of the pulses, in particular, the carotid and the femoral pulses, can identify underlying disease (Fig. 2.4). Diminished or absent distal pulses indicate peripheral vascular disease. The examiner should also auscultate for bruits over both carotids, over the femoral arteries, and in the abdomen. Abdominal auscultation should be performed, carefully listening for aortic or renal bruits, in the mid-abdominal area before abdominal palpation, which can stimulate increased bowel sounds. Distinguishing bruits from transmitted murmurs in the carotid and abdominal areas can be challenging. When this is a concern, carefully marching out from the heart using the stethoscope can be helpful. If the intensity of the murmur or bruit continually diminishes farther from the heart, it becomes more likely that this sound originates from the heart, rather than from a stenosis in the peripheral vasculature. Much information is available about the peripheral vascular examination, but by following the simple steps outlined herein, the examiner can gather most of the accessible clinical information.

Examination of the jugular venous pulsations is a commonly forgotten step. Jugular venous pressure, which correlates with right atrial

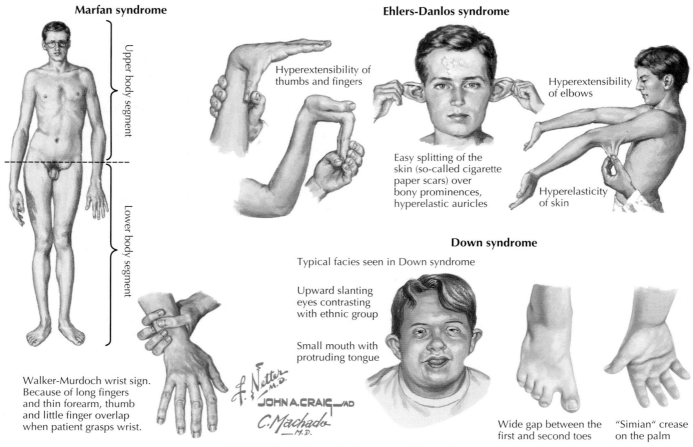

Marfan syndrome

Upper body segment

Lower body segment

Hyperextensibility of thumbs and fingers

Walker-Murdoch wrist sign. Because of long fingers and thin forearm, thumb and little finger overlap when patient grasps wrist.

Ehlers-Danlos syndrome

Hyperextensibility of elbows

Easy splitting of the skin (so-called cigarette paper scars) over bony prominences, hyperelastic auricles

Hyperelasticity of skin

Down syndrome

Typical facies seen in Down syndrome

Upward slanting eyes contrasting with ethnic group

Small mouth with protruding tongue

Wide gap between the first and second toes

"Simian" crease on the palm

FIG 2.3 Physical examination: general inspection.

pressure and RV diastolic pressure, should be estimated initially with the patient lying with the upper trunk elevated 30 to 45 degrees. In this position, at normal jugular venous pressure, no pulsations are visible. This correlates roughly to a jugular venous pressure of <6 to 10 cm. The absence of jugular vein pulsations with the patient in this position can be confirmed by occluding venous return by placing a fingertip parallel to the clavicle in the area of the sternocleidomastoid muscle. The internal and external jugular veins should partially fill. Although normal jugular venous pressure examination of the waveforms is less important, the head of the examination table can be lowered until the jugular venous pulsations are evident. When the jugular venous pulsations are visible at 30 degrees, the examiner should note the waveforms. It is possible to observe and time the *a* and *v* waves by simultaneously timing the cardiac apical impulse or the carotid impulse on the contralateral side. An exaggerated *a* wave is consistent with increased atrial filling pressures because of tricuspid valve stenosis or increased RV diastolic pressure. A large *v* wave generally indicates tricuspid valve regurgitation, a finding easily confirmed by auscultation.

Finally, it is important to palpate the precordium before cardiac auscultation. This is the easiest way to identify dextrocardia. Characteristics of the cardiac impulse can also yield important clues about underlying disease. Palpation of the precordium is best performed from the patient's right side with the patient lying flat. The cardiac apical impulse is normally located in the fifth intercostal space along the midclavicular line. Most examiners use the fingertips to palpate the apical impulse. It is often possible to palpate motion corresponding to a third or fourth heart sound. Use of the fingertips offers fine detail on the

size and character of the apical impulse. A diffuse and sustained apical impulse is consistent with LV systolic dysfunction. In contrast, patients with hypertrophic cardiomyopathy often have a hyperdynamic apical impulse. Thrills, palpable vibrations from loud murmurs or bruits, can also be palpated.

The RV impulse, if identifiable, is located along the left sternal border. Many clinicians prefer to palpate the RV impulse with the base of the hand, lifting the fingertips off the chest wall. In RV hypertrophy, a sustained impulse can be palpated, and the fingertips then can be placed at the LV impulse to confirm that the two are distinct. In patients with a sustained RV impulse, the examiner should again look for prominent *a* and *v* waves in the jugular venous pulsations.

Cardiac Auscultation

Hearing and accurately describing heart sounds is arguably the most difficult part of the physical examination. For this reason and because of the commonplace use of echocardiography, many clinicians perform a cursory examination. The strongest arguments for performing cardiac auscultation carefully are to determine whether further diagnostic testing is necessary and to correlate findings of echocardiography with the clinical examination so that in longitudinal follow-up, the clinician can determine the progression of disease without repeating echocardiography at each visit. In addition, as clinicians make more of these correlations, their skills in auscultation will become better, and their patients will be better served. With normal general cardiac physical examination results, the absence of abnormal heart sounds, and a normal electrocardiogram, the use of echocardiography for evaluation of valvular or

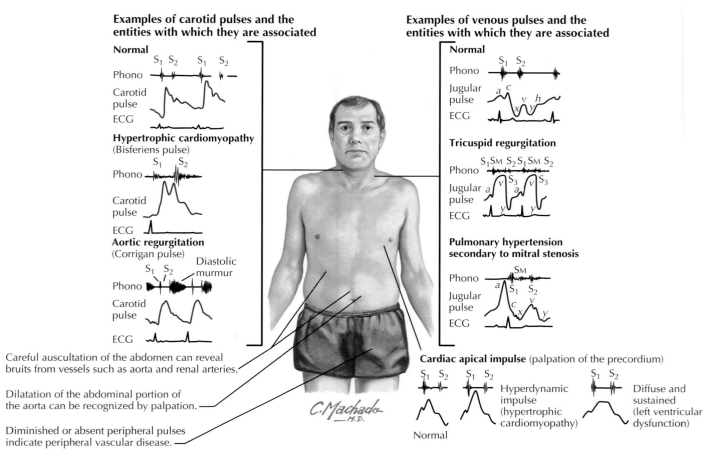

Examples of carotid pulses and the entities with which they are associated

Normal

Hypertrophic cardiomyopathy (Bisferiens pulse)

Aortic regurgitation (Corrigan pulse)

Careful auscultation of the abdomen can reveal bruits from vessels such as aorta and renal arteries.

Dilatation of the abdominal portion of the aorta can be recognized by palpation.

Diminished or absent peripheral pulses indicate peripheral vascular disease.

Examples of venous pulses and the entities with which they are associated

Normal

Tricuspid regurgitation

Pulmonary hypertension secondary to mitral stenosis

Cardiac apical impulse (palpation of the precordium)

Normal; Hyperdynamic impulse (hypertrophic cardiomyopathy); Diffuse and sustained (left ventricular dysfunction)

FIG 2.4 Important components of cardiac examination.

congenital heart disease is not indicated. Furthermore, if there are no symptoms of CHF or evidence of hemodynamic compromise, echocardiography is not indicated for assessment of LV function. Practice guidelines from cardiologists and generalists agree on this point, as do third-party insurers. It is neither appropriate nor feasible to replace a careful cardiovascular examination using auscultation with more expensive testing.

The major impact of echocardiography has been in the quantitative assessment of cardiovascular hemodynamics, that is, the severity of valvular and congenital heart disease. It is no longer necessary for the clinician to make an absolute judgment on whether an invasive assessment (cardiac catheterization) is needed to further define hemodynamic status or whether the condition is too advanced to allow surgical intervention based on history and physical examination. Instead of diminishing the role of cardiac auscultation, the advent of echocardiography has redefined it. Auscultation remains important as a screening technique for significant hemodynamic abnormalities, as an independent technique to focus and verify the echocardiographic study, and as an important means by which the physician can longitudinally follow patients with known disease.

There are several keys to excellence in auscultation. Foremost is the ability to perform a complete general cardiac physical examination, as described. The findings help the examiner focus on certain auscultatory features. Second, it is important to use a high-quality stethoscope. Largely dictated by individual preference, clinicians should select a stethoscope that has both bell and diaphragm capacity (for optimal appreciation of low-frequency and high-frequency sounds, respectively), fits the ears

comfortably, and is well insulated so that external sounds are minimized. Third, it is important to perform auscultation in a quiet environment. When skills in auscultation are developing, trying to hone these in the hall of a busy emergency department or on rounds while others are speaking is time poorly spent. In addition, taking the time to return to see a patient with interesting findings detected during auscultation, and repetition, are keys to becoming competent in auscultation.

The patient should be examined while they are in several positions: while recumbent, while in the left lateral decubitus position, and while sitting forward. Every patient is different, and by using all three positions, the examiner can optimize the chance that soft heart sounds can be heard. Likewise, it is important to listen carefully at the standard four positions on the chest wall (Fig. 2.5), as well as over the apical impulse and RV impulse (if present). It is also best to isolate different parts of the examination in time. Regardless of the intensity of various sounds, it is best always to perform the examination steps in the same chronological order so that the presence of a specific heart sound (e.g., loud murmur) does not result in failure to listen to the other heart sounds.

Listen for S_1 (the first heart sound) first. As with jugular venous pulsations, the heart sounds can be timed by simultaneously palpating the cardiac apical impulse or the carotid upstroke. Even the most experienced clinician occasionally needs to time the heart sounds. Is a single sound present, or is the first heart sound split? Is a sound heard before S_1, indicating an S_4? Next, listen to the second heart sound. Normally, the first component (A_2, the aortic valve closing sound) is louder than the second component (P_2, the pulmonic valve closing sound). A louder

Cardiac Auscultation: Precordial areas of auscultation

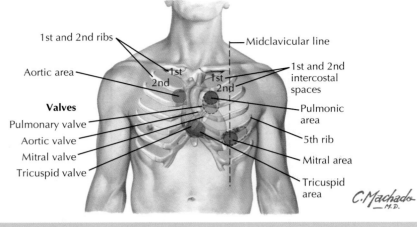

Diagrams of murmurs

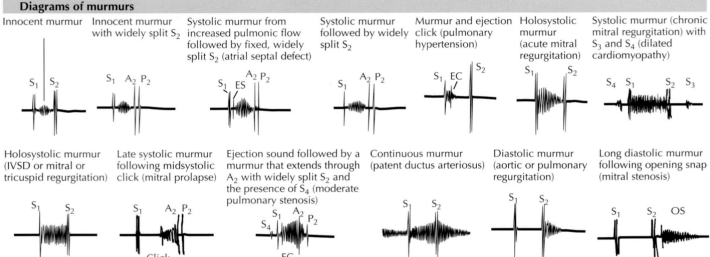

FIG 2.5 Cardiac auscultation: correlation of murmurs and other adventitious sounds with underlying pathophysiology. *EC,* Ejection click; *ES,* ejection sound; *IVSD,* intraventricular septal defect; *OS,* opening snap.

second component may indicate increased pulmonary pressure. A more subtle finding is a reversal of A_2 and P_2 timing that occurs with left bundle branch block and in some other circumstances. In addition, it is important to assess whether A_2 and P_2 are normally split or whether they are widely split with no respiratory variation—a finding that suggests an atrial septal defect. The examiner should then listen carefully for a third heart sound. An S_3 is often best heard over the tricuspid or mitral areas, and is a low-frequency sound. It is heard best with the bell and is often not heard with the diaphragm.

After characterizing these heart sounds, it is time to listen carefully for murmurs. Murmurs are classified according to their intensity, their duration, their location, and their auscultatory characteristics: crescendo, decrescendo, and blowing, among others. It is also important to note the site where the murmur is loudest and whether the murmur radiates to another area of the precordium or to the carotids. All of these features contribute to determining the origin of the murmur, the likelihood that it represents an acute or chronic process, and how it affects the diagnostic and therapeutic approaches. Most importantly, it is necessary for clinicians to judge whether a murmur represents cardiac disease or is innocent. Innocent murmurs, also termed "flow murmurs," are common in children.

More than 60% of children have innocent murmurs. Innocent murmurs become less common in adults; however, an innocent murmur can still be found into the fourth decade of life. Alterations in hemodynamics induced by pregnancy, anemia, fever, hyperthyroidism, or any state of increased cardiac output can produce an innocent murmur. These murmurs are generally midsystolic, heard over the tricuspid or pulmonic areas, and do not radiate extensively. They are often loudest in thin individuals. Innocent murmurs do not cause alterations in the carotid pulse and do not coexist with abnormal cardiac impulses or with other abnormalities, such as extra heart sounds (S_3 and S_4), in adults. A systolic murmur that shares auditory characteristics with the murmur of aortic stenosis is a common finding in older adults; however, carotid upstrokes are normal. This finding, aortic sclerosis, may necessitate confirmation by echocardiography. It represents sclerosis of the aortic leaflets but without significant hemodynamic consequence.

The characteristics of the most common and hemodynamically important murmurs are shown in Fig. 2.5. As noted, the murmur is defined not only by its auditory characteristics but also by the company it keeps. Often, the key to excellence in auscultation is being thorough in all aspects of the cardiovascular examination.

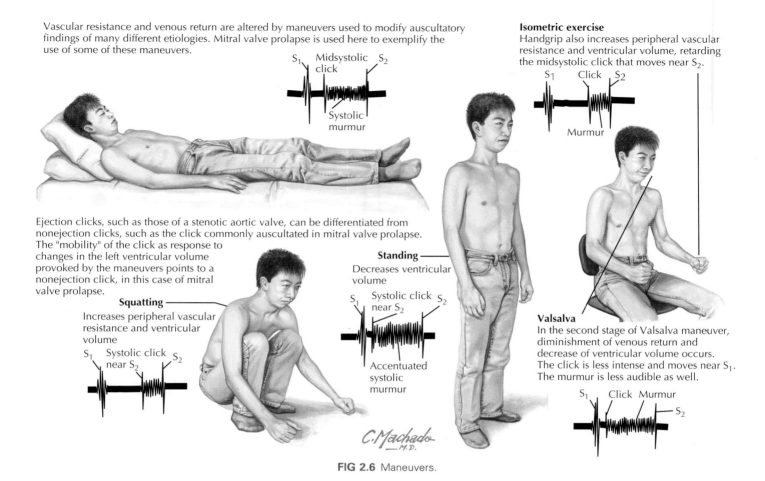

Vascular resistance and venous return are altered by maneuvers used to modify auscultatory findings of many different etiologies. Mitral valve prolapse is used here to exemplify the use of some of these maneuvers.

S_1 Midsystolic click S_2

Systolic murmur

Isometric exercise
Handgrip also increases peripheral vascular resistance and ventricular volume, retarding the midsystolic click that moves near S_2.

S_1 Click S_2

Murmur

Ejection clicks, such as those of a stenotic aortic valve, can be differentiated from nonejection clicks, such as the click commonly auscultated in mitral valve prolapse. The "mobility" of the click as response to changes in the left ventricular volume provoked by the maneuvers points to a nonejection click, in this case of mitral valve prolapse.

Squatting
Increases peripheral vascular resistance and ventricular volume

S_1 Systolic click near S_2 S_2

Standing
Decreases ventricular volume

S_1 Systolic click near S_2 S_2

Accentuated systolic murmur

Valsalva
In the second stage of Valsalva maneuver, diminishment of venous return and decrease of ventricular volume occurs. The click is less intense and moves near S_1. The murmur is less audible as well.

S_1 Click Murmur

S_2

C. Machado — M.D.

FIG 2.6 Maneuvers.

Maneuvers

No discussion of cardiac auscultation would be complete without the use of maneuvers to accentuate auscultatory findings. As shown in Fig. 2.6, patient positioning can alter peripheral vascular resistance or venous return, accentuating murmurs that are modulated by these changes. Murmurs associated with fixed valvular lesions change little with changes in position or the maneuvers illustrated in Fig. 2.6. Thus these maneuvers are most useful for diagnosing entities in which hemodynamic status affects murmurs. The two classic examples are the click and murmur of mitral valve prolapse, as shown, and the aortic outflow murmur of hypertrophic cardiomyopathy (not shown).

FUTURE DIRECTIONS

Handheld echocardiography machines can be carried on the shoulder and have a small transducer that can obtain echocardiographic images of sufficient quality to quantify murmurs and assess LV dysfunction. Although these portable echocardiographic machines have advantages and have been incorporated in medical school curricula at many institutions, they have not yet replaced the stethoscope, nor are they likely to do so.

The scope and role of a cardiac history and physical examination have changed. Today, the examination is performed beyond the clinic, with new advances in more accurate home blood pressure monitoring, high fidelity continuous blood pressure monitoring, and expansion to measuring vital signs at pharmacies, fire stations, and grocery stores. Today, it is believed that the role of the clinician is to use physical examination findings to establish the modifiable risk factors and previous probability of cardiovascular disease, whether CHD, valvular heart disease, or congenital heart disease, thereby determining the need for further testing and proper risk factor management. In the continual quest for improved noninvasive testing, it is likely that the skill of the clinician will continue to evolve as the interplay among history taking, physical examination, and diagnostic testing further develops.

ADDITIONAL RESOURCES

ACC/AHA Atherosclerosis Cardiovascular Disease Risk Calculator. Available at <http://www.cvriskcalculator.com>.
A website where you can enter patient-specific data to calculate the 10-year risk of cardiac event.
ACC/AHA Joint Guidelines. <http://www.americanheart.org/presenter.jhtml?identifier=3004542>. Accessed 22 February 2010.
Guidelines outlining the current opinion of experts from the American College of Cardiology and the American Heart Association for managing cardiovascular diseases.
American Heart Association. Heart Profilers. Available at: <http://www.americanheart.org/presenter.jhtml?identifier=3000416>. Accessed 22 February 2010.
Provides individual specific information based on the risk profile.

EVIDENCE

Diamond GA, Forrester JS. Analysis of probability as an aid in the clinical diagnosis of coronary-artery disease. *N Engl J Med.* 1979;300:1350–1358.
A classic discussion of the importance of pretest and posttest probabilities in interpreting any diagnostic testing.

Harvey WP. Cardiac Pearls [video recording]. Atlanta: Emory Medical Television Network; 1981.

This video recording is a timeless example of Dr. Harvey—a master clinician—and his approach to the evaluation of patients with cardiovascular disease.

Hurst JW, Morris DC. *Chest Pain*. Armonk, NY: Futura Publishing; 2001.

Drs. Hurst and Morris provide a sophisticated summary on the evaluation of patients with chest pain.

National Heart, Lung and Blood Institute. Third Report of the Expert Panel on Detection, Evaluation, and Treatment of High Blood Cholesterol in Adults (Adult Treatment Panel III) and ATP III Update 2004: Implications of Recent Clinical Trials for the ATP III Guidelines. Available at: http://www.nhlbi.nih.gov/guidelines/cholesterol. Accessed 10 November 2009.

An overview of the current recommendations regarding treatment of elevated lipids.

3

Genetics in Cardiovascular Disease

Fredy H. El Sakr, Xuming Dai, Cam Patterson, Marschall S. Runge

In 1953, Watson and Crick published their landmark paper on the molecular structure of nucleic acids and a particularly prescient comment was made: "It has not escaped our notice that the specific pairing we have postulated immediately suggests a possible copying mechanism for the genetic material."

The pace of technological innovation and our resulting understanding of the relationship of genetics to human disease continues to increase exponentially. Today, the ability to partially or completely sequence the genetic code of an individual is an inexpensive commodity, and the current and future impact of this knowledge continues to increase.

With this knowledge, our understanding of disease associations with the genetic code has become more complex, beyond simple assessment of various types of mutations leading to a certain phenotype. This is driven by an ever-increasing understanding of the interplay between genetic and environmental factors in disease. Today, in addition to easily understanding environmental factors important in cardiovascular disease (e.g., smoking, diet, exercise, and many others), it is apparent that the environment interacts with the genome in complex ways. Epigenetics, which is the study of changes in gene modification, or translation-altering gene expression, is now understood to be a mechanistic explanation, and possibly a therapeutic target for these environmental–genetic interactions (Fig. 3.1). One classic example of epigenetics in clinical medicine was the observation of children born to famished mothers during the Dutch Hunger Winter of 1944 to 1945. These children were observed in their sixth decade of life and were found to have higher rates of obesity and coronary artery disease (CAD). Further evaluation showed them to have decreased methylation of insulin-like growth factor-2, a factor known to be important in metabolism, energy use, and weight, compared with their genetically similar siblings. The increased understanding of factors that alter methylation, histone packaging, and noncoding RNA, to name a few, will lead to a stronger grasp of the correlation between disease and the genetic code. Because of the growing complexity and rapid pace of new information presented, the development of genetic specialists within each field has been paramount to assist healthcare providers in deciphering this information and its clinical implications.

The goal of this chapter is to introduce the clinically important principles of genetics and the application of these principles to clinical medicine, with particular emphasis on the genetics of cardiovascular diseases (Table 3.1). A brief glossary of the clinically important terms in this chapter is shown in Box 3.1.

GENETIC EVALUATION: SELECTED EXAMPLES

Cardiomyopathies

In the coming years, it is likely that genetic analysis will play an increasingly important role in understanding high-risk cardiovascular syndromes. Significant advances have been made in several cardiovascular phenotypes, as illustrated by the examples in this chapter.

Hypertrophic Cardiomyopathy

Cardiomyopathy is a term that refers to a heterogeneous group of diseases that affect the myocardium. Cardiomyopathies result from multiple etiologies, including ischemia, nonischemic causes (restrictive or infiltrative), and hypertrophy, each of which has subcategories. The study of familial trends and transmissible genetic abnormalities in cardiomyopathies has led to more detailed classification based not only on phenotypic appearance, but also on genetic alterations. In some cases, this knowledge is of importance for risk stratification and treatment.

A classic example is hypertrophic cardiomyopathy (HCM), which is defined as the presence of myocardial hypertrophy caused by myocardial disarray. HCM is a disease that affects 0.02% to 0.23% of the general population, and in some, but not all HCM patients, it results in symptomatic diseases due to left ventricular outflow obstruction and an increased risk for fatal arrhythmias, such as ventricular tachycardia. Current understanding of the genetic basis of HCM is complex (Fig. 3.2). Most cases are caused by autosomal dominant mutations in genes that encode proteins in the sarcomere. Beta-myosin heavy chain and myosin-binding protein C are the most common genes affected; however, other genes in the sarcomere protein, including troponins I and T, the tropomyosin α-1 chain, and myosin light chain-3 have also been implicated in HCM.

The specific genetic basis for HCM in a given family has allowed a much better understanding of the disease and its management.

For those with an identifiable genetic cause of HCM, genetic screening of family members allows for more focused disease surveillance and management at an early stage before symptoms develop. For those in the same family who lack the causative mutation, surveillance can be less frequent, or in some cases, not necessary. The treatment of left ventricular outflow obstruction is not driven by genetic mutations per se; however, combining pedigree–phenotype analysis with DNA sequence information can identify those with an increased risk of sudden cardiac death (SCD) and may be used for decision making in the use of implantable cardioverter-defibrillator. In addition, genetic testing can identify a subset of individuals with a positive genotype but a negative phenotype, which raises new clinical questions, such as whether these individuals should be excluded from participation of competitive sports, would benefit from a prophylactic defibrillator, and how often they should be screened for phenotypic HCM.

Genetic etiologies also underlie numerous autosomal recessive and X-linked metabolic causes of cardiomyopathy, such as Anderson-Fabry disease, mitochondrial cardiomyopathies, neuromuscular diseases, and infiltrative diseases. Certain drugs, such as anabolic steroids and tacrolimus, are also therapies that have been shown to be causes of HCMs.

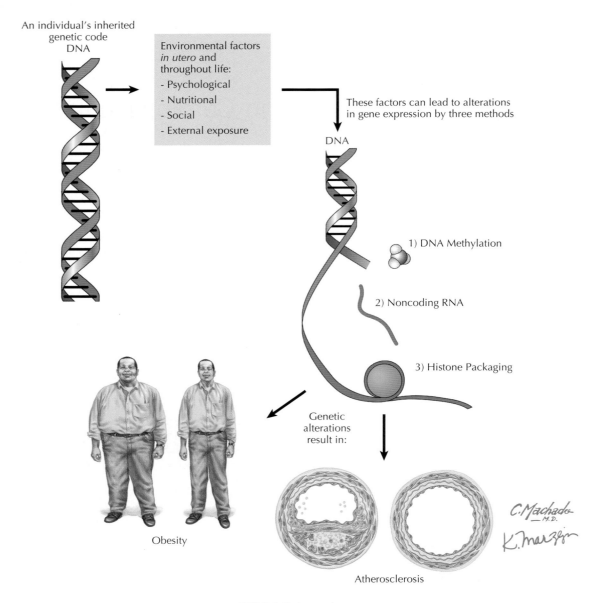

An individual's inherited genetic code
DNA

Environmental factors *in utero* and throughout life:
- Psychological
- Nutritional
- Social
- External exposure

These factors can lead to alterations in gene expression by three methods

DNA

1) DNA Methylation

2) Noncoding RNA

3) Histone Packaging

Genetic alterations result in:

Obesity

Atherosclerosis

FIG 3.1 Epigenetics.

Arrhythmogenic Diseases
Long QT Syndrome

Arrhythmogenic diseases result from heterogeneous causes that lead to atrial and ventricular tachyarrhythmias. Some of these disease processes overlap with structural heart diseases and cardiomyopathies, such as arrhythmogenic right ventricular dysplasia and left ventricular non-compaction, which predispose patients to fatal ventricular tachycardia and fibrillation. Although molecular causes of these complex phenotypes are only now being studied, much is known about these disease processes that phenotypically only affect the conduction system and spare the myocardium.

Long QT syndrome (LQTS) describes a group of diseases whose common phenotypic feature is an abnormal QT interval on the ECG. Usually patients with a corrected QT interval exceed the 99th percentile (>450 ms for men and 470 ms for women). QT prolongation is associated with SCD, presumably because of the propensity for polymorphic ventricular tachycardia (Torsades de pointes) when a premature ven-

tricular contraction occurs in the refractory period (prolonged in these cases. More than 200 mutations in 5 different genes (all coding for sodium or potassium channel proteins or their chaperones) have been reported to cause LQTS (Fig. 3.2; lower panel). Both autosomal-dominant and autosomal-recessive inheritance have been described for LQTS, which is the inheritance depending on the gene involved. Some forms of LQTS manifest only when a secondary cause of QT prolongation is present, such as electrolyte abnormalities, medications, or myocardial ischemia. The diagnosis of LQTS can be made by noninvasive (ECG) testing in most cases (except in the case of LQTS provoked by a secondary cause). For individuals from families with a history of SCD, careful analysis of the ECG is necessary, and provocative testing may be indicated in some circumstances. Nevertheless, the genetic basis for LQTS may be highly informative in terms of prognosis and as a guide to clinical therapy, as well as for identifying family members at risk for sudden death. More than 90% of all those with genotype-positive LQTS have genetic mutations in three main genes: *KLNQ1* (its mutation causing

TABLE 3.1 Select Examples of Diseases With Known Genetic Causes

Phenotype	Genetic Alteration (Most Common)	Functional Effect of Mutation	Method of Inheritance	Prevalence	Disease Characteristic
Cardiomyopathy					
HCM[a]	MYPBPC3, TNNI3, TNNT2, TPM1, MYL3	Sarcomere protein mutation leading to myocardial disarray	Autosomal dominant	0.02%–0.23%	LVH, LVOT obstruction, ventricular tachycardia
Fabry disease	GAL-A (GLA)	Loss of function of α-galactosidase-A in lysosomes, leading to build up of globotriaosylceramide in organs, including the heart	X-linked	0.0025%	LVH, systolic and diastolic dysfunction, coronary artery disease, conduction abnormalities, valvular dysfunction
ARVD	JUP, DSP, PKP2, DSMG2, DSC2, TGFβ3, TMEM43	Desmosome dysfunction leading to loss of electrical coupling between myocytes, leading to cell death with fibrofatty replacement and arrhythmias	Autosomal dominant	0.02%–0.05%	Fibrofatty replacement of RV myocytes. RV regional (early) or diffuse (late) disease. LV abnormalities can exist. Depolarization and repolarization abnormality leading to ventricular tachycardia and fibrillation
Familial DCM[a]	LMNA, MYH6, MYH7, MYPN, TNNT2, SCN5A, MYBPC3, etc.	Predominantly genes affecting stability of inner nuclear membrane, sarcomeric protein, or ion flux, though not exclusively	Variable	20%–35% of patients with idiopathic DCM	LV or biventricular dysfunction
Arrhythmia					
LQTS[a]			Autosomal dominant	0.014%–0.04%	Prolonged corrected QT >440 ms. Propensity VT/VF and SCD
Type 1	KCNQ1/KVLQT1	Mutation in α subunit of I_{Ks}			
Type 2	KCNH2/HERG	Mutation in α subunit of I_{Kr}			
Type 3	SCN5A	Mutation in α subunit of I_{NA}			
Brugada syndrome[a]	SCN5A, GPD1-L CACNA1c	Mutation in α subunit of I_{NA} Mutation in α subunit of I_{CA}	Autosomal dominant		Abnormal ECG with RBBB with characteristic cove-shaped ST elevation in leads V_1–V_3 without secondary causes. Propensity for VT/VF and SCD
Coronary Artery Disease					
Autosomal dominant familial hypercholesterolemia[a]	LDLR, APOB, PCSK9	Inability for LDL-R to LDL-C binding lead to diminished catabolism of LDL-C leading to elevated plasma levels of cholesterol	Autosomal dominant		Elevated LDL subparticles lead to accelerated atherosclerosis, leading to coronary artery disease

[a]Denotes only a select example of known genetic abnormalities.
ARVD, Arrhythmogenic right ventricular dysplasia; *DCM*, dilated cardiomyopathy; *HCM*, hypertrophic cardiomyopathy; *LDL-C*, low-density lipoprotein cholesterol; *LDL-R*, LDL receptor; *LV*, left ventricular; *LVH*, left ventricular hypertrophy; *LVOT*, left ventricular outflow tract; *RBBB*, right bundle branch block; *RV*, right ventricular; *SCD*, sudden cardiac death; *VT/VF*, ventricular tachycardia/ventricular fibrillation.

LQT1), *KCNH2* (LQT2), and *SCN5A* (LQT3). Additional minor genes, such as *KCNE1*, *KCNE2*, *CAV3*, *SCN4B*, *SNTA1*, *ANKB*, and *KCNJ2*, only account for approximately 5% of genotype-positive LQTS. Commercial genetic testing of all these LQTS genes are available at affordable costs. LQTS is an excellent example of a spectrum of diseases (which were once clustered together as a single entity) that will likely benefit from the principles of pharmacogenomics, which is the use of specific medications based on genotype.

Atherosclerosis

Atherosclerosis is the common pathology underlying a spectrum of arterial diseases, including coronary heart disease, ischemic stroke, aortic aneurysm, and peripheral arterial disease. Atherosclerosis continues to be a leading cause of morbidity and mortality in the Western world and a leading disorder seen by a broad range of physicians, and in its most extreme form, by cardiovascular specialists. The heritability of atherosclerotic coronary heart disease is approximately 50% to 60% with >10 monogenic causal genes and their mutations reported to cause familial atherosclerotic disease in a Mendelian pattern with variable penetrations. However, genetic and epigenetic factors that lead directly or indirectly to the accelerated process of atherosclerosis are vast and remain incompletely understood.

Recent studies of the genetics of atherosclerosis have made important advances in the identification of risk alleles for atherosclerosis, yet have

BOX 3.1   Terminology

Alleles: Copies of a specific gene. Humans have two alleles for each gene (one each from the biological father and mother). Alleles may have functional differences in their DNA sequence. A person with two identical copies of an allele is termed homozygous; a person with two different copies of an allele is called heterozygous.

Dominant mutation: A mutation in one allele of a gene that is sufficient to cause disease. More severe disease or lethality may result from a dominant mutation in both alleles of a gene.

Environmental effects: For this chapter, any potentially controllable influence on an individual. Examples are diet, exercise, air quality, a response to a prescribed or an over-the-counter medication, cigarette smoking, and alcohol use.

Genotype: The genetic makeup of an individual. Genotype can refer to specific genes or to the overall genetic profile.

Mutation: Changes in the DNA sequence of a gene that result in a gene product (protein) that has an altered sequence. For this chapter, mutations are considered to be changes in the DNA sequence of a gene that result in either loss of function or severely altered function.

Phenotype: The functional effects of genetic changes together with environmental influences. For instance, a person's appearance (body build, muscularity, hair color), the presence of measurable abnormalities that may reflect underlying disease processes, or other physical features demonstrate phenotypes. The list of measurable abnormalities is almost infinite, from blood pressure abnormalities to abnormal biochemical measurements (e.g., serum glucose levels) to ECG abnormalities reflecting ion channel abnormalities (as occur in LQTS) to coronary heart disease measured by angiography or endothelial dysfunction measured by forearm blood flow variability.

Polymorphism: An inherited variation in the DNA sequence of a gene that occurs at a greater frequency than would be expected of a mutation. Humans have thousands of polymorphisms, none of which are believed to be solely responsible for disease. Technically no different from mutations (a change in DNA sequence from "normal"), polymorphisms typically alter the gene product more subtly than mutations. It is believed that many human phenotypes result from the interplay between an individual's mix of polymorphisms and the environment.

Recessive mutation: A mutation that requires alterations in both alleles of a gene to cause disease (except in the case of mutations in the X and Y chromosomes).

LQTS, Long QT syndrome.

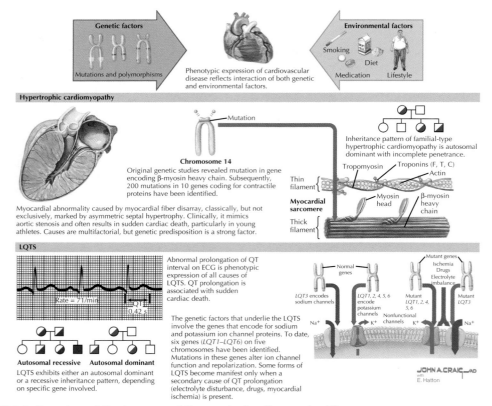

FIG 3.2 Genetic and Environmental Factors in Cardiovascular Disease. *LQTS*, Long QT syndrome.

also raised important questions about the usefulness of applying information about the presence of these risk alleles to clinical decision making. Using unbiased genome-wide association studies of genetic variants associated with atherosclerotic CAD, several groups simultaneously identified multiple highly correlated single nucleotide polymorphisms on chromosome 9 (9p21.3) that identified individuals at increased risk for developing coronary atherosclerosis. The immediate cross validation of this risk locus provided a high degree of certainty that it does incur increased risk of cardiovascular disease. The merits of screening individuals for these risk alleles are less certain. More than 50 single nucleotide polymorphisms have been identified to be associated with an increased risk of atherosclerotic CAD. For individuals who are known to have clinically significant atherosclerosis, knowledge of risk allele status is of little value, at least until or if specific therapies are developed for patients bearing these polymorphisms. For individuals concerned about their future risk of cardiovascular disease, it is unclear whether knowledge about risk allele status confers additional information beyond known clinical risk factors. Attempts to construct a genetic risk score to provide lifelong prediction of CAD risk, by taking a panel of genetic variants associated with increased risk of CAD, are at its early stage. Time and additional research will clarify these issues, but at present the clinical value of genetic testing for these risk alleles is not established, even if the tests are now easily available.

GENETICS IN PHARMACOLOGY

The genetic role in cardiovascular diseases has been essential, especially in the field of pharmacology. The identification of genetic and epigenetic associations with diseases has led to the development of medications in the prevention and treatment of cardiovascular diseases. An important and novel example is the development of a class of medications called proprotein convertase subtilisin/kexin type 9 (PCSK9) inhibitors. The binding of circulating low-density lipoprotein (LDL) cholesterol to LDL receptors, predominantly found in the liver, activates endocytosis of both the receptor and LDL cholesterol, with a resulting decrease in plasma LDL levels. PCSK9 is a protein that binds to LDL receptors and leads to the degradation of LDL receptors (Fig. 3.3). An important early finding was based on genetic analysis of French families with autosomal familial hypercholesterolemia. That study, and many since, have identified mutations that resulted in a gain of function to PCSK9, which led to elevated LDL levels in plasma. Two missense mutations that led to a loss of function of PCSK9 were found in a group of African Americans, which resulted in lower LDL levels. Based on these and more mechanistic studies, drug development to inhibit PCSK9 began. Currently, two novel monoclonal antibodies, evolocumab and alirocumab, are approved for use in humans with resistant hypercholesterolemia to lower LDL levels.

Genetics have also been used to evaluate individual response to medications currently in use. A common example is for dose adjustment of a common blood thinner, warfarin, a vitamin K antagonist used for a number of disease entities, such as prevention of strokes in atrial fibrillation and treatment of venous thromboembolism. Warfarin has a narrow therapeutic window, measured by the international normalized ratio. Polymorphisms in two alleles, CYP2C9 and VKORC1, have been studied in initiating, escalating, and maintenance doses of warfarin. Clinical data have shown a correlation of maintenance doses for warfarin with various genetic polymorphisms of the preceding alleles; however, routine clinical use continues to be of questionable importance. It is reasonable to anticipate that pharmacogenetic studies will lead to more precise use and dosage of a variety of cardiovascular drugs.

FUTURE DIRECTIONS

As our understanding of the roles that genetics and epigenetics play in cardiovascular diseases grows, our methods of classification and management will continue to evolve. Research on targeted therapy, stem cell replacement, and the use of angiogenic factors continues, while the role of epigenetics in all disease entities is a rapidly growing and promising field. As new factors in epigenetics are found, there is hope for development of novel risk stratification models and new medications. Across the world, cardiovascular scientists are focusing on "precision medicine" approaches for prevention and treatment strategies that take individual variability into account.

It is important to bear in mind that despite the rapid growth of available information and resources, we have much to learn. We now

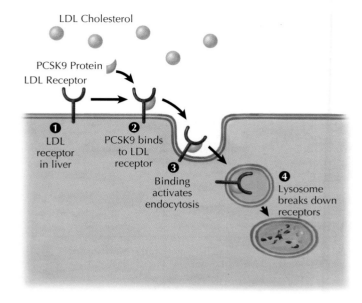

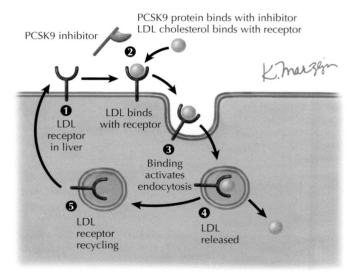

FIG 3.3 Proprotein Convertase Subtilisin/Kexin Type 9 (PCSK9). *LDL,* Low-density lipoprotein.

understand that relying solely on genetic abnormalities is not sufficient to make therapeutic decisions in most circumstances. As described previously, regarding the use of genetic evaluation of warfarin metabolism, and similarly seen in genetic testing for the use of clopidogrel, a common antiplatelet used for CAD, although genetic associations may be made, the clinical significance and importance must always be weighed against the cost and inconvenience of many such technologies. This is true to an even greater degree in more complex cardiovascular diseases.

It should be expected, and has already been clinically seen, that as the wealth of genetic and epigenetic information grows, the management of many disease entities will become more complex and require a multidisciplinary team approach. Dedicated centers for diseases (e.g., HCM) already exhibit such a model, with cardiologists, electrophysiologists, geneticists, physical therapists, and dieticians all intricately involved in managing each patient.

ADDITIONAL RESOURCES

McKusick VA. *Mendelian Inheritance in Man: A Catalogue of Human Genes and Genetic Disorders*. 12th ed. Baltimore: Johns Hopkins Press; 1998.

Dr. McKusick was the father of human genetics. His compendium on genetic causes of human diseases is a useful reference for anyone involved in the care of patients.

Watson JD. *Molecular Biology of the Gene*. 6th ed. Menlo Park, CA: Benjamin/ Cummings; 2007.

An excellent reference for students seeking to better understand biology at the molecular level.

Watson JD, Crick FH. Molecular structure of nucleic acids: a structure for deoxyribose nucleic acid. *Nature*. 1953;171:737–738.

A classic article describing the structure of DNA. Watson and Crick were awarded the Nobel Prize for this work.

EVIDENCE

Arad M, Seidman JG, Seidman CE. Phenotypic diversity in hypertrophic cardiomyopathy. *Hum Mol Genet*. 2002;11:2499–2506.

Describes the widely variable effects specific mutations have on cardiac development and the phenotype of HCM due to other genetic and environmental influences.

Bogardus C, Tataranni PA. Reduced early insulin secretion in the etiology of type 2 diabetes mellitus in Pima Indians. *Diabetes*. 2002;51(suppl 1): S262–S264.

One of the early descriptions of the mechanisms responsible for diabetes in the Pima Indian population.

Khoury MJ, McCabe LL, McCabe ER. Population screening in the age of genomic medicine. *N Engl J Med*. 2003;348:50–58.

Addresses issues related to the use of genetic tools in screening populations.

National Center for Biotechnology Information (home page on the Internet). Available at: <http://www.ncbi.nlm.nih.gov>. Accessed March 22 2010.

Provides valuable, constantly updated information on the genetics of human diseases.

Vincent GM. The long-QT syndrome: bedside to bench to bedside. *N Engl J Med*. 2003;348:1837–1838.

A useful review of the genes that have been implicated in LQTS, the mechanisms by which these genes cause QT prolongation, as well as diagnostic and therapeutic approaches to individuals with LQTS.

4

Effects of Exercise on Cardiovascular Health

Eileen M. Handberg, Richard S. Schofield, David S. Sheps

Although there has been a 25.3% decline in cardiovascular disease (CVD) mortality between 2004 and 2014, coronary heart disease (CHD) is still the leading cause of mortality and morbidity in the United States. It is estimated that >92 million American adults have ≥1 type of CVD. Physical inactivity is a global issue, identified by the World Health Organization (WHO) as the fourth leading risk factor for death, which leads to an estimated 3.2 million deaths annually. Individuals with a sedentary lifestyle have a relative risk of 1.9 for CHD compared with those with an active occupation and/or lifestyle. In a study of American adults with less than recommended aerobic physical activity, economic analyses indicated that inadequate physical activity was associated with an 11% of aggregate healthcare expenditures, accounting for $117 billion dollars per year. Statistics from the President's Council on Fitness, Sports, and Nutrition from 2017 indicate that only one in three adults achieve the 2008 Physical Activity Recommendations of 150 minutes of exercise weekly, and perhaps more alarming is that only one in three children are physically active every day.

A sedentary lifestyle is a modifiable risk factor for CHD, and the data support that it is never too late to change behavior and achieve health benefits. Even an increase in physical activity in mid or late life is associated with a decreased risk of death and disability. Epidemiological research has shown that physical activity lowers the risk of CHD, stroke, hypertension, metabolic syndrome (MS), and noninsulin–dependent diabetes mellitus. Physical activity also results in weight loss when combined with diet, improved cardiorespiratory fitness, and prevention of falls. The Physical Activity Guidelines Advisory Committee Report provided a comprehensive review of the exercise literature and the evidence of a lifetime benefit from regular exercise. These guidelines recommended that adults (ages 18–64 years) should exercise 150 min/week at moderate intensity or 75 min/week at vigorous intensity. This exercise should involve aerobic physical activity or an equivalent combination of moderate- and vigorous-intensity aerobic physical activity. Activities should be performed in episodes of at least 10 minutes in duration, and ideally should be spread across the week. In addition, muscle-strengthening activities that involve all major muscle groups should be performed on ≥2 days a week. The Physical Activity Guidelines Advisory Committee Report also recommended increasing the duration of weekly moderate-intensity physical activity to 5 hours/week for additional health benefits. Older adults are advised to follow the same guidelines.

These guidelines have not been adopted by the public to the extent that the authors would have desired based on the previously described statistics (only one in three adults achieve the recommended levels of physical activity). However, there has been a decrease in CVD mortality over the past 10+ years. The improvements in pharmacotherapy, reduced door-to-balloon times for acute myocardial infarction (MI), and other improvements in guideline-directed medical therapy have certainly played a role, but it could be hypothesized that any incremental increase in population-level physical activity also plays a role in reducing mortality and morbidity. The Advisory Committee has been reconvened and an updated activity recommendation is anticipated in 2018.

Increasing physical activity is extremely important, but achieving a higher level of fitness is even more important, especially for individuals who are at high risk for CHD or have experienced a cardiac event and require rehabilitation. Participating in a high-level exercise program, whether before or after a cardiac event, results in substantial improvement in cardiovascular (CV) risk factors, including resting blood pressure (BP), lipid levels, body composition, and insulin sensitivity. This chapter addresses specific issues related to exercise, primary and secondary prevention, and population health initiatives to improve physical activity among those at highest risk.

DEFINITIONS

Numerous terms are used in the literature in reference to exercise and physical activity. In this chapter, we use these terms as they are commonly defined. Physical activity is any bodily movement produced by contraction of skeletal muscle that increases energy expenditure above the basal level. Physical activity is generally categorized by mode, intensity, and purpose. Leisure activities are considered to be physical activities performed by a person that are not required as essential activities of daily living and are performed at the discretion of the person. Leisure activities include sports participation, exercise conditioning or training, and recreational activities, such as going for a walk, dancing, and gardening. Exercise is a subcategory of physical activity that is "planned, structured, and repetitive" and generally has a purpose to improve or maintain some aspect of physical fitness. Physical fitness is defined in many ways, but an accepted definition is "the ability to carry out daily tasks with vigor and alertness, without undue fatigue and with ample energy to enjoy leisure-time pursuits and meet unforeseen emergencies." There are many components to fitness, both performance and health related. Health-related fitness consists of cardiorespiratory fitness, muscle strength and endurance, body composition, flexibility, and balance. Because of the explosion of technology and mobile communications resulting in >1 billion smartphones and >165 million tablets shipped annually worldwide, there are now novel, evolving platforms for healthcare monitoring and delivery, and a new vocabulary related to this technology. The WHO defines mobile health (mHealth) as "medical and public health practice supported by mobile devices such as mobile phones, patient monitoring devices, personal digital assistants and other wireless devices."

PRIMARY PREVENTION

High levels of sedentary activity in adults are prevalent according to the 2015 National Health Interview Survey. One in three adults does not engage in leisure-time physical activity. Inactivity increases with age, in women, with Hispanic and black adults providing a large potential pool of the public to target for activity interventions to reduce CVD risk. There is a strong inverse relationship between physical activity and the risk of coronary disease and death. Across studies, there is an estimated 30% risk reduction in all-cause mortality, comparing the most physically active subjects with the least active subjects. Similar CV benefit from fitness also exists in both sexes and across different races and ethnic groups (Fig. 4.1). The inverse dose–response relation for total volume of physical activity is curvilinear, meaning that those with the lowest physical activity levels have the largest risk reduction with increased physical activity. Studies in men support a role for physical activity in reducing the risk of mortality. In nonsmoking, retired men, ages 61 to 81 years, who had other risk factors controlled, the distance walked daily at baseline inversely predicted the risk for all-cause mortality during a 12-year follow-up. Of 10,269 Harvard alumni born between 1893 and 1932, those individuals who began moderately vigorous sports between 1960 and 1977 had a reduced risk of all-cause and CHD-related death over an average of 9 years of observation compared

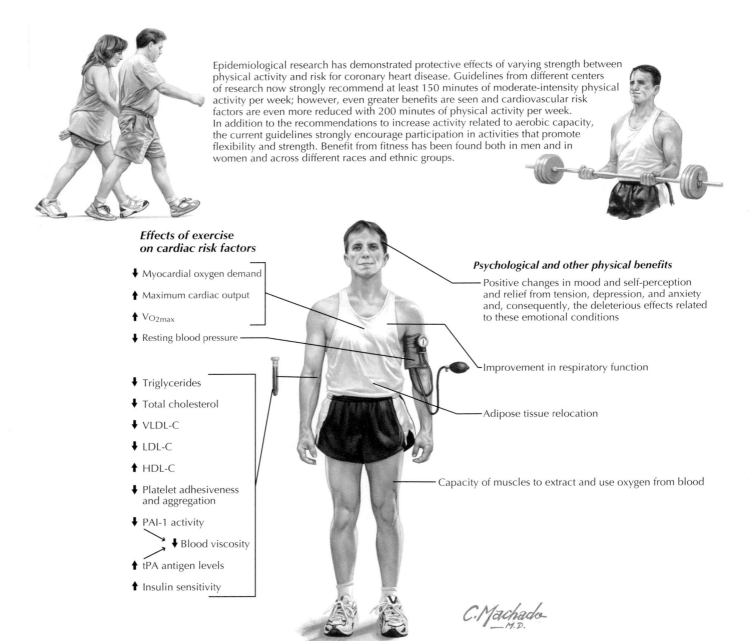

Epidemiological research has demonstrated protective effects of varying strength between physical activity and risk for coronary heart disease. Guidelines from different centers of research now strongly recommend at least 150 minutes of moderate-intensity physical activity per week; however, even greater benefits are seen and cardiovascular risk factors are even more reduced with 200 minutes of physical activity per week. In addition to the recommendations to increase activity related to aerobic capacity, the current guidelines strongly encourage participation in activities that promote flexibility and strength. Benefit from fitness has been found both in men and in women and across different races and ethnic groups.

Effects of exercise on cardiac risk factors

- ↓ Myocardial oxygen demand
- ↑ Maximum cardiac output
- ↑ V_{O2max}
- ↓ Resting blood pressure

- ↓ Triglycerides
- ↓ Total cholesterol
- ↓ VLDL-C
- ↓ LDL-C
- ↑ HDL-C
- ↓ Platelet adhesiveness and aggregation
- ↓ PAI-1 activity
  - → ↓ Blood viscosity
- ↑ tPA antigen levels
- ↑ Insulin sensitivity

Psychological and other physical benefits

Positive changes in mood and self-perception and relief from tension, depression, and anxiety and, consequently, the deleterious effects related to these emotional conditions

Improvement in respiratory function

Adipose tissue relocation

Capacity of muscles to extract and use oxygen from blood

Physical activity guidelines are targeted to increase physical activity to promote health, but they will not necessarily result in physical fitness and should not diminish the importance of achieving physical fitness.

FIG 4.1 Effects of Exercise on Cardiovascular Health: Primary Prevention. *HDL-C,* High-density lipoprotein cholesterol; *LDL-C,* low-density lipoprotein cholesterol; *PAI-1*; plasminogen activator inhibitor type 1; *tPA,* tissue plasminogen activator; *VLDL-C,* very low-density lipoprotein cholesterol; V_{O2max}, oxygen consumption.

with those who did not increase sports participation. This finding was independent of the effects of lower BP or lifestyle behaviors related to low cardiac risk, such as cessation of smoking and maintenance of lean body mass. Data on the leisure-time physical activity levels of men participating in the Multiple Risk Factor Intervention Trial (MRFIT) supported a reduction of risk for all-cause and CHD-related fatalities when leisure time was spent doing moderate or high (compared with low) levels of physical activity. The effect was retained when confounding factors, including baseline risk factors and MRFIT intervention group assignments, were controlled. Mortality rates for the high and moderate physical activity groups were similar. The Lipid Research Clinics Mortality Follow-up Study found that men with a lower level of physical fitness, as indicated by heart rate (HR) during phase 2 (submaximal exercise) of the Bruce Treadmill Test, were at significantly higher risk for death due to CV causes within 8.5 years compared with men who were physically fit.

The same benefits from physical activity accrue for women. In women, higher physical activity level was related to an improved health outcome in several longitudinal studies. The Iowa Women's Health Study observed 40,417 postmenopausal women for 7 years; moderate and vigorous exercise were associated with a reduced risk of death. This reduction of risk was present for all-cause mortality and specifically for deaths resulting from CV and respiratory causes.

Women who increase their frequency of activity from rarely or never to ≥4 times per week also have a reduced risk of death. The Women's Health Initiative (73,743 postmenopausal women) and the Nurses' Health Study (72,488 women aged 40–65 years) assigned subjects into quintiles based on energy expenditure. Age-adjusted risk decreased incrementally from the lowest to the highest energy expenditure group, was statistically significant when other CV risk factors were controlled, and was similar in white and black women. In addition, energy expenditure from vigorous exercise or walking and time spent walking were linked to a lowered risk for the development of CHD. This inverse relation between CHD risk and activity level was observed in groups of women with other high-risk factors, including smokers and women with high cholesterol levels, although it was not observed in hypertensive women. In one study of postmenopausal women, the odds ratios for nonfatal MI, adjusted for confounding factors, decreased across the second, third, and fourth highest quartiles of energy expenditure compared with the lowest quartile. Exercise equivalent to 30 to 45 minutes of walking 3 days/week decreased the risk for MI by 50%.

Studies show that in black and white men and women, lack of exercise is associated with a higher risk of 5-year all-cause mortality, independent of age, male sex, low income, BP, or a number of CV measures (left ventricular [LV] ejection fraction, abnormal ECG) or other physiological measures (e.g., glucose level, creatinine level). A community-based study of older adults (aged 65 years or older) with no history of heart disease showed that walking at least 4 hours weekly significantly reduced the risk of hospitalization due to CV disease events during the subsequent 4 to 5 years.

The epidemic of obesity in the United States has significantly affected the development of CHD, hypertension, diabetes, and other atherosclerosis risk factors. In 2011 to 2014, it was estimated that approximately 69% of the adult population aged older than 20 years was overweight or obese with a body mass index (BMI) of ≥25 kg/m^2. The prevalence of obesity differs across racial/ethnic and socioeconomic groups. Native Americans, African Americans, Hispanics, and Pacific Islanders have significantly higher BMIs compared with whites and Asian Americans. There is also a significant sex–ethnicity interaction. African American women have a much higher prevalence of obesity (BMI >30 kg/m^2) (57%) compared with Hispanic (46%) and white (38%) women. This holds true for men as well, although the prevalence is lower (38%, 39%, and 34%, respectively). The total estimated costs in 2008 related to obesity were $147 billion USD. There is a dose–response relationship between physical activity and weight loss, but in general, successful weight loss and maintenance is a complex issue, which includes caloric restriction, in addition to increased physical activity. Several studies have shown that anthropometric measures (BMI, waist circumference, waist-to-hip ratio) are associated with CHD risk factors and/or adverse events. The increased risk is partially explained by the milieu of insulin resistance, inflammation, and other atherosclerotic risk factors associated with obesity. Although weight loss is important and improves CV risk factors, the direct benefit of weight reduction alone on CV risk is not clear. However, physical activity reduces CV risk. A study of women being evaluated for suspected myocardial ischemia found that measures of increased BMI, waist circumference, waist-to-hip ratio, and waist-to-height ratio were not independently associated with coronary artery disease (CAD) or adverse CV events. Lower levels of self-reported physical fitness scores were associated with higher prevalence of CHD risk factors and angiographic CAD, and higher risk of adverse events during follow-up, independent of other risk factors. This supports the findings that fitness may be more important than overweight or obesity in women and men.

SECONDARY PREVENTION

Recent studies have conclusively demonstrated that exercise and fitness are as beneficial for patients with an established diagnosis of CHD as for those who do not have known CHD (Fig. 4.2). In subjects with higher levels of physical activity, there is a 20% to 35% lower risk for CVD, CHD, and stroke compared with those with the lowest levels of activity. In a large study of men with established heart disease, regular light to moderate activity (such as 4 hours/week of moderate to heavy gardening or 40 min/day of walking) was associated with reduced risk of all-cause and CV mortality compared with a sedentary lifestyle. Another large study assessed health status and physical fitness in men during two medical examinations scheduled approximately 5 years apart. Men who were unfit at both examinations (baseline and 5 years later) had the highest subsequent 5-year death rate (122/10,000 man-years). The death rate was substantially lower in initially unfit men who improved their fitness (68/10,000 man-years) and was lowest in the group who maintained their fitness from the first to the second examination (40/10,000 man-years). The mortality risk decreased approximately 8% for each minute that the maximal treadmill exercise time at the second examination exceeded the baseline treadmill time. These results were retained when subjects were stratified by health status, demonstrating that unhealthy and initially healthy individuals benefited from exercise fitness.

Exercise intervention experiments have documented better health and survival even in patients who have experienced an MI. In one randomized study, patients were enrolled in a rehabilitation program of three 30-minute periods of exercise weekly, whereas other patients—matched by age, sex, coronary risk factors, site and level of cardiac damage, and acute-phase complications—served as control subjects. At 9 years after the initial MI, the rate of death caused by acute MI and the frequency of angina pectoris were lower in the treatment group. In the National Exercise and Heart Disease Project, male post-MI patients were randomly assigned to a 3-year program of supervised regular vigorous exercise (jogging, cycling, or swimming) or to regular care not involving an exercise program. Subjects were reevaluated at 3, 5, 10, 15, and 19 years to determine total and CV-related mortality. A moderate advantage of the treatment versus control condition in reducing the risk of all-cause and CV death was seen at the first follow-up

It has been found that exercise of light to vigorous intensity (moderate to heavy gardening, jogging, cycling, swimming, etc.) and fitness are beneficial in patients with established diagnoses of coronary heart disease, including those who experienced a myocardial infarction, lowering mortality from acute myocardial infarction and frequency of angina pectoris, and increasing functional capacity and reduction of myocardial work.

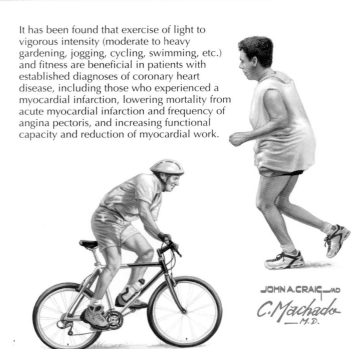

JOHN A. CRAIG—MD
C. Machado
—M.D.

Studies have also shown that intensive exercise on a regular basis associated with a low-fat, low-cholesterol diet may be associated with regression in atherosclerotic coronary lesions, an increase in myocardial oxygen consumption, and a decrease in stress-induced myocardial ischemia.

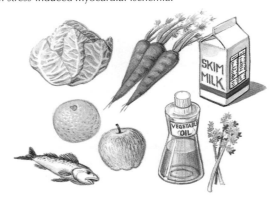

FIG 4.2 Secondary Prevention.

time point but diminished and eventually reversed as the time since baseline increased. This may indicate that the benefits of an intensive exercise program are time-limited or may be related to several other factors (see later discussion). Each metabolic equivalent unit by which the work capacity of the participant increased from the outset to the completion of the 3-year program resulted in an incremental reduction in total and CV-related mortality, which suggested that increasing exercise fitness did promote survival. Failure to observe a long-term benefit in the treatment group versus the control group might have resulted from crossover between the two groups during the protracted follow-up period, improvements in medical therapy (routine use of statins), and/or revascularization approaches.

A large meta-analysis of 10 randomized clinical trials of post-MI patients showed that cardiac rehabilitation (CR) with exercise reduced all-cause mortality by 24% and CV death by 25% versus that of control subjects. However, the risk of nonfatal recurrent MI did not differ between groups.

Exercise training plays an important role in post-MI rehabilitation. Significant increases in functional capacity (10%–60%) and reductions of myocardial work at standardized exercise workloads (10%–25%) have been observed after 12 weeks of post-MI CR. The Exercise in Left Ventricular Dysfunction Trial demonstrated that exercise training after an MI might also improve ventricular remodeling and LV function. The American Heart Association (AHA) guidelines on physical activity in secondary prevention after MI, bypass surgery, or clinical ischemia recommend that the maximal benefit occurs when an exercise–CR program is initiated at supervised facilities where symptoms, HR, and BP can be monitored. A symptom-limited exercise test is essential for all participants before starting an exercise program.

Limiting Coronary Atherosclerotic Progression

Several randomized intervention studies evaluated the influence of exercise training on progression of coronary atherosclerosis. In one study, patients with a history of stable angina were randomized to receive a behavioral intervention (≥2 hours/week of intensive exercise group training sessions, at least 20 min/day of exercise, and a low-fat, low-cholesterol diet) or usual care. After 1 year, 32% of the treatment group versus 9% of the control group had regression in atherosclerotic coronary lesions, and conversely, 48% of the control group versus 23% of the treatment group had progression of lesions. These differences were statistically significant. Other changes in the treatment group included reductions in weight, total cholesterol, and triglyceride levels, and increases in high-density lipoprotein cholesterol (HDL-C) levels, work capacity, and myocardial oxygen consumption. Stress-induced myocardial ischemia also decreased from the intervention, which was presumably attributable to enhanced myocardial perfusion. At the 6-year follow-up, the progression of CAD was significantly slowed in the treatment group compared with the control group. Retrospective analysis of exercise intensity and angiographic data revealed that eliciting a regression of coronary stenosis necessitated expenditure of at least 2200 kcal/week (equivalent to 5–6 hours of exercise).

In the Stanford Coronary Risk Intervention Project, patients received a behavioral risk reduction intervention or usual care. Intervention programs were similar to those in the aforementioned studies, but smoking cessation and pharmacological treatment of lipid profiles (according to established treatment guidelines) were added. Evaluation at 4 years after baseline revealed that the risk reduction intervention significantly improved levels of low-density lipoprotein cholesterol (LDL-C), apolipoprotein B, HDL-C, triglycerides, body weight, exercise capacity, cholesterol, and intake of dietary fat. These positive changes were not seen in the control group. The rate of coronary stenosis progression and the number of hospitalizations were also lower for the intervention group, although each group experienced the same number of deaths.

The Lifestyle Heart Trial used an intervention program to transform lifestyle behaviors, including a low-fat vegetarian diet, aerobic exercise, stress management training, smoking cessation, and group psychosocial support. Follow-up angiograms at 1 and 5 years after baseline showed an average relative decrease in stenosis of 4.5% and 7.9%. Conversely, individuals in the control group showed a 5.4% and 27.8% average relative worsening of stenosis. The 5-year risk of adverse cardiac events was also significantly greater in the control group.

Based on these findings, it is apparent that programs that introduce intensive measures to alter coronary risk–promoting behaviors, especially via exercise training and cholesterol reduction, can limit or even reverse the progression of coronary stenosis. Although the associated changes in coronary diameter were relatively small and therefore unlikely by themselves to explain the accompanying improvements in myocardial perfusion, improvements in vascular tone and reduction in the risk of plaque rupture might have contributed to the observed outcomes.

PHYSIOLOGY OF EXERCISE EFFECTS ON CARDIOVASCULAR HEALTH

Oxygen Supply and Demand

Ventilatory oxygen uptake is increased by exercise training via enhanced maximum cardiac output (blood volume ejected by the heart per minute, which determines the amount of blood delivered to exercising muscles) and the capacity of the muscles to extract and use oxygen from blood. Increased exercise capacity, in turn, favorably affects hemodynamic, hormonal, metabolic, neurological, and respiratory function. Exercise training reduces the myocardial oxygen demand associated with a given level of work, as represented by a decrease in the product of HR times systolic arterial BP, and allows persons with CHD to attain a higher level of physical work before reaching the threshold at which an inadequate oxygen level results in myocardial ischemia (Box 4.1).

Lipids

Exercise training regimens in general all favorably alter lipid and carbohydrate metabolism. The positive effect of a low-saturated fat, low-cholesterol diet on blood lipoprotein levels is enhanced by a strict regular exercise regimen in overweight adults. Training also influences adipose tissue relocation, which is believed to be important in lowering CV risk. Intense endurance training also enhances insulin sensitivity and has a highly salutary effect on fibrinogen levels in healthy older men.

The beneficial effects of exercise on lipids are at least part of the benefits that result in primary and secondary prevention of heart disease in the studies reviewed here. Kraus and colleagues examined the effects of graded exercise on serum cholesterol in sedentary and overweight adults with hyperlipidemia who completed a 6-month protocol. Comparing the three treatment exercise programs—high-amount, high-intensity exercise; low-amount, high-intensity exercise; and low-amount, moderate-intensity exercise—with control groups, all of the exercising groups showed improvements in plasma lipoprotein levels, including a decrease in very low-density lipoprotein cholesterol triglycerides and an increase in the size of LDL-C particles. Increased HDL-C levels and particle size occurred only in the high-amount, high-intensity group; the largest improvements in LDL-C measures were also seen only in this group. These effects were independent of weight loss, and higher amounts of exercise were associated with greater benefits in lipoproteins.

BOX 4.1   Benefits of Exercise Training

- Reduces all-cause mortality risk
- Reduces cardiovascular mortality risk
- May limit atherosclerotic progression
- Enhances oxygen uptake
- Reduces myocardial work
- Constructively alters lipid and carbohydrate metabolism
- Influences adipose relocation
- Enhances insulin sensitivity
- Reduces the conversion of HDL-C into LDL-C and VLDL-C
- May suppress platelet adhesiveness and aggregation
- Increases activity of mitochondrial enzymes
- Lowers blood pressure
- Improves functional capacity and peak oxygen consumption in heart failure

HDL-C, High-density lipoprotein cholesterol; *LDL-C,* low-density lipoprotein cholesterol; *VLDL-C,* very low-density lipoprotein cholesterol.

A recent meta-analysis supported the findings that volume of exercise exposure was the primary determinant of HDL-C change.

Mechanisms that link exercise with an improved lipoprotein profile may include increased lipoprotein lipase activity and reduced hepatic lipase activity, leading to HDL-C increases and decreased conversion of cardioprotective HDL_2 into smaller HDL_3 particles. Exercise reduces the conversion of HDL-C into LDL-C and very low-density lipoprotein cholesterol by decreasing serum concentrations of cholesterol ester transfer protein. It increases the conversion of HDL_3 to HDL_2 by increasing levels of serum lecithin cholesterol acyltransferase. LDL-C does not seem to be as responsive to exercise training as HDL-C and triglycerides.

Triglyceride levels are consistently and robustly affected in direct correlation to the total amount of exercise, similar to those changes seen in HDL-C (10–20 metabolic equivalent tasks—hours per week), although some reports suggest that women are more resistant to changes in triglycerides with exercise than men.

Metabolic Syndrome and Diabetes

MS is a cluster of metabolic risk factors that promote development of atherosclerotic CVD. Risk factors include atherogenic dyslipidemia, hypertension, elevated blood glucose, central adiposity, and proinflammatory and prothrombotic markers. Prospective studies have demonstrated a twofold increase in the relative risk of atherosclerotic events, and for those without diabetes, a fivefold increase in the risk for developing diabetes. There are several groups who have defined MS. The two most widely cited are the Adult Treatment Panel III (ATP III) and WHO criteria. The ATP III criteria for diagnosis of MS is the presence of any three of the following criteria: (1) waist circumference >40 inches in men and >35 inches in women, (2) triglycerides >150 mg/dL or drug treatment, (3) low HDL-C or drug treatment (<40 mg/dL in men; <50 mg/dL in women), (4) elevated BP or drug treatment (>130/85 mm Hg), and (5) fasting glucose >100 mg/dL or drug treatment. The WHO defines MS as insulin resistance, identified by one of the following: (1) type 2 diabetes, (2) impaired fasting glucose, (3) impaired glucose tolerance, (4) or for those with normal fasting glucose levels (<6.1 mmol/L), glucose uptake below the lowest quartile for the background population being investigated under hyperinsulinemic, euglycemic conditions; plus any two of the following: (1) antihypertensive medication and/or high BP (≥140 mm Hg systolic or >90 mm Hg diastolic), (2) plasma triglycerides >150 mg/dL, (3) HDL cholesterol <35 mg/dL in men or <39 mg/dL in women, (4) BMI >30 kg/m^2 and/or waist-to-hip ratio >0.9 in men and >0.85 in women, (5) urinary albumin excretion rate >20 µg/min or albumin-to-creatinine ratio >3.4 mg/mmol.

Regular physical activity is associated with a 30% to 40% lower risk for developing MS. There is an inverse dose–response association between level of activity and risk. The minimal amount of activity necessary to prevent MS ranges from 120 to 180 minutes of activity per week. These findings are consistent for both men and women. There have been no prospective trials to examine exercise training as a treatment to reverse MS.

Currently, it is estimated that 23.4 million Americans have been diagnosed with diabetes and that another 7.6 million are undiagnosed, and 81.6 million adults have prediabetes (fasting blood glucose of 100 to <126 mg/dL). There were 1.7 million new cases of diabetes diagnosed in 2012. Although mortality rates have declined in women and men with and without diabetes, the rates of CVD mortality are still twofold higher for those with diabetes compared with those without diabetes. Numerous large-cohort studies have demonstrated the benefit of physical activity in preventing type 2 diabetes. In the Nurses' Health Study, walking and vigorous activity were associated with a decreased risk for diabetes, with greater physical activity providing the most benefit. The estimate across studies is a 30% to 40% lower risk for developing type 2 diabetes for those with moderate levels of activity. The benefits are seen for both men and women, as well as young and old and for different races/ethnic groups. The data indicate that at least 120 to 150 minutes of moderate to vigorous physical activity are needed to significantly lower risk for diabetes.

Type 2 diabetes is associated with reduced exercise capacity, which is associated with cardiac and hemodynamic abnormalities. Exercise increases the activity of mitochondrial enzymes, which improves muscle energetics. Even modest levels of exercise increase insulin sensitivity and reduce visceral adipose tissue and plasma triglycerides. Women with diabetes who exercise moderately or vigorously for at least 4 hours/week have a 40% lower risk of developing coronary disease than those with lower exercise levels. Low physical activity in men with diabetes is an independent predictor for CHD. Several cohort studies have shown that CV fitness and physical activity levels are inversely correlated with mortality and/or CVD event rates in subjects with type 2 diabetes. In the Nurses' Health Study of 5000 diabetic women followed for 14 years, the relative risk for CV events decreased progressively with increasing weekly volume of moderate to vigorous activity. This relationship remained after adjusting for smoking, BMI, and other CV risk factors.

Blood Pressure

Maintaining a habitual exercise routine can lower systolic BP by as much as 5 to 15 mm Hg in patients with essential hypertension; mean reductions of 4 to 5 mm Hg systolic pressure and 3 to 5 mm Hg diastolic pressure are widely reported. Just as perseverance with an exercise program elicits a hypotensive response, detraining is associated with an increase in BP toward the pre-exercise level. Reductions in circulating norepinephrine level, plasma volume, and cardiac index parallel the reduction in BP and are probably involved in the antihypertensive consequences of exercise. Reduced systemic vascular resistance resulting from decreased sympathetic activity probably also affects BP.

The recommended targets for BP control have undergone revisions since the publication of the Eighth Joint National Committee (JNC-8). However, because of the change in methodology for review, sponsoring of the oversight group midway through the guideline development process, and recent publication of the results of the Systolic Blood Pressure Intervention Trial (SPRINT), the current recommended BP targets have been subjected to intense criticism and have resulted in confusion for patients. The guidelines were updated in the fall of 2017. Normal blood pressure is now defined to be <120/80. The previous threshold of >140/90 is now considered stage 2 hypertension.

ROLE OF EXERCISE TRAINING IN HEART FAILURE

Heart failure (HF) is a growing problem in the industrialized world and has reached epidemic proportions in the United States. Although the central effects of HF are pulmonary and peripheral vascular congestion, many patients believe that exercise limitation is the most troubling feature. Traditional therapies, such as angiotensin-converting enzyme inhibitors, β-blockers, spironolactone, and most recently, neprilysin inhibitors combined with angiotensin receptor blockers show impressive reductions in mortality with somewhat less significant improvement in functional capacity. Hence, there is a need for therapies targeted at improving functional capacity. Exercise training was once prohibited in HF patients out of concern for patient safety. However, it is now recognized as a therapeutic option for improving functional capacity in patients with HF (Fig. 4.3), with the most recent full revision of the American College of College/American Heart Association (ACC/AHA) HF guidelines made in 2013, which provided a class I recommendation

(level of evidence A) for exercise training (or regular physical activity) as being "safe and effective for patients with heart failure who are able to participate to improve functional status."

In HF, mechanical function and functional capacity do not always have a direct correlation. LV ejection fraction is a poor index of exercise capacity in patients with chronic HF; therefore other factors must contribute to exercise intolerance in HF. The physiological mechanisms for exercise intolerance in HF, albeit incompletely understood, help to explain the potential benefits of exercise training.

Among the factors contributing to exercise limitation are impaired LV systolic and diastolic function, baroreflex desensitization, sympathetic nervous system activation, impaired vasodilator capacity, skeletal muscle abnormalities, and abnormalities of pulmonary function. The emerging data on diastolic dysfunction indicates that this pathology results in disabling symptoms and activity intolerance, and has been labeled HF with preserved ejection fraction (HFpEF). Skeletal muscle abnormalities in patients with HF include atrophy of highly oxidative, fatigue-resistant (type I) muscle fibers; increased glycolytic, less fatigue-resistant (type II) muscle fibers; decreased mitochondrial oxidative enzyme concentration and activity; reduced mitochondrial volume and density; and reduced muscle bulk and strength. As HF progresses, patients become more physically limited because of pulmonary congestion and therefore reduce physical activity, causing a downward spiral in which cardiac limitation aggravates skeletal muscle deconditioning. The increases in circulating cytokines, part of the HF syndrome, further worsen muscle atrophy. Reduced peak skeletal muscle blood flow with exercise limitation also reduces shear stress and thereby depletes tissue vasodilator reserve.

Pulmonary abnormalities are also common in HF, including reduced lung volumes and respiratory muscle strength and endurance; increased airway resistance with reduced flow rates; reduced diffusion capacity as a result of alveolar edema; and increased ventilatory drive, minute ventilation, respiratory rate, and dead space-to-tidal volume ratio. The effects of training on these ventilatory abnormalities in patients with HF include reduction in minute ventilation, reduced perceived sense of dyspnea, and improved respiratory muscle function.

The well-documented, abnormal activation of neurohormones in chronic HF is associated with a poor prognosis. An exercise training program can correct the increased plasma levels of angiotensin II, aldosterone, arginine vasopressin, and atrial natriuretic peptide in chronic HF to near-control values. Decreased HR variability, which is markedly abnormal in patients with HF, is a further marker of sympathetic activation. A physical conditioning program can improve HR variability and endothelial dysfunction in patients with chronic HF.

Clinical trials of exercise training in HF show improvements in exercise time, functional capacity, and peak oxygen consumption. Exercise training seems to be safe and generally well tolerated in patients with HF with a reduced ejection fraction and HFpEF. One randomized trial found a reduction in cardiac events, an improvement in Minnesota Living with Heart Failure scores, and, most importantly, an improved survival rate in patients with HF who were randomized to exercise training. The HF-ACTION (Heart Failure–A Controlled Trial Investigating Outcomes of Exercise Training) study was sponsored by the National Institutes of Health and designed to test the hypothesis that patients with LV systolic dysfunction and New York Heart Association functional class II to IV symptoms who underwent exercise training in addition to usual care would have a 20% lower rate of death and hospitalization over 2 years compared with usual care. The results showed a balanced randomization of 2331 patients to exercise or usual care. Exercise consisted of a 36-week supervised training program followed by a home-based program. The mean follow-up was 2.5 years. The rates of all-cause mortality and all-cause hospitalizations combined were not significantly different between the two groups. Using a prespecified adjustment for

Once prohibited in heart failure, exercise training has only recently been recognized as a viable therapeutic option for improvement of functional capacity. Most of the abnormalities seen in HF can be improved or even reversed by exercise training.

Some of the abnormalities seen in HF that can be improved or even reversed by exercise training

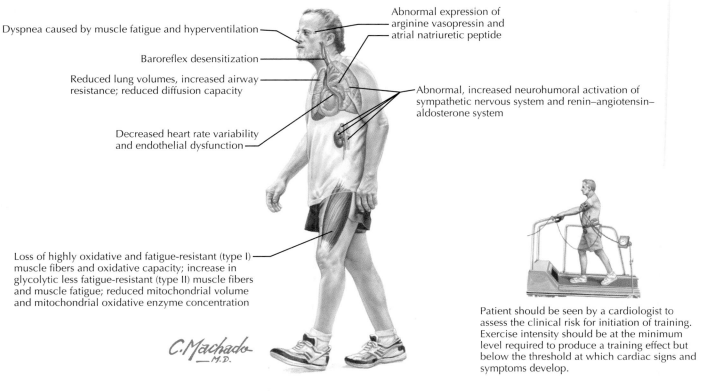

Dyspnea caused by muscle fatigue and hyperventilation

Baroreflex desensitization

Reduced lung volumes, increased airway resistance; reduced diffusion capacity

Decreased heart rate variability and endothelial dysfunction

Abnormal expression of arginine vasopressin and atrial natriuretic peptide

Abnormal, increased neurohumoral activation of sympathetic nervous system and renin–angiotensin–aldosterone system

Loss of highly oxidative and fatigue-resistant (type I) muscle fibers and oxidative capacity; increase in glycolytic less fatigue-resistant (type II) muscle fibers and muscle fatigue; reduced mitochondrial volume and mitochondrial oxidative enzyme concentration

Patient should be seen by a cardiologist to assess the clinical risk for initiation of training. Exercise intensity should be at the minimum level required to produce a training effect but below the threshold at which cardiac signs and symptoms develop.

FIG 4.3 Exercise Training in Heart Failure (HF).

prognostic factors, there was a significant reduction in the composite primary outcome by 11% (hazard ratio: 0.89; 95% confidence interval [CI]: 0.81–0.99; $P = 0.03$), and a composite of CV mortality–HF hospitalizations were reduced by 15% (hazard ratio: 0.85; 95% CI: 0.74–0.99; $P = 0.03$). Importantly, there were no differences in adverse events between the two groups, indicating that exercise training in this population was safe. There was also a statistically significant improvement in quality of life in the exercise training group. The findings of HF-ACTION offer good evidence for recommending exercise as a safe but modestly effective treatment for patients with HF.

Exercise training in patients with HF is best initiated within a traditional phase II (outpatient) CR program. Patients should be prescreened by a cardiologist to assess the clinical risk for training initiation. Most patients with New York Heart Association functional class II to IV symptoms can exercise safely; however, patients with unstable symptoms, recent MI, unstable angina, severe aortic stenosis, uncontrolled arrhythmias, significant hypotension (systolic BP <85 mm Hg), or acute myocarditis should be excluded. Chronotropic response may be blunted in patients with HF, so the level of perceived exertion and dyspnea should be used as a termination point and should be no higher than 11 to 14 on the Borg scale (light to somewhat difficult exertion). Patients with HF require prolonged warm-up and cool-down periods compared with healthy individuals and should avoid resistance training initially. Patients also should be counseled to avoid exercise after meals. The usual recommended activities, walking and cycling, arm ergometry (e.g., using arm motion, instead of leg motion, to peddle an upright stationary bicycle), and rowing, are well suited for individuals whose walking or cycling is limited by arthritis or conditions other than CV fatigue.

Exercise intensity should be at the minimum level needed to produce a training effect but below the threshold at which cardiac signs and symptoms develop. A baseline maximal oxygen consumption (MVo_2) study can be helpful in designing the exercise prescription but is not mandatory. Target intensity should begin at 40% of the MVo_2 and progress to 75% of the MVo_2 (roughly 70%–85% of peak HR) over 4 to 6 weeks. Initially, the frequency of exercise generally should be three times per week. MVo_2 plateaus when the frequency of exercise exceeds three to five sessions per week, and the injury rate increases exponentially. In frail or high-risk individuals, two sessions per week may also be effective for initial conditioning. The frequency of exercise should eventually increase to five sessions per week.

Exercise sessions should begin with a 10- to 15-minute warm-up and end with a 10- to 15-minute cool-down. The initial duration of exercise should be 10 to 20 minutes. Interval training may be required in markedly deconditioned patients, with 2 to 6 minutes of exercise alternating with 1 to 2 minutes of rest. Duration should increase gradually to 20 to 40 minutes per session. After 12 weeks, patients can proceed to unsupervised exercise and can consider light to moderate resistance training.

CARDIAC REHABILITATION

CR is a comprehensive intervention program that includes prescribed exercise, CV risk factor modification, education, counseling, and behavioral intervention for patients with CVD. Based on strong evidence from randomized clinical trials, it is recommended and reimbursable for patients with stable angina pectoris, post-MI, coronary revascularization, heart transplantation, and valve surgery, as well as HF. Despite this, the referral of patients to CR and the enrollment of those referred remains low. The reasons for this are multifactorial and include limited availability of programs for the volume of patients who qualify, especially patients in rural areas, frequency of visits requiring leave from work, transportation to sessions, lack of full reimbursement depending on healthcare plan, in addition to other financial or social issues. Telehealth programs and other mHealth applications (wearables, Internet-based support groups) have been under evaluation as potential solutions. The Million Hearts Program, as part of its second phase initiative, is targeting better use of CR to 80% of eligible patients because of the known risk reduction that can be achieved with these programs.

In 2007, the AHA and American Association of Cardiovascular and Pulmonary Rehabilitation established the core components of CR to include the following, which are all components of promoting cardiovascular health that have been outlined in this chapter:

- initial patient assessment
- nutrition counseling
- weight management
- BP management
- lipid management
- diabetes management
- tobacco cessation
- psychosocial management
- physical activity counseling and exercise training

CR, in addition to promoting to physiological health, improves psychological health. CR programs can help to identify and facilitate management of psychological issues related to acute and chronic disease states (e.g., anxiety and depression). The education regarding lifestyle changes provides understanding and allows for mastery of skills for successful self-management. There are also strong data that psychological benefits of exercise include positive changes in mood; relief from tension, depression, and anxiety; increased ability to cope with daily activities; and improved cognitive function. These benefits bring about positive changes in self-perception, well-being, self-confidence, and awareness, and may result in more health-promoting behaviors.

FUTURE DIRECTIONS

Increasing physical activity and exercise in patients at risk for and with CHD should be a primary intervention in all patients. The documented benefits for CV risk reduction, as well as reduction in the progression of (and in some cases normalization of) MS and type 2 diabetes, make this one of the most effective therapies in a practitioner's arsenal. It must be noted that the obstacles to convincing a patient to engage in regular exercise are significant and begin with patient motivation. Further research is needed to learn more about dosing of exercise and physical activity, as well as better methods to improve subject compliance and adherence to prescribed exercise. In addition, public policy changes are necessary to alter aspects of our society that promote sedentary habits in children and adults, which contribute to obesity, diabetes, and CHD progression. The emergence of mHealth technology will provide new platforms to make exercise interventions more available to an almost limitless number of people, allow a mechanism for monitoring, and perhaps allow for more population-wide intervention strategies to improve CV health. The next decade will be an exciting time as this technology evolves and becomes more facile, accurate, accepted, and incorporated into everyone's life.

EVIDENCE

Eijsvogels TM, Molossi S, Lee DC, et al. Exercise at the extremes: the amount of exercise to reduce cardiovascular events. *J Am Coll Cardiol.* 2016; 67:316.

Summarizes the available evidence for the relationship between exercise volumes and risk reduction in CV morbidity and mortality. Summarizes data comparing moderate-intensity exercise versus high-intensity exercise interventions and volumes of exercise in the athletic population and its associated risks.

Kokkinos P, Faselis C, Myers J, et al. Age-specific exercise capacity threshold for mortality risk assessment in male veterans. *Circulation.* 2014; 130:653.

Defines age-specific exercise capacity thresholds as a guide to assess mortality risk in veterans undergoing a clinical exercise test.

LeFevre ML, U.S. Preventive Services Task Force. Behavioral counseling to promote a healthful diet and physical activity for cardiovascular disease prevention in adults with cardiovascular risk factors: U.S. Preventive Services Task Force Recommendation Statement. *Ann Intern Med.* 2014;161:587.

Updates the U.S. Preventative Services Task Force recommendation on dietary counseling for adults with risk factors for CVD, calling for the referral of those overweight or obese or with additional CVD risk factors to intensive behavioral counseling to promote a healthful diet and physical activity for CVD prevention.

Pahor M, Guralnik JM, Ambrosius WT, et al. Effect of structured physical activity on prevention of major mobility disability in older adults: the LIFE study randomized clinical trial. *JAMA.* 2014;311:2387.

Reports findings on the impact of structured physical activity program compared with health education in reducing risk of major mobility disability in sedentary men and women aged 70 to 89 years.

Physical Activity Guidelines Advisory Committee. Physical Activity Guidelines for Americans Report, 2008. Washington, DC: U.S. Department of Health and Human Services; 2008.

These guidelines were written to provide the general public with evidence-based information on the effects of physical activity and to provide the recommended amount of physical activity by age group. Also discusses the benefits of following these recommendations.

Sharma K, Kass DA. Heart failure with preserved ejection fraction; mechanisms, clinical features, and therapies. *Circ Res.* 2014;115:79–96.

HFpEF is prevalent and challenging to manage. This provides an overview of the pathophysiology and treatment options, which are limited, but exercise training offers a potential treatment strategy that is under investigation.

Shiroma EJ, Lee IM. Physical activity and cardiovascular health: lessons learned from epidemiological studies across age, gender, and race/ethnicity. *Circulation.* 2010;122:743.

A review of the current data to explore the magnitude of the association between physical activity and CHD/CVD and to determine if there is a dose response and if physical activity can reduce the observed increased risk of CHD/CVD seen with increased adiposity.

Soares-Miranda L, Siscovick DS, Psaty BM, et al. Physical activity and risk of coronary heart disease and stroke in older adults: The Cardiovascular Health Study. *Circulation.* 2016;133:147.

Cohort analysis to examine the impact of regular physical activity in those older than 75 years of age.

Yancy CW, Jessup M, Bozkurt B, et al. 2013 ACCF/AHA guideline for the management of heart failure: executive summary. *Circulation.* 2013;128:e240–e327.

The ACC/AHA heart failure guidelines give a class I recommendation (level of evidence A) for exercise training (or regular physical activity) as being "safe and effective for patients with heart failure who are able to participate to improve functional status" and recommend CR, stating that it "can be useful in clinically stable patients with heart failure to improve functional capacity, exercise duration, health related quality of life and mortality" (class IIA, level of evidence B).

5

Cardiovascular Epidemiology and Risk Prediction Models

Eric P. Cantey, John T. Wilkins

Cardiovascular epidemiology studies the determinants and distribution of cardiovascular disease (CVD). The overarching goal of CVD epidemiology is to reduce the incidence and prevalence of CVD within the population. Cardiovascular epidemiology has provided vital bidirectional connections between basic mechanistic science and clinical research. Through these types of investigations, our understanding of the extent of CVD and its natural history, mechanisms, and underlying pathophysiology is expanding greatly, which provides opportunities for individual-level therapeutic strategies, as well as population-level approaches to reduce the incidence and burden of CVD.

PREVALENCE OF CARDIOVASCULAR DISEASE

CVD remains the leading cause of death for men and women in the United States, more than cancer and respiratory disease combined. Within the United States, most individuals have an approximately 30% chance of dying of CVD and a 66% lifetime risk of CVD. Fortunately, over the past 40 years, there have been significant and substantial reductions in CVD risk and age-adjusted mortality in the United States by approximately 40%. However, the burden of CVD in the United States and globally still remains massive.

Worldwide, CVD is the most common cause of death, accounting for an estimated 31% of all deaths. Although 22% of reductions in the CVD death rate have been observed, the total number of CVD deaths continues to increase because of population growth and aging of the population. The death rate varies widely across countries, with the highest death rates attributable to CVD in Russia and the lowest rates seen in Western Europe, North America, and Central America.

Similarly, there are substantial differences in CVD incidence, prevalence, and mortality rates seen across different geographic regions, race, ethnic, and socioeconomic groups within the United States. For example, the southeastern United States has a substantially higher incidence rate and mortality associated with stroke. African Americans have long had substantially higher age-adjusted rates of hypertension, stroke, heart failure, and coronary heart disease than age-matched whites in the United States.

EPIDEMIOLOGY OF CARDIOVASCULAR DISEASE RISK FACTORS

Epidemiological research has not only provided critical insights into the prevalence of CVD, but has also identified risk factors and patient characteristics that predict the presence and development of CVD. Several risk factors like sex, race, and age are nonmodifiable and enhance our understanding of the risk of an individual, but these factors are not useful as targets of therapy. In contrast, reducing the incidence and optimizing levels of modifiable risk factors is the mainstay of primary and secondary prevention efforts. The identification of modifiable risk factors led to multiple randomized controlled clinical trials that demonstrated the primacy of risk factor prevention and their management of CVD risk reduction.

Hypertension

The American Heart Association (AHA) defines ideal blood pressure as <120/80 mm Hg. Observational cohort studies have consistently demonstrated increased risk for stroke, heart attack, heart failure, and cardiovascular mortality across all age groups at blood pressures above this level. On average, every increase in the systolic blood pressure by 20 mm Hg or diastolic blood pressure by 10 mm Hg is associated with a doubling in the risk of death caused by stroke, coronary heart disease, or other vascular disease. Using JNC 7 guidelines, hypertension was defined as a systolic blood pressure greater than 140 mm Hg, a diastolic blood pressure greater than 90 mm Hg, or the use of blood pressure–lowering medications. In the fall of 2017, the AHA and ACC redefined hypertension as blood pressure greater than 130/80 mm Hg.

Using statistics that reflect JNC 7 guidelines, there are an estimated 85.7 million adults in the United States with hypertension. The prevalence of hypertension increases with age and varies by race. African Americans have substantially higher rates of hypertension than age-matched white Americans. Unfortunately, only 76% of those with hypertension are on antihypertensive medication, and only 54% have their blood pressure under adequate control.

Hyperlipidemia or Dyslipidemia

Higher levels of total cholesterol, low-density lipoprotein (LDL) cholesterol, and non–high-density lipoprotein (HDL) cholesterol are associated with increased risks for atherosclerotic cardiovascular disease (ASCVD). There is approximately a 50% higher ASCVD risk for every 40 mg/dL increase in total cholesterol. The association appears log-linear across higher levels of total cholesterol. Thus, total cholesterol and the atherogenic fractions LDL cholesterol and non-HDL cholesterol have become targets for therapy with lifestyle modification and pharmacotherapy. Conversely, across usual levels of HDL cholesterol, there is an inverse association with ASCVD risk.

Hyperlipidemia is commonly defined as total cholesterol levels >230 mg/dL. Within the United States, an estimated 28.5 million adults, or 11.9% of the population, are considered to have hyperlipidemia. Over the last 14 years, the prevalence of hyperlipidemia has decreased by approximately 7%. The most recent estimates of mean total cholesterol, LDL cholesterol, HDL cholesterol, and triglyceride levels in the United States are 196, 113, 53, and 103.5 mg/dL, respectively.

Tobacco Use

Cigarette smoking increases ASCVD risk twofold to fourfold. Cessation of tobacco products is associated with rapid changes in physiology and substantial reductions in CVD risk. Therefore, tobacco use has been a major target of public health campaigns. Because of these large efforts, tobacco use has been declining over the last 50 years from prevalence rates of 51% in men and 34% in women in 1965 to 16.7% in men and 13.7% in women in 2017.

Although the overall trend in tobacco use is promising, certain minority groups, including sexual and gender minorities, individuals with low socioeconomic status, disabled persons, and individuals with psychiatric illness, have not experienced the same decrease in prevalence rates that are seen in the overall population. Furthermore, recent increases in electronic cigarette use, particularly in adolescent populations, could result in increased tobacco use in younger age groups.

Diabetes

The AHA defines an ideal fasting glucose as <100 mg/dL. Currently, only 56% of adults in the United States meet this criterion. Diabetes is associated with a twofold to threefold increase in risk for coronary heart disease, stroke, peripheral artery disease, heart failure, and atrial fibrillation. It is also associated with a 6- to 8-year shorter life expectancy than is seen in nondiabetics.

The National Heart, Blood, and Lung Institute defines diabetes as a fasting blood sugar >125 mg/dL, and it defines prediabetes as a fasting blood sugar between 100 and 125 mg/dL. In a recent representative survey of the United States population, 23.4 million adults have diabetes and 7.6 million are not aware of having diabetes. Furthermore, 81.6 million have prediabetes. Of the cases of diabetes identified, 90% to 95% are classified as type 2 diabetes. In part because of the obesity epidemic, the prevalence of diabetes has been increasing over the last 10 to 15 years. African Americans and Hispanic Americans have substantially higher rates of diabetes than white Americans.

Obesity, Diet, and Physical Activity

The AHA defines an ideal body weight as a body mass index (BMI) of 18.5 to 25 kg/m^2. Obesity is defined as a BMI >30 kg/m^2, and overweight, which also confers an increased risk for CVD, is defined as a BMI between 25 and 30 kg/m^2. Obesity is a risk factor for CVD, including ASCVD, heart failure, stroke, venous thromboembolism, and atrial fibrillation, and a risk factor for other CVD risk factors, including dyslipidemia, hypertension, and diabetes. Obesity rates have slowly increased over the past several decades, with most recent prevalence rates reported in 2013 to 2014 as 37.7%. Women have a higher prevalence of both obesity and class III obesity, defined as BMI >40 kg/m^2, with prevalence rates of 40.4% and 9.9%, respectively. There is substantial regional variation in obesity prevalence rates, with higher levels observed in the Midwest and southeastern United States.

A central determinant of the obesity epidemic is caloric excess and physical inactivity. The AHA defines a healthy diet as one that is rich in fresh fruits, vegetables, whole grains, low-fat dairy, seafood, legumes, and nuts. This diet has consistently been found to reduce blood pressure, improve lipid fractions, and reduce risks for heart attack and stroke. Conversely, diets that are high in saturated fats and salt, and low in fruits and vegetables are associated with adverse changes in blood cholesterol and blood pressure, and likely increase ASCVD risk. Current estimates suggest that only 1.5% of adults consume an ideal healthy diet and that 678,000 deaths per year are attributable to a suboptimal diet.

Like obesity and dietary indiscretion, physical inactivity increases risks for CVD and CVD risk factors. Currently, the AHA recommends that adults perform at least 150 minutes of moderate intensity exercise per week or 75 minutes of vigorous activity a week plus 2 days of muscle strengthening. Individuals who meet these recommendations have been found to have a 30% to 40% lower risk for diabetes, a 30% to 40% lower mortality risk, and a 20% to 30% lower risk for coronary heart disease. Forty-four percent of adults meet the criteria specified by the AHA; however, 30% of adults do not engage in any physical activity. Women, older adults, African Americans, and Hispanics meet these requirements less frequently than other sex, race, and ethnic groups.

EFFORTS AT CARDIOVASCULAR DISEASE PREVENTION

Population and High-Risk Approaches to Cardiovascular Disease Risk Reduction

Cardiovascular risk has a bell-shaped distribution within the population. A high-risk approach targets individuals at the highest risk with aggressive risk reduction. This type of approach is currently recommended to determine which patients should receive statin therapy for primary prevention of ASCVD events. Because the relative benefits of statin medications are consistent across absolute levels of risk, the high-risk approach will result in the greatest absolute benefit in individuals at highest absolute risk.

In contrast, a population-level approach attempts to reduce risk factor levels in the population as a whole through optimization of population mean risk factor levels. Although this may seem counterintuitive, this approach often results in greater numbers of prevented events because there are much larger numbers of individuals around the mean value in a bell-shaped distribution. Therefore, most events occur within this portion of the population. To continue with the example of impact of cholesterol on ASCVD events, the risk of an individual for ASCVD with mean cholesterol levels is low because of the large denominator of people close to the mean. However, the risk for this segment of the population is still high. Therefore, even a modest decrease in the mean cholesterol concentrations would translate into a large number of prevented CVD events (Fig. 5.1).

High-risk and population-level approaches are not mutually exclusive: in fact, they are complimentary. Thus, CVD epidemiological efforts are aimed at reducing population-level burdens of risk factors and at identifying individuals at higher risk for aggressive primary prevention interventions.

INTRODUCTION TO RISK ESTIMATION

Individual risk factors are probabilistic and typically do not capture the complete ASCVD risk of an individual. Risk estimator equations have been developed to help clinicians determine which patients are in the highest risk groups and, therefore, who would benefit most from primary prevention interventions. The currently recommended use of 10-year and lifetime risk estimator for the management of dyslipidemia with statin medications provides an excellent example of the use of risk scores in clinical practice.

Defining Risk

It is important to understand the term risk is a construct and not a reality. For example, when risk factors of a patient confer a 50% 10-year risk of developing an ASCVD event, the patient in reality will either have the clinical event or not have the clinical event. Because of the inherent limitations in predicting the future, risk estimation is only a starting point when making decisions about initiation of primary prevention measures. Clinicians may need to consider other factors, including family history of CVD, subclinical CVD, and comorbid conditions, among others, to individualize risk estimation for patients and make decisions about the initiation of statin medications.

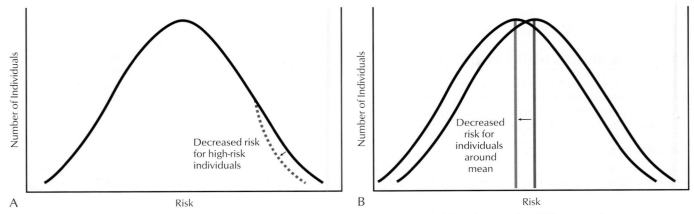

FIG 5.1 (A) A high-risk approach targets individuals at the high end of risk for intervention. This approach results in the greatest reduction of risk for those individuals, but does little to reduce the risk in the population as a whole. (B) A population-based approach aims to reduce the mean risk, albeit often by a modest amount, in the overall population. This approach can lead to large reductions in risk of coronary heart disease in a population because events actually occur in individuals near the mean level of risk in the population.

Currently recommended CVD risk assessment tools generate absolute risk estimates. Absolute risk represents the likelihood of an event occurring over a given unit of time. In contrast, relative risk is a metric of how much higher or lower the risk of an individual is compared to some referent level of risk (e.g., relative risk, hazard ratio, and odds ratio).

Absolute risk is chosen over relative risk for clinical risk estimation for multiple reasons. First, estimates of relative risk are dependent on the risk in the referent group, which can be inherently misleading. Second, studies have demonstrated that both patients and clinicians are poor at predicting true risk. Third, in terms of guideline-based recommendations for statin therapy in patients with dyslipidemia, the calculation of absolute risk for ASCVD events allows clinicians to directly compare the average expected benefits of statin therapy to the average expected harms of statin therapy. Therefore, quantifying absolute risk allows for a quantitative risk–benefit decision and improves communication between clinicians and patients.

An alternative approach to a risk-based approach, albeit a cumbersome and impractical approach, would be for a clinician to gather all of the clinical trials that examined the effect of statins as primary prevention for ASCVD and identify which trial identified their specific patient by its inclusion criteria. However, because of the nature of randomized clinical trials, which typically have strict inclusion and exclusion criteria, these studies are unlikely to ever include the complete spectrum of patients encountered in clinical practice.

Risk Score Generation

To apply risk scores appropriately in clinical practice, it is important to have an understanding of their development. Typically, risk scores are derived from cohort study datasets. When developing and using risk estimation equations, it is important that the individuals in the cohort(s) from which the score is derived are similar to the patients to whom the risk score is applied. If the baseline rates of risk factors or disease are substantially higher or lower than the population in which the risk score is applied, the risk score may underestimate or overestimate risk in such a population.

The accuracy and clinical usefulness of absolute risk estimates are sensitive to the time horizon over which they are intended to predict. Most CVD risk estimation scores use 10-year time horizons, because it is a convenient time interval that is easy to remember and understand.

Furthermore, it is also easier to develop robust estimates of risk over this time interval.

Although 10-year time horizons are clinically convenient and provide robust estimates of risk, they may lead to an incomplete understanding of CVD risk burden in some patients. This is best exemplified in a young woman with multiple risk factors for ASCVD. Although a risk score predicts a low 10-year risk of ASCVD events, this patient has a high lifetime risk for CVD. Thus, if only a 10-year risk estimate were communicated to such a patient, she may overestimate her cardiovascular health and not institute much needed lifestyle change. However, if she is informed of how her modifiable risk factors are increasing her risk well beyond the 10-year time horizon, she may improve adherence to healthy lifestyle modifications. The 2013 AHA risk calculator not only includes 10-year risk estimates of ASCVD events, but estimates lifetime risk for individuals younger than 64 years old, as well.

It is vital that risk calculators use outcomes that are important to both patients and clinicians. The ATP-III risk calculator estimated the risk of nonfatal and fatal myocardial infarction. Unquestionably, these are important outcomes. However, contemporary CVD epidemiological data have demonstrated that women, particularly young African American women, are at substantial risks for acute stroke, which was not accounted for by earlier versions of the risk calculator. In response, the 2013 AHA risk calculator was designed to estimate the risk for both fatal and nonfatal stroke, as well as myocardial infarction.

When choosing inputs for risk estimation calculators, researchers choose risk factors that are readily available in clinical practice and that enhance the ability of the statistical model to accurately predict risk. Because of the mathematics of statistical models, variables that are highly correlated tend to be redundant and rarely add substantially to the ability of a statistical model to accurately predict risk. However, it is critical to understand that a variable excluded from the risk estimation model may be of significant clinical importance. For example, obesity is not included in many ASCVD risk calculators despite its central role in CVD risk. Obesity is a major risk factor for the development of hypertension, diabetes, and dyslipidemia, and it is strongly associated with poor diet and a lack of exercise. Because of these associations, it does not add to risk prediction above and beyond blood pressure, the presence of diabetes, levels of HDL cholesterol and total cholesterol. However, when counseling a patient about ways to reduce their CVD risk, a clinician would be remiss to not discuss the importance of optimal body weight with a patient.

EVALUATION OF RISK SCORE PERFORMANCE

Discrimination and calibration are used to evaluate risk score performance. A rudimentary understanding of these concepts allows clinicians to identify risk scores that are most appropriate for their clinical practice and to integrate risk scores into the care of individual patients.

Discrimination

Discrimination refers to a risk estimator's ability to rank order individuals who will develop disease at a higher level of risk than those who will not develop disease. It is important to note that discrimination does not capture the accuracy of the absolute risk estimate. Statistically, the degree of correct discrimination is described by the c-statistic. The c-statistic is the area under the receiver-operating characteristic curve, or the plot of the sensitivity and 1-specificity of the outputs of the statistical model. Generally, c-statistics of <0.7 are considered poor discrimination, whereas c-statistics between 0.7 and 0.8 are considered adequate discrimination, and c-statistics >0.8 are excellent discrimination (Fig. 5.2). To describe discrimination in common language, a c-statistic of 0.8 means that 80% of the time the risk model ranked individuals who were more likely to have an event as being at higher risk than those who did not have an event and were therefore at lower risk. This metric partially describes the performance of the risk estimation equation when used as a population-wide screening test. It is not sensitive to risks that may be present in certain niche groups within the population (e.g., individuals with HIV, chronic inflammatory conditions, or those in the extreme distributions of CVD risk factors).

Calibration

Risk estimation is dependent on accurate absolute risk estimates, not just rank ordering. Calibration compares the estimated absolute risk for an event with the observed event rate in a population sample. When

risk estimators are applied to populations with different event rates, the risk calculators often require recalibration to avoid overestimating or underestimating risk. Thus, it is quite possible that a risk estimator may have a high c-statistic but is poorly calibrated for a given population. In many instances, risk estimation equations can be recalibrated to different populations, although this is not routinely done in clinical practice (Fig. 5.3).

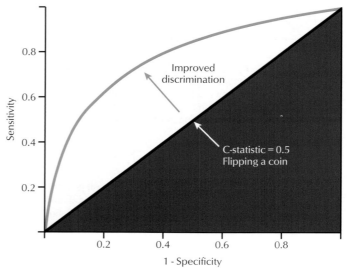

FIG 5.2 Receiving-Operating Characteristic Curve. Movement of the curve to the upper left of the figure represents improved discrimination, movement toward the line of unity represents worsened discrimination. The area under the curve *(shaded region)* is the c-statistic, which represents the ability of a prediction model to rank order individuals at high risk above individuals at lower risk.

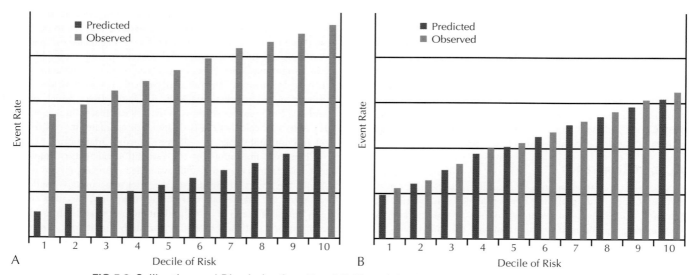

FIG 5.3 Calibration and Discrimination. (A and B) Plots of the risk predicted by a hypothetical risk estimation equation *(purple bars)* and the observed risk *(gray bars)* in deciles of coronary heart disease risk in a population sample. (A) The model *(purple bars)* appears to have excellent discrimination, as individuals at low risk appear to be consistently ranked below individuals at higher risk. However, the estimated absolute risk is significantly lower than the observed (presumably true) risk. Thus, (A) is an example of good discrimination, but poor calibration. (B) However, model B appears to have excellent discrimination and calibration because the absolute risk estimated and observed appear similar across all deciles of risk.

Risk Reclassification

When patients have an intermediate estimate of CVD risk, or a 10-year CVD risk of 4% to 7.5%, clinicians commonly use testing above and beyond what is included in the risk estimation equation to individualize the risk of CVD in the patient. For example, high coronary artery calcium scores identify individuals with high atherosclerotic burden. When high coronary artery calcium scores are added to an estimated intermediate 10-year risk of CVD, patients can appropriately be reclassified to a higher level of risk. Therefore, this test can help clinicians determine which patients may benefit from statin therapy and those who may not benefit from statin therapy in the near term.

INNOVATIONS AND FUTURE DIRECTIONS OF CARDIOVASCULAR DISEASE EPIDEMIOLOGY

Although great advances in CVD epidemiology have been achieved over the last 70 years, significant challenges remain. The burden of CVD and CVD risk factors remains high in the US population and worldwide. Thus, despite having identified the determinants of most CVD events, further improvements need to be made to reduce the prevalence of these risk factors. This will require advancements in population-level interventions (changes in food policy, smoking bans, and so on) and continued efforts to understand the underlying physiology that contributes to the development of incident risk factors. Collaborative efforts that compile large cohort, genomic, proteomic, and metabolomic data with the aim of understanding the physiological underpinnings of CVD are currently underway and will certainly be a continued focus of epidemiological research in the future. Similarly, the development of digital and remote sensing technologies and wearable devices will allow researchers opportunities for surveillance of physiological characteristics and health-related behaviors that may contribute to CVD risk.

ADDITIONAL RESOURCES

High Risk Versus Population Approach

Rose G. Sick individuals and sick populations. *Int J Epidemiol.* 2001;30(3):427–432.

This paper is an erudite discussion and comparison of the high-risk approach to identification of susceptible individuals to the population-based approach of understanding the determinants of disease in the population as a whole.

American Heart Association Risk Assessment Guidelines

Goff DC Jr, Lloyd-Jones DM, Bennett G, et al. American College of Cardiology/American Heart Association Task Force on Practice Guidelines. 2013 ACC/AHA guideline on the assessment of cardiovascular risk: a report of the American College of Cardiology/American Heart Association Task Force on Practice Guidelines. *Circulation.* 2014;129(25 suppl 2):S49–S73.

This paper provides updated clinical guidelines for cardiovascular risk assessment. This risk estimation equation provides sex- and race-specific 10-year and lifetime risks for fatal and nonfatal coronary heart disease and stroke.

American Heart Association Cholesterol Lowering Guidelines

Stone NJ, Robinson JG, Lichtenstein AH, et al. American College of Cardiology/American Heart Association Task Force on Practice Guidelines. 2013 ACC/AHA guideline on the treatment of blood cholesterol to reduce atherosclerotic cardiovascular risk in adults: a report of the American College of Cardiology/American Heart Association Task Force on Practice Guidelines. *Circulation.* 2014;129(25 suppl 2):S1–S45.

This paper provides the updated guidelines for cholesterol testing and treatment. These evidence-based guidelines address recommendations for screening and/ or detection.

American Heart Association Yearly Statistics Update

Benjamin EJ, Blaha MJ, Chiuve SE, et al. American Heart Association Statistics Committee and Stroke Statistics Subcommittee. Heart Disease and Stroke Statistics-2017 Update: a report from the American Heart Association. *Circulation.* 2017;135(10):e146–e603.

This publication from the American Heart Association is updated yearly, and it provides updates on domestic and global epidemiology of CVD and its risk factors.

EVIDENCE

Blood Pressure and Cardiovascular Mortality

Lewington S, Clarke R, Qizilbash N, Peto R, Collins R, Prospective Studies Collaboration. Age-specific relevance of usual blood pressure to vascular mortality: a meta-analysis of individual data for one million adults in 61 prospective studies. *Lancet.* 2002;360(9349):1903–1913.

This highly influential study of 1 million adults during 12.7 person-years quantifies the CVD risks associated with different levels of blood pressure across all age strata. Notably, it demonstrates a linear increase in risk for all blood pressures >120/80 mm Hg across all adult age groups.

Cholesterol and Cardiovascular Events

The Emerging Risk Factors Collaboration. Major lipids, apolipoproteins, and risk of vascular disease. *JAMA.* 2009;302(18):1993–2000.

This analysis quantifies the associations among major lipid fractions, apolipoproteins, and atherosclerotic CVD risk in 1.2 million cohort participants. This is an essential reference for understanding individual-level estimates of the associations between lipids and ASCVD risk.

Ideal Cardiovascular Health

Folsom AR, Yatsuya H, Nettleton JA, Lutsey PL, Cushman M, Rosamond WD, ARIC Study Investigators. Community prevalence of ideal cardiovascular health, by the American Heart Association definition, and relationship with cardiovascular disease incidence. *J Am Coll Cardiol.* 2011;57(16):1690–1696.

This paper outlined the community prevalence of ideal cardiovascular health, as defined by the AHA, and the strong association between achieved levels of ideal cardiovascular health and incident CVD. This is an essential read for anyone interested in understanding the impact of the prevention of CVD risk factors and the maintenance of ideal CVD health.

Validation of 2013 Risk Assessment Estimation Equation

Muntner P, Colantonio LD, Cushman M, et al. Validation of the atherosclerotic cardiovascular disease Pooled Cohort risk equations. *JAMA.* 2014;311(14):1406–1415.

This paper reports on the validation of the 2013 AHA pooled risk estimation equation in the REGARDS study. For this analysis, the authors used indexes of discrimination and calibration as discussed in this chapter.

Coronary Artery Calcium and Atherosclerotic Cardiovascular Disease Risk Prediction

Blaha MJ, Cainzos-Achirica M, Greenland P, et al. Role of coronary artery calcium score of zero and other negative risk markers for cardiovascular disease: the multi-ethnic study of atherosclerosis (MESA). *Circulation.* 2016;133(9):849–858.

This paper evaluates the impact of negative biomarkers, including coronary artery calcium, on risk prediction in the Multi-Ethnic Study of Atherosclerosis. These results suggest that a coronary artery calcium score of 0 in individuals at intermediate to low estimated CVD risk may help identify individuals who may not benefit from cholesterol-lowering therapy in the near-term.

Polonsky TS, McClelland RS, Jorgensen NW, et al. Coronary artery calcium score and risk classification for coronary heart disease prediction: the multi-ethnic study of atherosclerosis. *JAMA.* 2010;303(16):1610–1616.

This paper demonstrates the additive value of coronary artery calcium assessment for the prediction of ASCVD risk in the Multi-Ethnic Study of Atherosclerosis.

6

Stem Cell Therapies for Cardiovascular Disease

Gentian Lluri, Arjun Deb

Myocardial infarction and congestive heart failure are the leading causes of morbidity and mortality worldwide, despite great therapeutic achievements in the treatment of cardiovascular diseases. The inability of the heart to regenerate lost cardiac muscle, coupled with a robust fibrotic repair response, contribute to adverse ventricular remodeling and decline in postinjury cardiac function. Consequently, much of the research of the last three decades has focused on reducing the atherosclerotic burden of ischemic heart disease, reperfusion, and addressing the fibrotic changes associated with heart failure. After an ischemic insult and the formation of necrotic myocardium, the process of scar formation from the recruitment of activated cardiac fibroblasts leads to reduced cardiac pump function. However, in recent years, it has been convincingly shown that the heart has the ability to regenerate cardiomyocytes, albeit at a low rate (~0.3%–1% annually). These findings and our better understanding of stem cell biology are paving the way to a new area of research, with the main goal of regenerating cardiac tissue.

Two defining features of stem cells are their ability to self-renew and to differentiate to cells of a specific lineage under appropriate conditions. Recent observations have shed light on the existence of cardiac stem cells and extracardiac stem cells that are capable of leading to cardiomyocytes, smooth muscle cells, and endothelial cells. Such therapies are still experimental but hold great promise in potentially ushering in novel regenerative treatment strategies for heart disease.

STEM CELLS

Types of Stem Cells and Mechanisms of Benefit

Stem cells can be classified according to their level of potency. A totipotent stem cell, such as a fertilized zygote, can lead to an entire organism. A pluripotent cell, such as an embryonic stem (ES) cell, leads to cells from all three germ layers but is unable to generate an organism. Multipotent stem cells, such as mesenchymal stem cells (MSCs), can lead to different types of cells from the same cell germ layer, such as adipocytes, bone, or cartilage cells. Skeletal muscle myoblasts, endothelial progenitor cells, and bone marrow mononuclear cells (BN-MNCs) are other examples of multipotent stem cells that have been studied in cardiac regeneration.

The signaling pathways that drive stem cells into cardiomyocyte fate are areas of intense research; better understanding of these pathways can be used as valuable therapeutic tools in enhancing cardiac regeneration. Differentiation is the process by which stem cells can become cardiomyocytes, whereas transdifferentiation is a process in which a somatic cell adopts alternative cell fates (e.g., a fibroblast adopting an endothelial cell fate). Another process by which stem cells can alter cardiac function is fusion. When stem cells fuse with somatic cells (e.g., cardiomyocytes), the resulting cells have characteristics of both cell types; however, the extent to which any clinical benefit can be achieved from this process is currently unclear. Another mechanism by which

stem cells can enhance tissue regeneration is through a paracrine mechanism. After injection, stem cells are believed to release cytokines and/or growth factors that have physiological effects on other cells in the injured environment and affect repair. For instance, injection of MSCs into the injured heart affects the balance of Wnt signaling in the injured environment to modulate angiogenesis and fibrosis. Identification of key stem cell secreted molecules mediating pro-reparative effects on the injured heart may lead to development of new therapeutic strategies in which injection of key stem cell secreted molecules, rather than stem cells, may be sufficient to augment cardiac healing and obviate issues such as immune response, dose titration, and availability.

ES cells have the ability to give rise to any cell type of the organism, and under the appropriate conditions, can differentiate into cardiomyocytes. They originate from the inner cell mass of the blastocyst during development. Studies have shown that injection of ES cells leads to successful engraftment of them into the surrounding cardiac tissue, making this approach appealing. However, large-scale generation of ES cell–derived cardiomyocytes currently remains unrealistic, because this is a field still in its infancy and filled with several ethical and political challenges. Differentiation of bone marrow stem cells into functioning cardiomyocytes has been more challenging.

Bone marrow contains different types of progenitor stem cells, among which BM-MNCs and MSCs have been extensively studied. Injection of BM-MNCs into the diseased cardiac muscle leads to improvement of cardiac function. Although initial studies suggested that BM-MNCs transdifferentiated into myocytes, later studies suggested an indirect effect likely related to the paracrine effects of cells. A paracrine effect contributing to salutary effects on cardiac repair was confirmed for MSC injection after cardiac injury. In vitro studies suggested that these cells could also differentiate into beating cardiomyocytes, and these findings generated a lot of excitement that led to several preclinical studies. These studies suggested that injection of MSCs into the injured myocardium resulted in improved cardiac function despite the low number of mesenchymal-derived cardiomyocyte cells, which suggested a multifactorial effect similar to BM-MNCs.

The limited supply of ES cells and associated social challenges have led to other pathways to develop pluripotent stem cells. A type of cell that has attracted a lot of interest recently is the resident cardiac progenitor cell. The existence of these cells and their ability to differentiate into cardiomyocytes, as well as endothelial and smooth muscle cells, has shaken the long-standing belief that the heart is a fixed organ unable of regeneration. Several challenges remain to fully derive the potential benefits of these cells. First, different cell markers have been used to characterize these cells, and it is presently unclear if there are any biological differences between cells with different cell markers. Second, the number of these cells is small, and their role in normal cardiac function is not clear. However, injection of these cells into an infarcted heart leads to improvement of cardiac function. What makes these cells particularly attractive is their ability to differentiate into other cell types (e.g., endothelial and smooth muscle cells) because the regenerating cardiomyocytes will need new blood vessels and supporting cells to properly function. Also, use of these cells appears to avoid some of the ethical challenges that can arise with the ES cells. Their small number and the technical difficulties associated with successfully multiplying them have led to the development of other types and techniques, among which induced pluripotent stem cells merit special mention. These are ES cells derived from skin fibroblasts through genetic manipulation (through the overexpression of certain transcription factors). What makes this approach unique and revolutionary is the ability of skin fibroblasts to be reprogrammed into induced pluripotent stem cells that could be injected into an injured heart. Although this field and its technology are in their infancy, it holds great promise for future cardiovascular regeneration therapy.

Another type of stem cell that deserves special mention is the endothelial progenitor cell, especially for vascular regeneration. Injury of the vascular endothelium triggers a cascade of events that aims to reconstitute the endothelium via the proliferation of the remaining endothelial cells and differentiation of the endothelial progenitor cells. It is based on these premises that administration of endothelial progenitor cells might indirectly improve cardiac function by enhancing vasculature repair and angiogenesis.

Cardiospheres have also been tested in heart regeneration after myocardial infarction. Cardiospheres are three-dimensional multicellular structures from cardiac explant cultures in nonadhesive surfaces. It is currently believed that injected cardiospheres modulate scar formation via paracrine effects or secreted exosomes containing active molecules such as microRNA. The phase I clinical trial testing cardiospheres in humans did not show any left ventricular ejection fraction improvement; however, this trial did show a reduction of scar mass at 6 months and an increase in viable myocardium.

During this first wave of excitement, skeletal myoblasts have also been studied, with promising results in early tests, but with no significant benefit in clinical trials; therefore the use of these cells in cardiovascular regeneration is uncertain (Table 6.1).

Approaches to Stem Cell Administration, Technical Challenges, and Safety Concerns

The main two approaches of stem cell administration have been catheter-based intracoronary injection and surgical-based epicardial injection; each delivery method presents unique advantages and disadvantages. One factor to keep in mind when selecting the appropriate approach is to have an optimal environment for successful stem cell engraftment. For example, an intracoronary injection approach after revascularization is disadvantageous because the myocardial areas that need the most number of cells might have reduced blood flow and thus would receive less stem cells. Another factor to consider when selecting the optimal delivery method is the type of cells delivered. For example, certain stem cells (e.g., skeletal myoblasts) are larger; therefore they could lead to microvasculature obstruction and subsequent decreased blood flow. The epicardial injection delivery approach solves the problem of reduced delivery in poorly perfused areas, but cardiac perforation is a real risk, especially in the setting of inflamed and necrotic myocardium tissue. The inflamed cardiac microenvironment is also not optimal for engraftment of injected cells, and the first 4 days after infarction are associated with the least amount of cell engraftment. Focal delivery of stem cells also may not be sufficient in cases of global myocardial dysfunction, such as in nonischemic-dilated cardiomyopathy. Thus it is likely that the decision on what route of delivery to choose will depend on the cardiac condition that needs to be treated and the type of cells to be delivered.

From a safety standpoint, stem cells have been shown to be safe, but long-term data are lacking. Beyond the technical challenges and potential procedure-related complications, there are several specific concerns that need to be taken into consideration when discussing stem cell–based therapy. First, ventricular arrhythmias are a real concern with the newly differentiated and engrafted cells. This specific adverse effect has been observed with skeletal myoblasts, which are believed to be secondary to a lack of electromagnetic coupling with native cardiomyocytes. The second concern is noncardiac engraftment; if the route of administration is through the systemic circulation, then stem cells can also populate other organs; this has been seen in patients who have undergone stem cell injection. Localization of stem cells to other organs can have unpredictable effects, especially tumor angiogenesis or enhancement of malignancy.

Clinical Evidence of Stem Cell Therapy

There have been many trials involving thousands of patients and different types of stem cells injected into patients with different cardiac pathologies (for a more comprehensive list of selected trials, see Table 6.2). BM-MNCs have been evaluated in acute myocardial infarction and chronic myocardial ischemia. In post–acute myocardial infarction patients, the benefits of bone marrow cells were studied in randomized-controlled trials such as the BOne marrOw transfer to enhance ST-elevation infarct regeneration (BOOST) and Reinfusion of Enriched Progenitor cells And Infarct Remodeling in Acute Myocardial Infarction (REPAIR-AMI) trials. Both studies showed improvements in left

TABLE 6.1 Types of Stem Cells and Their Main Mechanism of Action in Cardiovascular Regeneration

Type of Stem Cells	Main Mechanism of Action
Embryonic stem cells	Differentiation
Mesenchymal stem cells	Paracrine/transdifferentiation
Bone marrow mononuclear cells	Paracrine/transdifferentiation
Endothelial progenitor cells	Differentiation
Skeletal myoblasts	Paracrine
Cardiospheres	Paracrine
Cardiac resident progenitor cells	Differentiation
Induced pluripotent stem cells	Differentiation

TABLE 6.2 Summary of Selected Trials of Stem Cell Therapy in Cardiovascular Disease

Name of Trial	Type of Cell Used	Indication
BOOST	BM-MNCs	Acute MI
REPAIR-AMI	BM-MNCs	Acute MI
PROTECT-CAD	BM-MNCs	Chronic myocardial ischemia
APOLLO	MSCs	Acute MI
PRECISE	MSCs	Chronic myocardial ischemia
MAGIC	Skeletal myoblasts	Chronic myocardial ischemia
SCIPIO	Cardiac stem cell	Post-MI LV dysfunction
CAUDECEUS	Cardiosphere-derived cells	Post-MI LV dysfunction

BM, Bone marrow mononuclear cells; *LV,* left ventricular; *MI,* myocardial infarction; *MSCs,* mesenchymal stem cells.

ventricular ejection fraction, and 1-year follow-up in REPAIR-AMI patients also showed a reduction in major adverse cardiovascular events. Patients with more severely impaired left ventricular function appeared to benefit the most according to subgroup analysis of these studies. Bone marrow stem cell therapy for chronic myocardial ischemia was also evaluated in several studies, including the Prospective Randomized Trial of Direct Endomyocardial Implantation of Bone Marrow Cells for Therapeutic Angiogenesis in Coronary Artery Disease (PROTECT-CAD) trial, as well as in a randomized-controlled, double-blind trial with improvement in the quality of life and cardiac perfusion. Although these findings are promising, for most of the studies, the left ventricular ejection fraction might not be the most accurate endpoint, and larger phase III clinical trials with significant primary endpoints (such as mortality, recurrent myocardial infarction, or stroke) will reveal the true impact of bone marrow stem cell therapies and their long-term safety.

MSCs also have been tested for stem cell therapy, but clinical data are scarce. The initial phase I clinical data used intravenous injection of these cells, which established their safety but did not show any cardiovascular benefit. However, the passage of these cells through the pulmonary circulation might have hampered any potential benefit of these cells in the coronary circulation and cardiac seeding. Subsequently, early nonrandomized studies showed that intracoronary injection of MSCs resulted in improvement of the left ventricular ejection fraction and symptoms. Another source of mesenchymal cells are adipose tissue–derived stem cells. The AdiPOse-derived stem ceLLs in the treatment of patients with ST-elevation myOcardial infarction (APOLLO trial assessed the safety of adipose tissue–derived cells and showed a significant reduction in infarct size and improved perfusion at 6 months in patients with acute myocardial infarction. The AdiPose-deRived stEm Cells In the treatment of patients with nonrevaScularizable ischEmic myocardium (PRECISE) trial evaluated the safety and benefits of these cells in chronic myocardial ischemia, which suggested an improvement in the functional status in patients treated with adipose tissue–derived stem cells.

After skeletal muscle injury, resident stem cells (satellite cells) contribute to skeletal muscle regeneration. Hence, there was an initial interest in the usefulness of skeletal myoblasts in cardiovascular regeneration. Although the early nonrandomized small studies suggested a clinical benefit, the most comprehensive trial was the randomized, double-blind, phase II Medical Research Council Adjuvant Gastric Infusional Chemotherapy (MAGIC) trial, which showed no benefit at 6 months. These cells were injected around the scar tissue in patients who underwent bypass surgery. The potential proarrhythmic and microembolization effects of myoblasts, although not fully understood, limited the excitement for these cells as potential source of stem cells in cardiovascular regeneration.

The recent findings that human cardiomyocyte renewal occurs naturally at a rate of 1% in the young and 0.3% in older adults led to the quest of identifying and characterizing these resident cardiac stem cells. The first challenge was to fully evaluate these cells; several subtypes of cells were described, based on the cell markers used to identify them. It is still not clear if these are cells of different subpopulations with distinct phenotypes or if they are part of the same subpopulation. The second challenge was to expand them, because their number is low in the heart. Despite these challenges, early-stage clinical studies, such as the Stem Cell Infusion in Patients with Ischemic cardiOmyopathy (SCIPIO) and CArdiosphere-Derived aUtologous stem CElls to reverse ventricUlar dySfunction (CADUCEUS) trials, established their safety and feasibility, as well as showed a reduction in infarct size. Further ongoing studies are needed to further elucidate any clinical benefit of these cells.

FUTURE DIRECTIONS OF STEM CELL THERAPY

After an exciting decade full of both reassuring and disappointing results, the future of stem cell therapy in cardiovascular disease is expected to grow even more. With the discovery of inducible pluripotent cells and their ability to differentiate into functional cardiomyocytes, a new field has been born in stem cell therapy. However, before applying these cells in clinical trials, certain crucial hurdles have to be resolved, especially safety concerns regarding their tumorigenicity (which has been observed in animal models). Furthermore, technology for upsizing to an effective number of induced pluripotent stem cells is needed.

In addition to the previously described stem cell approaches, the concept of pretreating the stem cells to enhance their therapeutic activity before injection has been tested in several trials. The idea is to improve any function that influences migration, engraftment, survival, differentiation, and other functions that can improve efficiency. The Enhanced Angiogenic Cell Therapy in Acute Myocardial Infarction (ENACT-AMI) trial tested the usefulness of overexpression endothelial nitric oxide synthase in endothelial progenitor cells, because it had previously been shown that a reduction of endothelial nitric oxide synthase limits the repair capability of endothelial progenitor cells in patients with hypertension and diabetes. Another trial is the Mesenchymal Stem Cells and Myocardial Ischemia (MESAMI) II trial, which is designed to pretreat MSCs with melatonin before injection. This approach is based on data that suggest that the melatonin hormone improves survival and the paracrine effects of MSCs. It is expected that many more trials will test different pretreatment methods to enhance the effects of stem cell therapy in cardiovascular regeneration.

Another technology that has not been applied to any clinical trials yet is nanotechnology. The harmful microenvironment after myocardial infarction has detrimental effects on survival and function of the newly transplanted stem cells. Therefore there has been a growing interest in designing biomaterials that can provide a supportive role for the transplanted cells within infarcted myocardium. Before any human trials can be planned, several potential questions need to be addressed, such as dosing, biodegradability, excretion of the byproducts, and any immunological incompatibility of these bio-nanomaterials.

SUMMARY

The initial excitement for stem cell cardiac tissue repair has been replaced by a consensus that this approach holds great promise, but further elaborate laboratory bench work, thoughtful and detailed description of these cells, and meticulous elucidation of the pathways through which these cells act are needed. Such knowledge will allow us to enable optimization and testing of this therapy at all levels. Despite all the challenges, we are given the task of taking this field to the next level so that it becomes routine therapy in clinical practice.

ADDITIONAL RESOURCES

Al-Rubeai M, Naciri M. *Stem Cells and Cell Therapy*. New York: Springer; 2014.

A detailed reference on the basics, therapeutic options, and processing of the stem cells.

Atala A, Lanza R. *Handbook of Stem Cells*. 2nd ed. London: Academic Press; 2013.

An outstanding and comprehensive textbook of stem cell science, history, and applications.

Cohen IS, Gaudette GR. *Regenerating the Heart: Stem Cells and the Cardiovascular System*. New York: Humana Press; 2011.

A complete reference of bench-to-bedside resources on the usefulness of stem cell therapy in cardiovascular regeneration.

EVIDENCE

Caplice NM, Deb A. Myocardial-cell replacement: the science, the clinic and the future. *Nat Clin Pract Cardiovasc Med.* 2004;1(2):90–95.

This article explores questions on the scientific basis, mechanism of action, and therapeutic evidence in the field of stem cell–based cardiovascular regeneration.

Chen C, Termglinchan V, Karakikes I. Concise Review: Mending a broken heart: the evolution of biological therapeutics. *Stem Cells.* 2017;35(5): 1131–1140.

This concise review focuses on the most recent advances in gene- and cell-based therapies in cardiovascular medicine.

Karra R, Poss KD. Redirecting cardiac growth mechanisms for therapeutic regeneration. *J Clin Invest.* 2017;127(2):427–436.

This article focuses on the stimulating endogenous factors that can emerge as regeneration therapies for cardiac repair.

Diagnostic Testing

7

Electrocardiography

Leonard S. Gettes, Eugene H. Chung

It is now >100 years since the Dutch physiologist Willem Einthoven recorded the first ECG in humans. Although the number of recording leads has increased from 3 leads to at least 12 leads, and the recording instruments have evolved into sophisticated automated digital recorders capable of recording, measuring, and interpreting the ECG waveform, the basic principles underlying the ECG are unchanged. The electrocardiograph is basically a voltmeter that records, from the body surface, the uncanceled voltage gradients created as the myocardial cells sequentially depolarize and repolarize.

The ECG is the most commonly used technique to detect and diagnose heart disease, and to monitor therapies that influence the electrical activity of the heart. It is noninvasive, virtually risk free, and relatively inexpensive. Since its introduction, a large database has been assembled correlating the ECG waveform recorded from the body surface to the underlying electrical activity of individual cardiac cells on the one hand, and to the clinical presentation of the patient on the other hand, thereby providing insight into the electrical behavior of the heart and its modification by physiological, pharmacological, and pathological events.

LEADS

Twelve leads are routinely used to record the body surface ECG: three bipolar limb leads labeled I, II, and III; three augmented limb leads labeled aVR, aVL, and aVF; and six chest leads labeled V_1 through V_6 (Fig. 7.1). In the bipolar limb leads, the negative pole for each of the leads is different. The chest leads are often referred to as "unipolar leads" because the negative pole is constant. It is created by the left arm, right arm, and left leg electrodes connected together to form a single lead that is referred to as the Wilson central terminal. The positive chest lead is an exploring lead that can be placed anywhere. In children, the routine ECG often includes leads placed on the right side of the chest in positions referred to as V_3R and V_4R. Similar right-sided chest leads are often used in adults to diagnose right ventricular infarction, and one or more leads placed on the back are sometimes used to diagnose posterior wall infarction.

The chest leads are relatively close to the heart and are influenced by the electrical activity directly under the recording electrode. This is in contrast to the limb leads in which the electrodes are placed outside of the body torso. Changes in the position of an individual chest lead or the relationship between the chest leads and the heart may cause significant changes in the ECG pattern. For instance, if the patient is in a sitting rather than a supine position, the relationship of the various chest leads to the heart will change, and the ECG waveform recorded by the chest leads could be altered. Similarly, if a chest lead is placed an interspace too high or too low, the ECG waveform recorded by that lead will change. For this reason, it is important that lead placement be consistent and reproducible when serial ECGs are recorded. In contrast, limb leads may be placed anywhere on the various limbs with little significant alteration of the ECG waveform. However, placing the limb leads on the body torso, which is often done during exercise testing and when patients are monitored in critical care areas, will affect the recorded waveform.

ELECTROCARDIOGRAPHIC WAVEFORM

The ECG waveform consists of a P wave, a PR interval, the QRS complex, an ST segment, and T and U waves. The relationship of these waveform components to the underlying action potentials of the various cardiac tissues and an example of normal 12-lead ECG are shown in Figs. 7.2A and 7.2B, respectively. The P wave reflects depolarization of the atria, the QRS complex reflects depolarization of the ventricles, and the ST segment and T wave reflect repolarization of the ventricles. The U wave occurs after the T wave and is believed to be an electromechanical event coupled to ventricular relaxation.

Depolarization of the sinus node occurs before the onset of the P wave, but its voltage signal is too small to be recorded on the body surface by clinically used ECG machines, and the event is electrocardiographically silent. Similarly, the electrical activity of the atrioventricular (AV) node and the His-Purkinje system, which occur during the PR interval, is electrocardiographically silent.

P Wave

The P wave is caused by the voltage gradients created as the atrial cells sequentially depolarize. The shape and duration of the P wave are determined by the sequence of atrial depolarization and the time required to depolarize the cells of both atria. The sinus node is located at the junction of the superior vena cava and the right atrium, and the direction of atrial depolarization during sinus rhythm—from right to left, from superior to inferior, and from anterior to posterior—reflects this geography. This results in a P wave that is characteristically upright or positive in leads I, II, aVL, and leads V_3 to V_6 (the leads in which the positive electrode is placed on the left side of the body), and inverted or negative in lead aVR (the lead in which the positive electrode is placed on the right side). In lead V_1, the P wave may be upright, biphasic, or inverted. The amplitude and duration of the normal sinus P wave may be affected by atrial hypertrophy and/or dilation and by slowing of interatrial and intraatrial conduction.

Impulses arising from an ectopic atrial focus are associated with P waves whose shape depends on the location of the focus. If the abnormal focus is located close to the sinus node, the sequence of atrial activation will be normal or nearly normal, and the P wave will resemble the normal sinus P wave. The more distant the ectopic focus is from the sinus node, the more abnormal will be the sequence of atrial activation and the configuration of the P wave. For instance, impulses originating in the inferior portion of the atrium or within the AV node will depolarize the atria in a retrograde, superiorly oriented direction and will

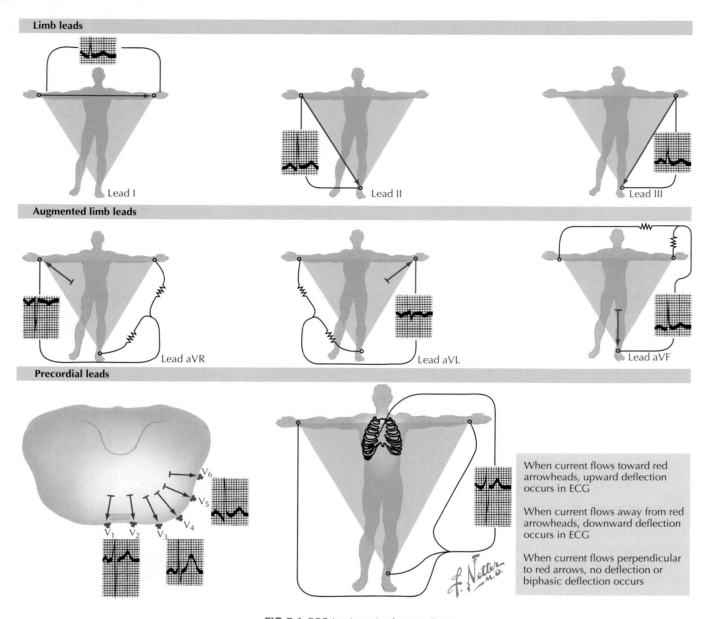

Limb leads

Lead I

Lead II

Lead III

Augmented limb leads

Lead aVR

Lead aVL

Lead aVF

Precordial leads

V₁ V₂ V₃ V₄ V₅ V₆

When current flows toward red arrowheads, upward deflection occurs in ECG

When current flows away from red arrowheads, downward deflection occurs in ECG

When current flows perpendicular to red arrows, no deflection or biphasic deflection occurs

FIG 7.1 ECG leads and reference lines.

be associated with the P waves that are inverted in leads II, III, and aVF and upright in lead aVR (Fig. 7.3).

PR Interval

The PR interval extends from the onset of the P wave to the onset of the QRS complex and includes the P wave and the PR segment (the segment from the end of the P wave to the onset of the QRS), which consist of atrial repolarization and depolarization of the AV junction, which, in turn, includes the AV node, the common His bundle, the two bundle branches (left and right) and the Purkinje fiber network. AV conduction is prolonged and may be blocked by factors that slow AV nodal conduction, such as a decrease in sympathetic tone or an increase in vagal tone, drugs that have these effects (e.g., digitalis and the β-adrenergic blocking agents), electrolyte abnormalities (e.g., hypokalemia), ischemia, and a variety of infectious, inflammatory, infiltrative, and degenerative diseases that affect the AV junction. As a result, the PR interval will be prolonged, or in severe cases when AV conduction

is completely blocked, the P waves will be dissociated from the QRS complex. The PR interval is shortened when impulses bypass the AV node and reach the ventricles via an AV nodal bypass tract to cause ventricular preexcitation (Wolff-Parkinson-White pattern).

QRS Complex

The QRS complex reflects ventricular depolarization. The interventricular septum is the first portion of the ventricle to be depolarized. It is activated by fibers from the left bundle branch, depolarizes from its left side to its right, and is responsible for the initial portion of the QRS complex. Thereafter, the impulse spreads through the His-Purkinje system and then depolarizes the ventricles simultaneously, from the endocardium to the epicardium and from the apex to the base. Because the left ventricle is three times the size of the right ventricle, its depolarization overshadows and largely obscures right ventricular depolarization. The normal QRS complex reflects this left ventricular dominance, and for this reason, the QRS complex is usually upright

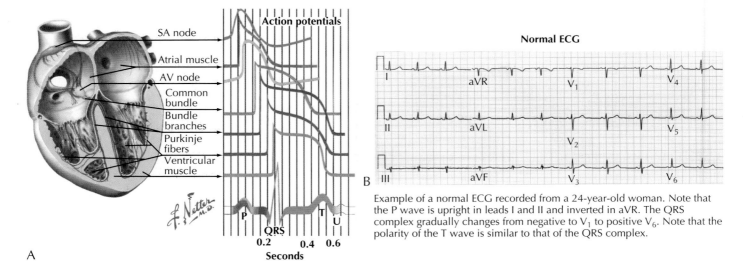

FIG 7.2 (A) Relation of action potential from the various cardiac regions to the body surface ECG. (B) Normal ECG.

Example of a normal ECG recorded from a 24-year-old woman. Note that the P wave is upright in leads I and II and inverted in aVR. The QRS complex gradually changes from negative to V_1 to positive V_6. Note that the polarity of the T wave is similar to that of the QRS complex.

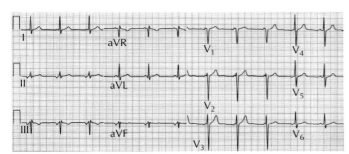

Electrocardiogram showing an ectopic atrial rhythm. It was recorded from a 59-year-old man. The polarity of the P wave is abnormal. It is inverted in leads II, III, and aVF and upright in lead aVR.

FIG 7.3 Ectopic atrial rhythm.

or positive in leads I, V_5, and V_6, the left-sided and more posterior leads, and negative or inverted in leads aVR and V_1, the right-sided and more anterior leads. It is only in situations such as right bundle branch block and significant right ventricular hypertrophy that the electrical activity associated with right ventricular depolarization is identified on the ECG.

The QRS complex is altered in both shape and duration by abnormalities in the sequence of ventricular activation. These include the bundle branch blocks (Fig. 7.4A), the fascicular blocks, ventricular preexcitation (Fig. 7.4B), nonspecific intraventricular conduction disturbances, and ventricular ectopic beats (Fig. 7.4C). The increase in QRS duration may range from a few milliseconds, as in the case of fascicular blocks, to >40 ms, as with bundle branch blocks. The fascicular blocks reflect conduction slowing in one fascicle of the left bundle and are characterized by a shift in the electrical axis and subtle changes in the initial portion of the QRS complex. Bundle branch blocks on the ECG reflect conduction slowing or interruption in the right or left bundle branch, and are usually caused by fibrosis, calcification, or congenital abnormalities involving the conducting system. They are associated with more pronounced abnormalities in the sequence of ventricular activation than are the fascicular blocks, and thus, with more significant changes in the QRS configuration. Intraventricular conduction abnormalities may also occur without a change in QRS configuration and reflect

slow conduction without a change in the sequence of activation. Such slowing may be caused by cardioactive drugs, an increase in extracellular potassium concentration, and diffuse fibrosis or scarring, which may occur in patients with severe cardiomyopathies.

The ECG criteria for the diagnosis of intraventricular conduction disturbances have been published. Important features include the following:

1. The fascicular blocks, by altering the initial portion of the QRS complex and the electrical axis in the frontal plane, may obscure the diagnosis of a previous myocardial infarction (MI) while causing other changes that can simulate an infarction.
2. Right bundle branch block does not affect the initial portion of the QRS complex, because activation of the interventricular septum and the left ventricle are unaffected. Thus the ECG changes of a previous MI or left ventricular hypertrophy can still be appreciated.
3. Left bundle branch block and ventricular preexcitation do affect the initial portion of the QRS complex. Thus the ECG changes associated with a previous MI and hypertrophy can be obscured, or as frequently occurs with ventricular preexcitation, can be mimicked.
4. Abnormalities in the sequence of depolarization are always associated with abnormalities in the sequence of repolarization. This results in secondary changes in the ST segment and T wave. This is particularly prominent in the setting of left bundle branch block and ventricular preexcitation (see Figs. 7.4A and 7.4B).
5. Changes in intraventricular conduction may be rate dependent and present only when the rate is above a critical level or after an early atrial premature beat. In this situation, it is referred to as rate-dependent aberrant ventricular conduction.
6. The shape and duration of the QRS complex of ectopic ventricular beats and of paced ventricular beats will be influenced by the site of the ectopic focus or the location of the pacemaker just as the shape and duration of atrial ectopic beats are influenced by their site of origin.

The amplitude of the QRS complex is subject to a variety of factors, including the thickness of the left ventricular and right ventricular walls, the presence of pleural or pericardial fluid, or an increase in chest wall thickness or body mass. QRS amplitude is also affected by age, sex, and race. For instance, younger individuals have greater QRS voltages than older individuals, and men have greater QRS voltages than women. In left ventricular hypertrophy, the amplitude of the R wave in the

Left bundle branch block

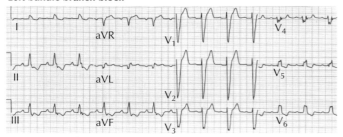

(**A**) Electrocardiogram showing left bundle branch block. It was recorded from a 73-year-old man. Note that the QRS complex is diffusely widened and is notched in leads V_3, V_4, V_5, and V_6. Note also that the T wave is directed opposite to the QRS complex. This is an example of a secondary T-wave change.

Ventricular preexcitation

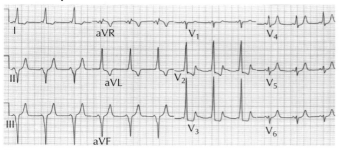

(**B**) ECG showing ventricular preexcitation. It is recorded from a 28-year-old woman. Note the short PR interval (0.9 seconds) and the widened QRS complex (0.134 seconds). The initial portion of the QRS complex appears slurred. This is referred to as a *delta wave*. This combination of short PR interval and widened QRS complex with a delta wave is characteristic of ventricular preexcitation. Note also that the T wave is abnormal, another example of a secondary T-wave change.

Ventricular premature beats

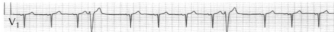

(**C**) Ventricular premature beats recorded from a 30-year-old man with no known heart disease.

ECG changes of LV hypertrophy

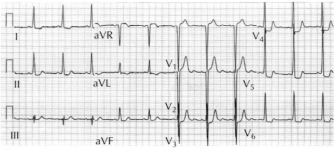

(**D**) Example of the ECG changes of LV hypertrophy. It is recorded from an 83-year-old woman with aortic stenosis and insufficiency. Note the increase in QRS amplitude, the slight increase in QRS duration to 100 ms, and the ST-segment and T-wave changes.

FIG 7.4 (A) Left bundle branch block. (B) Ventricular preexcitation. (C) Ventricular premature beats. (D) ECG changes of left ventricular (LV) hypertrophy.

left-sided leads (V_5 and V_6) and the S wave in the right-sided chest leads (V_1 and V_2) are increased. The duration of the QRS complex may increase, reflecting the increased thickness of the left ventricle, and there may be changes in repolarization that result in changes in the ST segment and the T wave (Fig. 7.4D). Right ventricular hypertrophy is more difficult to diagnose electrocardiographically. Initially, it causes cancellation of left ventricular forces, resulting in a decrease in S-wave amplitude in the right-sided leads V_1 and V_2 and a decrease in R-wave amplitude in the left-sided leads V_5 and V_6. With more advanced right ventricular hypertrophy, an increased R wave occurs in the right-sided leads, and a deeper S wave is seen in the left-sided leads. Pericardial and pleural effusions decrease QRS voltage in all leads; infiltrative diseases such as amyloidosis may also do the same.

ST Segment and T Wave

The ST segment and the T wave reflect ventricular repolarization. During the ST segment, the ventricular action potentials are at their plateau voltage, and only minimal voltage gradients are generated. For this reason, the ST segment is at the same voltage level as (i.e., is isoelectric with) the TP and PR segments, during which time the action potentials are at their resting levels, and there are no voltage gradients. The T wave is caused by the voltage gradients created as the ventricular cells rapidly and sequentially repolarize. If the sequence of repolarization was the same as the sequence of depolarization, the T wave would be opposite in direction to the QRS complex. However, the sequence of repolarization is reversed relative to the sequence of depolarization. As a result, the normal T wave is generally upright or positive in leads

with an upright or positive QRS complex (leads I, V_5, and V_6), and it is inverted or negative in leads with an inverted QRS complex (aVR and V_1) (see Fig. 7.2B).

Abnormalities in repolarization are manifested by elevation or depression of the ST segment and changes in polarity of the T wave. As mentioned previously, such changes may be secondary to intraventricular conduction disturbances, or they may be due to primary changes in repolarization, which occur as the result of electrolyte abnormalities or cardioactive drugs, or as the manifestation of diseases such as hypertrophy, ischemia, or myocarditis. Changes in T-wave polarity that occur in the absence of QRS and ST-segment changes are among the most difficult ECG abnormalities to interpret because they are nonspecific and may result from a variety of nonpathological as well as pathological causes. The following guidelines serve as an approach to interpreting T-wave abnormalities:

1. In general, T-wave amplitude should be ≥10% of the QRS amplitude.
2. Inverted T waves in lead I are always abnormal and usually indicative of underlying cardiac pathology.
3. Minor T-wave changes, such as T-wave flattening or slightly inverted T waves, particularly when they occur in the absence of known cardiac abnormalities or in populations at low risk for cardiac disease, are more likely to be nonspecific and nonpathological than more marked T-wave changes or T-wave changes that occur in the presence of cardiac disease.
4. Flat or inverted T waves often occur in association with rapid ventricular rates and in the absence of other ECG changes. These changes are nonspecific and not indicative of underlying cardiac disease.

Elevation or depression of the ST segment indicates the presence of voltage gradients during the plateau and/or resting phases of the ventricular action potential and are most often a manifestation of cardiac disease. Among the most common causes of ST-segment elevation are acute transmural ischemia and pericarditis. High serum potassium and acute myocarditis may also cause ST-segment elevation and simulate ischemia, although this is rare. A normal variant referred to as early repolarization is a fairly common cause of ST elevation, particularly in young males. These changes characteristically occur in the V leads, involve elevation of the junction of the ST segment with the end of the QRS complex, and may simulate acute ischemia or pericarditis.

Left ventricular hypertrophy, cardioactive drugs, low serum potassium, and acute nontransmural or subendocardial ischemia are the most common causes of ST-segment depression.

U Wave

The U wave follows the T wave, or may arise within the terminal portion of the T wave and be difficult to distinguish from a notched T wave. It is most easily seen in leads V_2 to V_4 and its amplitude is normally no more than one-third that of the T wave. An increase in U-wave amplitude is frequently associated with hypokalemia (Fig. 7.5A) and with some direct-acting cardiac drugs. Notching of the T wave resembling an increase in the U-wave amplitude and lengthening of the QT-U interval can also occur in patients with congenital long QT syndrome (Fig. 7.5B).

QT ABNORMALITIES

The QT interval is measured from the onset of the Q wave to the end of the T wave and is slightly longer in females than in males. Changes in the duration of the QRS complex, the ST segment, and/or the T wave alter the QT interval. The QT interval is rate dependent, reflecting the rate-dependent changes in the duration of the action potential. It shortens at faster heart rates and lengthens at slower rates. To accommodate this rate dependency, several correction factors have been applied to the measured QT interval and used to generate the corrected QT interval. The QT interval is also influenced by a variety of other factors, including (but not limited to) temperature, drugs, electrolyte abnormalities, neurogenic factors, and ischemia.

There is an extensive and ever-increasing list of drugs that lengthen the QT interval by prolonging the ST segment or the T wave, and it is often necessary to monitor the ECG when drugs recognized as having the potential for lengthening the QT interval are initiated. This is clinically important because lengthening of the QT interval after administration of these drugs may be a harbinger of a specific type of ventricular tachycardia (Torsades de pointes), which may progress to ventricular fibrillation.

Low serum potassium and low serum calcium are both associated with prolongation of the QT interval. However, their ECG patterns are different and distinctive. As mentioned previously, low potassium causes ST-segment depression, T-wave changes, a prominent U wave, and prolongation of the QT-U interval (Fig. 7.6A), whereas low calcium lengthens the ST segment, usually without causing significant T-wave changes (Fig. 7.6A). Marked elevations in serum potassium (usually >6.5 mM) may cause prolongation of the QRS complex. Increases in serum potassium and in serum calcium shorten the QT interval by shortening the ST segment. High potassium also shortens the duration of the T wave and makes it more symmetrical, giving it a tented or peaked appearance (Fig. 7.6B).

Abnormalities in one or more of the several genes that regulate the repolarizing currents are responsible for causing congenital long QT syndrome, a significant cause of ventricular arrhythmias that often lead to sudden cardiac death. The ECG changes associated with congenital long QT syndrome (see Fig. 7.5B) are often difficult to distinguish from those caused by low potassium (see Fig. 7.5A) and low calcium (see Fig. 7.6A).

Marked QT prolongation and deeply inverted T waves frequently occur within the first several days after an acute MI, particularly when the MI is due to occlusion of the left anterior descending coronary artery (Fig. 7.6C). This QT prolongation usually resolves within several days, although the T-wave inversion may persist for longer periods. Similar T-wave and QT-interval changes may also occur in the chest leads after an acute ischemic event but in the absence of an infarction. This particular ECG pattern usually indicates a severely but not totally obstructed proximal portion of the left anterior descending coronary artery.

Some neurological events, particularly intracranial hemorrhage and an increase in intracranial pressure, may cause T-wave inversion and dramatic lengthening of the QT interval, similar to that shown in Fig. 7.6C. When it occurs in this clinical setting, it is called the cerebrovascular accident pattern and is believed to represent an imbalance of sympathetic stimulation. These ECG changes generally resolve within a few days.

Changes associated with hypokalemia

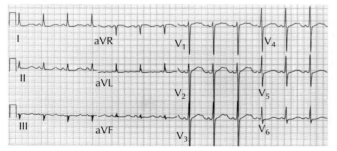

(**A**) Example of the changes associated with hypokalemia. It is recorded from a 44-year-old man who was receiving long-term thiazide therapy. The QT interval is prolonged due to the presence of a U wave, which interrupts the descending limb of the T wave and is of equal amplitude to the T wave. In this patient, the serum potassium concentration was 2.7 mM.

Congenital long QT syndrome

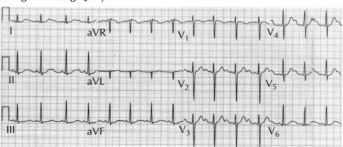

(**B**) Recorded from a 16-year-old girl with syncopal episodes that were documented to be due to rapid ventricular tachycardia. It is an example of long QT syndrome. The T wave is notched and prolonged in much the same way as was shown in the patient with hypokalemia. However, in this patient, the serum potassium concentration was normal.

FIG 7.5 (A) ECG changes associated with hypokalemia. (B) Congenital long QT syndrome.

ST-segment and QT-interval changes associated with hypocalcemia

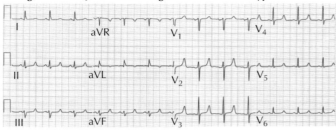

(**A**) ST-segment and QT-interval changes associated with hypocalcemia. It is recorded from a 53-year-old man with chronic renal disease. The ST segment is prolonged, but the T wave is normal. The QT interval reflects ST-segment lengthening and is prolonged.

Changes associated with hyperkalemia

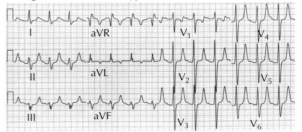

(**B**) Example of the ECG changes associated with hyperkalemia. It is recorded from a 29-year-old woman with chronic renal disease. The P wave is broad and difficult to identify in some leads. The QRS is diffusely widened (0.188 seconds) and the T wave is peaked and symmetrical. These changes are characteristic of severe hyperkalemia and, in this patient, the serum potassium concentration was 8.2 mM.

T-wave changes induced by a recent ischemic event

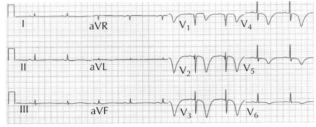

(**C**) T-wave changes induced by a recent ischemic event, recorded from a 70-year-old man. The QT interval is prolonged and the T waves are markedly inverted in the precordial leads (V₁ through V₆). These changes gradually evolved over several days, and coronary angiography recorded the day this tracing was taken revealed a subtotal occlusion of the left anterior descending coronary artery.

FIG 7.6 (A) Hypocalcemia. (B) ECG changes associated with hyperkalemia. (C) T-wave changes induced by a recent ischemic event.

ACUTE ISCHEMIA AND INFARCTION

Acute myocardial ischemia and infarction cause a series of metabolic, ionic, and pathological changes in the region supplied by the occluded coronary artery that cause characteristic changes in the ST segment, QRS complex, and T wave (Fig. 7.7A). The recognition of these changes permits the early diagnosis and prompt treatment—either thrombolytic therapy or percutaneous coronary revascularization—that can reverse ischemia and prevent the loss of myocardial cells and its sequelae.

The sequence of ECG changes associated with acute ischemia and infarction is as follows: (1) peaking of the T wave; (2) ST-segment elevation and/or depression; (3) development of abnormal Q waves; and (4) T-wave inversion.

Peaking of the T waves in leads overlying the ischemic region is the earliest ECG manifestation of acute transmural ischemia and is transient. It is infrequently seen because the ECG is usually not recorded early enough to permit its detection unless the patient is in a hospital setting when ischemia first begins. ST elevation and depression are the most frequently observed early changes and develop within minutes of the onset of the acute event. The ST changes are caused by voltage gradients across the border between the ischemic and nonischemic regions that result in an electrical current, referred to as an injury current, flowing across the ischemic border. Whether these injury currents cause ST elevation or depression depends on the extent and location of the ischemic zone and the relationship of the ECG electrodes to the ischemic zone. In general, electrodes that directly overlie a region

of transmural ischemia will record ST elevation, whereas all other electrodes will record ST depression or no change in the ST segment (Fig. 7.7B).

Subendocardial ischemia, such as that associated with subtotal coronary occlusion and which is often brought on by exercise in patients with flow-limiting coronary artery obstruction, does not extend to the epicardium. Thus none of the body surface leads lie directly over the ischemic region, and ST depression, rather than ST elevation, is recorded.

The development of abnormal Q waves indicates absent conduction through the infarcted region and may last indefinitely. Abnormal Q waves that mimic those associated with infarction may also occur in other settings, particularly hypertrophy of the interventricular septum and intraventricular conduction disturbances, most notably ventricular preexcitation.

The various ECG changes in the setting of an acute transmural ischemic event permit localization and an estimation of the extent of the ischemic or infarcted region and, by inference, identification of the occluded vessel.

ARRHYTHMIAS

The ECG is indispensable for the diagnosis of cardiac arrhythmias. For instance, abnormally rapid heart rates (>100 beats/min) may have multiple causes, including sinus tachycardia, atrial and AV nodal reentrant tachycardia (Fig. 7.8A), atrial flutter and atrial fibrillation

Myocardial ischemia, injury, and infarction

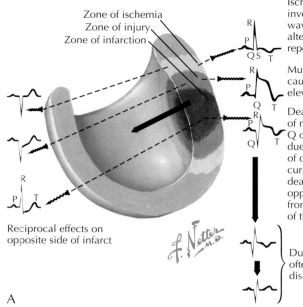

Zone of ischemia
Zone of injury
Zone of infarction

Ischemia causes inversion of T wave due to altered repolarization

Muscle injury causes ST-segment elevation

Death (infarction) of muscle causes Q or QS waves due to absence of depolarization current from dead tissue and opposing currents from other parts of the heart

Reciprocal effects on opposite side of infarct

During recovery (subacute and chronic stages) ST segment often is first to return to normal, then T wave, due to disappearance of zones of injury and ischemia

A

ST-segment changes associated with an acute ischemic event

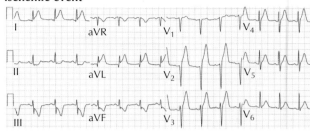

B

Example of ST-segment changes associated with an acute ischemic event. It is recorded from a 43-year-old man with chest pain. Note the ST-segment elevation in leads V₁, aVL, and V₂ through V₆, and the ST-segment depression in leads III and aVF.

FIG 7.7 (A) Myocardial ischemia, injury, and infarction. (B) ST- and T-wave segment changes associated with acute ischemic event.

Abnormal cardiac rhythms

AV nodal reentrant tachycardia

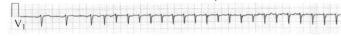

(A) Lead V₁ recorded from a patient with abnormal cardiac rhythms. This tracing shows the onset of AV nodal reentrant tachycardia in a 47-year-old man. There are three sinus beats followed by an atrial premature beat, which initiates a run of AV nodal reentrant tachycardia, with a rate of 170 beats/min.

Atrial fibrillation

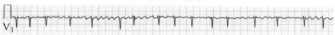

(B) Example of atrial fibrillation in a 50-year-old woman. Note the undulating baseline and the irregularly irregular QRS complexes, with a rate of 105 beats/min.

Ventricular tachycardia

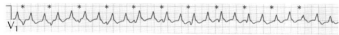

(C) Ventricular tachycardia with a rate of 150 beats/min from a 56-year-old man. The QRS complex is widened, and there is AV disassociation. The P waves, with an atrial rate of 73 beats/min, are marked with an asterisk.

Complete AV block

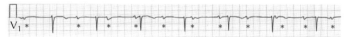

(D) Complete AV block from a 78-year-old woman. The atrial rate is 70 beats/min, and the ventricular rate is 46 beats/min. There is no relation between the P waves (marked with an asterisk) and the QRS complexes.

Irregular cardiac rhythms

Atrial premature beats

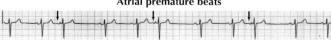

(E) Atrial premature beats (shown with an arrow) recorded from a 77-year-old man. In this example, there is an atrial premature beat after every two sinus beats. This is referred to as *atrial trigeminy*. Note that the shape of the premature P wave is different than that of the sinus P waves, reflecting its ectopic location.

Type I second-degree AV block

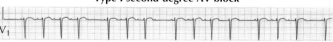

(F) Type I second-degree AV block with Wenckebach periodicity recorded from a 74-year-old man. There is progressive prolongation of the PR interval, followed by a blocked or nonconducted P wave. This leads to irregular groups of QRS complexes. In this example, there is 5:4 and 4:3 AV block. The atrial rate is 110 beats/min, and the ventricular rate is 90 beats/min.

FIG 7.8 (A) Atrioventricular (AV) nodal reentrant tachycardia. (B) Atrial fibrillation. (C) Ventricular tachycardia. (D) Complete AV block. (E) Atrial premature beats. (F) Second-degree AV block (type I).

(Fig. 7.8B), and ventricular tachycardia (Fig. 7.8C). The correct diagnosis is made by analysis of the rate and configuration of the P wave, its relation to the QRS complexes, and the shape and duration of the QRS complex. Abnormally slow heart rates (<50 beats/min) may also be caused by several entities, including sinus bradycardia, or sinoatrial or AV block (Fig. 7.8D). Again, the diagnosis can be established by noting the rate, regularity, and configuration of the P wave and QRS complexes, the relation of the P wave to the QRS complexes, and the PR interval.

Irregular rhythms may be due to atrial and ventricular premature beats (Figs. 7.8E and 7.4C), atrial fibrillation with a slow ventricular response, and incomplete (second-degree) sinoatrial or AV block (Fig. 7.8F).

SCREENING

The role of the ECG in the asymptomatic patient as a screening tool remains the subject of debate. Some pathological conditions, such left ventricular hypertrophy, the Wolff-Parkinson-White pattern (if antegrade conduction down the accessory pathway is evident), long QT, Brugada pattern, congenital complete heart block, and T-wave changes consistent with hypertrophic cardiomyopathy or arrhythmogenic right ventricular cardiomyopathy (ARVC) can be detected on a screening ECG. However, the specificity of the ECG to detect such conditions is highly variable, and the use of ECG screening in the general population, especially in asymptomatic individuals, raises concerns. A 2012 report from the U.S. Preventive Services Task Force advised against routine ECGs at rest or with exercise in asymptomatic low-risk subjects as a screening for coronary heart disease. ECG screening in specific patient groups may be more beneficial. The role of the ECG in preparticipation screening of competitive athletes has generated much interest in the last decade. Many of the conditions associated with sudden death in athletes, such as long QT syndrome and ARVC, have distinct ECG findings. In athletes, the definition of what is considered normal on a screening ECG continues to be refined. Areas of continued investigation include the impact of age, race, sex, and the type of training on normal variants on the ECG.

FUTURE DIRECTIONS

The ECG provides a window into the electrophysiological properties of the heart and their modification by physiological, pharmacological, and pathological factors. When correctly interpreted, it provides diagnostic and prognostic information that is of inestimable help in the diagnosis and treatment of patients with a wide variety of cardiac diseases. It is of particular importance in the diagnosis of myocardial ischemia and arrhythmias, and in the evaluation of patients with chest pain, heart murmurs, palpitations, shortness of breath, and syncope, and during the administration of drugs that are capable of prolonging the QT interval. It is also of help in identifying the site of "culprit" coronary artery obstructions, the site of origin of atrial and ventricular ectopic beats and rhythms, and the location of AV nodal bypass tracts. The use of the ECG recorded during daily activities and during stress further adds to its capabilities. The value of the ECG is greatly enhanced when pertinent patient information, such as symptoms, drug usage, and important laboratory findings, is provided to the reader. It is reasonable to anticipate that in the future, additional leads such as V_3R, V_4R, and V_{7-9} may be recorded and/or provided by computer reconstruction; that new analytical measurements, particularly those dealing with the QRS complex and the T wave, will be developed; and that the library of diagnostic and prognostic statements will be expanded. However, it is important to stress that the automated interpretations provided by computerized ECG systems now and in the future may be incomplete or inaccurate, particularly when the tracing is abnormal. For that reason, overreading by qualified personnel is essential.

ADDITIONAL RESOURCES

American Heart Association Electrocardiography and Arrhythmias Committee, Council on Clinical Cardiology; the American College of Cardiology Foundation; and the Heart Rhythm Society Endorsed by the International Society for Computerized Electrocardiology. Recommendations for the standardization and interpretation of the electrocardiogram.
This scientific statement is a six-part series of reports designed to update ECG standards and interpretation. The articles were published simultaneously in Circulation, Journal of the American College of Cardiology, and Heart Rhythm.

Part I
Kligfield P, Gettes LS, Bailey JJ, et al. The electrocardiogram and its technology. *Circulation.* 2007;115:1306–1324. *J Am Coll Cardiol.* 2007;49:1109–1127; *Heart Rhythm.* 2007;4:394–412.
This article emphasizes areas that have clinical relevance by focusing on the currently used computerized, automated technology.

Part II
Mason JW, Hancock EW, Gettes LS, et al. Electrocardiography diagnostic statement list. *Circulation.* 2007;115:1325–1332. *J Am Coll Cardiol.* 2007;49:1128–1135; *Heart Rhythm.* 2007;4:412–419.
Provides a set of diagnostic statements that are more concise and streamlined than the existing diagnostic statements, and should eliminate differences in the various systems currently in use.

Part III
Surawicz B, Childers R, Deal BJ, et al. Intraventricular conduction disturbances. *J Am Coll Cardiol.* 2009;53:976–981. *Circulation.* 2009;119(10):e235–e240.
This article reviews and updates standards for adults and children.

Part IV
Rautaharju PM, Surawicz B, Gettes LS, et al. ST segment, T and U waves and the QT interval. *J Am Coll Cardiol.* 2009;53:982–991. *Circulation.* 2009;119(10):e241–e250.
Focuses on the various components of repolarization, their electrophysiological basis, and ECG features.

Part V
Hancock EW, Deal BJ, Mirvis DM, et al. Electrocardiogram changes associated with cardiac chamber hypertrophy. *J Am Coll Cardiol.* 2009;53:992–1002. *Circulation.* 2009;119(10):e251–e261.
Reviews the various ECG criteria used to diagnose chamber hypertrophy in children and adults, and recommends changes to clarify statements currently in use.

Part VI
Wagner GS, MacFarlane P, Wellens H, et al. Acute ischemia/infarction. *J Am Coll Cardiol.* 2009;53:1003–1011. *Circulation.* 2009;119(10):e262–e270.
This final article in the series reviews the electrocardiographic manifestations of acute ischemia/infarction and suggests changes to permit identification of culprit lesion locations.

Consensus Statements on the Use of the ECG to Screen Various Populations for Potentially Lethal Cardiac Diseases
Drezner JA, Sharma S, Baggish A. International criteria for electrocardiographic interpretation in athletes. *Br J Sports Med.* 2017;1:1–28.
This statement represents the consensus of an international group of experts in sports cardiology, inherited cardiac diseases, and sports medicine. It provides opinion-based recommendations for ECG interpretation in athletes, linking specific ECG abnormalities and the secondary evaluation for conditions associated with sudden cardiac death.

Moyer VA. Screening for coronary heart disease with electrocardiography: U.S. Preventive Services Task Force recommendation statement. *Ann Intern Med.* 2012;157:512–518.
This is an update of a previous Task Force recommendation. It reviews new evidence on the benefits of ECG screening in asymptomatic adults to reduce the risk for coronary heart disease.

EVIDENCE

Chou TC, Surawicz B, Knilans TK, eds. *Chou's Electrocardiography in Clinical Practice.* 6th ed. Philadelphia: WB Saunders; 2008.
A complete text with excellent figures and extensive up-to-date references.

Gettes LS. *ECG tutor (CD-ROM).* Armonk, NY: Future Publishing; 2000.
This animated graphic CD-ROM illustrates the electrophysiological basis for the ECG and the interpretive approach.
Surawicz B. *Electrophysiologic Basis of ECG and Cardiac Arrhythmias.* Baltimore: Williams & Wilkins; 1995.
This book provides an in-depth correlation of basic electrophysiological phenomena to the waveform of the normal and abnormal body surface ECG.
Wellens HJJ, Gorgels PM, Doevendans PA. *The ECG in Acute Myocardial Infarction and Unstable Angina: Diagnosis and Risk Stratification.* Norwell, MA: Kluwer Academic Publishers; 2004.
An in-depth review and analysis of the ECG changes of acute ischemia and/or infarction and their use to predict the infarct-related artery, the size of the jeopardized myocardium, and the potential for reversibility.

8

Chest Radiography

Cody S. Deen, Andrew O. Zurick III, Park W. Willis IV

TECHNICAL ASPECTS

Chest radiography was one of the first clinical studies to use x-rays, which were discovered in 1895 by Wilhelm Conrad Roentgen. X-rays are typically generated by passing a current across a diode, which results in the generation of electrons. The electron beam is aimed at a metal anode, and the resultant interaction produces x-ray photons. The x-ray beam diverges as it exits from the x-ray tube and produces a conical-shaped beam. When x-rays are captured by film or a digital system, the divergence of the beam can lead to geometric distortion, which is a function of the distance from the x-ray source to the object and from the object to the detector. The further an object is from the radiation source, the less geometric distortion and clearer image that will be produced, but higher levels of energy and longer exposure times are required for adequate image production. More energy and longer exposure lead to an increase in radiation exposure for the patient. To balance the competing factors of geometric distortion and radiation exposure, 6 feet is considered the standard source-to-image distance for a typical posteroanterior (PA) and lateral chest x-ray. The radiation exposure of a standard PA and lateral chest x-ray at this distance is approximately 3 millirems or approximately 1/100 of the typical annual rate of celestial radiation for an individual. Because ionizing radiation causes a dose-dependent increase in the risk of genetic alteration and malignancy, as low as reasonably allowable principles of radiation safety are followed to minimize patient exposure.

Anatomic structures with different tissue compositions will produce varying degrees of absorption, blocking, and disruption of the x-ray photons, thereby producing shades of gray or contrast in the image. This contrast allows differentiation of fluid-filled structures (heart and great vessels) from air-filled lungs and the much denser bony structures of the thorax. The x-ray image is produced as x-ray photons strike and alter silver iodide crystals in the x-ray film. Alternatively, digital radiography (filmless technique) can produce images with a flat plate that directly converts incident photons to a digital signal.

The quality of the technique used in obtaining a chest radiograph can be appreciated after a quick survey of the film. The key components are a review of identification, inspiration, penetration, and rotation. Patient identifiers and radiographic markers should be noted. PA chest film should demonstrate the diaphragm along the eighth to tenth posterior rib space or the fifth to sixth anterior rib space. The film should have adequate penetration to allow the intervertebral disc space of the thoracic spine to be barely visualized but not overly penetrated, which would obscure bony details of the spine or identification of pathology within the pulmonary fields. Rotation should be evaluated by confirmation that the thoracic spine lies posterior to the sternum, and that the clavicles are at approximately the first anterior rib.

NORMAL ANATOMY

The chest x-ray can be useful at detecting structural abnormalities of the heart and great vessels and sequelae of cardiovascular disease. It is also frequently used to identify endotracheal tubes, central venous lines, pacemaker leads, and to evaluate for postprocedure complications (e.g., pneumothorax). To effectively use the chest x-ray for these purposes requires an understanding of the normal anatomy as it appears on a chest x-ray. In the PA projection (Fig. 8.1), the cardiac silhouette typically is <50% of the transverse diameter of the chest. The heart overlies the spine with roughly one-quarter of the heart at the right of the spine and three-quarters to the left of the spine. The right border of the heart is formed inferiorly by the right atrium and superiorly by the superior vena cava. Superimposed over the superior vena cava is the aortic arch. The arch traverses the chest and forms the most superior aspect of the left border of the cardiac silhouette (the aortic knob). The descending aorta usually can be visualized near midline from the aortic knob to the diaphragm. Inferior to the aortic knob is the left pulmonary artery, which is usually indistinguishable from the mediastinum. In some patients, the left atrial appendage may be found to be inferior to the pulmonary trunk. The inferior aspect of the cardiac silhouette is made up of the left ventricle as it rests on the diaphragm.

In the lateral projection (Fig. 8.2), the right ventricle can be found in the retrosternal space and is the most anterior chamber. Superiorly, the right atrium is present but usually not well visualized. The main pulmonary artery arises from the outflow tract of the right ventricle and courses superiorly and posteriorly. Superior to the pulmonary artery is the aortic arch, which continues as the descending aorta, and is visualized down to the diaphragm and forms the most posterior structure of the intrathoracic cavity.

CLINICAL USEFULNESS

The chest x-ray can be helpful in detecting a multitude of cardiovascular diseases, quick radiographic assessments after procedures, and for identifying various intracardiac and intravascular devices. Although the chest radiograph is frequently normal in coronary artery disease, calcifications of coronary arteries can be noted and correspond to advanced disease. When congestive heart failure is present, there may be evidence of chamber enlargement, increased pulmonary vascularity, and occasionally, pleural effusions. Aneurysmal segments of myocardium, especially if calcified, may also be distinguished by chest x-ray. The left ventricle normally has a blurry myocardial border due to cardiac motion during film exposure and the apical fat pad. Aneurysmal segments may appear as more distinct myocardial borders arising from the left ventricle.

Disease of the aorta may also be noted on a chest x-ray. Calcifications in the aorta suggest significant atherosclerotic disease. Enlargement

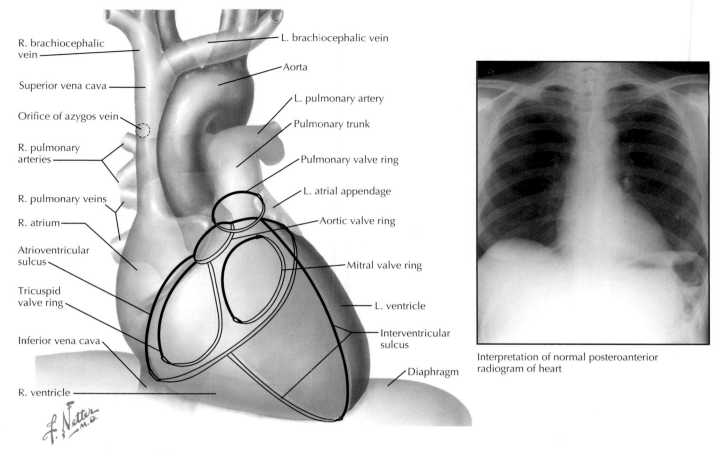

R. brachiocephalic vein

L. brachiocephalic vein

Aorta

Superior vena cava

L. pulmonary artery

Orifice of azygos vein

Pulmonary trunk

R. pulmonary arteries

Pulmonary valve ring

L. atrial appendage

R. pulmonary veins

Aortic valve ring

R. atrium

Atrioventricular sulcus

Mitral valve ring

Tricuspid valve ring

L. ventricle

Inferior vena cava

Interventricular sulcus

R. ventricle

Diaphragm

Interpretation of normal posteroanterior radiogram of heart

FIG 8.1 Posteroanterior chest radiograph with corresponding cardiovascular structures.

of the aorta can be present with ascending, arch, and descending aneurysmal segments. Aortic dissection may present as a widened mediastinum. A PA chest x-ray may suggest a widened mediastinum (note that the anteroposterior [AP] technique typically used for portable examination may lead to a false suggestion of a widened mediastinum). Dissection is suggested on an AP film if the mediastinum is >8 cm wide at the aortic knob or if aortic calcifications are displaced >1 cm from the border of the aorta.

A chest x-ray can be valuable in diagnosing valvular heart disease. In aortic stenosis, findings frequently include calcified aortic annulus, poststenotic aortic root dilation, and left ventricular hypertrophy. Clinically significant chronic aortic regurgitation can produce left ventricular enlargement. Mitral valve annulus calcifications can be present in mitral valve disease and are typically best seen on overpenetrated films. Mitral regurgitation can lead to left ventricular dilation, and mitral stenosis may lead to left atrial enlargement. Aortic and mitral annulus calcifications are best visualized on lateral radiographs. Left atrial enlargement is also best seen in the lateral examination, whereas left ventricular changes may be present in both PA and lateral images.

A variety of congenital defects may be suggested by the chest x-ray. Coarctation of the aorta may be suggested by "notching" of the third to ninth ribs because of collateral filling of the distal aorta via the internal mammary arteries. The figure three sign may also be present in coarctation, because the dilation of the left subclavian artery, dilation of the proximal aorta, and dilation of the distal aorta may resemble the number 3 on the chest x-ray. Tetralogy of Fallot typically presents with a boot-shaped heart due to right ventricular enlargement and may have a right-sided aortic arch. Dextrocardia and situs inversus may also be noted

from the standard chest x-ray, but left-sided or right-sided annotation markers are useful in confirming these lesions from a reversed normal film. The "scimitar sign," which is a curved radiodensity lateral to the right heart border, can be seen in anomalous pulmonary venous return.

Pericardial disease may also present with findings on chest x-ray. A globular-appearing cardiac silhouette, or "water bottle," appearance with pulmonary congestion is suggestive of pericardial effusion. Pericardial calcifications can be suggestive of chronic pericarditis. An eggshell calcification may be more suggestive of a chronic inflammatory cause, for which latent tuberculosis typically has a denser, irregular pattern of calcifications.

Portable chest x-ray examinations are frequently used in postprocedural care and to identify appropriate placement of devices. PA and lateral chest x-rays are used to ensure appropriate lead placement of implantable pacemakers and defibrillators. The leads should course under the clavicle and enter the superior vena cava. The right atrial lead typically will have an upward deflection as it inserts into the right atrial appendage. The right ventricular lead will typically be in the right ventricular apex. Complications from lead placement, such as a dislodged lead or a pneumothorax, can also be noted on a chest x-ray. Intraaortic balloon pump positioning is frequently checked with a portable chest x-ray. The superior radio-opaque marker should be at a level 2 cm above the carina. Central venous catheter and pulmonary artery catheter positioning can be evaluated on a chest x-ray. Central venous catheters should be positioned so that the catheter travels from the internal jugular or subclavian veins into the superior vena cava, with termination of the catheter tip at or above the junction of the superior vena cava and the right atrium. Pulmonary artery catheters typically will follow a

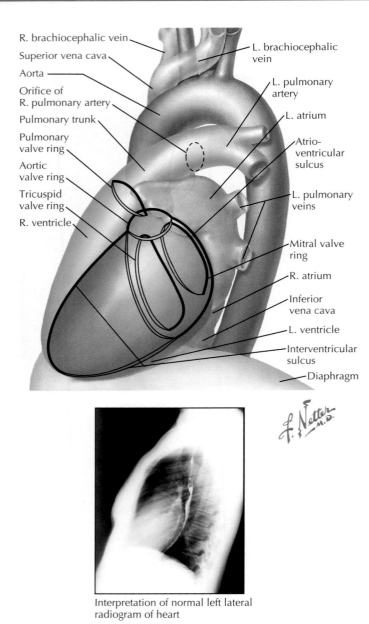

R. brachiocephalic vein

Superior vena cava

Aorta

Orifice of
R. pulmonary artery

Pulmonary trunk

Pulmonary
valve ring

Aortic
valve ring

Tricuspid
valve ring

R. ventricle

L. brachiocephalic
vein

L. pulmonary
artery

L. atrium

Atrio-
ventricular
sulcus

L. pulmonary
veins

Mitral valve
ring

R. atrium

Inferior
vena cava

L. ventricle

Interventricular
sulcus

Diaphragm

Interpretation of normal left lateral
radiogram of heart

FIG 8.2 Lateral chest radiographs with corresponding cardiovascular structures.

similar path through the central venous vasculature and then through the right atrium, right ventricle, the right ventricular outflow tract, and into the pulmonary artery. Proper positioning of the catheter should be no more than 1 cm past the mediastinal border in either the right or left pulmonary arteries.

Finally, chest x-rays may be used to identify unknown implantable cardiac devices in patients. The presence of coils in leads placed in the superior vena cava and right ventricular apex are seen in implantable cardioverter-defibrillator leads. The manufacturer of the device can be discerned from the chest x-ray by radio-opaque alphanumeric codes, header orientation, generator can shape, and configuration of the connector pins.

LIMITATIONS

The major benefits of chest radiography are that it is widely available, quick to perform, and relatively inexpensive. Although the usefulness of chest radiography is clearly beneficial in identifying pathology and monitoring procedural care, there are limitations to the technique. There is relatively poor differentiation of soft tissue structures, such as the myocardium, blood pool, and fluid collections. Alternative imaging techniques can easily distinguish between soft tissue types and provide more accurate evaluation of anatomy and gross pathology in cardiovascular disease.

ADDITIONAL RESOURCES

Baron MG. The cardiac silhouette. *J Thorac Imaging.* 2000;15:230–242.
Excellent review of the chest x-ray in evaluating the cardiac silhouette, with detailed information that can be obtained regarding the presence, nature, and severity of the disease, as well as prognosis.
Bettmann MA. The chest radiograph in cardiovascular medicine. Chapter 15. In: Mann DL, Zipes DP, Libby P, Bonow RO, eds. *Braunwald's Heart Disease: A Textbook of Cardiovascular Medicine.* 10th ed. Philadelphia: Saunders/Elsevier; 2008.
A comprehensive review of the usefulness of the chest x-ray in the evaluation of cardiovascular diseases.
Jacob S, Shahzad MA, Maheshwari R, et al. Cardiac rhythm device identification algorithm using x-rays: CaRDIA-X. *Heart Rhythm.* 2011;8(6):915–922.
A comprehensive review of identifying the manufacturers and the type of pacing and/or defibrillators, complete with detailed radiographic examples.
Website: https://www.med-ed.virginia.edu/courses/rad/cxr/.
Web site from the Department of Radiology, University of Virginia for aiding medical students and residents in evaluating imaging techniques for the chest radiograph, complete with a step-by-step tutorial and practicum.

9

Echocardiography

Thelsa Thomas Weickert, Andrew O. Zurick III, Park W. Willis IV

Echocardiography is a highly reproducible, safe, and widely available noninvasive imaging technique integral to the practice of modern clinical cardiology. With the use of high-frequency ultrasound to image cardiac and great vessel structure and blood flow, this method provides definitive anatomic and hemodynamic information crucial to the diagnosis and management of patients with a wide range of cardiac and vascular conditions. Although often considered a mature imaging technique, the technology and its applications continue to improve.

IMAGING METHODS AND CLINICAL APPLICATIONS

Transthoracic Echocardiography

A comprehensive transthoracic echocardiographic examination (TTE) includes the acquisition of standard two-dimensional (2D) and M-mode views of the intrathoracic structures complemented by continuous-wave and pulsed-wave spectral Doppler data and color flow Doppler imaging. Current commercial echocardiographic imaging systems also have tissue harmonic imaging capability that helps to enhance endocardial definition in patients with technically difficult TTE windows. In addition, tissue Doppler imaging (TDI), which is analogous to pulsed-wave Doppler assessment of blood flow velocity, is used to measure longitudinal myocardial motion. When combined with a comprehensive TTE examination, TDI can yield clinically useful information regarding diastolic ventricular function and cardiac filling pressures. Small, lightweight, and highly portable ultrasound systems are also available for bedside TTE imaging. Commonly referred to as "handheld" TTE devices, these instruments possess limited capability compared with standard echocardiographic equipment, but this technology continues to evolve. These devices are widely used for the rapid triage of patients in emergency department and intensive care unit settings.

Transthoracic 2D echocardiography is the foundation of the clinical echocardiographic examination. Tomographic images are obtained usually from four standard imaging "windows" on the chest wall, defined by the transducer position and image plane (Fig. 9.1). These are the parasternal, apical, subcostal, and suprasternal positions. It provides a reliable, portable, and reproducible evaluation of cardiac chamber sizes, myocardial thickness, ventricular contractile performance, valvular structure and function, the pericardium, and the great vessels. Doppler echocardiographic assessment of the direction and velocity of blood flow within the heart and great vessels is valuable for the detection and quantification of obstructive lesions and valvular regurgitation (Fig. 9.2).

M-mode echocardiography was the first application of ultrasound in cardiology. It provides both high spatial and temporal (time-related) resolution. Hence, it is especially valuable in the evaluation of mitral and aortic valve motion in dynamic and fixed left ventricular outflow obstruction, in the timing of mitral valve closure in aortic regurgitation, and in the assessment of pericardial disease.

Although coronary arteries cannot be reliably imaged by TTE, the method is nevertheless valuable in the assessment of known or suspected coronary artery disease (CAD). Echocardiographic evidence of segmental ventricular contractile dysfunction can be used to screen for acute or chronic ischemic myocardial injury or infarction, secondary to CAD. However, the diagnosis of CAD is not established by segmental wall motion abnormalities because these can also be caused by cardiac trauma, myocarditis, and infiltrative myocardial diseases. In addition, multivessel CAD can cause globally decreased ventricular contraction without segmental wall motion abnormalities, a circumstance that generally requires further evaluation.

TTE is used for the initial diagnostic evaluation and follow-up of patients with congenital and valvular heart disease, including the assessment of right ventricular systolic pressure and pulmonary arterial hypertension. Anatomic information about the nature of a congenital defect and its hemodynamic consequences, including the direction and magnitude of intracardiac shunts and estimation of pulmonary and systemic blood flow, can be estimated by 2D and Doppler techniques (Fig. 9.3).

Transthoracic 2D echocardiography provides a comprehensive picture of the valvular, subvalvular, and annular structures, and when 2D echocardiography is combined with Doppler ultrasound techniques, obstructive gradients can be accurately measured and the cross-sectional valve area can be estimated. Regurgitant valvular lesions can be accurately quantified by color flow Doppler imaging. Clinical decisions regarding medical therapy and operative intervention for patients with valvular disease are usually based on TTE 2D and Doppler echocardiographic data, supplemented by information from cardiac catheterization.

TTE is the primary tool for evaluating the presence and hemodynamic consequences of pericardial effusion. Two-dimensional imaging and a comprehensive Doppler examination can reliably identify patients with pericardial effusion and tamponade pathophysiology. TTE-guided pericardiocentesis can reduce procedural complications and improve therapeutic results. A thickened pericardium and typical hemodynamic alterations can alert the clinician to the diagnosis of pericardial constriction, but magnetic resonance imaging and catheterization are usually needed for full evaluation. Analysis of Doppler-measured ventricular inflow velocities and TDI can be useful in differentiating between pericardial constriction and infiltrative cardiomyopathy.

Transesophageal Echocardiography

A transesophageal echocardiographic examination (TEE) requires an ultrasound probe placed into the esophagus, posterior to the heart. Because of the decreased distance between the transducer and the heart, as well as the absence of interference from bone and lung tissue, the signal-to-noise ratio is more favorable with TEE than with TTE, and higher frequency transducers can be used to improve resolution. Therefore TEE image quality is generally superior to that of TTE, particularly

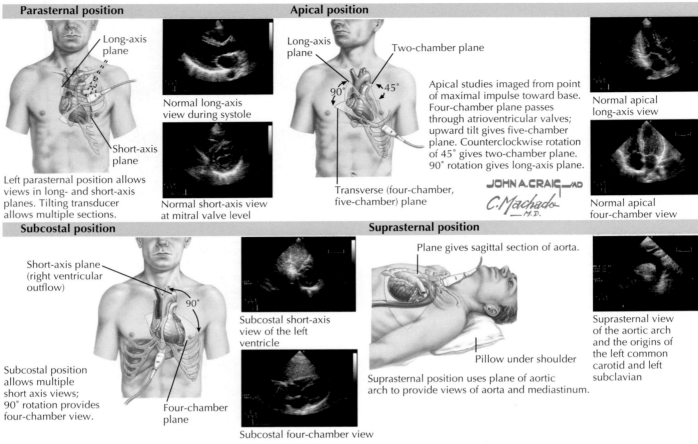

Parasternal position

Long-axis plane

Short-axis plane

Left parasternal position allows views in long- and short-axis planes. Tilting transducer allows multiple sections.

Normal long-axis view during systole

Normal short-axis view at mitral valve level

Apical position

Long-axis plane

Two-chamber plane

90°   45°

Apical studies imaged from point of maximal impulse toward base. Four-chamber plane passes through atrioventricular valves; upward tilt gives five-chamber plane. Counterclockwise rotation of 45° gives two-chamber plane. 90° rotation gives long-axis plane.

Transverse (four-chamber, five-chamber) plane

JOHN A. CRAIG__MD
C. Machado __M.D.

Normal apical long-axis view

Normal apical four-chamber view

Subcostal position

Short-axis plane (right ventricular outflow)

90°

Subcostal position allows multiple short axis views; 90° rotation provides four-chamber view.

Four-chamber plane

Subcostal short-axis view of the left ventricle

Subcostal four-chamber view

Suprasternal position

Plane gives sagittal section of aorta.

Pillow under shoulder

Suprasternal position uses plane of aortic arch to provide views of aorta and mediastinum.

Suprasternal view of the aortic arch and the origins of the left common carotid and left subclavian

FIG 9.1 Transducer positions in echocardiographic examination.

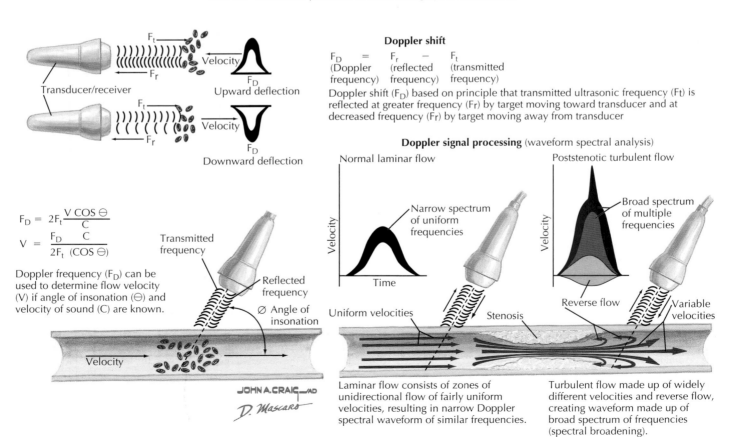

F_t Velocity F_r

Transducer/receiver

F_D
Upward deflection

F_t Velocity F_r

F_D
Downward deflection

Doppler shift

$$F_D = F_r - F_t$$
(Doppler   (reflected   (transmitted
frequency)   frequency)   frequency)

Doppler shift (F_D) based on principle that transmitted ultrasonic frequency (F_t) is reflected at greater frequency (F_r) by target moving toward transducer and at decreased frequency (F_r) by target moving away from transducer

Doppler signal processing (waveform spectral analysis)

Normal laminar flow

Narrow spectrum of uniform frequencies

Poststenotic turbulent flow

Broad spectrum of multiple frequencies

$$F_D = 2F_t \frac{V \cos \ominus}{C}$$
$$V = \frac{F_D}{2F_t} \frac{C}{(\cos \ominus)}$$

Doppler frequency (F_D) can be used to determine flow velocity (V) if angle of insonation ($\ominus$) and velocity of sound (C) are known.

Transmitted frequency

Reflected frequency

∅ Angle of insonation

Velocity

JOHN A. CRAIG__MD
D. Mascaro

Uniform velocities

Stenosis

Reverse flow

Variable velocities

Laminar flow consists of zones of unidirectional flow of fairly uniform velocities, resulting in narrow Doppler spectral waveform of similar frequencies.

Turbulent flow made up of widely different velocities and reverse flow, creating waveform made up of broad spectrum of frequencies (spectral broadening).

FIG 9.2 Principles of Doppler echocardiography.

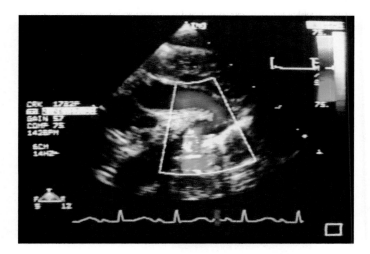

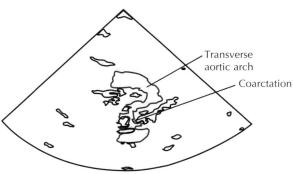

FIG 9.3 Coarctation of the aorta.

for posterior structures, including the pulmonary veins, left atrium, interatrial septum, and mitral valve. TEE is most commonly applied in the evaluation for suspected patent foramen ovale (PFO), atrial septal defects (ASDs), quantification of valvular regurgitation, valvular vegetations, left atrial or atrial appendage thrombus, and aortic disease. TEE is being used with increasing frequency in clinical cardiac electrophysiology before elective cardioversion and invasive procedures, including ablative therapy for atrial fibrillation (Fig. 9.4).

Stress Echocardiography

Exercise and pharmacological stress echocardiography enables evaluation of the heart at rest and during stress. The clinical usefulness of stress echocardiography depends on acquisition of high-quality TTE images of the left ventricle, in multiple planes, at maximal cardiac workload. With exercise stress, patients must be highly motivated not only to reach, but ideally exceed, a target heart rate, because cardiac workload falls rapidly with cessation of exercise. Repositioning of the subject and immediate poststress image acquisition usually requires 30 to 60 seconds, and test sensitivity falls when echocardiographic data are recorded at less than maximal workload. For these reasons, equivocal test results are fairly common with exercise stress (unless a recumbent bike is used). This is rarely a problem with pharmacological stress test (usually dobutamine) because patient repositioning is not necessary, and maximal cardiac workload can be maintained while image acquisition is completed. Pharmacological stress also has a technical advantage in that patients are not moving during the study; sequential images can be recorded as cardiac workload is gradually increased, and respiratory interference at peak stress is not a limiting factor.

Stress echocardiography is an accurate, noninvasive approach to detect the presence and extent of CAD. A stress-induced segmental wall motion abnormality usually indicates flow-limiting CAD. In addition to providing a useful approach for detecting obstructive CAD, stress echocardiography can be used to assess an area of myocardium at risk, for detection of myocardial viability, in risk stratification after myocardial infarction, and for evaluation of the results of coronary revascularization. Stress echocardiography is especially useful in detecting CAD in patients after heart transplantation, in those being considered for renal transplantation, and for preoperative evaluation of individuals undergoing vascular surgery. Exercise echocardiography is invaluable to the assessment of exercise-induced pulmonary hypertension, especially in the setting of mitral valve disease and evaluation of dynamic left ventricular outflow tract gradients in patients with hypertrophic obstructive cardiomyopathy. Low-dose dobutamine stress echocardiography plays an important role in the evaluation of asymptomatic or low gradient aortic stenosis (Fig. 9.5).

Contrast Echocardiography

Contrast echocardiography is now widely used to detect intracardiac and intrapulmonary shunts, to augment Doppler velocity signals, and to enhance endocardial border definition. Intravenous injection of agitated normal saline is most often used for opacification of the right heart, shunt detection, and augmentation of tricuspid regurgitant jets to allow more accurate estimation of right ventricular systolic pressure. Commercially available contrast agents, termed "microbubbles," are made of a high-molecular-weight gas encapsulated in a shell of phospholipid or protein. Modifications of the microbubble shell and gas properties have resulted in improved stability of these agents as they pass through the pulmonary circulation after intravenous injection, and high-quality imaging of the left heart chambers can be reliably obtained. Myocardial perfusion imaging with contrast echocardiography is not routinely used for clinical purposes.

Strain Imaging

Strain is an assessment of myocardial deformation with strain rate being the rate of myocardial deformation in time. It can be obtained from TDI or from the speckle tracking method. TDI can be used even in poor echocardiographic windows. Speckle tracking allows for assessment of longitudinal (global longitudinal strain), radial, and circumferential strain. There is an expanding role for strain imaging for the assessment of segmental wall motion abnormalities, cardiac dyssynchrony analysis, right ventricular function, infiltrative cardiomyopathies (e.g., amyloidosis) and monitoring of oncology patients on cardiotoxic drugs such as adriamycin or trastuzumab (Herceptin) (Fig. 9.6).

Intravascular Ultrasound and Intracardiac Echocardiography

The development of intravascular ultrasound (IVUS) and intracardiac echocardiography (ICE) techniques has extended the application of echocardiography and bridged traditional boundaries between noninvasive and invasive imaging methods. IVUS uses a miniaturized transducer on the end of a flexible, steerable catheter that is inserted into arteries, which allows in vivo ultrasound imaging of vascular anatomy from the inside of the artery. ICE relies on a catheter-like ultrasound probe that can be advanced to the right heart chambers via the femoral vein and inferior vena cava, and it also crosses the interatrial septum. ICE probe technology has evolved rapidly and is capable of high-resolution 2D echocardiography and a full complement of Doppler imaging modalities.

Intracoronary IVUS is commonly used in cardiac catheterization laboratories to delineate atherosclerotic plaque morphology, lesion

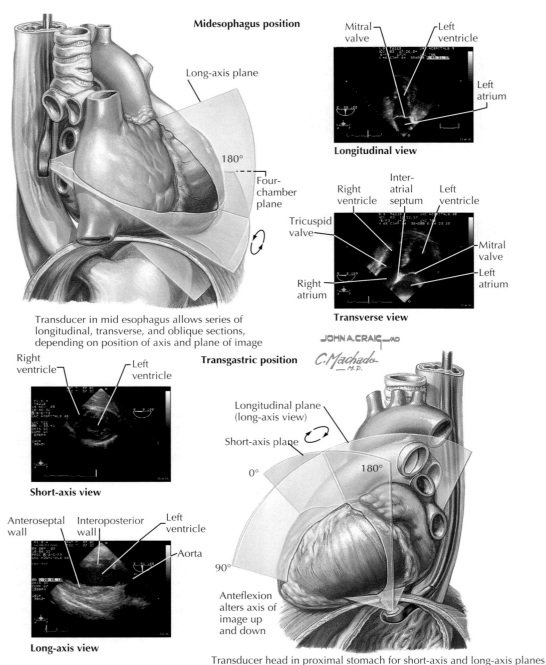

Midesophagus position

Long-axis plane

180°

Four-chamber plane

Transducer in mid esophagus allows series of longitudinal, transverse, and oblique sections, depending on position of axis and plane of image

Mitral valve — Left ventricle

Left atrium

Longitudinal view

Right ventricle — Inter-atrial septum — Left ventricle

Tricuspid valve

Mitral valve

Right atrium — Left atrium

Transverse view

JOHN A. CRAIG —MD

C. Machado —M.D.

Transgastric position

Right ventricle — Left ventricle

Short-axis view

Anteroseptal wall — Interoposterior wall — Left ventricle

Aorta

Long-axis view

Longitudinal plane (long-axis view)

Short-axis plane

0°   180°

90°

Anteflexion alters axis of image up and down

Transducer head in proximal stomach for short-axis and long-axis planes

FIG 9.4 Transesophageal echocardiography.

length, and obstruction severity when standard coronary angiographic and pressure data are ambiguous. Intracoronary IVUS can help guide percutaneous coronary intervention and stent implantation, and aid in the diagnosis of in-stent restenosis. ICE is also often used to monitor noncoronary interventional procedures in interventional electrophysiology and cardiac catheterization laboratories. ICE has proven useful for direct visualization of the pulmonary veins and left atrial appendage during invasive ablation procedures for atrial fibrillation. In addition, ICE is now used to assist with guidance of radiofrequency catheter ablation of atrial arrhythmias in the right side of the heart. ICE augments fluoroscopy through improving visualization of landmarks, ensuring endocardial contact, and assisting with transseptal puncture.

This technique is also useful in the prompt detection of procedural complications, including intracardiac thrombus formation, pericardial effusion, and pulmonary vein obstruction.

Three-Dimensional Echocardiography

Three-dimensional (3D) echocardiography, via either a transthoracic or transesophageal approach, can provide improved definition of spatial relationships between normal and abnormal cardiac structures and eliminate the need for cognitive reconstruction of image planes currently required for interpretation of standard 2D images.

Three-dimensional echocardiography has the potential to provide more accurate and reliable measurements of cardiac chamber dimensions

Exercise echocardiography

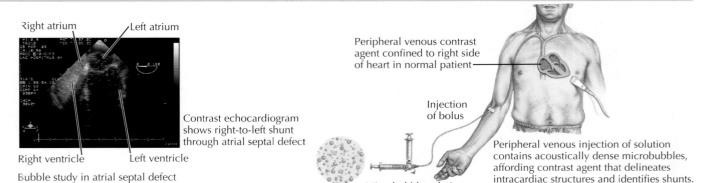

Left ventricle
Anteroseptal wall
Right ventricle
Aortic valve
Left atrium
Anterior leaflet mitral valve

Resting echocardiogram

Left ventricle
Anteroseptal wall
Inferoposterior wall

Baseline stress echocardiogram long axis

Left ventricle   Anteroseptal wall
Inferoposterior wall

Diastolic postexercise echocardiogram, long axis

Left ventricle   Anteroseptal wall
Inferoposterior wall

Systolic postexercise echocardiogram, long axis

Exercise performed to elicit ischemic signs and postexercise echocardiogram used to evaluate ventricular function, wall motion, and thickness. Often correlated with stress echocardiography

JOHN A.CRAIG—MD
C.Machado
—M.D.

Contrast echocardiography

Right atrium   Left atrium

Right ventricle   Left ventricle

Bubble study in atrial septal defect

Contrast echocardiogram shows right-to-left shunt through atrial septal defect

Peripheral venous contrast agent confined to right side of heart in normal patient

Injection of bolus

Peripheral venous injection of solution contains acoustically dense microbubbles, affording contrast agent that delineates intracardiac structures and identifies shunts.

Microbubble solution

FIG 9.5 Exercise and contrast echocardiography.

and function. This is especially true and probably most important when dealing with complex shapes such as the right ventricle or aneurysmal left ventricle because quantification by 2D methods, which rely on geometric assumptions about shape, are less accurate. Significant advances in ultrasound, electronic, and computer technology have made real-time–rendered 3D images more practical and potentially valuable in clinical practice. There is evidence to support the use of 3D echocardiography for quantification of left ventricular mass, volume, and ejection fraction, as well as in the measurement of the mitral valve area in patients with mitral stenosis (Fig. 9.7).

Interventional Echocardiography

Over the past decade, percutaneous catheter–based interventions of various structural heart disorders have expanded dramatically. This has led to an emerging new field of interventional echocardiography, especially with the addition of 3D imaging. Interventions involving percutaneous balloon mitral valvuloplasty, and percutaneous repair of the

mitral valve (MitraClip procedure) and the tricuspid valve heavily rely on both 2D and 3D TEE support. TEE is also useful in the cardiac catheterization laboratory to assist with transseptal puncture and for optimal percutaneous placement of closure devices in patients with PFO or ASD and left atrial appendage closure. Transcatheter aortic valve replacements have usually relied on TEE guidance; however, many centers are currently performing at least some cases with conscious sedation and TTE imaging. Although these procedures have expanded into use in the lower risk populations, TEE imaging will continue to play an important role in ensuring optimal outcomes.

LIMITATIONS

Although modern echocardiography imaging systems are sophisticated multimodality devices, echocardiography remains an operator-dependent technique. High-quality echocardiographic imaging requires a solid foundation of training in cardiac anatomy, cardiovascular physiology,

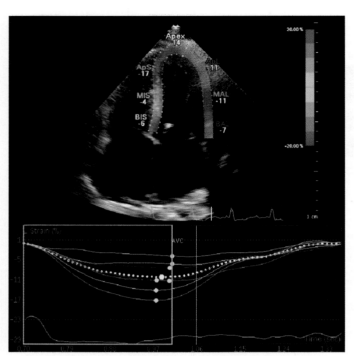

FIG 9.6 Abnormal myocardial strain pattern in a patient with amyloidosis.

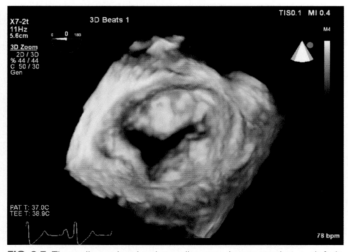

FIG 9.7 Three-dimensional echocardiogram demonstrating a cleft in the posterior leaflet of the mitral valve.

and pathophysiology. A working knowledge of ultrasound physics, as well as considerable technical skill, expertise, and patience of the physician or technician obtaining images, is essential. Even in trained hands, image acquisition is limited by obesity, chronic obstructive pulmonary disease, and patient discomfort; chest wall injuries or recent surgery can make TTE particularly challenging. Suboptimal images may be seen in up to 10% to 15% of all patients undergoing echocardiography. Because of this difficulty, contrast media have been used more widely to enhance endocardial definition.

TEE is limited in many clinical circumstances. Patients must be physically able, well-oriented, and sufficiently cooperative to follow simple commands to successfully swallow the ultrasound probe. Although generally well tolerated, TEE carries risks related to sedation and esophageal intubation; complications include esophageal perforation and aspiration of gastric contents.

FUTURE DIRECTIONS

Evolving technological improvements, increasing availability, and new clinical applications will fuel continued growth in the use of echocardiographic imaging. The ongoing explosion of new echocardiographic modalities will present the echocardiographer with constantly challenging questions regarding appropriate application of these methods to standard examination protocols. As the road to full automation of echocardiographic examinations progresses, excellent knowledge of cardiac anatomy and physiology, as well as good spatial imagination, are still required from the echocardiographer.

ADDITIONAL RESOURCES

Chu E, Kalman JM, Kwasman MA, et al. Intracardiac echocardiography during radiofrequency catheter ablation of cardiac arrhythmias in humans. *J Am Coll Cardiol.* 1994;24:1351–1357.

Prospective cohort study that evaluated the preliminary experience using ICE as an adjunct to fluoroscopy for guiding radiofrequency catheter ablation of right-sided atrial arrhythmias.

Hernández F, García-Tejada J, Velázquez M, et al. Intracardiac echocardiography and percutaneous closure of atrial septal defects in adults. *Rev Esp Cardiol.* 2008;61:465–470.

Retrospective study that reviewed 52 adult patients with ASD who underwent transcatheter closure using an Amplatzer occluder device under ICE monitoring. The authors concluded that ICE can be safely and effectively used in this setting.

Jamal F, Kukulski T, Sutherland GR, et al. Can changes in systolic longitudinal deformation quantify regional myocardial function after an acute infarction? An ultrasonic strain rate and strain study. *J Am Soc Echoardiogr.* 2002;15:723–730.

This longitudinal, case-controlled study of 40 patients was conducted to investigate the additional value of strain rate and strain versus myocardial velocity alone for the identification and quantification of regional asynergy following myocardial infarction. The authors concluded that strain rate and strain provided a better assessment of segmental dysfunction severity than myocardial velocities alone after myocardial infarction.

Lang RM, Mor-Avi V, Sugeng L, et al. Three-dimensional echocardiography. The benefits of the additional dimension. *J Am Coll Cardiol.* 2006;48: 2053–2069.

Well-written review article describing the usefulness of 3D echocardiography in clinical practice and advantages of the technique; the article includes discussion of available literature.

Lester SJ, Tajik AJ, Nishimura RA, et al. Unlocking the mysteries of diastolic function: deciphering the rosetta stone 10 years later. *J Am Coll Cardiol.* 2008;51:679–689.

A thorough and exceptionally well-written update on 2D echocardiographic and Doppler assessment of diastolic function.

Olszewski R, Timperley J, Szmigielski C, et al. The clinical applications of contrast echocardiography. *Eur J Echocardiogr.* 2007;8:S13–S23.

An excellent review of the literature with in-depth discussion of the clinical applications of contrast echocardiography.

Perk G, Kronzon I. Interventional echocardiography in structural heart disease. *Curr Cardiol Rep.* 2013;15:338. doi:10.1007/s11886-012-0338-y.

A review of the applications of interventional echocardiography in structural heart disease.

EVIDENCE

Cheitlin MD, Alpert JS, Armstrong WF, et al. ACC/AHA guidelines for the clinical application of echocardiography. *Circulation.* 1997;95:1686–1744.

Comprehensive document detailing evidence-based guidelines for appropriate application of echocardiography in a wide range of clinical circumstances.

Cheitlin MD, Armstrong WF, Aurigemma GP, et al. ACC/AHA/ASE 2003 guideline update for the clinical application of echocardiography. *Circulation.* 2003;108:1146–1162.

An update of original evidence-based guidelines for the use of echocardiography published in 1997. A relatively brief and concise document, it is best appreciated in the context of the original publication. (Cheitlin MD, Alpert JS, Armstrong WF, et al. Circulation. 1997;95:1686–1744.)

Douglas PS, Khandheria B, Stainback RF, et al. ACCF/ASE/ACEP/ASNC/ SCAI/SCCT/SCMR 2007 appropriateness criteria for transthoracic and transesophageal echocardiography. *J Am Coll Cardiol.* 2007;50:187–204.

Detailed review of the risks and benefits of TTE and/or TEE for several indications and in a wide range of clinical scenarios. Most data are presented in table format, making it a readily accessible and useful reference.

Douglas PS, Khandheria B, Stainback RF, et al. ACCF/ASE/ACEP/AHA/ ASNC/SCAI/SCCT/SCMR 2008 appropriateness criteria for stress echocardiography. *Circulation.* 2008;117:1478–1497.

This expert panel rated indications for stress echocardiography by the appropriateness method, combining expert clinical judgment with the scientific literature to evaluate risk and benefit. It covers most clinical situations faced by practicing physicians. The consensus recommendations are presented in a concise table format.

10

Stress Testing and Nuclear Imaging

Arif Sheikh, Faiq Shaikh

Stress ECG and stress imaging studies are widely used noninvasive procedures that provide important information on cardiac function and the presence of hemodynamically significant coronary artery disease (CAD). The correct use of stress testing is critically important for the cost-effective management of patients with known or suspected CAD. When the most appropriate procedure is performed, it provides important diagnostic and prognostic information that determines the optimal management strategy to be undertaken for that individual. Stress testing is also used in patients with known CAD to determine exercise "prescriptions" before cardiac rehabilitation (Fig. 10.1).

EXERCISE STRESS TESTING

Exercise stress testing (EST) involves subjecting a patient to increasing levels of exercise with continuous ECG monitoring for myocardial ischemia and arrhythmias. Although the sensitivity and specificity of stress ECG for the detection of CAD are low (range: 55%–75%) compared with more advanced testing (including the use of imaging), stress ECG is widely available, relatively inexpensive, and can provide important prognostic information about the patient. Generally, diagnostic treadmill stress testing is done on patients with a low or intermediate pretest likelihood of having CAD. However, EST can also be used in patients with known CAD to evaluate the effectiveness of current therapies, to ascertain overall functional capacity, to determine general prognosis, and/or to provide an exercise prescription. In children with congenital heart disease, EST can be used to quantify functional capacity.

The sensitivity of EST for detecting CAD is proportional to the heart rate (HR) achieved during exercise. Thus, in preparation for the study, patients are usually asked to transiently discontinue medications that affect HR response (e.g., β-blockers or calcium channel blockers). Patients should fast for at least 4 hours before the test. Exercise is done on a treadmill, or alternatively, using a bicycle ergometer. In special circumstances, arm ergometry and isometric hand exercises can be used. There are several different protocols for EST. All of them start exercise at a given rate and incline angle, and then gradually increase one or both parameters until an adequate HR and exercise endurance are achieved. Generally, exercise is continued until the patient reaches a target HR of at least 85% of the maximum predicted HR (MPHR) for the age of the patient (220 beats/min − age in years ± 10 to 12 beats/min). Studies that have correlated ECG changes with CAD generally involve reaching this target HR.

Once a patient reaches the target HR, they should continue to exercise until fatigued or until signs or symptoms develop. If a patient exceeds a double product (HR × systolic blood pressure) of 25,000 or attains an exercise level of at least 5 metabolic equivalents as a secondary target, the test may be considered adequate. Hemodynamic instability, gross ECG changes, or severe patient symptoms are also indications to terminate the procedure. At the end of exercise testing, the patient slowly reduces the intensity of exercise. Vigorous exercise results in increased blood flow and pooling in the extremities, and a "step-down" phase (low-level exercise) allows the patient to re-equilibrate before ceasing exercise. After exercise termination, patients are monitored in a supine position until they are no longer tachycardiac (i.e., HR <100 beats/min) if not back to baseline HR. Importantly, if there were any ECG changes or symptoms experienced by the patient during the study, posttest monitoring should be continued with any necessary treatments until these have been resolved, even if hemodynamics (HR and blood pressure) have returned to acceptable levels. The posttest monitoring serves to reveal any arrhythmias or ST-segment changes that may develop and that may be late signs of ischemic disease (Fig. 10.2).

The ECG must be interpreted with certain caveats. Although the standard 12-lead configuration can be used, in many instances, a modified 12-lead configuration is substituted. This involves placing limb leads more proximally than is done for a standard ECG (e.g., electrodes are placed on the shoulders rather than the arms). This modification results in ST-segment changes being accentuated and more easily detected during stress, but it is also a baseline stress ECG that differs from a supine ECG done with standard lead placement.

The presence of myocardial ischemia during the test is suggested if previously normal ST segments show flattened or downsloping depression >1 mm below the baseline in three consecutive beats. An important issue concerns ST-segment changes that can occur in some individuals simply because of the increased respiratory rate that accompanies exercise. A prestress or poststress ECG performed with hyperventilation should be done to allow comparison of ECG changes that are associated with an increased respiratory rate.

The prognostic information obtained from a treadmill stress test is often useful for deciding on the next diagnostic or therapeutic step for a given patient. Of the several methods used for prognosis after EST, the most widely used is the Duke Treadmill Score. The time of exercise, the presence (or absence) of ST-segment changes during the study, and patient symptoms are used to determine a score that correlates with event-free survival.

Bicycle-based studies use a comparable approach to provide similar information. The patient maintains a steady, pedaling rate over a period of time with regular increases in the intensity required for pedaling. At comparable HRs, a higher level of physiological stress (reflected by metabolic equivalents) is present in individuals walking on a treadmill than individuals pedaling a bicycle. However, the data available for comparing these two forms of exercise are limited. Caution should be used in translating clinical information between forms of exercise.

Contraindications to exercise include unstable coronary syndrome, decompensated heart failure (HF), severe obstructive valvular or hypertrophic cardiomyopathic disease, untreated life-threatening arrhythmias, and advanced atrioventricular block. Under certain circumstances, exercise testing under rigorously controlled conditions is performed

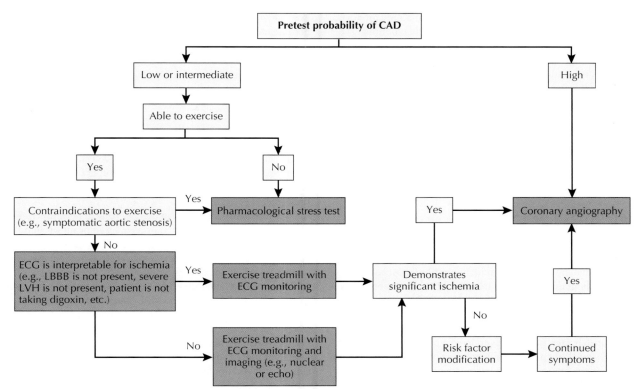

FIG 10.1 Evaluation for Hemodynamically Significant Coronary Artery Disease (CAD) in Clinically Stable Patients. *LBBB*, Left bundle branch block; *LVH*, left ventricular hypertrophy.

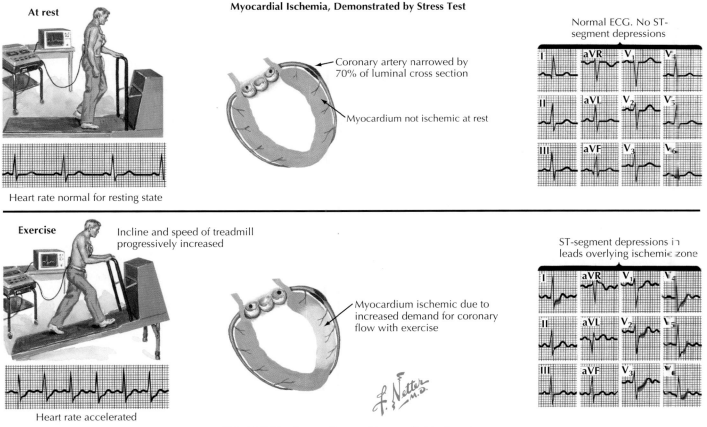

FIG 10.2 Testing to Detect Myocardial Ischemia.

on patients with aortic stenosis to determine their suitability for aortic valve replacement. Severe baseline hypertension (>220/120 mm Hg) or the presence of large arterial aneurysms are also contraindications, as are systemic illnesses such as acute pulmonary embolus and aortic dissection. Exercise studies should be used cautiously in individuals with an implantable cardiac defibrillator (ICD), particularly if their underlying ECG shows a prolonged QRS interval (due to an underlying bundle branch block or paced rhythm), because in this circumstance, the defibrillator may "recognize" the rapid HR induced by exercise as ventricular tachycardia. Arrhythmias such as uncontrolled atrial fibrillation may also make interpretation of exercise stress ECGs difficult or impossible, and patients with these arrhythmias should be considered for a stress imaging study.

CARDIAC STRESS IMAGING

Stress imaging studies combine either EST or an infusion of either dobutamine or a coronary vasodilator with imaging of the heart. Imaging can be accomplished by a variety of modalities; those most commonly used are echocardiography or nuclear imaging. MRI has also been used, and CT is being studied as a modality for stress imaging. Stress imaging is preferred over EST without imaging in several settings: (1) when the ECG is uninterpretable for myocardial ischemia; (2) when a patient is unable to adequately exercise (but can undergo a pharmacological stress imaging study); or (3) when a treadmill stress test is positive for ischemia in a low-risk patient, and correlation by imaging is preferred to cardiac catheterization. Individuals with an abnormal baseline ECG, particularly with ST-segment abnormalities, should be referred for a stress imaging study, because ECG changes in the setting of an abnormal baseline are far less specific for CAD. Patients with significant left ventricular hypertrophy on their baseline ECG or those taking digoxin have similar limitations for interpretation of ischemia with exercise. Stress imaging could be used as a primary modality, rather than ECG-only stress testing, in patients with an intermediate to high pretest likelihood of disease because of its higher sensitivity and specificity. Even with rapid advances in other modalities, stress imaging remains a highly effective and available modality to evaluate ischemia and function at present, and it is likely that this will be the case in coming years.

Myocardial Perfusion Imaging

Myocardial perfusion imaging (MPI) involves injection of a radiopharmaceutical that distributes throughout the myocardium in a manner dependent upon coronary blood flow. Images are obtained of the radiopharmaceutical distribution attained near peak stress and at rest. Changes in the distribution of the radiopharmaceutical can reflect comparable blood flow at rest and during stress, diminished blood flow with stress compared with rest (reflecting stress-induced ischemia), or diminished blood flow both with stress and at rest, which can be correlated with previous myocardial infarction (MI). Left ventricular function and ejection fraction (EF) and left ventricular size at rest and with stress can also be measured with this technique. The sensitivity of stress nuclear imaging for detection of hemodynamically significant CAD is 85% to 90%. The prognostic value of a negative stress nuclear imaging study is also excellent in otherwise low-risk to intermediate-risk patients.

Imaging can be done with SPECT or with PET. These systems offer different spatial resolution and use different tracers; however, the basic approach of stress perfusion and the functional images obtained are essentially the same.

Stress With Myocardial Perfusion Imaging

In stress with MPI, the radiopharmaceutical is injected when the patient is at the maximum level of coronary vasodilation, which occurs at peak exercise or pharmacological stress. Exercise stress is preferred for MPI because of the added prognostic information obtained from the hemodynamic response to exercise and functional tolerance. Exercise improves imaging characteristics of the tracers, leading to fewer artifacts and improved accuracy.

The same previously noted contraindications noted for EST apply to patients undergoing exercise MPI. Many of the limitations inherent in ECG-only exercise testing (e.g., left bundle branch block, pacing, atrial fibrillation, left ventricular hypertrophy, and baseline ST- and T-wave changes) can largely be overcome when using MPI. In general, the sensitivity and specificity of MPI for detection of CAD are better when coupled with exercise than when coupled with pharmacological stress. For this reason, if a patient is able to exercise, exercise MPI is preferred.

When patients are unable to exercise (due to poor functional capacity, orthopedic, or other factors) or have a significant left bundle branch block, MPI can be performed using pharmacological stress. Two general approaches are used in pharmacological stress testing: infusion with a coronary vasodilator or with dobutamine.

Dipyridamole, adenosine, and regadenoson are coronary vasodilators used in pharmacological stress MPI. Dipyridamole causes vasodilation by blocking endogenous adenosine breakdown and raising its levels. Adenosine can also be directly infused and is preferred in many centers over dipyridamole because it results in a more consistent serum adenosine level (and more consistent coronary vasodilatation) than does the infusion of dipyridamole. Adenosine infusion is associated with more symptoms than dipyridamole infusion, but these symptoms are short-lived because of its short half-life. Regadenoson acts more specifically on the coronary adenosine ($A_{2\alpha}$) receptors compared with the nonspecific vasodilation action of pure adenosine. Thus, it should have a lower risk of common side effects (e.g., bronchospasm, atrioventricular nodal blockade, and flushing), although these side effects can still be present.

Coronary vasodilators work by increasing blood flow except in areas where hemodynamically significant stenoses are present, precluding vasodilator-induced increased flow. A relative decrease in the intensity of the MPI signal indicates an inability to increase flow to that area of the myocardium, and therefore, the presence of flow-limiting CAD in the coronary artery supplying that area can be deduced.

The use of vasodilators is contraindicated in patients with active bronchospastic disease, and in those with advanced heart block or sick sinus syndrome without a pacemaker. In addition, patients taking aminophylline or theophylline must discontinue the use of these drugs before vasodilator pharmacological stress testing, because these drugs counteract the effects of these vasodilators. Similarly, caffeine intake within the previous 12 hours also blocks the effects of vasodilators. Regadenoson is associated with a lower seizure threshold and is often avoided in patients with a history of seizures. Some also avoid its use in end-stage renal disease. If a patient receiving vasodilators does have either bronchospasm or another side effect with drug infusion, these side effects can be mitigated by infusion of aminophylline or theophylline. It is rare that reversal of the effects of adenosine is required because of its short half-life.

If patients are able to perform submaximal exercise, a combination of a vasodilator with exercise can be performed. This protocol has the advantages of decreasing side effects and improving image quality by decreasing splanchnic tracer accumulation. Vasodilator-exercise protocols allow limited exercising of patients who are not able to attain target HRs. However, patients with contraindications to either exercise or vasodilators (see the preceding text) should not be considered for a combined stress study. In addition, vasodilator EST should not be performed in patients with a history of cerebrovascular and/or carotid disease, especially if walking is the exercise mode. Rapid loss of consciousness and collapse on the treadmill have been reported, due to cerebrovascular perfusion steal, which results from pharmacological vasodilation coupled with exercise (Fig. 10.3).

If patients are unable to exercise and also have contraindications to vasodilator stress, dobutamine pharmacological stress can be performed. Dobutamine is more often used for stress echocardiography than for stress MPI, and is similar to exercise in that it increases HR and myocardial contraction. It is administered as an incrementally increasing infusion rate until either the MPHR of the patient or the infusion rate is reached. Atropine can be used for HR augmentation if the target HR is still not reached with maximal dobutamine doses. Stress targets are similar to those for exercise, but it is important to note that because systolic blood pressure can remain constant or fall with dobutamine, whereas it rises with exercise, the double product (and thus, level of stress) associated with a given HR is less during dobutamine testing than with exercise testing. Some clinical variables, such as fatigue, which is useful in EST, are generally not useful with dobutamine administration.

The major contraindications to dobutamine and/or atropine stress MPI are the same as for EST, but also include the presence of narrow-angle glaucoma, and a history of prostatic enlargement and urinary obstruction. In addition, a relative contraindication to dobutamine and/or atropine stress MPI is a propensity for inducible arrhythmias.

Finally, less conventional stress methods such as cold pressor testing and mental stress are described in the literature. Mental stress testing is believed to induce a sympathoadrenal response that has similar effects on the coronary blood flow as the previously described methods, which induces the steal phenomenon and exposes perfusion defects. However, the exact mechanism is unknown. The mental stress test coupled with echocardiography may improve sensitivity of the test but not the specificity. Low sensitivity of the test can be due to inability to identify the stressors that may induce ischemia in a patient. Cold pressor testing is more often used when coronary vasospastic syndromes are suspected, and reduce blood flow to areas where such vasomotor dysfunction exists, thereby inducing ischemia.

An imaging protocol for acute chest pain involves administration of a radiopharmaceutical while the patient is having a chest pain syndrome. In a low-risk to intermediate-risk patient, a normal scan has a high negative predictive value for the absence of an acute coronary syndrome. This protocol has been used in emergency room settings in low-risk to intermediate-risk patients with otherwise undifferentiated chest pain and allows for safe discharge with outpatient follow-up.

Radiotracers

Thallium-201 (^{201}Tl) thallous chloride, a radioactive analogue of potassium, was the most commonly used tracer for myocardial perfusion for several decades. Although its use has declined with the advent of technetium-99m (^{99m}Tc)–based agents, it is still sometimes used as part of dual-isotope protocols and in viability imaging. Its relatively low energy results in images that lack resolution, although it has a higher myocardial extraction fraction compared with ^{99m}Tc-based agents. The two most commonly used ^{99m}Tc-based MPI agents are ^{99m}Tc-sestamibi (MIBI) and ^{99m}Tc-tetrofosmin. Images obtained with the two agents are comparable and have a higher resolution than images obtained using ^{201}Tl for cardiac imaging. MIBI demonstrates a slightly higher extraction fraction than tetrofosmin, although it results in a slightly higher radiation dose to the patient compared with tetrofosmin. A previously used ^{99m}Tc-based agent, teboroxime, demonstrated a substantially higher extraction fraction than the aforementioned agents, but its rapid washout from the myocardium limited its clinical usefulness. Teboroxime is no longer marketed in the United States.

The ^{99m}Tc-agents are the most commonly used SPECT radiopharmaceuticals. Several imaging protocols using these agents have been

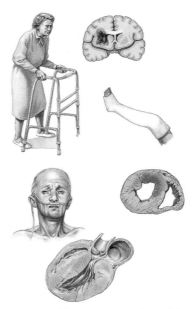

Patients unable to or contraindicated for exercise

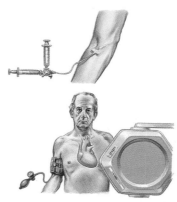

Tracer injection at peak vasodilation, then imaging after completion

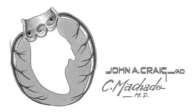

Myocardial perfusion at rest and peak vasodilation

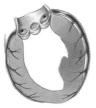

Vasodilator test: nonstress test

FIG 10.3 Pharmacological Stress Nuclear Testing.

developed. A commonly used protocol is the 1-day rest-stress, wherein a scan is performed following a low dosage tracer administration to the patient at rest. The second step in this protocol is to stress the patient (exercise or pharmacological stress), administering the resting dosage of the radiotracer at peak stress approximately three times, and then perform imaging again.

A variation of this protocol used in some nuclear laboratories for low-risk patients is the stress-rest study. In this case, stress images are obtained first. Resting images can be omitted if the stress images are completely normal, but can be performed on the same or subsequent day if needed. In the former, a lower dosage stress image is obtained followed by a higher dosage rest image. The disadvantage of this approach is that stress images are obtained at lower doses of radiotracer and thus may be of lower quality. A 2-day protocol administration of relatively high dosages of radiopharmaceutical is used for both rest and stress. This protocol allows for better image quality, especially in obese patients in whom high-quality images cannot otherwise be attained. The limitations of this study protocol are the higher radiation doses and the inconvenience of having the patient return on a subsequent day.

A dual-isotope protocol uses ^{201}Tl for the resting images followed by poststress images obtained with a ^{99m}Tc-based tracer. However, differences in spatial resolution between ^{201}Tl and ^{99m}Tc can sometimes complicate the interpretation of subtle findings. Imaging can also be performed using ^{201}Tl only. Because of the limitations of ^{201}Tl, the only feasible approach is to perform a stress-rest study. The entire study can be performed with a single injection of tracer, and one can obtain additional physiological and prognostic information (e.g., lung uptake) and an assessment of myocardial viability. However, these studies are not done frequently in most laboratories because they are associated with significantly higher radiation doses than those only using ^{99m}Tc-agents, are more time-consuming, and provide lower resolution images.

PET radiopharmaceuticals use positron-emitting radionuclides to create images. Rubidium-82 (^{82}Rb) chloride is a positron-emitting potassium analogue. It has the lowest extraction fraction of the clinically available PET radiopharmaceuticals ($\sim$60%). This extraction fraction is still higher than that of either sestamibi or tetrofosmin. The half-life of ^{82}Rb is short ($\sim$75 seconds). There are benefits and limitations for the use of ^{82}Rb because of its short half-life. The short half-life essentially precludes use of ^{82}Rb for exercise stress imaging. However, it facilitates obtaining images when the patient is truly at the peak of performance induced by pharmacological stress. For this reason, ^{82}Rb images can be used to accurately assess cardiac reserve, which are defined as the difference between left ventricular EF at rest and at peak stress. The short half-life of ^{82}Rb also facilitates obtaining pharmacological stress and resting images in a relatively short period of time. ^{82}Rb has a lower intrinsic spatial resolution than the other PET agents but is still far better than the SPECT tracers. ^{82}Rb is produced by a generator system, but this is quite expensive; for this reason, it is only available at some centers.

Nitrogen-13 (^{13}N) ammonia has a high extraction fraction ($\sim$83%), higher imaging resolution than ^{82}Rb, and a 10-minute half-life. It can be used for exercise nuclear imaging. Oxygen-15 ($[^{15}O]H_2O$) water is short-lived (half-life of 2 minutes) and possesses a high extraction fraction of approximately 95%. However, its freely diffusible nature means that ^{15}O is distributed into tissues adjacent to the myocardium, including the lungs and cardiac blood pool. For this reason, imaging is complicated, requiring sophisticated background subtraction techniques. Although both ^{13}N and ^{15}O have higher intrinsic spatial resolution than ^{82}Rb, they require generation in a cyclotron. Their short half-lives mean that these isotopes can only be used in facilities with an on-site cyclotron. For most institutions that perform PET myocardial imaging studies, ^{82}Rb is preferred for this logistic reason. Newer fluorine-18 (^{18}F)–labeled

perfusion tracers that would allow exercise imaging and do not require an on-site cyclotron are being developed and studied. The ^{18}F tracers have a high extraction fraction and the highest imaging resolution, making them attractive for the assessment of CAD.

PET tracers use protocols based on SPECT imaging. Because of its exceedingly short half-life, ^{82}Rb protocols can be either rest-stress (more common) or stress-rest. An entire ^{82}Rb study can be completed within 30 minutes. An advantage of PET tracers is that despite higher γ-emission energies, their radiation doses are comparably lower while delivering better images than the SPECT tracers.

There is increasing interest in stress first protocols in both SPECT and PET modalities. This allows significant radiation and costs reduction, as well as shortens the overall procedure time for the patient. The approach is more feasible with newer technologies, such as iterative image processing, attenuation correction, and cardiac-specific cameras because they can help eliminate many imaging artifacts. These technologies are not specifically reimbursed, but may significantly increase the cost of the procedure to the laboratory, which is a barrier to wider adoption. Nevertheless, the imaging community has dedicated itself to overall radiation dose reduction in an era of rising concerns about radiation exposures from diagnostic testing and healthcare cost containment.

With the variety of techniques available, it is important to choose the optimal imaging modality (SPECT vs. SPECT-CT vs. PET), tracer, stress modality, and imaging protocol, tailoring each for the specific patient situation to maximize the information obtained. For example, the overall prognosis of a normal stress MPI study is better in patients who exercised than in those who were evaluated with a vasodilator study. Careful attention should be paid to understanding the meaning of the results in the context of the history of the patient and how the study was performed. The study design also has to be weighed against the technological abilities of the stress laboratory, throughput, procedure costs, and the radiation exposure of the patient.

IMAGE INTERPRETATION

SPECT nuclear images are analyzed in three ways. The "raw" rotating image interpretation is a critical step that allows the reader to assess whether patient motion, attenuation artifacts (breast overlap, diaphragmatic interference, or other factors) must be considered in interpretation of the study. Occasionally, the presence of significant extracardiac findings such as breast or lung masses, thyroid or parathyroid nodules, and lymphadenopathy is seen on these raw images. The second step is to examine reconstructed images that are presented as "slices" of the myocardium. Using this set of images, it is possible to visualize myocardial perfusion in multiple axes to assess flow-limiting CAD (Fig. 10.4 and Table 10.1). The amount of ischemic or infarct burden can be quantified. By dividing the ventricle into segments (usually 17 or 20) and

TABLE 10.1	**Myocardial Perfusion Patterns**
Scan Finding	**Interpretation**
No perfusion defect on either stress or rest study	Normal
Perfusion defect at stress that is normal at rest	Ischemia
Perfusion defect both at stress and rest	Myocardial scar
Perfusion defect at rest but normal at stress	Probable artifact, consider subendocardial infarction (reverse redistribution)

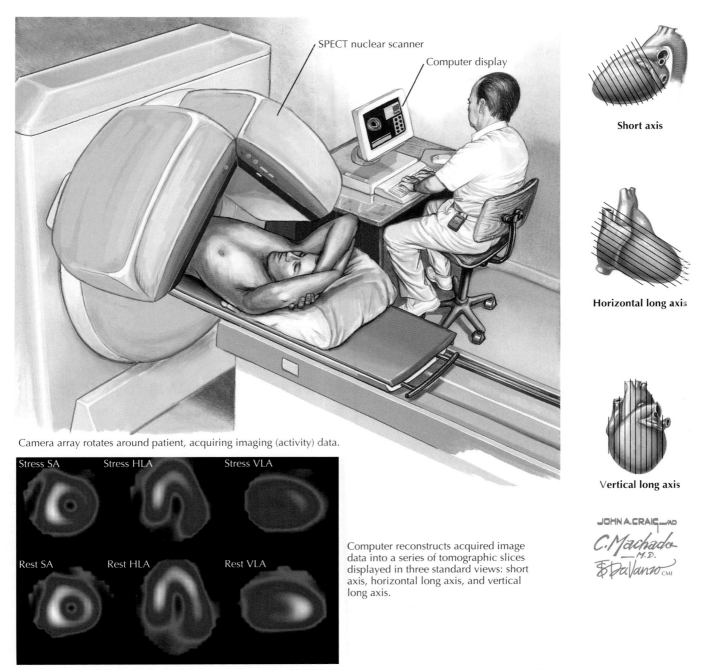

SPECT nuclear scanner

Computer display

Camera array rotates around patient, acquiring imaging (activity) data.

Short axis

Horizontal long axis

Vertical long axis

Stress SA   Stress HLA   Stress VLA

Rest SA   Rest HLA   Rest VLA

Computer reconstructs acquired image data into a series of tomographic slices displayed in three standard views: short axis, horizontal long axis, and vertical long axis.

JOHN A. CRAIG—AD
C. Machado
—M.D.
B. Pallanzo CMI

FIG 10.4 Stress Nuclear Imaging by SPECT. Lateral wall shows normal perfusion at rest, but decreased at stress consistent with ischemia. *HLA,* Horizontal long axis; *SA,* short axis; *VLA,* vertical long axis.

then deriving scores based on the extent and severity of segments affected by pathology, a quantitative assessment can be made that strongly correlates with patient outcomes. The summation of these data, the "sum score," can be compared in the rest and stress studies. Third, gated images can also be obtained and reviewed in a looped-cine method. These images allow determination of wall motion abnormalities, ventricular volumes, and left ventricular EFs. Analysis of wall motion also provides an independent means to assess apparent perfusion defects and confirm infarction, ischemia, or the presence of an artifactual perfusion abnormality.

Comparison of images obtained at stress with images obtained at rest makes it possible to determine if there is a relative decrease in flow

with stress. This reversible myocardial perfusion defect correlates with viable tissue in the distribution of a coronary artery with a significant stenosis and represents an ischemic territory. If a portion of the myocardium has limited perfusion at stress and at rest, this indicates that the myocardium with the nonreversible defect may represent an infarcted area.

Due to the higher isotope energies involved with PET imaging, its inherent attenuation correction, and the superior tracer characteristics of PET radiopharmaceuticals compared with the current ^{99m}Tc-based SPECT agents, PET images are of far superior quality and usefulness in the diagnosis of CAD in both obese and general patients. The approach to interpretation of PET imaging is similar to that described previously for SPECT imaging. Reconstructed perfusion and gated images are approached the same way, but no raw images are displayed because of the manner in which PET images are acquired. An important step to consider in PET is the alignment of the emission and transmission (the latter being CT in PET-CT or MR in PET-MR units) scans. By default, PET has an attenuation correction built in for the reconstruction of its final images. A misalignment between the two portions of the scan can result in serious artifacts, which can be misread if not recognized and/ or corrected. Although this can be frequently corrected by manual realignment of the images, occasionally, the relevant scan has to be repeated to obtain the correct data.

PET imaging also makes absolute quantification of myocardial blood flow and coronary flow reserve possible, which is useful for detection of endothelial dysfunction, and assessment of multivessel ischemia that might otherwise appear as normal stress imaging if ischemia is global and balanced.

ADVANCES AND INTEGRATION OF CARDIAC IMAGING

Numerous important innovations in cardiac nuclear imaging have improved the diagnostic performance of the field. More sophisticated processing using iterative reconstructive techniques has allowed for imaging and technological developments in the field of nuclear imaging, specifically for cardiac imaging. Some solutions involve using nuclear SPECT cameras and developing "cardiocentric" collimators. Other solutions have developed SPECT cameras specifically for cardiac imaging, where the patient sits upright, thus improving patient comfort. Other cardiac-specific cameras use multi-pinhole designs and are without moving parts. Newer cameras use cadmium zinc telluride high-efficiency, solid-state detectors, but these significantly increase the costs of these systems.

It is useful to consider nuclear imaging techniques (SPECT and PET) with newer cardiac imaging technologies such as cardiac MRI (CMRI) and cardiac CT angiography (CTA), because their use has increased dramatically within the last few years; there are advantages and disadvantages for each. CMRI is capable of generating exquisite images of cardiac structures, with a resolution far superior to nuclear techniques and without the need for ionizing radiation. This technology is also useful for viability assessment and nonischemic cardiomyopathies. The current major limitation to the use of CMRI in stress testing is its limited availability.

Cardiac CTA provides high-resolution images of coronary and other cardiac anatomy and pathology that are not possible with current nuclear techniques, with radiation doses somewhat comparable to SPECT imaging but higher than those of PET. Although its negative predictive value for the detection of CAD is excellent, its positive predictive value in determining disease severity is considerably lower. It is anticipated that as technology advances, cardiac CTA characterization of coronary anatomy will improve.

It is also possible that CT technology will be able to provide a combined scan that includes stress testing, viability assessment, and coronary anatomy, all in a reasonable time frame and with an acceptable radiation dose. However, there are limitations of these newer technologies. For patients with renal insufficiency who have a higher risk of allergic or nephropathic complications, nuclear tracers are preferred over studies that require intravenous contrast (either CT or MRI). MRI studies are generally contraindicated in patients with implanted cardiac rhythm devices (pacemakers and ICDs; coronary stents are not a contraindication for MRI). At present, CMRI and cardiac CTA are less widely available than nuclear studies.

Ultimately, the combination of imaging modalities may provide the greatest noninvasive information for cardiac patients. Combined modality imaging has proven to be useful for detection and prognostication in cancer patients. The idea of combining high-resolution images with physiological and/or functional measures is equally attractive for the assessment of CAD. The integration of CT into both SPECT and PET imaging devices can be useful for anatomic localization of perfusion defects and for attenuation correction, particularly in obese patients, and is important for PET perfusion studies.

Furthermore, the perfusion and/or metabolic information provided by SPECT or PET can be obtained sequentially, and then fused with structural information provided by CTA. This approach offers the potential advantage of evaluating both the extent and severity of atherosclerotic vascular disease and its effect on myocardial perfusion, and can also be of great use in distinguishing between flow-limiting coronary artery stenosis and microvascular disease.

Similarly, PET and MRI have been combined as a PET-MR device that also overcomes the major limitations of poor anatomic resolution in MPI, while overcoming the limited spatial coverage in stress MRI. Development of new tracers could expand the clinical potential of PET-MR imaging, which would allow highly specific assessment of vascular atherosclerosis, nonischemic cardiomyopathies, and HF. All these advancements have allowed the reduction of imaging time and tracer dosages, which leads to a decrease in overall patient radiation exposures.

OTHER USES OF CARDIAC NUCLEAR MEDICINE

Equilibrium Radionuclide Ventriculography (Multiple-Gated Acquisition Scan)

Multiple-gated acquisition (MUGA) scanning is an approach used to quantify both left and right ventricular function, based on images generated after the injection of ^{99m}Tc-labeled erythrocytes. The labeling procedure can be performed in vitro using a commercially available kit (UltraTag; Mallinckrodt, St. Paul, Minnesota), in vivo, or semi–in vitro. The in vitro method provides the highest labeling efficiency and best images, but it is the most laborious, time-consuming, and expensive technique. Once the circulating blood pool has been appropriately labeled, determination of wall motion abnormalities, left ventricular volumes, and EFs can be made. These measures are accurate, repeatable, and reproducible, and are often used for serial follow-up of EFs in patients who receive cardiotoxic drugs, particularly chemotherapeutic agents. In some cases, MUGA is used for the serial follow-up of HF patients.

An advantage of MUGA is the ability to do first-pass imaging, which allows evaluation of the right ventricle, as well as quantitative shunt analysis. Although the latter procedure is now predominantly done via echocardiography, the former is still sometimes used in select patient populations, such as congenital heart disease in the pediatric population, and in some cases, combined with standard myocardial perfusion scans as an approach to evaluating right ventricular function.

Stress MUGA scanning can be performed either with dobutamine or with an exercise ergometer bicycle that is attached to a seat or the bed on which the patient lies. It offers the ability to provide real-time EF imaging, as well as imaging of any wall motion abnormalities that develop during the study (Fig. 10.5). Like echocardiography, ischemic changes can be detected by evaluating wall motion changes from rest to stress. Newer approaches in MUGA include performing SPECT, which enables a more accurate separation of the ventricles from each of the other chambers (Fig. 10.5). Although in theory this should yield better ventricular volumes and EFs than planar estimates, it has not been validated like the planar techniques. For this reason and the emergence

Exercise ergometry

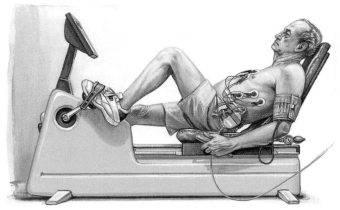

RBC tracer radiolabeling and injection

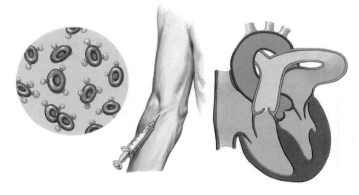

First-pass evaluation

JOHN A. CRAIG—MD
C. Machado—M.D.

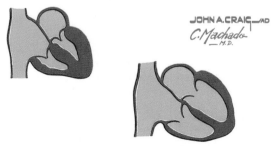

FIG 10.5 Multiple-Gated Acquisition (MUGA) and Stress-MUGA Scanning. *RBC,* Red blood cell.

of competing technologies such as echocardiography and MRI, this modality is rarely used.

Viability

Because more patients survive myocardial infarctions (MIs) as a result of advances in cardiology, detection of myocardial viability has become increasingly important. Identifying a hibernating myocardium that is still viable but chronically hypoperfused and ischemic is believed to be important for decision making with respect to revascularization. However, because no survival benefit has been shown with surgical intervention on areas identified as viable with imaging, this is less frequently done. Nevertheless, viability imaging is still occasionally done to answer specific questions and to manage difficult scenarios, in part because the advances

in viability assessment available since the original studies are believed to be far superior and of greater clinical benefit.

Because ^{201}Tl is a potassium analogue, its exchange across a membrane is a hallmark of a viable myocyte. Viability protocols make use of the ability of ^{201}Tl to undergo redistribution and involve imaging at baseline, following redistribution, and often following repeat injection of an extra dosage. Viable myocytes will take up ^{201}Tl for as long as 24 hours after injection. A newer approach has been to use administration of nitrates in conjunction with either ^{99m}Tc agents or ^{201}Tl. In theory, this approach causes vasodilation in areas that are otherwise hypoperfused at baseline, causing increased flow to those regions, and resulting in improved tracer uptake. The specificity of this procedure can be improved by obtaining gated images with graded dobutamine infusion during imaging.

Unlike ^{201}Tl, which is used as a perfusion marker for SPECT, ^{18}F, 2-deoxyglucose (FDG) is a marker of myocardial glucose metabolism that is imaged with PET. Myocardial uptake of FDG is facilitated by previous administration of glucose, often coupled with intravenous insulin administration to drive glucose use by viable cardiomyocytes. In conjunction with perfusion imaging, FDG imaging can provide useful information for the assessment of myocardial viability, and is generally favored more than SPECT techniques. In many cases, CMRI is preferred because of its better resolution and similar accuracy as PET, and because it also provides anatomic details that could be helpful in surgical planning. Nevertheless, PET can be used when MRI may be contraindicated due to the presence of metal and cardiac devices, which are frequent in this population of patients. An ideal approach would be to use PET-MR, which could provide the best viability assessment in a single imaging session. This is under further study.

FUTURE DIRECTIONS IN CLINICAL CARDIAC MOLECULAR IMAGING

Ventricular Dyssynchrony Assessment

Biventricular pacing has been shown to reduce symptoms in some patients with advanced HF, presumably by improving dyssynchronous left ventricular contraction. However, not all patients improve. It has been hypothesized that the patients who obtain maximal benefit are those who have the greatest restoration of synchronous contraction of the left ventricle. This has stimulated research focused on using nuclear imaging (SPECT-MPI or other modalities) to assess the effect of placing pacemaker leads in specific locations in the right and left ventricles. Comparison of synchrony at baseline and with pacing could facilitate optimization of lead placement and outcomes from biventricular pacing in this setting.

Ischemic Memory

Fatty acid (FA) imaging has been proposed as a sensitive and specific method to determine whether a patient presenting with a recent history of ischemic symptoms did indeed have an ischemic event. Although cardiac biomarkers such as creatinine kinase and cardiac troponins are sensitive indicators of myocardial necrosis, there is no current test to confirm if a recent event represented ischemia at a level insufficient to result in measurable levels of these cardiac biomarkers.

Under fasting, ischemic, or hypoxic conditions, FA metabolism is suppressed and glucose oxidation becomes increasingly important for myocardial energy production. This finding has led to the notion that alterations in FA metabolism could function as a sensitive marker for myocardial ischemia. Radiopharmaceuticals such as iodine-123 15-(p-iodo-phenyl)-3-R,S-methylpentadecanoic acid—an FA analogue—are being studied as a SPECT imaging agent. Because metabolic abnormalities usually persist long after the ischemic event has resolved, this type of radiotracer could be used to identify at-risk areas of myocardium long after the symptoms of angina have abated in patients, and flow has been restored, without having to repeat a stress test.

FDG with PET is another agent potentially capable of detecting recent ischemia, but may be more limited by practical limitations compared with FA imaging.

Cardiac Neurotransmission Imaging

Radioiodine-labeled ^{123}I-metaiodobenzylguanidine (mIBG) has been studied as a SPECT imaging agent based on the notion that cardiac receptors for neurotransmitters may be altered in certain disease states. Alterations in mIBG uptake may identify myocardium that is mechanically functional but highly sensitive to catecholamine stimulation and arrhythmogenic on that basis. mIBG has been studied in patients with idiopathic ventricular tachycardia and/or fibrillation, arrhythmogenic right ventricular dysplasia, and cardiac dysautonomias, including diabetic neuropathy and drug-induced cardiotoxicity. In conjunction with EF, brain natriuretic peptide, or some other variables, mIBG scanning has been reported to accurately predict patients who will benefit from ICD placement. Because of our current inability to distinguish between patients with low EFs who require defibrillation for ventricular tachycardia and/or fibrillation within 5 years of ICD placement and those who will not, plus the high cost of ICD implantation, more precision in determining patients at high risk and low risk, beyond assessment of left ventricular function, is an attractive concept.

Imaging with mIBG is an independent prognostic predictor of overall survival in patients with HF. When combined with other clinical variables, this could prove to be a strong modality in affecting management of patients with HF, in whom studies are ongoing.

Sarcoidosis and Other Inflammatory Pathology

Cardiac sarcoid causes focal granulomatous inflammation at various locations in the myocardium, which can result in electrical or functional cardiac disturbances. In patients with cardiac sarcoid, ^{201}Tl imaging shows patchy defects that presumably correspond to areas of scarring and/or inflammation. Because of the low resolution of ^{201}Tl images, small defects can be missed. Other SPECT tracers used include ^{67}Ga-citrate or ^{111}In-octreotide, which can detect areas of active inflammation in conjunction with a perfusion tracer. More recent uses of fasting FDG-PET have also been successful in detecting inflammatory lesions that have increased tracer uptake, and differentiating them from areas of scarring without uptake.

There is evidence to show that FDG-PET can better localize inflammatory etiologies such as endocarditis and myocarditis, which are both difficult diseases to diagnose. Additional studies have shown the ability to risk stratify aortic aneurysms; those that exhibit increased tracer localization are associated with a worse prognosis, and these patients likely need more immediate intervention.

Although clinical outcomes associated with MRI evaluations are very good, nuclear imaging offers the possibility of detecting lesions with active inflammation and those that respond to therapy. More recently, the introduction of the octreotide analogue PET radiotracers ^{68}Ga-DOTATATE, ^{68}Ga-DOTATOC, and ^{68}Ga-DOTANOC, offers the chance to develop this area even further, with the consideration of again combining the respective strengths with PET-MR imaging.

Cardiac Amyloidosis

The SPECT radioactive isotopes predominantly involved in cardiac amyloid include ^{99m}Tc–3-diphosphono-1, 2-propanodicarboxylic acid (^{99m}Tc-DPD) and ^{99m}Tc-pyrophosphate (^{99m}Tc-PYP), which can detect areas of calcification deposits, and ^{123}I-mIBG, which may detect cardiac denervation and autonomic dysfunction in cardiac amyloid. An important aspect is to be able to identify the main types of amyloid without cardiac biopsy: light chain (AL) and transthyretin (ATTR). Both ^{99m}Tc-labeled agents have been shown to discriminate well between the two forms, and can be used in lieu of an endocardial biopsy. This is important because correct identification of the type of disease leads to important differences in prognosis, and thus subsequent management of the disease. However, there is a need to identify the role of these tracers in tracking progression of disease and to monitor treatment response.

There are PET agents that are used for the detection of β-amyloid neural plaques for the assessment of Alzheimer disease. One of the agents, ^{18}F-florbetapir, has been studied in cardiac amyloidosis, and holds some promise in detecting the disease and potentially differentiating between the AL and ATTR variants. Further usefulness of this agent in these diseases is ongoing.

APPROPRIATE USE CRITERIA

The advances, developments, and improvements in cardiac nuclear imaging come with significant price tags that have a major impact on healthcare costs, as well as raising other issues, such as radiation exposure to the patient and other unwanted secondary drawbacks. To curb the previous practice of unnecessary testing, several medical boards have initiated campaigns and guidelines (such as Image Wisely) to aid clinicians in making evidence-based decisions. Appropriate use criteria in nuclear cardiology have been developed to risk stratify patients, with subsequent recommendations as to what tests should be considered. Hence, several previous practices, such as routine stress test imaging of patients in cardiac rehabilitation, are now discouraged. Other areas, such as HF, will need to be assessed as to whether any of the newer tools like mIBG imaging, assessment of sarcoid and amyloid, or even use of PET-MR, are cost-effective uses. As always, advanced imaging should be considered against the costs and benefits to the patient, and their treatment options and clinical prognosis.

ADDITIONAL RESOURCES

Hendel RC, Berman DS, Di Carli MF, et al. ACCF/ASNC/ACR/AHA/ASE/ SCCT/SCMR/SNM 2009 appropriate use criteria for cardiac radionuclide imaging: a report of the American College of Cardiology Foundation Appropriate Use Criteria Task Force, the American Society of Nuclear Cardiology, the American College of Radiology, the American Heart Association, the American Society of Echocardiography, the Society of Cardiovascular Computed Tomography, the Society for Cardiovascular Magnetic Resonance, and the Society of Nuclear Medicine. *Circulation.* 2009;119(22):e561–e587.
This article presents appropriateness criteria for MPI use.
Henzlova MJ, Duvall WL, Einstein AJ, et al. ASNC imaging guidelines for SPECT nuclear cardiology procedures: stress, protocols, and tracers. *J Nucl Cardiol.* 2016;23:606.
This article provides the official ASNC guidelines, from the technical aspects to the procedural methodologies.
Mann DL, Zipes DP, Libby P, et al. *Braunwald's Heart Disease: A Textbook of Cardiovascular Medicine.* 10th ed. Philadelphia: Elsevier; 2015.
This book provides a basic overview of stress testing and cardiac nuclear medicine.
Zaret B, Beller G. *Clinical Nuclear Cardiology: State of the Art and Future Directions.* 4th ed. Philadelphia: Elsevier; 2010.
In-depth overview of cardiac nuclear medicine, including protocols, indications, and future directions.
Ziessman HA, O'Malley JP, Thrall JH. *The Requisites: Nuclear Medicine.* Philadelphia: Elsevier; 2014. http://www.snmmi.org/ClinicalPractice/ content.aspx?ItemNumber=6414&navItemNumber=10790.
Overview of nuclear medicine techniques, including cardiac nuclear medicine.

EVIDENCE

Bateman TM, Heller GV, McGhie AI, et al. Diagnostic accuracy of rest/stress ECG-gated Rb-82 myocardial perfusion PET: comparison with ECG-gated Tc-99m sestamibi SPECT. *J Nucl Cardiol.* 2006;13(1):24–33.
This article discusses the diagnostic superiority of PET versus SPECT MPI.
Chang SM, Nabi F, Xu J, et al. Normal stress-only versus standard stress/rest myocardial perfusion imaging similar patient mortality with reduced radiation exposure. *J Am Coll Cardiol.* 2010;55:221–230.
This article discusses the development and advantages of stress-only imaging.

Jacobson AF, Senior R, Cerqueira MD, et al. Myocardial iodine-123 meta-iodobenzylguanidine imaging and cardiac events in heart failure. Results of the prospective ADMIRE-HF (AdreView Myocardial Imaging for Risk Evaluation in Heart Failure) study. *J Am Coll Cardiol.* 2010;55(20):2212–2221.
This trial shows the prognostic significance of mIBG imaging in chronic HF.
Nichols K, Saouaf R, Ababneh AA, et al. Validation of SPECT equilibrium radionuclide angiographic right ventricular parameters by cardiac magnetic resonance imaging. *J Nucl Cardiol.* 2002;9(2):153–160.
This paper discusses the development and validation of SPECT-MUGA.

11

Cardiac Computed Tomography and Magnetic Resonance Imaging

Andrew O. Zurick III, J. Larry Klein

The past decade has seen rapid development in cardiovascular imaging technologies coupled with novel clinical applications. Noninvasive cardiac imaging technologies currently allow for assessment of cardiac morphology, function, perfusion, and metabolism. Both cardiac computed tomography (CCT) and cardiac magnetic resonance (CMR) imaging have interesting and unique advantages compared with alternate imaging modalities. Understanding the applications and limitations of these modalities will permit their optimal and efficient use in the future.

CARDIAC COMPUTED TOMOGRAPHY

For decades, investigators sought to develop new technologies that would allow rapid noninvasive imaging of the heart. One such technology that has evolved rapidly in the past several decades has been CCT. CCT now permits visualization of the coronary arteries and lumen, as well as providing assessment of cardiac function, valvular structures, prosthetic materials, the pericardium, left atrial anatomy, congenital heart disease, pulmonary arterial and venous anatomies, and diseases of the aorta.

Technology of Cardiac Computed Tomography

Imaging the heart and coronary arteries with CT is an extremely challenging undertaking for several reasons, and requires more sophisticated hardware and software analysis tools than are required for imaging other body regions. Major difficulties arise because coronary arteries are relatively small moving structures with branches of interest in the range of 2 to 4 mm in diameter. The coronary arteries show rapid cyclic motion throughout the cardiac cycle—essentially moving in three dimensions with each heartbeat. Furthermore, when the subject breathes, the heart and vessels move within the chest due to diaphragmatic motion.

Several major advances in recent years have dramatically improved the resolution of CCT images. Improvement in scanner technology in the past 5 years includes increased Z-axis coverage, now up to 16 cm with some vendors, which means that the entire heart can be imaged in a single gantry rotation. In addition, gantry rotation speeds have also continued to improve; they currently approach 0.2 seconds per 360-degree rotation, which results in improved temporal resolution. ECG gating has also improved. These improvements have significantly decreased overall patient radiation exposure, which is now substantially less than traditional SPECT and is often less than 2 mSv. As the United States continues to deal with the obesity epidemic, vendors have started manufacturing CT scanners with increasingly larger bore diameters and table weight limits to better accommodate these patients.

Over its relatively short history, several different CT technologies have been used for cardiac imaging. Electron beam CT (EBCT), which was initially introduced in the mid-1970s, uses an electron source reflected onto a stationary tungsten target to generate x-rays, which allows for rapid scan times. EBCT is well suited for cardiac imaging because of its high temporal resolution (50–100 ms), with an estimated slice thickness of 1.5 to 3 mm and the ability to scan the heart in a single breath hold. The primary use of this technique was for coronary arterial vessel wall calcium volume and density, which generated a patient-specific score. Coronary calcium scores are independent of other traditional cardiac risk factors in the prediction of cardiac events, and as such, can be considered an excellent biomarker for the presence of coronary artery disease (CAD) and the risk of future cardiac events.

EBCT has since been largely supplanted by multidetector CT (MDCT) technology, which involves a mechanically rotated x-ray source within a cylindrical gantry with a collimated detector located 180 degrees opposite that permits the simultaneous acquisition of more data ("slices"). Collimator rows that measure 0.625 mm provide for markedly increased spatial resolution and for complete acquisition of data during one breath hold. However, what MDCT offers is improved spatial resolution to make coronary CT angiography (CTA) feasible.

Coronary CTA was initially performed using MDCT machines capable of obtaining only four to eight slices per scan. As technology has advanced, 256-slice (and higher) scanners are now available that allow acquisition of higher resolution images without the requirement for long breath holds or extremely slow heart rates. It is currently recommended that CTA be performed using a minimum 64-slice scanner. Newer technology allows up to 320 to 512 anatomic slices to be simultaneously acquired. With a minimal slice thickness of 0.6 mm, an entire heart can be imaged in a single heartbeat. Even with newer generation scanners, temporal resolution at its best now approaches 140 ms, and cannot reach what can be obtained routinely in a cardiac catheterization laboratory, which is closer to 33 ms. To overcome the necessity of a slow heart rate, one vendor has placed two x-ray sources in the scanner (termed dual-source imaging) at 90-degree angles to one another. This technology offers an improved temporal resolution even with heart rates approaching ≥100 beats/min.

Data Acquisition Techniques

In the past, for coronary CTA using a single x-ray source scanner, it was typically necessary to obtain images with heart rates at <65 beats/min. An oral or intravenous β-blocker usually was given to patients to slow the heart rate. Newer generation scanners have somewhat lessened these rigid low heart rate requirements, although the adage still holds when imaging the heart that slower tends to be better. Coronary CTA requires intravenous administration of a contrast agent to opacify the lumen of the coronary arteries. The intravenous contrast agents used for CTA carry the same dose-dependent risks in patients with renal dysfunction as contrast agents used for cardiac catheterization, as well as the risk of an allergic reaction to iodine. Respiratory motion is minimized by patient breath holds up to 10 seconds, depending on scanner generation and patient body size. Data acquisition varies somewhat based on scanner type. The most common data acquisition protocol uses a spiral mode involving continuous data acquisition during constant rotation of the x-ray tube while the patient is simultaneously and continually advanced on the table through the x-ray gantry. To minimize radiation exposure, data acquisitions can be performed in sequential mode (step and shoot). This involves acquisition of single transaxial slices sequentially as a patient is advanced stepwise through the scanner.

Excessive cardiac motion can lead to blurring of the contours of the coronary vessels. For this reason, a regular heart rate is necessary for optimal imaging of the coronary arteries. Relative contraindications to performing CTA include the presence of frequent ectopic beats or atrial fibrillation. Coordinating data acquisition and analysis to the cardiac cycle involves either prospective triggering or retrospective gating. In prospective triggering, data are acquired in late diastole, based on simultaneous ECG recordings. In retrospective gating, data are collected during the entire cardiac cycle. Postprocessing then allows only data from specific periods of the cardiac cycle to be used for image reconstruction.

Clinical Indications
Coronary Artery Calcium Score

Coronary artery calcium (CAC) has emerged as a robust marker of subclinical atherosclerosis. CAC scoring uses no contrast and readily detects calcium because of its high x-ray attenuation coefficient (or CT number) measured in Hounsfield units (HUs) (Fig. 11.1). The Agatston scoring system assigns a calcium score based on the maximal CT number and the area of calcium deposits. Recently, analysis of several large clinical data sets confirmed that the CAC score is a robust predictor of coronary events, particularly in the asymptomatic patient population, independent of traditional risk factors. In at least one study, the calcium score was more predictive than C-reactive protein and standard risk factors for predicting CAD events.

The coronary calcium score is derived by identifying coronary arterial tree segments that have attenuation characteristics (HU) greater than a certain value (100–130 depending on software and patient size) that correlate with the attenuation due to calcium. These calcified lesions are scored by size and density, with a weighting factor for increasing density. Discrete lesions are scored separately, and the density of calcium within each lesion is graded from 1 to 4 according to the HU. The sums of all the lesions are totaled to arrive at a single coronary calcium score. In general, the higher the score, the greater the amount of calcified plaque within the arterial tree. There is a positive correlation of cardiac events with this score. However, it is important to remember that exclusively noncalcified coronary artery plaques have been reported in up to 4% of asymptomatic patients.

The Multiethnic Study of Atherosclerosis (MESA) Group published a series of articles that suggests that the calcium score is an independent risk factor for cardiac events. Also, MESA's website (https://www.mesa-nhlbi.org/calcium/input.aspx) has the capacity to allow comparison of the calcium score of an individual patient against their large database. This score takes into account age, sex, and race, and generates a percentile compared with the database studies. The presence of a high calcium score may prompt clinicians to use more aggressive therapy as if they were reclassified into a higher risk group or to convince patients who are reluctant to take drugs (e.g., statins) to take their disease more seriously. Recent studies have shown that a zero CAC score demonstrated an annual event rate in asymptomatic subjects of only 0.11% (10-year risk of only 1.1%). Among asymptomatic patients, the incidence of abnormal nuclear stress testing is 1.3%, 11.3%, and 35.2% for calcium scores <100, 101 to 400, and >400, respectively. Studies that have looked at serial calcium scanning have noted that calcified plaque progression is significantly and independently associated with a worse overall prognosis.

Coronary Artery Imaging (Cardiac CT Angiography)

Chest pain is a common clinical problem and one of the most common complaints of individuals presenting for urgent medical evaluation. One of the most important, life-threatening causes of chest pain is CAD. Although cardiac catheterization is the best method to assess for the presence of hemodynamically significant obstructive CAD, it is impractical as a screening test. It is invasive and costly, can be especially dangerous in some patients, and when used broadly as a screening tool, it is performed on a substantial number of patients who have no significant CAD and/or whose chest pain is unrelated to cardiac causes. Approximately 10% to 25% of the patients who are referred for invasive coronary angiography are found to have normal coronary arteries or nonobstructive CAD. Furthermore, several meta-analyses have demonstrated poorer prognosis and increased numbers of hard cardiac endpoints with nonobstructive CAD compared with normal coronary arteries.

CT angiography (CTA) uses intravenous contrast to differentiate the vessel lumen from the vessel wall. In 2010, the American College of Cardiology and many other societies with interests in cardiac imaging put together recommendations of appropriateness criteria for the use of cardiac CTA (CCTA) that include appropriate (Box 11.1) and

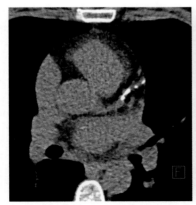
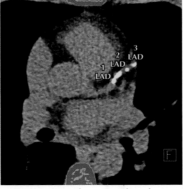

Artery	No. of lesions (1)	Volume [mm³] (3)	Equiv. mass [mg/cm³ CaHA] (4)	Score (2)
LM	0	0.0	0.00	0.0
LAD	3	181.9	43.32	247.6
LCX	0	0.0	0.00	0.0
RCA	0	0.0	0.00	0.0
Total	3	181.9	43.32	247.6

Example of coronary calcium scoring. Computer software utilized to determine Agatston score.

(1) Lesion is volume based
(2) Agatston score
(3) Isotropic interpolated volume
(4) Calibration factor 0.787

FIG 11.1 Coronary calcium scoring. *LAD*, Left anterior descending; *LCX*, left circumflex; *LM*, left main; *RCA*, right coronary artery.

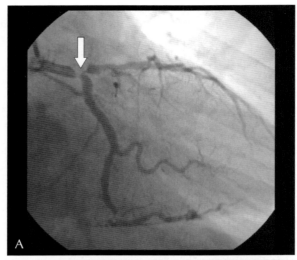

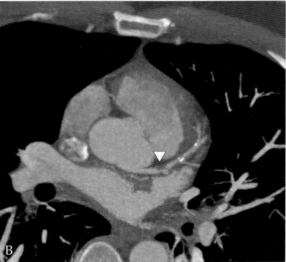

(A) Conventional coronary angiogram showing severe left main coronary artery disease (*arrow*) and (B) complementary coronary CT angiogram showing same left main lesion (*arrowhead*) with mixed calcified and noncalcified plaques.

FIG 11.3 Conventional diagnostic coronary angiogram and coronary CT angiogram.

BOX 11.1   Appropriate Indications for Cardiac CT

Detection of CAD (Symptomatic)
- Low/intermediate pretest probability of CAD
- Uninterpretable ECG or unable to exercise
- Evaluation of suspected coronary artery anomalies
- Uninterpretable or equivocal stress test (exercise, perfusion, or stress echo)

Structure and Function[a]
- Assessment of complex congenital heart disease, including anomalies of coronary circulation, great vessels, and cardiac chambers and valves
- Evaluation of coronary arteries in patients with new-onset heart failure to assess etiology
- Evaluation of cardiac masses
- Patients with technically limited images from transthoracic echocardiogram, MRI, or transesophageal echocardiogram
- Evaluation of pericardial conditions
- Evaluation of pulmonary vein anatomy before invasive radiofrequency ablation for atrial fibrillation
- Noninvasive coronary vein mapping before placement of biventricular pacemaker
- Noninvasive coronary arterial mapping, including internal mammary artery before repeat cardiac surgical revascularization
- Evaluation of suspected aortic dissection or thoracic aortic aneurysm
- Evaluation for suspected pulmonary embolism

[a]Preoperative planning for transcatheter structural heart interventions.
CAD, Coronary artery disease.

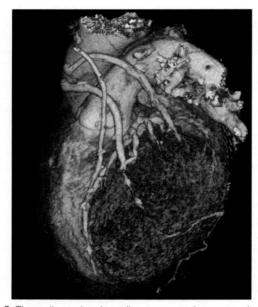

FIG 11.2 Three-dimensional cardiac computed tomography volume rendering showing patent bypass grafts.

inappropriate uses of this technology. The most common appropriate use is diagnostic study of patients presenting with chest pain who do not have significant ECG changes or elevated cardiac biomarkers, but who do have an intermediate probability of CAD (Fig. 11.2). At experienced centers with careful data acquisition, sensitivities range from 83% to 99% and specificities range from 93% to 98%, with remarkably high estimated negative predictive values (95%–100%), indicating

that CCTA may be used to reliably rule out the presence of significant flow-limiting coronary atherosclerotic disease. It should be pointed out that CCTA would be inappropriate for patients at high risk for or with other indications of cardiac ischemia, such as elevated biomarkers or significant ECG changes. Those patients should be referred immediately for invasive imaging. Currently, there is no indication for performing CCTA in asymptomatic patients. The appropriateness criteria definitively recommend against the use of CCTA in the asymptomatic population until further evidence suggests that it would positively affect outcomes.

Bypass graft imaging is more easily accomplished than coronary artery imaging because of the larger size of bypass grafts (particularly saphenous vein grafts) and less rapid movement of bypass grafts compared with native coronary arteries. The patency or occlusion of grafts can be determined by the presence or absence of distal target vessel contrast enhancement (Fig. 11.3). Imaging internal mammary grafts are often more difficult because of artifacts caused by metallic clips near the grafts. Imaging of coronary artery stents is challenging because of artifacts caused by metal that can obscure visualization of the coronary artery lumen. Studies that evaluated CCTA to assess in-stent restenosis have been somewhat disappointing, yielding sensitivities of 54% to 83%. Stents <3.0 mm in diameter are much more likely to be difficult to evaluate. An additional important application of CCTA is in patients with congenital abnormalities of their coronary arteries, including anomalous coronary artery origins and the presence of intramyocardial bridges (coronary arteries that, for a portion of their course, are not epicardial but rather covered by a layer of myocardial tissue).

The past several years have seen several new developments in CCTA technology that have focused not just on the coronary artery anatomy, but have also evaluated functional data simultaneously on the presence or absence of myocardial ischemia. There have been several publications in the past few years that have focused on the use of CCT for myocardial perfusion imaging, transluminal attenuation gradients, and corrected coronary opacification indexes and fractional flow reserve calculated from resting CCTA data.

Structural Heart Evaluation

Through appropriate timing of intravenous chamber contrast enhancement, extensive cardiac morphological and functional information can be obtained by CCT. Myocardial mass and ventricular function can be estimated with a high level of accuracy. CCT can also provide a detailed morphological picture of the left atrium and left atrial appendage anatomy, which is information that can be useful before planned catheter ablation for atrial fibrillation or device implantation in the left atrial appendage. Three-dimensional anatomic data obtained by CCT can be fused with electrical mapping data acquired in the electrophysiology laboratory, which greatly facilitates the procedure.

The past several years has seen an explosive growth in the use of transcatheter therapies for the treatment of valvular and structural heart disease. Advancement in transcatheter aortic valve replacement (Fig. 11.4) technology has relied heavily on appropriate aortic annular sizing data obtained with CCT. Studies have demonstrated that accurate three-dimensional aortic annular sizing assessment with CCT results in reduced paravalvular regurgitation, which has been associated with increased mortality following these procedures. In 2012, the Society of Cardiovascular Computed Tomography released guidelines for the use of CCT before TAVR. Furthermore, several new therapies on the horizon for mitral and tricuspid valve repair will also rely heavily on preprocedural CCT for accurate sizing and morphological assessment.

Congenital Heart Disease

Assessment of complex congenital heart disease, including anomalous coronary artery circulation, great vessels, cardiac chambers, and valves are all appropriate indications for CCT. Specific indications include shunt assessment, aortic geometry in coarctation or Marfan syndrome, partial or total anomalous pulmonary venous return, and pulmonary artery visualization in patients with cyanotic heart disease.

Evaluation of Intracardiac and Extracardiac Structures

In patients with technically limited images on echocardiography and who are unable to undergo MRI, CCT can be used to evaluate for cardiac mass (i.e., tumor, thrombus, or potentially vegetation). Pericardial diseases can also be evaluated using CCT by looking specifically for pericardial cysts, pericardial calcification that may be suggestive of constrictive pericarditis, or complications of cardiac surgery. Thickening of the pericardium (normal thickness is <4 mm) can be suggestive of an inflammatory process.

Evaluation of Thoracic Aorta and Pulmonary Artery Disease

In patients with suspected pulmonary embolism, CCT has both high sensitivity and specificity (>90%) for the diagnosis of proximal pulmonary embolism. Emboli can be visualized in the main pulmonary artery and as far distally as the segmental pulmonary artery branches. Evaluation of the pulmonary venous anatomy is useful before (and after) atrial fibrillation ablation to assess for pulmonary vein stenosis or pulmonary venous anomalies. CCT assessment of the aorta typically

Pre - TAVR

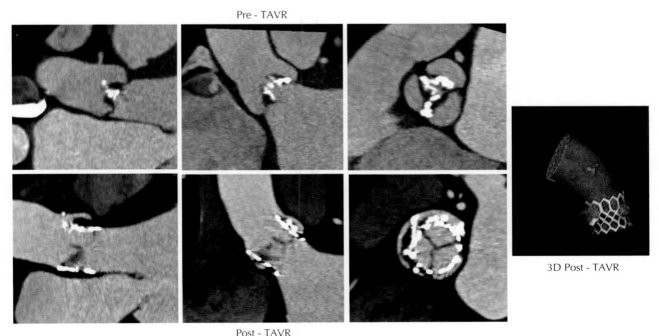

Post - TAVR

3D Post - TAVR

FIG 11.4 Cardiac CT images pretranscatheter and posttranscatheter aortic valve replacement (TAVR). *3D,* Three-dimensional.

requires contrast enhancement. Three-dimensional reconstruction can be useful diagnostically and also before planned endovascular repair. Typical indications for CCT in assessment of the aorta include aneurysm, dissection, and intramural hematoma.

Cardiac CT Limitations

CCT involves exposure to radiation and the potential for radiation-related risk (particularly related to the risk of cancer induction). Radiation exposure (effective dose) is quantified in millisieverts. Patient radiation doses are dependent upon tube current (milliamperes) and tube voltage (kiloelectron volts), as well as duration of radiation exposure and patient body size. Current generation CT scanners are now able to perform electrocardiographically gated cardiac imaging with 1 to 2 mSv. For comparison purposes, typical gated cardiac SPECT carries a similar radiation dose (effective dose: 10–15 mSv), whereas conventional coronary angiography carries a lower radiation dose (effective dose: 6 mSv) compared with CCT. ECG-correlated tube current modulation (reduction of tube current in systole) with retrospectively gated studies can reduce radiation exposure by 30% to 50%. Retrospectively gated studies have more recently been replaced by prospectively triggered studies that limit radiation exposure to a single portion of the cardiac cycle, further significantly decreasing overall patient radiation exposure. In addition, improvements in iterative reconstruction techniques have also been developed that also further reduce patient radiation exposure. Although the risk from radiation is relatively low, it does mean that CCT is not well suited for use as a screening test on a regular or repeated basis.

In addition, allergic contrast reactions have been reported in 0.2% to 0.7% of patients who receive nonionic contrast materials. In the absence of preexisting renal disease, the risk of renal dysfunction due to contrast administration is low.

Future Directions

It is estimated that nearly 60 million CT scans were performed in the United States in 2001, with growth estimated at 9% per year in the coming decade. Current CCT use has not constituted a broad replacement for conventional coronary angiography, but in appropriately selected patients, it may serve as a useful alternative. Dual-source CCT has improved temporal resolution, and 320-detector row coronary CTA now allows imaging of the entire heart in a single heartbeat. Combination cardiac PET/CT promises to provide additional information regarding cardiac morphology, perfusion, and metabolism. At present, CCT is not covered by many insurance carriers. Based on the results of ongoing clinical studies—demonstration of both efficacy and cost-effectiveness of CCT as a diagnostic modality—there may well be expanded coverage of CCT by insurers.

CARDIAC MAGNETIC RESONANCE IMAGING

CMR imaging has continued to advance as a robust cardiac noninvasive imaging technique. Through electromagnetic manipulation of biological hydrogen protons, CMR provides assessment of cardiac structure, function, perfusion, tissue characterization, blood flow velocity, cardiac masses, valvular heart disease, pericardial disease, and vascular disease. Continued improvements in hardware and pulse sequence design have allowed for improved image quality, speed of data acquisition, and reliability, further increasing the usefulness of CMR for clinical applications. CMR is similar to echocardiography in that neither uses ionizing radiation to acquire high-resolution images, which avoids the exposures inherent in invasive coronary angiography and SPECT imaging. CMR offers viewing cardiac motion in any view. In addition, the versatility of CMR permits imaging of a large field of view in nearly any plane, which allows for the assessment of both cardiac and noncardiac pathologies.

Technology of Cardiac Magnetic Resonance

MRI (including CMR) is based upon the electromagnetic manipulation of biological hydrogen protons. Hydrogen is the most abundant element present within the human body; it is present in all tissues, whether in water, adipose tissue, or soft tissue. Each water molecule contains two hydrogen nuclei with a single proton, and they behave like tiny magnets. Proton spins can be aligned by application of a powerful magnetic field in the $\beta(0)$ direction, because of the appropriate frequency via the Larmor equation ($f = \gamma\beta$, where f is the precessional frequency; β is the magnet field strength; and γ is the gyromagnetic ratio). A second radiofrequency electromagnetic field can then be briefly applied and then rapidly discontinued. As protons return to their original alignment after the electromagnetic field is turned off ("relaxation"), they generate a net magnetization that decays to its former position with energy loss in the form of a radio signal that can be detected with a radiofrequency antenna and quantified. Image tissue contrast depends on differences in the decay of net magnetization in the longitudinal plane (T_1) and transverse plane (T_2). Through the application of additional electromagnetic fields (gradient fields), radio waves coming from the body can be spatially encoded, which allows localization within an imaging plane.

Data Acquisition Sequences and Techniques

CMR uses two basic imaging sequences: spin echo ("dark blood") and gradient echo ("bright blood"). Spin-echo sequences are commonly used for multislice anatomic imaging, providing clear delineation of the mediastinum, cardiac chambers, and great vessels. Alternatively, gradient echo sequences are used more often for physiological assessment of function through cine acquisitions. Because of higher possible imaging speeds, gradient echo is more appropriately used for ventricular function and myocardial perfusion assessment, as well as valvular assessment. Phase contrast imaging (PCI) allows quantitative flow velocity and volume flow assessment. All cardiac and most vascular CMR sequences require cardiac ECG gating. Through data acquisition of segments at different phases of the cardiac cycle, a cine image loop can be created to track cardiac motion. Perfusion imaging, through the use of intravenous contrast agents, permits assessment of tissue vascularity. In the case of vasodilator stress perfusion imaging, assessment of myocardial ischemia is possible (Fig. 11.5). Inotropic stress imaging, typically with intravenous dobutamine, allows assessment of new regional wall motion abnormalities. Gadolinium-based contrast agents, chelated to other nontoxic molecules for clinical use, are commonly used for imaging the cardiovascular system.

Clinical Indications
Ventricular Function

CMR is highly accurate and reproducible, providing clinically useful measurements of cardiac wall thickness, chamber volumes, and systolic contractile function (Fig. 11.6). CMR is recognized as the gold standard for assessment of left and right ventricular function. Left ventricular ejection fraction, left ventricular end-diastolic volume, left ventricular end-systolic volume, stroke volume, cardiac output, and left ventricular mass can all be reliably quantified. Left ventricular diastolic function can also be reliably interrogated using PCI.

Aortic Disease

CMR has rapidly evolved into a clinically reliable, reproducible modality to evaluate the aorta and its primary branch vessels. Gadolinium-enhanced, three-dimensional CMR angiography is an extremely rapid

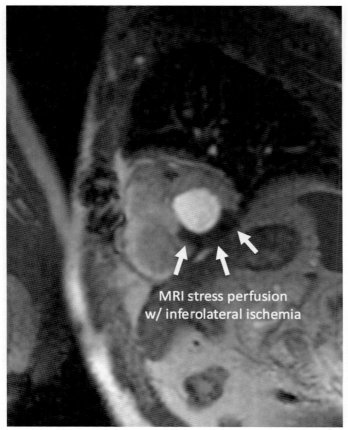

FIG 11.5 Cardiac magnetic resonance stress perfusion imaging, demonstrating inferolateral ischemia.

technique that can accurately depict aortic pathology. Serial monitoring of chronic aortopathy can be monitored safely, without continued radiation exposure, with CMR angiography.

Ischemic Heart Disease

CMR is the most sensitive cardiac imaging modality for assessment of myocardial viability and the extent of myocardial infarction. It is the imaging modality of choice for patients in whom there is a question about whether the myocardial tissue in the distribution of a planned revascularization is viable (Fig. 11.7). For this application, compared with nuclear imaging, CMR is much more sensitive in detecting subendocardial viability (and lack of viability), and obviously, CMR does not require radiation exposure for patients. Gadolinium is excluded from intact myocardial cell membranes and thus is useful in defining areas of infarction. Correlation with anatomic specimens suggests a sensitivity and specificity of >95%. Delayed hyperenhancement (DHE) protocols, which most often use phase sensitive inversion recovery imaging, are based on the high-signal intensity (bright) that results from T1 time shortening due to gadolinium contrast localization within scar tissue. Alternatively, first-pass perfusion images that appear hypointense are probably a combination of ischemic and infarcted tissues. The highest likelihood of recovery of contractility impairment exists when the transmural infarction extent, as assessed by DHE, is <50% transmural.

Cardiomyopathies

CMR is an important tool in the evaluation of dilated cardiomyopathy, hypertrophic cardiomyopathy, and infiltrative disorders. It provides

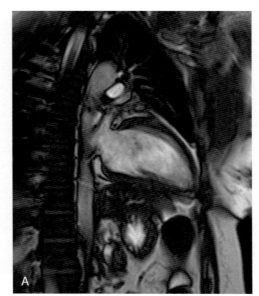

Two-chamber

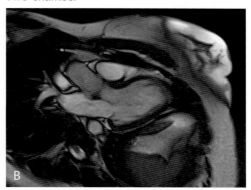

Three-chamber—LVOT view

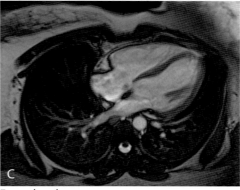

Four-chamber

FIG 11.6 MRI can generate images of the heart in multiple user-defined orientation. *LVOT*, Left ventricular outflow tract.

accurate assessment of ventricular function in patients with dilated cardiomyopathies. DHE CMR has a niche role in helping to differentiate heart failure related to dilated cardiomyopathy from CAD, although the distinction is not perfect. More than 10% of patients with dilated nonischemic cardiomyopathy have gadolinium enhancement that is identical in appearance to that seen in patients with CAD.

In hypertrophic cardiomyopathy, CMR can accurately localize hypertrophy, particularly when echocardiographic data are equivocal. Cine

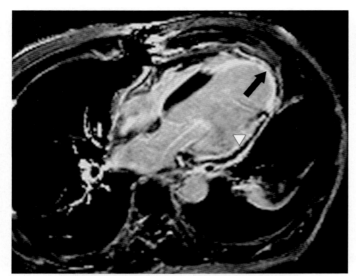

Example of a patient that has sustained a myocardial infarction and demonstrates an area of transmural scar at the apex (*arrow*) and nontransmural scar involving the lateral wall (*arrowhead*).

FIG 11.7 Cardiac magnetic resonance imaging: transmural and nontransmural scars.

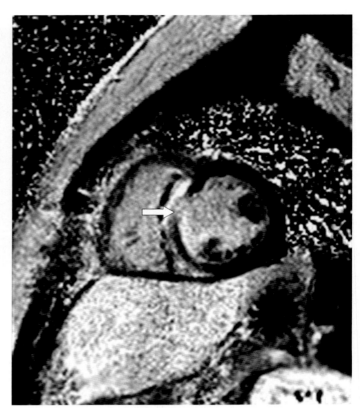

Patchy, nontransmural delayed hyperenhancement involving mid-septum and inferoseptum in a patient with cardiac sarcoidosis (*arrow*).

FIG 11.8 Sarcoidosis: CMR phase-sensitive inversion recovery.

images can also demonstrate systolic anterior motion of the anterior mitral valve leaflet and dynamic outflow tract obstruction, which are useful measures in selecting an optimal therapeutic approach in this patient population. More recent data indicate that increased DHE scar burden in patients with hypertrophic cardiomyopathy is correlated with increased risk of arrhythmia or sudden cardiac death. CMR also has a role in the evaluation of patients with suspected infiltrative cardiomyopathies. Sarcoidosis is an infiltrative granulomatous disease pathologically known to nonuniformly involve the myocardium. This patchy distribution tends to result in a moderate to high number of false-negative cardiac biopsy results. When an initial biopsy result is negative in patients with suspected cardiac sarcoidosis, the benefits of repeated biopsy procedures must be considered because of the risks inherent in this procedure. CMR DHE imaging can depict areas of interstitial changes and granulomatous disease (Fig. 11.8). In patients with a high pretest probability for cardiac sarcoid, CMR can potentially serve as a reliable screening tool, obviating the need for biopsy, particularly if the diagnosis of sarcoidosis has been confirmed by biopsy of noncardiac tissue. Amyloid infiltration in the myocardium may show diffusely increased signal intensity with DHE imaging sequences. In addition, the combination of ventricular hypertrophy without ECG concordance, atrial wall thickening, valve thickening, pericardial and pleural effusion, and restrictive diastolic filling pattern can collectively raise the clinical suspicion for infiltrative cardiac amyloidosis. CMR is also capable of confirming the diagnosis of arrhythmogenic right ventricular dysplasia, a diagnosis that historically is based on meeting several major and minor criteria. Use of contrast agents and DHE imaging may permit detection of fibro-fatty right ventricular free wall infiltration, regional right ventricular wall motion abnormalities, and assessment of indexed right ventricular volume, which are observations that increase specificity for this otherwise difficult diagnosis.

Pericardial Diseases

CMR permits assessment of pericardial effusion, constrictive pericarditis, pericardial cysts, and congenital absence of the pericardium. Normal pericardium thickness on CMR is 1 to 4 mm. Functional and structural abnormalities of the pericardium can be reliably assessed using CMR imaging. Pericardial DHE imaging has been demonstrated to correlate with active pericardial inflammation and neovascularization. In addition, free breathing cine imaging can demonstrate increased ventricular interdependence suggestive of constrictive pericarditis. Failure to see slippage between the visceral and parietal pericardial layers suggests fibrosis, scarring, or connections between these two normally separate tissue layers. CMR has also proven useful in the evaluation of pericardial cysts.

Valvular Heart Disease

CMR has become a valuable complementary technique for evaluating the severity of valvular heart disease. Through a combination of steady-state free precession and PCI, CMR can provide a comprehensive valvular assessment. Although echocardiography is capable of superior temporal resolution, is more accessible, and is less labor-intensive, CMR is capable of imaging flow in three dimensions (x, y, and z planes), which is more accurate for measuring absolute flow volumes and feasible in patients whose body habitus precludes obtaining optimal echocardiographic images. In valvular regurgitant lesions, PCI can provide exact quantifications of regurgitant volume and fraction. In patients with aortic stenosis, planimetry of the aortic valve provides accurate measurements rather than geometric estimations available via echocardiography and catheterization techniques. In addition, CMR provides accurate measurement of peak transstenotic jet velocities that are orthogonal to the valve, not merely across it.

Cardiac Masses

CMR is the imaging modality of choice for evaluation of cardiac masses because of its ability to perform tissue characterization. Spin-echo imaging provides excellent images for evaluation of the presence, extent, attachment site, and secondary effects of cardiac mass lesions. CMR has a proven role in the identification of intracardiac thrombi, primary and secondary cardiac tumors, and pericardial cysts (Fig. 11.9).

Congenital Heart Disease

CMR is an ideal imaging modality for the assessment of congenital heart disease by providing superior anatomic imaging coupled with functional interrogation and reproducibility. In the evaluation of great vessel abnormalities, CMR is the gold standard, particularly for conditions such as aortic coarctation. Through velocity mapping of the coarctation jet, a pressure gradient across the area of narrowing can be determined. Tetralogy of Fallot, including overriding aorta, membranous ventricular septal defect, right ventricular hypertrophy, and infundibular or pulmonary stenosis, can be completely characterized before and after correction. In addition, as is often the case with patients who required surgical tetralogy repair, CMR is an excellent tool for monitoring patients for progressive pulmonary valvular regurgitation and right ventricular dilation. CMR is also capable of reliably depicting anomalous coronary artery origins and their relation to other cardiac structures and the great vessels.

Coronary Artery Bypass Graft Imaging

Although coronary angiography remains the gold standard for evaluating coronary atherosclerotic disease, CMR may be used in the future for noninvasive assessment of the coronary arteries. The main limitations to CMR coronary angiography include limited spatial resolution, respiratory motion, rapid coronary motion (up to 20 cm/s in certain phases), and an inability to easily assess distal runoff. Quantification (and sometimes even detection) of coronary luminal stenosis remains challenging. Currently, this is an area of significant ongoing research. Coronary flow velocities can be estimated by CMR, and some centers are now using adenosine infusion with CMR to measure coronary flow as a diagnostic test for functionally important CAD. Anomalous coronary arteries can be identified using CMR. In particular, CMR is well suited to demonstrate the relationship of anomalous coronary arteries with other vascular structures (the aorta and main pulmonary artery) and thus, to make decisions on the need and timing of surgery.

Safety, Risks, and Contraindications

Because of the physical nature of CMR, magnetic field generation poses a risk to patients of moving metallic, ferromagnetic projectiles while physically inside the scanner. Care must be taken to ensure protocols are in place to minimize this risk. Most prosthetic heart valves, vascular stents (including coronary artery stents), and orthopedic implants are safe to be imaged using CMR, but CMR is currently contraindicated for patients with most implantable pacemakers and defibrillators. However, several device manufacturers have developed MR safe pacemakers that have been approved by the Food and Drug Administration. In all cases in which there is a question on device MRI safety, the website www.mrisafety.com is a robust source of compiled information on this topic.

Future Directions

CMR has advanced rapidly in the past decade, and the clinical applications for its use continue to evolve. Ultrafast imaging through improved magnet design will continue to improve the logistic constraints associated with CMR. CMR holds promise for further assessment and characterization of atherosclerotic plaque burden and composition, and research is active in this area.

Left atrial myxoma

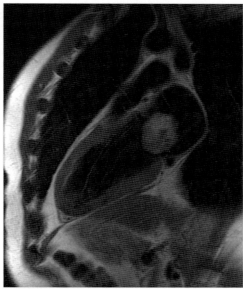

Dark blood

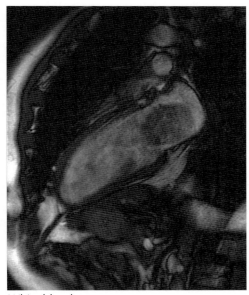

White blood

FIG 11.9 Cardiac MRI showing left atrial myxoma.

ADDITIONAL RESOURCES

Achenbach S. Computed tomography coronary angiography. *J Am Col. Cardiol.* 2006;48:1919–1928.
This paper is a thorough review of various issues concerning CT scanner technology, image acquisition and reconstruction, image interpretation, and potential clinical applications.
Finn PJ, Kambiz N, Vibhas D, et al. Cardiac MR imaging: state of the technology. *Radiology.* 2006;241:338–354.
This review covers some of the major milestones in CMR; it discusses some of its technical and diagnostic clinical uses.

EVIDENCE

Achenbach S, Delgado V, Hausleiter J, et al. SCCT expert consensus document on computed tomography before transcatheter aortic valve implantation (TAVI)/transcatheter aortic valve replacement (TAVR). *J Cardiovasc Comput Tomogr.* 2012;6:366–380.

Excellent review on the role of CT for imaging patients with severe aortic valve stenosis, with discussion of data acquisition protocols, assessment of access routes, predictors of vascular injury, and image processing and measurements.

Agatston AS, Janowitz WR, Hildner FJ, et al. Quantification of coronary artery calcium using ultrafast computed tomography. *J Am Coll Cardiol.* 1990;15:827–832.

Landmark cohort study that demonstrated the usefulness of ultrafast CT to detect and quantify CAC levels.

Arad Y, Goodman KJ, Roth M, et al. Coronary calcification, coronary disease risk factors, C-reactive protein, and atherosclerotic cardiovascular disease events: The St. Francis Heart Study. *J Am Coll Cardiol.* 2005;46:158–165.

Prospective, population-based study that demonstrated that the electron beam CT coronary calcium score predicts CAD events independently of standard risk factors more accurately than standard risk factors and C-reactive protein, and re-defines Framingham risk stratification.

Brenner DJ, Hall EJ. Computed tomography—an increasing source of radiation exposure. *N Engl J Med.* 2007;357:2277–2284.

This review article describes the use of CT, as well as the associated radiation doses and subsequent biological effects of ionizing radiation.

Cohen JD, Costa HS, Russo RJ. Determining the risks of magnetic resonance imaging at 1.5 tesla for patients with pacemakers and implantable cardioverter defibrillators. *Am J Cardiol.* 2012;110:1631–1636.

Single center retrospective review of 109 patients with pacemakers and defibrillators who underwent MRI imaging that resulted in no device or lead failures. A small number of clinically relevant changes in device parameter measurements were noted.

de Araujo Goncalves P, Rodriguez-Granillo GA, Spitzer E, et al. Function evaluation of coronary disease by CT angiography. *J Am Coll Cardiol Img.* 2015;8:1322–1335.

This review describes myocardial perfusion CT, the transluminal attenuation gradient, and corrected coronary opacification and fractional flow reserve computed from CTA.

Detrano R, Guerci AD, Carr JJ, et al. Coronary calcium as a predictor of coronary events in four racial or ethnic groups. *N Engl J Med.* 2008;358:1336–1345.

Landmark study evaluating large population-based sample consisting of men and women from multiple racial and ethnic groups using CT methods for measurement of CAC. Established that the coronary calcium score is a strong predictor of incident coronary heart disease and provides predictive information in addition to standard atherosclerotic risk factors.

Greenland P, Bonow RO, Brundage BH, et al. ACCF/AHA 2007 Clinical expert consensus document on coronary artery calcium scoring by computed tomography in global cardiovascular risk assessment and in evaluation of patients with chest pain: a report of the American College of Cardiology Foundation Clinical Expert Consensus Task Force (ACCF/AHA Writing Committee to Update the 2000 Expert Consensus Document on Electron Beam Computed Tomography) developed in collaboration with the Society of Atherosclerosis Imaging and Prevention and the Society of Cardiovascular Computed Tomography. *J Am Coll Cardiol.* 2007;49:378–402.

Clinical expert consensus document providing a current perspective on the role of CAC scanning by fast CT in clinical practice.

Hajime S. Magnetic resonance imaging for ischemic heart disease. *J Magn Reson Imaging.* 2007;26:3–13.

Extensive, thorough review article discussing the use of MRI in patients with ischemic heart disease.

Halliburton SS, Abbara S, Chen MY, et al. SCCT guidelines on radiation dose and dose-optimization strategies in cardiovascular CT. *J Cardiovasc Comput Tomogr* 2011;5:198–224.

Comprehensive overview of cardiovascular CT radiation dose standards and measurements, radiation risk, appropriate use criteria, dose optimization techniques, and dose monitoring.

Hecht H. Coronary artery calcium scanning. *J Am Coll Cardiol Img.* 2015;8:579–596.

Excellent review article that addresses the technology of coronary artery calcium scanning, prognostic data, cost-effectiveness, role of calcium progression, and need for serial scanning and limitations of the technology.

Kim RJ, Wu E, Rafael A, et al. The use of contrast-enhanced magnetic resonance imaging to identify reversible myocardial dysfunction. *N Engl J Med.* 2000;343:1445–1453.

Prospective cohort study evaluating contrast-enhanced MRI in patients with ventricular dysfunction before revascularization. Concluded that reversible myocardial dysfunction can be identified by contrast-enhanced MRI before revascularization. Of regions with greater than 50% hyperenhancement before revascularization, 90% failed to improve after revascularization was completed.

Krombach GA, Hahn C, Tomars M, et al. Cardiac amyloidosis: MR imaging findings and T1 quantification, comparison with control subjects. *J Magn Reson Imaging.* 2007;25:1283–1287.

Comparison study that looked specifically at the T_1 time of the myocardium in a patient with known amyloidosis compared with other individuals without known myocardial disease. It concluded that T_1 quantification may increase diagnostic confidence in patients with amyloidosis.

Oncel D, Oncel G, Tastan A, Tamci B. Evaluation of coronary stent patency and in-stent restenosis with dual-source CT coronary angiography without heart rate control. *AJR Am J Roentgenol.* 2008;191:56–63.

Prospective study evaluating in-stent restenosis and occlusion in a small patient cohort with known clinical CAD having all undergone prior coronary artery stent placement with dual-source CT. The accuracy of dual-source CT in the detection of in-stent restenosis and occlusion was reported at 96%.

Stein PD, Yaekoub AY, Matta F, Sostman HD. 64-slice CT for diagnosis of coronary artery disease: a systematic review. *Am J Med.* 2008;121:715–725.

Systematic review of all published trials that used 64-slice CT to diagnose CAD. Concluded that a negative 64-slice CT reliably excludes significant CAD with a reported negative predictive value of 96% to 100%.

Tandri H, Saranathan M, Rodriguez ER, et al. Noninvasive detection of myocardial fibrosis in arrhythmogenic right ventricular cardiomyopathy using delayed-enhancement magnetic resonance imaging. *J Am Coll Cardiol.* 2005;45:98–103.

Prospective study that evaluated 30 consecutive patients with known arrhythmogenic right ventricular disease using myocardial delayed-enhancement MRI. The study concluded that noninvasive detection of right ventricular myocardial fibro-fatty changes in arrhythmogenic right ventricular disease is possible with myocardial delayed-enhancement MRI and correlated well with histopathology and predicted inducible ventricular tachycardia on programmed electrical stimulation.

Taylor AJ, Cerqueira M, Hodgson J, et al. ACCF/SCCT/ACR/AHA/ASE/ASNC/NASCI/SCAI/SCMR 2010 Appropriate Use Criteria for Cardiac Computed Tomography: A Report of the American College of Cardiology Foundation Appropriate Use Criteria Task Force, the Society of Cardiovascular Computed Tomography, the American College of Radiology, the American Heart Association, the American Society of Echocardiography, the American Society of Nuclear Cardiology, the North American Society for Cardiovascular Imaging, the Society for Cardiovascular Angiography and Interventions, and the Society for Cardiovascular Magnetic Resonance.

Guideline paper reviewing appropriate use criteria for cardiac CT imaging.

Zurick AO, Bolen MA, Kwon DH, et al. Pericardial delayed hyperenhancement with Cardiac Magnetic Resonance Imaging in Patients with Constrictive Pericarditis Undergoing Surgical Pericardiectomy: A Case Series with Histopathological Correlation.

Retrospective cohort study that evaluated 25 patients with constrictive pericarditis that went on to surgical pericardiectomy. All patients underwent preoperative MRI imaging with assessment for pericardial delayed hyperenhancement. Patients with pericardial enhancement demonstrated greater fibroblastic proliferation, neovascularization, more prominent chronic inflammation and granulation tissue.

12

Diagnostic Coronary Angiography

David W. Lee, George A. Stouffer

The ability to directly visualize arteries with an injection of a radiopaque contrast agent was a seminal advance in the history of modern medicine and led directly to the development of the concept of transluminal angioplasty (first performed in 1964), coronary artery bypass grafting (CABG; first performed in 1967), percutaneous transluminal peripheral balloon angioplasty (first performed in 1974), and percutaneous coronary intervention (PCI; first performed in 1977). Coronary angiography enables direct visualization of the coronary arteries and provides essential information in the diagnosis and management of coronary artery disease (CAD) by defining the presence, location, and severity of coronary artery pathology. In addition, coronary angiography can be used to diagnose anomalous coronary arteries, spasm, myocardial bridging, fistulas, dissections, and aneurysms. This chapter focuses on coronary anatomy, preprocedural evaluation, technical aspects, and potential complications of diagnostic coronary angiography.

CORONARY ANATOMY

The right coronary artery (RCA) arises from the right coronary sinus and runs in the right atrioventricular (AV) groove (Fig. 12.1). The conus artery is typically the first branch that arises from the RCA and supplies the right ventricular outflow tract. The sinoatrial nodal and AV nodal branches also arise from the RCA and supply the sinus node and the AV node, respectively. Marginal branches usually arise from the mid-RCA and supply the right ventricular wall. The distal RCA gives rise to right posterolateral branches and the posterior descending artery (PDA) in 85% of cases (defined as right dominance). The PDA arises from the left circumflex (LCX) in 8% of cases (defined as left dominance), and from both the RCA and LCX in 7% of cases (defined as co-dominance). The PDA runs in the posterior interventricular groove and supplies the posterior aspect of the interventricular septum.

The left main coronary artery arises from the left coronary sinus and bifurcates into the left anterior descending (LAD) and LCX arteries (Fig. 12.1). In a minority of cases, the left main coronary artery trifurcates into the LAD artery, ramus intermedius artery, and LCX artery. The LAD artery runs in the anterior interventricular groove toward the apex of the heart and supplies the anterior wall of the left ventricle. Septal perforator branches arise from the LAD artery and supply the interventricular septum. Diagonal branches also arise from the LAD artery and supply the anterolateral wall of the left ventricle. The LCX artery runs in the left AV groove and provides obtuse marginal branches that supply the posterolateral wall of the left ventricle. As noted previously, in a minority of cases, the PDA will arise from the LCX artery.

There are many schemes for describing coronary anatomy: the Coronary Artery Surgery Study (CASS) classification, the Synergy Between PCI With Taxus and Cardiac Surgery (SYNTAX) classification, and the Bypass Angioplasty Revascularization Investigation (BARI) modification of the CASS map are some of the most widely accepted.

CORONARY ARTERY ANOMALIES

Coronary artery anomalies are typically a result of abnormal embryological development and are found in 1% to 1.5% of cases. Most coronary artery anomalies are clinically benign. The most common coronary artery anomaly is the presence of separate origins of the LAD and LCX arteries, which occurs in 0.4% to 1% of cases and may be associated with a bicuspid aortic valve. Clinically significant anomalies include a coronary artery originating from the opposite coronary sinus (e.g., left main coronary artery originating from the right coronary sinus), the presence of a single coronary ostium leading to a single coronary artery, a coronary artery coursing between the great vessels (e.g., between the aorta and pulmonary artery), and a coronary artery leading to decreased oxygenation of the myocardium (e.g., a coronary artery originating from the pulmonary artery or a coronary artery–ventricular fistula) (Fig. 12.2).

PREPROCEDURAL EVALUATION

Obtaining a history, physical examination, routine laboratory data (such as chemistry, complete blood count, and coagulation studies), a 12-lead ECG, and a transthoracic echocardiogram can provide valuable information for procedural planning. An accurate history can help determine patient candidacy for PCI and dual antiplatelet therapy in the event that the angiographic findings demonstrate obstructive CAD. Physical examination of the peripheral pulses can help plan the site of vascular access. Stress testing can be performed to risk stratify patients before coronary angiography and to help localize the area of myocardial ischemia.

Indications

The American College of Cardiology and American Heart Association have published guidelines on the indications for diagnostic coronary angiography (Table 12.1). Patients with acute coronary syndromes should undergo emergent or urgent diagnostic coronary angiography. In particular, patients with ST-elevation myocardial infarction (STEMI) should undergo emergent coronary angiography with the goal of establishing reperfusion with angioplasty within 90 minutes of clinical presentation. Patients who have a non-STEMI or unstable angina, and who are at intermediate or high risk for adverse events should undergo early coronary angiography within 24 to 72 hours. Patients with high-risk features (e.g., refractory angina, hemodynamic or electrical instability, or cardiogenic shock) should undergo coronary angiography within the first few hours of clinical presentation.

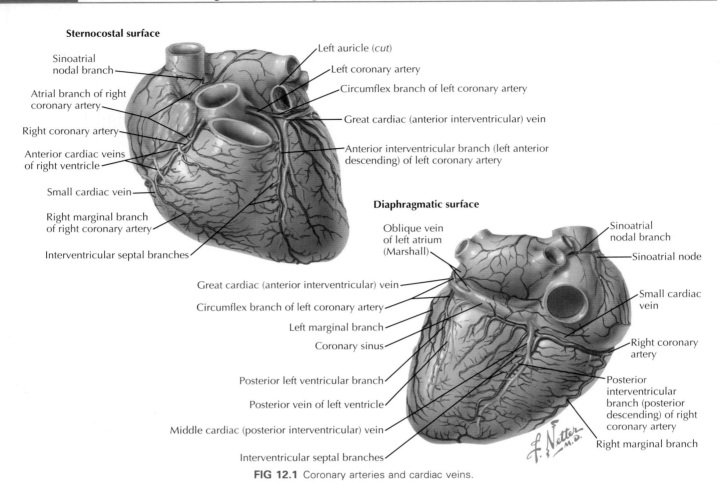

Sternocostal surface

Sinoatrial nodal branch

Atrial branch of right coronary artery

Right coronary artery

Anterior cardiac veins of right ventricle

Small cardiac vein

Right marginal branch of right coronary artery

Interventricular septal branches

Left auricle (*cut*)

Left coronary artery

Circumflex branch of left coronary artery

Great cardiac (anterior interventricular) vein

Anterior interventricular branch (left anterior descending) of left coronary artery

Diaphragmatic surface

Oblique vein of left atrium (Marshall)

Great cardiac (anterior interventricular) vein

Circumflex branch of left coronary artery

Left marginal branch

Coronary sinus

Posterior left ventricular branch

Posterior vein of left ventricle

Middle cardiac (posterior interventricular) vein

Interventricular septal branches

Sinoatrial nodal branch

Sinoatrial node

Small cardiac vein

Right coronary artery

Posterior interventricular branch (posterior descending) of right coronary artery

Right marginal branch

FIG 12.1 Coronary arteries and cardiac veins.

Patients with stable angina and certain clinical features may undergo coronary angiography without previous stress testing. For instance, patients who have symptoms highly typical of angina or patients who have symptoms with minimal or no exertion should be directly referred for coronary angiography without previous stress testing. Additional clinical features that may prompt referral for coronary angiography without previous stress testing include a history of myocardial infarction, previous percutaneous or surgical revascularization, and congestive heart failure.

CONTRAINDICATIONS

The only absolute contraindication to diagnostic coronary angiography is the lack of patient consent. There are many relative contraindications that can increase the risks of the procedure in patients with certain co-morbidities (Table 12.2). For example, acute renal failure or preexisting renal dysfunction, especially in patients with diabetes mellitus, can increase the risk of contrast-induced nephropathy. Electrolyte abnormalities and/or digitalis toxicity can increase the risk of arrhythmias during contrast injection. Active bleeding, severe thrombocytopenia, and/or severe coagulopathy from co-morbidities or medications (e.g., such as warfarin or the new anticoagulants) can increase the risk of vascular complications and/or bleeding risk in the setting of PCI. Decompensated heart failure, severe aortic stenosis, or uncontrolled hypertension can increase the risk of acute flash pulmonary edema and respiratory failure when the patient is required to remain supine during the procedure. Other relative contraindications include active infection, allergic reactions to iodinated contrast agents, severe peripheral vascular disease, pregnancy, and patient inability to cooperate.

PROCEDURAL TECHNIQUE

Diagnostic coronary angiography is routinely performed in a cardiac catheterization laboratory. Written informed consent must be obtained before the procedure. Patients should be informed of the indication, benefits, risks, and alternatives of coronary angiography. If there is a possibility of obstructive CAD that leads to PCI, patients should also be informed of the indication, benefits, risks, and alternatives of PCI before the procedure. Once in the cardiac catheterization laboratory, patients are prepared with antiseptic solution at the access site and draped in a sterile fashion. A time-out is performed with the physicians, nurses, and cardiovascular technologists to verify the patient, procedure, indication, access site, and any allergies. Sedatives with analgesics are then administered intravenously for conscious sedation.

Arterial Access

Arterial access can be obtained via percutaneous puncture of the common femoral artery (CFA), brachial artery, or radial artery (Fig. 12.3). Although the femoral approach is historically the most commonly used site for arterial access, the radial approach has become increasingly popular and may be the preferred strategy in patients with morbid obesity, decompensated heart failure, or severe peripheral artery disease.

The femoral approach requires the proper identification of anatomic landmarks before vessel puncture (Fig. 12.4). The fluoroscopic landmark for the optimal CFA entry site is generally considered to be the upper one-half or the upper one-third of the femoral head. In a study of 200 femoral angiograms, the CFA bifurcated below the center of the femoral head in 98% of patients, whereas in another study of 208 femoral

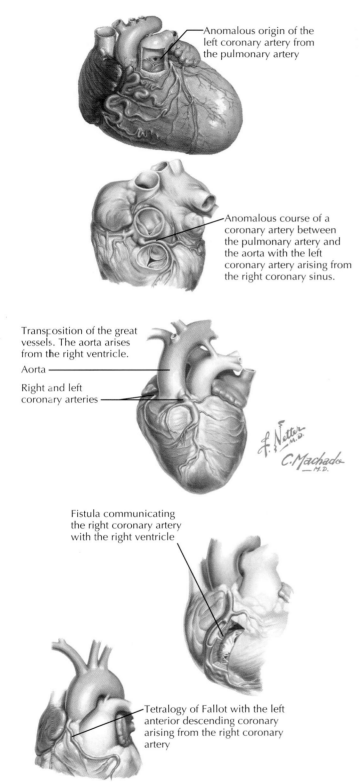

Anomalous origin of the left coronary artery from the pulmonary artery

Anomalous course of a coronary artery between the pulmonary artery and the aorta with the left coronary artery arising from the right coronary sinus.

Transposition of the great vessels. The aorta arises from the right ventricle.

Aorta

Right and left coronary arteries

Fistula communicating the right coronary artery with the right ventricle

Tetralogy of Fallot with the left anterior descending coronary arising from the right coronary artery

FIG 12.2 Congenital coronary artery anomalies.

bleeding). Risk factors for vascular complications are both clinical and anatomic, and include age, female sex, weight, uncontrolled hypertension, previous arteriotomy at the same site, type and level of anticoagulation, arterial sheath size, renal failure, concomitant venous sheath, peripheral vascular disease, prolonged sheath duration, and location of the arteriotomy. Arterial puncture below the femoral head may lead to an increased risk of vascular complications (e.g., an arteriovenous fistula, a pseudoaneurysm, or a hematoma).

The hand receives dual circulation from the radial artery and the ulnar artery through the superficial and deep palmar arches (Fig. 12.5). The Allen test assesses the patency of the arch circulation and involves the simultaneous compression of the radial and ulnar arteries at the level of the wrist for 1 to 2 minutes, which leads to pallor of the hand, followed by the release of ulnar compression. The spontaneous return of color to the hand in 5 to 10 seconds indicates patency of the palmar arch. Although theoretically attractive, the Allen test is less widely used now than previously because it has not been shown to correlate with outcomes. The optimal access site for the radial approach is the point of radial artery pulsation, palpated approximately 2 cm proximal to the radial styloid process. Vasospasm is a possible vascular complication of the radial approach because the radial artery is a small-caliber vessel with a relatively large muscular media. To prevent vasospasm, a vasodilator such as verapamil is routinely administered intra-arterially through the sidearm of the sheath after obtaining radial access.

Coronary Artery Cannulation

A standard 0.035-inch, J-tipped guidewire is introduced through the sheath in the access artery and advanced to the ascending aorta. The guidewire is used to guide the coronary catheter to the aortic root, and is always advanced before the catheter to prevent the proximal edges of the catheter from causing vascular damage. Once the proximal end of the catheter is positioned in the root, the guidewire is removed from the catheter and the catheter is connected to the manifold. When the pressure transducer connected to the manifold confirms an appropriate aortic pressure waveform, the catheter is flushed with heparinized saline and loaded with contrast. Using fluoroscopy, the catheter is advanced or withdrawn as it is being rotated until it engages the ostium of the coronary artery. During coronary artery cannulation, the catheter location and pressure tracing should be carefully monitored to ensure that the catheter tip is coaxial with the ostium of the coronary artery and is not either against the arterial wall or obstructing flow in the artery. Coronary angiography is performed with cineradiography during injection of contrast. The left and right coronary arteries are typically cannulated by different catheters (Figs. 12.6 and 12.7). Catheter selection depends on the access site, the coronary artery being investigated, the location of the coronary ostium, the diameter of the aortic root, and operator preference.

In patients with a history of CABG, all bypass conduits should be investigated. Saphenous vein grafts are anastomosed to the anterior wall of the ascending aorta above the sinuses of Valsalva. Several strategies can be used to assist with graft cannulation, including a review of previous postsurgical angiograms, identification of markers that were placed during surgery at the ostium of the saphenous vein grafts, and use of different views (left anterior oblique [LAO] to cannulate grafts to the RCA and right anterior oblique [RAO] to cannulate grafts to the left coronary system).

The left internal mammary artery (LIMA) is routinely used in surgical revascularization and typically arises anteriorly from the left subclavian artery, several centimeters distal to the vertebral artery (Fig. 12.8). A 0.035-inch guidewire is advanced through a catheter into the distal left subclavian artery either when the catheter is in the aorta or after it has been used to cannulate the left subclavian artery. The catheter is advanced into the subclavian artery and then slowly

angiograms, the bifurcation of the CFA occurred below the upper one-third of the femoral head in 99% of patients. The access site can be confirmed under fluoroscopy and/or vascular ultrasound can be used. Arterial puncture above the inguinal ligament may lead to an increased risk of bleeding complications (e.g., a hematoma or retroperitoneal

TABLE 12.1   American Heart Association/American College of Cardiology Foundation Guideline-Recommended Indications for Diagnostic Coronary Angiography

Evaluation of Patients With Stable Ischemic Heart Disease (Suspected or Known)
- Clinical characteristics and/or noninvasive test results that indicate a high likelihood of severe ischemic heart disease
- Intermediate-risk results on noninvasive testing and depressed left ventricular function (ejection fraction <50%)
- Intermediate-risk results on noninvasive testing, preserved left ventricular function (ejection fraction >50%), and decreased quality of life due to angina
- Abnormal results on noninvasive testing in high-risk occupation (e.g., pilot or bus driver)
- Inconclusive results on noninvasive testing
- CCS class III or IV angina, on medical therapy
- Successful resuscitation from sudden cardiac death
- Sustained (>30 sec) monomorphic ventricular tachycardia
- Nonsustained (<30 sec) polymorphic ventricular tachycardia

Evaluation of Patients With Non–ST-Elevation Acute Coronary Syndromes
- Non–ST-elevation acute coronary syndrome with refractory angina, recurrent angina, or ischemia at rest or with low-level activities, hemodynamic or electrical instability, congestive heart failure, or new or worsening mitral regurgitation
- Non–ST-elevation acute coronary syndrome with an intermediate or high risk for adverse clinical events
- Non–ST-elevation acute coronary syndrome with an initial low risk for adverse clinical events and subsequent high-risk results on noninvasive testing

Evaluation of Patients With STEMI
- STEMI and symptom onset within 12 h
- STEMI, symptom onset within 12 to 24 h, and clinical and/or ECG evidence of ongoing ischemia
- STEMI with hemodynamic or electrical instability, congestive heart failure, or cardiogenic shock, irrespective of symptom onset
- STEMI and successful resuscitation from out-of-hospital cardiac arrest, irrespective of symptom onset
- STEMI and intermediate or high-risk findings on noninvasive stress testing, irrespective of symptom onset

Evaluation of Patients With Heart Failure
- Evaluation of cardiogenic shock
- Evaluation of left ventricular systolic dysfunction
- Evaluation episodic congestive heart failure with normal left ventricular systolic function
- Evaluation before and after cardiac transplantation

Evaluation of Patients With Valvular Heart Disease
- Evaluation prior to TAVR, transcatheter balloon aortic valvotomy, or surgical aortic valve replacement or repair in patients with severe aortic stenosis
- Evaluation prior to surgical aortic valve replacement or repair in patients with severe aortic regurgitation
- Evaluation prior to transcatheter mitral valve repair or surgical mitral valve replacement or repair in patients with severe mitral regurgitation
- Evaluation prior to pulmonic or tricuspid valve surgery
- Evaluation of infective endocarditis with evidence of coronary embolization

Evaluation of Patients With Nonvalvular Structural Heart Disease
- Evaluation prior to congenital heart disease intervention in a patient with chest pain, ischemia by noninvasive testing, and/or multiple risk factors for CAD
- Evaluation of hypertrophic cardiomyopathy in patients who have angina despite medical therapy

Evaluation of Patients Before Noncardiac Surgery
- Evaluation prior to aortic surgery
- Intermediate- or high-risk results on noninvasive testing
- Equivocal results on noninvasive testing in intermediate– or high–clinical risk patients undergoing high-risk noncardiac surgery

CAD, Coronary artery disease; *CCS,* Canadian Cardiovascular Society; *STEMI,* ST-elevation myocardial infarction; *TAVR,* transcatheter aortic valve replacement.

withdrawn with gentle counterclockwise rotation (so that the catheter tip faces anteriorly) until it cannulates the LIMA.

Angiographic Views

Comprehensive evaluation of the coronary arteries requires angiography in multiple views to ensure that all vessel segments are visualized without foreshortening or overlap (see Fig. 12.6). Rotating the image intensifier to different positions around the patient allows images to be obtained in different views. Angiographic views consist of a specific projection (e.g., RAO, LAO, or anteroposterior [AP]), with a specific angulation toward the head or foot of the patient (designated as cranial or caudal,

respectively). The most common views for RCA angiography include the RAO projection, LAO projection, and AP projection with cranial angulation (see Figs. 12.6 and 12.7). The most common views for left coronary angiography include the RAO projection with cranial and caudal angulation, the LAO projection with cranial and caudal angulation, and the AP projection with cranial and caudal angulation.

Angiographic Analysis

The essential components of coronary angiographic analysis are listed in Table 12.3. The origin, caliber, course, and branches of all major

Text continued on p. 89

TABLE 12.2 Contraindications to Diagnostic Coronary Angiography

Absolute Contraindication	Relative Contraindications
• Patient refuses to consent to procedure	• Acute renal failure • Chronic kidney disease • Significant electrolyte abnormalities • Digitalis toxicity • Active bleeding • Severe thrombocytopenia • Severe coagulopathy • Uncontrolled hypertension • Decompensated heart failure • Severe aortic stenosis • Aortic valve endocarditis • Active infection • Acute stroke • Allergic reactions to iodinated contrast agents • Severe peripheral vascular disease • Pregnancy • Patients who are unable to cooperate

TABLE 12.3 Comprehensive Angiographic Analysis of Coronary Arteries

Normal Angiographic Findings	Abnormal Angiographic Findings

• Origin of major coronary arteries
• Caliber of coronary arteries
• Course of coronary arteries
• Branches originating from large- and medium-caliber coronary arteries
• Dominance (right, left, or co-dominance)
	• Coronary atherosclerotic plaque
	  • Presence
	  • Location
	  • Length
	  • Degree of narrowing (severity)
	  • Appearance (e.g., eccentricity, thrombus, calcification)
	  • Involvement of side branch
	  • Flow (e.g., TIMI grading scale)
	• Anomalous coronary arteries
	• Myocardial bridging of coronary arteries
	• Presence of collaterals
	• Presence of coronary fistulas
	• Presence of coronary dissections
	• Presence of coronary aneurysms
	• Presence of coronary vasospasm and response to nitroglycerin

TIMI, Thrombolysis in myocardial infarction.

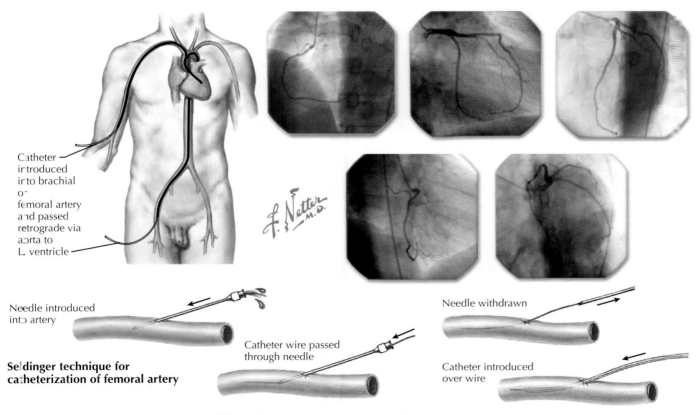

Catheter introduced into brachial or femoral artery and passed retrograde via aorta to L ventricle

Needle introduced into artery

Catheter wire passed through needle

Needle withdrawn

Catheter introduced over wire

Seldinger technique for catheterization of femoral artery

FIG 12.3 Left-sided heart catheterization.

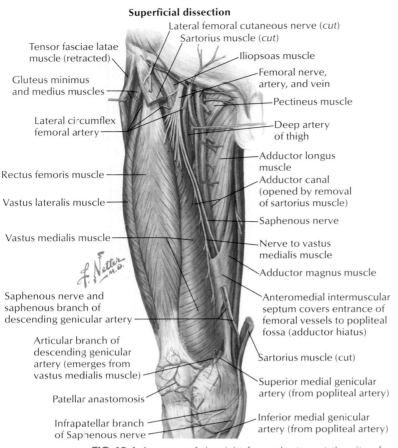

Superficial dissection

Tensor fasciae latae muscle (retracted)

Lateral femoral cutaneous nerve (*cut*)

Sartorius muscle (*cut*)

Iliopsoas muscle

Gluteus minimus and medius muscles

Femoral nerve, artery, and vein

Pectineus muscle

Lateral circumflex femoral artery

Deep artery of thigh

Rectus femoris muscle

Adductor longus muscle

Adductor canal (opened by removal of sartorius muscle)

Vastus lateralis muscle

Saphenous nerve

Vastus medialis muscle

Nerve to vastus medialis muscle

Adductor magnus muscle

Saphenous nerve and saphenous branch of descending genicular artery

Anteromedial intermuscular septum covers entrance of femoral vessels to popliteal fossa (adductor hiatus)

Articular branch of descending genicular artery (emerges from vastus medialis muscle)

Sartorius muscle (cut)

Superior medial genicular artery (from popliteal artery)

Patellar anastomosis

Infrapatellar branch of Saphenous nerve

Inferior medial genicular artery (from popliteal artery)

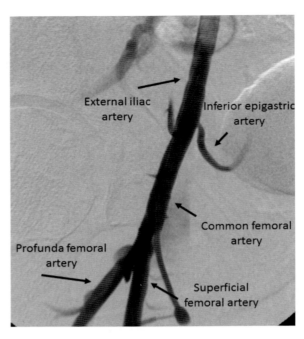

External iliac artery

Inferior epigastric artery

Profunda femoral artery

Common femoral artery

Superficial femoral artery

FIG 12.4 Anatomy of the right femoral artery at the site of vascular access. The image on the right was taken in an RAO projection via a sheath placed in the common femoral artery.

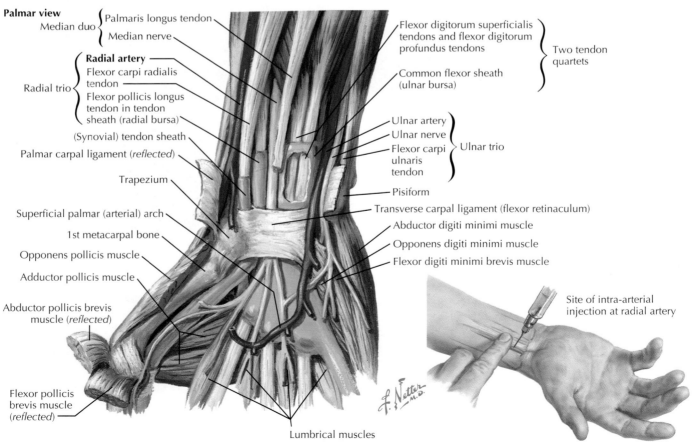

Palmar view

Median duo { Palmaris longus tendon

Median nerve

Flexor digitorum superficialis tendons and flexor digitorum profundus tendons } Two tendon quartets

Radial artery

Radial trio { Flexor carpi radialis tendon

Flexor pollicis longus tendon in tendon sheath (radial bursa)

Common flexor sheath (ulnar bursa)

(Synovial) tendon sheath

Ulnar artery

Ulnar nerve

Palmar carpal ligament (*reflected*)

Flexor carpi ulnaris tendon } Ulnar trio

Trapezium

Pisiform

Superficial palmar (arterial) arch

Transverse carpal ligament (flexor retinaculum)

1st metacarpal bone

Abductor digiti minimi muscle

Opponens pollicis muscle

Opponens digiti minimi muscle

Adductor pollicis muscle

Flexor digiti minimi brevis muscle

Abductor pollicis brevis muscle (*reflected*)

Site of intra-arterial injection at radial artery

Flexor pollicis brevis muscle (*reflected*)

Lumbrical muscles

FIG 12.5 Radial artery access.

Left coronary artery: Left anterior oblique view

Left coronary artery

Circumflex branch

Left anterior descending (anterior interventricular branch)

Diagonal branches of anterior interventricular branch

Atrioventricular branch of circumflex branch

Left marginal branch

Posterolateral branches

(Perforating) interventricular septal branches

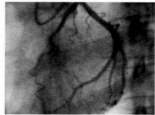

Arteriogram

Left coronary artery: Right anterior oblique view

Left coronary artery

Anterior interventricular branch (left anterior descending)

Circumflex branch

(Perforating) interventricular septal branches

Left marginal branch

Posterolateral branches

Diagonal branch of left anterior descending

Anterior interventricular branch

Atrioventricular branch of circumflex branch

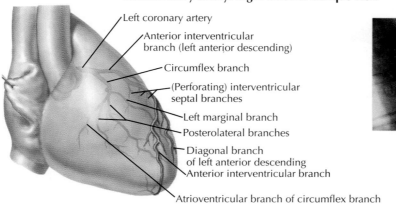

Arteriogram

Right coronary artery: Left anterior oblique view

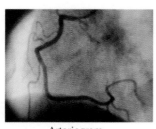

Arteriogram

SA nodal branch

Right coronary artery

AV nodal branch

Branches to back of left ventricle

Right marginal branch

Posterior interventricular branch (posterior descending artery)

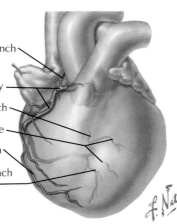

Right coronary artery: Right anterior oblique view

SA nodal branch

Conus (arteriosus) branch

Right coronary artery

Right marginal branch

AV nodal branch

Right posterolateral branches (to back of left ventricle)

Posterior interventricular branch (posterior descending artery)

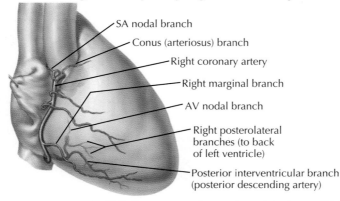

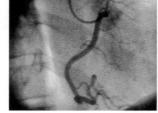

Arteriogram

FIG 12.6 Coronary arteries: angiographic views. *AV,* Atrioventricular; *SA,* sinoatrial.

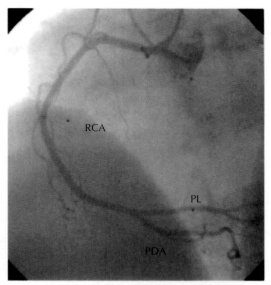

Angiogram of normal RCA and normal PL and PDA branches

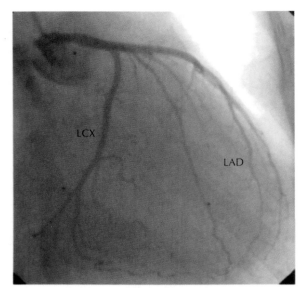

Angiogram of normal LAD coronary artery and LCX artery

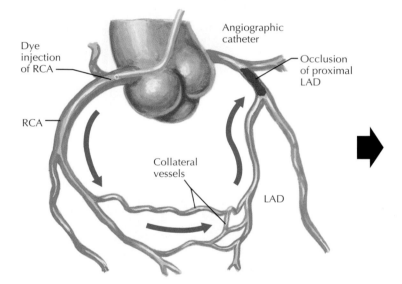

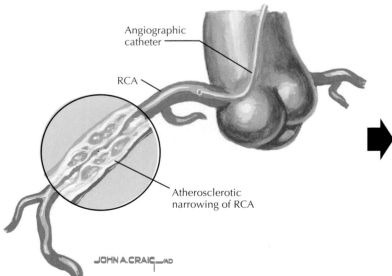

Angiogram demonstrating filling of LAD by dye injected into RCA via collateral vessels

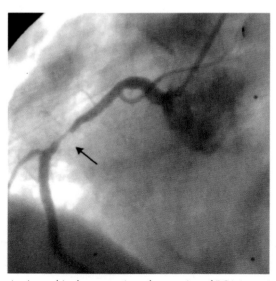

Angiographic demonstration of narrowing of RCA (*arrow*)

FIG 12.7 Normal and abnormal coronary artery findings on angiography. *LAD,* Left anterior descending; *LCX,* left circumflex; *PDA,* pulmonary descending artery; *PL,* posterolateral; *RCA,* right coronary artery.

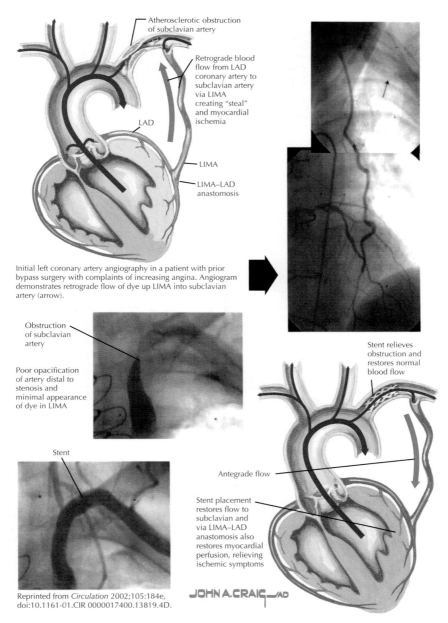

Atherosclerotic obstruction of subclavian artery

Retrograde blood flow from LAD coronary artery to subclavian artery via LIMA creating "steal" and myocardial ischemia

LAD

LIMA

LIMA–LAD anastomosis

Initial left coronary artery angiography in a patient with prior bypass surgery with complaints of increasing angina. Angiogram demonstrates retrograde flow of dye up LIMA into subclavian artery (arrow).

Obstruction of subclavian artery

Poor opacification of artery distal to stenosis and minimal appearance of dye in LIMA

Stent

Stent relieves obstruction and restores normal blood flow

Antegrade flow

Stent placement restores flow to subclavian and via LIMA–LAD anastomosis also restores myocardial perfusion, relieving ischemic symptoms

JOHN A. CRAIG_AD

Reprinted from *Circulation* 2002;105:184e, doi:10.1161-01.CIR 0000017400.13819.4D.

FIG 12.8 Left internal mammary artery *(LIMA)* and subclavian disease. *LAD,* Left anterior descending.

coronary arteries should be identified. The presence, location, severity, and appearance (e.g., eccentricity or calcification) of any atherosclerotic plaque in the major coronary arteries should be described. The severity of luminal narrowing can be quantified by comparing the minimal diameter of the narrowed coronary segment with that of an adjacent normal-appearing reference segment. Although experienced observers are able to visually estimate the degree of stenosis, the severity of the stenosis can be quantified using calipers or quantitative computer angiography. The flow in coronary arteries can be defined using the Thrombolysis In Myocardial Infarction (TIMI) flow grading scale. TIMI 3 flow describes normal flow with complete filling of the distal vessel. TIMI 2 flow describes delayed or sluggish flow with complete filling of the distal vessel. TIMI 1 flow describes faint flow beyond the stenosis with incomplete filling of the distal vessel. TIMI 0 flow describes a completely occluded artery with no distal flow beyond the lesion. The presence of anomalous arteries, myocardial bridging, fistulas,

dissections, aneurysms, and spasm should also be noted. In patients with a history of CABG, graft patency and the presence of competitive flow should be observed. In the setting of total occlusion of a coronary artery, prolonged cineradiography allows the capture of late-filling collateral circulation that may exist (Fig. 12.7). The collaterals can either originate from the occluded artery or a different coronary artery or bypass graft.

LIMITATIONS

Coronary angiography has several limitations in the evaluation of CAD. First, it produces a two-dimensional representation of three-dimensional coronary anatomy. As such, the severity of CAD may be underestimated. Second, coronary angiography delineates the vessel lumen but is unable to provide accurate information about the vessel wall. Angiographic findings of normal vessel lumen cannot exclude underlying disease

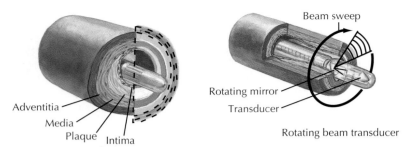

Differences in acoustic sensitivity allow discrimination of vessel wall components

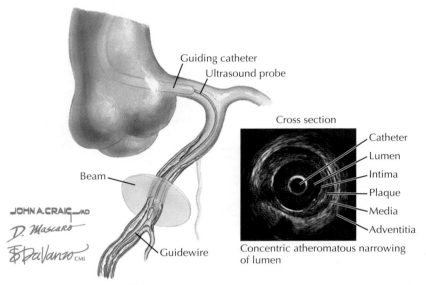

FIG 12.9 Intravascular ultrasound.

of the coronary endothelium. Furthermore, proper interpretation of stenosis severity involves identification of an appropriate reference segment with which to compare the diseased segment; this may prove to be difficult because of the possibility of inaccurate vessel wall delineation.

These limitations have led to advances in technology that can supplement coronary angiographic analysis. Fractional flow reserve (FFR) uses a pressure wire (coronary guidewire attached to a pressure transducer) to measure the intracoronary pressure distal to a stenosis, and compares this distal intracoronary pressure with aortic pressure at rest and during maximal coronary hyperemia (see Chapter 26). FFR is calculated based on this comparison, can help determine the hemodynamic significance of a lesion, and is clinically useful in the assessment of an angiographically intermediate lesion. Intravascular ultrasound (IVUS) uses a catheter with an ultrasound core to provide cross-sectional images in which the three layers (intima, media, and adventitia) of the vessel can be identified and characterized (Fig. 12.9). Optical coherence tomography (OCT) also uses an intracoronary catheter, but with an optical imaging core that provides high-resolution cross-sectional images. OCT and IVUS can be used to assess the size of the artery, the vascular wall and plaque composition, and burden, and can be used to assess and optimize PCI results.

COMPLICATIONS

The major complications that can occur during or immediately after coronary angiography include death, myocardial infarction, and stroke. The risk of major complications is 0.3%. Minor complications include coronary artery dissection, bleeding, vascular complications, arrhythmias, and contrast reactions. The risk of any of these complications is still <2%. Patient comorbidities that increase the risk of complications include acute coronary syndrome, left main CAD, shock, congestive heart failure, severe valvular disease, renal failure, peripheral vascular disease, increased age, and previous anaphylactoid reaction to contrast media. Complication rates from coronary angiography have remained remarkably consistent across registries from the 1980s. Complication rates from PCI have been the focus of more recent registry analysis.

FUTURE DIRECTIONS

Coronary angiography is an effective and safe diagnostic modality for the evaluation of CAD. It forms the basis for revascularization, including PCI and CABG. Newer techniques, better equipment, and the use of radial artery access have increased the safety and efficiency of the procedure. Recently developed diagnostic modalities such as FFR, OCT, and IVUS have supplemented the information provided by angiography.

ADDITIONAL RESOURCES

Amsterdam EA, Wenger NK, Brindis RG, et al. 2014 AHA/ACC guideline for the management of patients with non-ST-elevation acute coronary syndromes: a report of the American College of Cardiology/American Heart Association Task Force on Practice Guidelines. *J Am Coll Cardiol.* 2014;64:e139-e228.
This article outlines the clinical practice guidelines for the management of patients with non-STEMI.

Fihn SD, Gardin JM, Abrams J, et al. 2012 ACCF/AHA/ACP/AATS/PCNA/ SCAI/STS guideline for the diagnosis and management of patients with stable ischemic heart disease: a report of the American College of Cardiology Foundation/American Heart Association Task Force on Practice Guidelines, and the American College of Physicians, American Association for Thoracic Surgery, Preventive Cardiovascular Nurses Association, Society for Cardiovascular Angiography and Interventions, and Society of Thoracic Surgeons. *J Am Coll Cardiol.* 2012;60:e44-e164.
This article outlines the clinical practice guidelines for the diagnosis and management of stable ischemic heart disease.

Lotfi A, Jeremias A, Fearon WF, et al. Expert consensus statement on the use of fractional flow reserve, intravascular ultrasound, and optical coherence tomography: a consensus statement of the Society of Cardiovascular Angiography and Interventions. *Catheter Cardiovasc Interv.* 2014;83:509-518.
This article is an expert consensus statement on the use of adjunctive diagnostic modalities during coronary angiography, including FFR, IVUS, and OCT.

O'Gara PT, Kushner FG, Ascheim DD, et al. 2013 ACCF/AHA guideline for the management of ST-elevation myocardial infarction: a report of the American College of Cardiology Foundation/American Heart Association Task Force on Practice Guidelines. *J Am Coll Cardiol.* 2013;61:e78-e140.
This article outlines the clinical practice guidelines for the management of patients with STEMI.

Scanlon PJ, Faxon DP, Audet AM, et al. ACC/AHA guidelines for coronary angiography. A report of the American College of Cardiology/American Heart Association Task Force on practice guidelines (Committee on Coronary Angiography). Developed in collaboration with the Society for Cardiac Angiography and Interventions. *J Am Coll Cardiol.* 1999;33:1756-1824.
This article outlines the clinical practice guidelines for the use of coronary angiography.

EVIDENCE

Angelini P, Velasco JA, Flamm S. Coronary anomalies: incidence, pathophysiology, and clinical relevance. *Circulation.* 2002;105:2449-2454.
This review article describes various coronary anomalies.

Nissen SE, Yock P. Intravascular ultrasound: novel pathophysiological insights and current clinical applications. *Circulation.* 2001;103:604-616.
This review article describes the evidence and applications of IVUS during coronary angiography.

Pijls NH, de Bruyne B, Peels K, et al. Measurement of fractional flow reserve to assess the functional severity of coronary artery stenosis. *N Engl J Med.* 1996;334:1703-1708.
This study compares the use of FFR to various modalities of stress testing.

13

Left and Right Heart Catheterization

David W. Lee, Allison G. Dupont, Mark E. Boulware, George A. Stouffer

Right and left heart catheterization is the introduction of a catheter into the right heart and left heart chambers, respectively. Right and left heart catheterization provide key hemodynamic data that can be used to diagnose various cardiac disorders. Left heart catheterization also allows for the performance of left ventriculography to assess left ventricular (LV) systolic function and valvular function. This chapter focuses on the procedural techniques, data interpretation, and clinical applications of right and left heart catheterization.

RIGHT HEART CATHETERIZATION

Right heart catheterization generally involves the introduction of a balloon-tipped catheter into the right atrium (RA), right ventricle (RV), and pulmonary artery (PA). The use of an inflatable balloon on the tip enables rapid and safe passage of the catheter through the venous system and right heart chambers; this technique was developed in the 1970s by Dr. Harold Swan, Dr. William Ganz, and colleagues. A PA catheter has a port at the distal tip, a port that is approximately 30 cm proximal from the distal tip, an inflatable balloon at the distal tip, and a thermistor near the distal tip. The distal and proximal ports can be used to transduce pressure, or serve as access for fluids and medications. The balloon can be inflated to temporarily occlude the PA, which allows the distal port to transduce a "wedge" pressure. The thermistor can be used to measure the temperature change of fluid injected into the proximal port; this measurement is used in the calculation of cardiac output.

A comprehensive preprocedural evaluation that includes history, physical examination, routine laboratory data, a 12-lead ECG, and a transthoracic echocardiogram can help guide appropriate patient selection, procedural planning, and data interpretation.

Indications

The American College of Cardiology, the American Heart Association, the American College of Chest Physicians, the American Thoracic Society, the Society of Critical Care Medicine, and the American Society of Anesthesiologists have published guidelines and consensus statements on the indications for right heart catheterization. Box 13.1 lists the common indications for right heart catheterization. Although right heart catheterization is indicated for the diagnostic evaluation of many disease processes, there is much debate on the routine use of PA catheters to guide clinical management of critically ill patients. Several randomized trials have investigated the efficacy and safety of ongoing PA catheter-based clinical management in patients with heart failure, patients who have undergone high-risk noncardiac surgery, and patients with acute respiratory distress syndrome. These studies demonstrated that there is no improvement in survival, and that there is an increased risk of complications in patients randomized to PA catheter-based management. However, these studies have been criticized for their study design,

improper patient selection, and variably experienced physicians who performed the catheter placement and data interpretation. As a result, there is no clear consensus on whether PA catheters are beneficial or harmful for guiding clinical management over time.

Contraindications

There are several absolute contraindications to right heart catheterization. First, lack of informed consent. Patients with a terminal illness in whom an invasive hemodynamic evaluation will not affect treatment or prognosis should not undergo right heart catheterization. Patients with a mechanical prosthetic tricuspid or pulmonic valve are at risk for catheter entrapment within the valve apparatus, and should not undergo right heart catheterization. Finally, patients with right-sided endocarditis, thrombus, or intracardiac tumor should not undergo right heart catheterization. Relative contraindications to right heart catheterization include active infection, active bleeding, severe thrombocytopenia, severe coagulopathy, and underlying left bundle branch block (which increases the risk of complete heart block if the PA catheter causes a right bundle branch block).

Procedural Technique and Data Interpretation

Right heart catheterization can be performed in the cardiac catheterization laboratory, intensive care unit, or operating room. Central venous access can be obtained via percutaneous puncture of the common femoral vein, the internal jugular vein, the brachial vein, or the subclavian vein. Before the procedure, the patency of the access vein should be assessed by vascular ultrasound. The patient is then prepared and draped in the usual sterile fashion. After a time-out is performed and local anesthesia is administered, a needle is introduced into the access vein. A sheath is placed in the access vein by means of the modified Seldinger technique with ultrasound guidance.

A PA catheter is introduced into the venous sheath. When the PA catheter advances beyond the sheath, the distal balloon is inflated, and the PA catheter is advanced into the RA, the RV, and the main PA. Direct fluoroscopic visualization or pressure monitoring can be used to guide advancement of the PA catheter. The pressure waveform in each chamber is carefully examined and recorded before advancing the PA catheter into the next chamber. After the PA catheter has reached the main PA, it is advanced into a distal PA until it has occluded the distal PA. At this point, the pressure transduced from the distal port is defined as the pulmonary capillary wedge pressure (PCWP) and reflects the estimated left atrium (LA) pressure and the LV diastolic pressure (when there is no obstruction between the LA and LV). Once the PCWP is recorded, the balloon is deflated, and the PA catheter is withdrawn back into the proximal PA. Finally, blood samples are collected from the PA to measure the mixed venous saturation.

Right heart catheterization provides the following hemodynamic information through direct measurements and calculations based on

LV, Left ventricular; *MI*, myocardial infarction; *RV*, right ventricular.

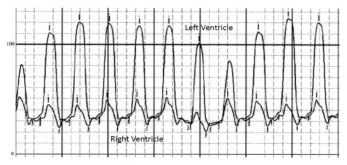

FIG 13.1 Hemodynamic findings in constrictive pericarditis. Simultaneous pressure tracings from the left ventricle and right ventricle. In this patient with constrictive pericarditis, there are elevated and equalized diastolic pressures and discordant right and left ventricular systolic pressures.

these measurements: ventricular preload (RA pressure is a reflection of RV preload, and PCWP is a function of LV preload), ventricular afterload (systemic vascular resistance and pulmonary vascular resistance), and cardiac output. These data can be used to evaluate various disorders, including shock, valvular disease, cardiomyopathy, pericardial disease (Fig. 13.1), and intracardiac shunts (Table 13.1).

The pressures in the vena cavae, RA, RV, PA, and PCWP position can be directly measured with the PA catheter. The mixed venous saturation can also be measured with the PA catheter. The cardiac output (CO) and cardiac index (CI) can be calculated by two methods: the thermodilution method and the Fick method. To calculate CO by the thermodilution method, a substance cooler than blood (typically, room temperature saline) is injected through the proximal port of the PA catheter. As the injected substance passes through the PA, the blood

temperature decreases, and this change is measured by the thermistor at the distal tip of the PA catheter. The change in the temperature over time is used to calculate the CO. The Fick principle, first described by Adolph Fick in 1870, states that the total uptake or release of a substance by an organ is the product of blood flow to that organ and the arteriovenous concentration of the substance. With the use of this principle, pulmonary blood flow can be determined with the arteriovenous difference of oxygen across the lungs and the oxygen consumption. Oxygen consumption can be assumed, but a more accurate measure of CO requires measurement of oxygen consumption. Direct measurement of oxygen consumption can be done with either a Water's hood or a metabolic cart. The CI can then be calculated to compare cardiac performance among patients of various sizes. CI is simply the CO divided by the body surface area (BSA): CI = CO/BSA.

The resistance across the systemic vasculature and the pulmonary vasculature can be calculated with the preceding hemodynamic information. Systemic vascular resistance (SVR) is a measure of systemic afterload. The equation for SVR is as follows: SVR = (MAP – CVP)/(CO × 80), where MAP is mean arterial pressure; CVP is central venous pressure; CO is cardiac output; and 80 is a correction factor to convert units for SVR to dynes/s/cm^5. The pulmonary vascular resistance (PVR) can be calculated in a manner similar to the SVR substituting (mean PA pressure – PCWP) in place of (MAP – CVP) in the preceding equation. The PVR is sometimes reported in Wood units, which is calculated as PVR = (mean PA pressure – PCWP)/80.

Complications

There are three categories of potential complications: (1) complications associated with central venous access (e.g., bleeding, infection, and pneumothorax); (2) PA catheter–associated complications; and (3) misinterpretation of the acquired data. Venous access complications related to PA catheter placement are not any different from those associated with any procedure that involves percutaneous access of central veins. Specific PA catheter–associated complications include the following. (1) Atrial and ventricular arrhythmias or complete heart block as the PA catheter is advanced through the right heart chambers. These rhythm disturbances are typically self-limited and resolve after changing the catheter position. As the PA catheter crosses the tricuspid valve, it can cause trauma to the right bundle, leading to right bundle branch block, which is usually transient. If the patient has a preexisting left bundle branch block and develops a PA catheter–induced right bundle branch block, the patient can develop transient complete heart block. For this reason, in patients with a left bundle branch block, temporary pacing capabilities should be readily available in the event that complete heart block occurs. (2) Direct damage to the tricuspid or pulmonic valve, catheter-associated endocarditis of either valve, and catheter-associated thrombus formation, which leads to an increased risk of pulmonary embolus and infarction. Pulmonary infarction can also occur from prolonged inflation of the balloon within a branch of the PA. (3) The complication with the highest mortality rate is rupture of a PA due to either overinflation of the distal balloon or repeated trauma to the PA. PA rupture is fatal in approximately 50% of cases. Although rare, this complication occurs most commonly in patients with PA hypertension. Other factors increasing the risk of PA rupture include advanced age, female sex, and frequent wedging of the balloon

LEFT HEART CATHETERIZATION

Left heart catheterization is distinct from coronary angiography which involves the cannulation and interrogation of the coronary arteries. Patients who undergo coronary angiography or right heart catheterization typically also undergo left heart catheterization as part of a

TABLE 13.1 Hemodynamic Profiles of Specific Clinical Situations

Clinical Situation	Catheterization Findings
Vasodilatory shock	Elevated CO, decreased SVR, decreased PCWP
Cardiogenic shock	Decreased CO, increased SVR, increased PCWP
Mitral stenosis	Increased LA pressure (PCWP) with a gradient between the LA (PCWP) and the LV (LVEDP) that persists throughout diastole, increased right heart pressures at rest and/or with exercise, prominent *a* wave on a RA tracing, decreased slope of *y* descent
Mitral regurgitation	Acute MR: elevated PCWP, elevated PA pressure, prominent *v* wave, hyperdynamic LV function; hemodynamics can mimic constrictive pericarditis, may have hypotension/shock
	Chronic, compensated MR: normal to mildly elevated right heart pressures, *v* wave less prominent, normal EF
	Chronic, decompensated MR: elevated PCWP, elevated PA pressure, elevated right heart pressures, decreased EF
Restrictive cardiomyopathy	PA systolic pressure may be >50 mm Hg, RV/LV systolic pressure concordant, RVEDP/LVEDP separation >5 mm Hg, pronounced *y* descent, RVEDP/RV systolic pressure <1/3, dip and plateau in RV pressure, Kussmaul sign absent
Constrictive pericarditis	Elevated RA pressure, elevated PCWP, PA systolic pressure usually <50 mm Hg, RV/LV systolic pressure discordant, RVEDP/LVEDP separation <5 mm Hg, pronounced *y* descent, RVEDP/RV systolic pressure >1/3, dip and plateau in RV pressure, Kussmaul sign present
Cardiac tamponade	Elevated diastolic pressures and equalization of end-diastolic pressures, *x* descent preserved or prominent and *y* descent small or absent on RA pressure tracing, no dip and plateau on RV pressure tracing, pulsus paradoxus
Dilated cardiomyopathy	Right and left heart filling pressures typically elevated, decreased CO and index, decreased mixed venous oxygen saturation, pulsus alternans (beat-to-beat variation in systolic pressure)
Hypertrophic obstructive cardiomyopathy	Spike and dome arterial pulse, systolic intraventricular pressure gradient, elevated LVEDP, Brockenbrough sign (aortic pulse pressure does not increase after PVC)
Aortic stenosis	Pressure gradient between the LV and aorta, elevated LVEDP, elevated PCWP, elevated PA pressures as resultant heart failure progresses, LV/aortic gradient decreases with reduction in preload, and pulse pressure increases after a PVC (negative Brockenbrough sign), Carabello sign (a rise in peak aortic systolic pressure by >5 mm Hg when a catheter is removed from the LV) in severe aortic stenosis
Aortic insufficiency	Wide pulse pressure, low aortic diastolic pressure, elevated LVEDP; in severe aortic insufficiency, the LV and aortic pressures will be equal at the end of diastole and there will be premature closure of the mitral valve during diastole.

CO, Cardiac output; *EF,* ejection fraction; *LA,* left atrium (atrial); *LV,* left ventricle (ventricular); *LVEDP,* left ventricular end-diastolic pressure; *MR,* mitral regurgitation; *PA,* pulmonary artery (arterial); *PCWP,* pulmonary capillary wedge pressure; *PVC,* premature ventricular contraction; *RA,* right atrium (atrial); *RV,* right ventricle (ventricular); *RVEDP,* right ventricular end-diastolic pressure; *SVR,* systemic vascular resistance.

comprehensive hemodynamic evaluation. The common indications for left heart catheterization include the evaluation of LV hemodynamics, LV systolic function, cardiomyopathy, valvular disease (e.g., aortic stenosis or mitral regurgitation), and intracardiac shunts (e.g., ventricular septal defects). The absolute contraindications for left heart catheterization include patient refusal, known or suspected LV thrombus, and mechanical prosthetic aortic valves. The relative contraindications for left heart catheterization include active bleeding, severe thrombocytopenia, severe coagulopathy, active infection, severe peripheral vascular disease, pregnancy, and patient inability to cooperate.

Procedural Technique and Data Interpretation

Left heart catheterization is routinely performed in the cardiac catheterization laboratory. Arterial access is obtained via percutaneous puncture of the common femoral artery, brachial artery, or the radial artery, as described in Chapter 18. A standard 0.035-inch, J-tipped guidewire is introduced into the access artery and is used to guide the catheter to the ascending aorta. The most common catheters that are used in left heart catheterization are the pigtail catheter and the Judkins right (JR) catheter. Each catheter requires a specific technique to cross the aortic valve and enter the LV. A pigtail catheter is rotated to make the pigtail resemble a "6" and is gently advanced until it pushes against the aortic valve and prolapses into the LV. When the JR catheter is used, the catheter is advanced several centimeters above the aortic valve and rotated so that the distal curve points between 4:00 and 6:00 o'clock. The guidewire is then advanced across the aortic valve, and the JR catheter is advanced into the LV over the wire. The typical radiographic

view for crossing the aortic valve is the right anterior oblique (RAO) projection.

Once the catheter has crossed the aortic valve, the distal end of the catheter is positioned in the mid-cavity of the LV. The guidewire is removed, and the catheter is connected to a manifold with a pressure transducer. The LV pressure waveform is carefully examined and recorded. In particular, the LV peak systolic pressure and the LV end-diastolic pressure are noted (Fig. 13.2). Right heart catheterization with simultaneous recording of right-sided pressures can help further define specific hemodynamic profiles (Table 13.1).

Left heart catheterization is also useful in determining the presence and etiology of a LV outflow tract pressure gradient. A pressure difference between the LV apex and the aorta can be caused by a fixed obstruction at the subvalvular, valvular, or supravalvular level; or by a dynamic obstruction of the LV outflow tract in patients with hypertrophic obstructive cardiomyopathy (Fig. 13.3). A pressure gradient can be measured by several methods: a "pullback" across the aortic valve in which the catheter is slowly retracted from the LV into the aorta; a recording of simultaneous LV and femoral arterial pressure (used as a surrogate for aortic pressure); and a recording of simultaneous LV and aortic pressure (with a dual-lumen catheter with one lumen in the LV and the other lumen in the aorta). In all of these methods, the location of the obstruction can be estimated by slowly retracting an end-hole catheter from the LV apex and noting where the pressure decreases. Dynamic LV outflow tract obstruction, which can occur in the setting of massive septal hypertrophy with or without systolic anterior motion of the mitral valve, can be provoked by means of various maneuvers that decrease either preload

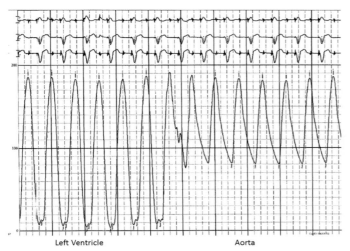

FIG 13.2 Pressure tracing during catheter pullback from the left ventricle to the aorta.

and/or afterload (e.g., Valsalva maneuver or administration of nitroglycerin), or that increase contractility (e.g., isoproterenol infusion or inducing a premature ventricular contraction).

After hemodynamic assessment, left ventriculography can be performed to estimate the LV ejection fraction, examine function of specific LV walls, measure the presence and severity of mitral regurgitation, and identify any ventricular septal defects. Left ventriculography is performed with cineradiography, and simultaneous power or manual injection of contrast. The typical angiographic views for left ventriculography are the RAO and the left anterior oblique (LAO) projections (Fig. 13.4). The RAO projection provides the best visualization of the inferior, apical, and anterior walls. The LAO projection provides the best visualization of the septal, lateral, and posterior walls, as well as the LV outflow tract and the aortic root. By convention, mitral valve regurgitation is quantified by observing the degree of opacification of the left atrium relative to the LV (Fig. 13.5). Mitral regurgitation is graded as follows:

1+: Contrast does not opacify the entire LA and clears with every heartbeat.

2+: The entire LA is faintly opacified to a degree less than that of the LV after several beats, and it is not cleared by a single beat.

3+: The LA is completely opacified, and the degree of opacification equals that of the LV.

4+: The LA is completely opacified in a single beat, and the opacification increases with each beat. In addition, in 4+ mitral regurgitation, contrast can be seen filling the pulmonary veins.

FUTURE DIRECTIONS

Right and left heart catheterizations have been used in the diagnosis of heart disease for >50 years. The procedural technique and equipment have advanced to the point in which it is a safe and effective procedure that is commonly used in cardiac catheterization laboratories. Current research efforts are focused on obtaining a better understanding of the natural history of hemodynamic changes in patients with congenital, valvular, and cardiomyopathic conditions, and in developing devices to treat structural heart disease. Examples of devices under development or in clinical use include percutaneous valves (aortic, mitral, and pulmonic), septal defect occluders (for atrial septal defects, patent foramen ovale, and ventricular septal defects), atrial appendage occluders (to reduce the risk of thromboembolism in patients with atrial fibrillation), and advanced intracardiac imaging devices (e.g., intracardiac echocardiography).

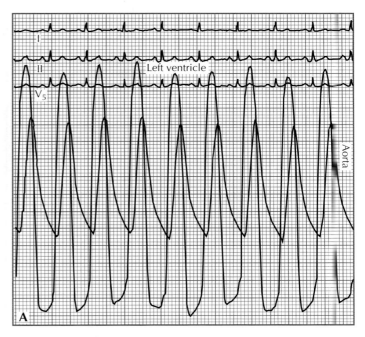

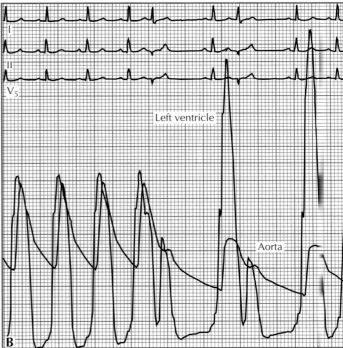

FIG 13.3 Simultaneous pressure tracings from the left ventricular apex and aorta in (A) aortic stenosis and (B) hypertrophic obstructive cardiomyopathy. In this patient with aortic stenosis, there is an approximate 40 mm Hg pressure change across the aortic valve. In the patient with hypertrophic obstructive cardiomyopathy, there is minimal pressure difference at baseline. After a premature ventricular contraction, the left ventricular systolic pressure exceeds aortic systolic pressure by >100 mm Hg. In the first sinus rhythm beat after a premature ventricular contraction, there is a decrease in aortic pulse pressure as compared with the last sinus beat before the premature ventricular contraction. This is known as the Brockenbrough-Braunwald-Morrow sign.

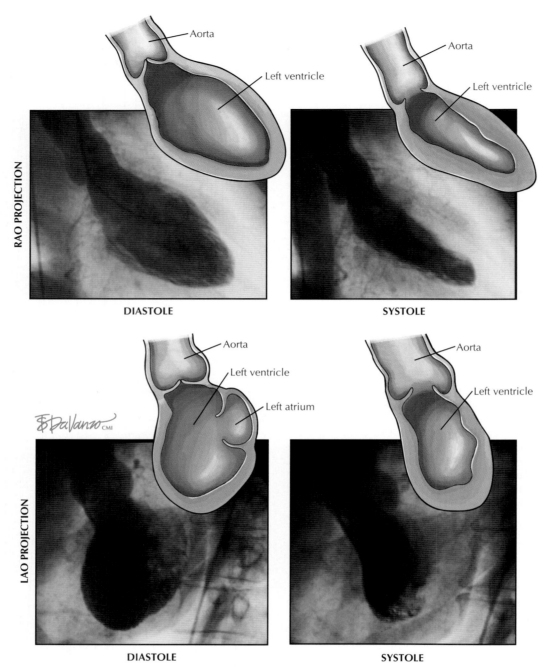

FIG 13.4 Measurement of Left Ventricular Function With Ventriculography. *LAO,* Left anterior oblique; *RAO,* right anterior oblique.

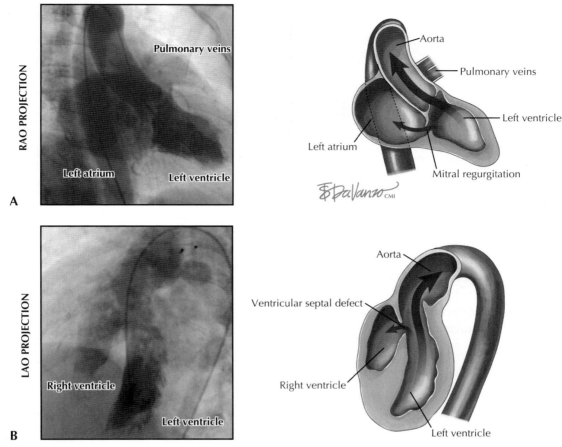

FIG 13.5 (A) Contrast injection into the left ventricle in a patient with severe mitral regurgitation (right anterior oblique *[RAO]* projection; note opacification of the left atrium and pulmonary veins). (B) Contrast injection into the left ventricle in a patient with a ventricular septal defect (left anterior oblique projection *[LAO]*; note that the right ventricle is opacified).

ADDITIONAL RESOURCES

American Society of Anesthesiologists Task Force on Pulmonary Artery Catheterization. Practice guidelines for pulmonary artery catheterization: an updated report by the American Society of Anesthesiologists Task Force on Pulmonary Artery Catheterization. *Anesthesiology.* 2003;99:988–1014.
Guidelines from the American Society of Anesthesiologists.

Bernard GR, Sopko G, Cerra F, et al. Pulmonary artery catheterization and clinical outcomes: National Heart, Lung, and Blood Institute and Food and Drug Administration Workshop Report. Consensus Statement. *JAMA.* 2000;283:2568–2572.
Consensus statement from the National Heart, Lung, and Blood Institute and Food and Drug Administration.

Mueller HS, Chatterjee K, Davis KB, et al. ACC expert consensus document. Present use of bedside right heart catheterization in patients with cardiac disease. American College of Cardiology. *J Am Coll Cardiol.* 1998;32:840–864.
Consensus statement from the American College of Cardiology.

Pulmonary Artery Catheter Consensus conference: consensus statement. *Crit Care Med.* 1997;25:910–925.
Consensus statement from members of the American College of Chest Physicians, the American Thoracic Society, the American College of Critical Care Medicine, the Society of Critical Care Medicine, the European Society of Intensive Care Medicine, and the American Association of Critical Care Nurses.

Stouffer GA, ed. *Cardiovascular Hemodynamics for the Clinician.* London: Blackwell Publishing; 2007.
This book provides an overview of normal cardiovascular hemodynamics and the hemodynamic changes found in various disorders, including valvular, congenital, myopathic, and ischemic heart disease.

EVIDENCE

Shah MR, Hasselblad V, Stevenson LW, et al. Impact of the pulmonary artery catheter in critically ill patients: meta-analysis of randomized clinical trials. *JAMA.* 2005;294:1664–1670.
A meta-analysis of studies that investigated clinical outcomes in patients who underwent right heart catheterization.

Swan HJ, Ganz W, Forrester J, et al. Catheterization of the heart in man with use of a flow-directed balloon-tipped catheter. *N Engl J Med.* 1970;283:447–451.
The original description of the balloon-tipped right heart catheter.

Vascular Biology and Risk Factors for Coronary Artery Disease

14

Angiogenesis and Atherosclerosis

Xuming Dai, Cam Patterson

Revascularization via coronary artery bypass surgery and percutaneous coronary intervention (PCI) remains the definitive therapy for patients with refractory ischemic heart disease, particularly when accompanied by left ventricular (LV) dysfunction. In particular, bypass surgery reduces mortality in patients with multivessel coronary artery disease and LV dysfunction. However, the surgery itself is invasive and is associated with significant mortality and morbidity. In fact, 37% of patients who undergo surgery are found to have one or more coronary vessels that are not technically suitable for bypass grafting. In addition, many patients are poor candidates for bypass based on their coronary anatomy, coexisting conditions, or the severity of their heart failure. Likewise, anatomic complications may make PCI (e.g., balloon angioplasty and stent implantation) a poor choice for many of these patients. Up to 10% to 30% of patients with angina pectoris and obstructive coronary artery disease who undergo cardiac catheterization cannot be treated with either coronary artery or PCI due to diffuse obstructive coronary artery disease. Therefore there is a substantial need for an alternative means of revascularization. The identification of endogenous pathways that regulate angiogenesis—the growth of new blood vessels from existing vessels—has fostered the intriguing hypothesis that if angiogenesis could be promoted in a controlled manner, endogenous pathways could be stimulated to augment blood vessel formation and revascularize tissues in myocardial ischemic zones.

MECHANISMS OF ANGIOGENESIS

Angiogenesis occurs by the budding of new blood vessels from existing vessels (Fig. 14.1). Inflammation and hypoxia are the two major stimuli for new vessel growth. Hypoxia regulates angiogenesis predominantly by activating transcription factors, hypoxia-inducible factors (HIF) 1 and 2, which, in turn, activate the angiogenesis gene expression cascades, including vascular endothelial growth factor (VEGF), platelet growth factor, angiopoietin 1 and 2, as well as stromal cell-derived factor 1α. Based on this concept, HIF-1 promotes sprouting of blood vessels and neovascularization by homing of stem cells and enhancing vascular endothelial cell proliferation. HIF-2 mediates vascular maintenance. Inflammation stimulates angiogenesis mainly by the secretion of inflammatory cytokines derived primarily from macrophages. In either of these events, the result is production of VEGF and other potent angiogenic peptides. VEGF interacts with specific receptors on endothelial cells that, in turn, activate pathways to break down the extracellular matrix and stimulate proliferation and migration toward an angiogenic stimulus and recruitment of stem cells, pericytes, and smooth muscle cells to establish the three-dimensional structure of a blood vessel. After making appropriate connections with the vascular system, the newly formed vessel is capable of maintaining blood flow and providing oxygen to the tissue in need.

Angiogenesis occurs in numerous circumstances, some of which are necessary for normal development and organ function. In other circumstances, angiogenesis is a maladaptive response to local injury or stress. During development, the formation of every organ system is dependent on angiogenic events; the cardiovascular system is the first organ system to function during embryogenesis. In women, the menstrual cycle is dependent on cyclic angiogenesis that is stimulated in part by reproductive hormones. However, most angiogenesis in adults occurs in pathological conditions or as a response to injury. Tumor growth and metastasis, diabetic vascular disease (including retinopathy), inflammatory arthritides, and wound healing are some of the processes that depend on angiogenesis. In addition, the invasion of ischemic tissues with new capillaries and the development of a collateral circulation to supply occluded vessels, which may occur in chronic obstructive coronary disease, are angiogenic processes.

ANGIOGENESIS AND ATHEROSCLEROSIS

The response to ischemia in organs such as the heart involves angiogenic events that increase perfusion to the compromised tissue. Thus it is ironic that atherosclerosis (the most common cause of myocardial ischemia) is itself an angiogenesis-dependent process. The possibility that neovascularization contributes to the pathophysiology of atherosclerosis surfaced when cinefluorography demonstrated the presence of rich networks of vessels surrounding human atherosclerotic plaques. Diffusion of oxygen and other nutrients is limited to 100 μm from the lumen of the blood vessel and is adequate to nourish the inner media and intimal layers in normal arteries. The media of arteries remains avascular until a critical width is achieved, beyond which vascularization is necessary for medial nutrition. As vessel wall thickness increases in the setting of vascular disease, proliferation of the vasa vasorum and intimal neovascularization is observed. Increased blood flow within atherosclerotic lesions is due to new growth of medial vessels and not to dilation of existing vessels. New vessels in atherosclerotic lesions form primarily by branching from the adventitial vasa vasorum.

Neovascularization may contribute to the clinical consequences of atherosclerosis by several mechanisms. Neovascularization provides a source of nutrients, growth factors, and vasoactive molecules to cells within the media and the neointima, which is evident from the association between neovascularization of atherosclerotic lesions and proliferation of adjacent smooth muscle cells. Intimal hemorrhage, which is associated with plaque instability, is due to rupture of the rich network of friable new capillaries surrounding lesions. Regulation of blood flow through plaque microvessels may contribute to the pathophysiology of vasospasm in advanced lesions. Vascular wall remodeling also seems to be related to neovascularization. Finally, neovascularization within human atherosclerotic lesions is associated with expression of adhesion molecules, which is strongly related to neointimal inflammatory cell recruitment. Increasingly, accumulating histopathological data have associated plaque angiogenesis with more rapidly progressive and unstable vascular disease. Microvessel density is greatest in vulnerable atheroma plaques characterized with marked macrophage infiltration of the fibrous cap, thin cap, and large lipid-rich core. The presence of angiogenesis

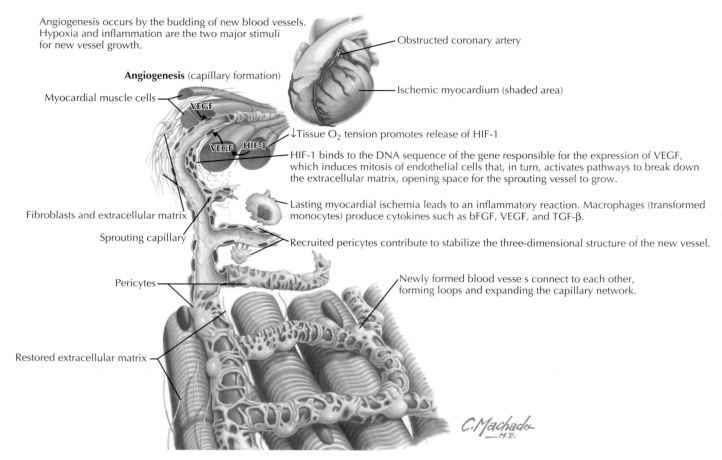

Angiogenesis occurs by the budding of new blood vessels. Hypoxia and inflammation are the two major stimuli for new vessel growth.

Angiogenesis (capillary formation)

Myocardial muscle cells

VEGF

VEGF HIF-1

Fibroblasts and extracellular matrix

Sprouting capillary

Pericytes

Restored extracellular matrix

Obstructed coronary artery

Ischemic myocardium (shaded area)

↓Tissue O₂ tension promotes release of HIF-1

HIF-1 binds to the DNA sequence of the gene responsible for the expression of VEGF, which induces mitosis of endothelial cells that, in turn, activates pathways to break down the extracellular matrix, opening space for the sprouting vessel to grow.

Lasting myocardial ischemia leads to an inflammatory reaction. Macrophages (transformed monocytes) produce cytokines such as bFGF, VEGF, and TGF-β.

Recruited pericytes contribute to stabilize the three-dimensional structure of the new vessel.

Newly formed blood vessels connect to each other, forming loops and expanding the capillary network.

FIG 14.1 Mechanisms of Angiogenesis. *bFGF*, Basic fibroblast growth factor; *HIF-1*, hypoxia inducible factor; *TGF-β*, transforming growth factor beta; *VEGF*, vascular endothelial growth factor.

at the base of the plaque has been independently correlated with plaque rupture, underscoring the potential for a direct contributory role of neovascularization in this process. Antiangiogenesis therapy is understandably an attractive concept that targets inhibition of microvessel formation and/or function within atherosclerotic plaque. Although >300 angiogenesis inhibitors have been identified and >80 are being tested in clinical studies for cancer therapy, the greatest concern regarding the use of angiogenesis inhibitors to treat atherosclerosis is the potential aggravation of preexisting myocardial ischemia caused by inhibition of beneficial angiogenesis in the setting of ischemic heart disease.

ANGIOGENESIS AND ISCHEMIC HEART DISEASE

Refractory coronary ischemia, particularly in patients with decreased LV function who may not be candidates for revascularization, remains a difficult clinical problem. Recognition of angiogenesis as an endogenous mechanism for perfusion of ischemic tissues raises the possibility that angiogenic factors or cells that produce them might be therapeutic tools for patients with refractory ischemia. Angiogenesis seems to be amenable to gene therapy approaches. Although gene therapy may induce angiogenesis and improve perfusion in a wide spectrum of animal models of ischemia, thus far the usefulness of these approaches in humans has been limited. New vessel growth is a process that occurs over weeks to months (precluding single-dose therapies). However, after new vessels form, they are not likely to regress if they are conduit vessels; therefore long-term therapy may not be necessary. Gene delivery by plasmids and adenoviruses can be directed to occur within this "angiogenic

window," raising hope for angiogenic gene therapies in chronic ischemic syndromes.

Gene therapy approaches to deliver VEGF to patients with ischemic coronary and peripheral vascular diseases have progressed, albeit not at the rates hoped for based on initial investigations in the 1990s. The use of angiogenic gene therapy still has tremendous potential for patients with refractory ischemic heart disease who otherwise have no options. Because angiogenesis is a new mechanism for treating this disease, it should be additive to the effects of pharmacological agents (β-blockers, aspirin, and nitrates). The possibility of the creation of new, long-lived conduit vessels offers the potential for a "cure" because these new vessels could provide relief long after the effects of VEGF or other angiogenic factors have dissipated.

However, it is not yet clear that angiogenesis, which predominantly involves the formation of new capillaries, creates vessels with the capacity to significantly increase blood flow to ischemic tissues. Uncontrolled capillary growth may cause hemangioma formation, which would not be beneficial and might be deleterious. Few data are available that allow prediction of the appropriate dose, location, and duration of angiogenic gene therapy. In therapy for myocardial ischemia, required invasive approaches are associated with appreciable morbidity. Despite predictions of side effects based on diseases with known angiogenic components, little is known about side effects of angiogenic therapies in humans. Of greatest concern is the possibility that angiogenic therapies will accelerate or unmask occult tumors or metastases, because it is well known that tumor growth is an angiogenesis-dependent process. Worsening diabetic neovascular complications, especially diabetic retinopathy,

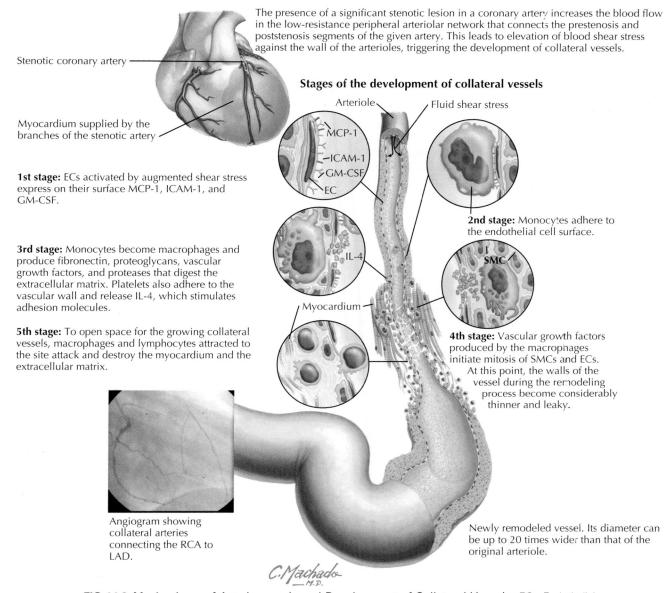

The presence of a significant stenotic lesion in a coronary artery increases the blood flow in the low-resistance peripheral arteriolar network that connects the prestenosis and poststenosis segments of the given artery. This leads to elevation of blood shear stress against the wall of the arterioles, triggering the development of collateral vessels.

Stenotic coronary artery

Myocardium supplied by the branches of the stenotic artery

Stages of the development of collateral vessels

Arteriole Fluid shear stress

MCP-1
ICAM-1
GM-CSF
EC

1st stage: ECs activated by augmented shear stress express on their surface MCP-1, ICAM-1, and GM-CSF.

2nd stage: Monocytes adhere to the endothelial cell surface.

3rd stage: Monocytes become macrophages and produce fibronectin, proteoglycans, vascular growth factors, and proteases that digest the extracellular matrix. Platelets also adhere to the vascular wall and release IL-4, which stimulates adhesion molecules.

IL-4

SMC

5th stage: To open space for the growing collateral vessels, macrophages and lymphocytes attracted to the site attack and destroy the myocardium and the extracellular matrix.

Myocardium

4th stage: Vascular growth factors produced by the macrophages initiate mitosis of SMCs and ECs. At this point, the walls of the vessel during the remodeling process become considerably thinner and leaky.

Angiogram showing collateral arteries connecting the RCA to LAD.

Newly remodeled vessel. Its diameter can be up to 20 times wider than that of the original arteriole.

C. Machado
M.D.

FIG 14.2 Mechanisms of Arteriogenesis and Development of Collateral Vessels. *ECs,* Endothelial cells; *GM-CSF,* granulocyte macrophage colony-stimulating factor; *ICAM-1,* intercellular adhesion molecule 1; *IL-4,* interleukin-4; *LAD,* left anterior descending artery; *MCP-1,* monocyte chemotactic protein 1; *RCA,* right coronary artery; *SMCs,* smooth muscle cells.

are also a concern, because of the prevalence of diabetes in patients with severe atherosclerotic disease.

Early clinical trials in angiogenesis have produced results that are variably interpreted, depending on the views of those reviewing these studies. Small, but statistically significant, improvements in pain-free exercise duration have been demonstrated in angiogenesis trials involving the coronary vasculature (with chest pain as the limiting symptom) and the peripheral vasculature (in patients with limiting claudication). These data support the concept of clinical angiogenesis. An opposing view is that because the improvements are modest, these studies have fallen short of demonstrating an important clinical benefit; moreover, thus far, no studies have shown an effect on mortality or major morbidity.

Whether angiogenesis is an effective approach, how and when to apply angiogenic agents, and the possible side effects of angiogenic stimulants are still under investigation. Long-term studies are necessary to definitively exclude adverse consequences (e.g., tumor promotion).

VASCULOGENESIS AND ARTERIOGENESIS: ALTERNATIVES TO ANGIOGENESIS

New vessel growth in chronic ischemic syndromes is an attractive idea. Fortunately, more than one mechanism exists to create new blood vessels. Angiogenesis is the creation of blood vessels from sprouts off the existing vessels. In contrast, vasculogenesis is the creation of de novo blood vessels by differentiation of new blood cells. Endothelial cell precursors in the bone marrow and circulating in the bloodstream can integrate into developing vessels and contribute to vessel growth in a manner similar to the vasculogenesis of embryonic development. The therapeutic potential of these cells has not been tested, but they can be recruited from bone marrow and may be a means to accelerate endogenous revascularization in patients with ischemia.

In contrast to angiogenesis, arteriogenesis or collaterogenesis is the recruitment of existing vessels to increase their capacity and consequent blood flow to ischemic tissue (Fig. 14.2). Arteriogenesis represents the maturation of vessels that exist but that may not contribute significantly to regional blood flow until properly stimulated. Most collateral vessels visualized by arteriography are probably vessels that have undergone arteriogenesis instead of angiogenesis. Because arteriogenesis creates capacitance vessels, this process is more likely to increase blood supply in a way that substantially affects tissue perfusion. The proteins that affect arteriogenesis are distinct from those that regulate angiogenesis. VEGF does not seem to be important for arteriogenesis, whereas macrophage-derived factors are necessary. The therapeutic potential of arteriogenesis has not been tested, but because of the role of arteriogenesis in collateral formation in patients with chronic myocardial ischemia, arteriogenesis represents another potential therapeutic tool for the creation of new blood vessels in patients with refractory angina.

FUTURE DIRECTIONS

Despite the range of therapies for patients with coronary atherosclerosis, there is still a large population of patients who are not adequately treated or in whom revascularization by bypass surgery or PCI is not feasible because of coronary anatomy or other comorbidities. The creation of new blood vessels to increase tissue perfusion is one way to alleviate myocardial ischemia. The challenge is to determine the best way to increase tissue perfusion with minimal side effects. Angiogenic agents such as VEGF and stem cell transplantation have the lead in the development of novel therapeutic agents and approaches, although their overall benefit remains unproven. It is likely that other therapies designed to stimulate vasculogenesis and arteriogenesis will be evaluated in this patient population. Treatments designed to enhance blood vessel growth are being tested on patients with otherwise refractory disease, but eventually these approaches could be applied to any patient with ischemic heart disease and could even obviate the need for revascularization procedures in a significant cohort of patients.

ADDITIONAL RESOURCES

Folkman J. Angiogenesis. *Annu Rev Med.* 2006;57:1–18.

This review provides a broad overview of the role of angiogenesis in a variety of physiological and pathological processes, including cardiovascular diseases.

Freedman SB, Isner J. Therapeutic angiogenesis for coronary artery disease. *Ann Intern Med.* 2002;136:54–71.

This review summarizes potential roles for targeting angiogenesis therapeutically to treat or prevent complications of atherosclerosis.

Henning RJ. Therapeutic angiogenesis: angiogenic growth factors for ischemic heart disease. *Future Cardiol.* 2016;12(5):585–599.

This paper reviewed the paracrine mechanisms of angiogenesis and clinical trials that explored the effectiveness of therapeutic angiogenesis in ischemic heart disease.

EVIDENCE

Doyle B, Caplice N. Plaque neovascularization and antiangiogenic therapy for atherosclerosis. *J Am Coll Cardiol.* 2007;49(21):2073–2080.

This review summarizes the mechanisms and impact of neovascularization in atherosclerosis and discusses the concept of antiangiogenic therapy of atherosclerosis using angiogenesis inhibitors.

Hou L, Kim JJ, Woo YJ, Huang NF. Stem cell-based therapies to promote angiogenesis in ischemic cardiovascular disease. *Am J Physiol Heart Circ Physiol.* 2016;310(4):H455–H465.

This review summarizes the current status of using stem cells as therapeutic angiogenesis for treatment of ischemic limb and heart disease.

Virmani R, Kolodgie FD, Burke AP. Atherosclerotic plaque progression and vulnerability: angiogenesis as a source of intraplaque hemorrhage. *Arterioscler Thromb Vasc Biol.* 2005;25:2054–2061.

This review discusses the specific role of intraplaque angiogenesis in plaque destabilization via its effect on enhancing hemorrhages within atherosclerotic lesions, and the potential adverse consequences of enhancing angiogenesis as a therapeutic strategy for cardiovascular diseases.

15

Hypertension

Alan L. Hinderliter, Raven A. Voora, Romulo E. Colindres

Hypertension, or high blood pressure (BP), is a major risk factor for atherosclerotic cardiovascular disease (Box 15.1). Despite advances in the understanding of the pathophysiology, epidemiology, and natural history of hypertension, as well as improvements in therapy, many patients with hypertension are undiagnosed or inadequately treated. Hypertension remains an important contributor to coronary events, heart failure, stroke, and end-stage kidney disease.

BP is a continuous variable, and any BP level chosen to define hypertension is arbitrary. For years, hypertension was generally defined as an office systolic BP ≥140 mm Hg or diastolic BP ≥90 mm Hg when averaged over multiple measurements and visits. The 2017 Guideline for the prevention, detection, evaluation, and management of high blood pressure in adults, however, proposes a new classification of blood pressure. Hypertension is defined as a BP ≥130/80 mm Hg; stage 1 hypertension is a BP of 130–139/80–89 mm Hg; and stage 2 hypertension is a BP ≥140/90 mm Hg. A BP <120/80 mm Hg is considered normal, and a BP of 120–129/<80 is classified as elevated.

More than 100 million people in the United States have hypertension, and BP is controlled in less than one-half of this population. The percentage of patients with controlled hypertension is even lower in many Western countries and is <10% in developing countries; these are disappointing figures because of the available medications and education of the public and physicians about the risks of high BP. Because hypertension is a worldwide problem and a major cardiovascular risk factor, its prevention and treatment should be a high public health priority.

ETIOLOGY AND PATHOGENESIS

Hypertension is a disorder of BP regulation that results from an increase in cardiac output, or most often, an increase in total peripheral vascular resistance. Cardiac output is usually normal in established essential hypertension, although increased cardiac output plays an etiologic role. The phenomenon of autoregulation explains that an increase in cardiac output causes persistently elevated peripheral vascular resistance, with a resulting return of cardiac output to normal. Fig. 15.1 shows mechanisms that can cause hypertension. Inappropriate activation of the renin-angiotensin system, decreased renal sodium excretion, and increased sympathetic nervous system activity, individually or in combination, are probably involved in the pathogenesis of all types of hypertension. Hypertension also has genetic and environmental causes; the latter includes excess sodium intake, obesity, and stress. The inability of the kidney to optimally excrete sodium, and thus regulate plasma volume, leads to a persistent increase in BP whatever the etiology.

Many older adults with elevated BP have isolated systolic hypertension, which is a systolic pressure that is ≥130 mm Hg with a normal diastolic pressure. Stiffening of large arteries and increased systolic pulse wave velocity elevate systolic BP, increase myocardial work, and decrease coronary perfusion.

CLINICAL PRESENTATION

Most patients with early hypertension have no symptoms attributable to high BP. However, long-term BP elevation often leads to hypertensive heart disease, atherosclerosis of the aorta and peripheral vessels, cerebrovascular disease, and chronic kidney disease.

Left ventricular hypertrophy (LVH) is the principal cardiac manifestation of hypertension. Increased left ventricular (LV) mass can be identified by echocardiography in nearly 30% of unselected hypertensive adults and in most patients with long-standing, severe hypertension. LVH is more prevalent in men and more common in black individuals than in white individuals with similar BP values. Increasing age, obesity, high dietary sodium intake, and diabetes are also associated with cardiac hypertrophy.

Increased ventricular afterload resulting from elevated peripheral vascular resistance and arterial stiffness is considered the principal determinant of myocardial hypertrophy in patients with hypertension. Hemodynamic overload stimulates increases in myocyte size and the synthesis of contractile elements. Fibroblast proliferation and deposition of extracellular collagen accompany these cellular changes and contribute to ventricular stiffness and myocardial ischemia. A growing body of evidence suggests that angiotensin II and aldosterone, independent of pressure overload, stimulate this interstitial fibrosis (Fig. 15.2).

Clinical consequences of hypertensive heart disease include heart failure and coronary heart disease (CHD). More than 90% of patients with heart failure have hypertension, and data from the Framingham Heart Study suggest that high BP accounts for almost one-half of the population burden of this disorder. Treating hypertension reduces the risk of heart failure by nearly 50%. Heart failure develops because of the myocyte hypertrophy and ventricular fibrosis that characterize hypertensive LVH. As illustrated in Fig. 15.3, the early functional manifestations of LVH include impaired LV relaxation and decreased LV compliance. Although the ejection fraction is preserved initially, diastolic dysfunction often results in increased filling pressures, leading to pulmonary congestion. This mechanism accounts for the symptoms observed in approximately 40% of hypertensive patients with heart failure. If excessive BP levels persist, myocyte loss and fibrosis contribute to ventricular remodeling and contractile dysfunction. Compensatory mechanisms, including remodeling of the peripheral vasculature and activation of the sympathetic nervous and renin-angiotensin systems, accelerate the deterioration in myocardial contractility. Ultimately, decompensated cardiomyopathy and heart failure from systolic dysfunction develop.

CHD is approximately twice as prevalent in hypertensive individuals as in normotensive individuals of the same age. CHD risk increases in

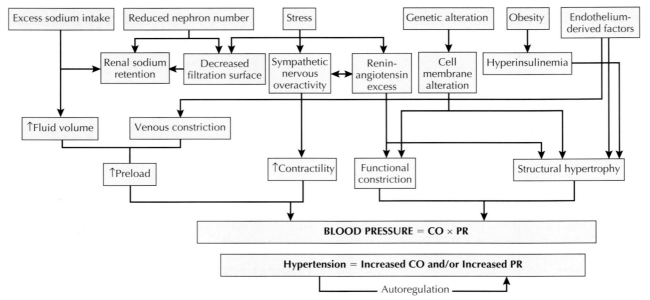

FIG 15.1 Factors Involved in the Control of Blood Pressure. *CO*, Cardiac output; *PR*, peripheral resistance. (With permission from Kaplan NM. *Kaplan's Clinical Hypertension*. 8th ed. Philadelphia: Lippincott Williams & Wilkins; 2002. p 63.)

BOX 15.1   Hypertension as a Risk Factor for Cardiovascular Disease

- High BP accelerates atherogenesis and increases the risk of cardiovascular events by twofold to threefold.
- Levels of systolic BP and diastolic BP are associated with cardiovascular events in a continuous, graded, and apparently independent fashion. This relation is closer for systolic BP than for diastolic BP.
- Every 20-mm Hg increase in systolic BP above 115 mm Hg results in a doubling of mortality from CHD and stroke.
- Hypertension often occurs in association with other atherogenic risk factors, including dyslipidemia, glucose intolerance, and obesity, which in combination with high BP dramatically increase the risk of cardiovascular events.

BP, Blood pressure; *CHD*, coronary heart disease.

BOX 15.2   Identifiable Causes of Hypertension

Renal
    Renal parenchymal disease
    Renal vascular disease
Endocrine
    Hypothyroidism or hyperthyroidism
    Adrenal disorders
    Primary hyperaldosteronism
    Cushing syndrome
    Pheochromocytoma
Exogenous hormones
    Glucocorticoids
    Mineralocorticoids
    Sympathomimetic agents
    Erythropoietin
Coarctation of the aorta
Sleep apnea
Neurological disorders
    Elevated intracranial pressure
    Quadriplegia
Acute stress
    Perioperative
    Hypoglycemia
    Alcohol withdrawal
Drugs and medications
    Alcohol
    Cocaine
    Nicotine
    Nonsteroidal antiinflammatory agents
    Immunosuppressive agents (cyclosporine, tacrolimus)

---

a continuous and graded fashion with both systolic BP and diastolic BP. A reduction in diastolic BP of 5 mm Hg with drug therapy decreases the incidence of myocardial infarction (MI) by approximately 20%. Multiple factors contribute to the enhanced risk of CHD associated with high BP: atherosclerotic narrowing of epicardial coronary arteries is accelerated; coronary arteriolar hypertrophy, reduced myocardial vascularity (rarefaction), and perivascular fibrosis limit coronary arterial flow reserve and predispose the LV to ischemia; and impaired coronary endothelial function increases coronary tone. MI and chronic ischemia contribute to LV dysfunction, increasing the risk of heart failure and cardiovascular death.

DIFFERENTIAL DIAGNOSIS

Approximately 95% of patients with elevated arterial pressure have hypertension of unknown etiology, which is known as essential hypertension. The remaining 5% have an identifiable cause of secondary hypertension (Box 15.2). Although relatively few patients have secondary hypertension, identification of these patients is important, because their

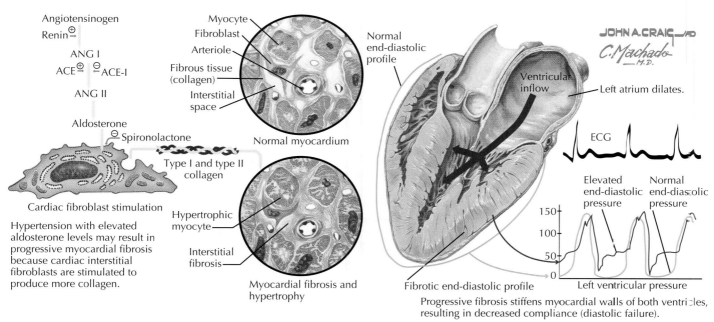

FIG 15.2 Myocardial Fibrosis. *ACE*, Angiotensin-converting enzyme; *ACE-I*, angiotensin-converting enzyme inhibitor; *ANG I*, angiotensin I; *ANG II*, angiotensin II.

BOX 15.3 Indications for Considering Testing for Identifiable Causes of Hypertension

- Sudden onset or worsening hypertension at age younger than 30 years or onset of diastolic hypertension at age older than 55 years
- Target organ damage at presentation
  - Serum creatinine concentration >1.5 mg/dL
  - Left ventricular hypertrophy determined by electrocardiography
- Presence of features indicative of secondary causes
  - Hypokalemia
  - Abdominal bruit
  - Labile pressures with tachycardia, sweating, and tremor
  - Family history of kidney disease
- Hypertension resistant to ≥3 drugs

---

hypertension can often be cured or significantly ameliorated by an interventional procedure, a specific drug therapy, or stopping a culprit drug.

Identifiable causes of hypertension should be sought in the initial history, physical examination, and laboratory studies. Further diagnostic evaluation for secondary hypertension causes is pursued when the presentation is atypical for essential hypertension or when the initial evaluation suggests an identifiable cause (Box 15.3).

DIAGNOSTIC APPROACH

Objectives of the initial evaluation of a hypertensive patient include confirmation of hypertension, evaluation of the presence and extent of target organ disease, identification of cardiovascular risk factors and coexisting conditions that influence prognosis and therapy, as well as exclusion or detection of identifiable causes of elevated BP. These goals can usually be achieved with a comprehensive history, a thorough physical examination, and selected laboratory studies (Box 15.4).

Detection and diagnosis of hypertension begin with accurate office measurements of BP. Measurements should be acquired at each encounter, with follow-up determinations at intervals based on the initial level. Accurate equipment and proper technique, as described in Box 15.5, are critical. Measurement in the upper arm with an oscillometric device is preferred over auscultatory methods, and automated office BP measurement (AOBP)—the use of an automated device that measures BP repeatedly in the absence of a healthcare professional—is optimal. Before treatment with medication is initiated, high BP should be confirmed with measurements outside the office setting. Ambulatory BP monitoring (ABPM) (Box 15.6), a technique by which BP is measured over the course of a typical day using a small, portable machine worn by the patient, is the best method for diagnosing hypertension. Confirmation of high BP with home BP monitoring (HBPM) (Box 15.7), with measurements acquired systematically using a validated, automated device, is also acceptable. Both ABPM and HBPM are more reproducible, correlate more closely with target organ damage, and are more predictive of cardiovascular events than measurement of BP in the office. Approximately 20% of patients believed to have hypertension on the basis of office measurements have lower BP outside the office setting and do not require medical therapy. Conversely, some patients have "masked" hypertension, with high BP for most of the day despite normal office levels.

MANAGEMENT AND THERAPY

The principal goal of hypertension treatment is to reduce the risk of cardiovascular morbidity and death. The treatment approach is determined not only by the level of BP, but also the presence of other major cardiovascular risk factors and target organ damage. Lower risk patients with mild BP elevations may benefit from a period of observation and lifestyle modification, using medical therapy if the average BP exceeds 140/90 mm Hg over months of monitoring. The 2017 Hypertension Guideline recommends a medication treatment threshold of 130/80 mm Hg in patients with a high absolute risk of cardiovascular

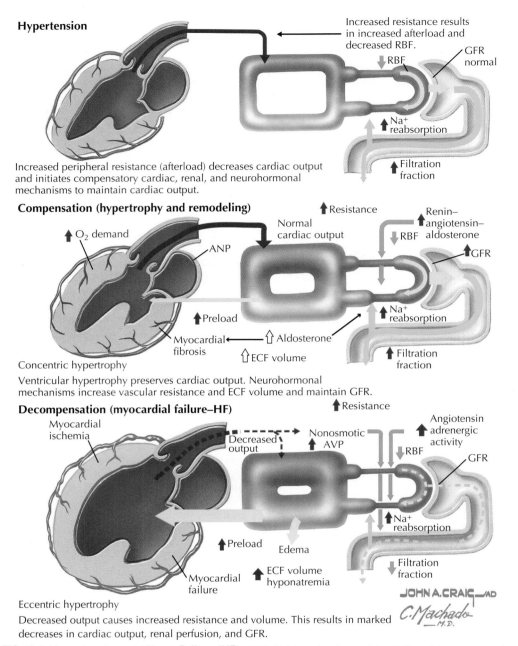

Hypertension

Increased resistance results in increased afterload and decreased RBF.

↓RBF

GFR normal

↑Na+ reabsorption

↑Filtration fraction

Increased peripheral resistance (afterload) decreases cardiac output and initiates compensatory cardiac, renal, and neurohormonal mechanisms to maintain cardiac output.

Compensation (hypertrophy and remodeling)

↑Resistance

↑O₂ demand

ANP

Normal cardiac output

Renin– angiotensin– aldosterone

↓RBF

↑GFR

↑Preload

Myocardial fibrosis

⇧Aldosterone

⇧ECF volume

↑Na+ reabsorption

↑Filtration fraction

Concentric hypertrophy

Ventricular hypertrophy preserves cardiac output. Neurohormonal mechanisms increase vascular resistance and ECF volume and maintain GFR.

Decompensation (myocardial failure–HF)

↑Resistance

Myocardial ischemia

Decreased output

Nonosmotic ↑AVP

Angiotensin adrenergic activity

↓RBF

GFR

↑Preload

Edema

↑Na+ reabsorption

Myocardial failure

↑ECF volume hyponatremia

↑Filtration fraction

Eccentric hypertrophy

Decreased output causes increased resistance and volume. This results in marked decreases in cardiac output, renal perfusion, and GFR.

JOHN A. CRAIG—MD
C. Machado —M.D.

FIG 15.3 Hypertension and Heart Failure (HF). *ANP,* Atrial natriuretic peptide; *AVP,* arginine vasopressin; *ECF,* extracellular fluid; *GFR,* glomerular filtration rate; *Na,* sodium; *RBF,* renal blood flow.

events—that is, those with clinical cardiovascular disease (coronary heart disease, heart failure, or stroke), diabetes, chronic kidney disease (stage 3 or higher or stage 1 or 2 with albuminuria [≥300 mg/d, or ≥300 mg/g albumin-to-creatinine ratio]), or a calculated 10-year atherosclerotic vascular disease risk exceeding 10%. A treatment threshold of 140/90 mm Hg is reasonable in individuals with confirmed hypertension but lower cardiovascular risk. A target BP <130/80 mm Hg is recommended in most patients. However, in selected patients at high risk, a goal systolic BP of <120 mm Hg may be appropriate.

Lifestyle modifications are an important component of therapy for high BP. All patients with hypertension, high-normal BP, or a strong family history of hypertension should be encouraged to adopt the measures outlined in Box 15.8. These lifestyle changes are proven to lower

BP and may reduce the need for drug therapy, enhance the effectiveness of antihypertensive drugs, and favorably influence other cardiovascular risk factors. Other measures, including smoking cessation and reduced intake of saturated fats, may further reduce cardiovascular risk.

Pharmacological treatment of hypertension reduces the incidence of heart failure, stroke, and MI, and decreases the mortality rate due to cardiovascular causes in middle-aged and older adults. Drug therapy is indicated if lifestyle modifications do not bring BP into the desired range within a reasonable period of time. Thiazide diuretics, angiotensin-converting enzyme (ACE) inhibitors, angiotensin-receptor blockers (ARBs), and calcium antagonists are appropriate first-line agents. Thiazide diuretics and calcium antagonists are preferred in black patients who do not have a specific indication for an ACE inhibitor or ARB. In many

BOX 15.4 Appropriate History, Physical Examination, and Laboratory Tests

Comprehensive History
- Assessment of the duration and severity of elevated BP and the results of previous medication trials
- Evaluation for the presence of diabetes, hypercholesterolemia, tobacco use, and other cardiovascular risk factors
- Identification of a history or symptoms of target organ disease, including CHD and heart failure, cerebrovascular disease, peripheral vascular disease, and renal disease
- Assessment of symptoms indicating identifiable causes of hypertension
- Identification of the use of drugs or substances that may raise BP
- Evaluation of lifestyle factors (e.g., diet, leisure-time physical activity, and weight gain) that may influence BP control
- Assessment of psychosocial and environmental factors, such as family support, income, and educational level, that influence the efficacy of antihypertensive therapy
- Identification of family history of hypertension or CVD

Physical Examination
- Careful measurement of BP
- Measurement of height and weight
- Funduscopic examination for hypertensive retinopathy
- Examination of the neck for carotid bruits, elevated jugular venous pressure, and thyromegaly
- Examination of the heart for abnormalities of the apical impulse or the presence of extra heart sounds or murmurs
- Examination of the abdomen for bruits, enlarged kidneys, and other masses
- Examination of the extremities for diminished arterial pulsations or peripheral edema

Laboratory Studies
- Complete blood count
- Serum concentrations of potassium, calcium, creatinine, thyroid-stimulating hormone, HbA_{1c}, fasting glucose, triglycerides, total cholesterol, HDL-C, and LDL-C
- Urinalysis for blood, protein, glucose, and microscopic examination
- Electrocardiography

BP, Blood pressure; *CHD*, coronary heart disease; *CVD*, cardiovascular disease; *HbA$_{1c}$*, glycosylated hemoglobin; *HDL-C*, high-density lipoprotein cholesterol; *LDL-C*, low-density lipoprotein cholesterol.

BOX 15.5 Measurement of Blood Pressure in the Office

- Measurements should be made by a trained provider with a validated device equipped with an appropriately sized cuff.
- Use of an oscillometric device is preferred; AOBP—the use of an automated device that measures BP repeatedly in the absence of a healthcare professional—is optimal.
- The patient should be seated for 5 minutes with the feet on the floor and the arm at heart level before any measurements.
- Caffeine, exercise, and smoking should be avoided for at least 30 minutes.
- An average of ≥2 measurements acquired on ≥2 occasions should be used to estimate an individual's BP.
- Standing BP should be measured in older patients and in patients with postural symptoms.
- Patients should be provided with verbal and written reports of BP values.

AOBP, Automated office blood pressure measurement; *BP*, blood pressure.

BOX 15.6 Ambulatory Blood Pressure Monitoring

- Validated monitors that measure BP on the upper arm with a cuff of the appropriate size should be used for ambulatory monitoring.
- The cuff should be applied to the nondominant arm unless the measured BP is 10 mm Hg higher in the dominant arm.
- The device should record data for 24 hours, with a measurement frequency of once every 15 to 30 minutes during the day and every 15 to 60 minutes at night.
- Daytime and night-time periods should ideally be defined using a patient-reported diary.
- The BP monitoring report should include individual values; average values over 24 hours, as well as average daytime and night-time readings; the percentage of successful readings; and the "dipping" percentages.
- Criteria for a successful ambulatory BP monitoring study include at least 70% of the successful readings, with 20 successful daytime and 7 successful night-time readings.
- Hypertension is defined as an ambulatory awake BP ≥130/80 mm Hg or ambulatory 24-hour BP ≥125/75 mm Hg.

BP, Blood pressure.

BOX 15.7 Home Blood Pressure Monitoring

- Validated oscillometric monitors that measure BP in the upper arm with a cuff of the appropriate size should be used for home monitoring.
- The patient should be seated for 5 minutes with the feet on the floor and the arm at heart level before any measurements.
- Caffeine, exercise, and smoking should be avoided for at least 30 minutes.
- Two or three readings should be taken in the morning (before medications) and in the evening over the course of a week before the patient's office visit.
- At least 12 readings should be acquired for making clinical decisions; average systolic and diastolic BPs should be calculated, excluding the first day's readings.
- Hypertension is defined as a home BP ≥130/80 mm Hg.

BP, Blood pressure.

BOX 15.8 Lifestyle Modifications for Prevention and Treatment of Hypertension

- Weight loss if overweight. All overweight hypertensive patients should be enrolled in a monitored weight reduction program, with a goal body mass index of <25 kg/m^2.
- Dietary modification. An eating plan that emphasizes fruits, vegetables, low-fat dairy products, and whole grains, and minimizes saturated fats and sweets (the DASH diet) is recommended.
- Limitation of dietary sodium intake. Daily sodium intake should not exceed 2400 mg.
- Regular aerobic physical activity. Sedentary individuals should be encouraged to engage in regular aerobic exercise, with a goal of 30 to 60 minutes of moderate intensity dynamic exercise 4 to 7 days per week.
- Moderation of alcohol intake. Patients with high blood pressure who drink alcohol should be counseled to limit their daily intake to two standard drinks for men and one standard drink for women.

patients, the choice of a drug is influenced by comorbid conditions. Table 15.1 lists agents that are preferred or relatively contraindicated in specific circumstances.

Many patients with hypertension have established cardiovascular disease, and their treatment regimen should include medications that control symptoms, slow disease progression, and prevent cardiovascular events. Treatment strategies for patients with ischemic heart disease or heart failure are addressed in Chapters 19 and 29.

TABLE 15.1 Choice of Antihypertensive Agent Based on Coexistent Illness

Characteristics	Specific Drugs
Indications	
Diabetes mellitus with renal or cardiovascular disease	ACE-I or ARB
Heart failure	ACE-I or ARB, β-blocker, diuretic, aldosterone antagonist
Myocardial infarction	ACE-I or ARB, β-blocker, aldosterone antagonist
Chronic coronary heart disease	ACE-I or ARB, β-blocker
Chronic kidney disease	ACE-I or ARB
Contraindications	
Pregnancy	ACE-I, ARB, direct renin inhibitor
Chronic kidney disease[a]	Potassium-sparing agent
Peripheral vascular disease[a]	β-blocker
Gout[a]	Thiazide diuretic
Depression[a]	β-blocker, central α-agonist
Reactive airway disease[a]	β-blocker
Second- or third-degree heart block	β-blocker, non-dihydropyridine calcium antagonist
Hepatic insufficiency	Labetalol, methyldopa

[a]Relative contraindication.
ACE-I, Angiotensin-converting enzyme inhibitor; *ARB,* angiotensin-receptor blocker.

In brief, β-blockers and ACE inhibitors mitigate symptoms and prolong survival in patients with CHD or LV dysfunction. ARBs are an effective alternative in patients with heart failure who cannot tolerate ACE inhibitors. Aldosterone antagonists are beneficial in patients with LV dysfunction or a history of MI. Calcium antagonists are useful adjuncts in patients with angina or hypertension that cannot be controlled by β-blockers and ACE inhibitors. The optimal therapy for patients with heart failure with preserved ejection fraction is not well established and is under investigation; agents that treat LV systolic dysfunction, especially aldosterone antagonists, seem to be useful. Lowering BP with any of the first-line drugs leads to LVH regression.

The optimal target BP in patients with isolated systolic hypertension and chronic ischemic heart disease is controversial. In general, lower values of systolic BP are associated with better outcomes. However, myocardial perfusion occurs almost exclusively in diastole, and excessive lowering of diastolic BP in patients with obstructive coronary disease could theoretically result in ischemia and increase the risk of coronary events. Several studies have suggested a J-shaped relationship between diastolic BP and coronary risk, with an increase in events as diastolic BP is lowered to <80 mm Hg. These observations have led some experts to caution against aggressive BP lowering in patients with isolated systolic hypertension and ischemic heart disease.

In general, therapy with antihypertensive drugs should be initiated at low doses to minimize side effects. Long-acting formulations with 24-hour efficacy are preferred over shorter acting agents because of greater patient adherence to once-daily dosing regimens and more consistent BP control throughout the day. Based on patient response, the dose of the initial agent can be slowly titrated upward, or a small dose of a second agent can be added. Most patients with hypertension require multiple drugs for optimal BP control. Effective drug combinations use medications from different classes and result in additive BP-lowering effects, while minimizing dose-dependent adverse effects. Thiazide diuretics potentiate the effect of ACE inhibitors, ARBs, and calcium antagonists; other useful combinations include calcium antagonists and ACE inhibitors or ARBs. A combination of an ACE inhibitor or ARB plus a thiazide diuretic and calcium antagonist is often effective in patients who require three drugs. Recommended combinations of antihypertensive medications are illustrated in Fig. 15.4.

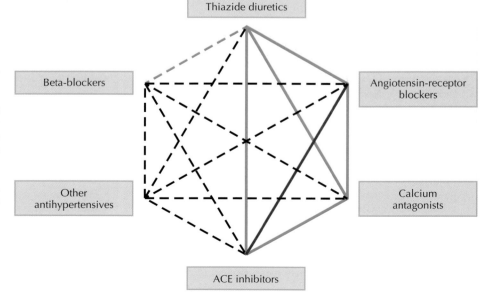

FIG 15.4 Combinations of Classes of Antihypertensive Drugs. *Green continuous line,* preferred combination; *green dashed line,* useful combination (with some limitations); *black dashed lines,* possible but less well-tested combinations; *red continuous line,* not recommended combination. *ACE,* Angiotensin converting enzyme. (With permission from Giuseppe Mancia M, Fagard R, Narkiewicz K, et al. 2013 ESH/ESC Guidelines for the management of arterial hypertension. *J Hypertens* 2013;31:1281–1357; Fig. 4, p. 1315.)

Resistant hypertension is defined as a properly measured BP that remains above goal despite the adherence of patients to a regimen of three optimally dosed antihypertensive agents of different classes, one of which is a diuretic. The true prevalence of resistant hypertension is not known, but it is probably present in approximately 15% of treated patients with hypertension. These patients are more likely to have target organ damage and are at greater risk of stroke, MI, heart failure, and chronic kidney disease compared with patients who have more easily controlled hypertension. Referral to a hypertension specialist should be considered for in-depth evaluation and treatment. Aldosterone antagonists are the most effective agents for lowering BP in patients with resistant hypertension who are already on a three drug regimen. Several device-based interventions, including renal denervation, carotid baroreceptor activation, and an arteriovenous coupler device are under investigation, but none of these technologies are currently approved for use in the United States.

Lowering BP is but one mechanism by which cardiovascular risk can be reduced in hypertensive patients. Irrespective of baseline cholesterol levels, statin therapy is recommended to reduce the incidence of MI and stroke in patients at intermediate or high risk of cardiovascular events. Low-dose aspirin also reduces cardiovascular event rates in selected patients.

FUTURE DIRECTIONS

Future research and public health initiatives should clarify the efficacy and cost-effectiveness of various methods of measuring BP (AOBP, ABPM, and HBPM) in the initial evaluation and subsequent management of patients with high BP; determine the most useful agents for alleviating symptoms and improving longevity in patients with hypertension and heart failure with preserved ejection fraction; develop more effective drugs for treating older adults with isolated systolic hypertension; provide better strategies to improve patient awareness of and adherence to lifestyle modifications and medication regimens; and test the efficacy of device-based methods for treatment of high BP.

ADDITIONAL RESOURCES

2013 AHA/ACC guideline on lifestyle management to reduce cardiovascular risk: a report of the American College of Cardiology/American Heart Association Task Force on Practice Guidelines. *J Am Coll Cardiol.* 2014;63:2960–2984.

This rigorous, evidence-based guideline provides recommendations for dietary patterns, nutrient intake, and levels and types of physical activity that are useful in the management of hypertension and hypercholesterolemia.

2013 AHA/ACC guideline on the assessment of cardiovascular risk: a report of the American College of Cardiology/American Heart Association Task Force on Practice Guidelines. *J Am Coll Cardiol.* 2014;63:2935–2959.

This document describes the development of the multivariable risk equations for the prediction of 10-year risk of atherosclerotic cardiovascular disease used in the 2017 Hypertension Guideline.

2017 ACC/AHA/AAPA/ABC/ACPM/AGS/APhA/ASH/ASPC/NMA/PCNA guideline for the prevention, detection, evaluation, and management of high blood pressure in adults: a report of the American College of Cardiology/American Heart Association Task Force on Clinical Practice Guidelines. *Hypertension.* 2018;71:e13–e115.

This comprehensive guideline will have a major influence on the evaluation and management of high blood pressure in the United States. Important features of the document include a new classification of BP, defining hypertension as a BP ≥130/80 mm Hg; an emphasis on out-of-office blood pressure measurement in diagnosing hypertension and assessing the effects of therapy; and endorsement of a BP treatment threshold and target of 130/80 mm Hg in patients at high risk of cardiovascular events.

ACC/AHA Pooled Cohort Equations risk calculator: http://tools.acc.org/ASCVD-Risk-Estimator/.

This tool, available online and as a cell phone app, can be used to estimate the 10-year risk of atherosclerotic cardiovascular disease in adults with no clinical history of cardiovascular disease.

Detailed Summary from the 2017 Guideline for the prevention, detection, evaluation, and management of high blood pressure in adults. http://professional.heart.org/idc/groups/ahamah-public/@wcm/@sop/@smd/documents/downloadable/ucm_497446.pdf.

This is a succinct summary of the 2017 Hypertension Guideline.

European Society of Hypertension practice guidelines for ambulatory blood pressure monitoring. *J Hypertens.* 2014;32:1359–1366.

This is a concise summary of the important aspects of using ABPM in clinical practice.

Hypertension Canada's 2017 Canadian hypertension guidelines for risk assessment, prevention, and treatment of hypertension in adults. *Can J Cardiol.* 2016;33:557–576.

Hypertension Canada's Canadian Hypertension Education Program Guidelines Task Force provides annually updated, concise, evidence-based recommendations to guide the evaluation and treatment of hypertension.

Kaplan NM, Victor RG. *Clinical Hypertension.* 11th ed. Philadelphia: Wolters Kluwer; 2014.

This is a thorough, detailed, yet succinct, eminently readable textbook on clinical hypertension authored by Drs. Kaplan and Victor. The book is updated every 4 years and reflects the vast clinical experience and wisdom of the authors and offers up-to-date references on all topics.

Screening for high blood pressure in adults: U.S. Preventive Services Task Force recommendation statement. *Ann Intern Med.* 2015;163:778–786.

This report reviews the evidence in support of screening for hypertension, and examines the diagnostic accuracy of different methods for confirming a diagnosis of hypertension. Measurements of BP outside of the clinical setting, preferably with ambulatory blood pressure monitoring, are recommended for diagnostic confirmation before starting treatment.

EVIDENCE

The ALLHAT Officers and Coordinators for the ALLHAT Collaborative Research Group. Major outcomes in high-risk hypertensive patients randomized to angiotensin-converting enzyme inhibitor or calcium channel blocker vs. diuretic: The Antihypertensive and Lipid-Lowering treatment to prevent Heart Attack Trial (ALLHAT). *JAMA.* 2002;288:2981–2997.

This is the largest double-blind trial ever undertaken in hypertensive patients and strongly influenced the treatment recommendations in the United States. The trial compared treatment with amlodipine or lisinopril with a reference drug chlorthalidone and found no advantage of newer drugs over a thiazide-type diuretic in preventing fatal CHD or nonfatal MI.

Blood Pressure Lowering Treatment Trialists' Collaboration. Effects of different blood-pressure-lowering regimens on major cardiovascular events: results of prospectively-designed overviews of randomized trials. *Lancet.* 2003;362:1527–1535.

This classic set of prospectively designed overviews with data from 29 randomized trials examined the comparative effects of different BP-lowering regimens and the benefits of targeting lower BP goals on the risk of major cardiovascular events and death. The overall conclusion was that treatment with any commonly used regimen reduces the risk of major cardiovascular events, and that greater reductions in BP produce greater reductions in risk.

Piper MA, Evans CV, Burda BU, Margolis KL, O'Connor E, Whitlock EP. Diagnostic and predictive accuracy of blood pressure screening methods with consideration of rescreening intervals: a systematic review for the U.S. Preventive Services Task Force. *Ann Intern Med.* 2015;162:192–204.

This systematic review of ambulatory and home blood pressure monitoring in comparison to office blood pressure provides the basis for the U.S. Preventive Services Task Force recommendation to perform out-of-office measurements to confirm the diagnosis of hypertension.

Reboussin DM, Allen NB, Griswold ME, Guallar E, Hong Y, Lackland DT, Miller ER 3rd, Polonsky T, Thompson-Paul AM, Vupputuri S. Systematic review for the 2017 ACC/AHA/AAPA/ABC/ACPM/AGS/APhA/ASH/ASPC/NMA/PCNA guideline for the prevention, detection, evaluation, and management of high blood pressure in adults: a report of the American College of Cardiology Foundation/American Heart Association Task Force on Clinical Practice Guidelines. *Hypertension.* 2018;71:e116–e135.

This systematic review examined self-monitored vs office-based measurement of blood pressure, targets of blood pressure lowering during anti-hypertensive therapy, and first-line antihypertensive drug class comparisons. The results informed the development of the 2017 Hypertension Guideline.

SPRINT Research Group. A randomized trial of intensive versus standard blood pressure control. *N Engl J Med.* 2015;373:2103–2116.

This landmark trial examined appropriate targets for systolic BP to reduce cardiovascular morbidity and mortality among persons at increased cardiovascular risk but without diabetes. Targeting a systolic BP <120 mm Hg compared with a BP <140 mm Hg, resulted in lower rates of fatal and nonfatal major cardiovascular events and death from any cause.

16

Management of Lipid Abnormalities

Phil Mendys, Golsa Joodi, Sidney C. Smith, Jr., Ross J. Simpson, Jr.

The management of lipid disorders in reducing the risk of coronary heart disease (CHD) has evolved in the past few years. There are a number of factors that account for these changes—the introduction of the 2013 American Heart Association/American College of Cardiology (AHA/ACC) guideline report on cholesterol management and a series of clinical trials on nonstatin therapies (notably, several trials involved the cholesteryl ester transfer protein inhibitors [CETPis] for high-density lipoprotein [HDL] elevation), as well as the introduction of proprotein convertase subtilisin/kexin type 9 (PCSK-9) therapies. The aforementioned 2013 recommendations are a key resource because of their evidence-based approach to patient care. They have simplified both the treatment approach to lipids and challenging issues such as dose titration, as well as achieving a specific and perhaps unreachable "target" lipid value. Of great importance, they allow for discretion on the part of the provider to engage with the patient in shared decision making and as stated, "Guidelines attempt to define practices that meet the needs of patients in most circumstances and are not a replacement for clinical judgment."

For most individuals at risk for CHD, elevated serum lipid levels—specifically, elevated low-density lipoprotein cholesterol (LDL-C)—are the dominant modifiable risk factor. The importance of lifestyle modification, inclusive of diet and exercise, cannot be understated in the coordinated effort to reduce vascular disease risk. A case example of individuals at high vascular risk are those determined to have the metabolic syndrome (Fig. 16.1). Together with appropriate medical management, therapeutic lifestyle modification represents an important and effective approach to overall patient management.

LDL-C levels are strongly associated with atherosclerosis and CHD events. Insights from genetic, epidemiological, and multiple clinical trial data reinforce the belief that LDL-C is a necessary and sufficient cause of atherosclerosis, and therefore, most emphasis is placed on lowering LDL-C. There appears to be a consistent graded reduction in risk in CHD events associated with lowering of LDL-C levels with drug and diet therapy. The 2013 AHA/ACC guidelines summarize the evidence base for lowering LDL-C with statins within four distinct patient groups based on their future risk for cardiovascular events. These groups are described as follows (Fig. 16.2):

- individuals with known clinical atherosclerotic cardiovascular disease (ASCVD);
- individuals with primary elevations of LDL-C to >190 mg/dL, typically seen in genetic dyslipidemia;
- individuals with diabetes, aged 40 to 75 years, with LDL-C of 70 to 189 mg/dL without clinical ASCVD; and
- patients without clinical ASCVD or diabetes with LDL-C of 70 to 189 mg/dL and an estimated 10-year ASCVD risk of >7.5%.

These statin guidelines are fundamental to lipid management, and additional guidance on nonstatin therapies are now available through a 2017 Focused Update from the ACC Expert Consensus Decision Pathway. This update provides expert guidance on individuals who respond inadequately to statin therapy or may not be able to tolerate maximum doses of statins. Drugs such as ezetimibe and the PCSK-9 inhibitors offer an important option of additional lowering of LDL-C and reducing cardiovascular risk. Alternative therapies, which include likely referral to a lipid specialist, other agents such as mipomersen or lomitapide, or LDL apheresis may also be considered for selected patients.

ASSESSMENT

Standard laboratory lipids measured by β-quantification consist of total cholesterol, triglycerides (TGs), and HDL-C levels as direct measurements, and LDL-C as estimated from the Freidewald equation. Direct measurement of LDL-C levels, particle size, and particle density are performed by ultracentrifugation, gradient gel electrophoresis, and nuclear magnetic resonance. Although measurement of apolipoprotein B and these other measures of LDL-C may provide additional information on lipid lipoprotein characteristics, detailed clinical studies that indicate the usefulness of drugs that target these individual lipid components are not available. For this reason, the usefulness of these measures may be of limited value because they rarely change management decisions for most patients. LDL-C measurement is the standard for evaluating risk and monitoring lipid therapy. For patients being considered for long-term therapy, two fasting measurements of the lipoprotein profile, taken at least 1 week apart, should be obtained to support a clinical decision.

The fasting TGs are also important to monitor, because elevated TGs (>200 mg/dL) may mask residual risk in the form of very low-density lipoprotein and other remnant cholesterol particles, which are also considered atherogenic.

The goal of therapy then is to match the intensity of LDL-C lowering with individual patient risk; for example, an individual with known ASCVD would be managed with a high-intensity statin that provides a ≥50% reduction in LDL-C. Patients at lower risk may be managed with a more modest LDL-C reduction approach, with the recognition there will be some variation in response according to the dose provided. The benefits of therapy must be considered in the context of safety to avoid possible adverse events in all patients.

HDL-C has been the subject of intense epidemiological and clinical investigation. HDL-C levels are influenced by lifestyle factors, such as diet, exercise, alcohol intake, obesity, and smoking, as well as specific drug therapy (e.g., diuretics and anabolic steroids). Of these factors, exercise, estrogens, and alcohol increase HDL-C, yet the possible benefits of these influences are unproven and not endorsed as preventive strategies. Moreover, recent clinical trials, including the use of niacin and CETPi, on raising HDL-C have been proven to have limited clinical usefulness.

Interest in clinical trials with niacin preparations dates back >40 years to the results of the Coronary Drug Project. As a therapeutic

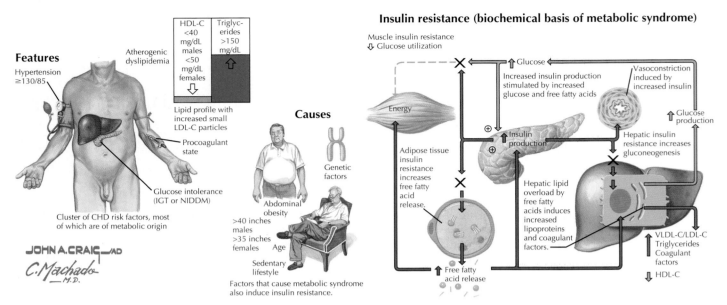

FIG 16.1 Metabolic Syndrome. *CHD*, Coronary heart disease; *HDL-C*, high-density lipoprotein cholesterol; *IGT*, impaired glucose tolerance; *LDL-C*, low-density lipoprotein cholesterol; *NIDDM*, non–insulin-dependent diabetes mellitus; *VLDL-C*, very low-density lipoprotein cholesterol.

intervention, niacin has multiple effects on serum lipoproteins (including LDL-C, TGs, and HDL-C), yet recent trials, including the Atherothrombosis Intervention in Metabolic syndrome with Low-HDL and High Triglycerides (AIM-HIGH) and Heart Protection Study 2-Treatment of HDL to Reduce the Incidence of Vascular Events (HPS₂ THRIVE) revealed no benefit outcomes and the potential for harm.

More recently, the option of using CETPis to raise HDL-C have been studied. The prototype agent, torcetrapib, increased HDL-C by >50%, together with 15% to 20% lowering of LDL-C, yet the investigation was terminated early due to an increase in cardiovascular and overall mortality in the treatment group. It is likely that an off-target effect on electrolytes and blood pressure elevations produced untoward toxicity. An alternate approach to CETP inhibition in the form of dalcetrapib, which had no apparent off-target effects similar to torcetrapib, had more modest effects on HDL-C and LDL-C. The early outcomes study, dal-OUTCOMES, was terminated due to clinical futility. The most recent attempt to demonstrate efficacy with a CETPi used evacetrapib, which had a potent effect on HDL-C and other presumably beneficial effects on other lipid biomarkers; LDL-C and lipoprotein(a) [Lp(a)] showed no evidence of benefit in the primary endpoint of vascular events. However, another outcome trial that used anacetrapib, which had similar dramatic effects on HDL-C, LDL-C, and Lp(a), showed modest but significant benefit. Taken together, these trials suggest that CTEP inhibition and drugs to raise HDL-C is not a major pathway to improving cardiovascular outcomes. However, although the implications of HDL-C as a target of treatment remains unresolved, the usefulness of HDL-C as an important predictor of cardiovascular risk remains unchallenged.

TGs are important plasma lipids found in varying concentrations in all plasma lipoproteins. The relationship between plasma TGs and CHD is still unclear due to the lack of specific randomized clinical trials demonstrating benefit outcomes. Recent epidemiological analyses suggest that elevated TGs, or so-called remnant lipoproteins, are a contributor to residual risk of ASCVD. Elevations in TGs in the range of 200 to 500 mg/dL should be interpreted as a component of residual risk, and may obscure our interpretation of LDL-C values from

laboratory assessments. In this context, using advanced diagnostic parameters of apolipoprotein B or LDL particles (via nuclear magnetic resonance) is comparable in association with clinical outcomes to assess risk for CVD when questions arise on standard laboratory analyses.

Patients with genetic disorders of lipid metabolism or familial hypercholesterolemia (FH) are at particularly high risk for coronary artery disease. These individuals present with premature atherosclerotic heart disease, a strong family history of coronary disease, and represent a significant clinical challenge to healthcare providers. The prevalence of HeFH, which is a heterozygote FH with baseline LDL-C levels ≥190 mg/dL, in the general population is believed to occur in 1 in 250 individuals based on recent population data. Such patients are a priority treatment group according to the current treatment guidelines. The introduction of PCSK-9 inhibitors and the attendant science on LDL receptor regulation have provided significant insights into epidemiological and clinical considerations in addressing the challenges of FH. FH often remains underdiagnosed and undertreated until after a primary coronary event. Historically, the treatment approach has been limited to a combination of statins and other oral therapies or plasma apheresis. The advent of newer treatment strategies, including mipomersen lomatipide, and PCSK-9 inhibitors (evolocumab and alirocumab), hold much promise for this patient population.

MANAGEMENT AND THERAPY

Therapeutic Lifestyle

The proof of efficacy of statin and other drugs is built on effective lifestyle modification, such as healthy diet and physical activity, which are generally a part of randomized trials combined with these agents (Fig. 16.3). Patients should receive dietary counseling by a trained physician, nurse, or nutritionist. As in previous clinical recommendations, the recent AHA/ACC guidelines continue to emphasize the importance of lifestyle modification (i.e., adhering to a heart healthy diet, regular exercise habits, avoidance of tobacco products, and maintenance of a healthy weight) as a critical component of health promotion and ASCVD risk reduction before and in concert with cholesterol-lowering drug

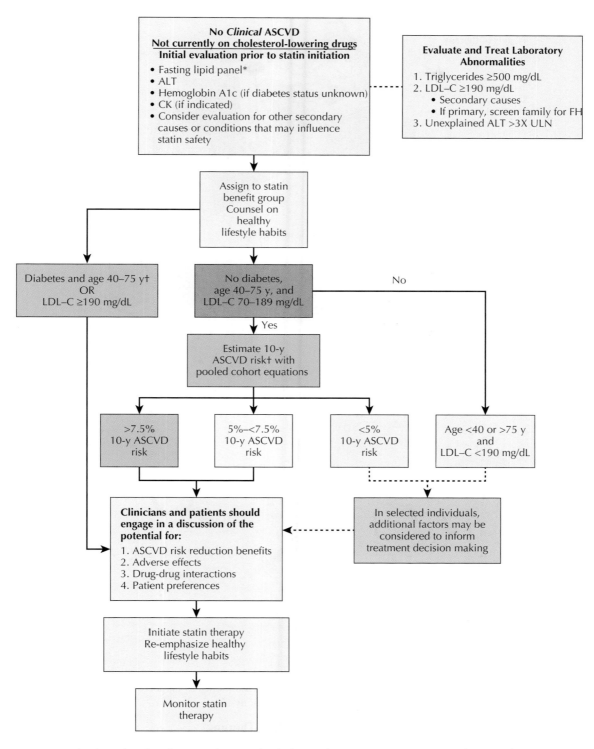

*Fasting lipid panel preferred. In a nonfasting individual, a nonfasting non-HDL–C >220 mg/dL may indicate genetic hypercholesterolemia that requires further evaluation or a secondary etiology. If nonfasting triglycerides are >500 mg/dL, a fasting lipid panel is required.

†The Pooled Cohort Equations can be used to estimate 10-year ASCVD risk in individuals with and without diabetes.

FIG 16.2 Algorithm for Management of Lipid Goals. *CAD,* Coronary artery disease; *HDL-C,* high-density lipoprotein cholesterol; *LDL-C,* low-density lipoprotein cholesterol. (Reused with permission from Stone NJ, Robinson JG, Lichtenstein AH, et al. 2013 ACC/AHA guideline on the treatment of blood cholesterol to reduce atherosclerotic cardiovascular risk in adults. *Circulation.* 2014;129[25 Suppl 2]:S1–45.)

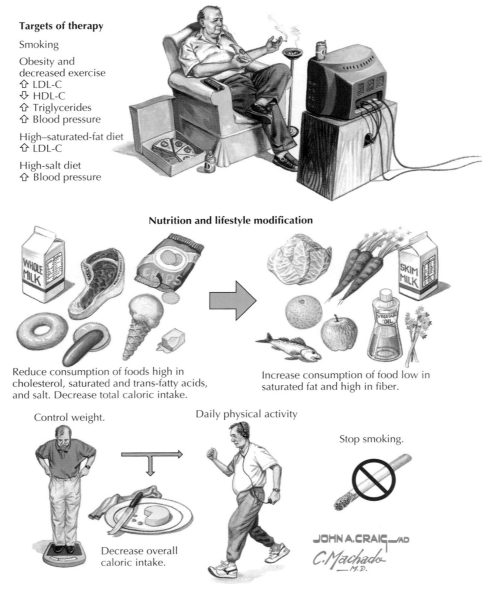

Targets of therapy

Smoking

Obesity and
decreased exercise
⇧ LDL-C
⇩ HDL-C
⇧ Triglycerides
⇧ Blood pressure

High–saturated-fat diet
⇧ LDL-C

High-salt diet
⇧ Blood pressure

Nutrition and lifestyle modification

Reduce consumption of foods high in
cholesterol, saturated and trans-fatty acids,
and salt. Decrease total caloric intake.

Increase consumption of food low in
saturated fat and high in fiber.

Control weight.

Decrease overall
caloric intake.

Daily physical activity

Stop smoking.

FIG 16.3 Nonpharmacological Therapy for Management of Lipid Goals. *HDL-C*, High-density lipoprotein cholesterol; *LDL-C*, low-density lipoprotein cholesterol.

therapies (Fig. 16.3). The 2013 Lifestyle Management Work Group Guideline for lifestyle recommendations for healthy adults identified patterns of nutrition rather than specific diets such as the Dietary Approach to Stop Hypertension (DASH) or Mediterranean diets. These "patterns" include an emphasis on intake of fruits, vegetables, and whole grains. Sources of proteins should include low-fat dairy products, poultry, fish, and legumes, as well as limited intake of sweets, sugar-sweetened beverages, red meats, and overall calorie intake from saturated fat. Plant stanols/sterols (2 g/day) and up to 25 mg of soluble fiber have been suggested to aid in lowering LDL-C, either alone or in conjunction with appropriate pharmacotherapy.

Physical activity is addressed in the 2008 Physical Activity Guidelines for Americans as a key to healthy aging. Although the 2013 AHA/ACC Lifestyle Management Guideline suggest 2.5 hours per week of moderate intensity exercise and promote physical activity, an individual approach

should be outlined to support as much physical activity as abilities and conditions allow.

Drug Therapy

Although all treatment options are not considered as first-line treatment, there are various options that affect LDL-C and TG levels through different mechanisms of action (Fig. 16.4). The 2013 ACC/AHA practice guidelines provide an evidence-based drug treatment framework for treatment of LDL-C and reducing cardiovascular risk. These recommendations are based on a comprehensive review of randomized clinical trials of statins. They emphasize the intensity of statin treatment based on the risk of the patient as an initial approach to patient care. High-intensity treatment with statins to achieve an LDL-C reduction of ≥50% and moderate intensity to achieve a reduction of 30% to 50% in LDL-C is recommended based on the risk group of the patients. The decision

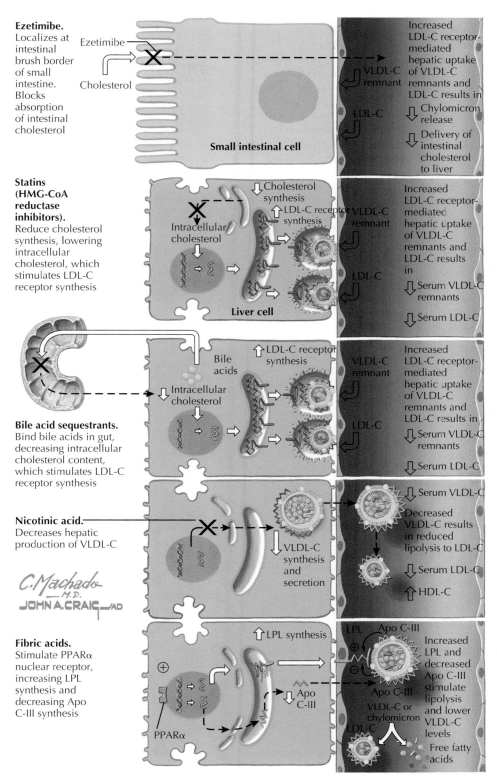

FIG 16.4 Mechanism of Action of Lipid-Lowering Drugs. *Apo C-III*, Apolipoprotein C-III; *HDL-C*, high-density lipoprotein cholesterol; *HMG-CoA*, 3-hydroxy-3-methylglutaryl coenzyme A; *LDL-C*, low-density lipoprotein cholesterol; *LPL*, lipoprotein lipase; *PPARα*, peroxisome proliferator activator receptor α; *VLDL-C*, very low-density lipoprotein cholesterol.

to treat and the amount of LDL-C reduction is based on the baseline risk of the patient within the four treatment groups. Shared decision making with the individual patient is emphasized (see Fig. 16.2).

Although the aggregate of randomized clinical trials with statins suggest a graded and direct association between treated LDL-C and reduced cardiovascular events, the available data do not support specific targets for treatment goals. However, it is believed that even in patients who are currently managed by effective doses of statins, additional cardiovascular events might be reduced by more aggressive LDL-C lowering. The recent results of the ezetimibe plus statin IMProved Reduction of Outcomes: Vytorin Efficacy International Trial (IMPROVE-IT) showed a modest but significant reduction in cardiovascular events with addition of this nonstatin therapy.

The PCSK-9 inhibitors may introduce important options for patient management because they share the ability to increase LDL-C receptor activity with statins and produce dramatic reductions in LDL-C. Added to statin therapy, they can reduce LDL-C by an additional 50% to 60% and produce treatment levels well below current levels that can generally be achieved with statins alone. The results of large outcome studies show great promise, and a recent study level meta-analysis suggested improved all-cause mortality and fewer myocardial infarction events, as well as a possible reduction in cardiovascular mortality. Potentially serious adverse events associated with PCSK-9 inhibition appear to be low.

Practical Considerations

Despite the extensive data supporting the safety and efficacy of statins to lower LDL-C, many patients may not tolerate statin therapy in doses necessary to achieve optimal outcomes. This may be in part due to patient concern about drug safety and the poor understanding of patients about the risks and benefits of statins. Medication adherence is often a multi-faceted issue, and interventions to improve statin adherence must be individualized to the patient. "De-prescribing" in older adults based on considerations of polypharmacy, as well as defined risk and benefit may also be appropriate. However, for all patients, the decision to treat should be accompanied by information to support a clear understanding for the patient to appreciate the benefits and risks of the options of their care.

FUTURE DIRECTIONS

Additional diagnostic tests to more precisely define the risk of patients developing CHD events and to better characterize their lipid profiles are being developed. These include blood tests to assess new risk factors and quantitative measurements to assess early atherosclerotic disease. Diagnostic tests include the high-sensitivity C-reactive protein assay to measure chronic inflammation, assessment of lipid particle size and density, electron beam tomography to assess calcium scores in the coronary arteries, carotid Doppler ultrasound to test intima-media thickness ratios, and the ankle-brachial index for assessment of peripheral vascular disease. The combination of new diagnostic tests to better identify individuals at risk for CHD events and expanded therapies to treat dyslipidemia should result in major advances in the prevention of the epidemic of CHD.

EVIDENCE

ACC Writing Committee. 2016 ACC expert consensus decision pathway on the role of non-statin therapies for LDL-cholesterol lowering in the management of atherosclerotic cardiovascular disease risk. *J Am Coll Cardiol.* 2016;68(1):92–125.
Updated summary of treatment options supporting the original guidelines.
DiBartolo BA, Duong M, Nicholls SJ. Clinical trials with cholesterol ester protein inhibitors. *Curr Opin Lipidol.* 2016;27:545–549.
An overview of a treatment class that did not provide improved outcomes.
Eckel RH, et al. 2013 AHA/ACC guideline on lifestyle management to reduce cardiovascular risk. *Circulation.* 2013;00:1–46.
An important adjunct to medical management is well described in this reference.
Gidding SA, Champagne MA, Ferranti SD, et al. The agenda for familial hypercholesterolemia: a scientific statement from the American Heart Association. *Circulation.* 2015;132:2167–2192.
Our knowledge for genetic dyslipidemias continues to expand as summarized in this statement.
Hassan M. HPS2-THRIVE, AIM-HIGH and dal-OUTCOMES: HDL-cholesterol under attack. *Glob Cardiol Sci Pract.* 2014;37:235–240.
Important insights on the lack of benefit associated with the use of niacin.
Lloyd-Jones DM, et al. 2017 Focused update of the 2016 ACC expert consensus decision pathway on the role of non-statin therapies for LDL-cholesterol lowering in the management of atherosclerotic cardiovascular disease risk. *J Am Coll Cardiol.* 2017;70:1785–1822.
Provides important guidance on the use of nonstatin therapies—a practical guide for clinicians.
Navarese EP, Kolodziejczak M, Schulze V. Effects of proprotein convertase subtilisin/kexin type 9 antibodies in adults with hypercholesterolemia: a systematic review and meta-analysis. *Ann Intern Med.* 2015;163:40–51.
A preamble to what is anticipated with novel therapies such as PCSK-9 inhibitors.
Nordestgaard BG. Triglyceride-rich lipoproteins and atherosclerotic cardiovascular disease: new insights from epidemiology, genetics, and biology. *Circ Res.* 2016;118:547–563.
Although LDL-C remains a focus of lipid management, elevated triglyceride levels must also be interpreted.
O'Keefe JH, DiNicolantonio JJ, Lavie CJ. Statins, ezetimibe, and proprotein convertase subtilisin-kexin type 9 inhibitors to reduce low-density lipoprotein cholesterol and cardiovascular events. *Am J Cardiol.* 2017;119:565–571.
An important overview of evidence-based lipid-lowering therapies.
Pearson TA, Mensah GA, Alexander RW, et al. AHA/CDC Scientific Statement. Markers of inflammation and cardiovascular disease: application to clinical and public health forum: a statement for healthcare professionals from the Centers for Disease Control and Prevention and the American Heart Association. *Circulation.* 2003;107:499–511.
An appreciation on the role of inflammation in vascular disease and cardiac events.
Stone NJ, Robinson J, Lichtenstein AH, et al. 2013 ACC/AHA guideline on the treatment of blood cholesterol to reduce atherosclerotic cardiovascular risk in adults: a report of the American College of Cardiology/American Heart Association Task Force on Practice Guidelines. *Circulation.* 2013;00:1–85.
An important update supported by evidence to help reduce cholesterol and vascular disease risk.

17

Diabetes and Cardiovascular Events

Matthew A. Cavender

ETIOLOGY AND PATHOGENESIS

Diabetes mellitus is the resultant state of insulin deficiency that causes elevated blood glucose. The etiologies of this insulin deficiency can broadly be classified as either type 1 or type 2 diabetes. Type 1 diabetes is characterized by an autoimmune process that results in β-cell dysfunction and inadequate insulin production. This form of diabetes frequently presents during childhood or adolescence, and requires insulin supplementation due to the inadequate production of insulin by the pancreas.

Type 2 diabetes (T2DM) is more common in adults and is characterized by insulin resistance. Because most adult patients have T2DM, it is this group that will be the focus of this chapter. All of the mechanisms that underlie the development of insulin resistance have not been fully elucidated. It is likely that the disease is caused by the interaction of multiple different factors, including genetic, environmental, and lifestyle factors, all of which contribute to the development of the disease. It is clear that obesity plays a central role and decreases the body's responsiveness to insulin. This decrease in the response to insulin is known as insulin resistance, and patients with insulin resistance are considered to have prediabetes. In patients with prediabetes, higher levels of insulin are required to maintain glucose homeostasis. These increased demands on the pancreas place the insulin-producing β cells under stress. Ultimately, the pancreas is no longer able to produce enough insulin to maintain euglycemia, and thus, hyperglycemia results. These patients are considered to have progressed from prediabetes to T2DM. In patients with longstanding and poorly controlled T2DM, insulin production can fall, exacerbating the insulin deficiency and excess hepatic glucose production, which results in physiology that can resemble T1DM.

The presence of T2DM increases the risk of multiple adverse health events, including death. Broadly speaking, diabetes complications can be divided into those that are microvascular or macrovascular in origin (Fig. 17.1). Microvascular disorders include retinopathy (diabetes remains a leading of blindness), nephropathy (which can lead to end-stage renal disease), and neuropathy. Macrovascular complications from diabetes refer to those events that are predominately seen in larger caliber vessels and include myocardial infarction, stroke, and peripheral arterial disease. Patients with diabetes are at considerably higher risk of atherosclerosis and ischemic events.

Multiple biological mechanisms link diabetes and atherosclerosis. The higher burden of atherosclerosis seen in patients with diabetes is related partially to the direct effects of hyperglycemia. Hyperglycemia increases the proliferation of vascular smooth muscle cells that causes vascular beds to have diffusely diseased vessels and decreased capacity for delivery of blood (Fig. 17.2). Hyperglycemia also results in oxidative stress and the formation of reactive oxygen species, which, in turn, promote lipid oxidation, endothelial damage, inflammation, and progression of lipid-rich plaques. Finally, alterations in lipid metabolism and the association of hypertension and obesity that occur frequently in patients with diabetes also contribute to the development of atherosclerosis and the increased risk of cardiovascular events seen in this population.

In addition, it is becoming increasingly clear that patients with diabetes are also at increased risk of heart failure. The relationship between diabetes and heart failure has been known for some time; however, it was believed that diabetes predominately increased the risk for ischemic cardiomyopathies secondary to the higher rates of coronary artery disease seen in this population. Although coronary artery disease remains a significant risk factor for heart failure, it has been shown that the relationship between diabetes and heart failure is independent of the presence of atherosclerosis. In the REduction of Atherothrombosis for Continued Health (REACH) registry, which is a large international registry of patients with either established atherosclerosis or at high risk for atherosclerosis, patients with previous myocardial infarction or stroke had higher rates of heart failure than patients without established cardiovascular disease. However, the presence of diabetes resulted in a similar relative increase in the risk of heart failure, regardless of whether patients had a previous ischemic event or only had risk factors for heart failure. Patients with diabetes are at risk for heart failure with preserved ejection fraction, and this form of heart failure occurs independently from coronary artery disease. Although diabetes also increases the risk of other events (e.g., infections), preventing microvascular, macrovascular, and heart failure complications are the dominant goals of the current therapies for diabetes.

EPIDEMIOLOGY

The prevalence of diabetes is increasing across the world. In 1980 it was estimated that 108 million people had diabetes, and that is affected approximately 4.3% of the world's population. Over the past 25 years the rate of diabetes has grown exponentially, such that in 2014 it was estimated that diabetes was present in 422 million people worldwide and affected approximately 9% of men and 8% of women. Although some of this increase is believed to be secondary to aging of the population, overall increases in the prevalence of obesity are thought to be a considerable driver for the more than fourfold increase in prevalence. The incidence rate of diabetes is expected to continue to climb, and some studies have suggested that >700 million people may have diabetes by 2025.

There are multiple risk factors for the development of diabetes, including genetic predisposition, caloric intake and/or diet, and physical activity (or the lack thereof). All of these issues factor into the risk of developing diabetes. Ultimately, the rates of T2DM are closely linked with the presence of obesity. Most increases in the prevalence of diabetes are at least somewhat linked with the increasing incidence of obesity. Although diabetes and obesity are increasing in the United States, the rates of diabetes are increasing at the highest absolute rate in the

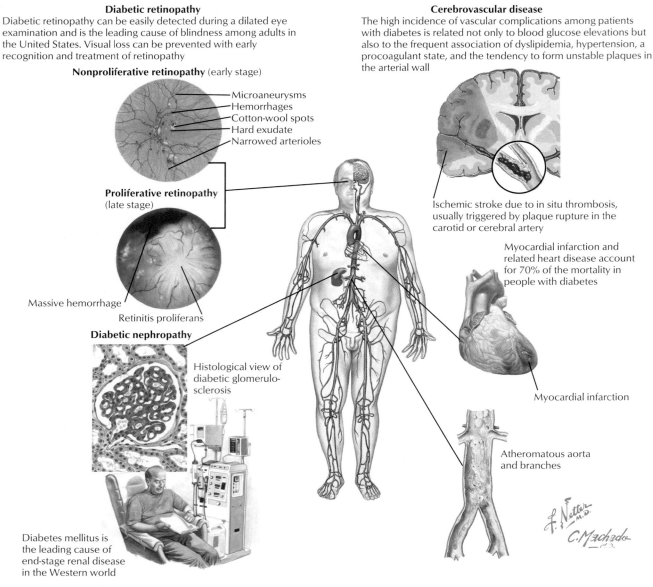

Diabetic retinopathy
Diabetic retinopathy can be easily detected during a dilated eye examination and is the leading cause of blindness among adults in the United States. Visual loss can be prevented with early recognition and treatment of retinopathy

Nonproliferative retinopathy (early stage)

—Microaneurysms
—Hemorrhages
—Cotton-wool spots
—Hard exudate
—Narrowed arterioles

Proliferative retinopathy
(late stage)

Massive hemorrhage

Retinitis proliferans

Diabetic nephropathy

Histological view of diabetic glomerulo-sclerosis

Diabetes mellitus is the leading cause of end-stage renal disease in the Western world

Cerebrovascular disease
The high incidence of vascular complications among patients with diabetes is related not only to blood glucose elevations but also to the frequent association of dyslipidemia, hypertension, a procoagulant state, and the tendency to form unstable plaques in the arterial wall

Ischemic stroke due to in situ thrombosis, usually triggered by plaque rupture in the carotid or cerebral artery

Myocardial infarction and related heart disease account for 70% of the mortality in people with diabetes

Myocardial infarction

Atheromatous aorta and branches

FIG 17.1 Diabetes mellitus and its complications: microvascular and macrovascular complications.

developing world. This increase appears to be due, at least in part, to the increase of high caloric diets and decreases in energy use as these societies move from predominately agrarian to more industrialized ways of life. Efforts to prevent the increase in the prevalence of diabetes are focused on the developing world because these increases are contributing significantly to the overall increase in the incidence of diabetes.

Patients with diabetes have higher rates of death compared with patients without diabetes. When evaluating the reasons for the differential rates of death, the largest contributor to the excess in deaths in patients with diabetes are cardiovascular events. Thus, targeting cardiovascular events is likely the most effective strategy to improve outcomes in patients with diabetes. Although rates of cardiovascular complications are declining, both in the general population and in patients with diabetes, the large increases in the number of patients with obesity and diabetes may threaten the long-term decreases in the cardiovascular event rate.

CLINICAL PRESENTATION

The duration of diabetes and degree of glycemic control with diabetes is a significant predictor of future diabetes complications. Previous studies have shown that glycosylated hemoglobin (HbA_{1c}), which is a marker of glucose levels over the previous 3 months, predicts cardiovascular events in patients both with and without established diabetes. The duration of diabetes is also a significant independent predictor of future diabetes complications. Thus, identification of patients at risk for diabetes, prediabetes, and new-onset diabetes allows for intensified therapy that may mitigate the risk of long-term complications from diabetes.

The American Diabetes Association (ADA) has identified some important risk factors associated with the development of diabetes: lack of physical activity; patients of African American, Latino, Native American, Asian American, Pacific Islander race or ethnicity; patients with a family history of diabetes (particularly those with first-degree

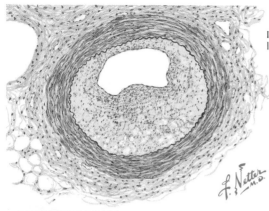

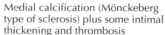

Intimal proliferation (atherosclerosis); lumen greatly reduced

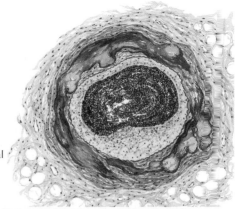

Medial calcification (Mönckeberg type of sclerosis) plus some intimal thickening and thrombosis

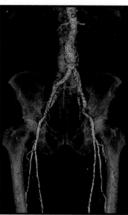

CT angiogram of the abdominal aorta shows the infrarenal abdominal aorta is mildly ectatic. There is a stenosis at the origin of the left internal iliac artery.

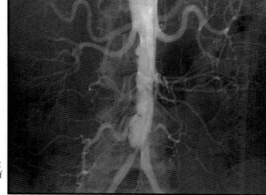

Aortogram showing advanced atheromatous disease involving the infrarenal abdominal aorta with multiple areas of ulceration. Tight atheromatous stenosis involving the origin of the right common iliac artery.

FIG 17.2 Atherosclerosis in diabetes.

relatives who have diabetes); women previously diagnosed with gestational disease; patients with hypertension; patients with low high-density lipoprotein cholesterol (<35 mg/dL) and/or high triglycerides (>250 mg/dL); patients with evidence of insulin resistance (HbA$_{1C}$ ≥5.7%); patients with impaired glucose tolerance (glucose of 140–199 mg/dL on a 2-hour glucose tolerance test) or impaired fasting glucose (100–125 mg/dL); patients with severe obesity; patients with acanthosis nigricans and/or polycystic ovarian syndrome; patients with hypertension (≥140/90 mm Hg or on treatment); and patients with a known cardiovascular disease are all independent predictors of having diabetes.

Current guidelines recommend screening for diabetes in patients who are overweight and/or obese and have at least one of the previously mentioned risk factors for diabetes. The diagnosis of diabetes requires the presence of at least one of four different clinical findings: (1) fasting plasma glucose of ≥126 mg/dL; (2) oral glucose tolerance test (with equivalent of 75 g anhydrous glucose dissolved in water) with a 2-hour postprandial glucose of ≥200 mg/dL; (3) HbA$_{1C}$ ≥6.5%; or (4) random plasma glucose of ≥200 mg/dL.

Patients are considered to have prediabetes if the HbA$_{1c}$ is between 5.7% and 6.4% (additional criteria for prediabetes include fasting plasma glucose between 100 and 124 mg/dL or glucose tolerance test with 2-hour glucose between 140 and 199 mg/dL). Patients with prediabetes are at increased risk of developing diabetes over time, and patients with tests closer to the upper range for prediabetes have a greater risk than patients with test results that are closer to the lower range. Patients with diabetes should be encouraged to begin exercise programs, work to lose weight, initiate therapies designed to modify cardiovascular risk factors, and reduce the risk of cardiovascular events. Previous studies have found

that exercise and weight loss are particularly efficacious in reducing the risk of developing diabetes.

MANAGEMENT AND THERAPY

The management of patients with diabetes depends upon whether patients have prediabetes and/or insulin sensitivity or if they have developed T2DM. The goals of therapy for patients with prediabetes focus on improving risk factor control and preventing the progression from insulin resistance to diabetes. Current recommendations focus on therapies shown to improve insulin sensitivity. Exercise and weight loss improve insulin sensitivity and have been shown to be effective strategies to reduce the risk of progression to diabetes. In a trial of 3234 patients with elevated fasting and postload plasma but without diabetes, patients randomized to lifestyle modification programs with goals of ≥7% weight loss and 150 minutes of physical activity per week had lower incidence of diabetes. In this same study, patients randomized to metformin also had lower rates of diabetes compared with patients who had usual care. However, the incidence of new-onset diabetes was lowest in those patients who received lifestyle interventions. Thus, in patients with prediabetes, lifestyle modifications and metformin form the foundation of current treatment recommendations. In patients with prediabetes who have had a stroke or transient ischemic attack, treatment with pioglitazone has been shown to be effective in reducing the progression to diabetes and decreasing the risk of future stroke or myocardial infarction.

In patients with established diabetes, the goals of therapy focus on the prevention of the microvascular and macrovascular complications of diabetes. Early identification of retinopathy through diabetic eye

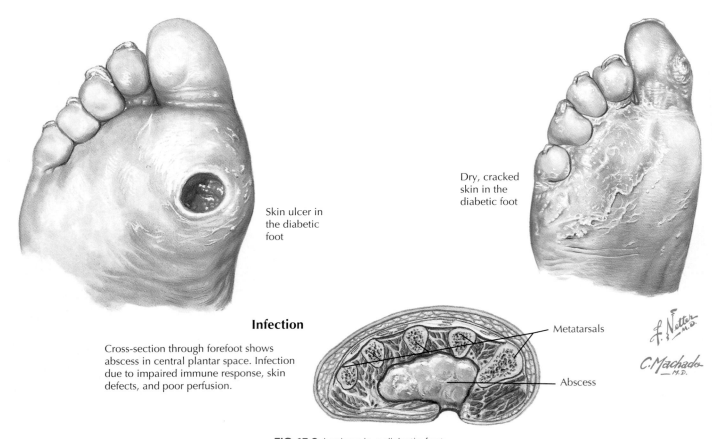

Skin ulcer in the diabetic foot

Dry, cracked skin in the diabetic foot

Infection

Cross-section through forefoot shows abscess in central plantar space. Infection due to impaired immune response, skin defects, and poor perfusion.

Metatarsals

Abscess

FIG 17.3 Lesions in a diabetic foot.

examinations, detection of nephropathy with urine microalbumin, and diabetic foot examinations to identify neuropathy and its complications are the cornerstones for preventing microvascular complications (Fig. 17.3). Glycemic control and glucose-lowering drugs are particularly important in preventing the microvascular complications of diabetes. In the United Kingdom Prospective Diabetes Study (UKPDS), microvascular events such as diabetic nephropathy were reduced with intensive glucose control. Although this study was performed in an era in which there were limited drugs for diabetes, and cardiovascular risk factors were not as aggressively controlled, there is a continued role for glycemic control in reducing microvascular complications.

The impact of glucose control on cardiovascular and other macrovascular events remains less clear. Previous studies have shown a clear association between the degree of glycemic control and the risk for cardiovascular events; yet, there are less data on whether glycemic control can reduce the risk of cardiovascular events. In the UKPDS trial, patients randomized to intensive glucose lowering had evidence of lower rates of myocardial infarction. However, this benefit was not seen during the initial trial, and only became evident after 10 years of follow-up. Similar studies, such as the Action to Control Cardiovascular Risk in Diabetes (ACCORD) trial, the Veterans Affairs Diabetes Trial (VADT), and Action in Diabetes and Vascular Disease: Preterax and Diamicron MR Controlled Evaluation (ADVANCE) trial, which randomized a more contemporary cohort of patients either to an intensive or routine glucose-lowering strategy, also did not show lower rates of either cardiovascular death or myocardial infarction. When pooled together in a meta-analysis, these studies suggested that intensive glycemic control likely does reduce myocardial infarction.

Current treatment guidelines for the treatment of diabetes recommend metformin as a first-line therapy for lowering glucose in patients with diabetes. Metformin is effective in lowering blood glucose, and a small trial has provided some evidence, albeit with a small number of events, that it may also reduce cardiovascular events. It remains the first-line therapy based upon the long history of use that has provided observational evidence of safety and efficacy with regard to glucose control. Although there is limited evidence for reductions in cardiovascular events, metformin is widely available and affordable, making it a reasonable choice for the initial treatment of patients with diabetes.

Most patients with diabetes will either have such poorly controlled glucose when diagnosed with diabetes that they will require more than one drug or will have progression of diabetes over time, making further therapies necessary. Current treatment guidelines support the concept of individualizing diabetes therapy based on individual patient factors. In patients at risk of cardiovascular disease, using therapies that have been shown to reduce cardiovascular risk should take a precedence over those therapies that have only been found to be effective in improving glucose control.

Sodium/Glucose Cotransport-2 Inhibitors

Currently, drugs from two different classes have been shown to be effective in reducing cardiovascular events in patients with diabetes. The sodium/glucose cotransport-2 inhibitors (SGLT-2i) have been shown to reduce cardiovascular events in patients with diabetes with either established atherosclerosis or who are at high risk for developing cardiovascular disease. These drugs work by inhibiting the SGLT-2 cotransporter, which is found in the proximal tubule of the kidney. When functioning normally, this cotransporter serves to re-uptake glucose that has been filtered by the kidney. Inhibition of this cotransporter results in glycosuria, which causes a mild osmotic diuretic effect and reductions in blood pressure and weight.

Thus far, two large cardiovascular outcome trials found that treatment with empagliflozin (Empagliflozin Cardiovascular Outcome Event Trial in Type 2 Diabetes Mellitus Patients—Removing Excess Glucose [EMPA-REG]) and canagliflozin (Canagliflozin Cardiovascular Assessment Study [CANVAS]) reduces major cardiovascular events, as well as hospitalization for heart failure and progression of renal disease. In the Comparative Effectiveness of Cardiovascular Outcomes (CVD-REAL) study, a large observational study of 1.4 million patients with diabetes from six different countries, patients with diabetes initiated on SGLT-2i had a lower risk of death and hospitalization for heart failure, which provided further support for the role of SGLT-2i in the treatment of patients with diabetes. These drugs were the first class of drugs designed specifically to lower glucose that were found to be effective in reducing the risk of cardiovascular disease. Because of the nature of these drugs, it seems unlikely that the beneficial effects were related to reductions in glucose control. The exact mechanism by which these drugs improved cardiovascular outcomes remains unclear, but might be secondary to effects on weight, blood pressure, and progression of renal disease.

Glucagon-Like Peptide–1 Agonists

Some agonists of glucagon-like peptide–1 (GLP-1) have also been shown to improve outcomes in patients with diabetes. The physiological role of GLP-1 is to help maintain glucose homeostasis and glycogen storage. The ingestion of food results in the release of GLP-1, which lowers plasma glucose by increasing insulin secretion and glycogen storage. Agonists of GLP-1 and dipeptidyl peptidase IV (DPP-IV) inhibitors (drugs that block the breakdown of GLP-1, which results in higher levels of biologically active GLP-1), have been found to be effective in lowering plasma glucose. Two specific GLP-1 agonists, liraglutide and semaglutide, have been shown to reduce cardiovascular events in patients with diabetes. These benefits have not been seen with other GLP-1 agonists or with DPP-IV inhibitors. In the Liraglutide Effect and Action in Diabetes: Evaluation of cardiovascular outcome Results (LEADER) trial, patients treated with liraglutide had a lower risk of cardiovascular death, myocardial infarction, or stroke (13.0% vs. 14.9%; hazard ratio [HR]: 0.87; 95% confidence interval [CI]: 0.78–0.97), with consistent effects on cardiovascular death (4.7% vs. 6.0%; HR: 0.78; 95% CI: 0.66–0.93), myocardial infarction (HR: 0.86; 95% CI: 0.73–1.00; P = 0.046), and stroke (HR: 0.86; 95% CI: 0.71–1.06). Semaglutide is a longer acting GLP-1 agonist that was studied in a small randomized clinical trial that also showed reductions in cardiovascular events.

The exact mechanism by which liraglutide and semaglutide reduce major cardiovascular events has not been fully elucidated. GLP-1 receptors have been found in a variety of different cardiovascular tissues. Animal models suggest that GLP-1 agonists may activate molecular pathways that are important for myocardial survival. Human studies with intravenous GLP-1 at a pharmacological dose found improvements in left ventricular function, maximum oxygen uptake, and physical performance in subjects with congestive heart failure, as well as reductions in blood pressure in patients with hypertension. These studies raise the potential for a nonglycemic mechanism of cardiovascular benefit.

Hypertension Control

In addition to the SGLT-2i and GLP-1 agonists, patients with diabetes and established cardiovascular disease should have aggressive cardiovascular risk factor modification. Patients with blood pressures >120 mm Hg (systolic) or >80 mm Hg (diastolic) should increase exercise, lose weight, and decrease salt intake. Results from a large meta-analysis of 40 trials of antihypertensive therapy have found that the pharmacological treatment of hypertension is most beneficial in patients with diabetes who have a baseline blood pressure of >140 mm Hg. There are some studies that have suggested achieving a goal blood pressure of 130 mm Hg rather than 140 mm Hg, which could result in a small reduction in the percentage of cardiovascular events and stroke. However, current FDA guidelines recommend the initiation of antihypertensive therapy for patients with blood pressures >140 mm Hg (systolic) or >90 mm Hg (diastolic).

Lipid-Lowering Therapy

Lipid-lowering therapy is an important aspect in the prevention of cardiovascular disease in patients with diabetes. In patients with diabetes and established cardiovascular disease, lowering low-density lipoprotein cholesterol (LDL-C) to extremely low levels reduces the risk of cardiovascular events. In the Improved Reduction of Outcomes: Vytorin Efficacy International Trial (IMPROVE-IT), patients with an acute coronary syndrome were randomized to either simvastatin 40 mg/ezetimibe 10 mg or simvastatin 40 mg. Patients with diabetes who were treated with ezetimibe had lower rates of cardiovascular death, myocardial infarction, unstable angina that required hospitalization, coronary revascularization, or stroke at 7 years (45.5% vs. 40.0%; HR: 0.86; 95% CI: 0.78–0.94). The effects of ezetimibe in patients with diabetes was greater than in patients without diabetes (P value [interaction] = .02). Further reductions in cardiovascular events have also been shown with proprotein convertase subtilisin/kexin type 9 (PCSK9) inhibitors, which have been studied for use, in addition to statins. In the Further Cardiovascular Outcomes Research with PCSK9 Inhibition in Subjects with Elevated Risk (FOURIER) trial, patients treated with evolocumab, a PCSK9 inhibitor, had a mean LDL-C of 30 mg/dL and significantly lower rates of cardiovascular events. Although there are no specific trials in patients with diabetes, in the FOURIER trial, a large proportion of patients had diabetes (37%). Taken together, these studies suggest that patients with diabetes benefit from aggressive lowering of LDL-C.

Current guidelines recommend that intensive statin therapy should be used for all patients with diabetes and known cardiovascular disease or those with risk factors for cardiovascular disease who are younger than 75 years old. Moderate intensity statins should be used in patients 40 to 75 years old without risk factors for cardiovascular disease. Because of the data on ezetimibe and PCSK9 inhibitors when used in addition to statin medications, it is highly likely that future guidelines may move toward recommendations that support a low goal LDL-C in patients with diabetes.

Antiplatelet Medications

Antiplatelet therapy reduces the risk of future cardiovascular events in patients at high risk of cardiovascular disease without established atherosclerosis and in patients with established atherosclerosis. Aspirin is recommended for long-term use in patients with diabetes who have had either a previous ischemic event or known atherosclerosis. The benefit of aspirin in patients with diabetes who have no evidence of atherosclerosis is less clear. As such, current recommendations support the use of aspirin in patients with a 10% risk of cardiovascular disease during the next 10 years of follow-up. Traditionally, patients with diabetes who are 50 years or older are considered to be at increased risk if they have at least one other cardiovascular risk factor (family history of early atherosclerosis, hypertension, smoking, dyslipidemia, or albuminuria). In those patients with diabetes who are younger than 50 years old and have no cardiovascular risk factors, aspirin therapy is not recommended.

Following a myocardial infarction, lifelong aspirin and additional antiplatelet therapy with a P2Y$_{12}$ inhibitor for at least 1 year is indicated. Because of the high rate of recurrent cardiovascular events in patients with diabetes, this population has particular benefit from more intensive antiplatelet therapy with ticagrelor and prasugrel. Although patients in clinical practice are often treated with only 12 months of dual antiplatelet therapy, patients with diabetes should be considered for long-term therapy. Patients with diabetes in the Prevention of Cardiovascular Events in Patients with Prior Heart Attack Using Ticagrelor Compared to Placebo on a Background of Aspirin–Thrombolysis in Myocardial Infarction 54 (PEGASUS-TIMI 54) trial, which evaluated the usefulness of long-term ticagrelor in patients 1 to 3 years after an acute myocardial infarction, had lower rates of cardiovascular events, including cardiovascular death. This supports longer duration or more intensive antiplatelet therapy in patients with diabetes and a previous myocardial infarction.

FUTURE DIRECTIONS

There have been significant advances in the care of patients with diabetes that have resulted in an overall decline in the rates of cardiovascular events. However, these improvements are threatened by the prevalence of diabetes with an increasing overall number of cardiovascular events. Future efforts to improve outcomes in patients with established T2DM will focus on methods to more accurately prevent diabetes. Current prevention strategies focus mostly on risk stratification by identifying events that have already occurred (e.g., previous myocardial infarction). Moving forward, using cardiovascular biomarkers such as high-sensitivity troponin or B-type natriuretic peptide may allow more accurate prediction of which patients are at highest risk of future cardiovascular events and who could benefit from more intensive therapies.

New pharmacotherapies such GLP-1 agonists and SGLT-2i have been shown to reduce cardiovascular risk in patients with diabetes and established cardiovascular disease. Further work is needed to understand whether these same cardiovascular benefits can be seen in patients without established cardiovascular disease and possibly even in patients with only prediabetes. In addition, it will important to better understand the mechanism of action in these drugs to explore additional targets that could provide further benefit, and so that clinicians can better understand how to most effectively use these therapies.

ADDITIONAL RESOURCES

Cavender MA, Steg PG, Smith S, et al. Impact of diabetes mellitus on hospitalization for heart failure, cardiovascular events, and death: outcomes at 4 years from the Reduction of Atherothrombosis for Continued Health (REACH) Registry. *Circulation.* 2015;132(10):923–933.

Well-characterized observational study describing the rates of cardiovascular events in patients with T2DM. Highlights the high rates of heart failure in patients with T2DM and identifies T2DM as an independent risk factor.

Cavender MA, White WB, Jarolim P, et al. Serial measurement of high sensitivity troponin I and cardiovascular outcomes in patients with type 2 diabetes mellitus in the EXAMINE Trial. *Circulation.* 2017;135(20):1911–1921.

More than 90% of patients with T2DM have detectable levels of high-sensitivity troponin, and changes over time predict future cardiovascular events.

Chatterjee S, Khunti K, Davies MJ. Type 2 diabetes. *Lancet.* 2017;389(10085):2239–2251.

Excellent review of T2DM.

Gregg EW, Li Y, Wang J, et al. Changes in diabetes-related complications in the United States, 1990-2010. *N Engl J Med.* 2014;370:1514–1523.

This study identifies myocardial infarction as a common cardiovascular event in patients with T2DM, but it shows that the incidence of diabetes complications and myocardial infarction have declined over time.

Knowler WC, Barrett-Connor E, Fowler SE, et al. Reduction in the incidence of type 2 diabetes with lifestyle intervention or metformin. *N Engl J Med.* 2002;346(6):393–403.

This randomized clinical trial provides evidence for interventions in patients with prediabetes that can reduce the risk of progressing to T2DM.

Kosiborod M, Cavender MA, Fu AZ, et al. Lower risk of heart failure and death in patients initiated on SGLT-2 inhibitors versus other glucose-lowering drugs: the CVD-REAL Study. *Circulation.* 2017;doi:10.1161/CIRCULATIONAHA.117.029190.

This observational study finds an association between SGLT-2i use and a lower risk of cardiovascular events that supports the use of these agents in clinical practice.

Marso SP, Daniels GH, Brown-Frandsen K, et al. Liraglutide and cardiovascular outcomes in type 2 diabetes. *N Engl J Med.* 2016;375(4):311–322.

Liraglutide, a GLP-1 agonist, reduces cardiovascular events in patients with T2DM.

Neal B, Perkovic V, Mahaffey KW, de Zeeuw D, Fulcher G, Erondu N, Shaw W, Law G, Desai M, Matthews DR. Canagliflozin and cardiovascular and renal events in type 2 diabetes. *N Engl J Med.* 2017;doi:10.1056/NEJMoa 1611925.

Canagliflozin reduces cardiovascular events, including heart failure, in patients with T2DM.

Scirica BM, Bhatt DL, Braunwald E, Raz I, Cavender MA, Im K, Mosenzon O, Udell JA, Hirshberg B, Pollack PS, Steg PG, Jarolim P, Morrow DA. Prognostic implications of biomarker assessments in patients with type 2 diabetes mellitus at high cardiovascular risk. *JAMA Cardiol.* 2016;1(9):989–998.

High-sensitivity troponin can identify subgroups of patients with T2DM at high risk of cardiovascular events.

Zinman B, Wanner C, Lachin JM, et al. Empagliflozin, cardiovascular outcomes, and mortality in type 2 diabetes. *N Engl J Med.* 2015;373(22):2117–2128.

Dapagliflozin reduces cardiovascular events, including heart failure, in patients with T2DM.

18

Cardiovascular Effects of Air Pollutants

Weeranun D. Bode, Wayne E. Cascio

Cardiovascular disease risk factors—including hypertension, lipid abnormalities, diabetes mellitus, obesity, physical inactivity, and tobacco use—provide targets for the prevention or progression of heart disease. Yet, these risk factors account for only approximately 50% to 75% of cases of ischemic heart disease and cardiac events. Air pollution is an environmental factor that contributes independently and modifies the known cardiovascular risk factors. The World Health Organization estimates that >7 million premature deaths each year can be attributed to urban outdoor and indoor air pollution caused by the burning of solid fuels. However, the effects of air pollutants on the cardiovascular system are generally not appreciated by patients or their healthcare providers. This chapter reviews the links between air pollution and cardiovascular disease, describes plausible physiological mechanisms accounting for these effects, and provides an educational resource for physicians and patients to avoid exposure to air pollution and to decrease risk when exposure is inevitable.

HISTORY

During the 20th century, three notable extreme air pollution episodes focused the attention of the public and governments on the adverse public health impact of air pollution. These events occurred in the Meuse Valley, Belgium; Donora, Pennsylvania; and London, England, as a consequence of weather conditions that trapped combustion products and other pollutants from coal fires, vehicles, power plants, and industrial emissions in the air. The best known of these events was the Great London smog. In 1952, a cold air inversion trapped combustion products of the entire city of 8.3 million persons and its industry, resulting in an extreme air pollution episode that claimed >10,000 lives. During this event, daily mortality increased nearly fourfold, and the mortality rate remained significantly higher than usual for several weeks after the air pollution event resolved. Surprisingly, the additional deaths that continued to mount were not explained solely by pulmonary disease, but instead most deaths were attributed to cardiovascular etiologies.

These important historical events had a profound impact on local and governmental responses to air pollution and contributed significantly to the passing of the Clean Air Act (CAA) in the United States in 1970, which has been updated and modified several times since. Through the CAA, the U.S. Environmental Protection Agency (EPA) has statutory responsibility to regulate ambient air pollutants, including particulate matter (PM), sulfur dioxide (SO_2), nitrogen dioxide (NO_2), carbon monoxide (CO), ozone (O_3), and lead. The levels of permissible air pollutants are established by the doses at which a measurable health risk is anticipated, allowing for an adequate margin of safety. This risk assessment is based on scientific data updated every 5 years and published as the U.S. National Ambient Air Quality Integrative Science Assessment. Although urban air pollution continues to be a significant challenge, the overall quality of air in the United States has improved

continuously since the implementation of the CAA. The improvement in air quality has translated into decreased overall mortality and cardiopulmonary mortality associated with exposure to air pollutants. Yet, despite the remarkable progress made in air quality, health risks of air pollution remain. Intermittent increases in air pollution pose challenges, particularly in vulnerable and sensitive groups, such as older adults, those with low socioeconomic positions, and in individuals with cardiovascular disease, obesity, and diabetes mellitus.

PARTICULATE MATTER

Airborne PM is not a single compound but a mixture of materials that have a carbonaceous core and associated constituents, such as organic compounds, acids, metals, crustal components, and biological materials, including pollen, spores, and endotoxins. Combustion processes, such as those in vehicles and power plants, account for most human-generated PM. Importantly, particles generated by mechanical processes, wind-blown dust, and wildfires also contribute to the mass of PM.

Particles are classified based on their size. Ultrafine particles have an equivalent aerodynamic diameter of <0.1 μm (approximately one one-thousandth the diameter of a human hair). Fine particles ($PM_{2.5}$) have a diameter of ≤2.5 μm. Coarse particles (PM_{10}) have a diameter between 2.5 and 10 μm. Only particles <10 μm in diameter are respirable (Fig. 18.1). Ultrafine and fine particles are more likely to be produced by combustion, whereas the coarse particles are more likely to contain crustal and biological material. Outdoor PM readily penetrates into homes and buildings, depending on building stock and the use of air conditioning and heating; thus, increases in outdoor PM can result in increased indoor levels of PM. Cooking, smoking, dusting, and vacuuming also contribute to indoor PM, although not much is known about cardiovascular effects induced by exposure to indoor sources of air pollution in the United States. The U.S. national air quality standard for the allowable level of $PM_{2.5}$ averaged over 24 hours is 35 μg/m³, and the annual average is 12 μg/m³. The standard for PM_{10} averaged over 24 hours is 150 μg/m³.

Particle size appears to have an impact on the health effects of PM, with $PM_{2.5}$ having a stronger association with adverse cardiovascular outcomes than that of PM_{10}, presumably due to deeper penetration of fine particles into the lung. PM air pollution, which has the most data for $PM_{2.5}$, is associated with acute coronary syndrome (unstable angina and myocardial infarction), deep venous thrombosis, rhythm disturbances, stroke, and worsening of heart failure.

The cardiovascular effects associated with PM exposure can be categorized as short-term and long-term. Short-term exposure over a few hours to weeks can trigger cardiovascular disease that can be related to higher mortality and nonfatal events. The strongest evidence is for ischemic heart disease events, especially myocardial infarction and heart failure hospitalizations. Long-term exposure over a few years increases

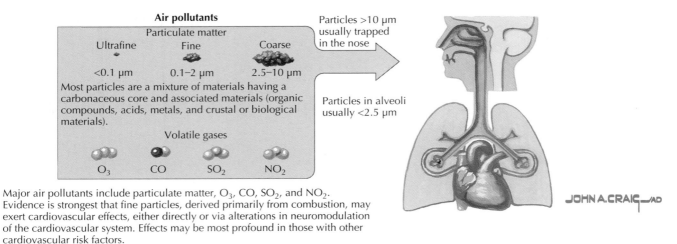

Major air pollutants include particulate matter, O_3, CO, SO_2, and NO_2. Evidence is strongest that fine particles, derived primarily from combustion, may exert cardiovascular effects, either directly or via alterations in neuromodulation of the cardiovascular system. Effects may be most profound in those with other cardiovascular risk factors.

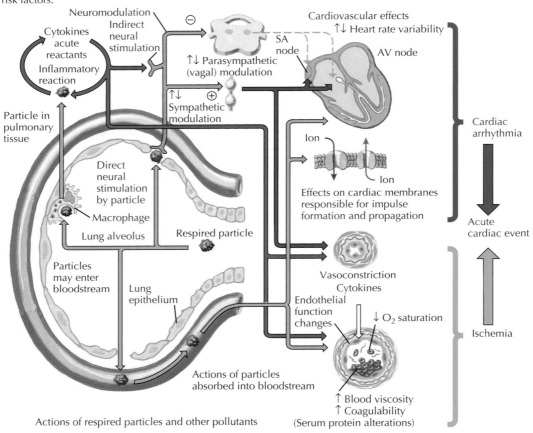

FIG 18.1 Cardiovascular Effects of Air Pollutants. *AV,* Atrioventricular; *CO,* carbon monoxide; *NO₂,* nitrogen dioxide; *O₃,* ozone; *SA,* sinoatrial; *SO₂,* sulfur dioxide.

cardiovascular mortality even more than short-term exposure, and decreases life expectancy.

The causal link between inhaled particles depositing on respiratory surfaces and cardiovascular health effects has been a topic of investigation for the past two decades. Exposure to PM can increase heart rate and blood pressure, and can decrease oxygen saturation within hours. PM also affects pulmonary oxygen transport and neural modulation of the sinus node and the vascular system, although the magnitude of these changes is small. An increase in heart rate might be caused by an increase in sympathetic input to the heart or a decrease in

parasympathetic input. Exposure to PM decreases cardiac vagal input, as suggested by a decrease in heart rate variability (HRV). Yet, the association between changes in HRV and ambient PM concentrations is inconsistent. Whether the differences relate to the chemical composition of PM, other associated pollutants, age, sex, genetic background, concurrent cardiac disease, medications, or the HRV methodology is not known. It is also not known whether change in HRV associated with PM exposure represents an independent measure of risk.

Many epidemiological studies that investigated the associations between air particle pollution and cardiovascular mortality and morbidity in single cities and multiple cities throughout the world showed concordance that ambient air particle pollution is associated with increased cardiovascular mortality and hospitalizations. Two of the most notable studies were the National Morbidity, Mortality and Air Pollution Study and the Air Pollution and Health: A European Approach Project. These studies addressed the effects of air pollution in many U.S. and European cities, and showed that air particle pollution was associated with an increased relative risk of cardiovascular mortality, ranging from 0.4% to 1.5% for each 20 μg/m^3 increase in PM$_{10}$. Likewise, other epidemiological studies linked exposure to PM, particularly traffic-related particles, to the onset of myocardial infarction or hospitalization for acute coronary syndrome, stroke, rhythm disturbances, and heart failure, which were associations that were stronger among individuals with underlying cardiac disease.

Long-term effects of air pollution were established in three important cohort studies: the Harvard Six-Cities Study, the American Cancer Society Study, and the Women's Health Initiative Observational Study. In contrast to previous studies, these studies investigated the long-term health effects of fine PM for several years in multiple cities, characterized by a large gradient in the concentration and types of air pollution. These studies showed a positive association between PM$_{2.5}$ and sulfate, and cardiopulmonary mortality and cardiovascular events. Subjects who resided in the most heavily polluted of the Harvard six cities lived on average 2 years less than those who resided in the least polluted city, after potential confounding and effect-modifying factors were taken into consideration.

There are at least three possible mechanisms by which PM induces changes in cardiac physiology: a neural reflex from afferents in the lung that interact with PM directly or indirectly through associated pulmonary inflammation; secondary effects of inflammatory cytokines and acute-phase reactants produced systemically and in the lung, as well as coagulation proteins; and direct effects of particles or adsorbed soluble constituents of PM on cardiac membrane currents responsible for impulse formation and repolarization. The observations that inhalation of fine-particulate air pollution and O$_3$ causes arterial vasoconstriction, and that sympathetic activation reduces endothelium-dependent, flow-mediated vasodilation, provide a mechanistic link between the changes in HRV and the changes in vascular reactivity, which are known risks for cardiac events. Because sudden shifts in neural input to the heart may be arrhythmogenic, changes in HRV imply changes in neural input to the heart as a mechanism of arrhythmia. Such changes would be expected to increase the risk of cardiovascular events secondary to thrombosis and arrhythmias.

The effects of long-term exposure to fine particulate air pollution have been inferred from linking cardiovascular risk factors and estimates of air pollution exposure to the cause of death in epidemiological studies. These observational studies showed that fine particulate air pollution increased the rate of mortality from cardiopulmonary causes. The risk of cardiopulmonary mortality was most strongly associated with fine particles compared with larger particles. Although the mechanisms are unknown, possible explanations of the risks include acceleration of atherosclerosis progression secondary to increased oxidative stress or systemic inflammation, and modulation of factors that enhance coronary plaque instability or electrical instability. Data are emerging that show that PM accelerates atherosclerosis in humans and in animal models of long-term PM exposure, although the effect is probably indirectly mediated through increased inflammation and oxidant stress. For instance, high-sensitivity C-reactive protein (hs-CRP) correlates with cardiac events. The liver produces CRP in response to the cytokines interleukin (IL)-1, IL-6, and tumor necrosis factor-α. Measurement of cytokines, and even hs-CRP, may provide a mechanism to assess cardiovascular risk in response to PM exposure. Because of the complexity

of the mechanisms that regulate initiation and progression of atherosclerosis, and the complex constituents of PM, proof of a causal effect of PM on the development of atherosclerosis will be a challenge. Yet, the Multi-Ethnic Atherosclerosis Study substudy, MESA Air, did show an association between long-term exposure to PM$_{2.5}$ and NO$_2$ and coronary artery calcium accumulation.

It is possible that PM has a direct effect on cardiac autonomic function, on cardiac repolarization, or on both, and that PM increases an individual's susceptibility to myocardial ischemia and to ventricular fibrillation during regional myocardial ischemia. Long-term exposure to airborne PM might initiate cellular signaling that affects the expression of the cellular proteins that are important to electrical impulse formation and conduction in the heart. Potential protein targets include structural proteins, as well as voltage-gated and ligand-gated channels, and ion exchangers. Thus, cardiac deaths associated with exposure to PM are likely to result from interaction of the direct effects of PM on vascular function, cardiac electrophysiology, autonomic regulation, and/or coronary thrombosis in individuals at high risk for sudden cardiac death.

Exposure to secondhand tobacco smoke is a reasonable model for understanding how exposure to PM mediates changes in the cardiovascular system and contributes to cardiac events. Acute exposure activates platelets and decreases endothelial function in humans, whereas long-term exposure accelerates the formation of atherosclerosis.

Sulfur Dioxide

SO$_2$ is a gas produced by coal-burning power plants, smelters, refineries, pulp mills, and food-processing plants. Typical ambient air reactions include formation of sulfuric acid (acid rain) and sulfates. A positive correlation exists between SO$_2$ levels and hospital admissions, the mortality rate in older adults, and the presence of cardiovascular disease. It is often difficult to separate the contributions of individual components of air pollution and to attribute them to health effects. For example, in one study, the total mortality rate was estimated to increase by 5% for each 0.038 parts per million (ppm) increase in SO$_2$; yet, the effects were no longer significant when respirable particles were included in the statistical model. Thus, SO$_2$ is likely to be a surrogate marker of PM because of the common sources of SO$_2$ and PM. The U.S national air quality standard for the allowable level of SO$_2$ averaged over 1 hour is 75 ppb.

Nitrogen Dioxide

NO$_2$ and nitric oxide (NO) are reactive gases produced by gasoline and diesel fuel combustion, electric power generation, chemical manufacturing, soil emission (including fertilizers), and solid waste disposal. NO$_2$ is also a major indoor air pollutant produced by gas stoves and gas heaters. Both gases are critical components of the photo-oxidation cycle and O$_3$ formation. NO is also produced endogenously at levels that can exceed 1 ppm. It is a mediator and a strong vasodilator and bronchodilator. The ultimate fate of NO$_2$ and NO in ambient air and biological fluids is the formation of nitrite and nitrate.

NO$_2$ is primarily associated with long-term respiratory effects. Children and adults with existing respiratory diseases are at increased respiratory risk from NO$_2$ inhalation. Healthy individuals have shown slightly reduced cardiac output when inhaling NO$_2$ during exercise. Increased levels of NO$_2$ and black carbon are positively associated with arrhythmias. A positive significant association also exists between NO$_2$ and an increased risk of myocardial infarction. Numerous epidemiological studies have linked elevated levels of NO$_2$ to coronary heart disease. Prolonged exposure of coronary heart disease patients to NO$_2$ has been shown to correlate with reduced HRV. Daily exposure to NO$_2$, particularly in older adults, was significantly associated with daily emergency department visits for ischemic heart disease. The U.S. national air quality standard for the allowable level of NO_2 averaged over 1 hour is 100 ppb, and averaged over a year is 53 ppb.

Carbon Monoxide

CO is produced by combustion. When inhaled, CO binds avidly to hemoglobin, thereby reducing the capacity of blood to deliver oxygen to the tissues. Within tissue, CO may bind to cytochrome P-450, cytochrome oxidase, and myoglobin, which affects intracellular function. Individuals most susceptible to these effects have flow-limiting coronary disease.

A study of the long-term health effects of CO exposure in a comparison of bridge and tunnel workers showed that the relative risk of coronary artery disease was greater in tunnel workers. Prolonged exposure to CO and attendant carboxyhemoglobin (COHb) concentration in excess of 10% increased heart rate, systolic blood pressure, red blood cell mass, and blood volume. CO has been implicated in atherogenesis and in increased risk of myocardial infarction. In general, controlled exposure to CO reduces the time to onset of electrocardiographic evidence of exercise-induced ischemia and angina in individuals with ischemic heart disease, and increases the frequency of ventricular arrhythmias during exercise. These effects occur at COHb levels as low as 2.9%. The baseline COHb in healthy nonsmokers is 0.5% to 1.0%. Prolonged exposure to 9 ppm CO would produce a blood COHb level of approximately 2%. Thus, the U.S. national air quality standards for CO (35 ppm averaged over 1 hour and 9 ppm averaged over 8 hours) should provide protection even for a sensitive population with ischemic heart disease.

Ozone

O_3 is a secondary air pollutant formed in the atmosphere by photochemical reactions involving primary pollutants, volatile organic compounds, and NOs. The U.S. national ambient air quality standard for ground-level O_3 is 0.07 ppm averaged over 8 hours. Exposure to O_3 irritates mucous membranes, decreases lung function, increases the reactivity of airways, and causes airway inflammation. Consequently, O_3 exposure can cause symptoms of chest pain and decreased exercise capacity. Initial epidemiology studies that showed associations between PM and mortality were not able to reproducibly show similar relationships between O_3 and mortality, primarily because there is a close correlation of these two pollutants in many cities. However, several epidemiology studies showed associations between exposure to O_3 and increased mortality and morbidity. In one study, an increase in O_3 of 21.3 ppb increased the cardiovascular disease mortality rate by 2.5% and the respiratory disease mortality rate by 6.6%; the effect of O_3 was independent of that of other pollutants. Whether O_3 and PM affect the cardiovascular system by similar or different mechanisms remains unknown.

AIR POLLUTION EFFECTS ON CONGENITAL HEART DISEASE

There are several case-control and retrospective studies that have investigated the association of maternal exposure to air pollution and the risk of congenital heart disease. Each study focused on a different air pollutant. Higher levels of $PM_{2.5}$ exposure were associated with an increased risk of nonisolated truncus arteriosus, total anomalous pulmonary venous return, coarctation of the aorta, and interrupted aortic arch, as well as any critical isolated and nonisolated congenital heart defect in Florida. The exposure to the 90th percentile of SO_2 in Italy was associated with an increased prevalence of congenital heart disease and ventricular septal defects. CO, NO, and black smoke exposure in Northeast England were associated with congenital heart disease. Mechanisms linking air pollution to congenital heart disease remain extremely challenging to study, mainly due to the difficulty in estimating the net effect of environmental pollution in comparison to underlying comorbidities and individual lifestyle factors in pregnant mothers.

WHAT PATIENTS CAN DO TO PROTECT AGAINST CARDIOVASCULAR EFFECTS OF AIR POLLUTION

Patients with heart disease should be made aware of the increased risk associated with exposure to air pollution and educated about strategies to decrease exposure. Patients can reduce their exposure and risk by decreasing their time outdoors when air pollutants are at concentrations believed to impart a health risk and/or by decreasing the intensity of outdoor physical activity. For example, if a patient usually jogs, exercising indoors in an air-conditioned environment can be recommended. If an alternative and acceptable indoor location is not available, one should walk instead of jog. Outdoor PM contributes to indoor PM. When conditions are severe (e.g., wood smoke secondary to a wildfire), activities should be restricted indoors as well, and consideration should be given to using high-efficiency particulate air filter air cleaners to reduce indoor PM levels. PM and NO_2 are typically elevated in the morning and afternoon when automotive and truck traffic increases during rush hour commutes. O_3 concentration increases in the heat of the day, and therefore, is highest in the midday and in the summer months. In general, patients can reduce exposure by the following: limiting exercise outdoors in the afternoons when air pollutant concentrations are high; exercising indoors or away from roadways; closing doors and windows, and using air conditioning; seeking out air quality reports and forecasts; and using the Air Quality Index (AQI) to guide outdoor activities. The AQI provides a national standard for reporting daily air quality and providing anticipated health effects for the quality reported. The AQI can be reviewed daily in the local media or on the EPA website.

In some areas of the United States, state and local environmental agencies in cooperation with the EPA provide a service, EnviroFlash (http://www.enviroflash.info/), that provides air quality alerts by email. Patients can customize reports so that they are notified of only those conditions that would pose a health risk for their specific clinical condition.

FUTURE DIRECTIONS

More information is needed to establish the cardiovascular health effects of specific pollutants. The dose-dependence of these effects is key for determining air quality standards. Environmental concentrations of air pollutants vary widely, as do their sources and toxicities. Source apportionment is important for identifying origins of the various PM constituents so that health effects might be linked to specific PM constituents and sources.

Many questions remain about the cardiovascular effects of air pollutants. Does the interaction of air pollutants lead to additive, synergistic, or decreased health effects? Do the signaling pathways responsible for short-term and long-term health effects differ? Why do older adults and individuals with prevalent cardiovascular and pulmonary disease, diabetes, and hypertension have a greater susceptibility to the effects of air pollution? What is the role of PM-induced systemic inflammation in the development and progression of atherosclerotic vascular disease? To what extent does gene–environment interaction determine the health effects of air pollution exposure? Further investigation is needed to answer these questions.

ADDITIONAL RESOURCES

AIRNow. Available at: http://www.epa.gov/airnow. Accessed January 3, 2017.

A U.S. EPA-supported website providing an overview of air quality in the United States. Includes the AQI, which provides information about the level of anticipated health risk for any reported level of air quality. Several other learning and information resources are available.

Brook RD, Franklin B, Cascio W, et al. Air pollution and cardiovascular disease: a statement for healthcare professionals from the expert panel on population and prevention science of the American Heart Association. *Circulation.* 2004;109:2655–2671.

American Heart Association (AHA) scientific statement compiled by experts in the field that provides a comprehensive review of the literature before 2004.

Brook RD, Rajagopalan S, Pope A III, et al. Particulate matter air pollution and cardiovascular disease: an update to the scientific statement from the American Heart Association. *Circulation.* 2010;121:2331–2378.

AHA scientific statement compiled by experts in the field that provides a comprehensive review of the literature between 2004 and 2010.

Gold DR, Mittleman MA. New insights into pollution and the cardiovascular system 2010 to 2012. *Circulation.* 2013;127:1903–1913.

A contemporary review about the cardiovascular effects of air pollution.

Kaufman JD, Adar SD, et al. Association between air pollution and coronary artery calcification within six metropolitan areas in the USA (the Multi-Ethnic Study of Atherosclerosis and Air Pollution): a longitudinal cohort study. *Lancet.* 2016;388:696–704.

Longitudinal study showing a positive association between long-term exposure to $PM_{2.5}$ and NO_2 and the accumulation of coronary artery calcium.

National Ambient Air Quality Standards (NAAQS) Table. Available at: http://www.epa.gov/criteria-air-pollutants/naaqs-table. Accessed January 3, 2017.

A U.S. EPA-supported website providing National Ambient Air Quality Standards for six principal pollutants.

U.S. Environmental Protection Agency. Available at: http://www.epa.gov. Accessed January 3, 2017.

The U.S. EPA home page providing the portal to science and technology, laws and regulations, and health information, including continuing medical education programs related to air pollution.

EVIDENCE

Chen Y, Craig L, Krewski D. Air quality risk assessment and management. *J Toxicol Environ Health A.* 2008;71:24–39.

Comprehensive review of the effects of air pollution on health, with a good discussion of the health effect of gases.

Dockery DW, Pope CA III, Xu X, et al. An association between air pollution and mortality in six U.S. cities. *N Engl J Med.* 1993;329:1753–1759.

Large-cohort study that included six U.S. cities characterized by long-term follow-up, and gradients in air pollutants that were specifically designed to investigate the association between air pollutants and mortality. This was the first large-cohort study that provided a quantitative assessment of the impact of air pollution on mortality.

Dominici F, Peng RD, Bell ML, et al. Fine particulate air pollution and hospital admission for cardiovascular and respiratory diseases. *JAMA.* 2006;295:1127–1134.

Ambitious and comprehensive study of the short-term cardiovascular and respiratory health effects of air pollution across the United States in the Medicare population.

Miller KA, Siscovick DS, Sheppard L, et al. Long-term exposure to air pollution and incidence of cardiovascular events in women. *N Engl J Med.* 2007;365:447–458.

The Women's Health Initiative cohort was used to investigate the effects of air pollution on postmenopausal women. The findings were consistent with those of the Harvard Six-Cities Study and the American Cancer Society Study and indicated that increases in $PM_{2.5}$ were associated with an increased risk of cardiovascular death. The study also supported the hypothesis that increases in $PM_{2.5}$ were correlated with cardiovascular events.

Pope CA III, Burnett RT, Thun MJ, et al. Lung cancer, cardiopulmonary mortality, and long-term exposure to fine particulate air pollution. *JAMA.* 2002;287:1132–1141.

This large, longitudinal American Cancer Society Study was used to test the hypothesis that air particle pollution is associated with an increase in cardiopulmonary mortality. Like the Harvard Six-Cities Study, this study showed a positive association between long-term exposure to inhaled PM and an increase in cardiopulmonary mortality and lung cancer.

Pope CA III, Muhlestein JB, May HT, et al. Ischemic heart disease events triggered by short-term exposure to fine particulate air pollution. *Circulation.* 2006;114:2443–2448.

This paper describes the adverse cardiovascular health impact of short-term exposure to air pollution in the Wasatch Front area of Utah. A case-crossover design was used to demonstrate that increased ambient $PM_{2.5}$ was associated with an increase in acute coronary syndrome, as defined by unstable angina and myocardial infarction.

Coronary Heart Disease

19

Stable Coronary Artery Disease

Venu Menon

Advances in pharmacotherapy and revascularization strategies have dramatically improved the short-term and long-term outcomes for patients with atherosclerotic coronary artery disease (CAD). At the same time, the worldwide incidence of atherosclerosis and CAD has also increased, largely driven by significant increases in obesity and type 2 diabetes mellitus. As a result, atherosclerotic CAD will remain a major public health issue for the foreseeable future.

Patients with atherosclerotic CAD can present to healthcare providers in many different ways. This chapter focuses on chronic stable angina. Other clinical presentations of atherosclerotic CAD (acute coronary syndromes [ACSs], congestive heart failure, sudden cardiac death, and cardiogenic shock) are described in separate chapters (Chapters 20, 21, 24, 28, 29, and 44).

ETIOLOGY AND PATHOGENESIS

In contrast to oxygen extraction by skeletal muscle, oxygen use by cardiac tissue is near maximal, even at rest (Fig. 19.1). The heart responds to the need for increased cardiac output by increasing heart rate and contractility, both of which increase wall stress and myocardial oxygen requirements. This need for increased myocardial oxygen cannot be met by increasing the efficiency of oxygen extraction, and thus must be met by increasing coronary blood flow. If a significant flow-limiting epicardial stenosis is present, coronary blood flow is maintained by compensatory dilatation of the coronary bed beyond the obstruction. This diminishes coronary flow reserve and results in an inability to meet oxygen requirements as myocardial demand increases, creating a supply-demand mismatch. Symptoms of angina reflect myocardial ischemia and arise when the blood supply to a region of the heart cannot increase sufficiently to match myocardial oxygen demand. Ischemia can be elicited by treadmill or bicycle exercise testing (or using pharmacological vasodilator stress), and may be measured as loss of systolic thickening on echocardiography, diminished perfusion on SPECT, ST-segment depression on the surface ECG, and provocation of angina or its equivalent.

Increased vasoreactivity may also result in decreased myocardial blood flow with or without increased demand. Vasoreactivity seems to be responsible for some of the circadian, seasonal, and emotional components associated with angina. The other major biological mechanism that results in myocardial ischemia is sudden spontaneous rupture or erosion of an atherosclerotic plaque in a coronary artery, which results in sudden diminished blood flow and ACSs, as discussed in Chapters 20 and 21.

CLINICAL PRESENTATION

Chronic stable angina is characterized by angina that occurs with increased oxygen demand. Symptoms can be provoked by exertion,

heavy meals, or emotional distress. Symptoms tend to be reproducible and usually have been present over many months or longer. These symptoms most commonly result from fixed coronary stenoses (Fig. 19.2). Chest discomfort is typically described as a pressure or tightness, or discomfort over the left precordium, although many individuals with myocardial ischemia do not manifest classic symptoms. The discomfort may radiate along the ulnar aspect of the left arm and is often accompanied by shortness of breath, nausea, and diaphoresis (Fig. 19.3). Symptoms may also radiate or be isolated to the throat, jaw, interscapular region, and epigastrium. Radiation below the umbilicus and to the occiput is uncharacteristic, as are symptoms that are well localized to a fingertip, as provoked by palpation and movement, or relieved by lying down. Typically, stable anginal pain lasts for more than a few minutes and <10 minutes, is associated with exertion or other stresses, and is relieved by rest or the use of sublingual nitroglycerin within 1 to 2 minutes. Angina can occasionally be mistaken as indigestion, accounting for a delay in presentation or treatment. It is important to understand that atypical presentations of angina can occur in any patient but are more common in individuals with diabetes, women, and older adults. In these individuals, it is important to further evaluate any exertion-related symptoms that may reflect an inability to increase myocardial oxygen delivery, including significant dyspnea on exertion, new or worsened fatigue with exertion, or similar symptoms.

DIFFERENTIAL DIAGNOSIS

The quality of chest pain is similar to that experienced in the setting of acute unstable angina or acute myocardial infarction (MI). In that setting, it is usually more intense and prolonged, but the difference may be subjective. An important difference is that the pain associated with an acute MI is usually unremitting, although it may wax and wane in severity. Angina, or any symptoms that reflect a limitation of myocardial oxygen demand, may also reflect non–coronary artery etiologies, including severe aortic valve stenosis, hypertrophic cardiomyopathy, and microvascular dysfunction. Other cardiovascular causes of chest pain to be considered include pericarditis, aortic dissection, and pulmonary embolism. These may be difficult to distinguish from angina based on the history and physical examination, and often require further diagnostic evaluation. The most common noncardiac causes of angina-like pain are gastrointestinal conditions, such as gastroesophageal reflux disease, esophageal spasm, peptic ulcer disease, biliary disease, and pancreatitis. Of these, gastroesophageal reflux disease is most commonly encountered. Pleuritis or chest pain related to other lung pathology may also present in this manner. Cervical disk disease, costochondral syndromes, and shingles may also mimic angina. Chest discomfort is also a common manifestation in patients with panic disorder, but this remains a diagnosis of exclusion.

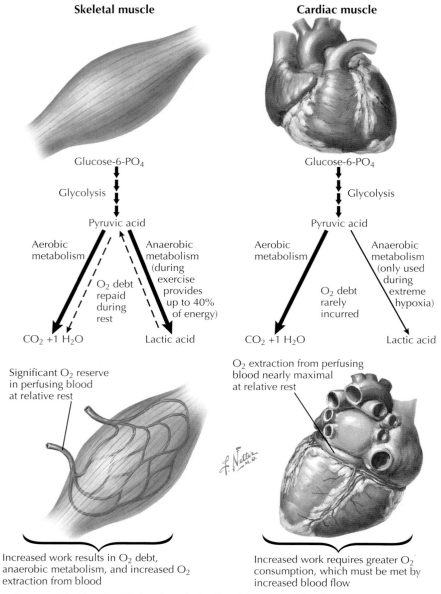

Skeletal muscle   **Cardiac muscle**

Glucose-6-PO_4 Glucose-6-PO_4

Glycolysis   Glycolysis

Pyruvic acid   Pyruvic acid

Aerobic   Anaerobic   Aerobic   Anaerobic
metabolism   metabolism   metabolism   metabolism
                       (during   (only used
              O_2 debt   exercise O_2 debt   during
              repaid   provides   rarely   extreme
              during   up to 40%   incurred   hypoxia)
              rest   of energy)

CO_2 +1 H_2O Lactic acid CO_2 +1 H_2O Lactic acid

Significant O_2 reserve O_2 extraction from perfusing
in perfusing blood   blood nearly maximal
at relative rest   at relative rest

Increased work results in O_2 debt,   Increased work requires greater O_2
anaerobic metabolism, and increased O_2 consumption, which must be met by
extraction from blood   increased blood flow

FIG 19.1 Oxygentilization in Skeletal and Cardiac Muscles. *CO₂,* Carbon dioxide; *H₂O,* water; *O₂,* oxygen; *PO₄,* phosphate.

Because the mortality and morbidity associated with CAD is higher than many noncardiac causes of angina-like symptoms, it is important to be thorough and thoughtful before dismissing CAD as the underlying cause of symptoms of an individual.

DIAGNOSTIC APPROACH

A history suggestive of angina mandates diagnostic and prognostic evaluations. The urgency of treatment is guided by the initial presentation and clinical evaluation. A history of new-onset angina, accelerating angina, angina at a low exertional threshold, and angina at rest are indicators for instability and warrant urgent attention. In individuals with previously stable angina, it is important to evaluate noncardiac causes of increased oxygen demand (anemia, hyperthyroidism, severe emotional stress, and so on) as a potential inciting agents. Physical examination during a routine consultation is unlikely to be rewarding,

but the clinician should look for clinical evidence of left ventricular (LV) dysfunction (resting tachycardia, laterally displaced apical impulse, an LV S_3, rales, jugular venous distention, positive hepatojugular reflex, pedal edema). In addition to evaluating the status of traditional cardiac risk factors (hypertension, smoking status, hyperlipidemia, diabetes), it is important to inquire about a history of claudication, stroke, and transient ischemic attack, and carefully screen for manifestations of atherosclerotic disease (audible bruits, asymmetrical pulses, palpable aneurysms, ankle-brachial index). The presence of atherosclerosis in any of these areas heightens the likelihood of underlying CAD. The examiner should also look for physical and biochemical signs of the metabolic syndrome (Box 19.1), as well as stigmata of hereditary hyperlipidemic conditions (Fig. 19.4).

The next steps in the diagnostic approach should be based on the pretest likelihood of disease. The interplay of traditional risk factors and genetic traits affects the development of atherosclerosis (Fig. 19.5). Patients

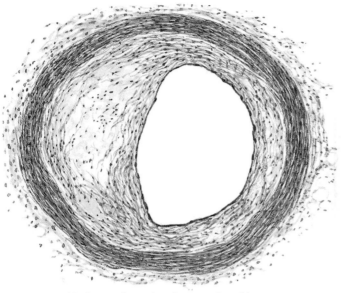

Moderate atherosclerotic narrowing of lumen

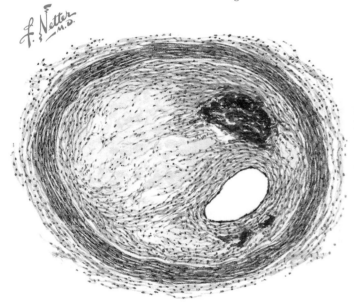

Almost complete occlusion by intimal atherosclerosis with calcium deposition

FIG 19.2 Types and Degrees of Coronary Atherosclerotic Narrowing or Occlusion.

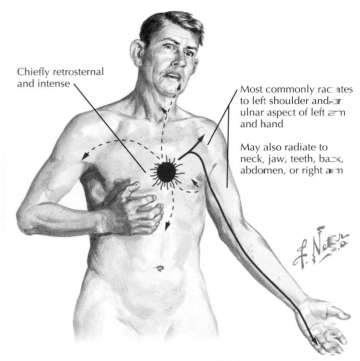

Chiefly retrosternal and intense

Most commonly radiates to left shoulder and/or ulnar aspect of left arm and hand

May also radiate to neck, jaw, teeth, back, abdomen, or right arm

FIG 19.3 Pain of Myocardial Ischemia.

BOX 19.1   Signs of the Metabolic Syndrome

- Abdominal obesity
  - Men >102 cm (>40 in)
  - Women >88 cm (>34.5 in)
- Blood pressure >130/85 mm Hg
- Fasting glucose >110 mg/dL
- HDL-C
  - Men <40 mg/dL
  - Women <50 mg/dL
- Triglycerides >150 mg/dL

HDL-C, High-density lipoprotein cholesterol.

---

with typical angina, multiple risk factors, and/or impaired LV function with a high likelihood of disease should be considered for diagnostic coronary angiography. Patients with a low pretest likelihood of disease and obvious noncardiac etiology should be reassured, without further additional cardiac testing, and provided appropriate consultation.

Rather than falling into the high-risk or low-risk categories, most patients have an intermediate likelihood of epicardial CAD. In these individuals, stress testing is useful for further risk stratification (Fig. 19.6). Patients with a normal resting ECG may be referred for standard exercise treadmill testing. However, as discussed elsewhere (Chapter 10), the diagnostic accuracy of exercise stress testing is limited. For this reason, evaluation with concomitant nuclear perfusion and/or

stress echocardiographic imaging studies is often preferred. It should be noted that the inability to perform adequate exercise by itself is a major indicator of adverse prognosis. This subset of patients may be referred for pharmacological stress testing with SPECT, PET, or MRI. Alternatively, CT angiography for anatomic definition may also be considered in middle-aged individuals when active CAD is suspected and renal dysfunction is not an issue.

Patients with typical symptoms and/or high pretest probability of disease should be referred for diagnostic coronary angiography. Subjects with severe segmental LV dysfunction and absence of inducible ischemia should be evaluated to determine whether the myocardium is scarred or viable. Low-dose dobutamine echocardiography, thallium-dipyridamole imaging, PET, and MRI may all be used to assess viability. Evidence of viability should lead to referral for angiography, with the goal of attempting revascularization whenever feasible. Patients with low-risk findings on noninvasive testing may be treated medically with risk counseling and adequate follow-up.

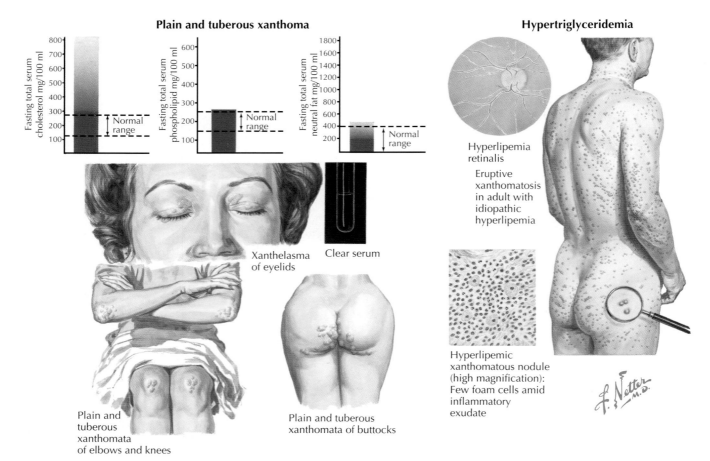

Plain and tuberous xanthoma

Xanthelasma of eyelids

Clear serum

Plain and tuberous xanthomata of elbows and knees

Plain and tuberous xanthomata of buttocks

Hypertriglyceridemia

Hyperlipemia retinalis

Eruptive xanthomatosis in adult with idiopathic hyperlipemia

Hyperlipemic xanthomatous nodule (high magnification): Few foam cells amid inflammatory exudate

FIG 19.4 Hypercholesterolemic Xanthomatosis.

MANAGEMENT AND THERAPY

Optimum Treatment

The treatment goals in patients with chronic stable angina are to prolong and improve quality of life. Optimal medical therapy (OMT) most often involves use of β-blockers, angiotensin-converting enzyme (ACE) inhibitors, statins, antiplatelet therapy, and lifestyle modifications (Fig. 19.7). This combined approach can markedly reduce angina and slow the progression of CAD.

Smoking cessation should be emphasized, and referral to cessation programs should be provided. Smoking cessation alone is more likely to reduce future cardiac risk than any combination of medications and revascularization procedures. Patients should also be educated about the beneficial effects of physical exercise.

In patients with stable coronary disease, the selection of antihypertensive therapy can be tailored to concurrently reduce blood pressure and relieve angina symptoms. People with diabetes should attain tight glucose control, and drugs that have proven cardiovascular benefits should be used preferentially. The value of weight reduction must be stressed when appropriate. Patients should be educated about the warning signs of MI and stroke, the prompt use of aspirin and nitroglycerin, and access to the emergency medical system.

Antiplatelet Therapy

All patients with atherosclerotic CAD should receive antiplatelet therapy. The cost and effectiveness of aspirin makes it the treatment of choice.

The Swedish Angina Pectoris Aspirin Trial (SAPAT) found that stable angina patients who received 75 mg of daily aspirin had a 4% absolute risk reduction in cardiovascular events compared with placebo. Similarly, a collaborative meta-analysis suggested a 34% proportional reduction in nonfatal MI and a 26% reduction in nonfatal MI or death with antiplatelet therapy over placebo in high-risk patients. Clopidogrel is an appropriate alternative in patients with a contraindication to aspirin.

The Clopidogrel for High Atherothrombotic Risk and Ischemic Stabilization Management and Avoidance (CHARISMA) trial evaluated dual antiplatelet therapy with aspirin and clopidogrel in patients with either clinically evident cardiovascular disease or multiple cardiovascular risk factors. Clopidogrel, in addition to aspirin, did not significantly reduce cardiovascular events in the overall population, although subgroup analysis demonstrated a reduction in death, MI, or stroke in patients with established cardiovascular disease.

All patients should be on dual antiplatelet therapy for 12 months after an ACS. The decision to continue with dual antiplatelet therapy in the long term should be guided by the individual ischemic and bleeding risk of the patient and may be assessed with a risk calculator like the Dual Antiplatelet Therapy (DAPT) score. In patients with high ischemic risk and low bleeding risk, continuation of dual antiplatelet therapy with aspirin and either clopidogrel or low dosage ticagrelor may be considered. A combination of low-dose antithrombotic rivaroxaban with low-dose aspirin was also recently proven to improve cardiovascular risk, including mortality reduction in patients with stable angina, but at the price of increasing bleeding risk.

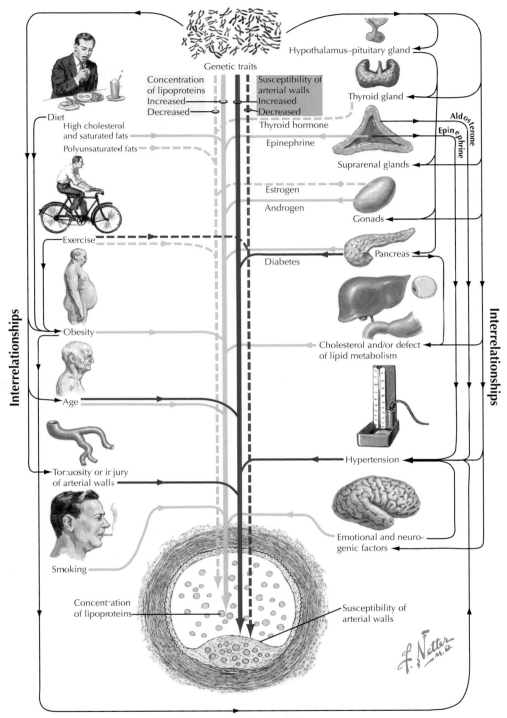

FIG 19.5 Cardiac Risk Factors.

Beta-Blockade

In the absence of contraindications, all patients with symptomatic CAD and/or previous MI should be prescribed a β-blocker. In the Beta Blocker Heart Attack Trial (BHAT), β-blockade with propranolol reduced the risk of recurrent nonfatal reinfarction and fatal coronary heart disease from 13% in the placebo group to 10% in the treatment group. In trials of stable angina, β-blockers were superior to calcium antagonists in reducing angina, although rates of cardiac death and MI were similar between the two.

Angiotensin-Converting Enzyme Inhibitors

All patients with established CAD and LV dysfunction should be prescribed an ACE inhibitor. In three large postinfarction trials, the mortality rate was lower with ACE inhibitors compared with placebo. High-risk patients with preserved LV function also seemed to derive benefit. In the Heart Outcomes Prevention Evaluation (HOPE) trial, the use of ramipril in subjects older than 55 years of age with preserved LV function significantly reduced the primary end points of MI, stroke, and cardiac death. For individuals who cannot tolerate treatment with an

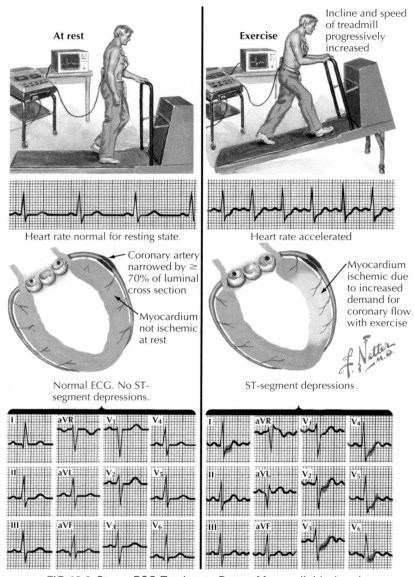

At rest

Heart rate normal for resting state

Coronary artery narrowed by ≥ 70% of luminal cross section

Myocardium not ischemic at rest

Normal ECG. No ST-segment depressions.

Exercise

Incline and speed of treadmill progressively increased

Heart rate accelerated

Myocardium ischemic due to increased demand for coronary flow with exercise

ST-segment depressions

FIG 19.6 Stress-ECG Testing to Detect Myocardial Ischemia.

ACE inhibitor due to side effects, treatment with an angiotensin-II receptor blocker should be considered. Although the data are not as strong as with ACE-inhibitor therapy, angiotensin-II receptor blockers probably have long-term benefits in this population.

Nitrates

Nitrates are endothelium-independent vasodilators that reduce myocardial ischemia and improve coronary blood flow. When used effectively in patients with stable angina, they improve exercise tolerance and increase the anginal threshold. Patients with frequent episodes of angina should be treated with long-acting oral nitrate therapy or with transdermal patches. If a transdermal patch is used, it is important to ensure a nitrate-free interval. Tachyphylaxis (loss of drug efficacy) occurs in patients without nitrate-free intervals in their treatment regimen. Patients with angina should also be supplied with sublingual tablets or spray for breakthrough angina.

Ranolazine

Ranolazine is a novel agent approved for treatment of chronic angina. Ranolazine is a sodium channel blocker believed to treat angina by

ultimately decreasing intracellular calcium and myocardial work. Unlike other antianginal medications, ranolazine does not alter heart rate or blood pressure. However, efficacy of ranolazine remains uncertain. The Ranolazine in Patients with Incomplete Revascularization after Percutaneous Coronary Intervention (RIVER-PCI) trial randomized patients at high risk for chronic angina to ranolazine versus placebo, and found that ranolazine did not reduce subsequent symptom driven hospitalizations or revascularizations.

Treatment of Hyperlipidemia

All patients should receive dietary counseling and instructions for weight reduction and increased physical activity. Current evidence suggests that all patients with elevated cardiovascular risk derive benefit from statin treatment irrespective of their measured lipid profile. The American Heart Association and American College of Cardiology (ACC/AHA), together with the United States Preventative Services Task Force, advocate using global cardiovascular risk profiles to guide statin therapy. Current cholesterol guidelines recommend high-intensity statin therapy for individuals aged 21 to 71 years with a history of coronary disease, a

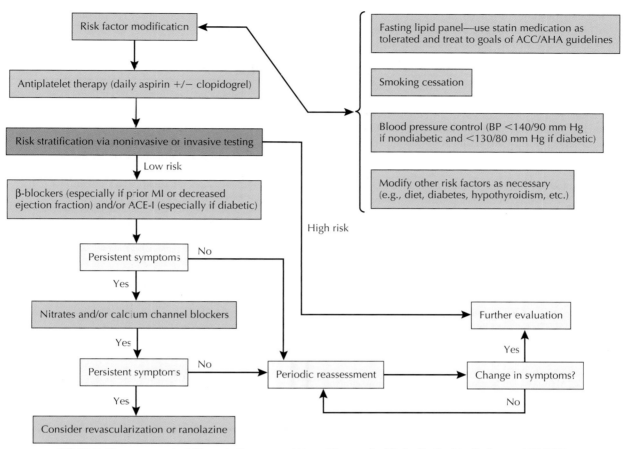

FIG 19.7 Management of Chronic Coronary Artery Disease in Clinically Stable Patients. *ACC/AHA,* American College of Cardiology/American Heart Association; *ACE-I,* angiotensin-converting enzyme inhibitor; *BP,* blood pressure.

10-year cardiovascular risk ≥7.5%, or anyone with low-density lipoprotein cholesterol (LDL-C) ≥190 mg/dL. Moderate intensity statin is recommended for individuals aged older than 75 years with a history of coronary disease, a 10-year cardiovascular risk >7.5%, or with diabetes with a <7.5% 10-year cardiovascular risk. The pooled cohort risk model used to calculate cardiovascular risk can be found on the ACC/AHA and United States Preventative Services Task Force websites. The model uses age, sex, race, total cholesterol, high-density lipoprotein cholesterol (HDL-C), systolic blood pressure, diastolic blood pressure, treatment for hypertension, diabetes, and smoking status to assess cardiovascular risk. In a meta-analysis that combined the results from three secondary prevention trials and two primary prevention trials, treatment with a statin resulted in a 31% reduction in major coronary events and a 21% reduction in all-cause mortality rates. In circumstances of hypertriglyceridemia, fibrates or niacin may be considered, although there is little trial evidence that shows reduction in major adverse cardiovascular events with these classes of medications. Trials have failed to show cardiovascular benefit with niacin in patients with a high risk of coronary disease or in high-risk patients with HDL <40 mg/dL.

Data from recent trials suggested the need for intensification of LDL targets and goal-directed care. Ezetimibe provides incremental cardiovascular risk reduction when added to statin therapy. In the Improved Reduction of Outcomes: Vytorin Efficacy International Trial (IMPROVE-IT), when added to simvastatin, ezetimibe lowered LDL-C from 69.9 to 53.2 mg/dL, and modestly reduced death from cardiovascular causes, major coronary events, or nonfatal stroke from 34.7% to 32.7% in

patients with recent ACS over a long duration of follow-up. Proprotein convertase subtilisin/kexin type 9 (PCSK9) inhibitors are a new class of lipid-lowering medications. Currently indicated for patient with hereditary hyperlipidemia or in patients with known coronary disease who are intolerant of statin therapy, these medications markedly lower LDL levels when added to high-dose statin therapy. In the Further Cardiovascular Outcomes Research with PCSK9 Inhibition in Subjects with Elevated Risk (FOURIER) trial, evolocumab administered subcutaneously either 140 mg every 2 weeks or 420 mg monthly reduced LDL levels in high-risk patients on statin therapy to a median of 30 mg/dL. This lipid modification was noted to be safe and was associated with a 15% relative risk reduction on the composite endpoint of cardiovascular death, MI, stroke, hospitalization for unstable angina, or coronary revascularization over 2.2 years.

INDICATIONS FOR REVASCULARIZATION

Revascularization in the setting of stable CAD is indicated to improve anginal symptoms and prolong life. The benefits of revascularization on longevity are greatest in patients with left main stenosis, three-vessel disease, or two-vessel disease with involvement of the proximal left anterior descending artery. Patients with LV dysfunction derive more benefit but also have a higher risk at the time of the procedure. The decision to revascularize with percutaneous coronary intervention (PCI) or coronary artery bypass graft (CABG) is guided by patient characteristics and preference, anatomic characteristics, presence of diabetes, and degree of LV dysfunction. In general, in patients with multivessel disease, CABG provides greater long-term freedom from angina compared with PCI, with less need for repeat revascularization. However, CABG may be associated with greater periprocedural mortality, stroke, and cognitive decline, whereas PCI is limited by anatomic challenges that result in incomplete revascularization and need for additional future procedures. Patients with diabetes and multivessel disease should preferentially have CABG. In the Future Revascularization Evaluation in Patients with Diabetes Mellitus: Optimal Management of Multivessel Disease (FREEDOM) trial, CABG was superior to PCI at 5 years, with a reduction in both death and MI, but with a higher incidence of stroke.

The Clinical Outcomes Utilizing Revascularization and Aggressive Drug Evaluation (COURAGE) trial enrolled patients with chronic angina, stable CAD suitable for PCI, and inducible myocardial ischemia, and compared OMT to PCI. An LV ejection fraction <30% was an exclusion criterion. PCI did not reduce all-cause death or MI compared with OMT alone. However, this study was criticized for high rates of crossover, strict exclusionary criteria, and low rates of drug-eluting stent use. Data from the COURAGE trial and other studies led many to suggest that although PCI could be effective for ischemia driven symptom improvement, it might not confer added benefit over OMT alone for the prevention of death or MI. The ongoing International Study of Comparative Health Effectiveness With Medical and Invasive Approaches (ISCHEMIA) trial will inform us greatly about the benefits of revascularization in this setting.

At present, ACC/AHA class I indications for PCI are symptom control, single-vessel and double-vessel disease with a large ischemic burden or left ventricular dysfunction, or sustained ventricular tachycardia, and restenosis. Those with clinical angina refractory to medical therapy should be offered PCI.

Revascularization may help to restore some degree of LV function in select patients with CAD. It is important to consider LV function and to assess myocardial viability when recommending for or against revascularization. The Surgical Treatment for Ischemic Heart Failure (STICH) trial randomized 1212 patients with CAD and ejection fractions <35% to CABG compared with medical therapy alone. At 10 years, performance of CABG was associated with 16% reduction in all-cause mortality. Although the STICH viability trial used dobutamine echo and SPECT, it showed no benefits for viability identification. More accurate assessment with PET and MRI have been proposed as ways to identify dysfunctional but viable myocardium that will respond favorably to revascularization.

Advances in functional evaluation of coronary disease may help to identify lesions likely to benefit from revascularization. Fractional flow reserve (FFR) invasively measures the indexed pressure gradient across a fixed coronary lesion. FFR is calculated by (pressure proximal to lesion)/(pressure distal to lesion). The Fractional Flow Reserve versus Angiography for Multivessel Evaluation 2 (FAME 2) trial found that among patients with stable coronary disease, PCI applied to lesions with FFR of ≤0.8 had a reduced composite endpoint of death, nonfatal MI, and urgent revascularization.

FUTURE DIRECTIONS

Noninvasive identification and quantification of atherosclerosis with CT, intravascular ultrasound, FFR, carotid intimal thickness measurements, and endothelial vasoreactivity blur the traditional distinction between primary and secondary prevention of CAD. Biomarker, genetic, and proteomics research will allow prognostication with increasing accuracy as new therapeutic targets for plaque stabilization and regression are translated from bench to bedside. Advances in angiogenesis

and stem cell transfer will potentially revolutionize therapy. A wonderful voyage lies ahead.

EVIDENCE

AIM-HIGH investigators. Niacin in patients with low HDL cholesterol levels receiving intensive statin therapy. *N Engl J Med.* 2011;365:2255–2267.
Among patients with cardiovascular disease, there was no incremental clinical benefit from the addition of niacin to statin therapy, despite improvements in HDL cholesterol and triglyceride levels.
Antithrombotic Trialists Collaboration. Collaborative meta-analysis of randomized trials of antiplatelet therapy for prevention of death, myocardial infarction, and stroke in high risk patients. *BMJ.* 2002;324:71–86.
Meta-analysis of randomized trials using antiplatelet agents to prevent high risk vascular events such as MI, stroke, or vascular death. Aspirin or other antiplatelet agents are protective in most types of patients with increased risk of occlusive vascular events, and absolute benefit outweighs risk of major extracranial bleeding.
BHAT investigators. The beta-blocker heart attack trial. *JAMA.* 1981;246:2073–2074.
Early randomized, double-blind, multicenter trial of propranolol versus placebo shortly after MI. Trial study early after demonstrating significant mortality benefit of β-blockers compared with placebo.
COURAGE Investigators. Optimal medical therapy with or without PCI for stable coronary disease trial has affected practice protocols. *N Engl J Med.* 2007;356(15):1503–1516.
Influential study that enrolled patients with chronic stable angina on OMT with CAD who were amenable to PCI. In stable CAD patients with relatively preserved LV function, PCI did not reduce the risk of death, MI, or other major cardiovascular events when added to OMT.
The FAME 2 Investigators. Fractional flow reserve-guided PCI vs medical therapy in stable coronary disease. *N Engl J Med.* 2012;367:991–1001.
The FAME 2 trial randomized patients with stable coronary disease with at least one coronary lesion with FFR ≤0.80 with PCI versus optimum medical therapy. Patients who underwent PCI decreased the likelihood of urgent revascularization in the future.
Flather MD, Yusuf S, Keber L, et al. Long-term ACE-inhibitor therapy in patients with heart failure or left ventricular dysfunction: a systematic overview of data from individual patients. *Lancet.* 2000;355:1575–1581.
Prospective analysis of use of ACE inhibitors after MI in five long-term randomized trials. The benefits of ACE inhibitors were lower rates of death, reinfarction, and readmission for heart failure. Benefits were identified over the entire range of ejection fractions found in the study participants.
Fourier Steering Committee and Investigators. Evolocumab and clinical outcomes in patients with cardiovascular disease. *N Engl J Med.* 2017;376:1713–1722.
When added to statin therapy, evolocumab significantly lowered LDL levels with reduction in cardiovascular events.
The FREEDOM Trial Investigators. Strategies for multivessel revascularization in patients with diabetes. *N Engl J Med.* 2012;367:2375–2384.
Randomized, multicenter trial comparing DES stents to CABG in patients with diabetes. At 5 years, CABG was superior to PCI with reduced death, myocardial infarction, but more strokes.
Heidenreich PA, McDonald KM, Hastie T, et al. Meta-analysis of trials comparing beta-blockers, calcium antagonists, and nitrates for stable angina. *JAMA.* 1999;281:1927–1936.
To compare the relative efficacy and tolerability of treatment with β-blockers, calcium antagonists, and long-acting nitrates for patients who had stable angina, β-blockers had similar efficacy and fewer adverse effects compared with calcium channel blockers in randomized trials of patients with chronic stable angina.
HOPE investigators. Effects of an angiotensin-converting-enzyme inhibitor, ramipril on cardiovascular events in high-risk patients. *N Engl J Med.* 2000;342:145–153.
Assesses the role of an ACE inhibitor in patients who were at high risk for cardiovascular events but who did not have LV dysfunction or congestive heart failure.

The patients enrolled typically had vascular disease or diabetes and one additional risk factor. Ramipril reduced the rates of death, MI, and stroke compared to placebo.

HPS2-Thrive Collaborative Group. Effects of extended-release niacin with laropiprant in high-risk patients. *N Engl J Med.* 2014;371:203–212.

Among participants with atherosclerotic vascular disease, the addition of extended-release niacin-laropiprant to statin-based LDL cholesterol-lowering therapy did not significantly reduce the risk of major vascular events but did increase the risk of serious adverse events.

IMPROVE-IT investigators. Ezetimibe added to statin therapy after acute coronary syndromes. *N Engl J Med.* 2015;372:2387–2397.

When added to simvastatin, ezetimibe resulted in incremental reduction in LDL-C, and reduction in subsequent myocardial infarctions.

RIVER-PCI investigators. Ranolazine in patients with incomplete revascularisation after percutaneous coronary intervention (RIVER-PCI): a multicentre, randomised, double-blind, placebo-controlled trial. *Lancet* 2016;387:136–145.

Ranolazine did not reduce need for future revascularization or hospitalizations for management of ischemia among patients with known coronary disease.

SAPAT investigators. Double-blind trial of aspirin in primary prevention of myocardial infarction in patients with stable chronic angina pectoris. The Swedish Angina Pectoris Aspirin Trial (SAPAT) Group. *Lancet.* 1992;340:1420–1425.

Early randomized trial showing that in patients with chronic stable angina, aspirin reduced cardiovascular events compared with placebo alone.

The STICH Investigators. Coronary-artery bypass surgery in patients with ischemic cardiomyopathy. *N Engl J Med.* 2016;374:1511–1520.

At 10 years of follow-up in patients with ischemic cardiomyopathy, performance of CABG reduced mortality and cardiovascular hospitalization were compared with medical therapy.

The STICH Investigators. Myocardial viability and survival in ischemic left ventricular dysfunction. *N Engl J Med.* 2011;364:1617–1625.

The STICH trial randomized patients with ischemic cardiomyopathy with LV ejection fractions of ≤35% to CABG versus OMT and showed reductions in all-cause mortality at 10 years. Among the 1212 patients randomized into the trial, 601 underwent an assessment of myocardial viability (primarily stress ech and SPECT). After adjusting for confounding, stress testing could not identify patients likely to live longer after CABG.

20

Non–ST-Elevation Acute Coronary Syndrome

Eric H. Yang

DEFINITION AND EPIDEMIOLOGY

Acute coronary syndrome (ACS) is a term used to describe a group of clinical syndromes included with acute myocardial ischemia. Unstable angina (UA), non–ST-segment elevation myocardial infarction (NSTEMI), and STEMI are included in this group of syndromes. Because the pathophysiology and management of patients with UA and NSTEMI are similar, these two groups are further subclassified as non–ST-segment elevation ACS (NSTE-ACS).

It is estimated that 1.4 million patients present with ACS per year in the United States. The median age of presentation is 68 years of age, and the male-to-female ratio is approximately 3:2. Seventy percent of ACS patients present with NSTE-ACS, and the remaining 30% present with STEMI. This chapter focuses on the diagnosis and management of patients with NSTE-ACS.

PATHOPHYSIOLOGY

The pathogenesis of NSTE-ACS is sudden plaque rupture followed by thrombus formation and partial occlusion of coronary blood flow (Fig. 20.1). These plaques consist of atherosclerotic lesions with lipid-rich cores and a fibrous cap. Previous angiographic studies and recent investigations involving intravascular ultrasound have demonstrated that plaque rupture is more related to the thickness of the fibrous cap than the amount of the lipid-rich core. Atherosclerotic lesions with thin fibrous caps are more prone to plaque rupture than those with thicker caps. Thus, plaque rupture that results in ACS is more likely to occur in lesions with <50% luminal stenosis due to less developed and thinner fibrous caps.

Other less frequent etiologies of ACS include coronary artery spasm secondary to endothelial dysfunction or administration of vasoconstricting agents, spontaneous coronary artery dissection, and thromboembolism.

CLINICAL PRESENTATION AND DIFFERENTIAL DIAGNOSIS

Common symptoms of NSTE-ACS include sudden onset of retrosternal chest pain with radiation to the neck, jaw, and/or arms. The pain typically occurs at rest or with minimal exertion, and last for ≥10 minutes. For those with previous anginal pain, NSTE-ACS angina may occur with less exertion, greater frequency and/or intensity, and for a longer duration. Associated symptoms include diaphoresis, nausea, and dyspnea. Approximately 30% of patients may present with atypical symptoms, which include fatigue, epigastric discomfort, and pleuritic chest pain.

The clinical manifestations of myocardial ischemia can be mimicked by many other processes. Musculoskeletal disorders involving the cervical spine, shoulder, ribs, and sternum can result in nonspecific chest discomfort and even pain syndromes that are similar to angina pectoris. Symptoms from gastrointestinal causes, including esophageal reflux with associated spasm, peptic ulcer disease, and cholecystitis, are often indistinguishable from angina. Intrathoracic processes such as pneumonia, pleurisy, pulmonary embolism, pneumothorax, aortic dissection, and pericarditis can also produce chest discomfort. Finally, panic attacks and hyperventilation are neuropsychiatric syndromes that can be mistaken for ACS.

DIAGNOSTIC APPROACH

History and Physical

NSTE-ACS is an initial clinical diagnosis based on the history obtained from the patient. Typical symptoms include chest pain and/or pressure with radiation to the shoulders, neck, arm, or jaw. The discomfort is usually sudden in onset, occurs at rest, and lasts >10 minutes. Some patients, including women and patients with diabetes, may present with "atypical" symptoms, including nausea, fatigue, emesis, or syncope. A careful evaluation of bleeding risks and history, medical compliance, and upcoming elective procedures is also important in determining if patients are potential candidates for long-term dual antiplatelet therapy.

The physical examination in NSTE-ACS patients focuses on evaluating for signs of hemodynamic instability and heart failure because these findings identify a higher risk group. Signs of heart failure include jugular venous distention, pulmonary congestion (rales), and hypotension. A careful assessment of peripheral pulses is also important for accessing potential access sites in patients in whom an invasive strategy is being considered.

Electrocardiogram

The resting ECG is a key component of the evaluation of patients with suspected ACS and should be performed within 10 minutes of the patient's arrival to the emergency department. Because the initial ECG may be normal in patients with ACS, serial ECGs at 15- to 30-minute intervals should be performed in all patients with suspected ACS. ECG findings consistent with NSTE-ACS include ST depression, T-wave inversion, and transient ST-elevation (Fig. 20.2). It is important to note that a normal ECG does not rule out a diagnosis of ACS and occurs in 5% to 15% of patients who present with ACS.

Biomarkers of Myocardial Damage

The biochemical markers of myocardial necrosis, creatine kinase (CK), and its relatively cardiac-specific MB isoenzyme (CK-MB), as well as cardiac troponins T and I, are also essential in the diagnosis and prognosis of patients with ACS. These markers become detectable after myocyte necrosis causes the loss of cell membrane integrity, which eventually allows these intracellular macromolecules to diffuse into the peripheral circulation.

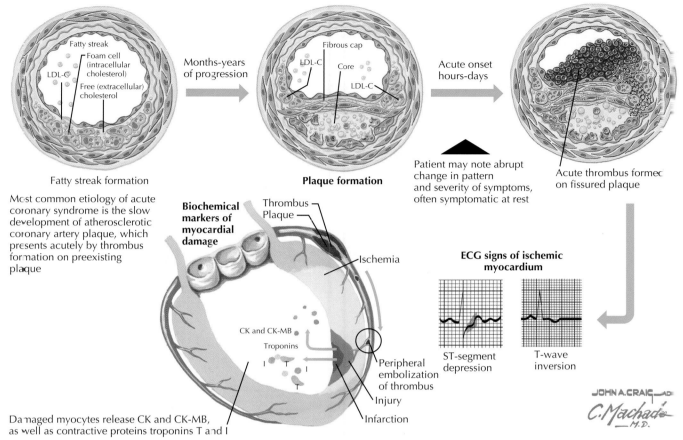

Fatty streak formation

Most common etiology of acute coronary syndrome is the slow development of atherosclerotic coronary artery plaque, which presents acutely by thrombus formation on preexisting plaque

Plaque formation

Patient may note abrupt change in pattern and severity of symptoms, often symptomatic at rest

Acute thrombus formed on fissured plaque

Biochemical markers of myocardial damage

ECG signs of ischemic myocardium

ST-segment depression

T-wave inversion

Damaged myocytes release CK and CK-MB, as well as contractive proteins troponins T and I

JOHN A. CRAIG
C. Machado
M.D.

FIG 20.1 Pathophysiology of Acute Coronary Syndromes. *CK*, Creatine kinase; *CK-MB*, creatine kinase-MB isoenzyme; *LDL-C*, low-density lipoprotein cholesterol.

In the past, CK and CK-MB were the primary biochemical markers used to evaluate patients with chest pain. However, several properties of CK and CK-MB limit their predictive value, including their presence at low levels in the blood under normal conditions and their presence in noncardiac sources. Therefore, in most centers, cardiac troponins have become the preferred markers of myocardial necrosis due to their increased sensitivity and specificity for myocardial damage. It should be noted that in chronic renal failure, severe hypertension, and in other less well-understood settings, there are patients in whom troponin concentrations are chronically elevated. It is important to note that an initial normal troponin level does not rule out ACS, and that all patients with a clinical suspicion of ACS need serial biomarker measurements. A rise and fall pattern in cardiac troponin is typically considered to be consistent with ACS.

MANAGEMENT AND THERAPY

The four key components of managing patients with NSTE-ACS include (1) risk stratification, (2) selection of overall management strategy, (3) antiplatelet and anticoagulation therapy, and (4) antiischemic therapy.

Risk Stratification

Because NSTE-ACS can exist in a heterogenous group of patients, proper risk stratification is essential in choosing the appropriate level of management for NSTE-ACS patients. Unstable patients should be considered the highest risk group and includes those with angina refractory to optimal medical management, signs or symptoms of hemodynamic

instability, and sustained ventricular tachycardia or fibrillation. More stable patients can be risk stratified based on clinical and laboratory findings.

The Thrombolysis in Myocardial Infarction (TIMI) risk score is a commonly used risk stratification tool and can be easily and quickly implemented in the assessment of NSTE-ACS patients. The score consists of seven 1-point risk indicators based on historical and clinical data evaluated in the Efficacy and Safety of Subcutaneous Enoxaparin in Non–Q-Wave Coronary Events (ESSENCE) and Thrombolysis in Myocardial Infarction 11 (TIMI 11) clinical trials. The seven factors and the associated risk scores are shown in Table 20.1.

The Global Registry of Acute Coronary Events (GRACE) risk model is another commonly used risk stratification model for NSTE-ACS patients. It is a more complicated model that includes multiple patient variables and findings. Unlike the TIMI risk score, the model cannot be completed at the bedside without the assistance of web-based or smart-phone tools. The web-based application is available at http://www.outcomes-umassmed.org/grace (accessed July 2017).

Selection of Overall Management Strategy

Once patients are risk-stratified, an overall management strategy should be selected. The four management strategies are discussed in the following sections.

Immediate Invasive Strategy

Patients are brought emergently (within 2 hours of presentation) to the cardiac catheterization laboratory for possible revascularization.

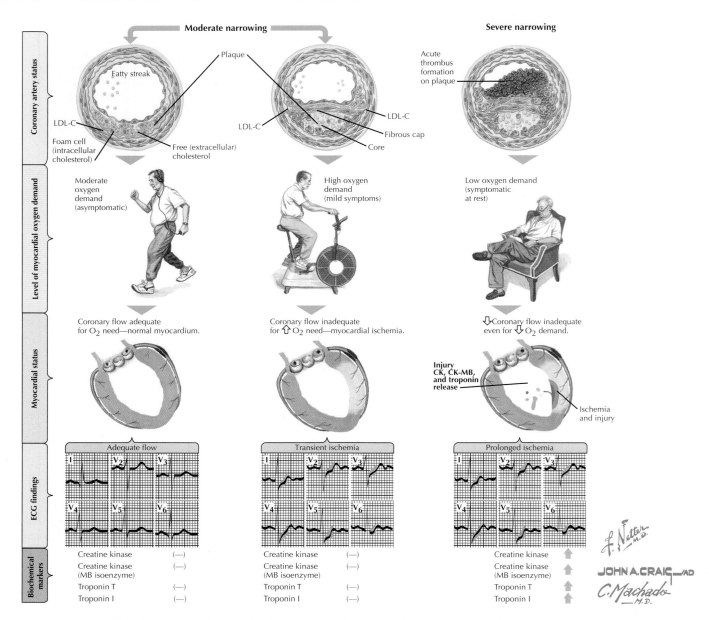

FIG 20.2 Risk Stratification for Patients With Coronary Heart Disease. *CK,* Creatine kinase; *CK-MB,* creatine kinase-MB isoenzyme; *LDL-C,* low-density lipoprotein cholesterol.

TABLE 20.1 **Thrombolysis in Myocardial Infarction Risk Score**		
	Risk of Adverse Cardiac Event[a]	
Risk Factors	**# of risk factors**	**% risk**
Age >65	0–1	4.7
>3 risk factors for CAD	2	8.3
Previous coronary stenosis >50%	3	13.2
>2 anginal event in past 24 h	4	19.9
Aspirin use in past 7 days	5	26.2
ST segment changes	6–7	41
Positive cardiac markers		

[a]Myocardial infarction, cardiac-related death, and/or persistent ischemia. *CAD,* Coronary artery disease.

This strategy is reserved for the highest risk NSTE-ACS patients and includes those with any of the following: angina refractory to optimal medical management, signs or symptoms of hemodynamic instability, and sustained ventricular tachycardia or fibrillation.

Early Invasive Strategy

Patients undergo cardiac catheterization in a nonemergent manner, but within 24 hours of presentation. NSTE-ACS patients who do not meet the criteria for an immediate invasive strategy and have a GRACE risk score >140, significant temporal changes in troponin levels, or significant new ST depression on ECG should be considered for an early invasive strategy.

Delayed Invasive Strategy

Patients who do not meet the criteria for an immediate or early invasive strategy but are at intermediate risk can undergo cardiac catheterization in a delayed manner (25–72 hours from presentation). Intermediate risk patients include those with a TIMI risk score ≥2, a GRACE risk score of 109 to 140, and those with reduced ejection fractions (<0.40).

Ischemia-Guided Strategy

Low-risk patients who do not meet criteria for any of the previously described invasive strategies should undergo an ischemia-guided management strategy. These patients are evaluated for ischemia with image-based stressed testing. Those with significant ischemia are then considered for possible further invasive management, whereas those with minimal or no ischemia are managed in a more conservative manner.

Antiplatelet and Anticoagulation Therapy

Because the pathophysiological mechanism of NSTE-ACS is plaque rupture with subsequent intracoronary thrombus formation, antiplatelet therapy and anticoagulation are the essential components of medical management. All patients suspected of NSTE-ACS should be managed with upfront dual antiplatelet therapy and anticoagulation regardless of their initial management strategy (invasive driven vs. ischemia driven).

Dual Antiplatelet Therapy

Aspirin. Aspirin is a nonreversible inhibitor of cyclooxygenase-1 and prevents the synthesis of thromboxane, which is an activator of platelets. An initial loading dose of 162 to 325 mg of nonenteric-coated aspirin should be given to all patients suspected of having NSTE-ACS. A subsequent maintenance dose of 81 mg should be used thereafter because previous studies have demonstrated that lower dose aspirin is as effective as 325 mg of aspirin in preventing future cardiac events and is associated with lower bleeding risks. Providers should not use enteric-coated aspirin in the acute setting due its delayed and reduced absorption.

P2Y$_{12}$ receptor inhibitors. In addition to aspirin, all patients suspected of NSTE-ACS should be treated with a P2Y$_{12}$ receptor inhibitor. Dual antiplatelet therapy is recommended for at least 1 year in all NSTE-ACS patients regardless of the management strategy (medical management alone vs. percutaneous coronary intervention [PCI] with bare metal or drug-eluting stents). Currently, there are three oral P2Y$_{12}$ receptor inhibitors available in the United States.

Clopidogrel. Clopidogrel is an indirect, irreversible inhibitor of the P2Y$_{12}$ receptor. The need for conversion of clopidogrel to its active metabolite results in a slower onset of action (3–6 hours). A loading dose of 600 mg should be given, followed by a daily maintenance dose of 75 mg.

Prasugrel. Similar to clopidogrel, prasugrel is an indirect, irreversible inhibitor of the P2Y$_{12}$ receptor. However, the conversion of prasugrel to its active metabolite is more rapid and less variable than clopidogrel. A loading dose of 60 mg followed by a daily maintenance dose of 10 mg is recommended. Prasugrel should not be used in patients with a history of cerebrovascular events and should also not be used until coronary angiography has been performed. It is therefore not considered an "upfront" agent to be used in the initial management of NSTE-ACS patients, but rather as an alternative to clopidogrel in the postangiography management of patients who undergo an invasive management strategy.

Ticagrelor. Ticagrelor is a direct acting, reversible inhibitor of the P2Y$_{12}$ receptor. Unlike clopidogrel and prasugrel, ticagrelor does not need to be converted to an active metabolite and thus has a quicker onset of action. A loading dose of 180 mg followed by a maintenance dose of 90 mg twice a day should be used. Ticagrelor is chemically similar in structure to adenosine and a significant number of patients (approximately 10%–15%) experience dyspnea while on the medication.

Intravenous Glycoprotein IIb/IIIa Receptor Inhibitors

The glycoprotein (GP) IIb/IIIa receptors are responsible for the cross linking of platelets to fibrinogen. In the past, GP IIb/IIIa receptor inhibitors were the mainstay of management in high-risk NSTE-ACS patients. However, with the increasing use of upfront dual antiplatelet therapy, routine use of GP IIb/IIIa inhibitors has greatly decreased. Currently, tirofiban and eptifibatide are recommend for use only in patients who did not receive dual antiplatelet therapy and are undergoing an invasive strategy.

Anticoagulation

Initiation of systemic anticoagulation, together with the previously mentioned antiplatelet therapy, is essential in the initial management of NSTE-ACS patients. Contrary to the belief of many providers, upfront anticoagulation is necessary in all patients suspected of having NSTE-ACS even if there is an initially normal ECG or troponin assay. Four anticoagulants can be used.

Unfractionated heparin. Unfractionated heparin (UHF) is the most commonly used systemic anticoagulant therapy in NSTE-ACS due to its fast onset of action, relatively low cost, and universal availability. It is recommended to give an initial loading dose of 60 IU/kg (maximum 4000 IU) followed by an infusion rate of 12 IU/kg per hour (maximum 1000 IU/hour) that is adjusted per a standardized nomogram.

Low-molecular-weight heparin. Compared with UFH, low-molecular-weight heparin (LMWH) possesses increased antifactor Xa activity in relation to antifactor IIa (antithrombin) activity. LMWH can be administered subcutaneously, and its anticoagulant effect is more predictable than that of heparin. Unlike UHF, LMWHs do not require routine monitoring per a standardized nomogram. Enoxaparin is the only LMWH shown to be superior to UHF in the treatment of patients with ACS and is the LMWH of choice for ACS patients. A dose of 1 mg/kg subcutaneously every 12 hours is the standard dosing regimen. For patients with a creatinine clearance of <30 mL/min, a reduced dosing regimen of 1 mg/kg subcutaneously per day should be used. For patients undergoing an immediate invasive strategy, UHF is still the preferred agent over enoxaparin.

Bivalirudin. Bivalirudin is a reversible direct thrombin inhibitor that has been studied in patients who have undergone PCI for ACS. In ACS patients who have been treated with upfront dual antiplatelet therapy and who have undergone PCI, bivalirudin was shown to be as effective as UFH + GP IIb/IIIa inhibition and was associated with a lower risk of bleeding. However, the risk of stent thrombosis was higher in the bivalirudin arm, and bivalirudin was ineffective in the subgroup of NSTEMI patients who were not treated with upfront dual antiplatelet therapy. Thus, bivalirudin should only be used in NSTE-ACS patients undergoing an immediate or early invasive strategy who are treated with upfront dual antiplatelet therapy. A loading dose of 0.10 mg/kg followed by an infusion of 0.25 mg/kg per hour is the recommended dosing strategy in patients with normal renal function. Unlike UFH and LMWH, bivalirudin can be used in patients with heparin-induced thrombocytopenia (HIT).

Fondaparinux. Fondaparinux is an Xa inhibitor that can be given subcutaneously and does not require routine monitoring. It can be used in patients with HIT and has been demonstrated to be effective in the management of NSTE-ACS patients undergoing an ischemia-guided strategy. In patients who underwent an invasive strategy, fondaparinux was associated with a higher risk of catheter thrombosis. To avoid this increased thrombosis risk, all patients treated with upfront fondaparinux should be given additional UFH at the time of cardiac catheterization. Fondaparinux should only be used in patients with normal renal function. A dose of 2.5 mg subcutaneously once per day is recommended.

Antiischemic Therapy
Nitrates

Nitrates reduce myocardial oxygen demand and increase coronary blood flow by reducing preload via peripheral vasodilation and endothelium-independent dilation of the epicardial coronary arteries. NSTE-ACS patients who are hemodynamically stable should receive antiischemic therapy with short-acting nitrates. Nitrates should not be used in patients with right ventricular ischemia or those who have recently used a phosphodiesterase-5 inhibitor.

Beta-Adrenergic Blockers

Beta-blockers are frequently used in patients presenting with NSTE-ACS. They decrease myocardial oxygen demand by decreasing the heart rate, contractility, and systemic blood pressure. A large randomized study in ACS patients demonstrated that intravenous β blockade should be avoided and that β-blockers (oral or intravenous) should not be administered in ACS patients with signs of heart failure or shock.

Non-Dihydropyridine Calcium Channel Blockers

Verapamil and diltiazem are non-dihydropyridine (NDHP) calcium channel blockers that can be used in NSTE-ACS patients who are unable to take β-blockers due to allergy or a history of reactive airway disease. These agents reduce heart rate, contractility, and blood pressure, and thus reduce overall myocardial oxygen demand. Non-dihydropyridine calcium channel blockers should not be used in patients with signs of heart failure or who are in shock.

FUTURE DIRECTIONS

The use of high-sensitivity troponin assays will assist with the earlier detection and risk stratification of patients with suspected NSTE-ACS.

An earlier diagnosis may result in improved outcomes and more efficient triage of patients presenting with chest pain. In addition, the use of handheld, bedside, point-of-care troponin assays may also result in improved diagnosis and risk stratification.

ADDITIONAL RESOURCES

Amsterdam EA, Wenger NK, Brindis RG, et al. 2014 AHA/ACC guideline for the management of patients with non–ST-elevation acute coronary syndromes. *Circulation.* 2014;130:e344–e426.
American College of Cardiology Guidelines on management of NSTE-ACS.

Apple FS, Sandoval Y, Jaffe AS, Ordonez-Llanos J. Cardiac troponin assays: guide to understanding analytical characteristics and their impact on clinical care. *Clin Chem.* 2017;63:73–81.
Review on the use of biomarkers in NSTE-ACS.

Corcoran D, Grant P, Berry C. Risk stratification in non-ST elevation acute coronary syndromes: risk scores, biomarkers and clinical judgment. *Int J Cardiol Heart Vasc.* 2015;8:131–137.
Review discussing the role of risk stratification.

Eisen A, Giugliano RP, Braunwald E. Updates on acute coronary syndrome: a review. *JAMA Cardiol.* 2016;1:718–730.
Recent review article on NSTE-ACS.

Elgendy I, Kumbhani D, Mahnoud A, Wen X, Bhatt D, Bavry A. Routine invasive versus selective invasive strategies for non-ST-elevation acute coronary syndromes: an updated meta-analysis of randomized trials. *Catheter Cardiovasc Interv.* 2016;88:765–774.
Review on treatment strategies in NSTE-ACS.

21

ST-Elevation Myocardial Infarction

Michael Bode, Christoph Bode

The diagnosis of acute coronary syndrome (ACS) is based on findings ranging from clinical presentation on ECG and/or biochemical findings to pathological characteristics. Patients with ACS include those whose clinical presentations cover the following range of diagnoses: unstable angina, non–ST-elevation myocardial infarction (NSTEMI), and ST-elevation MI (STEMI). An estimated 220,000 STEMI events per year occur in the United States.

ETIOLOGY AND PATHOGENESIS

The initial event in formation of an occlusive intracoronary thrombus is rupture or ulceration of an atherosclerotic plaque. Plaque rupture results in exposure of circulating platelets to the thrombogenic contents of the plaque, such as fibrillar collagen, von Willebrand factor, vitronectin, fibrinogen, and fibronectin. Adhesion of platelets to the ulcerated plaque, with subsequent platelet activation and aggregation, leads to thrombin generation, conversion of fibrinogen to fibrin, and further activation of platelets, as well as vasoconstriction, due in part to platelet-derived vasoconstrictors. This prothrombotic milieu promotes propagation and stabilization of an active thrombus that contains platelets, fibrin, thrombin, and erythrocytes, which results in occlusion of the infarct-related artery (Fig. 21.1A). Upon interruption of antegrade flow in an epicardial coronary artery, the zone of myocardium supplied by that vessel immediately loses its ability to perform contractile work (Fig. 21.1B). Abnormal contraction patterns develop: dyssynchrony, hypokinesis, akinesis, and dyskinesis. Myocardial dysfunction in an area of ischemia is typically complemented by hyperkinesis of the remaining normal myocardium due to acute compensatory mechanisms, including increased sympathetic nervous system activity. Etiologies other than plaque rupture are far less common and include coronary artery spasm (which is often due to cocaine), thromboembolism in the setting of atrial fibrillation or a mechanical heart valve, and hypercoagulable states that lead to intracoronary thrombus formation.

CLINICAL PRESENTATION

Typical prodromal symptoms are present in many patients but not in all patients who present with an acute MI. Of these, chest discomfort, which resembles classic angina pectoris but occurs at rest or with less activity than usual, is the most common symptom. The intensity of MI pain is variable, usually severe, and in some instances intolerable. Pain is prolonged, usually lasts >30 minutes, and frequently lasts for hours. The discomfort is typically described as constricting, crushing, oppressing, or compressing. The pain is usually retrosternal, frequently spreading to both sides of the anterior chest, with predilection for the left side. In some instances, pain of an acute MI may begin in the epigastric area and simulate a variety of abdominal disorders. In other patients, MI discomfort radiates to the shoulders, neck, jaw, or back (Fig. 21.2). In some patients, particularly older adults, an MI is manifested clinically not by pain but by symptoms of acute left ventricular (LV) failure and chest tightness, or by marked weakness or frank syncope. These symptoms may be accompanied by diaphoresis, nausea, and vomiting.

Numerous findings may be present in the patient who presents with an acute MI. LV dysfunction may also result in pulmonary edema, hypotension, and decreased peripheral perfusion with cool extremities and mottling. In addition, patients with acute mitral valve regurgitation may present with marked evidence of LV dysfunction and may have an audible holosystolic murmur upon presentation. A third heart sound usually reflects severe LV dysfunction with elevated filling pressures. Marked jugular venous distention and *v* waves consistent with tricuspid regurgitation are evident in right ventricular infarction.

DIFFERENTIAL DIAGNOSIS

The pain of an acute MI may simulate the pain of acute pericarditis, which is usually associated with some pleuritic features and aggravated by respiratory movements and coughing. Pleural pain is typically sharp, knifelike, and aggravated in a cyclic fashion by each breath. These features distinguish pleural pain from the deep, dull, steady pain of an acute MI. Pulmonary embolism generally produces pain laterally in the chest, is often pleuritic, and may be associated with hemoptysis. Pain from acute dissection of the aorta is usually localized in the center of the chest or back, is extremely severe, persists for many hours, often radiates to the back or lower extremities, and reaches maximal intensity shortly after onset of the pain. Often, one or more major arterial pulses are absent. Pain arising from the costochondral and chondrosternal articulations is characterized by marked localized tenderness. The pain of an acute MI, particularly of an inferior MI, may also simulate the pain of esophageal spasm, peptic ulcer disease, or stress gastritis.

DIAGNOSTIC APPROACH

Electrocardiographic Findings

A pattern of ST-segment elevation, especially with associated T-wave changes and ST depression in another anatomic distribution ("reciprocal changes"), combined with chest pain persisting >20 minutes is highly indicative of STEMI (Fig. 21.3). To meet the ECG criteria for STEMI, the ST segment must be elevated in at least two contiguous leads by >0.2 mV in leads V_2 and V_3 in men (0.15 mV in women) and/or by >0.1 mV in other leads. Patients with ACS are also considered to have a STEMI in the absence of ST-segment elevation if a new left bundle branch block (LBBB) or a true posterior MI is present. Many factors limit the ability of ECGs to diagnose and localize an MI; these include the extent of the myocardial injury, the age of the infarct, conduction defects, previous infarcts or acute pericarditis, changes in electrolyte concentrations, and the administration of cardioactive drugs. In

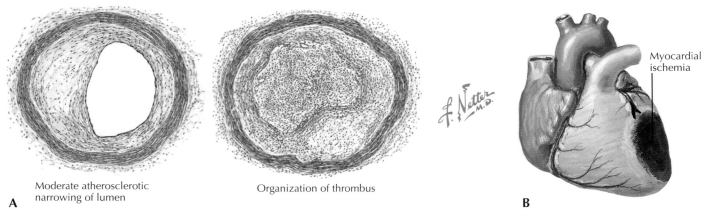

A Moderate atherosclerotic narrowing of lumen

Organization of thrombus

Myocardial ischemia

B

FIG 21.1 (A) Pathophysiology of Acute Myocardial Ischemia. (B) Myocardial Ischemia.

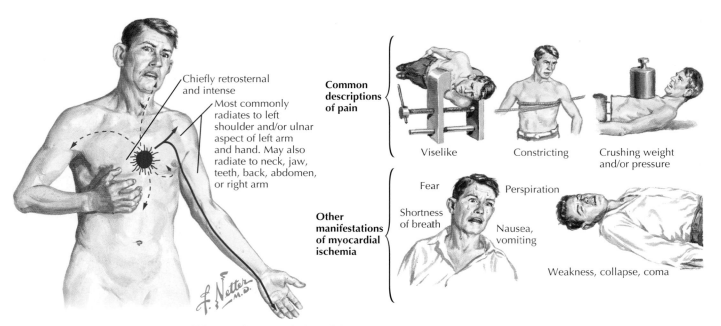

Chiefly retrosternal and intense

Most commonly radiates to left shoulder and/or ulnar aspect of left arm and hand. May also radiate to neck, jaw, teeth, back, abdomen, or right arm

Common descriptions of pain

Viselike　　Constricting　　Crushing weight and/or pressure

Other manifestations of myocardial ischemia

Fear　　Perspiration
Shortness of breath　　Nausea, vomiting

Weakness, collapse, coma

FIG 21.2 Characteristics of Chest Pain in Myocardial Ischemia.

addition, some patients with an acute MI do not have significant ST changes because of the location of the infarction. For these reasons, even in the absence of STEMI ECG criteria, severe myocardial ischemia necessitating therapy may be present. With an appropriate clinical history, it may be necessary to pursue further diagnostic testing to rule out acute MI.

Serum Cardiac Markers

Before cardiac markers can be detected in serum, the myocyte cell membrane has to have disintegrated. Because this disintegration process takes time, serum markers are not useful for early detection of an acute MI. However, serum markers are proof of an established MI and useful indicators of risk. Established serum markers used to diagnose an acute MI are creatine kinase (CK) and CK isoenzymes (CK-MB fraction), myoglobin, and cardiac-specific troponins (troponin I and troponin T). The smaller molecule myoglobin is released quickly from infarcted myocardium but is not cardiac-specific. Therefore, elevations

of myoglobin that may be detected early after the onset of infarction require confirmation with a more cardiac-specific marker, such as troponin I or troponin T. The troponins are the most specific markers in clinical use but may be elevated in other cardiac and noncardiac conditions in the absence of myocardial ischemia.

Other Imaging

In STEMI patients who present with cardiogenic shock, echocardiography can be useful in detecting correctable mechanical causes for low cardiac output—for instance, the presence of a new ventricular septum defect or papillary muscle dysfunction—and distinguishing these from global LV dysfunction. MRI can permit early recognition of an MI and an assessment of the severity of ischemic insult; however, MRI is currently not used clinically in STEMI patients at most medical centers. With emphasis on early reperfusion, the use of imaging techniques is extremely limited in the setting of an acute STEMI because of the time necessary for these studies.

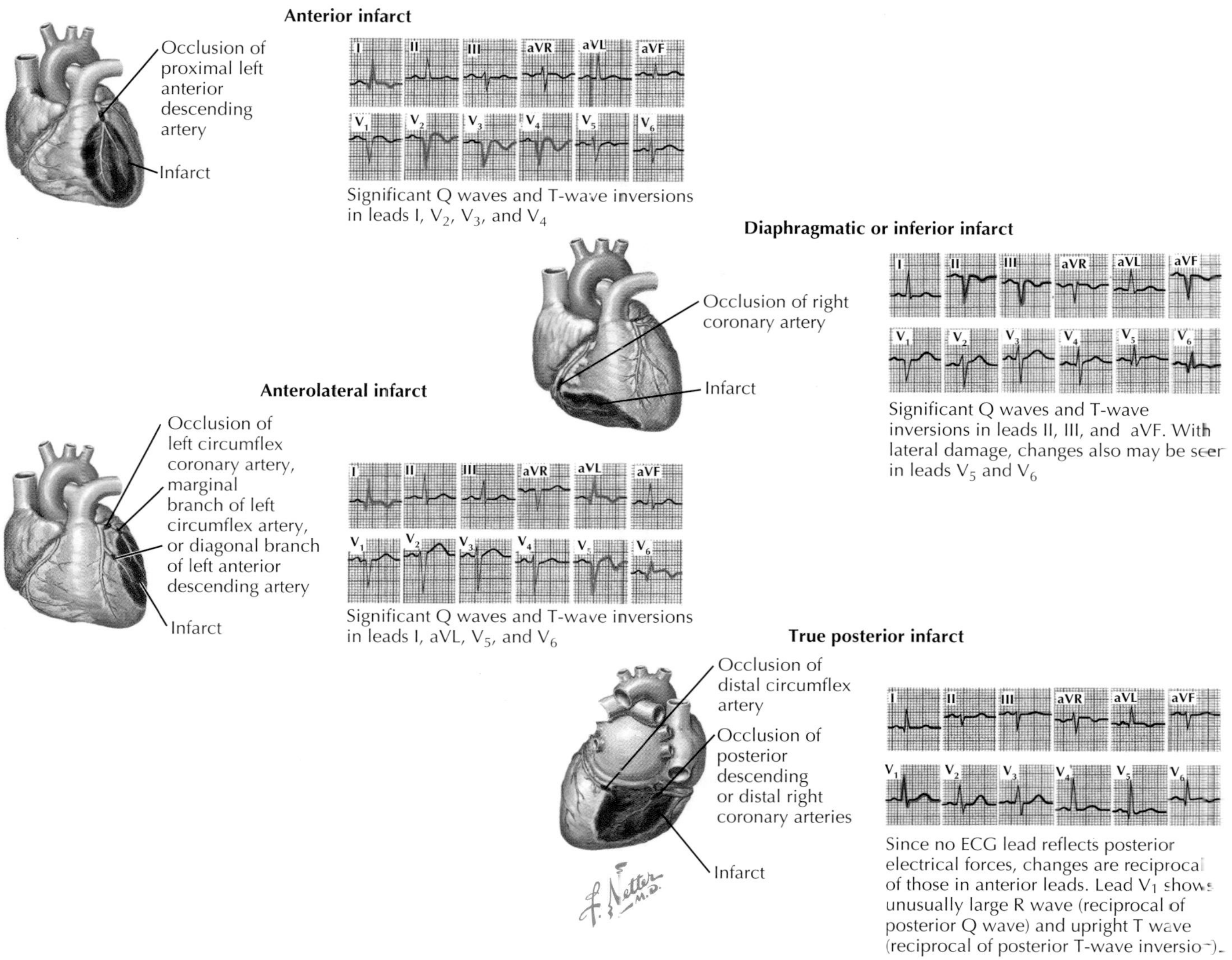

Anterior infarct

Occlusion of proximal left anterior descending artery

Infarct

Significant Q waves and T-wave inversions in leads I, V_2, V_3, and V_4

Anterolateral infarct

Occlusion of left circumflex coronary artery, marginal branch of left circumflex artery, or diagonal branch of left anterior descending artery

Infarct

Significant Q waves and T-wave inversions in leads I, aVL, V_5, and V_6

Diaphragmatic or inferior infarct

Occlusion of right coronary artery

Infarct

Significant Q waves and T-wave inversions in leads II, III, and aVF. With lateral damage, changes also may be seen in leads V_5 and V_6

True posterior infarct

Occlusion of distal circumflex artery

Occlusion of posterior descending or distal right coronary arteries

Infarct

Since no ECG lead reflects posterior electrical forces, changes are reciprocal of those in anterior leads. Lead V_1 shows unusually large R wave (reciprocal of posterior Q wave) and upright T wave (reciprocal of posterior T-wave inversion).

FIG 21.3 ECG Localization of ST-Elevation Myocardial Infarction.

MANAGEMENT AND THERAPY

Optimum Treatment

Several treatment options lower the mortality in acute STEMI (Fig. 21.4). These options include early reperfusion with percutaneous coronary intervention (PCI) or thrombolytic therapy, and administration of aspirin with a $P2Y_{12}$ receptor blocker, anticoagulant therapy, β-blockers, angiotensin-converting enzyme inhibitors, and statins. Other therapies for acute STEMI include the use of nitrates, and antiarrhythmic agents; however, the data supporting use of these therapies are less compelling. Nonsteroidal antiinflammatory drugs other than aspirin increase the risk of cardiovascular events and should be discontinued.

Reperfusion is by far the most effective treatment. PCI is the treatment of choice for patients with acute STEMI (Fig. 21.5). PCI is more effective than thrombolytic therapy because it achieves both higher infarct-related artery patency rates and more often results in Thrombolysis In Myocardial Infarction (TIMI) grade 3 flow (Fig. 21.6). PCI also has advantages over thrombolytic therapy in terms of the rates of short-term mortality, bleeding complications (including intracranial

hemorrhage), and stroke. The benefit of primary angioplasty with regard to the rates of mortality, reinfarction, and recurrent ischemia continues over long-term follow-up. Early intervention has the additional advantage of angiographic definition of the coronary vessels, which allows early risk stratification and identification of patients at particularly high or low risk for recurrent MI or cardiovascular compromise. The use of stents in primary angioplasty adds further benefits, addressing the frequent problem of restenosis and the need for repeat revascularization. The use of drug-eluting stents is advocated in the treatment of STEMI patients because of the reduced risk of restenosis associated with drug-eluting stents. Mechanical reperfusion is superior to thrombolysis, even if longer transport times to a specialized center must be accepted. Current guidelines suggest that primary PCI leads to improved outcomes over thrombolytic therapy if a patient with an acute MI can be transported to a PCI-capable facility within 90 minutes or be transported to a facility without PCI capability and then be transferred to a PCI-capable facility within 2 hours of first medical contact.

Until PCI became the standard of care in hospitals with interventional cardiology programs, thrombolytic therapy was the best available reperfusion therapy. In communities without interventional capabilities

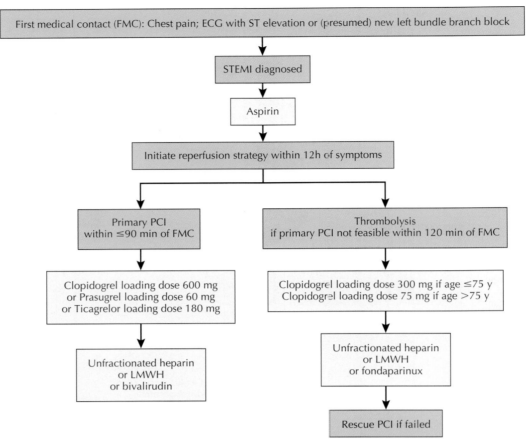

FIG 21.4 Optimum Treatment of ST-Elevation Myocardial Infarction (STEMI). *LMWH*, Low-molecular-weight heparin; *PCI*, percutaneous coronary intervention. See AHA/ACC STEMI Guidelines 2013 for complete classification and level of evidence recommendations.

where there are long transport times to an appropriate facility, thrombolytic therapy is indicated in patients who present with acute STEMI within 12 hours of symptom onset and no contraindications. Administration of thrombolysis does not require specialized facilities or staff, and these agents can be administered with minimal time delay. Numerous large clinical trials have associated the use of thrombolytic therapy with preservation of LV function, limitation of infarct size, and a highly significant reduction in the mortality rate. Failure to achieve complete restoration of normal coronary flow, which may occur in only 45% to 60% of patients, represents a severe efficacy limitation of this therapy. Even after successful reperfusion, reocclusion, and thus reinfarction, occurs in up to 20% of patients. Therefore, only approximately 25% of patients treated with thrombolytic therapy achieve the ideal outcome of rapid and sustained normalization of flow in the infarct-related artery. Finally, fibrinolytic therapy is limited by contraindications to its use, which affects up to 30% of patients, and a risk of lethal or intracranial hemorrhage of approximately 1%.

Adjunctive Therapy

Adjunctive antiplatelet and antithrombotic therapy are cornerstones of the treatment of STEMI. The antiischemic potency of the adjunctive therapy is based on its anticoagulatory effects and must be balanced against the bleeding risk to the respective patient. Aspirin, an irreversible antagonist of the arachidonic acid pathway of platelet activation, reduces mortality and is the first-choice antiplatelet drug that every patient who experiences STEMI should receive as soon as possible independent from the planned revascularization strategy. Antagonists

of the adenosine phosphate ($P2Y_{12}$) receptor responsible for platelet activation, such as clopidogrel, prasugrel, and ticagrelor, decrease ischemic events and reduce mortality in STEMI patients who undergo PCI. Clopidogrel is a prodrug and must be metabolized in the liver to be activated, resulting in a delayed onset of action. To achieve effective levels of platelet inhibition as fast as possible, a loading dose of 600 mg clopidogrel is recommended in the American College of Cardiology/American Heart Association (ACC/AHA) guidelines followed by a maintenance dose of 75 mg/day. Alternatively, the newer and slightly more potent agents prasugrel and ticagrelor can be used.

The traditional antithrombotic drug in ACS patients is unfractionated heparin. Newer anticoagulants have been developed to circumvent the disadvantages of heparin, which include high interindividual variability in antithrombotic response, the need for close monitoring of the effect, and the risk of heparin-induced thrombocytopenia, a potentially life-threatening side effect. Low-molecular-weight heparins have—as a result of their decreased binding to endothelial cells and plasma proteins—a more predictable antithrombotic effect than unfractionated heparin, and thus, doses can usually be given as weight-adjusted without further monitoring. Heparin or low-molecular-weight heparins should be used independently from the revascularization strategy. A direct antithrombin, bivalirudin, was approved for STEMI patients who undergo interventional revascularization; this was based on the finding that it was associated with lower bleeding risk compared with heparin given with glycoprotein (GP) IIb/IIIa antagonists. However, more recent studies have shown comparable bleeding risks compared with heparin alone, but have also found higher rates of early stent thrombosis with

Performance of percutaneous coronary intervention: stent deployment

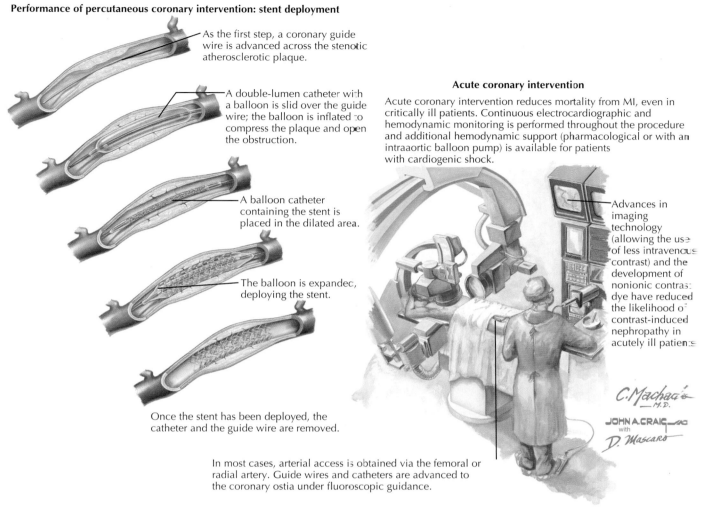

As the first step, a coronary guide wire is advanced across the stenotic atherosclerotic plaque.

A double-lumen catheter with a balloon is slid over the guide wire; the balloon is inflated to compress the plaque and open the obstruction.

A balloon catheter containing the stent is placed in the dilated area.

The balloon is expanded, deploying the stent.

Once the stent has been deployed, the catheter and the guide wire are removed.

In most cases, arterial access is obtained via the femoral or radial artery. Guide wires and catheters are advanced to the coronary ostia under fluoroscopic guidance.

Acute coronary intervention

Acute coronary intervention reduces mortality from MI, even in critically ill patients. Continuous electrocardiographic and hemodynamic monitoring is performed throughout the procedure and additional hemodynamic support (pharmacological or with an intraaortic balloon pump) is available for patients with cardiogenic shock.

Advances in imaging technology (allowing the use of less intravenous contrast) and the development of nonionic contrast dye have reduced the likelihood of contrast-induced nephropathy in acutely ill patients

FIG 21.5 Acute Percutaneous Coronary Intervention in the Management of Myocardial Infarction (MI) with ST-Elevation.

bivalirudin, in addition to higher cost. Thus, heparin is preferred over bivalirudin in most cases. GP IIb/IIIa receptor antagonists are occasionally used in patients who undergo primary PCI and who have a large thrombus burden or no reflow.

Patients who receive fibrinolysis as the primary reperfusion strategy should receive antiplatelet therapy with aspirin and a 300-mg clopidogrel loading dose if aged 75 years or younger or a 75-mg clopidogrel loading dose if aged older than 75 years. In addition, these patients should receive anticoagulant therapy with enoxaparin, fondaparinux if at higher bleeding risk, or unfractionated heparin if PCI is possible.

Hemodynamic Disturbances and Arrhythmias

LV dysfunction remains the most important predictor of death after survival of the acute phase of STEMI. In patients with STEMI, heart failure is characterized by systolic dysfunction or by both systolic and diastolic dysfunction. LV diastolic dysfunction can lead to pulmonary venous hypertension and pulmonary congestion; systolic dysfunction can result in markedly depressed cardiac output and cardiogenic shock. Mortality rates in patients with acute STEMI increase with the severity of hemodynamic deficits.

Mechanical causes of heart failure may occur in acute STEMI, including free wall rupture, pseudoaneurysm, rupture of the interventricular

septum, or rupture of a papillary muscle. Arrhythmias may occur in an MI as a consequence of electrical instability. Sinus bradycardia, sometimes associated with atrioventricular block and hypotension, may reflect augmented vagal activity. Ischemic injury can produce conduction block at any level of the atrioventricular or intraventricular conduction system.

Other complications after an acute MI are recurrent chest discomfort, ischemia, and infarction. Furthermore, pericardial effusion, pericarditis, and Dressler syndrome may also occur. An LV aneurysm develops in less than 5% to 10% of patients with STEMI (especially patients with an anterior MI). The mortality rate is up to six times higher in patients with LV aneurysm than in patients without aneurysms. Death in patients with an LV aneurysm is often sudden and presumably related to ventricular tachyarrhythmias, which frequently occur with aneurysms.

MEDICAL THERAPY TO IMPROVE OUTCOMES

Several medical therapies have been shown to improve outcomes after STEMI. Randomized trials of patients with a previous MI have shown that prolonged antiplatelet therapy leads to a 25% reduction in the risk of recurrent infarction, stroke, or vascular death. All patients after STEMI should receive indefinite therapy with aspirin and 1 year of a P2$_{12}$

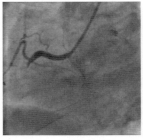

Coronary angiogram of an occluded RCA (STEMI inferior).

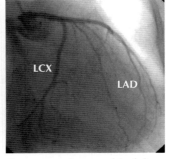

Coronary angiogram of the left coronary system.

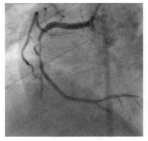

Coronary angiogram of the same RCA after recanalization by balloon angioplasty.

Angiographic catheter

RCA

Atherosclerotic narrowing of RCA

Anatomy of the right coronary stenotic lesion.

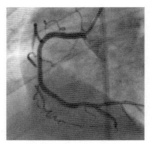

Coronary angiogram after stent placement.

JOHN A. CRAIG—AD

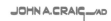

FIG 21.6 Recanalization of an Occluded Right Coronary Artery (RCA). *LAD,* Left anterior descending; *LCX,* left circumflex; *STEMI,* ST-elevation myocardial infarction.

inhibitor, regardless of the chosen reperfusion strategy. Indefinite angiotensin-converting enzyme inhibitor therapy is recommended for patients with clinically evident congestive heart failure; a moderate decrease in global ejection fraction (≤40%); or a large, regional wall motion abnormality. Patients with preserved LV function may also benefit from long-term therapy with an angiotensin-converting enzyme inhibitor. Meta-analyses of trials of oral β-adrenoceptor blockers have shown a 20% reduction in long-term mortality rates, probably due to a combination of the antiarrhythmic effect (prevention of sudden cardiac death) and prevention of a reinfarction. Note that the administration of β-adrenoceptor blockers must be carefully considered in patients with risk of LV failure or cardiogenic shock. If initially contraindicated, patients should be re-evaluated before discharge for initiation of β-blocker therapy. Mineralocorticoid receptor antagonists have been shown to reduce mortality in patients with LV ejection fractions of ≤40% and heart failure or diabetes. High-intensity statin therapy has been shown to reduce major adverse cardiovascular events after STEMI. All of the preceding therapies should be initiated in-hospital before discharge if not contraindicated. Early discharge within 3 to 5 days in uncomplicated patients who have undergone reperfusion therapy is considered safe.

SECONDARY PREVENTION

The concept of secondary prevention of reinfarction and death after recovery from an acute MI includes lifestyle modification, cessation of smoking, and control of hypertension, diabetes mellitus, and cholesterol. All patients should be evaluated for referral to cardiac rehabilitation because it comprehensively addresses all of the aforementioned risk factor modifications and has been shown to reduce all-cause and cardiovascular mortality.

Amiodarone may improve survival after an MI in the presence of significant arrhythmias in patients with preserved LV function. Implantable cardioverter-defibrillators offer a nonpharmacological approach for prevention of cardiac arrest from ventricular arrhythmias and should be considered in patients with ischemic cardiomyopathy with a reduced LV ejection fraction of ≤35% and who are in New York Heart Association (NYHA) functional classes II to III. These patients should be on guideline-directed optimal medical therapy and should be evaluated at least 40 days after MI and >3 months after revascularization before implantation of a device.

FUTURE DIRECTIONS

Patients who survive the initial course of an acute MI are at increased risk because of coronary artery disease and its complications. It is imperative to reduce this risk and expand preventive therapies to patients at risk who have yet to undergo a cardiac event. Special attention needs to be given to inpatient STEMI events because recognition is often challenging, and outcomes are worse compared with outpatient STEMIs.

ADDITIONAL RESOURCES

Aboufakher R. ECG in STEMI: Importance and Challenges. https://www.heart.org/idc/groups/heart-public/@wcm/@mwa/documents/downloadable/ucm_467056.pdf. Accessed July 2017.
A free presentation on the AHA website that provides a good review of ECG diagnosis of STEMI.
Braunwald E. *Heart Disease. A Textbook of Cardiovascular Medicine.* 10th ed. Philadelphia: WB Saunders; 2014.
An excellent textbook that covers not only the topic of acute MI extensively, but also most other topics in cardiology.
Mercader M. *STEMI: 3-Minute Diagnosis, 90-Minute Reperfusion: Saving Time, Saves Lives.* 1st ed. CreateSpace Independent Publishing Platform; 2014.
A textbook that explains the diagnosis of STEMI in a comprehensive way and is a good learning tool for students and residents.
Moscucci M. *Grossman & Baim's Cardiac Catheterization, Angiography and Intervention.* 8th ed. Philadelphia: Lippincott Williams & Wilkins; 2013.
An advanced textbook about the principles and techniques of cardiac catheterization.
O'Rourke R. *Hurst's The Heart.* 13th ed. New York: McGraw-Hill Education; 2011.
A standard reference work that covers acute MI and other topics in cardiology.

EVIDENCE

2013 ACCF/AHA guideline for the management of ST-elevation myocardial infarction: a report of the American College of Cardiology Foundation/American Heart Association Task Force on Practice Guidelines.
Current guidelines of ACC and AHA for management of STEMI with detailed recommendations and level of evidence for each recommendation.

Cavender M, Sabatine M. Bivalirudin versus heparin in patients planned for percutaneous coronary intervention: a meta-analysis of randomised controlled trials. *Lancet.* 2014;384(9943):599–606.

A metaanalysis that compares the effects of heparin and bivalirudin based regimens in MI.

Grines CL, Browne KF, Marco J, et al. A comparison of immediate angioplasty with thrombolytic therapy for acute myocardial infarction. The Primary Angioplasty in Myocardial Infarction Study Group. *N Engl J Med.* 1993;328(10):673.

A trial that demonstrated the superiority of primary angioplasty over fibrinolysis in terms of mortality, reinfarction, and intracranial bleeding.

ISIS-2 (Second International Study of Infarct Survival) Collaborative Group. Randomised trial of intravenous streptokinase, oral aspirin, both, or neither among 17,187 cases of suspected acute myocardial infarction: ISIS-2. *Lancet.* 1988;2(8607):349.

The first trial that showed the importance of aspirin after acute STEMI. Aspirin led to a 23% reduction in vascular mortality.

O'Gara PT, Kushner FG, Ascheim DD, et al. 2013 ACCF/AHA guideline for the management of ST-elevation myocardial infarction: a report of the American College of Cardiology Foundation/American Heart Association Task Force on Practice Guidelines. *Circulation.* 2013;127(4): e362.

ACC/AHA guidelines on how to treat patients with STEMI.

Thygesen K, Alpert JS, Jaffe AS, et al. Third universal definition of myocardial infarction. *Circulation.* 2012;126(16):2020.

The official definition of MI.

22

Percutaneous Coronary Intervention

Thomas D. Stuckey, Bruce R. Brodie

Percutaneous coronary intervention (PCI) has undergone a dramatic transformation since its introduction in the 1970s. In the early 1990s, coronary stenting revolutionized PCI, improving procedural results and dramatically reducing the need for emergency coronary artery bypass graft surgery (CABG). The introduction of drug-eluting stents (DESs) in the 2000s greatly reduced the frequency of late repeat revascularization compared with bare metal stents (BMSs), and second-generation DESs have further improved stent deliverability and have reduced the risk of stent thrombosis. The introduction of new devices and adjunctive pharmacology have enabled the treatment of more complex lesions and have increased safety. Today, PCI has become an integral part of the treatment of patients with coronary artery disease (CAD) by saving lives and improving quality of life.

PERFORMANCE OF PERCUTANEOUS CORONARY INTERVENTION

Procedure and Equipment

PCI is performed in cardiac catheterization laboratories with the same radiographic equipment used for diagnostic coronary arteriography. Arterial access is generally obtained via the femoral or radial artery (Fig. 22.1). Although femoral access has been the most widely used approach historically, radial access is increasingly preferred and is taught at most training centers. Advantages of the radial approach include infrequent access site bleeding, earlier ambulation, improved patient satisfaction, lower cost, and trends toward reduced mortality. Disadvantages are the significant learning curve, the potential for radial artery occlusion, and the inability to use this site for larger catheters, as well as patients with upper extremity renal access needs and those who require hemodynamic support.

Interventional guide catheters are slightly larger than diagnostic catheters to accommodate balloons, stents, and other devices, although improved catheter design has led to smaller transradial guide catheters capable of delivering stents in straightforward cases. After visualization of the coronary artery and the target lesion via arteriography, and after full anticoagulation, a coronary guide wire is advanced across the lesion and positioned in the distal vessel. A small double-lumen catheter with a distal balloon is passed over the guide wire and positioned at the lesion. Pre-dilatation with the balloon is often performed before stenting to open the obstruction by fracturing and compressing plaque. Today, coronary stenting is an integral part of virtually all angioplasty procedures. The undeployed stent is mounted on a second balloon catheter and is passed over the guide wire to the target lesion, where the balloon is inflated to expand and deploy the stent (Fig. 22.2). A high-pressure balloon catheter is then usually used to fully expand the stent. With continued improvements in devices, it is increasingly common to insert and deploy stents without pre-dilatation.

Following PCI by means of the femoral approach, the femoral sheath is removed once the activated clotting time has returned to baseline.

Hemostasis has traditionally been achieved with manual compression, but the use of closure devices has gained popularity, and provides immediate hemostasis in suitable patients and allows for earlier ambulation. Radial sheaths can generally be removed immediately after the procedure while the patient is still anticoagulated, and hemostasis is achieved with pressure maintained via a secured compression device.

Adjunctive Pharmacological Therapy

All patients undergoing PCI receive aspirin before the procedure and full anticoagulation during the procedure to prevent thrombus formation on intravascular devices. Traditionally, heparin has been used as the anticoagulant of choice with the addition of platelet glycoprotein IIb/IIIa inhibitors in high-risk patients, including those who present with acute coronary syndromes (ACSs), in whom the risk of a periprocedural infarction and ischemic events is increased. With the development of more rapid acting and potent oral antiplatelet agents, bivalirudin or heparin monotherapy without glycoprotein IIb/IIIa inhibitors has become the standard in most centers. Bivalirudin has the significant advantage of a short half-life, with a resultant reduction in both access and nonaccess site bleeding. However, heparin monotherapy has the advantage of lower cost, and in patients treated with radial access and those with lower bleeding risk, the value of bivalirudin in preference to heparin alone remains unproven.

With DESs, it may take months for struts to become completely covered with endothelium, and this may predispose patients to thrombus formation and stent thrombosis. Late stent thrombosis (ST) that occurs as long as a year after DES deployment has been a major concern with DESs, although the improved healing characteristics of second-generation DESs have reduced the risk of ST and allowed for a shorter duration of dual antiplatelet therapy (DAPT). Current guidelines call for a minimum of 6 months of DAPT (usually aspirin plus clopidogrel) in patients who receive DESs for stable coronary indications, and a minimum of 1 year in patients treated for an ACS. Guidelines recommend newer, more potent antiplatelet agents (prasugrel or ticagrelor) in patients with ACS, which overcome residual high platelet reactivity noted in some patients treated with clopidogrel. A longer duration of DAPT is suggested in some high-risk patients, such as those with previous myocardial infarction (MI) or first-generation stents (paclitaxel-eluting), who have acceptable bleeding risk.

Outcomes With Percutaneous Coronary Intervention

With the availability of new-generation DESs, greater operator experience, better imaging systems, and improved adjunctive therapies, outcomes of PCI procedures have improved dramatically. With proper patient selection and when performed by experienced operators, procedural success can be expected in >95% of patients. The risk of complications, such as coronary artery dissection with vessel occlusion or vessel perforation, is now a rarity in the catheterization laboratory.

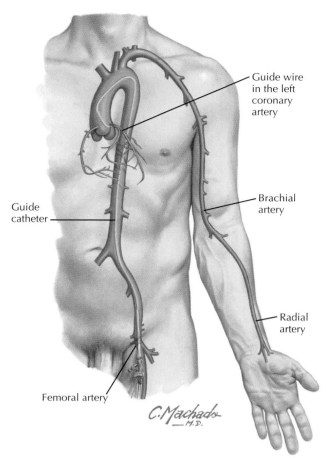

Guide wire in the left coronary artery

Guide catheter

Brachial artery

Radial artery

Femoral artery

FIG 22.1 Percutaneous Coronary Intervention: Vascular Access.

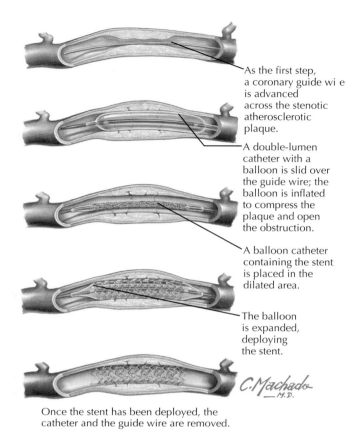

As the first step, a coronary guide wire is advanced across the stenotic atherosclerotic plaque.

A double-lumen catheter with a balloon is slid over the guide wire; the balloon is inflated to compress the plaque and open the obstruction.

A balloon catheter containing the stent is placed in the dilated area.

The balloon is expanded, deploying the stent.

Once the stent has been deployed, the catheter and the guide wire are removed.

FIG 22.2 Performance of Percutaneous Coronary Intervention Stent Deployment.

With improved safety, PCI is now often performed in hospitals without on-site surgery and has been demonstrated to be safe when there is strict adherence to careful patient selection and a well-organized strategy for emergency transfer to a designated high-volume center when needed.

Operator experience is mandatory for these procedures to be performed safely. The American Heart Association (AHA)/American College of Cardiology (ACC) guidelines for PCI recommend that PCI be performed only in institutions that do >400 PCI procedures per year and by operators who each perform >75 PCI procedures per year.

Restenosis was a major limitation of balloon angioplasty before the routine use of intracoronary stents, but the introduction of BMSs in the late 1980s greatly reduced restenosis rates. The addition of DESs—coated with a thin polymer carrying immunosuppressive or antiproliferative drugs that are released over time to prevent neointimal hyperplasia—dramatically reduced restenosis rates. The need for late repeat revascularization at 6 months decreased from 15% to 20% with BMSs to 5% to 7% with DESs. New-generation DESs are now the stents of choice in most patients undergoing PCI, because they have reduced restenosis rates, and because they have also reduced rates of late and very late ST compared with BMSs and first-generation DESs.

With these advances, many patients who previously required CABG can now be effectively treated in the catheterization laboratory. Although it is still an effective means of treating patients with complex coronary disease, CABG is now only necessary in a smaller percentage of patients.

Procedural Complications

The most frequent complications with PCI relate to the arterial access site. Bleeding and hematomas with the femoral approach occur in 3%

to 5% of patients but can usually be managed conservatively, and only occasionally necessitate blood transfusions or surgical intervention. Pseudoaneurysm formation at the access site occurs in <1% of patients and can usually be managed with ultrasound-guided compression and/or thrombin injection. Retroperitoneal hemorrhage is rare but may be life-threatening, particularly if unrecognized, and may necessitate surgical intervention. Radial artery occlusion may occur after transradial procedures, but these are virtually always asymptomatic because of the dual blood supply of the hand.

Cardiac complications are surprisingly infrequent. Balloon inflations and stent deployment occasionally result in embolization of atheromatous debris to the distal coronary bed, sometimes with thrombus formation and myocardial damage, but the resultant MIs are usually small and well tolerated. Ischemia-induced arrhythmias, including ventricular tachycardia and ventricular fibrillation, can usually be managed successfully with drug therapy and/or cardioversion. PCI-induced coronary dissection and/or thrombotic occlusion can result in Q-wave MI, emergency CABG, and occasionally death, but with contemporary PCI techniques and experienced operators, these complications are rare.

ADJUNCTIVE DEVICES

High-Speed Rotational Atherectomy

High-speed rotational atherectomy uses a diamond-coated burr rotating at high speed to fragment plaque into small particles that are absorbed downstream (Fig. 22.3). Used primarily to treat heavily calcified lesions, ostial lesions, and bifurcation lesions, rotational atherectomy is usually combined with stenting.

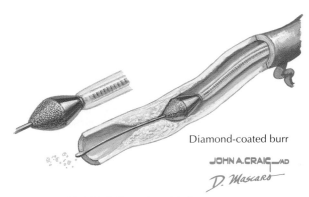

Diamond-coated burr

JOHN A. CRAIG _AD
D. Mascaro

FIG 22.3 Rotational Atherectomy.

Orbital Atherectomy

Orbital atherectomy received Food and Drug Administration approval in 2014 and has now become commonplace in many catheterization laboratories. This technique uses an orbiting eccentric diamond-coated crown on the end of a drive shaft powered by a pneumatic drive console. It is approved for the treatment of calcified coronary lesions and has similar limitations to rotational atherectomy, including an increased risk of coronary dissection, particularly in small or tortuous vessels.

Devices to Protect Against Distal Embolization

Friable plaque and thrombus that develop in saphenous vein grafts following CABG are prone to distal embolization during coronary intervention. Several devices protect against distal embolization, the most common of which are coronary filters (Fig. 22.4). The coronary filter, which is attached to a coronary guide wire and contained within a sheath, is positioned in the vein graft distal to the lesion. Stenting is then performed over the coronary guide wire proximal to the filter. Atherosclerotic and thrombotic debris, dislodged during stent deployment, are caught in the filter rather than embolizing downstream to the microvascular circulation, where it could potentially cause myocardial damage. After completion of the stent procedure, the filter is removed with a retrieval sheath. Distal protection devices have been shown to reduce periprocedural MI when used with PCI in saphenous vein grafts.

Devices to Remove Thrombus

Thrombus is frequently present at the site of obstructive coronary lesions, especially in patients with ST-segment elevation MI (STEMI) and other ACSs, and may embolize into the distal coronary bed during PCI, possibly compromising outcomes. The most commonly used thrombectomy devices are aspiration devices, which have a lumen for passage of the device over a coronary wire and a second lumen with a distal opening that is used for manual aspiration of thrombotic material. These devices are frequently used to treat STEMI patients who have a large thrombus burden. However, multiple randomized trials of aspiration thrombectomy in STEMI have failed to show benefit, and aspiration thrombectomy may be associated with an increased risk of stroke. Although aspiration thrombectomy is still used, guidelines have downgraded its indications, and the frequency of use in STEMI patients has declined.

The rheolytic thrombectomy device, which uses backward injected saline jets to create suction, is a powerful tool for managing vessels with a large thrombus burden.

Intravascular Ultrasound and Optical Coherence Tomography

Intravascular ultrasound (IVUS) and optical coherence tomography (OCT) are modalities that allow for intraluminal visualization of coronary

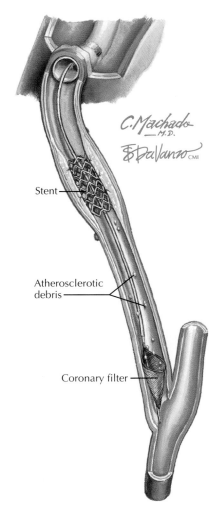

C. Machado M.D.
B DaVanzo CMI

Stent

Atherosclerotic debris

Coronary filter

FIG 22.4 Distal Protection Device: Filter Used for Saphenous Vein Graft Intervention.

arteries. IVUS is performed with a transducer that is passed over a coronary guide wire into the coronary artery. IVUS uses high-frequency sound waves (ultrasound) to visualize atherosclerotic plaque and the vessel wall, and provides diagnostic information not available from coronary angiography alone (Fig. 22.5). It is used before PCI to evaluate lesion severity and vessel size, to help determine the need for adjunctive devices, and to help size stents. After PCI, IVUS is frequently used to assess the adequacy of stent deployment and to ensure complete stent apposition to the vessel wall. OCT uses near–infra-red light, rather than ultrasound, to produce intravascular images, and provides higher resolution and better surface detail than IVUS, whereas IVUS demonstrates better penetration and better visualization of the media. OCT is particularly effective at demonstrating fine stent detail and visualization of thrombus, but requires the use of an additional contrast agent for visualization. Many laboratories use both to optimize procedural outcomes.

Cutting Balloon

The cutting balloon provides an alternative to standard balloon angioplasty for the treatment of technically difficult lesions, such as lesions within a stent, at sites of arterial bifurcation, at ostia of coronary arteries, and in small coronary arteries. The most commonly used cutting balloon has three cutting blades, or atherotomes, that cause a controlled dissection.

Intravascular ultrasonography

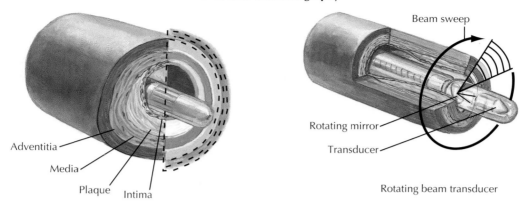

Differences in acoustic sensitivity allow discrimination of vessel wall components

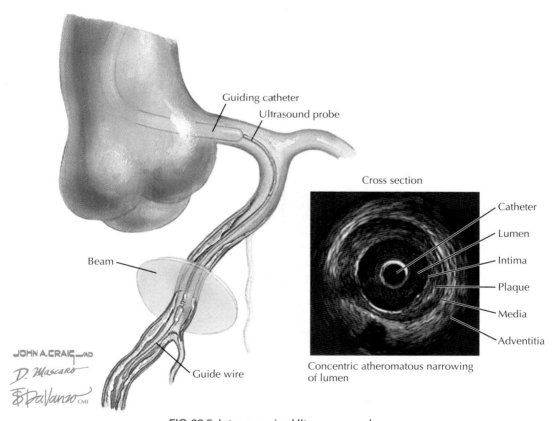

FIG 22.5 Intravascular Ultrasonography.

Fractional Flow Reserve

Fractional flow reserve (FFR) is a technique used to assess the physiological significance of intermediate coronary stenoses. A pressure transducer wire, which can also be used as a coronary guide wire, is introduced into the coronary artery and passed across the stenosis. FFR is calculated as the ratio of the pressure measured distal to the stenosis by the flow wire to the pressure proximal to the stenosis in the guiding catheter obtained during intravenous infusion of adenosine to maximize coronary flow. An FFR of <0.75 to 0.80 is considered abnormal and is associated with a higher likelihood of benefit from revascularization, and is now used as justification for intervention. Instant wave-free ratio is a modification of FFR that measures the pressure gradient across a lesion during a specific period in diastole without the use of vasodilating agents. This technique has shown promise and can be performed without the expense, time, and discomfort of pharmacological stress, and has good correlation with FFR.

INDICATIONS

Coronary revascularization with PCI can provide symptomatic relief from angina for patients with obstructive CAD and may improve survival in selected patients. Indications for PCI have been outlined in the AHA/ACC/Society for Coronary Angiography and Interventions guidelines for PCI. The decision to perform PCI involves weighing the likelihood of procedural success and long-term benefits against the risks of the procedure, and comparing PCI against alternative strategies of medical therapy and CABG. The likelihood of procedural success and late benefit with PCI is highly dependent on lesion and patient selection, as well as operator and institutional experience.

Patient Selection

Patients with obstructive CAD who are asymptomatic or have only mild angina, and who have no or minimal ischemia during stress testing, can often be treated medically. However, asymptomatic patients who have significant myocardial ischemia during stress testing and severe obstructive CAD at catheterization are at high risk of cardiovascular morbidity and should be considered for revascularization with either PCI or CABG.

Patients with stable angina and significant obstructive CAD in one or two vessels generally have improved symptoms and a better quality of life when treated with PCI compared with medical therapy. However, PCI does not reduce the frequency of death or reinfarction in most patients with stable angina. PCI is generally preferred as the revascularization strategy over CABG in patients with single- or double-vessel CAD if the lesions are suitable for PCI. Scoring systems derived from randomized trials are now available (e.g., Syntax score) to assist in patient selection for PCI versus CABG.

In patients with multivessel disease, both CABG and PCI are options. Most trials that compared PCI with CABG have shown higher rates of stroke with CABG but less need for repeat revascularization, and have shown similar rates of death and MI with both procedures. Whether to choose CABG or PCI depends on the presence of comorbid disease that may affect surgical risk, lesion characteristics that may affect PCI outcome, and patient preference, as well as weighing the initial risk and morbidity of open heart surgery against the increased need for repeat revascularization procedures after PCI. Diabetic patients with multivessel disease generally have better survival rates with CABG than with PCI.

Patients who present with ACS, unstable angina, or non-STEMI, can benefit significantly from an invasive strategy with a reduction in major events (death or MI) compared with medical therapy alone. An invasive strategy consists of urgent evaluation with coronary angiography followed by triage to PCI, CABG, or medical therapy, depending on the coronary anatomy and coexisting medical conditions.

Patients with STEMI derive the greatest benefit from PCI. PCI for patients with STEMI (primary PCI) has become the preferred reperfusion strategy when it can be performed by experienced personnel in a timely fashion. Primary PCI has special advantages in patients with cardiogenic shock and in patients who are ineligible for fibrinolytic therapy. Recently, there has been a nationwide effort to reduce time to treatment with PCI so that most STEMI patients can now be treated with primary PCI. STEMI patients who are treated with fibrinolytic therapy, but in whom reperfusion fails, as evidenced by persistent chest pain and lack of ECG ST-segment resolution, are candidates for rescue PCI, which can improve outcomes. PCI performed within hours or a few days after successful fibrinolytic therapy may reduce the frequency of recurrent ischemic events.

With improved primary and secondary prevention, better medical treatment, and more sagacious patient selection, the need for revascularization and the frequency of revascularization with either PCI or CABG has declined in recent years. This has been driven primarily by a reduction in the need for revascularization in patients with stable angina.

Coronary Lesion Selection

Coronary artery lesion characteristics are an important factor in deciding whether patients should be treated with PCI, CABG, or medical therapy. Complex coronary lesions include very long lesions, lesions with excessive tortuosity or calcification, extremely angulated lesions, some bifurcation lesions, ostial lesions, degenerative vein grafts, small vessel size, and chronic total occlusions. The presence of such lesions can make PCI more difficult and can compromise short- and long-term outcomes. When there are complex coronary lesions and the likelihood of a favorable outcome with PCI is reduced, other alternatives, such as medical therapy or CABG, may become more attractive.

Lesions in saphenous vein grafts after CABG are characterized by diffuse, friable plaque and thrombus, and have an increased frequency of distal embolization with PCI. Focal lesions in vein grafts can usually be treated with stenting using distal protection to prevent distal embolization (described previously), but diffuse degenerative lesions in multiple saphenous vein grafts are often best treated with repeat CABG when the native coronary vessels remain good targets.

Previously, the standard treatment strategy for lesions of the left main coronary artery has been CABG. However, improved PCI techniques and the availability of DESs have made stenting of left main coronary artery lesions feasible. Recently completed randomized studies have yielded mixed results, but have confirmed the safety of left main intervention, particularly in patients with less complex anatomy. It is likely that treatment of left main lesions with PCI will increase, and left main stenting is now supported in clinical guidelines.

Treatment of chronic total occlusions has dramatically improved with new devices, better procedural techniques, and new treatment algorithms. Success rates now approach 90% in experienced hands with the hybrid technique, a strategy that takes advantage of multiple approaches—anterograde, retrograde, and subintimal reentry—in a well-defined protocol honed over a decade with experienced operators.

FUTURE DIRECTIONS

New-generation stent designs, with decreased strut thickness, improved polymers, and better drug delivery have significantly reduced early, late, and very late stent thrombosis. New designs of metallic-based stents now include bioabsorbable polymers, polymer-free stents, and polymer and/or drugs limited to the abluminal surface. Bioabsorbable stents, which allow for restoration of vasomotor reactivity and improved endothelial function, are currently being evaluated in multiple clinical trials. Early challenges with stent delivery and stent thrombosis have largely been overcome and will be met with continued innovations in materials science and engineering. New stent designs and strategies to address challenging subsets like bifurcation lesions are also under active investigation. Additional developments include technical advances in radial catheter design and strategies to reduce operator lead use and radiation exposure, such as robotic catheter manipulation. Continued advances in adjunctive pharmacology are also anticipated. Together, these approaches offer the promise of continued improved outcomes for patients who undergo PCI.

ADDITIONAL RESOURCES

2016 ACC/AHA Focused Update on Duration of Dual Antiplatelet Therapy in Patients with Coronary Artery Disease. *J Am Coll Cardiol.* 2016;68:1082–1115.
Excellent update of decision making in the use and duration of DAPT in patients with CAD.
2011 ACCF/AHA/SCAI 2005 Guideline for Percutaneous Coronary Intervention. *J Am Coll Cardiol.* 2011;58:e44–e122.
Provides the current standard of care for the selection of patients for PCI and the use of adjunctive therapies with PCI.
ACCF/SCAI/STS/AATS/AA/ASNC. 2012 Appropriate use criteria for coronary revascularization. *J Am Coll Cardiol.* 2012;59:857–881.
Provides detailed guidelines for the selection of patients for coronary revascularization with either PCI or CABG.
Samady H, Fearor WF, Yeung AC, King SB III, eds. *Interventional Cardiology.* New York: McGraw-Hill; 2017.
Provides an excellent general reference for PCI and interventional cardiology.

23

Coronary Artery Bypass Surgery

Timothy Brand, Audrey Khoury, Kristen A. Sell-Dotin, Thomas G. Caranasos
Michael E. Bowdish, Sharon Ben-Or, Michael R. Mill, Brett C. Sheridan

Cardiovascular disease is the leading cause of death of both sexes in the United States and all industrialized nations, and is increasingly becoming an important cause of death in developing countries. According to the Centers for Disease Control and Prevention, approximately 600,000 people die annually in the United States as a result of cardiac disease; 150,000 of them are aged younger than 65 years. In 2017, approximately 790,000 Americans presented with a myocardial infarction (MI). Of these, approximately 525,000 were new MIs, and approximately 210,000 were recurrent MIs. Acute and chronic coronary syndromes result in inadequate delivery of oxygen to the myocardium and subsequent disturbances in oxidative metabolism. Insufficient coronary flow of nutrients to myocardial cells results in angina. If prolonged, myocardial ischemia leads to myocardial cell death. The most straightforward solution to this interruption of blood flow through coronary arteries is to bring new or additional blood flow through alternative pathways, thus bypassing the obstructed coronary arteries. The development of coronary artery bypass graft (CABG) surgery was fostered by this understanding.

ETIOLOGY AND PATHOGENESIS

The presence of risk factors for atherosclerosis—advanced age, genetic predisposition, male sex, hypertension, diabetes mellitus, renal disease, hyperlipidemia, and cigarette smoking—all result in a propensity for the normally thin intima of coronary arteries to increase in both thickness and smooth muscle cell content. This earliest stage of atherosclerosis is caused by the proliferation of smooth muscle cells; the formation of a tissue matrix of collagen, elastin, and proteoglycan; and the accumulation of intracellular and extracellular lipids. Thus, the first phase of atherosclerotic lesion formation is focal thickening of the intima with an increased presence of smooth muscle cells and the extracellular matrix. Intracellular lipid deposits also accumulate. Next, lesions called fatty streaks form. A fatty streak is an accumulation of intracellular and extracellular lipids that are visible in diseased segments of affected arteries. As the lesion evolves, a fibrous plaque can form from continued accumulation of fibroblasts that cover proliferating smooth muscle cells that are laden with lipids and cellular debris. Plaques progress in complexity as ongoing cellular degeneration leads to ingress of blood constituents and calcification. The necrotic core of the plaque may enlarge and become calcified. Hemorrhage into the plaque may disrupt the smooth fibrous surface, causing thrombogenic ulcerations. Clot organization on the plaque surface often occludes, or nearly occludes, the arterial lumen, further decreasing blood flow (see also Chapter 14).

Just as the rapidity of atherosclerotic lesion formation varies from individual to individual, the presentation of ischemic heart disease also varies. Objective evidence of myocardial ischemia is identified with concurrent coronary angiographic evidence of flow-limiting atherosclerotic lesions. The need for surgical treatment usually arises from presentation of an individual with an acute coronary syndrome and multivessel coronary artery disease (CAD) or with stable but debilitating angina. Examples of indications for urgent CABG include postinfarction angina, ventricular septal defect, acute mitral regurgitation, free wall rupture, and/or cardiogenic shock in patients admitted to the hospital with acute MI. Each of these acute conditions warrants surgical intervention and revascularization.

DIFFERENTIAL DIAGNOSIS

The differential diagnosis of myocardial ischemia includes atherosclerotic and nonatherosclerotic causes of epicardial coronary artery obstruction. Nonatherosclerotic causes include congenital anomalies, myocardial bridges, vascularities, aortic dissection, aortic valve stenosis, granulomas, tumors, and scarring from trauma, as well as vasospasm and embolism. Many of these entities may also be indications for CABG.

Other diseases that mimic angina include esophagitis due to gastrointestinal reflux, peptic ulcer disease, biliary colic, visceral artery ischemia, pericarditis, pleurisy, thoracic aortic dissection, and musculoskeletal disorders.

DIAGNOSTIC APPROACH

Although patients with ischemic heart disease present with a spectrum of clinical urgency, diagnostic evaluation relies on objective evidence of ischemia, assessment of disease burden, and determination of whether the coronary anatomy is amenable to surgical revascularization. The diagnostic approach begins with a complete history and extensive physical examination (see Chapter 2). It is important to note that the physical examination is an insensitive tool and may not assist in the diagnosis of chronic ischemic heart disease. Many patients with chronic ischemic heart disease have no physical findings related to the disease, and even when present, physical findings are often not specific for CAD. Because coronary atherosclerosis is common, any physical finding suggestive of heart disease should raise the suspicion of chronic ischemic heart disease.

Diagnostic evaluation includes multiple approaches. Laboratory studies should be performed to assess for the presence of cardiac risk factors, such as diabetes mellitus, hyperlipidemia, renal insufficiency, hepatic insufficiency, and hyperthyroidism. Electrocardiography can document myocardial ischemia during chest pain or with physiological or pharmacological stress testing. A stress test may also be used to detect CAD or assess the functional importance of coronary lesions. Test results are positive if the patient has signs or symptoms of angina pectoris with typical ischemic ECG changes. The predictive value of the ECG for detecting myocardial ischemia varies in different clinical settings, but the sensitivity and specificity of ECG are typically <70%. The predictive value of stress testing is improved by combining ECG with nuclear or echocardiographic imaging. In individuals who cannot exercise, stress can be induced by administration of the synthetic catecholamine dobutamine, which mimics exercise. Vasodilator drugs such as dipyridamole and adenosine are often used to accentuate flow variations that can occur in individuals with CAD. With vasodilation, these drugs also can cause increased heart rate, increased stroke volume, and an increase in myocardial oxygen demand. Wall motion abnormalities at rest or with stress may be assessed by transthoracic echocardiography, nuclear imaging, or by MRI (see Chapters 10 and 11).

The gold standard for evaluating coronary anatomy to determine the suitability for surgical revascularization is coronary angiography. Coronary angiography allows accurate assessment of coronary atherosclerosis, including quantification of disease location and severity. Studies on the relationship between coronary artery stenoses and myocardial ischemia support the notion that lesions that reduce the cross-sectional area of the coronary artery by ≥70% (50% in diameter) significantly limit flow, especially during periods of increased myocardial oxygen demand. If detected, such lesions are considered compatible with symptoms or other signs of myocardial ischemia. Because atherosclerosis is not uniform, coronary angiography is, to a certain degree, imprecise. The cross-sectional area of the coronary artery at the point of atherosclerotic lesion must be estimated by two-dimensional diameter measurements in several planes. When compared with autopsy findings, stenosis severity is usually underestimated by coronary angiography.

In addition, coronary angiography does not consider that serial coronary artery lesions may incrementally reduce flow to distal beds by more than is predicted by any single lesion. A series of apparently insignificant lesions may reduce myocardial blood flow substantially.

In choosing a diagnostic approach, noninvasive stress testing is performed first in evaluating patients with suspected coronary atherosclerosis, as long as they have not presented with an unstable coronary syndrome. Although the risks of both stress testing and coronary angiography are low, in patients with stable angina, or in patients being assessed following MI, the risk of stress testing is lower than that of coronary angiography. Mortality rates for stress testing average 1 per 10,000 patients compared with 1 per 1000 for coronary angiography. The physiological demonstration of myocardial ischemia and its extent form the basis of the therapeutic approach, regardless of coronary anatomy. Mildly symptomatic patients who have small areas of ischemia at intense exercise levels have an excellent prognosis and are usually treated medically, particularly if left ventricular (LV) function is normal or near normal. Knowledge of coronary anatomy is not necessary to make this therapeutic decision. For this reason, in stable patients, noninvasive assessment of myocardial ischemia and its extent is appropriate before considering coronary angiography.

Patients with profound symptoms of myocardial ischemia during minimal exertion are more likely to have severe diffuse multivessel coronary atherosclerosis or obstruction of the left main coronary artery. The likelihood that revascularization will be required is high, and coronary angiography should be performed as soon as possible. Patients with severe unstable angina should not undergo stress testing because of the increased risk in this population. Coronary angiography is recommended as the initial diagnostic study in these patients. Patients with angina or evidence of ischemia in the early post-MI period are considered to be unstable angina patients, and likewise, should also undergo coronary angiography instead of stress testing. Other indications for coronary angiography include situations in which noninvasive testing will be inaccurate, such as for many patients with left bundle

---

BOX 23.1   Indications for Coronary Artery Bypass Surgery

- Left main coronary disease
- Triple-vessel disease with normal or diminished ejection fraction
- Two-vessel disease with involvement of the proximal left-sided anterior descending coronary artery with normal or diminished ejection fraction
- Unstable (crescendo) angina
- Post–myocardial infarction angina
- Life-threatening ventricular arrhythmias with >50% left main disease or triple-vessel disease
- Acute coronary occlusion after percutaneous coronary intervention
- Persistent symptoms despite maximal medical therapy
- Coronary artery disease and the need for heart surgery for other indications (i.e., valve replacement surgery)
- Mechanical complications of acute myocardial infarction
- Ventricular septal defect
- Acute mitral regurgitation
- Free wall rupture
- Cardiogenic shock

Data from Brown ML, Sundt TM, Gersh BJ. Indications for revascularization. In: Cohn LH, ed. *Cardiac Surgery in the Adult*. New York: McGraw Hill; 2007.

---

branch block on ECG or those who are unable to exercise and difficult to image noninvasively.

MANAGEMENT AND THERAPY

With an indication for surgical myocardial revascularization, management evolves into an issue of timing (emergent, urgent, or elective) and surgical approach (traditional revascularization with cardioplegic arrest and cardiopulmonary bypass [CPB] support vs. off-pump CABG [OPCABG]) (Box 23.1; Fig. 23.1 and Fig. 23.2). The merits of percutaneous revascularization versus surgical revascularization in specific patient presentations are discussed in Chapters 19 to 22. The decision to proceed with CABG emergently is made when coronary angiography confirms the diagnosis of occlusive CAD with hemodynamic instability and/or ongoing myocardial ischemia despite intensive medical treatment. Although the increased myocardial perfusion that results from placement of an intraaortic balloon pump (IABP) can be useful in the short term, patients who require an IABP for control of myocardial ischemia should undergo revascularization as soon as safely possible. Urgent procedures are performed during the same hospital admission secondary to unstable symptoms and severely obstructed coronary anatomy. Patients with stable angina patterns, hemodynamic stability, and less threatening coronary anatomy may undergo elective CABG. A 2017 propensity score-matched analysis compared the clinical outcomes between patients who underwent early CABG (within the first 48 hours of admission) and those who underwent delayed CABG (after 48 hours of admission), and results showed no significant difference in in-hospital mortality (Ha 2017). In patients with acute MI pretreated with platelet $P2Y_{12}$-receptor antagonists (prasugrel or ticagrelor) who require urgent CABG, it is difficult to balance ischemia and bleeding risk. Preoperative platelet reactivity assays may identify those who recover platelet function in less than the recommended washout period of 5 to 7 days (Orvin 2017), and thus prevent delaying CABG.

Optimum Treatment

The gold standard for CABG is complete myocardial revascularization. CABG often allows more complete revascularization than is possible

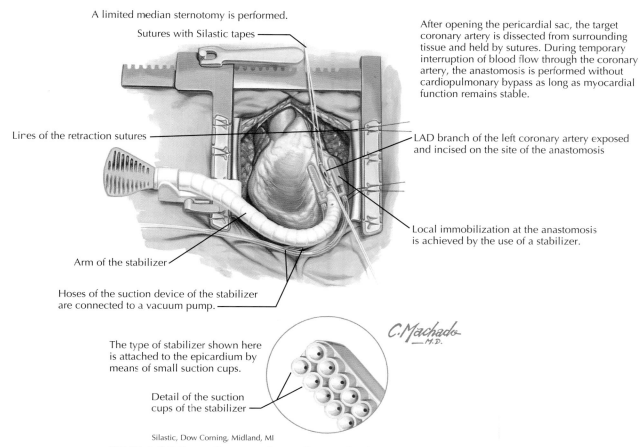

A limited median sternotomy is performed.

Sutures with Silastic tapes

After opening the pericardial sac, the target coronary artery is dissected from surrounding tissue and held by sutures. During temporary interruption of blood flow through the coronary artery, the anastomosis is performed without cardiopulmonary bypass as long as myocardial function remains stable.

Lines of the retraction sutures

LAD branch of the left coronary artery exposed and incised on the site of the anastomosis

Arm of the stabilizer

Local immobilization at the anastomosis is achieved by the use of a stabilizer.

Hoses of the suction device of the stabilizer are connected to a vacuum pump.

The type of stabilizer shown here is attached to the epicardium by means of small suction cups.

Detail of the suction cups of the stabilizer

Silastic, Dow Corning, Midland, MI

FIG 23.1 Off-Pump Coronary Artery Bypass Grafting. *LAD*, Left anterior descending.

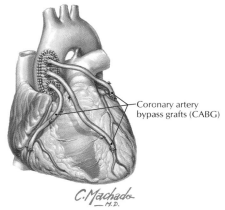

Coronary artery bypass grafts (CABG)

FIG 23.2 Coronary Bypass.

using percutaneous coronary revascularization approaches. CABG is traditionally performed with an arrested, still heart with circulatory support provided by CPB. CPB systems include a pump (most commonly a roller pump), a membrane oxygenator, and an open reservoir. Operating on the arrested heart permits careful examination of diseased vessels and selection of optimal sites for anastomosis of grafts to coronary vessels as small as 1.5 mm in diameter.

Initial studies suggested that because of the potential detrimental effects of circulatory support with CPB, the widespread use OPCABG would result in improved outcomes and less end-organ injury, including

fewer neurological, pulmonary, and renal sequelae. Subsequent studies then demonstrated that when surgery was conducted as expeditiously as possible and CPB time was minimized, outcomes for conventional CABG versus OPCABG were virtually identical. However, in 2017, results from the Randomized On/Off Bypass Follow-up Study (ROOBY F-) demonstrated lower rates of 5-year survival and event-free survival in subjects randomized to OPCABG compared with on-pump CABG (Shroyer 2017). These results were supported by findings from other randomized trials and a 2012 Cochrane systematic review.

Obtaining optimal outcomes for CABG involves attention to several important technical details. The traditional surgical revascularization technique involves placement of an aortic cross-clamp on the ascending aorta to control the surgical field. Cross-clamping the aorta results in myocardial ischemia. To minimize myocardial injury, the heart is protected both by the use of cardioplegia solutions and by cooling the heart to reduce metabolic demand. Blood and crystalloid cardioplegia are both used, with indications for each determined by surgeon preference and the presence or absence of acute ischemia. Hypothermic (4°C) oxygenated blood and cardioplegic solutions are administered by both anterograde and retrograde approaches to rapidly cool the heart. Hypothermic systemic perfusion provides enhanced right-sided ventricular protection, in that retrograde cardioplegia via the coronary sinus may provide limited delivery to the right ventricle. Retrograde cardioplegia is of importance, particularly in patients with impaired right-sided ventricular function, proximal right coronary artery occlusion, prolonged ischemic times, or when right-sided ventricular metabolic demand is increased. Because ventricular stretch impairs postoperative ventricular function, an LV vent can be used to decompress the LV if it distends during CPB. Following completion of anastomoses, approximately 100 mL of crystalloid cardioplegia solution at 4°C is delivered through each graft to the myocardium if inadequate myocardial protection is a concern. Cardioplegic redosing via the aortic root or coronary sinus is performed every 20 minutes throughout the cross-clamp period and is accompanied by strict vigilance to topical cooling, which ensures adequate maintenance of tissue hypothermia during the cross-clamp period. Novel cardioplegic solutions have different dosing protocols but the principle of diastolic arrest and cooling are tantamount to myocardial protection no matter what type of solution is used.

After cross-clamp application and inducement of cardioplegia, distal anastomoses are performed first. The vessels on the inferior surface of the heart (right coronary artery, posterior descending artery, LV branch) are grafted before other vessels. Then, proceeding in a counterclockwise direction, grafts are placed as needed for the posterior marginals, the middle marginals, the anterior marginals, the ramus intermedius, the diagonals, and, last, the left-sided anterior descending artery. The internal mammary artery anastomosis to the left anterior descending artery (or alternately, to the most important distal target) is performed last. Proximal anastomoses are then performed with the formation of aortotomies that are subsequently enlarged with a 4-mm punch. If the ascending aorta has substantial atherosclerotic disease (detected either by inspection or transesophageal echocardiography), embolic risk is minimized by the procedure being performed without a cross-clamp. Many surgeons place stainless-steel washers (that can be visualized by fluoroscopy) on the proximal graft anastomotic sites to assist with later catheterizations. Once proximal and distal anastomoses are completed, the aorta and grafts are de-aired with subsequent removal of the aortic clamp. This initiates myocardial reperfusion, and preparations are made for weaning the patient from CPB.

The heart is allowed to reperfuse in an unloaded beating state as electrolyte, acid-base, and hematocrit values are corrected and inotropic agents are started, if indicated. In general, the need for inotropic agents is determined by preoperative or intraoperative factors. Preoperative factors include advanced age, low ejection fraction, high pulmonary artery pressures, high LV end-diastolic pressure, or high central venous pressures. Intraoperative factors that prompt the need for inotropic assistance include incomplete revascularization, severe distal disease, prolonged CPB or cross-clamp times, poor myocardial protection, and poor LV contractility seen by visual inspection after cross-clamp removal. Intraoperative transesophageal echocardiography can be helpful in determining the need for inotropic agents after weaning from CPB.

An alternative approach to traditional CABG is to operate on the beating heart—so-called OPCABG. The placement of stabilizing devices on the targeted coronary artery makes this technique technically feasible (see Fig. 23.1, bottom). The coronary artery is briefly occluded (10–20 minutes), or intracoronary shunts are used to allow anastomosis of the graft to the coronary artery distal to the atherosclerotic obstruction. The targeted coronary artery is stabilized, and blood pressure is aggressively controlled with volume and inotropic agents delivered during anesthesia. OPCABG requires continued communication with the anesthesiologist throughout the procedure. Although hemodynamically and technically more challenging, this procedure allows for pulsatile anterograde flow through the coronary artery and systemic circulation without the added insults of hypothermia, CPB, and the obligatory proinflammatory blood–artificial surface interface.

Minimally invasive surgery is another less widely adapted technique. In brief, this approach incorporates the concept of OPCABG with a limited-access incision. A limited left-sided anterolateral thoracotomy is performed through the fourth intercostal space without resection or dissection of the ribs. After opening of the pericardial sac, the target coronary artery is dissected from the surrounding tissue and held by sutures at a short distance proximal and distal to the anastomosis that was snared over a piece of pericardium for temporary interruption of blood flow. The anastomosis is performed without CPB as long as myocardial function remains stable. A stabilizer permits local immobilization at the anastomosis site. This procedure has less usefulness than the other procedures because minimal exposure limits options with hemodynamic instability and multivessel disease. In most cases, this technique limits the surgeon to the use of the internal mammary artery, and usually, grafting of the left anterior descending coronary artery. Thus, minimally invasive CABG is most appropriate for single-territory myocardial revascularization.

Avoiding Treatment Errors

Avoiding treatment errors in CABG is multifactorial. An initial important issue is to determine the suitability of a given patient for CABG. Second, CABG requires meticulous attention to surgical technique. In addition, conduit choice is vital to long-term patency of grafts, and ultimately, long-term survival. For instance, the use of an internal mammary artery is superior to the use of vein grafts alone. In addition, survival is improved with bilateral internal mammary grafting as opposed to left internal mammary artery and vein grafting. Saphenous vein grafts (SVGs) do not have the same longevity as arterial grafts, and SVG failure is associated with significant adverse cardiac outcomes and mortality. Medical management for prevention of SVG failure includes antiplatelet therapy, anticoagulant therapy, lipid-lowering therapy, and gene therapy (McKavanagh 2017). Although multiple arterial grafting is more technically challenging, multiple studies have demonstrated that multiarterial CABG has better outcomes than single arterial CABG (Tomoaki 2017). Finally, excellent postoperative care is a necessity for success in any cardiac surgical program.

FUTURE DIRECTIONS

As noted, recent studies showed that patients who underwent OPCABG might have lower rates of 5-year survival and event-free survival than those who have undergone traditional on-pump CABG. The potential disadvantage of OPCABG is incomplete myocardial revascularization or compromised distal conduit–coronary anastomosis due to the increased technical difficulty of operating on the moving heart. For all CABG subtypes, revascularization should not be compromised. Conversion from off- to on-pump may be necessary to complete revascularization. In unusual situations, such as an extensively calcified (porcelain) aorta, OPCABG may be preferred because it may result in less manipulation of the aorta, potentially decreasing the risk of aortic emboli or stroke (Shroyer 2017). Additional studies investigating longer term post-CABG outcomes are warranted.

With the rapidly growing incidence of heart failure and a limited number of donors for heart transplantation, techniques to improve LV function in the context of myocardial revascularization have evolved. Surgical restoration of normal LV shape and volume following MI has gained widespread appeal. The National Institutes of Health is sponsoring a multicenter, prospective, randomized trial to examine the influence of LV endo-aneurysmorrhaphy and CABG on morbidity and mortality rates compared with medical treatment or CABG alone.

Advances in robotic technology, off-pump multivessel techniques, and closed-chest CPB systems have prompted exploratory use of remote CABG techniques. One study compared percutaneous intervention to limited access beating-heart minithoracotomy single-vessel coronary revascularization for proximal left-sided anterior CAD. The results were favorable for this hybrid surgical, less invasive approach.

The ultimate goal for robotic CABG is complete multivessel revascularization using an off-pump approach without sternotomy or even minithoracotomy. This requires that conduit harvesting, conduit preparation, target vessel preparation, control, and anastomosis are all performed remotely from a master control unit. Although two-vessel CABG has been successfully performed with this approach in Europe, limitations remain. Although robotic CABG is associated with longer CPB and cross-clamp times, a recent study demonstrated no significant difference in long-term outcomes (perioperative mortality, MI, and stroke rates) between robotic CABG and traditional CABG (Kofler 2017). New technologies in facilitated anastomotic devices, integrated real-time imaging, and guidance control systems will be mandatory to realize the vision of robotic multivessel CABG.

Finally, recent progress in the field of percutaneous coronary intervention led to a 2017 meta-analysis of multiple randomized controlled trials and observational studies comparing the outcomes of drug-eluting stents and CABG for left main CAD. Although there were no significant differences in mortality, MI, and stroke, drug-eluting stents were associated with an increase in repeat revascularization (Takagi 2017). Future studies are warranted to further investigate the long-term benefits of CABG versus percutaneous coronary intervention and CABG versus hybrid revascularization, which is a strategy that involves contemporary coronary stents and a left internal mammary artery graft.

ADDITIONAL RESOURCES

Ha LD, Ogunbayo G, Elbadawi A, et al. Early versus delayed coronary artery bypass graft surgery for patients with non-ST elevation myocardial infarction. *Coron Artery Dis.* 2017;doi:10.1097/MCA.0000000000000537.
A study evaluating the important concept of surgical timing following acute myocardial infarction.
Hillis LD, Smith PK, Anderson JL, et al. 2011 ACCF/AHA Guideline for Coronary Artery Bypass Graft Surgery: a report of the American College of Cardiology Foundation/American Heart Association Task Force on Practice Guidelines. *J Am Coll Cardiol.* 2011;58:e123–e210.
A comprehensive examination of the data surrounding CABG. Also provides state-of-the-art recommendations regarding indications, treatment, risks, and outcomes. Vital reference for anyone involved caring for patients with CAD.
Kofler M, Stastny L, Reinstadler SJ, et al. Robotic versus conventional coronary artery bypass grafting: direct comparison of long-term clinical outcome. *Innovations.* 2017;12(4):239–246.
No difference was noted in long-term outcomes when comparing conventional CABG to robotic approach.

McKavanagh P, Yanagawa B, Zawadowski G, et al. Management and prevention of saphenous vein graft failure: a review. *Cardiol Ther.* 2017;6:203–223.
Review of surgical and medical therapies to prevent vein graft failure.
Orvin K, Barac YD, Kornowski R, et al. Monitoring platelet reactivity during prasugrel or ticagrelor washout before urgent coronary artery bypass grafting. *Coron Artery Dis.* 2017;28:465–471.
Good demonstration of platelet function testing used in the perioperative setting.
Shroyer AL, Hattler B, Wagner TH, et al. Five-year outcomes after on-pump and off-pump coronary-artery bypass. *N Engl J Med.* 2017;377:623–632.
A 5-year follow-up of the ROOBY-FS clinical trial, with improved survival fo patients receiving conventional CABG compared with off-pump procedures.
Takagi H, Ando T, Umemoto T, et al. Drug-eluting stents versus coronary artery bypass grafting for left-main coronary artery disease. *Catheter Cardiovasc Interv.* 2018;91:697–709.
Meta-analysis of randomized trials comparing PCI with CABG in patients wit. left main coronary artery disease.
Tomoaki S. Optimal use of arterial grafts during current coronary artery bypass surgery. *Surg Today.* 2017;doi:10.1007/s00595-017-1565-z.
Review of surgical techniques and data to support the utilization of arteric conduits.

EVIDENCE

Loop FD, Lytle BW, Cosgrove DM, et al. Influence of the internal mammary artery graft on 10 year survival and other cardiac events. *N Engl J Med.* 1986;314:1–6.
Study from the Cleveland Clinic showing superiority of internal mammary arte. grafting versus all-vein grafting.
Lytle BW, Blackstone EH, Sabik JF, et al. The effect of bilateral internal thoracic artery grafting on survival during 20 postoperative years. *Ann Thorac Surg.* 2004;78:2005–2014.
Study from the Cleveland Clinic showing superiority of bilateral internal mamma y artery grafting at 20 years.
Puskas JD, Kilgo PD, Lattouf OM, et al. Off-pump coronary artery bypass provides reduced mortality and morbidity and equivalent 10-year survival. *Ann Thorac Surg.* 2008;86:1139–1146.
Study from Emory University analyzing outcomes of OPCABG.

24

Cardiogenic Shock After Myocardial Infarction

Venu Menon, Jay D. Sengupta, Joseph S. Rossi

Cardiogenic shock (CS) is characterized by hypotension and end-organ hypoperfusion as a result of low cardiac output. CS remains the most common cause of death after presentation with a myocardial infarction (MI). This clinical state occurs in up to 10% of patients hospitalized with acute MI and remains the leading cause of death during hospitalization. The incidence of CS has decreased only slightly over time, and the mortality rate remains high, at approximately 50% despite advances in interventional and pharmacological management. For patients with ischemic etiology following MI, early recognition and treatment with revascularization and mechanical circulatory support (MCS) improves prognosis and allows for stabilization while considering options for a durable left ventricular assist device (LVAD) and heart transplantation in selected refractory cases.

ETIOLOGY

CS that occurs as a consequence of acute MI is most commonly secondary to severe left ventricular (LV) dysfunction. This may result from a large-index MI or from acute injury in patients with previous LV dysfunction. In the SHOCK (Should We Revascularize Occluded Coronaries for Cardiogenic Shock) trial, predominant LV failure accounted for four of five of all such cases. Approximately one-third of the patients enrolled in the study had evidence of a previous MI.

Several unique clinical entities may also present with acute hemodynamic collapse. Mechanical complications associated with shock include acute mitral regurgitation related to papillary muscle dysfunction or rupture, ventricular septal rupture (VSR), or free-wall rupture. Right ventricular (RV) failure due to RV infarction in isolation or in combination with LV failure can also present in this manner. The clinician should also be aware of iatrogenic shock that results from inappropriate administration of medications (e.g., β-blockers). Occult hemorrhage due to procedure-related complications or in conjunction with therapy using antithrombotic, antiplatelet, and fibrinolytic agents can also cause hypotension and shock.

DIFFERENTIAL DIAGNOSIS

Several nonischemic and extracardiac etiologies must be considered in patients with hypotension and suspected CS. Acute myocarditis secondary to infections or toxins can lead to the development of CS within hours of the first signs of illness. Takotsubo cardiomyopathy (also known as stress cardiomyopathy or apical ballooning syndrome) is another cause of acute LV dysfunction, typically in response to emotional or physical stress, and can present as CS. The differential diagnosis should also include acute aortic dissection, which can be associated with acute aortic valve regurgitation, coronary artery dissection, aortic rupture, and tamponade. Cardiac tamponade can also present secondary to a focal myocardial hematoma after cardiac surgery or trauma or from a circumferential pericardial effusion from malignancy, infarction, or infection. A pulmonary embolism may cause volume and pressure overload of the RV and obstruction of RV outflow, which can lead to hemodynamic collapse. Myocardial depression secondary to septic shock must also be excluded. Acute aortic or mitral valve insufficiency from degenerative disease or bacterial endocarditis can also present with the hemodynamic findings of CS.

PATHOGENESIS

Predominant Left Ventricular Failure

CS is traditionally defined as an unsupported systolic blood pressure of <90 mm Hg with normal to elevated LV filling pressures and evidence of end-organ hypoperfusion. In the setting of acute MI, this is due to plaque rupture and/or thrombosis, which results in acute myocardial dysfunction with decreased cardiac output on the basis of inadequate LV stroke volume. Hypotension can then lead to further reduction in coronary perfusion pressure and further worsening of myocardial ischemia. There may also be cardiac ischemia due to fixed flow-limiting stenoses in nonculprit epicardial coronary arteries remote from the infarct-related vessel. Ischemia thus begets ischemia, which results in a progressive spiral of hemodynamic collapse, culminating with death. In this traditional paradigm of CS, vasoconstriction from falling cardiac output was believed to be the major mechanism by which the neurohormonal system compensates for hypotension. The recognition that many patients have unexpected vasodilation and low systemic vascular resistance in this setting has led to modification of this conceptual design. Observational evidence suggests that inflammatory cytokines, such as interleukin-6, interleukin-1, and tumor necrosis factor-α, are elevated in patients with CS to the same levels seen in patients in a septic state. These findings suggest that MI may result in a systemic inflammatory response syndrome as previously observed with infection or trauma that results in myocardial depression and hypotension independent of ischemic necrosis (Fig. 24.1). These findings are also of importance when considering the diagnostic evaluation of CS patients and optimal therapy (see the following).

Right Ventricular Failure

RV dysfunction commonly occurs when there is infarction of the territory supplied by the acute marginal branches of the right coronary artery (Fig. 24.2). This typically results in hypotension with clear lung fields and is often accompanied by bradyarrhythmic complications, including high-grade atrioventricular block and even complete heart block. ST-segment elevation in right-sided ECG leads V_3 and V_4 is a specific finding for RV infarction. A right-sided ECG should be obtained in all patients presenting with an acute inferior MI and in any patients suspected of having RV infarction. With RV infarction, the right-sided filling pressures become acutely elevated, because there is reduced forward

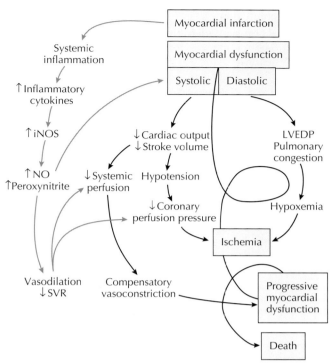

FIG 24.1 Classic Paradigm of Cardiogenic Shock With Recent Observation That Inflammatory Mediators Contribute to a Vicious Cycle of Hypotension and Further Ischemia. *iNOS,* Inducible nitric oxide synthase; *LVEDP,* left ventricular end-diastolic pressure; *NO,* nitric oxide; *SVR,* systemic vascular resistance. (Adapted from Hochman JS. Cardiogenic shock complicating acute myocardial infarction: expanding the paradigm. *Circulation.* 2003;107;2998–3002.)

flow through the pulmonary circulation into the left side of the heart. Elevation in RV end-diastolic pressure may also negatively affect LV filling by causing a "bowing" of the interventricular septum into the LV cavity. As a result, the LV is underfilled, and cardiac output further reduced. Reperfusion of the right coronary artery improves RV function, restores conduction, and can often result in normalization of hemodynamics.

Mitral Regurgitation

The anatomy of the mitral valve as depicted in Fig. 24.3 reveals how mitral leaflet closure depends on papillary muscle function. Each mitral valve leaflet is connected by chordae tendineae to both the posteromedial and anterolateral papillary muscles. The posteromedial papillary muscle is at greater risk from ischemic damage, because it often has a single blood supply from the posterior descending artery, whereas the anterolateral papillary muscle usually receives dual blood supply from the left anterior descending and circumflex arteries. Consequently, inferior and posterior MIs are more likely to cause papillary muscle dysfunction and/or rupture and resultant severe mitral regurgitation. Additional risk factors for papillary muscle rupture include age, female sex, first MI, hypertension, and single-vessel disease. When acute papillary muscle rupture occurs, the jet of mitral regurgitation is typically eccentric and directed away from the affected flail mitral leaflet. In contrast, chronic ischemic mitral regurgitation often results from a restricted posterior mitral leaflet with a resultant central or posteriorly directed jet of mitral regurgitation.

The prognosis of acute severe mitral regurgitation from papillary muscle rupture is poor, with three-quarters of patients dying within

24 hours and only 6% surviving >2 months. The severity of mitral regurgitation results in marked elevations in left atrial and pulmonary capillary wedge pressures, which leads to pulmonary edema and hypoxia. In the SHOCK Registry, despite having a higher mean LV ejection fraction, the cohort of patients with acute severe mitral regurgitation had similar in-hospital mortality with patients who had LV failure. There was a trend toward improved in-hospital survival in patients who underwent surgical repair in addition to revascularization compared with those treated with revascularization alone (40%–71%; *P* = 0.003). Ischemic mitral regurgitation in the setting of an acute MI may be difficult to recognize initially. For this reason, it is critical to keep this potential diagnosis in mind in the evaluation of MI patients with CS. At present, it is still recommended that these patients undergo surgery to repair or replace the mitral valve, coupled with urgent or emergent revascularization.

Ventricular Septal Rupture

CS due to VSR complicating acute MI has a mortality rate of >75%. Classically described as a late complication, it can also present early. The median time from MI to VSR was only 16 hours in the SHOCK Registry. Both anterior and inferior MIs can give rise to VSR. Inferior infarctions cause septal rupture in the basal inferior septum that are complex and serpiginous, and usually extend into the RV. In contrast, anterior infarctions are more likely to cause rupture in the apical septum. As with ischemic mitral regurgitation and/or papillary muscle rupture, the mainstay of management for peri-MI VSR is surgical; however, mortality remains high in patients who have surgery. Outcomes with apical septal VSR are better than with inferoseptal VSR because the surgical technique is simpler. Endovascular devices are being increasingly used in this situation, especially in patients who are not believed to be surgical candidates. Recently, the Amplatzer Post-Infarct Muscular VSD Occluder (St. Jude Medical, Minneapolis, Minnesota) was approved for this purpose under a humanitarian device exemption by the Food and Drug Administration (FDA).

Free-Wall Rupture

Cardiac rupture is a catastrophic complication of MI. Predisposing factors include advanced age, first MI, and female sex. Three types have been described from a series of 50 autopsies in 1975. Type I rupture occurs typically within 24 hours after MI and is characterized by a slit through a normal thickness infarct. Type II rupture occurs more often in posterior infarcts and is a localized erosion of the infarcted myocardium. Type III rupture is most commonly seen in anterior infarcts and occurs in severely expanded, thinned, and dilated infarcts. Rupture usually results in sudden death due to acute cardiovascular collapse. In some patients, the rupture may be contained to form a pseudoaneurysm. The treatment in both cases is emergency cardiac surgery for those patients who can be stabilized adequately to make surgery a feasible option.

It is likely that the incidence of both VSR and free-wall rupture decreased first with the routine use of thrombolytic therapy and further with the use of percutaneous coronary intervention (PCI) in acute MI. However, both are still seen, and must be diagnosed and treated early for there to be any reduction in mortality from these mechanical complications of MI.

CLINICAL PRESENTATION AND DIAGNOSTIC APPROACH

The clinical signs and symptoms of CS derive from the underlying pathophysiology. Patients presenting with MI complain of chest pain. Recurrent chest pain may imply ongoing ischemia or reinfarction but

Coronary Arteries: Arteriographic Views

Right coronary artery: left anterior oblique view

Right coronary artery: right anterior oblique view

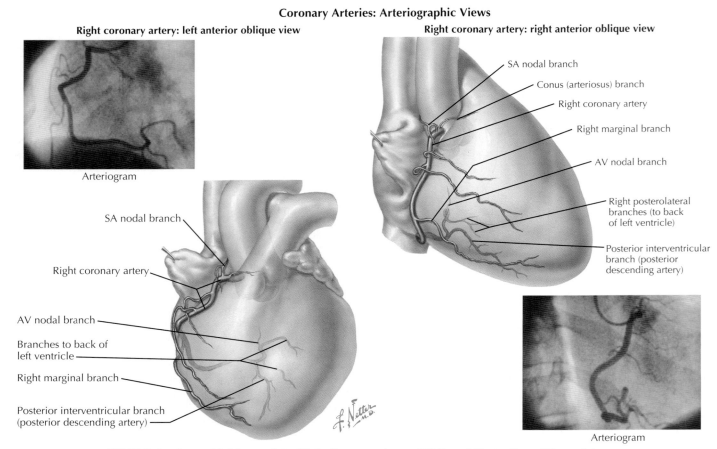

Arteriogram

SA nodal branch
Conus (arteriosus) branch
Right coronary artery
Right marginal branch
AV nodal branch
Right posterolateral branches (to back of left ventricle)
Posterior interventricular branch (posterior descending artery)

SA nodal branch
Right coronary artery
AV nodal branch
Branches to back of left ventricle
Right marginal branch
Posterior interventricular branch (posterior descending artery)

Arteriogram

FIG 24.2 Angiographic Views of the Right Coronary Artery (RCA) and Illustration of Normal Areas Perfused by the RCA. *AV,* Atrioventricular; *SA,* sinoatrial.

Heart in diastole: viewed from base with atria removed

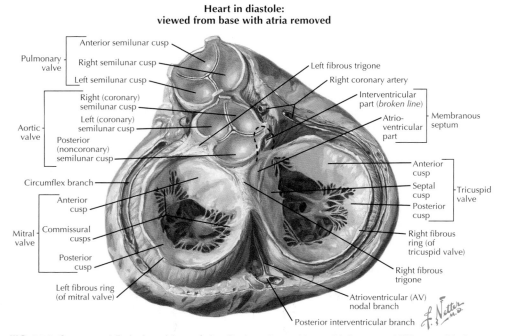

Pulmonary valve
- Anterior semilunar cusp
- Right semilunar cusp
- Left semilunar cusp

Aortic valve
- Right (coronary) semilunar cusp
- Left (coronary) semilunar cusp
- Posterior (noncoronary) semilunar cusp

Left fibrous trigone
Right coronary artery
Interventricular part (*broken line*)
Atrio-ventricular part
Membranous septum

Circumflex branch

Mitral valve
- Anterior cusp
- Commissural cusps
- Posterior cusp

Anterior cusp
Septal cusp
Posterior cusp
Tricuspid valve

Right fibrous ring (of tricuspid valve)

Right fibrous trigone

Left fibrous ring (of mitral valve)

Atrioventricular (AV) nodal branch

Posterior interventricular branch

FIG 24.3 Structural Relationships of the Pericardium, Heart, Valves, and Fibrous Skeleton.

may also reflect mechanical complications such as papillary muscle rupture, VSR, or free-wall rupture. Symptoms associated with ischemia include nausea, emesis, restlessness, and agitation. End-organ hypoperfusion associated with the redistribution of blood to vital organs by selective vasoconstriction results in cool and clammy peripheries. There may also be evidence of decreased urine output and mental status changes.

The elevated LV filling pressures give rise to pulmonary edema, and resultant dyspnea and tachypnea with associated bilateral rales on physical examination. Often, the development of respiratory failure can be sudden and dramatic. Laboratory evaluation may demonstrate evidence of acute kidney and liver dysfunction, as well as lactic acidosis.

Cardiopulmonary examination may give clues into the etiology of hemodynamic collapse. A diffuse point of maximal impulse, loud S_3 gallop, and elevated jugular venous pressure with rales on lung examination are specific findings associated with underlying heart failure. A new holosystolic murmur would lend suspicion for mitral regurgitation (although in the acute setting the murmur may be difficult to detect due to shorter duration and decreased intensity often noted in cases of acute mitral regurgitation), VSR, or RV failure with functional tricuspid regurgitation as a result of RV dilatation and volume overload. A precordial thrill may help to differentiate VSR. Evidence of hypotension with reduced pulse pressure, pulsus paradoxus, and distant heart sounds could indicate the presence of tamponade physiology related to free-wall rupture.

Echocardiography is a powerful diagnostic tool in patients who present after MI. In CS, this imaging modality can provide detailed information about the etiology and supplement findings from the history and physical examination. The echocardiogram can provide information regarding LV and RV size and function, as well as the presence of valvular and structural complications.

MANAGEMENT AND THERAPY

Optimum Treatment

The management of CS after an MI revolves around early reperfusion of the occluded coronary artery, with a goal of complete revascularization in the setting of severe multivessel coronary artery disease. Coronary angiography followed by revascularization is preferred over fibrinolytic therapy (Fig. 24.4). In the SHOCK trial, a strategy of early revascularization resulted in 132 lives saved at 1 year per 1000 patients treated compared with initial medical therapy followed by no or late revascularization as clinically determined. The benefit was noted in patients younger than 75 years of age, and the survival benefits persisted at long-term follow-up. In the setting of shock, the time window for benefit with revascularization is greater than that established with primary reperfusion for ST-elevation MI (STEMI). The SHOCK trial enrolled patients within 36 hours of their index MI, and patients throughout the time window benefited. Certain patients aged older than 75 years also seemed to derive benefit from revascularization in observational registries when selected by experienced physicians. The modality of revascularization should be guided by the extent and severity of coronary artery disease. PCI with stent implantation should be used in patients with single-vessel and two-vessel disease amenable to revascularization. In addition to opening the infarct-related artery, multivessel PCI should strongly be considered for other severely stenotic lesions in the acute setting. Patients with severe obstruction in three coronary vessels or severe left main trunk stenosis may be considered for emergency bypass surgery, especially if PCI is not feasible.

A Swan-Ganz catheter (SGC) for hemodynamic monitoring is a useful tool in CS. There is no evidence for survival benefit in patients with an SGC when independently studied; however, it is useful for

Acute coronary intervention reduces mortality from MI, even in critically ill patients. Continuous electrocardiographic and hemodynamic monitoring is performed throughout the procedure, and additional hemodynamic support (pharmacological or with mechanical circulatory support) is available for patients with cardiogenic shock.

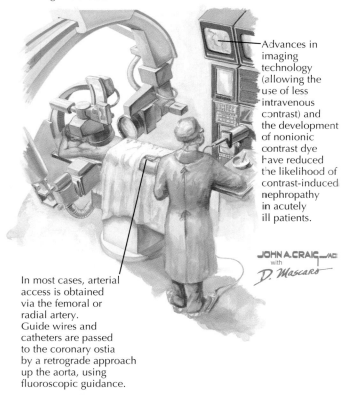

Advances in imaging technology (allowing the use of less intravenous contrast) and the development of nonionic contrast dye have reduced the likelihood of contrast-induced nephropathy in acutely ill patients.

JOHN A. CRAIG—AD
with
D. Mascaro

In most cases, arterial access is obtained via the femoral or radial artery. Guide wires and catheters are passed to the coronary ostia by a retrograde approach up the aorta, using fluoroscopic guidance.

FIG 24.4 Acute Coronary Intervention.

diagnosis and management. When the cause of hypotension is unclear, the SGC can confirm the presence of reduced cardiac output, with elevated intracardiac filling pressures distinguishing cardiogenic from alternative etiologies for shock. The presence of RV failure, papillary muscle rupture, and VSR can be further characterized by SGC hemodynamic patterns. In addition, the hemodynamic response to mechanical circulatory support and medication changes can be followed closely in real time.

MCS is another important adjunctive measure in CS management. The intraaortic balloon pump (IABP) (Fig. 24.5) has historically been the predominant treatment for initial management. It functions by inflating in diastole and deflating in systole as triggered by ECG or a pressure waveform during the cardiac cycle. The IABP creates a vacuum effect during systole that reduces afterload on the LV. During diastole, the IABP augments diastolic blood pressure, theoretically increasing coronary perfusion pressure. The current American College of Cardiology/American Heart Association guidelines support the use of IABPs as a stabilizing measure in CS.

Recently, the Impella family of devices (Abiomed Inc, Danvers, Massachusetts) have gained popularity due to superior hemodynamic support in patients with CS, and currently, the Impella device is the only MCS therapy with an FDA-approved indication for the treatment of CS. The Impella devices use an axial flow pump that moves blood directly from the inlet cannula in the LV to the ascending aorta. At high flow rates, the negative pressure at the inlet cannula can move the device toward the apex or against a papillary muscle. This can result in local turbulence and hemolysis, and impede flow through the mechanism, which can limit hemodynamic support. The Impella devices provide a range of cardiac output from 2.5 to 5 L/min. The device often requires repositioning with echo guidance after insertion, which can usually be performed at bedside with good results. The Impella RP device can be used for RV support and has received FDA approval under a humanitarian device exemption.

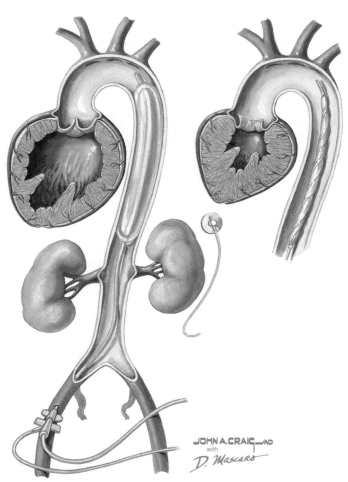

FIG 24.5 Intraaortic Balloon Counterpulsation Pump.

Numerous other devices are available for use in early stabilization as a bridge to recovery, often with simultaneous evaluation for durable LVAD placement or heart transplantation. The use of veno-arterial extracorporeal membrane oxygenation (ECMO) in the cardiac catheterization laboratory is gaining popularity, and the TandemHeart devices (CardiacAssist Technologies, Pittsburgh, Pennsylvania) are also used at select centers. Because of the poor prognosis of patients presenting with CS, the use of MCS therapies should be considered in the context of patient comorbidities and long-term prognosis. The relative hemodynamic limitations of various MCS strategies are summarized in Table 24.1.

The expression of inducible nitric oxide synthase may play an important role in the genesis and outcome after shock. However, in multicenter randomized trial testing, the nitric oxide synthase inhibitor L-N(G)-monomethyl arginine did not show reduction in mortality from CS.

The general approach to a patient with MI and CS is to stabilize the oxygenation, blood pressure, and rhythm while proceeding urgently to coronary angiography. Once the anatomy of the obstructive coronary artery disease is determined, the approach to revascularization can be decided. When cardiac catheterization is not readily accessible, fibrinolytic therapy may be considered for reperfusion in STEMI and early shock within 3 hours of initial symptom onset. All patients who receive pharmacological reperfusion in the setting of CS and acute MI should be transferred to a center with cardiac catheterization and coronary care unit capabilities (Fig. 24.6). A recent position statement produced by the American Heart Association Council on Clinical Cardiology emphasized the correlation of case volume with survival among hospitalized patients with CS, and early transfer to a PCI capable center with MCS capabilities should be considered in all patients.

Avoiding Treatment Errors

Patients with large infarct territories or hemodynamic instability after an MI benefit from monitoring in an intensive care setting to diagnose complications and guide management. Early identification of mechanical complications facilitates appropriate candidates for mechanical support and/or surgical intervention. Caution must be applied with routinely used medications to avoid iatrogenic shock. Patients with RV infarction are notoriously sensitive to reductions in preload. The administration of nitroglycerin in such cases may result in hypotension and exacerbation of ischemia. Similarly, patients with RV infarct may require a surprisingly high volume of fluid replacement (several liters) to achieve hemodynamic stability. Fluid replacement must be individualized in these patients, mean blood pressure must be monitored to be certain sufficient fluid has been given, and the patient must be followed carefully for evidence of fluid overload by physical examination and measurement of oxygen saturation. A patient with large infarct territory

TABLE 24.1	**Comparison of Short-Term Mechanical Circulatory Support Strategies for Cardiogenic Shock**				
	IABP	**Impella 2.5/CP**	**Impella 5.0**	**TandemHeart**	**ECMO**
Cardiac output support (L/min)	<1.0	Up to 2.5 Up to 3.8 (CP)	Up to 5.0	Up to 4.0	>4.5
Access	Femoral artery 7–8 Fr	Femoral artery 13–14 Fr	Surgical cutdown 22 Fr	Arterial outflow 15 Fr Venous inflow 21 Fr	Arterial outflow 16–19 Fr Venous inflow 19–23 Fr
Mechanism	Aortic counterpulsation	Axial flow pump	Axial flow pump	Centrifugal flow pump	Centrifugal flow pump
Surgical insertion	No	No	Yes	No	Not required
Limitations	Rhythm dependent	Hemolysis, pump movement within LV cavity can limit flow	Hemolysis, pump movement within LV can limit flow	Requires transseptal puncture for LA inflow	Oxygenator required; femoral insertion may require anterograde perfusion catheter

ECMO, Extracorporeal membrane oxygenation; *IABP,* intraaortic balloon pump; *LA,* left atrium; *LV,* left ventricle.

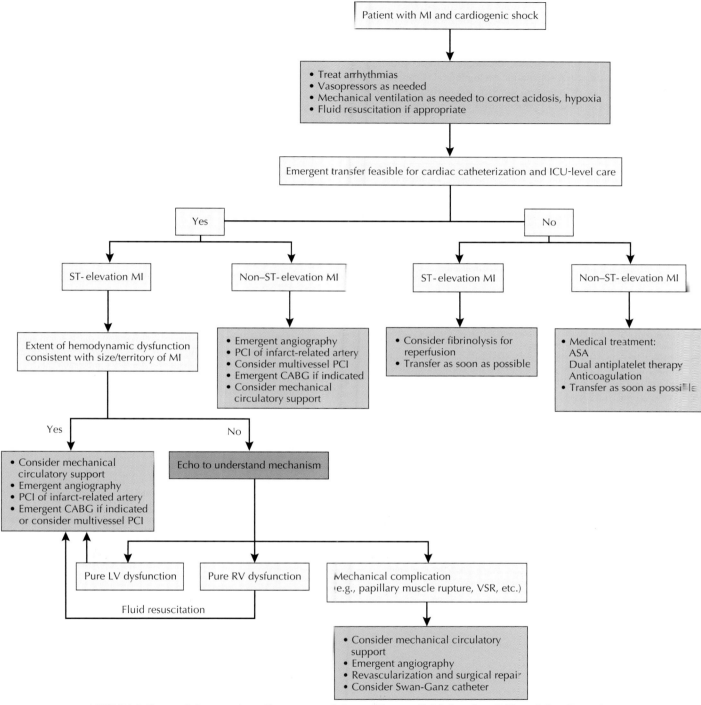

FIG 24.6 General Approach to Treatment of Acute Myocardial Infarction (MI) and Cardiogenic Shock. *ASA,* Aspirin; *CABG,* coronary artery bypass graft surgery; *IABP,* intraaortic balloon counterpulsation pump; *ICU,* intensive care unit; *LV,* left ventricular; *PCI,* percutaneous coronary intervention; *RV,* right ventricular; *VSR,* ventricular septal rupture.

and severe LV dysfunction can develop tachycardia to maintain adequate cardiac output. The administration of a β-blocker may result in reduced cardiac output and hemodynamic collapse in these patients. In the COMMIT (Clopidogrel and Metoprolol in Myocardial Infarction) Trial, early β-blockade in patients with acute MI was associated with an increase in CS. Overly aggressive use of angiotensin-converting enzyme inhibitors may also lead to iatrogenic hypotension.

FUTURE DIRECTIONS

Patients with persistent shock despite revascularization have poor prognosis. Eligible patients may be considered for cardiac transplantation. Selection of patients for mechanical support in CS is challenging. The possibility of ventricular recovery with revascularization alone must be weighed against prompt establishment of adequate cardiac output to prevent end-organ dysfunction. As more data become available with percutaneous LVADs, it will be easier to select patients who will benefit from early intervention. Smaller devices will be developed to provide good augmentation of cardiac output while minimizing the risk of vascular complications. Although mechanical support is most commonly used as a bridge to cardiac transplantation, technological advancements will allow for greater use of long-term support, or so-called destination therapy, with a durable LVAD in patients who are not candidates for transplantation.

ADDITIONAL RESOURCES

Aymong ED, Ramanathan K, Buller CE. Pathophysiology of cardiogenic shock complicating acute myocardial infarction. *Med Clin N Am.* 2007;91:701–712.
Thorough overview of pathophysiology and cellular pathways that propagate hypotension during CS after MI.
Chen EW, Canto JG, Parsons LS, et al. Relation between hospital intra-aortic balloon counterpulsation volume and mortality in acute myocardial infarction complicated by cardiogenic shock. *Circulation.* 2003;108:951–957.
Overview of data using IABP counterpulsation to stabilize patients with CS.
Hochman JS. Cardiogenic shock complicating acute myocardial infarction: expanding the paradigm. *Circulation.* 2003;107:2998–3002.
Editorial overview of the implications of data from the SHOCK Registry and appropriate application to clinical practice.
van Diepen S, Katz JN, Albert NM, et al. Contemporary management of cardiogenic shock: a scientific statement from the American Heart Association. *Circulation.* 2017;136:e232–e268.
Most recent scientific update on the evidence-based management of cardiogenic shock.
Vlodaver Z, Edwards JE. Rupture of ventricular septum or papillary muscle complicating myocardial infarction. *Circulation.* 1977;55:815–822.
Historical primary pathological description of papillary muscle and VSR complicating MI and leading to CS.

EVIDENCE

Becker AE, van Mantgem JP. Cardiac tamponade: a study of 50 hearts. *Eur J Cardiol.* 1975;15:349–358.
An original pathological characterization of post-MI complications.
Fox KA, Steg PG, Eagle KA, et al. Decline in rates of death and heart failure in acute coronary syndromes, 1996–2006. *JAMA.* 2007;297:1892–1900.
Statistical analysis of numerical trends over time in mortality and complications from ACS.

Gianni M, Dentali F, Grandi AM, et al. Apical ballooning syndrome or Takotsubo cardiomyopathy: a systematic review. *Eur Heart J.* 2006;27:1523–1529.
Overview of a recently diagnosed entity found among patients who present with a clinical picture similar to ACS but who have normal coronary arteries and characteristic and reversible LV dysfunction.
Hochman JS, Sleeper LA, Webb JG, et al. Early revascularization in acute myocardial infarction complicated by cardiogenic shock. *N Engl J Med.* 1999;341:625–634.
Landmark study that contains primary data for early revascularization in patients with CS.
Menon V, Webb JG, Hillis LD, et al. Outcome and profile of ventricular septal rupture with cardiogenic shock after myocardial infarction: a report from the SHOCK Trial Registry. Should we emergently revascularize occluded coronaries in cardiogenic shock? *J Am Coll Cardiol.* 2000;36(3 supplA):1110–1116.
Primary evidence-based analysis on subset of patients in the SHOCK Registry who have ventricular septal defect and discussion of appropriate management options.
O'Gara PT, Kushner FG, Ascheim DD, et al. 2013 ACCF/AHA guideline for the management of ST-elevation myocardial infarction. *J Am Coll Cardiol.* 2013;61:e78–e140.
Evidence-based and committee-driven guidelines on the standard of care for management of patients with STEMI.
Reynolds HR, Hochman JS. Cardiogenic shock: current concepts and improving outcomes. *Circulation.* 2008;117:686–697.
Overview and commentary of the evidence-based approach to CS.
Thompson CR, Buller CE, Sleeper LA, et al. Cardiogenic shock due to acute severe mitral regurgitation complicating acute myocardial infarction: a report from the SHOCK Trial Registry. *J Am Coll Cardiol.* 2000;36(3 supplA):1104–1109.
Primary evidence-based analysis on subset of patients in the SHOCK Registry who had mitral regurgitation and discussion of appropriate management options.
TRIUMPH Investigators. Effect of tilarginine acetate in patients with acute myocardial infarction and cardiogenic shock: the TRIUMPH Randomized Controlled Trial. *JAMA.* 2007;297(15):1711–1713.
Study that evaluated a novel medication that may affect clinical practice relating to CS complicating MI.
Wei JY, Hutchins GM, Bulkley BH. Papillary muscle rupture in fatal acute myocardial infarction: a potentially treatable form of cardiogenic shock. *Ann Intern Med.* 1979;90(2):149–152.
Original recognition of the consequences and potential targets for therapy in patients with papillary muscle rupture after an MI.

25

Congenital Coronary Anomalies

Tiffanie Aiken, Michael R. Mill, Sharon Ben-O

Unfortunately, presentation with cardiac arrest or sudden cardiac death is a common manifestation of congenital coronary anomalies. This clinical relevance underpins the necessity of understanding the anatomy and presentation of congenital coronary anomalies and their treatment options. The two primary congenital coronary anomalies, anomalous connection of the left coronary artery from the pulmonary artery (ALCAPA) and anomalous connection of a main coronary artery to the aorta, as well as two entities associated with coronary artery anomalies—coronary artery fistulas and anomalous coronary circulation—are the focus of this chapter (Fig. 25.1).

It was initially believed that the two main coronary arteries arise from separate ostia within the sinuses of Valsalva. However, current embryological information suggests the proximal coronary arteries grow from the peritruncal area into the aorta, and a single orifice is individually formed for the left and right coronary arteries. The left coronary artery (LCA) then divides into the left anterior descending artery, which traverses the anterior interventricular groove, and into the left circumflex coronary artery, which courses into the left atrioventricular groove. Normally, the right coronary artery (RCA) originates anteriorly from the right aortic sinus and courses along the right atrioventricular groove, commonly giving rise to the posterior descending artery.

ANOMALOUS CONNECTION OF THE LEFT CORONARY ARTERY FROM THE PULMONARY ARTERY

ALCAPA is a rare congenital anomaly, usually an isolated lesion, that occurs from 1 in 30,000 to 1 in 300,000 live births (Fig. 25.2). The clinical spectrum of ALCAPA is also known as Bland-White-Garland syndrome. Infants with myocardial ischemia typically present with failure to thrive, profuse sweating, dyspnea, pallor, and atypical chest pain upon eating or crying, usually at between 4 and 6 weeks of age. By 2 to 3 months of age, heart failure is apparent, and patients have persistent tachypnea and tachycardia. Malignant arrhythmias leading to sudden cardiac death are the most extreme presentation of myocardial ischemia in ALCAPA. During the neonatal period, high pulmonary vascular resistance ensures anterograde flow from the pulmonary artery through the LCA. However, as this resistance diminishes, there is an eventual reversal of flow, with left-to-right shunting through the pulmonary artery. The result is the phenomenon of "coronary steal," with left ventricular (LV) perfusion becoming dependent on collateral circulation from the RCA.

Because infantile circulation has little or no coronary collateral development, ALCAPA leads to severe myocardial ischemia, with resultant LV dysfunction and dilation. Dilation of the LV is due not only to the effects of ongoing myocardial ischemia but also to mitral valve regurgitation, because papillary muscle ischemia is common in

ALCAPA. Without surgical intervention and correction of the anomaly, 90% of patients die by age 1 year. Patients who survive to adulthood, secondary to the presence and formation of collateral circulation, may remain asymptomatic despite subclinical, ongoing ischemia. Arrhythmic sudden death purportedly occurs in 80% to 90% of patients by 35 years of age.

Although ALCAPA is rare, a high index of suspicion should be present for infants presenting with signs of myocardial ischemia or dysfunction, or for adolescents presenting with syncope, chest pain, or cardiac arrest after strenuous exercise. Dilated cardiomyopathy and endocardial fibroelastosis are two conditions with clinical signs that are difficult to distinguish from ALCAPA. All three conditions may present with cardiomegaly, mitral regurgitation that results in an apical pansystolic murmur and apical gallop rhythm, and ECG evidence of myocardial ischemia and LV hypertrophy. If an enlarged RCA with global hypokinesis and LV dilation are revealed with two-dimensional and pulsed Doppler echocardiography, ALCAPA must be considered in the differential diagnosis. The gold standard in diagnosing ALCAPA is cardiac catheterization and cineangiography. Hemodynamic data show a low cardiac output despite elevated filling and pulmonary arterial pressures. Magnetic resonance angiography has emerged as a noninvasive diagnostic tool, with similar sensitivity and specificity in comparison to cardiac catheterization. Pulsed and color-flow Doppler examination may delineate a left-to-right shunt. The degree of mitral regurgitation and LV function can be assessed using a left ventriculogram in addition to illustrating coronary anatomy. Coronary angiography also assists in excluding other anatomic etiologies for ischemia and ventricular dysfunction.

Surgical correction remains the gold standard of therapy and is necessary in all patients with ALCAPA due to risk of further myocardial ischemia and subsequent death. Important changes in technique have resulted in improved outcomes. Surgical repair involves direct reimplantation of the anomalous LCA into the aorta by transferring it with a button of the pulmonary artery (Fig. 25.3). There are several options to customize the surgical approach to overcome anatomic challenges of the length and course of the LCA for reimplantation. They include the Tunnel operation and/or Takeuchi repair, LCA translocation, and subclavian-to-LCA anastomosis. In adults in whom reimplantation is more technically challenging, bypass grafting with the left internal thoracic artery is an equally effective approach. If LV function does not improve following revascularization, cardiac transplantation may be indicated.

After reestablishment of a two-coronary system, the previously dilated RCA will generally return to normal size, and the intercoronary collateral network that developed before surgery will regress. Operative mortality for all surgical techniques has markedly decreased. Operations resulting in a two-coronary system have been reported to have a mortality rate of 0% to 14%, and represent a vast improvement compared

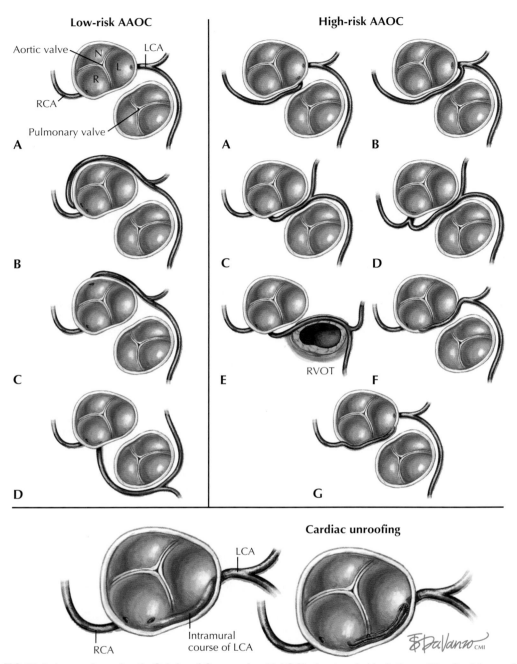

FIG 25.1 Anomalous Aortic Origin of Coronaries (AAOC): Anatomic Variations. The Positions of the Anatomic Right (R), Left (L), and Non (N) Coronary Cusps Are Shown. *LCA,* Left coronary artery; *RCA,* right coronary artery; *RVOT,* right ventricular outflow tract.

with the mortality rates reported in the early 1980s (75%–80%). One study of long-term survival reported no late deaths in 21 patients with a range of 2 months to 18 years of follow-up and a total of 145 patient-years of follow-up. No differences in LV function or the late mortality rate have been shown comparing the various reimplantation or revascularization techniques used today. Although the previous approach of directly ligating the anomalous coronary was abandoned because of poor outcomes, it is suggested as an option to help stabilize a critically ill patient before revascularization is undertaken.

ANOMALOUS AORTIC CONNECTION OF CORONARIES

Anomalous aortic origin of coronaries (AAOC) presents much more variably than ALCAPA and is characterized by coronary arteries with anomalies of aortic connection involving courses, stenoses, and compression. Some individuals have myocardial ischemia and can present with sudden death, but in others, this can be an entirely asymptomatic incidental finding at the time of cardiac catheterization or coronary

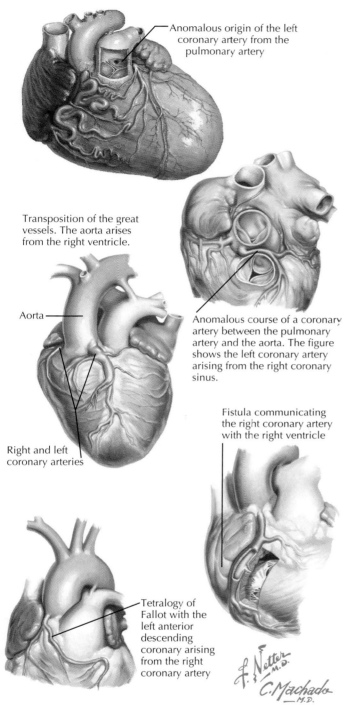

Anomalous origin of the left coronary artery from the pulmonary artery

Transposition of the great vessels. The aorta arises from the right ventricle.

Aorta

Right and left coronary arteries

Anomalous course of a coronary artery between the pulmonary artery and the aorta. The figure shows the left coronary artery arising from the right coronary sinus.

Fistula communicating the right coronary artery with the right ventricle

Tetralogy of Fallot with the left anterior descending coronary arising from the right coronary artery

FIG 25.2 Congenital Coronary Artery Anomalies.

Surgical correction is indicated in individuals who present with significant symptoms. In asymptomatic individuals, if the LCA arises from the right coronary sinus and courses between the aorta and the pulmonary artery, surgical intervention is indicated because the risk of sudden cardiac death is high in this group. However, if the RCA arises from the left aortic sinus and is nondominant, such an entity may be benign.

Prevalence of an anomalous course of a coronary artery between the pulmonary artery and aorta (ACCBPAA) is unknown, due to a lack of consistent pathognomonic and clinical features. Current estimates range from 0.1% to 0.3% of the general population. One review of 126,595 cardiac catheterizations revealed an incidence of 1.15%, constituting 87% of all coronary artery anomalies within this series. The most important review of this abnormality described sudden death in 59% of the 242 patients. The diagnosis should be considered in young patients with exercise-induced myocardial ischemia, aborted sudden death, or sudden death. It has recently been suggested that screening of first-degree relatives with echocardiography be performed because of potential familial link. Transthoracic echocardiography with color Doppler will provide valuable information, such as evaluation of heart function, identification of both coronary artery connections, and demonstration of the direction of blood flow within the aortic wall. Despite coronary angiography remaining the gold standard to accurately delineate the anatomy and exclude other associated coronary disease, it is not preferred in children. In those cases, noninvasive imaging with CT and MRI may be used to identify the coronary artery connections and/or confirm diagnosis.

Surgical intervention is indicated in patients with an interarterial and intramural course of the anomalous coronary artery, with signs and/or symptoms of myocardial ischemia or ventricular arrhythmias. Asymptomatic patients with anomalous connection and course of the left main coronary artery should also undergo surgical intervention due to a high risk of sudden death. Choice of surgical technique will depend on specific morphological details, as determined by preoperative imaging. The preferred procedure for patients with an interarterial and intramural course of the anomalous coronary artery is the unroofing procedure. A transverse aortotomy is essential to assess the coronary ostia. If the anomalous coronary artery arises from the opposite sinus, it is necessary to detach the aortic valve commissure. The slitlike ostium, which is characteristic of AAOC and partially responsible for ischemic symptoms, is opened along its longitudinal axis, and a portion of the common wall between the aorta and the coronary artery is excised, with reapproximation of the intimal surfaces. The valve commissure is subsequently resuspended with a pledgeted suture. This unroofing procedure creates a neo-ostium and obliterates the intramural course of the coronary artery.

Other surgical options include revascularization with an internal mammary artery or a saphenous vein bypass graft, direct reimplantation, or reconstruction of the orifice. However, an important issue to consider is that revascularization may lead to competitive flow between the bypass graft and the native circulation, thus increasing the likelihood of bypass graft failure. The advantage of reimplantation is that competitive flow is not an issue, because a single conduit vessel provides flow to the myocardium in that distribution. Even so, reimplantation may be more technically difficult because kinking may occur, or there may be insufficient tissue to create a button around the orifice.

CORONARY ARTERY FISTULAS

Coronary artery fistulas make up almost one-half of all congenital coronary anomalies. They are defined as communications with right-sided (arteriovenous fistula) or left-sided (arterio-arterial fistula) cardiac

artery imaging. The reasons for this variable presentation involve subtle differences in the anatomy and course of the anomalous coronary artery (see Fig. 25.2). The major anomalies of connection that are potentially serious include attachment of the RCA to the left sinus of Valsalva, attachment of the left main coronary artery to the right sinus of Valsalva, attachment of one or both major coronary arteries to the posterior noncoronary or nonfacing sinus of Valsalva, and lastly, a single coronary artery with only one aortic orifice and main stem that divides to supply branches to the entire heart.

Surgical correction of ALCAPA

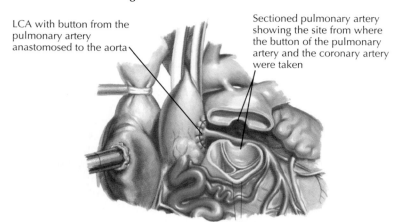

LCA with button from the pulmonary artery anastomosed to the aorta

Sectioned pulmonary artery showing the site from where the button of the pulmonary artery and the coronary artery were taken

The technique involves direct reimplantation of the anomalous LCA into the aorta by transferring it with a button of pulmonary artery. Seen here: Variation with transection of the pulmonary artery

Technique to close fistula from RCA to RV and plication of coronary aneurysm

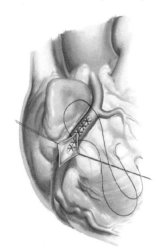

The aneurysmal coronary artery is opened and the fistula is sutured. The coronary artery is closed and the aneurysm is repaired by plication.

Arterial repair of transposition of the great arteries—First steps

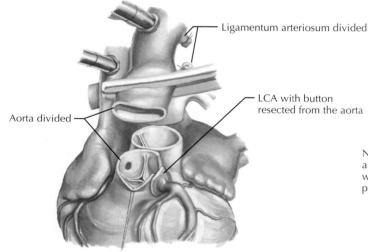

Ligamentum arteriosum divided

Aorta divided

LCA with button resected from the aorta

The aorta and the pulmonary artery are transected. The cut of the aorta is slanted and above the sinuses of the Valsalva. The pulmonary artery is divided above its valve at the same level of the transection of the aorta. Sinuses of the aorta and pulmonary artery are excised to translocate the coronary ostia from the pulmonary artery to the neoaorta. Pericardium is utilized to reconstruct the neopulmonary artery sinuses.

Arterial repair of transposition of the great arteries—Last steps

Coronary arteries anastomosed to neoaorta

Distal pulmonary artery

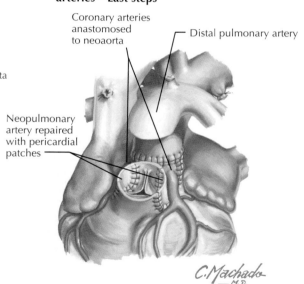

Neopulmonary artery repaired with pericardial patches

C.Machado
—M.D.

FIG 25.3 Surgical Procedures for Correction of Congenital Coronary Artery Anomalies. *ALCAPA,* Anomalous origin of the left coronary artery from the pulmonary artery; *LCA,* left coronary artery; *RCA,* right coronary artery; *RV,* right ventricle.

structures, and result in either a left-to-right or left-to-left shunt. The most common fistula is the RCA communicating with the RV. However, fistulas involving the LCA may have an aberrant connection with either heart chamber, the pulmonary artery or vein, the coronary sinus, or a central vein. Patients rarely present with symptoms during infancy and are frequently diagnosed in early adulthood. Often asymptomatic, fistulas are most commonly discovered during evaluation for a murmur. However, it is not uncommon for patients with a fistula to present with symptoms secondary to congestive heart failure or myocardial ischemia due to coronary steal.

Echocardiography can reveal the origin of the fistula, the chamber in which it drains, and the presence of enlargement or hypertrophy of any of the cardiac chambers. Color-flow Doppler is still used to demonstrate the fistula, and MRI has emerged as a noninvasive tool to diagnose and depict the anatomy of the coronary arterial fistula. However, the gold standard remains cardiac catheterization, selective coronary angiography, and aortography for definitive diagnosis, and planning surgical repair or coil occlusion. In addition, CT angiography is preferred in cases of adults and young children who do not require hemodynamic measurements for management decisions.

Intervention prevents ventricular volume overload and resulting congestive heart failure. Transcatheter coil embolization can be used to embolize the fistula and avoid the morbidities associated with cardiopulmonary bypass and sternotomy. However, these management options are limited to highly selected patients; therefore, the preferred option is surgical closure. It is suggested that all symptomatic patients undergo closure, even those with very small fistulas, because of the natural progression of fistulas to enlarge. In addition, moderate to large fistulas in asymptomatic patients are recommended to have elective surgical closure. If the fistula arises from the distal end of the coronary artery, ligation may be performed without cardiopulmonary bypass. Before permanent ligation, a trial occlusion of the affected coronary artery at the distal site should be performed to observe for signs of ischemia. If signs of myocardial ischemia are absent, ligation may then be performed. If the fistula arises from the midportion of a coronary artery, cardiopulmonary bypass with cardioplegic arrest allows the surgeon to open the abnormal coronary artery and to oversew the fistula at that point. If coronary artery luminal compromise occurs, bypass grafting may be warranted. In other instances, the fistulous tract may be closed internally via access through the involved cardiac chamber (see Fig. 25.3).

CORONARY ARTERY ANOMALIES ASSOCIATED WITH CONGENITAL HEART DISEASE

Several important forms of congenital heart disease are associated with coronary artery anomalies, and this can have major implications for surgical repair. Coronary artery anomalies are particularly important in patients with tetralogy of Fallot, transposition of the great arteries (TGA), and pulmonary atresia with an intact ventricular septum (see Fig. 25.2).

Coronary artery anomalies are reported in 1% to 10% of patients with tetralogy of Fallot. Most commonly, this involves a large coronary artery crossing the RV outflow tract just below the pulmonary valve. These anomalies include origin of the left anterior descending artery from the RCA, a large conus branch across the RV outflow tract, a paired anterior descending coronary artery off the RCA, and an origin of both coronary arteries from a single left ostium. In each situation, the potential exists for damage to or severing of the coronary artery during a right ventriculotomy to correct RV outflow tract obstruction.

In pulmonary artery atresia with an intact ventricular septum, embryonic sinusoids within the RV may persist and communicate with the epicardial coronary arteries in several ways. Usually this occurs in patients with diminutive RV chambers and severe RV hypertrophy. The communications may feed one or both coronary arteries, and may be associated with proximal or distal coronary stenosis, or both, at the insertion site of the fistulous communications. In some patients with coronary stenosis, the coronary fistulous connections are sufficiently developed to produce an RV-dependent coronary circulation. Angiography of the RV cavity is required to demonstrate retrograde filling of one or more coronary arteries via the fistulous connection. Coronary angiography can determine whether the LV myocardium is normally perfused or whether substantial segments are perfused from the RV through the myocardial sinusoids. In this circumstance, perfusion of parts of the LV from the RV must be identified before surgical repair. Importantly, correction of the RV outflow tract obstruction that is present in tetralogy of Fallot results in a reduced pressure within the RV, which can mean decreased perfusion pressure for the sinusoid LCA branches, decreased perfusion of the LV, and ultimately, myocardial ischemia and/or infarction during surgery.

Patients who have pulmonary artery atresia with an intact ventricular septum usually require an early systemic-to-pulmonary shunt, and if

the tricuspid valve and RV chamber have growth potential, surgical relief of the pulmonary atresia. If the RV is miniscule, a Fontan procedure is the definitive treatment. However, if the myocardium is perfused via the RV through the sinusoids because of stenotic coronary arteries, then a systemic RV must be preserved as part of the Fontan operation. Cardiac transplantation may be the only option for patients with pulmonary artery atresia with an intact ventricular septum.

The treatment for patients with a simple dextroposed-TGA (D-TGA) with a ventricular septal defect is an arterial switch operation during the neonatal period (see Fig. 25.3). In D-TGA, both in its simple form and with a ventricular septal defect, the aorta arises from the RV, and the pulmonary artery arises from the LV. Until the 1970s, the preferred surgical management was an atrial switch. However, over time dilation decreased ejection fraction, tricuspid insufficiency, and dysrhythmias were observed, indicating dysfunction of the RV. Subsequently, the preferred procedure has been the arterial switch, with observed operative survival rates near 100%. During the arterial switch procedure, the coronary arteries are transferred from the anterior semilunar valve to the posterior valve, together with reversing the location of the great vessels to the appropriate ventricles. The success of the operation depends on the transfer of the coronary arteries without compromising the blood supply of the coronary circulation. Seven different coronary artery patterns are recognized in patients with a D-TGA, but normal anatomy is present in 60% to 70% of patients. Although certain unusual coronary artery patterns were formerly associated with an increased mortality rate, the specific coronary artery anatomy has become less important because surgical experience with this operation has improved technical approaches and overall outcomes. The presence of an intramural coronary artery, a segment of coronary artery that courses within the wall of the aorta without a separate layer of adventitial tissue between the coronary artery and the aorta, remains a difficult challenge. Although follow-up angiography after the arterial switch operation shows varying coronary artery abnormalities in approximately 10% of patients, most patients are asymptomatic.

FUTURE DIRECTIONS

Several issues of anomalous coronary arteries remain to be explored, including, but not limited to, choosing the best noninvasive diagnostic imaging technique, particularly in children; further pathophysiological characterization of myocardial perfusion in patients with anomalous coronary arteries; and defining indications for percutaneous intervention in adults who have symptomatic coronary disease in anomalous coronary vessels.

The preferred diagnostic imaging modality for characterization of coronary ostia anomalies and course is cardiac CT angiography (CCT). The structure and course of the coronary artery is anatomically illustrated, in addition to the adjacent structures. However, CCT can fail to reveal smaller distal portions of coronary arteries and their branches, as well as the distal insertion of smaller fistulae. In addition, an optimal imaging protocol has yet to be determined in children. Multidetector-row CT (MDCT) coronary angiography is useful in assessing coronary abnormalities in pediatric patients, with accurate diagnostic image quality. Origin and course of the vessel, in addition to the presence or absence of compression of luminal narrowing is explicitly displayed. However, compared with invasive coronary angiography, MDCT cannot serve as an alternative due to the lack of a therapeutic role. Free-breathing, ECG-triggered, navigator-gated, T2-prepared, three-dimensional coronary MR angiography does not require injection of a contrast agent due to contrast between the coronary arteries and surrounding tissue. However, this modality is problematic in young children due to the long examination time and low spatial resolution. Lastly, dual-source

CT uses two x-ray tubes positioned 90 degrees to each other, allowing the scan time to be cut in half. Furthermore, it can be used with different energies of x-rays generated from each tube, which creates a differential change in attenuation of biological tissues at different energy levels that can then be processed to subtract certain material from the images.

Further investigation is warranted into regional myocardial flow reserve in survivors of ALCAPA related to its underlying pathology (i.e., endocardial and subendocardial fibrosis, damage to the papillary muscles, patchy myocardial necrosis, dilation of the ventricle, mitral incompetence, LCA hypoplasia of the media, distal stenosis, and hypoplasia of the RCA). Physiological issues will also require further definition with regard to myocardial perfusion after treatment in long-term survivors of this often lethal condition.

As stated, the use of the arterial switch operation for TGA has resulted in significantly improved outcomes. However, complications in patients who were treated with the atrial switch are now being found, predominantly because of dysfunction of the RV, tricuspid valve, and the baffle itself. Surgical management is challenging with these patients, who eventually require a heart transplantation.

Anomalous coronary arteries have a reported frequency of approximately 1.33% in nonselected patients undergoing coronary angiography; therefore, it can be predicted that adults who have anomalous coronary arteries will present with symptomatic coronary artery disease in these vessels later in life. Because this anatomy may offer unique challenges for interventional cardiologists, specific indications for percutaneous intervention remain to be defined in this area of improving interventional technology.

ADDITIONAL RESOURCES

Boxt LM, Abbara S. Cardiac computed tomography. In: *Cardiac Imaging: The Requisites.* 4th ed. Philadelphia, PA: Elsevier; 2016:143–199.
Overview of cardiac CT.
Brothers JA, Gaynor J. Surgery for congenital coronary artery anomalies. In: Yuh DD, Vricella LA, Yang SC, Doty JR, eds. *Johns Hopkins Textbook of Cardiothoracic Surgery.* 2nd ed. New York, NY: McGraw-Hill; 2014.
Comprehensive overview of coronary anomalies in children.
Kouchoukos NT, Blackstone EH, Hanley FL, Kirklin JK. Congenital anomalies of the coronary arteries. In: *Kirklin/Barratt-Boyes Cardiac Surgery: Morphology, Diagnostic Criteria, Natural History, Techniques, Results, and Indications.* 4th ed. Philadelphia: Elsevier/Saunders; 2013:1643–1671.
Comprehensive overview of coronary anomalies.
Zaer NF, Amini B, Elsayes KM. Overview of diagnostic modalities and contrast agents. In: Elsayes KM, Oldham SA, eds. *Introduction to Diagnostic Radiology.* New York, NY: McGraw-Hill; 2014.
Overview of diagnostic radiology.

EVIDENCE

Dodge-Khamati A, Mavroudis C, Backer C. Anomalous origin of the left coronary artery from the pulmonary artery: collective review of surgical therapy. *Ann Thorac Surg.* 2002;74:946–955.
Review of surgical therapy for anomalous origin of the left coronary artery from the pulmonary artery.
Goo HW. Coronary artery imaging in children. *Korean J Radiol.* 2015;16(2):239–250.
Review of coronary artery imaging in children.
Gulati R, Reddy VM, Culbertson C, et al. Surgical management of coronary artery arising from the wrong sinus, using standard and novel approaches. *J Thorac Cardiovasc Surg.* 2007;134:1171–1178.
Review of the surgical management of coronary arteries arising from the wrong sinus.
Hoffman JI. Abnormal origins of the coronary arteries from the aortic root. *Cardiol Young.* 2014;24(5):774–791.
Review of anomalous aortic origin of coronaries.
Hutchison SJ, Merchant N. Coronary artery anomalies of origin and course. In: *Principles of Cardiac and Vascular Computed Tomography.* Philadelphia: Elsevier/Saunders; 2015:108–142.
Description of use of cardiac CT in coronary artery anomalies of origin and course.
Juan C-C, Hwang B, Lee P-C, Meng C-CL. Diagnostic application of multidetector-row computed tomographic coronary angiography to assess coronary abnormalities in pediatric patients: comparison with invasive coronary angiography. *Pediatr Neonatol.* 2011;52(4):208–213.
Comparison between MDCT coronary angiography and invasive coronary angiography in the ability to assess coronary abnormalities in pediatric patients.
Karimi M, Kirshbom PM. Anomalous origins of coronary arteries from the pulmonary artery: a comprehensive review of literature and surgical options. *World J Pediatr Congenit Heart Surg.* 2015;6(4):526–540.
Review of surgical options for anomalous origin of the left coronary artery from the pulmonary artery.
Loukas M, Germain AS, Gabriel A, John A, Tubbs RS, Spicer D. Coronary artery fistula: a review. *Cardiovasc Pathol.* 2015;24(3):141–148.
Review of coronary artery fistulas.
Mavroudis C, Mavroudis CD, Jacobs JP. Repair techniques for anomalous aortic origins of the coronary arteries. *Cardiol Young.* 2015;25(8):1546–1560.
Review of surgical therapy for anomalous aortic origins of the coronary arteries.
Yamanaka O, Hobbs RE. Coronary artery anomalies in 126,595 patients undergoing coronary angiography. *Cath Cardiovasc Diag.* 1990;21:28–40.
Description of the frequency of coronary anomalies in a patient population undergoing coronary angiography.

26

Coronary Hemodynamics and Fractional Flow Reserve

George A. Stouffer

BASIC PRINCIPLES OF CORONARY BLOOD FLOW

Myocardial cell contraction and relaxation are aerobic processes that require oxygen. Determinants of myocardial oxygen demands include preload, afterload, heart rate, contractility, and basal metabolic rate. Other than basal metabolic rate, these are factors that influence stroke volume. Systolic wall tension uses approximately 30% of myocardial oxygen demand. Wall tension itself is affected by intraventricular pressure, afterload, end-diastolic volume, and myocardial wall thickness.

The coronary arteries are the first vessels to branch off the aorta, and through them the heart receives approximately 5% of the cardiac output when the body is at rest, or 250 mL/min. Under basal conditions, the myocardium extracts approximately 75% of delivered oxygen (Fig. 26.1). The myocardium has a basal metabolic requirement that is approximately 15 to 20 times that of resting skeletal muscle and approximately equal to that of skeletal muscle under severe acidotic conditions. The heart has the highest oxygen consumption per tissue mass of all human organs and the highest arterial-venous difference in oxygen concentration of any major organ. The oxygen saturation in the coronary sinus is one of the lowest in the body.

Because there is minimal ability for the heart to increase oxygen extraction, and the heart has limited capacity for anaerobic metabolism, increased metabolic demands of the heart are met primarily via increases in coronary blood flow. In the absence of obstructive epicardial coronary artery disease (CAD), coronary blood flow is primarily controlled by changes in resistance in the small arteries and arterioles (microvasculature) that play an important role in myocardial perfusion in general and in regional and transmural distribution. The presence of hemodynamically significant epicardial disease leads to a reduction in microvascular resistance at baseline so that coronary blood flow is maintained and thus limits the ability of the myocardium to increase flow in response to increased demand.

Coronary blood flow primarily occurs during diastole. Flow in the left coronary artery has a greater diastolic predominance than the right coronary artery because the compressive forces of the right ventricle (underlying a portion of the right coronary artery) are less than those of the left ventricle (Fig. 26.1). At least 85% of coronary flow in the left anterior descending artery occurs in diastole, whereas right coronary artery blood flow is more or less equal in systole and diastole. The predominance of flow during diastole exacerbates myocardial ischemia during tachycardia. With increased heart rates, oxygen supply is reduced (because diastole is shortened), whereas demand increases.

The heart has the ability to maintain coronary blood flow in the presence of varying perfusion pressures (termed autoregulation). Autoregulation maintains consistent coronary flow over a range of perfusion pressures from 60 to 150 mm Hg. In the setting of maximum vasodilation of coronary resistance vessels, coronary blood flow is no longer autoregulated and varies linearly with perfusion pressure. The ability of autoregulation to maintain flow when perfusion pressures are decreased is especially important in the presence of epicardial coronary stenoses.

CORONARY FLOW RESERVE

The ratio of maximal coronary flow to resting coronary blood flow is termed coronary flow reserve (CFR) (Fig. 26.2). Coronary blood flow is primarily controlled by release of local metabolites (e.g., adenosine or nitric oxide). Hypoxia is a more potent coronary vasodilator than either hypercapnia or acidosis. Neural influences on coronary blood flow are relatively minor. In clinical medicine, maximal coronary blood flow is achieved by intracoronary or intravenous administration of the potent microcirculation vasodilator, adenosine. Other agents that have been used to increase coronary flow include papaverine, regadenoson, nitroglycerin, and contrast dye.

The physiological principle underlying the clinical use of CFR is that the ratio of maximal blood flow to basal blood flow will decrease with progressive obstruction of the lumen of an epicardial coronary artery by atherosclerosis. CFR can be measured using an 0.014-inch guidewire with a 12-MHz piezoelectric transducer mounted on its tip. A wire is placed in the coronary artery of interest distal to the lesion and phasic spectral blood flow velocity is measured. It is assumed that there are minimal changes in coronary diameter, thus enabling velocity to be used in place of flow (flow = velocity × area). Measurements of blood velocity under basal conditions are taken, and then the patient is given a hyperemic stimulus (generally adenosine), velocity is remeasured, and CFR is calculated.

Although the Doppler wire has great theoretical advantages, it is not widely used because of several important limitations. First, conditions other than atherosclerosis can affect CFR. These include factors that raise basal coronary blood flow (e.g., fever, hypoxia, tachycardia, anemia, or ventricular hypertrophy) and factors that impair vasodilatory responses of the microvasculature (e.g., ventricular hypertrophy or diabetes mellitus). Second, accurate measurements are dependent upon correct positioning of the Doppler flow wire. The transducer should be pointing away from the vessel wall and into the flow stream to avoid vessel wall artifacts. Gray-scale signal amplitude and peak velocity can be used as indicators of proper positioning. Third, there is a lack of consensus on what value of CFR is consistent with a hemodynamically significant lesion. In various clinical studies, CFR cutoff values between 1.6 and 2.5 were used to determine ischemia-causing lesions.

Because CFR cannot discriminate between epicardial lesions and microvascular dysfunction, the concept of "relative CFR" (rCFR) was developed. This approach requires that CFR be measured in a coronary artery without epicardial disease to interpret the value of CFR in an artery with epicardial disease. If CFR is abnormal in the artery without disease, this result implies an impaired microvasculature. The use of rCFR has several caveats, including the requirement for a vessel without

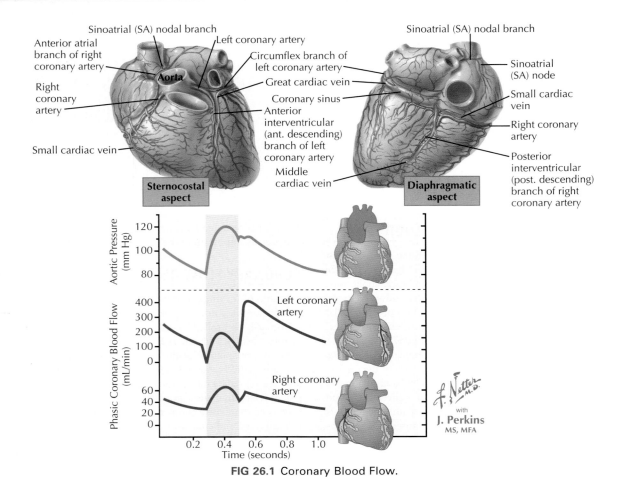

FIG 26.1 Coronary Blood Flow.

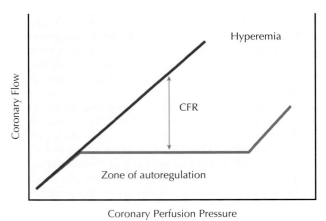

FIG 26.2 Coronary Flow Reserve (CFR).

significant epicardial disease and the assumption that microvasculature function is consistent across different vascular beds (an obvious problem in cases of previous myocardial infarction [MI]).

FRACTIONAL FLOW RESERVE

The basic principle of fractional flow reserve (FFR) is that when resistance is constant, changes in pressure are proportional to changes in

flow. The concept of using the pressure gradient as a technique to assess stenosis severity has existed since the early days of endovascular intervention. It is of historical interest that the original description of percutaneous transluminal coronary angioplasty by Gruentzig reported a decrease in translesional pressure gradients from 58 to 19 mm Hg in the 32 patients in whom percutaneous transluminal coronary angioplasty was successful. Early attempts to measure pressures distal to a stenosis were hampered by the use of fluid-filled tubes, which, because of their size, increased the translesional gradient. The advent of a pressure transducer mounted on a 0.014-inch angioplasty wire overcame these difficulties and enabled the introduction of the concept of pressure-derived FFR.

The concept of pressure as a surrogate for flow requires review of Ohm's law: flow = pressure/resistance. From a theoretical standpoint, several assumptions have to be made to simplify the equations from

$$FFR = \frac{(P_d - P_v)/R_{min}}{(P_a - P_v)/R_{min}}$$

to

$$FFR = \frac{P_d}{P_a}$$

but if those assumptions are met, FFR correlates with maximum myocardial blood flow in the presence of a stenosis divided by the theoretical maximum flow in a normal vessel (i.e., the absence of any stenosis).

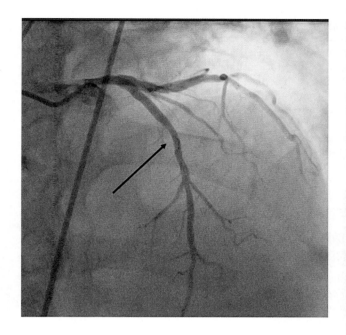

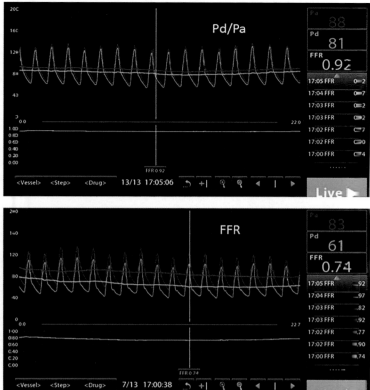

FIG 26.3 Clinical Use of Fractional Flow Reserve (FFR). Coronary angiography was obtained in the left anterior descending coronary artery of a 57-year-old man with chest pain. There was diffuse disease in the left anterior descending artery with Pa/Pd = 0.92. FFR was obtained with intravenous administration of adenosine with Pa/Pd = 0.74. Wire pullback showed that most of the pressure drop was in the mid-portion of the left anterior descending artery at the site demarcated by the arrow.

Under maximum arteriolar vasodilatation, the resistance imposed by the normal myocardial bed is minimal, and blood flow is proportional to driving pressure. Thus, FFR represents that fraction of normal maximum flow that is achievable in the presence of epicardial coronary stenosis. This index is independent of heart rate, systemic blood pressure, or myocardial contractility. The measurement and clinical use of FFR depends on two important assumptions: maximal hyperemia in the target vessel has been obtained, and there is negligible coronary venous pressure. In practical terms, FFR is obtained by simultaneously measuring the mean aortic pressure (from the distal tip of a coronary catheter) and coronary pressure distal to a stenosis (from the pressure transducer of the guidewire distal to a lesion) at maximal hyperemia (Fig. 26.3).

Key Clinical Studies of Fractional Flow Reserve

Initial studies were performed to determine the appropriate threshold of FFR for identifying patients who would benefit from revascularization compared with FFR with noninvasive stress testing. Pijls et al. performed bicycle stress tests, thallium scintigraphy, and stress echocardiography in 45 consecutive patients with chest pain and moderate coronary stenosis. In the 21 patients with FFR <0.75, all had at least one stress test with a positive result. Using a cutoff of 0.75 for FFR produced a sensitivity of 88%, specificity of 100%, and accuracy of 93% in this population. Furthermore, after revascularization of patients with FFR <0.75, all of the positive stress test results reverted to normal. Subsequent studies (most noticeably, the Fractional Flow Reserve versus

Angiography for Multivessel Evaluation [FAME] studies) modified the FFR threshold to 0.80, which is used in clinical practice today.

FAME studied FFR versus angiography in determining lesions that needed revascularization in patients with multivessel CAD. In this study, 1005 patients with multivessel CAD were randomized to undergo percutaneous coronary intervention (PCI) guided by angiography or guided by FFR. Patients in the angiography group received drug-eluting stents in all significant lesions, whereas those in the FFR group received stents only if FFR was ≤0.80. The event rate at 1 year for the combined primary endpoint of death, nonfatal MI, and repeat revascularization was 13.3% in the angiography group versus 13.2% in the FFR-guided group (F = 0.02). There was also a significant reduction in the number of stents placed in the FFR group.

In FAME 2, PCI significantly reduced major adverse cardiovascular events compared with optimal medical therapy alone. Eight hundred eighty-eight patients with stable ischemic heart disease referred for PCI with at least one lesion with FFR ≤0.8 were randomized to PCI plus optimal medical therapy versus optimal medical therapy alone. The primary outcome of death, MI, or urgent revascularization occurred in 12.7% of patients in the medical therapy group and in only 4.3% of the PCI plus medical therapy group at 1 year (hazard ratio [HR]: 0.32 95% confidence interval [CI]: 0.19–0.53). It should be noted that the event rate was largely driven by the need for urgent revascularization.

Other scenarios in which FFR was shown to be useful include left main lesions, nonculprit lesions in the setting of acute coronary syndromes (ACSs), tandem lesions, and bifurcation lesions.

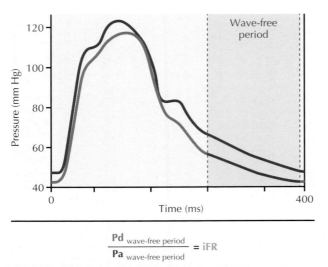

$$\frac{Pd_{\text{wave-free period}}}{Pa_{\text{wave-free period}}} = iFR$$

FIG 26.4 Instantaneous Wave-Free Ratio (iFR). (Image from Nijjer SS, Sen S, Petraco R, et al. Improvement in coronary haemodynamics after percutaneous coronary intervention: assessment using instantaneous wave-free ratio. *Heart* 2013;99:1740–1748.)

INSTANTANEOUS WAVE-FREE RATIO

The instantaneous wave-free ratio (iFR) is a measurement of the hemodynamic significance of a coronary artery stenosis that relies on comparison of pressures during diastole in the absence of hyperemia. It is measured during the wave-free period of mid to late diastole when flow during the cardiac cycle is the highest and the microcirculatory resistance is the lowest (Fig. 26.4). During this period, pressure and flow velocity are linearly related, allowing pressure ratios to be used to determine the limitation to flow of a lesion. Unlike FFR assessment, hyperemia (and thus adenosine) is not required.

The DEFINE-FLAIR and iFR-SWEDEHEART were two large studies (2492 and 2037 patients, respectively) in which patients with intermediate lesions were randomized to the use of FFR or iFR to determine hemodynamic significance. Most patients had stable angina, but patients with ACS could also be enrolled if flow reserve measurement was used to assess hemodynamic significance of nonculprit lesions. For FFR, hyperemia was induced with either intracoronary or intravenous adenosine. Revascularization was performed only if iFR was ≤0.89 or if FFR was ≤0.80. The primary endpoint in both studies was the rate of a composite of death from any cause, nonfatal MI, or unplanned revascularization within 12 months after the procedure. In the DEFINE-FLAIR study, the primary endpoint occurred in 78 of 1148 patients (6.8%) in the iFR group and in 83 of 1182 patients (7.0%) in the FFR group ($P = 0.78$). In iFR-SWEDEHEART, the primary endpoint event occurred in 68 of 1012 patients (6.7%) in the iFR group and in 61 of 1007 (6.1%) in the FFR group ($P = 0.53$). The rate at which PCI was performed was lower in the iFR group in both studies. The conclusion from both studies was that an iFR-guided revascularization strategy was noninferior to an FFR-guided revascularization strategy with respect to the rate of major adverse cardiac events at 12 months among patients with stable angina or ACS.

COMPUTED TOMOGRAPHY–FRACTIONAL FLOW RESERVE

Techniques with computational fluid dynamics have been developed to measure lesion-specific FFR from coronary CT angiography (CCTA).

These techniques involve creating three-dimensional models of pressure and flow within the aortic root and epicardial arteries with the equations by Navier-Stokes both at rest and during simulated maximal hyperemia. CT-FFR is based on three underlying assumptions: (1) coronary flow at rest is proportional to myocardial mass; (2) resistance of the microcirculation at rest is inversely but not linearly proportional to vessel size; and (3) the microcirculation reacts predictably to maximal hyperemia in patients with normal coronary flow. No additional radiation or intravenous contrast is necessary for FFR-CT, although high-quality CCTA is necessary, and the images must be free of artefacts. Small studies have shown that CT-FFR improves the diagnostic accuracy of CCTA. However, FFR-CT is time-consuming, available in only select centers, and is applicable to a limited population. In one study, even after excluding patients with high body mass indexes, atrial fibrillation, and who underwent previous PCI or coronary artery bypass graft procedures, CT-FFR could not be calculated in 13% of patients due to insufficient image quality.

LIMITATIONS OF FRACTIONAL FLOW RESERVE AND INSTANTANEOUS WAVE-FREE RATIO

From a theoretical standpoint, several assumptions have to be made to derive the equations for FFR and iFR, including that venous pressure and resistance are negligible. It is important also to remember that FFR has a continuous and independent relationship with clinical outcomes rather than a defined threshold value. Basing clinical decisions that use a continuous biological variable, such as iFR or FFR, in a dichotomous manner (i.e., above a threshold vs. below a threshold) introduces a rigidity that can negatively affect patient care. Evidence of this has been provided by studies that showed a gradient in major adverse outcomes in patients with FFR >0.80. Lastly, FFR and iFR do not measure microvasculature function. Microvasculature dysfunction can contribute to myocardial ischemia and has been reported in patients with previous MI and CAD risk factors.

EVIDENCE

Davies JE, Sen S, Dehbi H-M, et al. Use of the instantaneous wave-free ratio or fractional flow reserve in PCI. *N Engl J Med.* 2017;doi:10.1056/NEJMoa1700445.

The DEFINE-FLAIR was a study of 2492 patients randomized to FFR versus iFR. Results showed that coronary revascularization guided by iFR was noninferior to revascularization guided by FFR with respect to the risk of major adverse cardiac events at 1 year. Unfortunately, there were no data on symptom relief.

De Bruyne B, et al. Fractional flow reserve–guided PCI for stable coronary artery disease. *N Engl J Med.* 2014;371(13):1208–1217.

The FAME 2 study randomized 888 patients with stable, multivessel CAD with at least one lesion with an FFR <0.8 to either FFR-guided PCI with drug-eluting stents plus optimal medical therapy (OMT) or to OMT alone. Patients with FFR >0.8 were entered into a registry, prescribed OMT, and followed. The study was prematurely stopped after an interim analysis revealed a statistically significant decrease in unplanned hospitalization, which led to urgent revascularization in the FFR-PCI arm (1.6% vs. 11.1%; hazard ratio, 0.13; 95% CI, 0.06–0.30; P <0.001).

Götberg M, Christiansen EH, Gudmundsdottir IJ, et al. Instantaneous wave-free ratio versus fractional flow reserve to guide PCI. *N Engl J Med.* 2017;doi:10.1056/NEJMoa1616540.

Two large, randomized studies that compared the use of FFR to iFR in clinical decision making.

Gruentzig AR, Senning A, Siegenthaler WE. Non-operative dilation of coronary artery stenosis. *N Engl J Med.* 1979;301:61–68.

The original description of balloon angioplasty in which pressure gradients across a coronary stenosis were measured before and after dilation.

Johnson NP, Toth GG, Lai D, et al. Prognostic value of fractional flow reserve: linking physiologic severity to clinical outcomes. *J Am Coll Cardiol.* 2014;64:1641–1654.

Two retrospective studies that showed that FFR between 0.81 and 0.85 was associated with a higher event rate than FFR >0.85.

Masrani Mehta S, Depta JP, Novak E, et al. Association of lower fractional flow reserve values with higher risk of adverse cardiac events for lesions deferred revascularization among patients with acute coronary syndrome. *J Am Heart Assoc.* 2015;4(8):e002172. doi:10.1161/JAHA.115.002172.

In a study population of 674 patients (816 lesions) in whom revascularization was deferred based on FFR values >0.80, lower FFR values among ACS patients with coronary lesions deferred revascularization based on FFR were associated with a significantly higher rate of adverse cardiac events, whereas this association was not observed in non-ACS patients.

Pijls NH, De Bruyne B, Peels K, et al. Measurement of fractional flow reserve to assess the functional severity of coronary-artery stenoses. *N Engl J Med.* 1996;334:1703–1708.

One of the early descriptions of FFR in which it was correlated with noninvasive stress testing.

Pijls NH, van Schaardenburgh P, Manoharan G, et al. Percutaneous coronary intervention of functionally nonsignificant stenosis: 5-year follow-up of the DEFER Study. *J Am Coll Cardiol.* 2007;49:2105–2111.

The DEFER study randomized 325 patients with stable, single-vessel coronary artery disease without evidence of documented ischemia to either undergo PCI or to defer PCI. Subjects were allocated to three study groups: "defer" (no PCI, FFR ≥0.75), "reference" (PCI performed, FFR <0.75), and "perform" (PCI performed, FFR ≥0.75). The 5-year outcome of cardiac death or acute MI occurred at a rate of 3.3% in the defer group, 7.9% in the perform group, and 15.7% in the reference group.

Tonino PA, De Bruyne B, Pijls NH, et al. Fractional flow reserve versus angiography for guiding percutaneous coronary intervention. *N Engl J Med.* 2009;360:213–224.

The FAME study randomized 1005 patients with stable multivessel CAD to angiography versus an FFR-guided strategy for PCI. The primary endpoint of major adverse cardiac events (including death, MI, repeat revascularization) occurred in 91 patients (18.3%) in the angiography group and in 67 patients (13.2%) in the FFR-guided group (relative risk: 0.72; 95% CI: 0.54–0.96; P = 0.02).

Myocardial Diseases and Cardiomyopathy

27

Epidemiology of Heart Failure: Heart Failure With Preserved Ejection Fraction and Heart Failure With Reduced Ejection Fraction

Adam W. Caldwell, Patricia P. Chang

Over the last few decades, heart failure (HF) has emerged as a true epidemic, with an estimated global prevalence of 38 million patients. HF affects 6.5 million American adults, with nearly 1 million new cases annually. HF can be due to multiple different etiologies, and there are numerous identifiable risk factors. HF is the most common cause of hospitalization for patients 65 years and older in high-income countries. The prevalence and incidence of HF in middle- and low-income countries is increasing, leading to rising costs and the global burden of HF.

DEFINITIONS

The American Heart Association/American College of Cardiology Foundation (AHA/ACCF) define HF as a "complex clinical syndrome that results from any structural or functional impairment of ventricular filling or ejection of blood," with a variety of symptoms, including dyspnea, edema, malaise, and decreased exercise tolerance. Cardiomyopathies are a group of diseases that affect the myocardium and frequently lead to HF, but should not be used interchangeably with the term HF. The term congestive heart failure is no longer preferred because patients may present with a variety of symptoms and not strictly volume overload.

HF can be divided into two broad categories: HF with reduced ejection fraction (HFrEF) and HF with preserved ejection fraction (HFpEF). This terminology supplants the terms systolic HF and diastolic HF, respectively. In the past, there have been multiple different definitions and variable left ventricular ejection fraction (LVEF) cutoffs used in clinical trials and guidelines for HFrEF ($\leq$35%, <40%, and $\leq$40%) and HFpEF (>40%, >45%, >50%, and $\geq$55%). The most recent consensus guidelines from the ACC, AHA, Heart Failure Society of America (HFSA), and separate guidelines from the European Society of Cardiology (ESC) have attempted to provide some uniformity. Both groups define HFrEF as a LVEF of $\leq$40% and HFpEF as a LVEF of $\geq$50%. Per the ACC/AHA/HFSA guidelines, a LVEF of 41% to 49% is borderline HFpEF, considered similar in many respects to patients with HFpEF. Patients with previously diagnosed HFrEF who have recovered to a LVEF of >40% are categorized as improved HFpEF and represent a group that has not been well studied.

According to nomenclature from the ESC, HF with a LVEF of 40% to 49% is termed HF with mid-range EF (HFmrEF). To meet the ESC definitions of the HFpEF or HFmrEF, patients must have elevated natriuretic peptide levels in addition to HF symptoms and either relevant structural heart disease or diastolic dysfunction.

HF is further classified based on either symptoms or stages (Table 27.1). The frequently used New York Heart Association functional classification system divides HF into four classes based on symptoms. The ACC/AHA system has four distinct stages that incorporate risk factors, structural heart disease, and symptoms. The ACC/AHA stages were devised to identify patients at risk for HF to help guide preventative measures. To prevent progression of HF, interventions are aimed at modifying risk factors for stage A and treating structural heart disease for stage B. Once the patient becomes symptomatic and progresses to stages C and/or D, therapies are aimed at reducing morbidity and mortality.

CAUSES OF HEART FAILURE

There are multiple etiologies for HF, but a large proportion is secondary to ischemic heart disease. The prevalence of coronary artery disease (CAD) in new HF cases has been estimated to be as high as 68%. HF secondary to CAD is frequently referred to as ischemic cardiomyopathy, which results from compromised circulation of approximately two-thirds of the coronary blood supply. The nonischemic cardiomyopathy label represents all the other diverse etiologies of HF (Box 27.1).

PREVALENCE

The prevalence of HF in the United States is estimated at 6.5 million American adults based on National Health and Nutrition Examination Survey (NHANES) data from 2011 to 2014. Despite many advances in the care of patients with cardiovascular disease and increased awareness of risk factors, it is estimated that HF prevalence will increase by 46% from 2012 to 2030, to >8 million Americans with HF. This prediction is largely due to an aging population and the increased burden of HF in older adults because HF prevalence increases with age. For example, between 2011 and 2014, the prevalence of HF in men was 0.3%, 1.4%, 6.2%, and 14.1% at ages 20 to 39, 40 to 59, 60 to 79, and 80+ years, respectively. Prevalence rates were similar in woman, increasing from 0.5% at age 20 to 39 years to 13.4% for age 80+ years. Overall, HF prevalence is similar between the sexes, affecting 2.3% of men and 2.6% of women in 2012. Over the past decade in the United States, prevalence continues to rise despite the incidence of HF leveling off (Fig. 27.1

The prevalence of HFpEF is also increasing. Among the Get With the Guidelines-Heart Failure Registry patients, 49.8% had HFrEF, 13.7% had borderline HFpEF, and 36.5% had HFpEF between 2005 and 2010. The proportion of patients hospitalized for HFpEF exacerbations increased from 33% to 39% over this time, whereas the proportion of HFrEF hospitalizations decreased.

INCIDENCE

The incidence of HF has been estimated from multiple population studies and also increases with age. Between 2005 and 2013, there were

TABLE 27.1   Comparison of the ACC/AHA Stages of HF and the NYHA Functional Classification of HF

ACC/AHA Stage	Corresponding NYHA Functional Class	Examples	Therapies
A. At risk for HF, with no symptoms or evidence of structural heart disease	None	Hypertension, diabetes, family history of HF, cardiotoxic medication use, alcohol use	Modifying risk factors for HF
B. Structural heart disease, but no HF symptoms	I: Asymptomatic	Left ventricular hypertrophy, previous myocardial infarction, dilated left ventricle, valvular heart disease	Treating structural heart disease
C. Structural heart disease with previous or current HF symptoms	II: Symptomatic with moderate exertion III: Symptomatic with minimal exertion IV: Symptoms at rest	HF symptoms at rest or with exertion, patients undergoing treatment for current or previous HF symptoms	Evidence-based HF medications, diuretics
D. Refractory HF, needing specialized interventions	IV: Symptoms at rest	Patients with frequent hospitalizations, requiring advanced HF therapies	Evidence-based HF medications, diuretics, inotropic, or mechanical support, transplantation evaluation, hospice

ACC/AHA, American College of Cardiology/American Heart Association; *HF,* heart failure; *NYHA,* New York Heart Association.
Data from Hunt SA, Abraham WT, Chin MH, et al. ACC/AHA 2005 guideline update for the diagnosis and management of chronic heart failure in the adult: a report of the American College of Cardiology/American Heart Association Task Force on Practice Guidelines (Writing Committee to Update the 2001 Guidelines for the Evaluation and Management of Heart Failure): developed in collaboration with the American College of Chest Physicians and the International Society for Heart and Lung Transplantation: endorsed by the Heart Rhythm Society. *Circulation.* 2005;112(12):e154–e235; Yancy CW, Jessup M, Bozkurt B, et al. 2013 ACCF/AHA guideline for the management of heart failure: a report of the American College of Cardiology Foundation/American Heart Association Task Force on practice guidelines. *Circulation.* 2013;128(16):e240–e327; Dolgin M, Fox AC, Gorlin R, Levin RI, New York Heart Association. Criteria Committee. Nomenclature and criteria for diagnosis of diseases of the heart and great vessels. 9th ed. Boston: Lippincott, Williams, and Wilkins; 1994; and Criteria Committee, New York Heart Association. Diseases of the heart and blood vessels. Nomenclature and criteria for diagnosis. 6th ed. Boston: Little, Brown, and Co.; 1964:114.

BOX 27.1   Major Etiologies of Heart Failure

Ischemic heart disease
Hypertensive heart disease
Valvular disease
Congenital heart disease
Dilated cardiomyopathy: idiopathic or familial
Genetic: hypertrophic cardiomyopathy, arrhythmogenic right ventricular cardiomyopathy, left ventricular noncompaction, myopathies, ion-channel disorders
Endocrine/metabolic: obesity, diabetes, thyroid disease
Toxic: alcoholic, cocaine-induced, drug/chemotherapy, nutritional deficiencies
Tachycardia-induced
Inflammatory/infectious: HIV, Chagas disease, viral, myocarditis, rheumatological/connective tissue disease, hypersensitivity myocarditis
Infiltrative: amyloidosis, sarcoidosis, hemochromatosis
Stress-induced (Takotsubo) cardiomyopathy
Peripartum cardiomyopathy

960,000 new HF cases annually based on community surveillance in the Atherosclerosis Risk In Communities (ARIC) study. The incidence rate was approximately 5 cases per 1000 person-years in men and 3 cases per 1000 person-years in women in the Framingham Heart Study (FHS), from 1950 to 1999. Older adults have a higher rate, at nearly 10 cases per 1000 people after age 65 years. The lifetime risk of HF is 20% for people older than 40 years, and is higher among those with hypertension or obesity compared with those without HF. In an older adult cohort from the Health, Aging, and Body Composition (Health

ABC) Study, in patients aged 70 to 79 years in the late 1990s and early 2000s, the incidence of HF was 13.6 cases per 1000 person-years over 7 years. Incidence was not different between sexes for this older adult population, whereas earlier estimates from 1980 to 2003 in the FHS showed that HF incidence doubled in men every 10 years from age 65 to 85 years and tripled for women between ages 65 to 74 and 75 to 84 years. Incidence rates were even higher in those aged 75 years or older based on data from Kaiser Permanente from 2000 to 2005 (52.4 cases per 1000 person-years in men and 47.9 per 1000 person-years in women).

Race also affects HF incidence, with several studies showing that black patients are more likely to develop HF, especially in young adulthood and middle age. In the Coronary Artery Risk Development in Young Adults (CARDIA) study, HF at younger than 50 years was more common among blacks than whites. In the ARIC cohort study, the age-adjusted incidence of HF between 1987 and 2002 was highest for black men (9.1 per 1000 person-years), followed by black women (8.1 per 1000 person-years), then white men (6.0 per 1000 person-years), and lowest for white women (3.4 per 1000 person-years). Annual incidence rates for acute decompensated HF showed a similar trend in the ARIC study communities between 2005 and 2009. Although the rates of acute decompensated HF secondary to HFrEF and HFpEF were similar (53% and 47%, respectively), black men had more HFrEF events (70%). Racial differences in acute decompensated HF incidence diminished with increasing age in the ARIC study. The Multi-Ethnic Study of Atherosclerosis (MESA) also showed that African Americans had the highest incidence rate of HF (4.6 per 1000 person-years), followed by Hispanics (3.5 per 1000 person-years), whites (2.4 per 1000 person-years), and Chinese Americans (1.0 per 1000 person-years). The higher incidence of HF in African Americans was secondary to an increased prevalence of diabetes, hypertension, and socioeconomic factors.

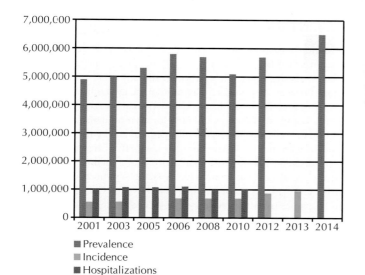

FIG 27.1 Heart Failure Prevalence, Incidence, and Hospitalizations in the United States. Based on data from Heart Disease and Stroke Statistics: 2003, 2006, 2008, 2010, 2013, 2014, 2015, 2016, 2017 updates (from the journal *Circulation*). Prevalence estimates are based on the National Health and Nutrition Examination Survey (NHANES) of adults aged 20 years or older. Incidence estimates of HF from 2001 through 2012 are from NHANES (aged 20 years or older); the 2013 estimate is from the Atherosclerosis Risk In Communities Study (aged 55 years or older). Hospitalization estimates are from the National Hospital Discharge Survey/National Center for Health Statistics and the National Heart, Lung, and Blood Institute (all ages).

Over time, the burden of HF secondary to HFpEF has become more evident. Approximately 55% of patients in Olmsted County, Minnesota, who had incident or prevalent HF had HFpEF based on echocardiography. Between 2005 and 2009 in the ARIC communities, white women had the highest proportion of acute decompensated HFpEF events (54.4%), followed by black women (43.2%), then white men (33.0%), and black men (25.9%).

Over the past two decades, the incidence of HF might have decreased. In Olmsted County, the age- and sex-adjusted incidence decreased from 315.8 per 100,000 in 2000 to 219.3 per 100,000 in 2010, which equaled a reduction of 37.5% over the decade. Both HFrEF and HFpEF showed decreased incidence over this time, but it was greater for HFrEF (−45.1% compared with −27.9%), which was likely due to better treatment of ischemic heart disease and myocardial infarction. Women also had a greater decline in HF incidence compared with men (−43% vs. −29%).

MORTALITY

Despite many advances in HF therapy over the last several decades, mortality remains extremely high. One in eight deaths in the United States has HF listed on the death certificate. Thirty-day, 1-year, and 5-year mortality rates after hospitalization for HF were high, at 10.4%, 22%, and 42.3%, respectively, in the ARIC study. The FHS showed that HF survival increased for both men and women over four decades, from 1950 to 1999; however, a patient diagnosed with HF in the 1990s still had a mortality of >50% at 5 years. Olmsted County showed similar results between 1979 and 2000, with 5-year adjusted survival improving from 43% to 52%. Despite the nominal improvements in survival, most of the survival gains were in men and younger patients, with little or no improvement in women and older patients. In Olmsted County between 1987 and 2001, survival was slightly better for those with HFpEF compared with those with HFrEF (29% vs. 32% at 1 year; 65% vs. 68% at 5 years). In addition, the survival rate for HFpEF did not change significantly over the study period, whereas HFrEF showed increased survival. In the older adult cohort of the Health ABC Study, those with HF had a significantly increased annual mortality (18%) versus the standard annual mortality (2.7%).

Mortality for hospitalized patients has improved. For Medicare patients in the 2000s, in-hospital morality decreased by 38%, 30-day mortality decreased by 16.4%, and 1-year mortality decreased by 13%. However, there may be racial differences according to the ARIC Study, with African Americans having significantly increased fatality compared with Caucasians, 5 years after a HF hospitalization.

RISK FACTORS

There are multiple risk factors for HF, including many of the traditional risk factors for heart disease. The NHANES follow-up study found that CAD carried a 62% population attributable risk (PAR), which was the highest among the examined risk factors, followed by cigarette use (17% PAR) and hypertension (10% PAR). Male sex, low physical activity, obesity, lack of high school education, and diabetes also carried increased risk for HF. The FHS identified hypertension as a major contributor to the development of HF, together with CAD. Follow-up studies with updated hypertension definitions have suggested that the PAR for HF from hypertension could be as high as 40% in men and 60% in women. In the FHS, >75% of patients diagnosed with HF had underlying hypertension, and the lifetime risk of HF was double for hypertensive patients. In Olmsted County from 1979 to 2002, hypertension was the most common risk factor for HF (66% of patients) followed by smoking (51%). Over this period, the PAR for hypertension increased from 15% to 29%. The PAR for obesity also more than doubled, from 8% to 17%, but the PARs for CAD, smoking, and diabetes did not change. Conversely, modifiable risk factors, including normal body weight, nonsmoking, exercise, moderate alcohol intake, and consumption of breakfast cereal and fruits and/or vegetables, were associated with decreased lifetime risk of HF in the Physicians Health Study.

Many biomarkers have also been identified as independent risk factors for HF, such as B-type natriuretic peptide (BNP), urine albumin/creatinine ratio, elevated serum γ-glutamyl transferase, increased hematocrit, white blood cell count, C-reactive protein, and troponin, as shown in the FHS and ARIC studies. N-terminal pro-BNP provides additional prognostic information based on the MESA study.

Risk factors for HFpEF can be similar to but are often distinct from risk factors for HFrEF. Older age, diabetes, and valvular disease were risk factors for both HFpEF and HFrEF in the Framingham cohort. Higher body mass index, smoking, and atrial fibrillation were predictors of HFpEF. In Olmsted County, HFpEF was associated with older age, female sex, and no history of myocardial infarction. HFpEF was also more likely in those with a history of hypertension, atrial fibrillation, and kidney disease. Laboratory values, including pro-BNP and troponin also tended to be lower.

HOSPITALIZATIONS AND COSTS

HF is the most common hospital admission diagnosis for patients older than 65 years, and there were >1 million hospital discharges for HF in 2010 alone. HF hospitalizations have steadily climbed over the last few decades, and most hospitalizations occur in patients older than 65 years. In Olmsted County, 83.1% of 1077 patients with HF were hospitalized at least once, and 43% were hospitalized at least 4 times. HF accounted for 16.5% of admissions, whereas 61.9% of hospitalizations were due to noncardiac causes. Hospitalization rates were similar for HFpEF and HFrEF. In addition to hospitalizations, there were an estimated 1.77 million physician office visits for HF in 2010 and >550,000 emergency room visits for HF in 2011.

Because of the high prevalence, incidence, and hospitalization rates for HF, the associated healthcare costs are also high. The elevated incidence of HF hospitalizations in the older adult population puts increased strain on Medicare/Medicaid. The AHA estimated the overall cost for HF in 2012 was $30.7 billion, with more than two-thirds of this amount due to direct medical costs. The cost for HF is projected to grow to almost $70 billion by 2030, increasing by nearly 127%.

GLOBAL BURDEN

The estimated 38 million HF patients worldwide is likely an underestimate because it does not include patients with asymptomatic disease. Until recently, the true global prevalence and incidence of HF was difficult to ascertain because most epidemiological studies were conducted in developed nations. With ischemic heart disease as the leading cause of death worldwide at 15.7% of age-standardized deaths, more attention has been focused on better identifying the burden of heart disease and HF in middle- and low-income nations. For men, HF prevalence is highest in North America, Oceania, and Eastern Europe. Women have the highest prevalence in Oceania, North America, and North Africa/Middle East. HF prevalence was lowest for both men and women in sub-Saharan Africa, but the prevalence is rising, with almost one-half of patients with newly diagnosed cardiovascular disease having HF.

Risk factors for HF vary by region and socioeconomic status as noted by the Global Burden of Disease Study. Ischemic heart disease is most prevalent in Europe and North America but rare in sub-Saharan Africa. In developing nations, hypertension, rheumatic heart disease, cardiomyopathy, and myocarditis contribute a large proportion of HF cases. Although it is uncommon in developed nations, rheumatic heart disease occurs more frequently in South Asia and sub-Saharan Africa, with 470,000 new cases per year worldwide. Chagas disease remains a major etiology of HF in South America, with 40% of patients with this disease developing DL. South American patients are less likely to have CAD, chronic obstructive pulmonary disease, and diabetes compared with North American patients. HF secondary to cardiomyopathies, including HIV-related cardiomyopathy, idiopathic-dilated cardiomyopathy, peripartum cardiomyopathy, and endomyocardial fibrosis are common in sub-Saharan Africa. Uncorrected congenital heart disease also likely leads to many HF cases in lower income countries.

HF contributes to a growing proportion of global health expenditures. In African hospitals, HF is the most frequent diagnosis for patients admitted with heart disease. HF patients are also more likely to be younger in Africa compared with Western nations (age 52 years vs. 70–72 years). South American and Asian countries show similar trends. Earlier onset of HF can contribute to high economic and social costs when patients are unable to work or act as caregivers.

There is still much to be learned about the epidemiology of HF globally. Many regions and populations, including minorities and women in developing nations are underrepresented in these studies. The impact of ethnic differences on HF are not fully understood. The diagnosis of HFpEF is absent in many of the currently available studies because most were conducted before the recent focus on this subtype. Additional research in developing nations may enable better identification of preventative measures for HF.

PREVENTION

Prevention measures for HF (ACC/AHA stage A) largely consist of aggressively treating risk factors for HF, including hypertension, CAD, diabetes, obesity, metabolic syndrome, and any other modifiable risk factors. Prevalence estimates for asymptomatic LV dysfunction, or stage B patients, vary. For example, prevalence estimates were 5% for asymptomatic systolic dysfunction and 36% for asymptomatic diastolic dysfunction in the FHS. The severity of asymptomatic LV dysfunction also correlates with the risk of developing incident HF, with systolic dysfunction associated with more risk than diastolic dysfunction. In the MESA trial, the prevalence of asymptomatic LV systolic dysfunction was highest in African Americans (2.6%) compared with whites, Chinese Americans, and Hispanics (overall prevalence 1.7%). Early recognition and treatment of patients with asymptomatic LV dysfunction, particularly those with a history of myocardial infarction or systolic LV dysfunction, will be critical to decrease the prevalence of HF in the future.

FUTURE DIRECTIONS

HF remains a growing problem with increasing prevalence in the United States and worldwide. In developed nations, an aging population will continue to burden the healthcare system with HF patients. Traditional risk factors for HF are becoming more prevalent in developing nations, which will likely cause further increases in global HF incidence. With high healthcare use, the economic burden of HF is staggeringly high. Although there has been some mortality improvement with evidence-based HF therapies, overall mortality remains high, and there are no therapies that decrease mortality in HFpEF. Aggressive measures targeting preventable risk factors for patients with asymptomatic disease, in addition to novel therapies to improve mortality for symptomatic patients, particularly for HFpEF, are desperately needed.

ADDITIONAL RESOURCES

American Heart Association. Heart and Stroke Statistics. https://www .heart.org/HEARTORG/General/Heart-and-Stroke-Association-Statistics _UCM_319064_SubHomePage.jsp.
The American Heart Association website for current heart and stroke statistics.
Sliwa K, Stewart S. Heart failure in the developing world. In: Mann DL, Felker GM, eds. *Heart Failure: A Companion to Braunwald's Heart Disease.* 3rd ed. Philadelphia, PA: Elsevier; 2015.
A comprehensive overview of HF epidemiology in developing nations.

EVIDENCE

Benjamin EJ, Blaha MJ, Chiuve ST, et al. Heart disease and stroke statistics – 2017 update: a report from the American Heart Association. *Circulation.* 2017;135(10):e146–e603.
The most recent statistics about HF and other cardiovascular diseases, compiled by the AHA, in conjunction with the Centers for Disease Control and Prevention, the National Institutes of Health, and other government agencies.
Heidenreich PA, Albert NM, Allen LA, et al. Forecasting the impact of heart failure in the United States: a policy statement from the American Heart Association. *Circ Heart Fail.* 2013;6(3):606–619.
Statement that estimates the future prevalence and burden of HF in the United States.
Yancy CW, Jessup M, Bozkurt B, et al. 2013 ACCF/AHA guideline for the management of heart failure: a report of the American College of Cardiology Foundation/American Heart Association Task Force on practice guidelines. *Circulation.* 2013;128(16):e240–e327.
The most recent HF guidelines and definitions from the ACC and AHA.

28

Management of Acute Heart Failure

Olivia N. Gilbert, Jason N. Katz

DEFINITIONS AND EPIDEMIOLOGY

The term acute decompensated heart failure (ADHF) encompasses an array of disease processes related to inefficient cardiac function with compromised hemodynamics and/or volume status. Although ADHF has historically been treated on an inpatient basis, there are increasing trends to intervene on an outpatient basis. Accordingly, admissions for HF have decreased over time. One study that examined epidemiological trends of HF found an approximate 27% reduction in HF admission rates from 2001 to 2009 in the United States. These trends are also true internationally due to improved risk factor control (e.g., hypertension and ischemic heart disease) and implementation of guideline-directed medical therapies.

Despite reductions in ADHF-related hospitalizations, HF-related costs are increasing. In 2013, the American Heart Association released a policy statement "Forecasting the Impact of Heart Failure in the United States" that estimated HF-related expenditures to be $31 billion and predicted doubling of that amount by 2030, mostly related to hospitalizations. Because HF increases with age, affecting up to 10% of those aged older than 65 years, this is particularly relevant to the Medicare population. Accordingly, ADHF is the most common reason for hospitalization in this group and consumes more Medicare dollars than any other diagnosis.

ETIOLOGY AND PATHOGENESIS

Heart failure hospitalizations can be broadly divided into one-half being caused by HF with a preserved left ventricular ejection fraction (HFpEF) of ≥40% and one-half being caused by HF with a reduced left ventricular ejection fraction (HFrEF). Understanding the specific mechanism that contributed to the presentation of ADHF in an individual patient due to HFpEF or HFrEF is critical to guide therapy. Most patient hospitalizations can at least be partially attributed to a particular cause, including cardiac ischemia, tachycardia, uncontrolled hypertension, renal disease, respiratory disease, as well as medical and dietary nonadherence.

Initiation of negative inotropic medications (e.g., calcium channel blockers and β-blockers) and therapies that increase salt retention (e.g., steroids, nonsteroidal antiinflammatory drugs, and thiazolidinediones) also need to be considered as triggers for ADHF. Finally, substance abuse (e.g., alcohol, cocaine, and methamphetamines) should be considered as a cause for decompensation. Once reversible etiologies of ADHF are identified, it is hoped that their specific treatment will result in improvement of HF (e.g., reperfusion strategies in cardiac ischemia, antiarrhythmic medications for tachycardia, or education for pharmacological and dietary nonadherence).

Regarding the pathophysiology of HFrEF, reduction in inotropy results in a downward shift of the Frank-Starling curve, such that the same blood volume results in decreased cardiac output (Fig. 28.1). With decompensated HF, acute compensatory mechanisms include increased heart rate (by activation of the sympathetic nervous system) and increased blood volume (by activation of the renin-angiotensin-aldosterone system), which allows for similar stroke volume to be achieved (Fig. 28.2). Physiologically, this is accomplished through increased renal renin release, which acts to increase levels of angiotensin II. Angiotensin II then stimulates release of aldosterone from the adrenal cortex and antidiuretic hormone from the pituitary gland, both of which results in increased fluid retention.

CLINICAL PRESENTATION

Dyspnea is the most common symptom of ADHF. However, this is relatively nonspecific because there are numerous disorders that can cause this. Orthopnea is the most reliable in terms of ability to predict true volume overload. Although there are numerous physical examination findings common to HF, the third heart sound and jugular venous distention are the most specific for diagnosing HF, and increased jugular venous distention has been validated to correlate with elevated pulmonary capillary wedge pressure (PCWP).

DIAGNOSTIC APPROACH

The symptoms, physical examination, laboratory work, chest x-ray, and ECG of the patient are all essential to ADHF workup. In the acute setting, the main purpose of the ECG is to rule out reversible causes of HF presentations, such as ischemia, or differential diagnoses such as right HF or pericardial disease. All patients presenting with ADHF should have a chest x-ray to evaluate for cardiomegaly or pulmonary edema, as well as to exclude differential causes for the presentation of the patient. Echocardiography should be performed in all those presenting with a new diagnosis of ADHF and in those with an established diagnosis if there is a significant change in their clinical status.

If the patient has a permanent pacemaker or an implantable cardioverter-defibrillator, this should be interrogated by the cardiology team to exclude arrhythmias that could contribute to the presentation of the patient. This is particularly critical when an implantable cardioverter-defibrillator shock is involved. The CardioMEMS device (Abbott Laboratories, Abbott Park, Illinois) is also an increasingly relevant technology for evaluating those with ADHF; it is a small pressure sensor implanted directly into the pulmonary artery (PA) that can assess volume status. Using these technologies, patients can be increasingly monitored from home and receive intervention before development of ADHF. Those patients whose impedance or PA pressure measurements fail to respond to outpatient interventions may warrant hospitalization for more aggressive intervention, such as with intravenous diuretics or inotropes.

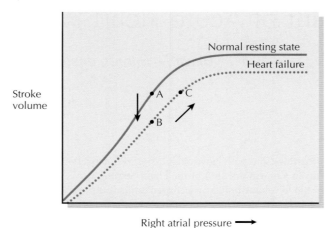

FIG 28.1 The Frank-Starling Curve Represents the Relationship Between Stroke Volume and Preload. As pertains to decompensated heart failure, decreased inotropy results in a downward shift in the curve, and a compensatory increase in blood volume results in an upward movement along the same curve to achieve a similar stroke volume of a normal heart.

MANAGEMENT

Triage

The decision to hospitalize a patient for ADHF and what level of care they warrant if hospitalized is a complex decision-making process. Shared variables of risk among registries include elevated heart rate, decreased systolic blood pressure, elevated blood urea nitrogen, elevated serum creatinine, and decreased serum sodium. Accordingly, clinicians may use these markers to aid in making decisions about whether it is appropriate to treat patients as inpatients or as outpatients. Extrapolating on this concept of risk stratification, algorithms have been created to help clinicians distinguish between true HF and similarly presenting entities. An example of one of these is the ProBNP Investigation of Dyspnea in the Emergency Department (PRIDE) Algorithm (Table 28.1 and Fig. 28.3).

Another classic diagnostic aid is to categorize patients based on volume status (wet or dry) to estimate intracardiac filling pressures and also by perfusion status (warm or cold) to estimate cardiac output. Indicators of poor perfusion include fatigue, impaired mentation, symptomatic hypotension, pulsus alternans, renal dysfunction, and cool extremities. As previously discussed, indicators of elevated congestion include complaints such as orthopnea and physical examination findings, such as increased jugular venous distention, third heart sound, and lower extremity swelling.

Based on these factors, each patient can be categorized into one of four categories: warm and dry, warm and wet, cold and dry, or cold and wet. According to this categorization, those who are warm and dry are in a well-compensated state and have the best survival outcomes.

Response to Decreased Blood Volume and Pressure

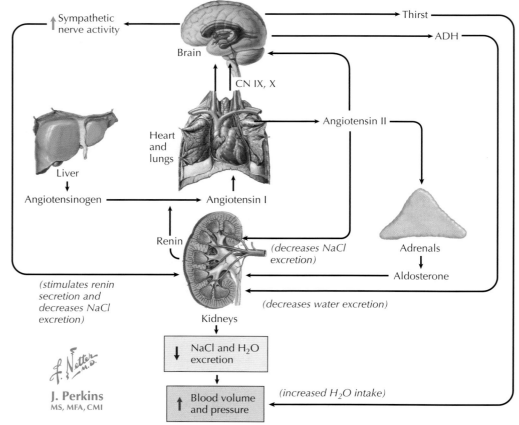

FIG 28.2 Compensatory Mechanisms in Decompensated Heart Failure. *ADH,* Antidiuretic hormone; H_2O, water; *NaCl,* sodium chloride.

TABLE 28.1 PRIDE Acute Congestive Heart Failure Score

Predictor	Points
Elevated NT-proBNP	4
Interstitial edema on chest x-ray	2
Orthopnea	2
Absence of fever	2
Current loop diuretic use	1
Age >75 yr	1
Rales on lung examination	1
Absence of cough	1

NT-proBNP, NT–pro-brain natriuretic peptide; *PRIDE*, ProBNP Investigation of Dyspnea in the Emergency Department.
A score of >7 has a high predictive accuracy for the diagnosis of acute congestive heart failure.
Reused with permission from Baggish AL, Cameron R, Anwaruddin S, et al. A clinical and biochemical critical pathway for the evaluation of patients with suspected acute congestive heart failure: the ProBNP Investigation of Dyspnea in the Emergency Department (PRIDE) algorithm. *Crit Pathw Cardiol* 2004;3:171–176.

Also, those who are wet (cold or warm) are at higher risk of death. If volume status is unclear in an individual based on laboratory work and physical examination, echocardiography can be helpful. Alternatively, placement of an invasive hemodynamic monitor with a PA catheter would be appropriate. Because most patients presenting with decompensated HF are in the warm and wet category, we focus our attention on that category.

Warm and Wet Patients With Hypertension

Preliminary treatment of warm and wet individuals with hypertension is vasodilatory therapy. Reduction of preload relieves pulmonary vascular congestion. Reduction of afterload improves cardiac output because there is less resistance to forward flow. Two agents that reduce both preload (venous flow) and afterload (arterial flow) are intravenous nitroglycerin and nitroprusside. Although nitroglycerin paste can be used, therapeutic benefits can be achieved more rapidly with intravenous administration.

Nitroglycerin is rarely associated with methemoglobinemia, and nitroprusside can result in cyanide toxicity, released as a byproduct. Because of this, nitroprusside is contraindicated in patients with impaired renal or hepatic function, both of which can affect cyanide clearance.

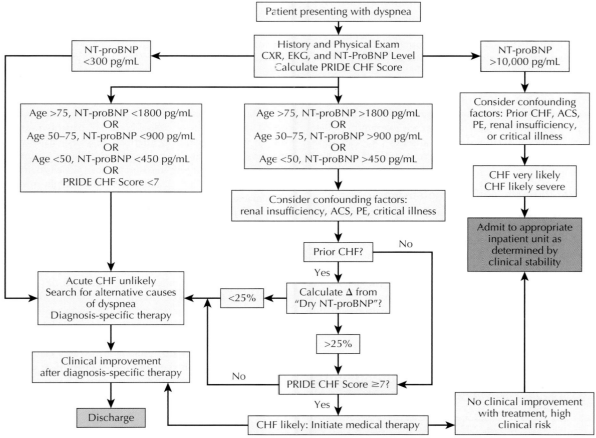

FIG 28.3 A Proposed Algorithm for NT–pro-Brain Natriuretic Peptide (NT-proBNP) and Clinically Guided Evaluation and Triage of Patients With Suspected Acute Congestive Heart Failure (CHF). *ACS*, Acute coronary syndrome; *CXR*, chest x-ray; *EKG*, electrocardiography; *PE*, pulmonary embolism; *PRIDE*, ProBNP Investigation of Dyspnea in the Emergency Department. (Reused with permission from Baggish AL, Cameron R, Anwaruddin S, et al. A clinical and biochemical critical pathway for the evaluation of patients with suspected acute congestive heart failure: the ProBNP Investigation of Dyspnea in the Emergency Department (PRIDE) algorithm. *Crit Pathw Cardiol* 2004;3:171–176.)

In addition, there is a risk of the coronary steal phenomenon with nitroprusside, in which blood flow favors more compliant blood vessels. Because of this, nitroprusside should be avoided in patients with ischemic heart disease. Finally, nesiritide, which is a synthetic B-type natriuretic peptide, has both vasodilatory and diuretic effects. However, avid support for its use has been hindered by concern of worsening renal function.

If evidence of volume overload remains, despite treatment of hypertension with vasodilatory therapy, diuretic therapy is indicated. However, this should be done thoughtfully because administration of furosemide has been shown to have vasoconstrictive effects that can decrease cardiac output by increasing arterial resistance to flow. Furthermore, as shown previously with our Frank-Starling curves, reduction in preload with less blood volume can result in a decrease in cardiac output.

The main class of diuretics used in decompensated HF are the loop diuretics, which prevent reabsorption of sodium in the loop of Henle. These include furosemide, torsemide, and bumetanide, which vary in terms of their bioavailability and pharmacodynamic potency (Table 28.2). Loop diuretic dosing should be the lowest possible to achieve the desired effect. If escalating doses of diuretic are required, particularly with ADHF, options include transitioning from bolus dosing to a continuous drip (for furosemide and bumetanide), switching to a more potent diuretic (from furosemide to torsemide or bumetanide), or changing to a different class of diuretic, such as a thiazide diuretic. Thiazide diuretics such as metolazone act downstream of the loop diuretics by blocking sodium reabsorption in the distal convoluted tubule (Fig. 28.4). To optimize the effects of furosemide (with a half-life of 2 hours), metolazone (with a half-life of 9 hours) is often administered before furosemide to maximize simultaneous blockade of the loop of Henle and the distal convoluted tubule.

Overall, by addressing mean arterial pressure with vasodilatory agents and central venous pressure (CVP) with diuretics, we are able to optimize organ perfusion pressure, which is defined as the difference between mean arterial pressure and CVP. This is particularly relevant to cardiac and renal function during ADHF, when elevation of CVP can affect cardiac and renal perfusion, which results in troponin and creatinine elevation, respectively.

Warm and Wet Patients With Normotension

The approach to normotensive individuals with decompensated HF again focuses on diuresis and vasodilatation but with greater emphasis on the former than the latter. Accordingly, rather than using intravenous agents to target blood pressure, oral agents such as angiotensin-converting enzyme inhibitors, hydralazine, and long-acting nitroglycerin can be used to achieve maximally tolerated afterload reduction. The goal should be to increase doses as high as tolerated without causing significant hypotension or symptoms (e.g., lightheadedness or syncope). If the patient fails to respond to this approach—either with ongoing fluid

retention or worsening renal function—reduction of home β-blockade is reasonable, as is invasive hemodynamics with placement of a PA catheter for adjunctive inotropic therapy.

PA catheters are placed through the internal jugular vein (either right or left) and pass through the right atrium and the right ventricle before resting in the PA. When the balloon tip of this catheter is inflated, it floats into the pulmonary capillary wedge position. An extraordinary amount of information can be obtained from these catheters, including right atrial pressure, right ventricular pressure, PA pressure, PCWP, systemic vascular resistance (SVR), as well as cardiac output and the cardiac index. Normal values are shown in Fig. 28.5.

Right atrial pressure, which is equivalent to CVP or right ventricular preload, is indicative of elevated right-sided filling pressures. PCWP and PA diastolic pressure, which are equivalent to left atrial pressure or left ventricular end-diastolic pressure in the absence of mitral stenosis or pulmonary vascular disease, are indicative of elevated left-sided filling pressures. Depending on the predominance of right-sided filling pressures versus left-sided filling pressures, right-sided HF versus left-sided HF can be further clarified and addressed through diuresis and/or afterload reduction. Cardiac output can be used to justify the use of inotropic agents, and afterload can be used to justify the use of vasodilators. Notably, it is not implausible that inotropic agents could be used to address cardiac output simultaneous to the use of vasodilators to decrease SVR.

Comprehension of the appropriate use of the three inotropes used to treat decompensated HF requires understanding of the receptors they target. Alpha-1 (α1) and α2 receptors facilitate peripheral vasoconstriction; β1 receptors increase heart rate and cardiac contractility; β2 receptors result in peripheral vasodilatation; and dopamine can also cause peripheral vasodilatation, particularly in the renal vasculature. Dobutamine and dopamine each act through their own combination of these receptors.

Dobutamine acts mostly on β-receptors, with a greater emphasis on β2 than β1. This is desirable for HF patients to increase cardiac output without increasing afterload. Risks associated with its use are increased tachyarrhythmias. In addition, although rare, prolonged high-dose infusions can result in eosinophilic hypersensitivity, characterized by eosinophilia, skin rash, and possible eosinophilic myocarditis. Long-term maintenance infusions may be subject to tachyphylaxis, necessitating dose uptitration over time. In addition, dobutamine may not be as effective for individuals with chronic HF, which can be associated with β-adrenergic receptor desensitization. If end organ perfusion fails to respond to dobutamine, a second agent such as milrinone or dopamine can be considered.

Depending on the dose of dopamine used, different receptors are recruited. At low doses of 1 to 3 μg/kg per minute, dopamine receptors are activated, and the predominant effect is increased renal perfusion, although the use of dopamine to augment renal function has not been clinically validated. At moderate doses of 2 to 5 μg/kg per minute, β receptors are also recruited, resulting in increased inotropy; chronotropy vasodilatation may also coexist. At high doses of >5 μg/kg per minute, α receptors are also activated, which increases vasoconstriction, mean arterial pressure, and SVR. Hence, low- and moderate-dose dopamine can be used to augment diuresis through inotropy and vasodilation, and high-dose dopamine can be used to treat hypotension. Similar to dobutamine, dopamine can result in arrhythmias and has a more limited potency in those with chronic HF.

As a phosphodiesterase inhibitor, milrinone increases levels of cyclic adenosine monophosphate by inhibiting its metabolism. This results in increased inotropic and lusitropic effects in the myocardium, as well as vasodilatory effects in the peripheral and pulmonary vasculature. Because it does not act on the β-receptors, it can be more effective for

TABLE 28.2   Pharmacological Comparison of Loop Diuretics

	Furosemide	Torsemide	Bumetanide
Relative PO potency	1	2x	40x
PO/IV conversion	2:1	1:1	1:1
Oral bioavailability	50%–60%	80%	60%–90%
Onset of action	PO 30–60 min	PO 60 min	PO 30–60 min
	IV 5 min	IV 10 min	IV 3 min
Half-life	1–2 h	3–4 h	1 h

IV, Intravenously; *PO,* per os.

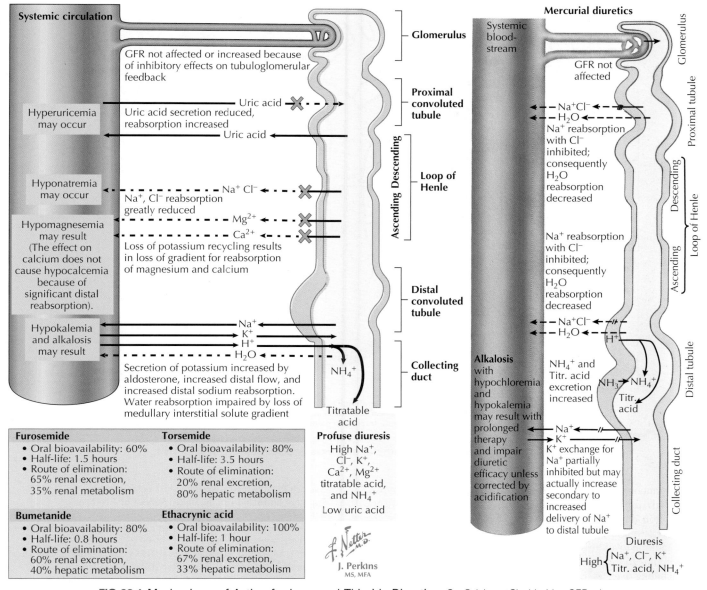

FIG 28.4 Mechanisms of Action for Loop and Thiazide Diuretics. *Ca,* Calcium; *Cl,* chloride; *GFR,* glomerular filtration rate; *H,* hydrogen; *H₂O,* water; *K* potassium; *Na,* sodium; *NaCl,* sodium chloride; *NH₃,* ammonia; *NH₄,* ammonium.

augmentation of cardiac output than dobutamine or dopamine in individuals with chronic HF. Because it acts via a different mechanism, milrinone can also be used in combination with β-adrenergic agents. An important consideration with milrinone is that its vasodilatory effects can result in hypotension in 10% of patients. Thus, it should not be used for increasing blood pressure. Also, its half-life is significantly longer than dopamine or dobutamine (2 hours compared with 2 minutes), particularly so in the setting of renal dysfunction (which can increase the half-life up to 18 hours). Finally, although it is also associated with development of arrhythmias, the baseline heart rate tends to be less elevated than with dobutamine or dopamine.

Cold Patients, Dry or Wet

In general, decompensated HF with signs of low cardiac output warrants treatment in an intensive care unit setting with invasive hemodynamic monitoring, and inotropic or mechanical vascular support.

Nondurable mechanical circulatory support (MCS) is reasonable as a "bridge to recovery" or a "bridge to decision," regarding whether a particular patient is an appropriate candidate for a durable left ventricular assist device or transplantation. Traditionally, nondurable MCS included intraaortic balloon pumps and extracorporeal membrane oxygenation. Recently approved devices include the TandemHeart percutaneous ventricular assist device (LivaNova, London, United Kingdom) and the Impella device (Abiomed, Inc., Danvers, Massachusetts). Alternatively, patients may be appropriate candidates to proceed directly with a left ventricular assist device or transplantation without needing nondurable MCS.

Discharge Planning

Transitioning patients from intravenous diuretics and/or inotropes should involve thoughtful consideration of previous, current, and anticipated home dosages of medications. Once weaned from inotropes,

NORMAL SATURATIONS (O₂) AND PRESSURE

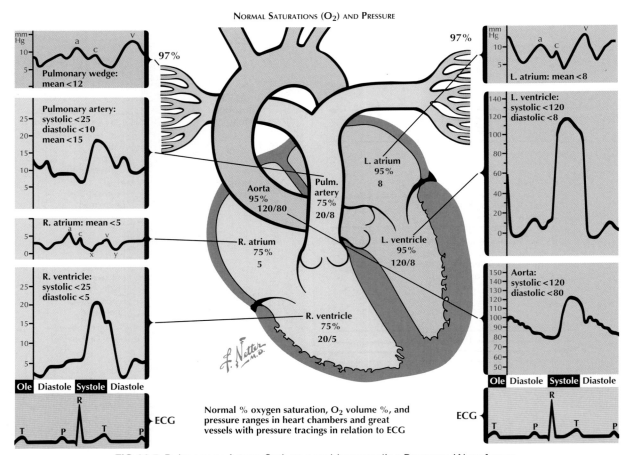

FIG 28.5 Pulmonary Artery Catheter and Intracardiac Pressure Waveforms.

extreme caution should be taken when re-initiating HF medical therapies, particularly β-blockade. Depending on the severity of the patient's hypotension during hospitalization, initiation of β-blockade in the after-care setting should be a strong consideration.

In addition to addressing individual causes for ADHF, admission is an ideal time to focus on comorbidities that can worsen the status of HF, including diabetes, iron deficiency anemia, and obstructive sleep apnea. It is also important to address adherence. Adherence to medical therapies, low-salt diet, and physical activity can be difficult to gauge. Poor adherence has been shown to correlate with worse clinical outcomes and increased healthcare costs. Hence, self-empowering education is a vital part of management of this chronic medical disease.

Because of a mortality risk of up to 20% and readmission risk of up to 30% at 6 months, transition of patients to home is a delicate process. Accordingly, current guidelines recommend that all patients admitted with ADHF follow-up within 7 to 14 days in person and/or within 3 days by telephone. In addition, it is recommended to use biomarkers and risk prediction tools to stratify those with the highest possibility for poor outcomes and to justify resource intensive strategies intended to improve clinical outcomes.

ADDITIONAL RESOURCES

Feldman D, Pamboukian SV, Teuteberg JJ, et al. The 2013 International Society for Heart and Lung Transplantation Guidelines for mechanical circulatory support: executive summary. *J Heart Lung Transplant.* 2013;32:157–187.
These guidelines provide current recommendations for use of MCS based on evidence-based data and consensus opinion.

Heidenreich PA, Albert NM, Allen LA, et al. Forecasting the impact of heart failure in the United States. *Circ Heart Fail.* 2013;6:606–619.
This policy statement by the American Heart Association examines current and projected costs related to HF.
Lindenfeld J, Albert NM, Boehmer JP, et al. HFSA 2010 Comprehensive Heart Failure Practice Guideline. *J Card Fail.* 2010;16:e1–e194.
These guidelines provide current recommendations for treatment of HF based on evidence-based data and consensus opinion.
Rihal CS, Naidu SS, Givertz MM, et al. 2015 SCAI/ACC/HFSA/STS clinical expert consensus statement on the use of percutaneous mechanical circulatory support devices in cardiovascular care. *J Am Coll Cardiol.* 2015;65:2140–2141.
These guidelines provide current recommendations for the use of percutaneous MCS based on evidence-based data and consensus opinion.
Yancy CW, Jessup M, Bozkurt B, et al. 2013 ACCF/AHA guideline for the management of heart failure. *Circulation.* 2013;128:e240–e327.
These guidelines provide current recommendations for treatment of HF based on evidence-based data and consensus opinion.

EVIDENCE

Baggish AL, Cameron R, Anwaruddin S, et al. A clinical and biochemical critical pathway for the evaluation of patients with suspected acute congestive heart failure: the ProBNP Investigation of Dyspnea in the Emergency Department (PRIDE) algorithm. *Crit Pathw Cardiol.* 2004;3:171–176.
Based on the prospective data obtained from the PRIDE study, this article suggested a pathway for the use of NT–pro-brain natriuretic peptide to distinguish presentations for HF from alternative diagnoses.

Chen J, Dharmarajan K, Wang Y, Krumholz HM. National trends in heart failure hospital stay rates, 2001 to 2009. *J Am Coll Cardiol.* 2013;61:1078–1088.

This study analyzed trends in HF hospital stays and mortality.

Fonarow GC, Abraham WT, Albert NM, et al. Factors identified as precipitating hospital admissions for heart failure and clinical outcomes: findings from OPTIMIZE-HF. *Arch Intern Med.* 2008;168: 847–854.

This study analyzed specific reasons for hospitalization in 48,612 patients enrolled in the Organized Program To Initiate life-saving treatMent In hospitaliZEd patients with Heart Failure (OPTIMIZE-HF) registry and concluded that precipitating factors could be identified in most of the cases.

Nohria A, Tsang SW, Fang JC, et al. Clinical assessment identifies hemodynamic profiles that predict outcomes in patients admitted with heart failure. *J Am Coll Cardiol.* 2003;41:1797–1804.

This classic study defined four hemodynamic classes of patients and correlated worse outcomes in those individuals who were volume overloaded.

O'Connor CM, Hasselblad V, Mehta RH, et al. Triage after hospitalization with advanced heart failure: the ESCAPE (Evaluation Study of Congestive Heart Failure and Pulmonary Artery Catheterization Effectiveness) risk model and discharge score. *J Am Coll Cardiol.* 2010;55:872–878.

This study analyzed risk factors for mortality and rehospitalization in 423 patients enrolled in the ESCAPE trial to create a risk model and score to be used for risk assessment following hospitalization for ADHF.

29

Management of Chronic Heart Failure

Hannah Bensimhon, Carla A. Sueta

Heart failure (HF) is a complex clinical syndrome that can result from any structural or functional cardiac disorder that impairs the ability of the ventricle to fill with (HF with preserved ejection fraction; HFpEF) or eject (HF with reduced ejection fraction; HFrEF) blood. Most commonly, HF results from myocardial muscle dysfunction with accompanying dilation and/or hypertrophy of the left ventricle (LV), remodeling, and neurohormonal activation. However, abnormalities of the valves, pericardium, endocardium, heart rhythm, and conduction can also cause HF.

ETIOLOGY AND PATHOGENESIS

Coronary artery disease (CAD) is the single most common cause of HF, accounting for 50% of cases. Patients with a previous myocardial infarction (MI) can develop both systolic dysfunction and diastolic impairment due to interstitial fibrosis and scar formation. Hibernating myocardium due to severe CAD can also cause HFrEF, which is potentially reversible with revascularization. Idiopathic cardiomyopathy, hypertension, and valvular heart disease are common causes. Familial cardiomyopathies may account for up to one-third of cardiomyopathies believed to be idiopathic. Other etiologies of dilated cardiomyopathy include thyroid disease, chemotherapy, myocarditis, HIV infection, diabetes, alcohol, cocaine, connective tissue disease, systemic lupus erythematosus, peripartum cardiomyopathy, and arrhythmias. Hypertrophic and restrictive cardiomyopathies are less common. It is crucial to identify the cause of HF because the degree of reversibility, and hence, the progression and management of HF depend on the etiology. Treatment of uncontrolled hypertension, thyroid disease, tachycardia, and active ischemia may result in significant improvement in LV function.

Heart Failure With Reduced Ejection Fraction

HFrEF, also called systolic heart failure, has been variously defined as an EF of <40% to 50%. Most clinical trials include patients with an EF ≤40%; therefore, specific pharmacological therapy is recommended in these patients. The initial insult, most often due to ischemia or increased pressure or volume load, results in a reduction in cardiac output that triggers activation of the renin-angiotensin-aldosterone system (RAAS), which results in salt and water retention. Declining blood pressure activates the sympathetic nervous system and increases endogenous hormones that result in systemic vasoconstriction. The short-term benefit of vasoconstriction—increased perfusion of critical organs—is followed by worsening HF due to chronically increased LV afterload. There is a compensatory increase in the A-type natriuretic peptide (ANP) and brain natriuretic peptide (BNP), which bind to NP receptors and generate diuresis, natriuresis, and myocardial relaxation and antiremodeling. ANP and BNP also inhibit renin and aldosterone secretion. Unfortunately, many of these beneficial peptides and bradykinin are degraded by neprilysin to inactive metabolites. The newest drug approved for treatment of HFrEF, Entresto (sacubitril/valsartan), is a combination of an angiotensin receptor blocker (ARB) and a neprilysin inhibitor.

LV remodeling, a maladaptive response, results in myocyte lengthening with a subsequent increase in chamber volume. Myocyte hypertrophy occurs, along with myocyte loss due to apoptosis or necrosis, and fibroblast proliferation and fibrosis (Fig. 29.1). The heart remodels eccentrically, becoming less elliptical, and more spherical and dilated. The mitral valve annulus often becomes dilated, which results in mitral regurgitation and further increased wall stress resulting in worsening HF.

Heart Failure With Preserved Ejection Fraction

HFpEF, previously referred to as diastolic heart failure, accounts for ≥50% of HF cases, is challenging to diagnose, and is often a diagnosis of exclusion. Several criteria have been proposed, including symptoms and/or signs of HFpEF (EF ≥50%), objective evidence of other underlying cardiac structural and/or functional abnormalities, and elevated BNP/proBNP levels. Patients with an intermediate EF (41%–49%) are often grouped with HFpEF. Ischemic heart disease and hypertension are the most common causes of isolated HFpEF. Compared with HFrEF patients, hospitalizations and deaths in patients with HFpEF are more likely to be noncardiovascular.

Typically, the ventricular size is normal in HFpEF. However, ventricular dilation can occur due to mitral or aortic valve regurgitation, or a high-output state (anemia or thiamine deficiency). Hypertrophic and restrictive cardiomyopathies, and constrictive pericarditis can result in a clinical presentation consistent with HFpEF. HFpEF is generally characterized by a normal end-diastolic volume, myocyte hypertrophy, and increased wall thickness that results in concentric remodeling compared with the increased end-diastolic volume and eccentric remodeling seen in HFrEF (Fig. 29.2). There is an increased extracellular matrix, abnormal calcium handling, and neurohormonal activation. These pathophysiological changes result in impaired ventricular relaxation, high LV diastolic pressure, high left atrial filling pressures, and resulting HF symptoms and signs.

CLINICAL PRESENTATION

Signs of HF include pulmonary congestion, edema, or inadequate organ perfusion. Symptoms include dyspnea on exertion, exercise intolerance, orthopnea, paroxysmal nocturnal dyspnea, cough, chest pain that may or may not represent angina, weakness, fatigue, edema, nocturia, insomnia, depression, and weight gain. Patients with end-stage disease may also complain of nausea, abdominal pain, oliguria, confusion, and weight loss. Physical examination should include assessment of jugular venous

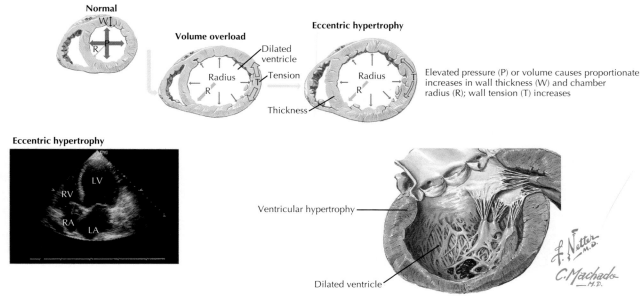

FIG 29.1 Cardiac Remodeling Secondary to Volume Overload. *LA,* Left atrium; *LV,* left ventricle; *RA,* right atrium; *RV,* right ventricle.

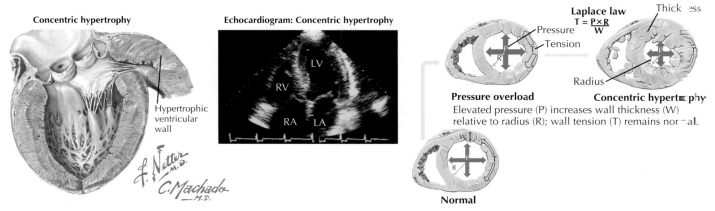

FIG 29.2 Heart Failure With Preserved Ejection Fraction Due to Hypertension. *LA,* Left atrium; *LV,* left ventricle; *RA,* right atrium; *RV,* right ventricle.

pressure, rales, wheezing, pleural effusion, displaced point of maximal intensity, right ventricular heave, increased intensity of P_2, S_3, and S_4, murmurs, hepatomegaly, hepatojugular reflux, low-volume pulses, and peripheral edema. Patients with end-stage disease may also exhibit pulsus alternans, tachycardia, ascites, cool, pale extremities, and cachexia.

The clinical presentation of HFrEF and HFpEF may be indistinguishable (Fig. 29.3). The cardiac silhouette may be enlarged in both, with cardiomegaly due to ventricular dilation in HFrEF and from hypertrophy in HFpEF. An assessment of LV function is essential for determining the optimal approach to treatment.

Differential Diagnosis

The difficulty in diagnosing HF lies in its vague symptoms and examination mimickers (Box 29.1). Symptoms of dyspnea and exercise intolerance can be attributed to many diagnoses. Sodium-avid states of nephrosis and cirrhosis, as well as pericardial disease, can present with similar findings of jugular venous distention, hepatomegaly, and edema.

BOX 29.1   Differential Diagnosis

Myocardial ischemia
Pulmonary disease
Sleep-disordered breathing
Obesity
Deconditioning
Thromboembolic disease
Anemia
Hepatic failure
Renal failure
Hypoalbuminemia
Venous stasis
Depression
Anxiety and hyperventilation syndromes

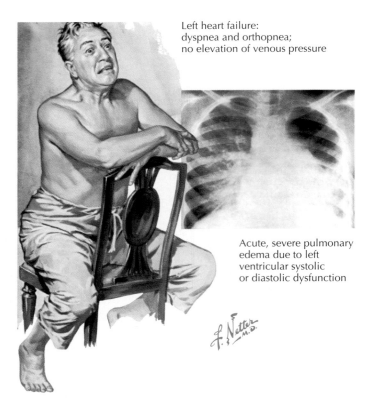

Left heart failure: dyspnea and orthopnea; no elevation of venous pressure

Acute, severe pulmonary edema due to left ventricular systolic or diastolic dysfunction

FIG 29.3 Left Heart Failure and Pulmonary Edema.

DIAGNOSTIC APPROACH

The diagnosis is made by taking a careful history, performing a directed examination, assessing cardiac structure and function, and laboratory evaluation. Transthoracic echocardiography (TTE) is the method of choice for cardiac examination. Information on chamber volumes, systolic and diastolic function, wall thickness, valve function, and pulmonary hypertension is readily determined. Measurement of natriuretic peptides, which correlate with elevated filling pressures, is a useful initial diagnostic test. Although an elevated BNP and/or proBNP level does not rule out pulmonary causes of dyspnea, normal levels argue against HF as the predominant cause. Although levels are generally higher in HFrEF, these tests cannot distinguish between HFrEF and HFpEF. Other conditions can cause elevated levels, including pulmonary hypertension, cor pulmonale, pulmonary embolism, critical illness, and renal dysfunction; obese patients may have normal levels. Initial laboratory evaluation should also include electrolytes, estimated glomerular filtration rate, hemoglobin, white blood cell count, glucose, glycosylated hemoglobin, lipids, albumin, liver function tests, urinalysis, thyroid-stimulating hormone, ferritin, and serum transferrin. Additional diagnostic tests should be considered when there is a clinical suspicion of a particular pathology, including genetic testing. Laboratory results, together with ECG, cardiac x-ray, and pulmonary function testing, will eliminate most noncardiac diagnoses.

Cardiac MRI is the best alternative cardiac imaging modality for patients with a nondiagnostic TTE and is the method of choice in patients with complex congenital heart disease. MRI provides an accurate assessment of size, mass, and function of both ventricles. It can be useful in clarifying myocardial viability and identifying infiltrative disease. Its usefulness is enhanced by gadolinium contrast, but this should not be used in patients with moderate to severe kidney disease. The presence of pacemakers and defibrillators is typically a contraindication for MRI, although new devices and protocols are in development.

Ischemic heart disease should be evaluated in every patient, because revascularization of a hibernating myocardium can result in significant improvement in systolic function. Focal wall motion abnormalities most commonly indicate CAD, but not always. Global LV dysfunction does not rule out an ischemic etiology. Testing options include cardiac catheterization and exercise or pharmacological echocardiographic or nuclear stress testing, CT angiography, MRI, and PET. Patients with left bundle branch block should not be evaluated with stress echocardiography because the conduction delay can result in a false-positive result.

Determining New York Heart Association (NYHA) classification is important for prognosis, as an indication for medical therapies and device placement, and as an evaluation of response to treatment.

MANAGEMENT AND THERAPY

It is critical to identify the cause and type of HF to determine the specific treatment and specific pharmacological therapy that will result in the best outcome. Next, it is important to correct precipitating factors, including ischemia, dietary nonadherence, uncontrolled hypertension, atrial fibrillation (AF), hypoxemia, thyroid disease, anemia, and medication nonadherence. An algorithm for management of symptomatic HFrEF is presented (Fig. 29.4).

Revascularization should be considered in ischemic patients, even with marked systolic dysfunction. The National Institutes of Health–sponsored STICH (Surgical Treatment for Ischemic Heart Failure) trial randomized patients with significant CAD (left anterior descending or multivessel disease) disease and EF ≤35% to coronary artery bypass grafting plus optimal medical therapy (OMT) versus OMT alone. Revascularization + OMT resulted in a significant decrease in death or cardiovascular hospitalization. Although there was no total mortality benefit at 5 years, the extension STICHES study found that coronary artery bypass grafting plus OMT significantly reduced mortality at 10 years. All patients with CAD should be treated with aspirin unless there is a contraindication. Patients who have had percutaneous intervention should also receive a P2Y12 inhibitor. We recommend a statin in ischemic patients. One of two trials reported a reduction in hospitalization in ischemic patients. The effect of withdrawal of a statin is unknown. There are no data to support statin therapy in nonischemic patients.

Pharmacological Treatment for Heart Failure With Reduced Ejection Fraction
Drugs That Reduce Mortality

An ACEI or ARB are recommended in all HFrEF patients. These drugs result in improved survival and decreased hospitalizations in patients in NYHA classes II to IV and asymptomatic NYHA class I post-MI patients. They also prevent and delay hospitalization in nonischemic NYHA class I patients. Providers should aim for target doses used in clinical trials (Table 29.1). In chronic stable NYHA classes II to III patients who tolerate an ACEI or ARB, replacement by an angiotensin receptor neprilysin inhibitor (ARNI), Entresto (sacubitril/valsartan combination), is now recommended to further reduce morbidity and mortality. In the PARADIGM-HF (Prospective Comparison of ARNI with ACEI to Determine Impact on Global Mortality and Morbidity in Heart Failure) trial, patients who tolerated enalapril 10 mg twice daily and who were already receiving a β-blocker with elevated BNP/proBNP levels were randomized. Entresto was found to be superior to enalapril; it reduced the composite endpoint of cardiovascular death and/or HF hospitalization by 20%, as well as total mortality by 16%. An algorithm for replacing an ACEI or ARB is provided (Fig. 29.5). An

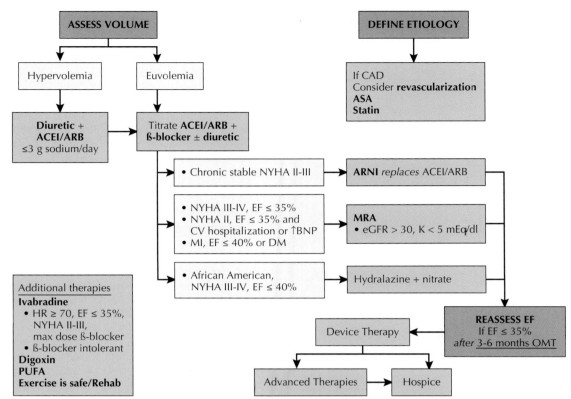

FIG 29.4 Management of Symptomatic Heart Failure With Reduced Ejection Fraction. *ACEI,* Angiotensin-converting enzyme inhibitors; *ARB,* angiotensin receptor blockers; *ARNI,* ARB neprilysin inhibitor combination; *ASA,* aspirin; *BNP,* brain natriuretic peptide; *CAD,* coronary artery disease; *CV,* cardiovascular; *DM,* diabetes; *EF,* ejection fraction; *eGFR,* estimated glomerular filtration rate; *HF,* heart failure; *HR,* heart rate; *MI,* myocardial infarction; *MRA,* mineralocorticoid receptor antagonists; *NYHA,* New York Heart Association; *OMT,* optimal medical therapy; *PUFA,* n-3 polyunsaturated fatty acids.

ARNI is contraindicated in patients with a history of angioedema, in patients currently taking an ACEI within 36 hours of the last dose of an ACEI because of the risk of angioedema, or in patients with severe hepatic impairment. Contraindications to ACEI/ARB/ARNI also include moderate to severe aortic stenosis, bilateral renal artery stenosis, and hyperkalemia (potassium >5.5 mmol/L). ACEIs can cause intractable cough, and rarely, angioedema. Although rare, angioedema has been reported with ARBs. In patients with significant renal dysfunction and hyperkalemia (potassium >5.5 mmol/L), the combination of isosorbide dinitrate and hydralazine is an alternative, although it is not as effective as ACEI therapy.

Beta-blockers should be added to ACEI/ARB therapy in all HFrEF patients. These drugs reduce mortality and hospitalization in NYHA class II to IV patients and in asymptomatic patients post-MI. Beta-blockers improve EF, which appears to be dose-dependent. Beta-blockers are also recommended to prevent and/or delay HF in nonischemic NYHA class I patients. Providers should aim for target doses used in clinical trials (Table 29.1). Contraindications include severe reactive airway disease in patients receiving inhaled daily β-agonists, severe bradycardia, or advanced heart block. Beta-blockers should be started at a low dose and titrated every 2 weeks. Most patients require diuretic therapy during β-blocker initiation and may require an increased diuretic dose to prevent or treat congestion. Beta-blockers should not be initiated or titrated in patients who demonstrate volume overload; diurese these patients first. Side effects (fatigue, weight gain, diarrhea) are more common with the first few doses. If patients have difficulty tolerating the drug, dose titration can be slowed by increasing the time between

titrations, increasing the dose by a smaller amount, or taking a once daily drug at night. Although target doses should be the goal, lower doses also confer a mortality and morbidity benefit. Studies indicate that at least 80% of patients can tolerate β-blocker therapy. ACEI/ARB and β-blocker uptitration can be alternated, rather than titrating ACEI/ARB to the target dose before adding a β-blocker. Beta-blockers can be safely added during hospitalization once the patient is euvolemic.

Mineralocorticoid receptor antagonists (MRAs) should be added to ACEI/ARB/ARNI and β-blocker therapy in NYHA classes III to IV patients, or class II patients if they have had previous cardiovascular hospitalization or elevated BNP/proBNP, and in post-MI patients (EF <40% or diabetic). Therapy should only be initiated if potassium is <5 mmol/L, serum creatinine is ≤2.5 mg/dL, and creatinine clearance is >30 mL/min. Hyperkalemia is common, occurring in 25% to 33% of patients, especially in diabetic and older patients. Regular monitoring is necessary. Potassium and renal function should be reassessed at least 1 week and 1 month after initiation or change in dose. Do not use a combination of ACEI + ARB + MRA because of the high risk of hyperkalemia.

The combination of isosorbide dinitrate and hydralazine added to ACEI/ARB and β-blocker therapy provides an additional mortality and morbidity benefit in NYHA classes III to IV African American patients.

Additional Therapies

Diuretics are prescribed in most patients to alleviate fluid overload. Because they activate the RAAS, the minimal effective dose should be prescribed. In patients with severe HF, combination therapy (loop diuretic

TABLE 29.1   Drug Therapy for Heart Failure With Reduced Ejection Fraction

Medication	Daily Starting Dose	Daily Target Dose
Angiotensin-Converting Enzyme Inhibitors		
Enalapril	2.5 mg twice	10 mg twice
Lisinopril	2.5–5 mg once	20–40 mg once
Ramipril	1.25–2.5 mg once	10 mg once
Trandolapril	1 mg once	4 mg once
Captopril	6.25 mg 3 times	50 mg 3 times
Perindopril	2 mg once	8–16 mg once
Fosinopril	5–10 mg once	40 mg once
Quinapril	5 mg twice	20 mg twice
Angiotensin Receptor Blockers		
Valsartan	20–40 mg twice	160 mg twice
Candesartan	4–8 mg once	32 mg once
Losartan	25 mg once	150 mg once
Angiotensin Receptor Neprilysin Inhibitor		
Valsartan sacubitril	26–51/24–49	103/97
β-blockers		
Bisoprolol[a]	1.25 mg once	10 mg once
Carvedilol[a]	3.125 mg twice	25–50 (>85 kg) mg twice
Metoprolol succinate ER[a]	12.5–25 mg once	200 mg once
Metoprolol tartrate	12.5–25 twice	100 mg twice
Carvedilol-CR[a]	10 mg once	80 mg once
Mineralocorticoid antagonists		
Spironolactone	12.5–25 mg once	25–50 mg once
Eplerenone	12.5–25 mg once	25–50 mg once
Nitrate + Hydralazine		
Isosorbide dinitrate[b]	10–20 mg 3 times	40–60 mg 3 times
Hydralazine[b]	10–25 mg 3 times	75–100 mg 3 times
Bidil (20 mg/37.7 mg)	1/2–1 tablet 3 times	2 tablets 3 times
Digoxin	0.125 mg once	0.125 mg once
Ivabradine	2.5–5 mg twice	7.5 twice

[a]Preferred β-blockers.
[b]If not on an angiotensin-converting enzyme inhibitor, angiotensin receptor blocker, or receptor neprilysin inhibitor, target daily doses are Isordil (isosorbide dinitrate) 160 mg in divided doses and hydralazine 300 mg in divided doses.
ER, Extended release.

and hydrochlorothiazide or metolazone) can be used, but potassium and magnesium levels must be carefully monitored.

A newer therapy, ivabradine, can be added if EF ≤35% and heart rate is >70 beats/min despite a targeted dose of β-blockers, or in patients with a contraindication to β-blockers. Ivabradine slows heart rate by inhibition of the funny current (*If*) specific to the sinoatrial node. This drug reduces hospitalizations and HF mortality (not all-cause mortality). Ivabradine is contraindicated in decompensated HF, if blood pressure is <90/50 mm Hg, and cannot be given to patients with pacemakers, sick sinus syndrome, sinoatrial block, or first-degree atrioventricular block unless a pacemaker is present.

Digoxin reduces hospitalizations and improves symptoms but confers no survival benefit. Higher serum concentration (≥1.2 ng/mL) is associated with mortality. Low-dose therapy is recommended, with a target concentration of <1 ng/mL. Consider adding therapy to patients in NYHA class IV who are hypotensive. Digoxin dose should be reduced by half and monitored closely if amiodarone or warfarin is initiated. Digoxin does not control exercise heart rate in AF. Use cautiously in older adults and patients with renal dysfunction.

In one clinical trial, n-3 polyunsaturated fatty acid (PUFA) was shown to reduce mortality in patients in NYHA classes II to IV.

Nitrates reduce preload and are prescribed as antianginal agents. Amlodipine and felodipine are not recommended as routine therapy but can be used to treat hypertension and angina that is unresponsive to β-blockers and nitrates. Clinical trials have demonstrated a neutral effect of these agents on mortality.

Pharmacological Therapy of Heart Failure With Preserved Ejection Fraction

To date, there is no drug that has been shown to reduce mortality in HFpEF. Guidelines recommend the following: control of systolic and diastolic blood pressure; diuretics for congestion; consideration of revascularization in CAD patients with symptoms attributable to ischemia; and management of AF. ARBs, ACEIs, β-blockers, calcium channel blockers, and MRAs all cause regression of LV hypertrophy. Agents that reduce preload, such as diuretics and nitrates, which can also be used to treat ischemia, are also commonly prescribed. Small studies have demonstrated a benefit of daily moderate exercise.

Spironolactone has been shown to reduce HF hospitalizations (without effect on total mortality) in patients with HFpEF (LVEF ≥45%) in TOPCAT (Treatment of Preserved Cardiac Function Heart Failure with an Aldosterone Antagonist Trial). The composite endpoint (cardiovascular mortality, aborted cardiac arrest, or HF hospitalization) was significantly reduced only in the subgroup of patients from the Americas compared with those from Eastern Europe, although this was not a prespecified analysis.

Device Therapy for Heart Failure
Implantable Cardioverter-Defibrillators and Cardiac Resynchronization Therapy

Implantable cardioverter-defibrillators (ICD) and cardiac resynchronization therapy (CRT) devices should be considered in HFrEF patients receiving OMT (ACEI/ARB/ARNI + β-blocker + MRA) for 3 to 6 months (Fig. 29.4). It is important to reassess LV function after reaching target or maximum tolerated doses before device implantation. Improvement in LV function may occur, obviating the indication for device placement.

ICD implantation should only be considered for patients with a life expectancy of at least 1 year. ICDs are indicated in all patients who have recovered from a ventricular arrhythmia that caused hemodynamic instability. ICD placement also reduces mortality in patients in NYHA classes II to III, EFs of ≤35%, whether ischemic (>40 days post-MI, >90 days postrevascularization) or nonischemic, and in class I ischemic patients with an EF ≤30%.

A wearable ICD may be considered for patients at risk of sudden cardiac death for a limited period or as a bridge to an implanted device. Most data have come from observational studies, but there is an ongoing randomized controlled trial called VEST (Vest Prevention of Early Sudden Death Trial) that is currently studying wearable ICDs.

CRT reduces mortality and hospitalization, modestly increases EF, and improves quality of life in approximately 70% of symptomatic patients with EFs of ≤35% and a QRS duration of ≥130 ms. One trial suggested harm in cases of QRS duration of <130 ms. Regardless of NYHA class, CRT is recommended for patients with an indication for ventricular pacing to reduce morbidity.

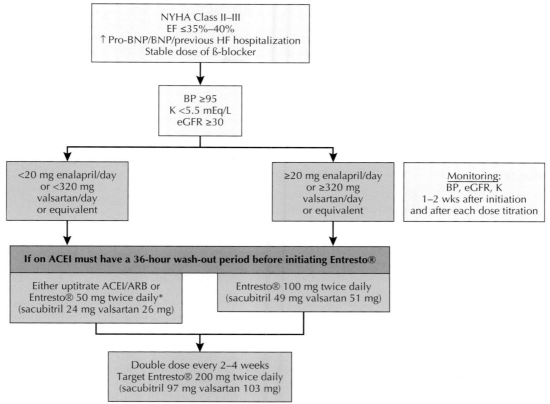

FIG 29.5 Replacement of ACEI/ARB With ARNI. *ACEI*, Angiotensin-converting enzyme inhibitors; *ARB*, angiotensin receptor blockers; *ARNI*, ARB neprilysin inhibitor combination; *BNP*, brain natriuretic peptide; *BP*, blood pressure; *EF*, ejection fraction; *eGFR*, estimated glomerular filtration rate; *HF*, heart failure; *NYHA*, New York Heart Association.

Fluid Monitoring Devices

Monitoring of pulmonary artery pressure using a wireless implantable hemodynamic monitoring system (CardioMems [Abbott Laboratories, Abbott Park, Illinois]) may be considered in symptomatic patients with previous HF hospitalization. The CHAMPION (The CardioMEMS Heart Sensor Allows Monitoring of Pressure to Improve Outcomes in NYHA Class III Heart Failure Patients) trial found a significant reduction in readmission rates in both HFpEF and HFrEF patients at 6 and 18 months.

Treatment of Co-morbid Disease

Aggressive management of hypertension, diabetes mellitus, obstructive sleep apnea, and depression is part of routine care. Treatment of AF in patients with HFrEF with either rate control or rhythm control results in similar outcomes. In a substudy of one trial, β-blockers significantly reduced mortality in AF. Common antiarrhythmic agents include amiodarone with thyroid and liver function monitoring every 6 months, and sotalol and dofetilide with dosing based on renal function. The CASTLE-AF (Catheter Ablation vs. Standard conventional Treatment in patients with LEft ventricular dysfunction and Atrial Fibrillation) trial reported a significant decrease in the combined and individual endpoints of mortality and hospitalization for worsening HF in 397 patients who had symptomatic paroxysmal or persistent atrial fibrillation, who had left ventricular ejection fraction (LVEF) of 35% or less, and who had refused or failed medical therapy. However, only 13% of eligible patients were randomized, those who did not

survive the 5-week run-in medication maximization phase were excluded, and 12.5% of patients who were randomized to ablation were lost to follow-up, limiting generalizability.

Nonpharmacological Strategies

Daily exercise, salt restriction (<3 g/day), fluid restriction, and daily weight measurements should all be in the care plan of the patient. Obese HF patients benefit from weight loss, and all HF patients benefit from smoking cessation and reduced alcohol intake, or if they have alcoholic cardiomyopathy, complete abstention. Every patient should receive an annual flu shot. Patients and their families should be educated about the symptoms and signs of the disease, prognosis, medications, and when to contact a health professional.

Advanced Directives and Palliative Care

Because of the high morbidity and mortality associated with HF, discussions with patients regarding prognosis and goals, including living wills and healthcare power of attorney, should be considered a key component of standard care. The World Health Organization defines palliative care as prevention and relief of suffering, promoting the best quality of life for patients and their families. Palliative care can be initiated when patients are diagnosed. As illness progresses, the ratio of palliative care to life-prolonging care gradually increases. Ultimately life-prolonging care may be discontinued according to the patient's wishes or when the harm of treatment outweighs its benefit. At this point, transition to hospice care is common.

Advanced Therapies

Consider referral to an HF specialist if the patient remains severely limited on OMT, does not tolerate medication uptitration, may be a candidate for a clinical trial, or may be a candidate for transplantation (refractory HF, EF <25%, without significant comorbid disease, compliant, psychologically stable with good social support), or for an LV assist device (bridge to cardiac transplantation and/or recovery, or as destination therapy). Long-term inotrope infusion with dobutamine or milrinone may be administered in transplantation-listed patients who have ICDs or as palliative therapy in end-stage patients.

Avoiding Treatment Errors

Concomitant administration of an ACEI, ARB, and MRA is not recommended because of the increased danger of hyperkalemia. In patients receiving RAAS inhibitors, including ARNI, regular monitoring of potassium and renal function is strongly recommended.

Routine administration of nonsteroidal agents is not recommended in patients with HF due to increased risk for fluid retention, worsening renal function, and increased mortality and morbidity. Nifedipine, verapamil, and diltiazem should not be used in patients with HFrEF because of their negative effect on contractility. Avoid prescribing thiazolidinediones because these agents have been associated with increased incidence of HF. Anticoagulation is not recommended in patients with chronic HF without AF, a previous thromboembolic event, or a cardioembolic source.

FUTURE DIRECTIONS

HF is a disease state with great heterogeneity, which complicates treatment strategy. Identifying more precise HF phenotypes in HFpEF will result in more targeted therapies and improvement in patient outcomes. Currently, patients with EFs of 41% to 49% are not well studied, and clinical trials are needed to guide treatment. The tremendous hope of stem cell therapies may be realized with the development of a synthetic version that could confer stability and reduce some of the risks associated with these therapies. Disease prevention by aggressive modification of risk factors and early detection will continue to have an enormous impact on cardiovascular disease leading to HF.

ADDITIONAL RESOURCES

Heart Failure Society of America http://www.hfsa.org.
Contains helpful information about HF for health professionals, patients, and their families.

EVIDENCE

McMurray JJ, Packer M, Desai AS, et al. PARADIGM-HF Investigators and Committees. Angiotensin–neprilysin inhibition versus enalapril in heart failure. *N Engl J Med.* 2014;371:993–1004.
This trial randomized 8399 patients with symptomatic HFrEF (LVEF <35%–40%), elevated BNP/proBNP, on a stable β-blocker, and who tolerated enalapril 10 mg twice daily to LCZ696 (valsartan sacubitril) or enalapril. The LCZ696 group had a reduction in the primary outcome of cardiovascular/HF hospitalization (21.8% vs. 26.5%; number needed to treat = 21). Total mortality was also significantly decreased (17.0% vs. 19.8%; number needed to treat = 36).

Ponikowski P, Voors AA, Anker SD, et al. 2016 ESC guidelines for the diagnosis and treatment of acute and chronic heart failure: the Task Force for the diagnosis and treatment of acute and chronic heart failure of the European Society of Cardiology (ESC). Developed with the special contribution of the Heart Failure Association (HFA) of the ESC. *Eur J Heart Fail.* 2016;18:891–975.
These guidelines provide current recommendations for treatment of HF based on evidence-based data and consensus opinion.

Swedberg K, Komajda M, Böhm M, et al. on behalf of the SHIFT Investigators. Ivabradine and outcomes in chronic heart failure (SHIFT): a randomized placebo-controlled study. *Lancet.* 2010;376:875–885.
This trial randomized 6558 patients with symptomatic HFrEF (NYHA classes II–IV; LVEF ≤35%) and a hospitalization for HF within the preceding year, as well as a resting heart rate of ≥70 beats/min despite maximally tolerated medical therapy (i.e., ACE/ARB, β-blocker, MRA) to ivabradine versus placebo. Ivabradine use was associated with a 5% absolute reduction in HF hospitalization (29% vs. 24%) and a 2% absolute reduction in HF mortality (3% vs. 5%).

Yancy CW, Jessup M, Bozkurt B, et al. 2013 ACCF/AHA guideline for the management of heart failure: a report of the American College of Cardiology Foundation/American Heart Association Task Force on Practice Guidelines. *J Am Coll Cardiol.* 2013;62:e147–e239.
These guidelines provide 2013 recommendations for treatment of HF based on evidence-based data and consensus opinion.

Yancy CW, Jessup M, Bozkurt B, Butler J, et al. 2016 ACC/AHA/HFSA focused update on new pharmacological therapy for heart failure: an update of the 2013 ACCF/AHA guideline for the management of heart failure: a report of the American College of Cardiology/American Heart Association Task Force on Clinical Practice Guidelines and the Heart Failure Society of America. *J Am Coll Cardiol.* 2016;68:1476–1488.
These guidelines provide current updated recommendations for treatment of HF based on evidence-based data and consensus opinion.

30

Hypertrophic Cardiomyopathy

John S. Douglas, Jr.

ETIOLOGY AND PATHOGENESIS

Approximately 700,000 individuals in the United States have hypertrophic cardiomyopathy (HCM), a monogenetic disorder that results in hypertrophy of the left ventricle (LVH) without another cardiac or systemic cause. HCM results from 1 of >1500 different mutations of genes that encode sarcomeric proteins. The mutation is transmitted in an autosomal dominant Mendelian pattern, such that 50% of direct descendants are gene-positive. Phenotypic expression of the gene results in myocyte hypertrophy and disarray, and hypertrophy of the LV that frequently involves the basal septum (Fig. 30.1). Individuals with similar genomes may have markedly different phenotypes. This phenotypic heterogeneity limits the predictive value of family history and genetic testing. In one-third of probands (clinical HCM), development of septal hypertrophy results in LV outflow tract (LVOT) obstruction at rest that is most often associated with systolic anterior motion (SAM) of the anterior leaflet of the mitral valve. The cause of SAM has been the subject of considerable debate, but contemporary explanations suggest that multiple factors are responsible, including a narrow LVOT due to septal hypertrophy, an anteriorly positioned mitral valve apparatus, and longer than usual mitral valve leaflets. The anterior mitral leaflet functions as a sail, increasingly obstructing the LVOT as it approaches and contacts the septum. This phenomenon results in the classical findings of hypertrophic obstructive cardiomyopathy (HOCM): a late systolic murmur, a bifid arterial waveform, and a posteriorly directed jet of mitral regurgitation. In one-third of probands, there is no LVOT gradient at rest, but LVOT obstruction can be induced by physiological provocation during the strain phase of the Valsalva maneuver, during exercise, or by inhaled amyl nitrite (Fig. 30.2). In the remaining one-third of probands, there is no LVOT gradient at rest or with provocation. LVOT obstruction has important implications. Prognosis is worse in the presence of obstruction, and treatment of symptomatic patients varies, depending on the presence of LVOT obstruction. Other factors that play important roles in the pathophysiology of HCM patients include stiffening of the thickened LV, which results in reduced LV filling, increased LV end-diastolic pressure, and increased left atrial size. Left atrial dilation promotes the development of atrial fibrillation. An eccentric jet of mitral regurgitation results from failure of coaptation of the anterior and posterior mitral valve leaflets caused by SAM. There is a positive correlation between the degree of SAM-related LVOT obstruction and the amount of mitral regurgitation. The amount of myocyte disarray and myocardial fibrosis is also important to determine clinical outcome. There is an increased risk of sudden cardiac death (SCD) associated with these findings. Development of thin-walled LV apical aneurysms has been reported in approximately 5% of HCM patients treated in referral centers. These patients appear to have a substantially increased risk of SCD and thromboembolic stroke.

CLINICAL PRESENTATION

The most common clinical presentation of HCM is the development of dyspnea or fatigue related to diastolic dysfunction with or without LVOT obstruction and mitral regurgitation. Typical anginal symptoms due to myocardial ischemia are relatively common due to myocardial blood flow supply–demand mismatch. Increased oxygen demand caused by LVH and adverse loading conditions occur in the face of compromised coronary blood flow due to medial hypertrophy of the coronary arteries and high LV end-diastolic pressure. Development of exercise-induced presyncope or syncope is a less frequent but important presentation in patients with LVOT obstruction. The timing of symptom onset relative to the age of the patient is highly variable. Clinical presentation of middle age or older adult patients reporting recent onset of symptoms is not unusual. In a small minority of individuals with HCM, the first recognized "symptom" is SCD, usually during exercise. This is the basis for attempting to identify and protect patients at high risk for arrhythmic death and for pre-participation screening of competitive athletes.

DIFFERENTIAL DIAGNOSIS

In 9 of 10 individuals there is evidence of LVH on ECG. Although the absence of LVH on ECG reduces the probability of HCM, its presence is quite nonspecific. Causes of LVH that must be excluded include systemic hypertension, valvular heart disease, and congenital disorders (e.g., subvalvular membranes, coronary fistula, and coarctation of the aorta).

DIAGNOSTIC APPROACH

History and Physical Examination

Heart failure symptoms, effort-related chest pain, syncope, or family history of HCM can be critical in initiating an evaluation leading to a diagnosis of HCM. Physical examination is rarely of assistance in patients without LVOT obstruction, but can be quite helpful in patients with HOCM. The carotid upstroke is brisk, and a bifid carotid waveform may be present. Cardiac auscultation that reveals a systolic murmur accentuated with a Valsalva maneuver or standing, and attenuated with squatting or isometric handgrip are important clues to the diagnosis of HOCM.

Electrocardiogram

Although the ECG is rarely normal in individuals with HCM, there is no pattern specific for HCM. LVH with secondary ST-T wave abnormalities is the norm (see Fig. 30.1). The degree of LVH on ECG does not correlate well with the amount of hypertrophy on echocardiography. Although T-wave changes may occur in any patient with HCM, giant

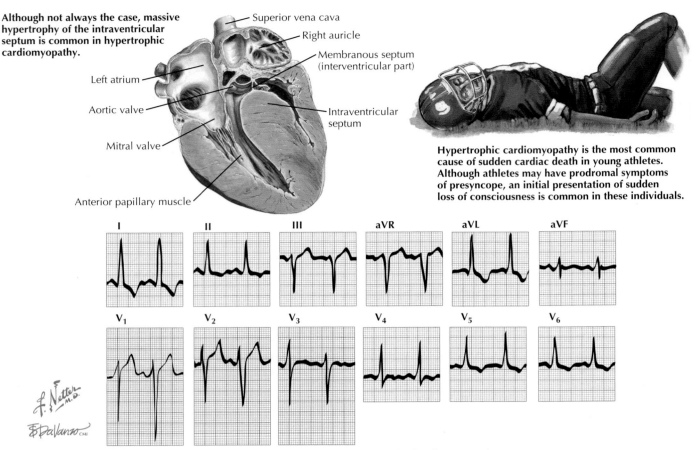

Although not always the case, massive hypertrophy of the intraventricular septum is common in hypertrophic cardiomyopathy.

Superior vena cava

Right auricle

Membranous septum (interventricular part)

Left atrium

Aortic valve

Intraventricular septum

Mitral valve

Anterior papillary muscle

Hypertrophic cardiomyopathy is the most common cause of sudden cardiac death in young athletes. Although athletes may have prodromal symptoms of presyncope, an initial presentation of sudden loss of consciousness is common in these individuals.

FIG 30.1 Sudden Death in Hypertrophic Cardiomyopathy.

T-wave inversion across the precordium has been noted to occur in individuals with apical hypertrophy and may be an important clue to the presence of this variant. Abnormal Q waves that occur most often in the inferior lateral leads are observed in a substantial minority of patients. Ambulatory ECG monitoring may be helpful in patients with palpitations, presyncope, or syncope by identifying patients with atrial or ventricular arrhythmias. A finding of atrial fibrillation, even a single time, is an important predictor of subsequent stroke and is an indication for anticoagulation with warfarin. Approximately 25% of individuals with HCM develop atrial fibrillation. Ventricular arrhythmias, particularly nonsustained ventricular tachycardia (VT), may be a prelude to more serious arrhythmic events.

Echocardiography

Transthoracic two-dimensional echocardiography is the primary imaging technique for the evaluation of individuals with suspected HCM. It is also used to monitor young individuals who are known to be gene positive, phenotype negative (G+P–) for the development of phenotypic manifestations, to follow the progress of HCM in affected asymptomatic individuals, and to monitor the response to treatment in symptomatic patients treated medically or with septal reduction strategies. Its safety and wide availability make it the ideal modality for evaluation of individuals of any age at almost any location. LV wall thickness can be measured, and the presence of LVOT obstruction can be determined at rest and with physiological and/or pharmacological provocation. In individuals with no resting LVOT obstruction, exercise echocardiography is also recommended. Exercise echocardiography is safe, provides

quantification of exercise capabilities, and is a physiological reproduction of what is happening in everyday life. Exercise-induced LVOT obstruction, blood pressure responses to exercise, and development of exercise-induced ventricular arrhythmias can be assessed. Contrast echocardiography is useful to exclude an apical aneurysm. Transesophageal echocardiography is not often needed but can be helpful when transthoracic echocardiography imaging is not optimal; it can also identify anomalous chordal attachments, subvalvular membranes, and papillary muscle abnormalities.

Cardiac Magnetic Resonance Imaging

In the past decade, cardiac magnetic resonance imaging (CMR) has been an increasingly important imaging tool in the diagnosis, treatment, and risk stratification of individuals with HCM. Advantages over echocardiography include more reliable detection of the location and extent of hypertrophy, including sites not well seen by echocardiography (e.g., the apex or posterior septum). In addition, delayed gadolinium enhancement distribution and extent (a measure of myocardial fibrosis) provides important prognostic information for risk of SCD. Delayed enhancement of ≥15% of LV mass conveys a twofold increase in risk of SCD. In some HCM centers, CMR is routinely performed in patients with HCM. CMR is expected to play a larger role in HCM imaging in the future.

Genetic Testing

HCM is the most common heritable heart disease, and in most adults, it results from mutations of genes encoding sarcomeric proteins (see

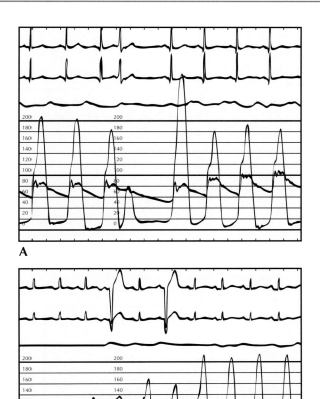

A

B

FIG 30.2 Left Ventricular Outflow Tract (LVOT) Pressure Gradient. (A) Simultaneous LV and aortic pressure tracings showing a resting LVOT pressure gradient of >100 mm Hg. Note the bifid arterial wave form and Brockenbrough-Braunwald-Morrow sign (postextrasystolic potentiation) with augmented LV pressure and pressure gradient. In the original description, the pulse pressure decreased but the criterion was later modified by these authors to include instances in which the pulse pressure failed to decrease, as illustrated here. (B) Performance of a Valsalva maneuver results in increased LV filling pressures, large LVOT pressure gradient, and a bifid arterial waveform.

Chapters 3 and 32). Genetic testing is most helpful in screening first-degree family members of an HCM patient with a known pathological mutation. Family members without the gene can be excluded from subsequent follow-up testing. Family members who test positive for the gene can be appropriately counseled and treated if symptomatic. Individuals who are gene positive but who do not have other manifestations of HCM should undergo periodic cardiac evaluation. This is particularly important in younger individuals in whom a yearly echocardiography may be advisable. Although participation in some sporting activities may be permitted in G+P− individuals, there is general agreement that G+P+ individuals should avoid competitive athletics. Because the conversion from P− to P+ can occur in middle life, periodic testing should extend into this phase of life. Genetic testing is less useful in the isolated individual who is suspected of having HCM because approximately one-half of HCM patients have a mutation that has not been previously reported. Genetic testing with the hope of providing

prognostic information is also less useful because of the highly variable phenotypic expression of a given genome that is perhaps related to modifier genes and environmental factors.

Cardiac Catheterization

Imaging with echocardiography and CMR in selected cases is usually adequate for diagnosis and management of younger patients with HCM. In symptomatic adults, cardiac catheterization may be required to rule out coronary atherosclerosis and is useful to quantitate LVOT obstruction at rest and with maneuvers that alter loading conditions and LV contractility (see Fig. 30.2).

MANAGEMENT AND THERAPY

There are three primary goals in the management of patients with HCM: (1) symptom relief by lifestyle changes and medications, and septal reduction in drug-refractory patients; (2) sudden death prevention by avoidance of intense exercise and by primary and secondary use of ICDs; (3) stroke prevention by anticoagulation in patients with apical aneurysms and/or atrial fibrillation.

Symptom Relief

Asymptomatic individuals with HCM do not generally require medical therapy. In symptomatic patients with LVOT obstruction, lifestyle changes, including avoidance of dehydration, alcohol consumption, and the splanchnic pooling that accompanies a large meal can be helpful. Beta-blocking drugs are recommended for the treatment of symptoms (angina or dyspnea) in patients with obstructive or nonobstructive HCM and who have a class I indication in the 2011 American College of Cardiology/American Heart Association guidelines statement (Fig. 30.3). Beta-blockers reduce LVOT obstruction primarily during exercise and have favorable effects on LV filling and coronary supply–demand mismatch by prolonging diastole. Verapamil also has a class I indication for patients who do not respond to β-blockers or who do not tolerate them. In patients with LVOT obstruction who do not respond to these class I drugs, disopyramide, an antiarrhythmic with negative inotropic effect, may be effective and has a class IIa indication.

In patients whose symptoms remain refractory to medical therapy, septal reduction strategies have proved to be highly effective. The surgical myectomy pioneered by Dr. Glenn Morrow more than 50 years ago has been modified by extended muscular resection. In HCM centers of excellence such as the Mayo Clinic, Toronto General Hospital, and Emory University, septal myectomy alone has proved to be highly effective in correcting LVOT obstruction, reducing mitral regurgitation, relieving symptoms, and yielding long-term outcomes similar to that expected in the general population. These results suggest that concomitant mitral valve surgery is rarely needed in the treatment of the mitral regurgitation typically seen in HOCM and related to SAM. That is, an effective myectomy treats both LVOT obstruction and SAM-related mitral regurgitation.

Alcohol septal ablation is a catheter-based procedure introduced by Sigwart >20 years ago. By injection of alcohol through a balloon catheter positioned in a septal perforating artery, an infarction of the hypertrophied basal septum is induced (Fig. 30.4). Alcohol injection and resultant septal hypokinesis immediately reduce or abolish the LVOT pressure gradient, SAM, and mitral regurgitation in most patients. Thinning of the septum over time frequently produces a result similar to that achieved surgically (Fig. 30.4F). Disadvantages of alcohol ablation compared with surgical myectomy include heart block that requires permanent pacing in 5% to 20% of patients and that septal artery anatomy limits the ability to target the precise area resected by the surgeon. CMR studies suggest that alcohol injection may cause transmural infarction

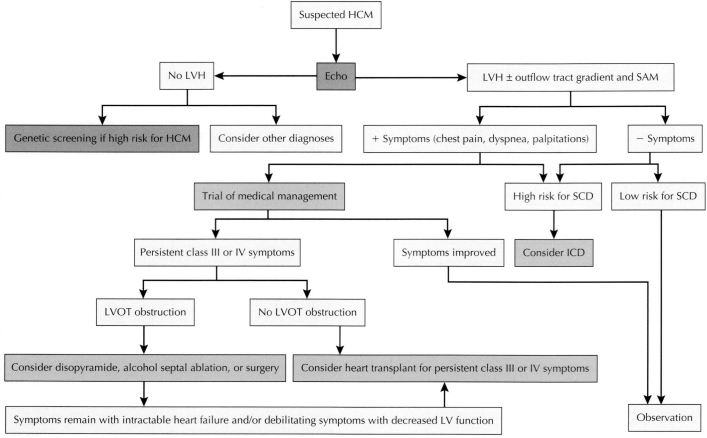

FIG 30.3 Diagnostic Algorithm for Suspected Hypertrophic Cardiomyopathy (HCM). *ICD,* Implantable cardiac-defibrillator; *LV,* left ventricle; *LVH,* LV hypertrophy; *LVOT,* LV outflow tract; *SAM,* systolic anterior motion; *SCD,* sudden cardiac death.

of the septum or infarction of the right side of the septum. Experienced operators have learned to select, where possible, septal arteries originating from diagonal branches or septal branches from the left anterior descending artery that supply the left side of the septum. Use of transthoracic echocardiography during alcohol ablation is essential to identify septal artery supply of sites distant from the septum (e.g., papillary muscles) that should be avoided. The fact that a septal scar is generated by alcohol septal ablation is an additional concern in a patient population with a baseline increased risk of arrhythmic sudden death. These facts and the more limited duration of follow-up of alcohol ablation–treated patients contributed to the recommendations put forth in the 2011 guideline statement in which a class IIa indication was given to myectomy and to alcohol septal ablation when surgery is contraindicated or high risk. Selection of alcohol septal ablation over myectomy by a well-informed patient is a class IIb indication. It is important to note that there are no randomized controlled trials of myectomy versus alcohol septal ablation, and none are expected. In general, there remains a trend toward referral of younger patients for surgical myectomy; older patients and those with comorbidities are referred to alcohol septal ablation. Septal myectomy is a technically demanding operation that requires expertise that is not widely available. Recent data from >5000 patients who underwent myectomy in the United States reported a 5.2% in-hospital mortality. This is in contrast to the reports from HCM centers of excellence of a surgical mortality of <1%. Since the publication of the 2011 guideline statement, increasing use of alcohol septal ablation, especially in Europe, has permitted long-term follow-up data

to be accumulated on large numbers of alcohol septal ablation–treated patients. Although there remain some concerns, the overall results point to favorable long-term safety after alcohol septal ablation. Observational studies indicate 5-year outcomes of alcohol septal ablation–treated patients are similar to the age- and sex-matched general population. Several meta-analyses of patients following myectomy and alcohol septal ablation indicate similar symptom relief and long-term survival. As a result of these observations, the 2014 European HCM guideline statement gives equal class I status to myectomy and alcohol septal ablation in treatment of drug refractory patients. Either procedure may be selected by a well-informed patient.

PREVENTION OF SUDDEN CARDIAC DEATH

The 2011 ACC/AHA and 2014 European HCM guideline statements provide recommendations for prevention of SCD primarily caused by ventricular fibrillation (VF) or VT. Lifestyle changes to exclude competitive athletes and ICD implantation in high-risk patients are the primary strategies. Class I indications for ICD implantation include previous cardiac arrest, VF, or hemodynamically significant VT. Class II indications include sudden death due to HCM in a first-degree relative, maximal LV wall thickness ≥3 cm, and recent unexplained syncope. Nonsustained VT or abnormal blood pressure during exercise when accompanied by other risk factors are also class II. The presence of delayed gadolinium enhancement on CMR, a measure of myocardial fibrosis recently recognized as an important risk factor for SCD, is not

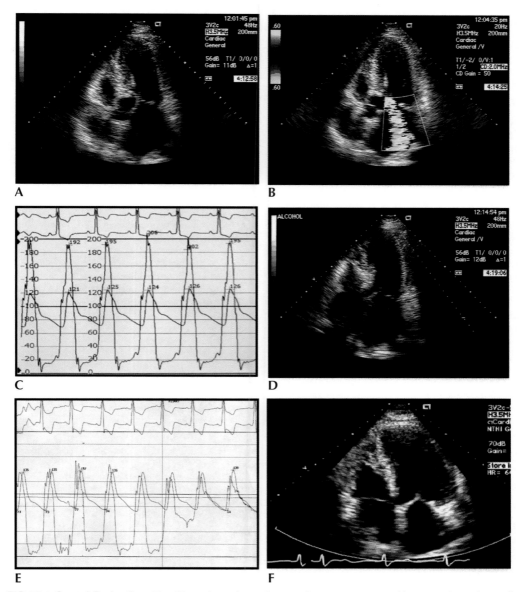

FIG 30.4 Septal Reduction. The (A) resting echocardiogram demonstrates septal hypertrophy and systolic anterior motion (SAM) with septal contact. An eccentric jet of (B) severe mitral regurgitation and (C) large left ventricular outflow tract (LVOT) pressure gradient were present. (D) Injection of agitated contrast into the first septal perforating branch followed by alcohol-produced basal septal brightening. (E) The LVOT pressure gradient was abolished immediately. (F) An echocardiogram 6 months later revealed reduction in basal septal thickness and no SAM. The echocardiographic results are similar to that achieved with myectomy. The patient became completely asymptomatic and had no mitral regurgitation or LVOT pressure gradient.

addressed in the 2011 or 2014 guideline statements. Please see Chapter 44 for further discussion of the use of ICDs.

There has been considerable controversy as to whether ECGs should be used for pre-participation screening of young athletes (Fig. 30.1). The American Heart Association guidelines do not recommend that ECGs be used because of high false-positive rates. However, recent studies performed in >10,000 young soccer players in the English Football Association indicated that updates to the "Refined Seattle Criteria" reduced the overall abnormal ECG rate to 2.1% while detecting >96% of serious cardiac pathology. These findings will likely lead to widespread use of ECGs in pre-participation screening of young athletes (see Chapter 42).

FUTURE DIRECTIONS

More cost effective diagnostic tools are needed to evaluate individuals with suspected HCM and for pre-participation screening of young athletes. HCM is an orphan disease that has been treated with old drugs developed for other diseases and applied to the treatment of HCM without randomized controlled trials. Pharmacological research of novel agents targeting intracellular pathways in HCM is underway and has promise to normalize energy homeostasis and reduce diastolic dysfunction and arrhythmogenesis. Studies are also underway with the aim of attenuating the phenotypic expression of HCM in GP+/P− individuals, and initial pilot trials show promise.

ADDITIONAL RESOURCES

Maron BJ, Roberts WC. The father of septal myectomy for HCM, who also had HCM. The unbelievable story. *J Am Coll Cardiol.* 2016;67:2900–2903.
This is a "must read."

Rowin EJ, Maron BJ, Haas TS, et al. Hypertrophic cardiomyopathy with left ventricular apical aneurysm: implications for risk stratification and management. *J Am Coll Cardiol.* 2017;69:761–773.
This study provides new insights into the subset of patients with hypertrophic cardiomyopathy and apical aneurysms.

Singh K, Qutub M, Carson K, et al. A meta analysis of current status of alcohol septal ablation and surgical myectomy for obstructive hypertrophic cardiomyopathy. *Catheter Cardiovasc Interv.* 2016;88:107–115.
This is the most recent meta-analysis comparing alcohol septal ablation and myectomy.

Steggerda RC, Geluk CA, Brouwer W, et al. Basal infarct location but not larger infarct size is associated with a successful outcome after alcohol septal ablation in patients with hypertrophic obstructive cardiomyopathy. *Int J Cardiovasc Imaging.* 2015;31:831–839.
Cardiac MR is an important tool for understanding alcohol septal ablation outcomes.

Veselka J, Jensen MK, Liebregts M, et al. Long-term clinical outcome after alcohol septal ablation for obstructive hypertrophic cardiomyopathy. *Eur Heart J.* 2017;37:1517–1523.
An important long-term follow-up of >1000 patients following alcohol septal ablation.

EVIDENCE

Elliott PM, Anastasakis A, Borger MA, et al. 2014 European Society of Cardiology guidelines on diagnosis and management of HCM. *Eur Heart J.* 2014;35:2733–2799.
The European guidelines are a bit more current than the American College of Cardiology/American Heart Association guidelines.

Feldman DN, Douglas JS, Naidu SS. Indications for and individualization of septal reduction therapy. In: Naidu SS, eds. *Hypertrophic Cardiomyopathy.* London, United Kingdom: Springer-Verlag; 2015:207.
This is one chapter from a very comprehensive book focusing on HCM.

Gersh B, Maron BJ, Bonow RO, et al. 2011 ACCF/AHA guideline for the diagnosis and treatment of HCM. *J Am Coll Cardiol.* 2011;58:e212.
This important guideline statement summarizes the North American approach to HCM.

Maron BJ, Casey SA, Chan RH, et al. Independent assessment of the European society of cardiology sudden death risk model for HCM. *Am J Cardiol.* 2015;116.
An important look at sudden death prevention.

Maron BJ, Ommen SR, Semsarian C, et al. Hypertrophic cardiomyopathy: present and future, with translation into contemporary cardiovascular medicine. *J Am Coll Cardiol.* 2014;64:83–99.
This is a good summary of current understanding of HCM.

31

Restrictive Cardiomyopathy

Thomas M. Bashore

ETIOLOGY AND PATHOPHYSIOLOGY

The variety of disease states that may result in a restrictive cardiomyopathic process are summarized in Box 31.1. Myocardial fibrosis, myocardial infiltration by specific proteins, endomyocardial scarring, and cardiac muscle hypertrophy all may contribute to diastolic dysfunction. Recent genetic studies have found a substantial number of patients with "idiopathic" restrictive cardiomyopathy (CM) caused by mutations in genes that have traditionally been associated with hypertrophic CM (HCM), some dilated CMs, and noncompaction. The finding of TNN13 mutations in some patients suggests a causal relationship with idiopathic restrictive CM, and this variant may be especially important in children and young adults who have especially severe disease. A working group with the European Society of Cardiology (ESC) has proposed a revised classification to include recognition of some of these genetic variants to include familial restrictive CM associated with sarcomeric protein gene mutations, such as with troponin I (restrictive CM ± HCM) and familial amyloidosis (transthyretin or apolipoprotein). Other identifiable causes include some desminopathies and associated systemic diseases, such as pseudoxanthoma elasticum, hemochromatosis, Fabry disease, and glycogen storage diseases.

Restrictive CM encompasses a spectrum of endomyocardial disease and is characterized by variable degrees of diastolic dysfunction out of proportion to systolic dysfunction. The ventricle is not dilated, but filling is impaired. Survival is poor in most patients. Hypertrophy may or may not be present except in infiltrative disorders, in which it is a constant. Restrictive CM is much less common than dilated or HCM outside the tropics, but remains a frequent cause of death in Africa, South and Central America, India, and Asia due to a high number of endomyocardial fibrosis cases in these regions.

Clinically, restrictive CM is often confused with constrictive pericarditis. Restrictive CM was originally described in 1961 as constrictive CM. This was later changed to the more accurate term, restrictive CM, in recognition of the primary myocardial nature of the problem. Differentiating between the two is a challenge but is important because of the implications for prognosis and treatment. Restrictive CM and constrictive pericarditis can also both be present in the same patient, further complicating the diagnosis and therapeutic decision-making. Because constrictive pericarditis is eminently more treatable than restrictive CM, the distinction is critical.

Restrictive CM is to be distinguished from secondary heart failure due to diastolic dysfunction and normal left ventricular (LV) systolic function (so-called heart failure with preserved ejection fraction [HFpEF]). HFpEF encompasses a mixed group of clinical diseases associated with valvular heart disease, pericardial disease, and right heart failure. It is related to pathological LV hypertrophy secondary to diseases such as aortic stenosis, systemic hypertension, and increased systemic arterial stiffness, and is particularly common in older adults.

Noninfiltrative Causes

Idiopathic restrictive CM is associated with patchy endomyocardial fibrosis, increased cardiac mass, and enlarged atria (Fig. 31.1). It is a rare condition. It is more common in older adults, but may be seen in children. In adults, 5-year survival is approximately 64%, and unfortunately, mortality may be even higher in children. Occasionally, the CM is accompanied by skeletal muscle myopathy, and in some patients, a clear familial component is definable. There are data that reveal increased myofilament sensitivity to calcium, as well as an increase in desmin and collagen accumulation. However, idiopathic restrictive CM is also found in families with no skeletal muscle involvement, and as an autosomal dominant disorder in patients with Noonan syndrome. Conduction system disease such as atrioventricular (AV) block may also be present, and conduction disease often precedes clinical myocardial dysfunction.

Infiltrative Causes

In adults, the most common variety of restrictive CM is due to amyloidosis. The diastolic dysfunction is due to the deposition of unique, twisted, β-pleated sheets of fibrils formed by various proteins (Fig. 31.1B). Although 25 different amyloidogenic proteins have been found, 3 are important for cardiac involvement. They are defined by their precursor proteins, primary AL (light chain) amyloidosis, secondary (AA) amyloidosis, or familial or senile (ATTR) amyloidosis. AL amyloidosis is caused by deposition of an amyloid protein composed of portions of an immunoglobulin light chain (designated AL for light chain–associated amyloidosis) produced by a monoclonal population of plasma cells. AL amyloidosis may or may not be the consequence of multiple myeloma. Cardiac involvement occurs in up to 50% of patients. AA amyloidosis is caused by the production of a nonimmunoglobulin protein and termed AA (for amyloid-associated) disease. Fragments of serum amyloid A, an acute phase reactant, are responsible. A β-2 reactive protein has been noted in dialysis patients. Cardiac involvement is rare (5%) in AA amyloid, and the protein may be associated with a variety of chronic inflammatory processes (e.g., rheumatoid arthritis). In ATTR amyloidosis, the protein consists of wild-type (nonmutant) or mutated transthyretin (TTR). TTR is a small protein produced in the liver. Wild-type TTR is responsible for senile systemic amyloidosis and frequently results in small amounts of cardiac amyloid deposition. One-quarter to one-third of individuals aged older than 80 year have evidence of this deposition. Most of the time there is little clinical heart failure, although atrial arrhythmias are common. Some mutations in the gene for TTR are more likely to result in a restrictive CM, whereas others are more likely to present with neurological or renal involvement. Mutant TTR is the main cause for familial amyloidosis. Familial amyloidosis is four times more common in blacks than in whites. An identified mutation, Val122Ile, is present in 3% to 4% of those of African descent and is associated with late-onset restrictive CM. Less common mutations include β-2 microglobulin dialysis-related amyloidosis and atrial natriuretic peptide amyloidosis. More than 80 mutations have been described. Mutant ATTR amyloid has a better prognosis than AL amyloid.

Regardless of the specific etiology, the overall size of the LV chamber is normal or small, and at least early in the disease, systolic function is mostly preserved even in individuals with significant diastolic dysfunction. The greater the myocardial thickness, the more amyloid is present, and the worse the prognosis.

Patients with cardiac amyloid present with severe diastolic dysfunction and predominantly right-sided heart failure. Later, there may be progressive loss of LV systolic function and pulmonary congestion. Amyloid deposits in the atria can produce a markedly thickened interatrial septum and loss of atrial function. Many patients experience arrhythmia and/or conduction system disease. Bradycardia is common, especially in ATTR amyloidosis; pacemaker implantation is often required. Ventricular arrhythmias may occur, but some observational data suggest that implantable cardioverter-defibrillators may not prolong life because many die from electromechanical dissociation. In patients with AL amyloid, atrial fibrillation and/or atrial contractile dysfunction can result in intracardiac thrombus, and these patients are at risk for thromboembolism. Small vessel disease in amyloidosis may manifest as purpura or angina. Periorbital purpura may occur with coughing or minor trauma. Macroglossia is evident in many with AL amyloid. Leg or jaw pain suggests vascular amyloidosis as well.

Amyloid deposits can also involve the pericardium with resultant pericardial effusions, and these may be large at times. Peripheral neuropathy is common, and orthostatic hypotension may be a major

A. Idiopathic cardiomyopathy

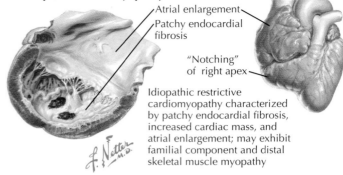

Atrial enlargement
Patchy endocardial fibrosis
"Notching" of right apex

Idiopathic restrictive cardiomyopathy characterized by patchy endocardial fibrosis, increased cardiac mass, and atrial enlargement; may exhibit familial component and distal skeletal muscle myopathy

B. Amyloidosis

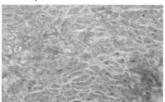 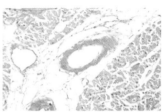

Focal deposition of amyloid around muscle cells of heart with dead myocardial fibers

Perivascular amyloid deposits in myocardium (×40)

Amyloidosis is the most common form of restrictive cardiomyopathy. Characterized by deposition of amyloid protein throughout the myocardium, causing thickening and diastolic dysfunction

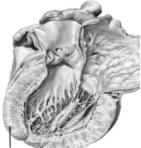

Thickened myocardium

C. Sarcoidosis

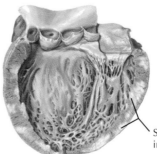 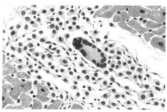

Granuloma with giant cell in heart wall

Scattered sarcoid granulomas in myocardium

Sarcoidosis exhibits myocardial involvement in a small percentage of patients with the systemic disease. Granulomas in myocardium lead to diastolic dysfunction, congestive heart failure, heart block, ventricular arrhythmias, and sudden cardiac death.

FIG 31.1 Idiopathic and Infiltrative Causes of Restrictive Cardiomyopathy.

A. Becker disease

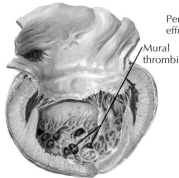

Peastricardial effusion

Mural thrombi

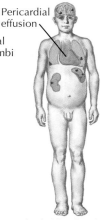

Endomyocardial fibrosis (Becker disease) occurs most commonly in Africa. Pericardial effusions are common. Fibrous endocardial lesions often involve AV valves. Myocardium shows a thick layer of collagen over loose connective tissue. Mural thrombi are common.

Multiple bland embolic infarctions (lung, spleen, brain, kidney); enlarged heart with episodic failure (enlarged liver, ascites, edema, episodic fever)

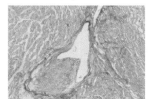

Verrucous lesions on thickened, edematous endocardium

Hyalinized polypoid protrusion into lumen of subendocardial vein

B. Löffler endocarditis

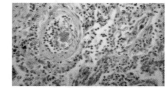

Acute eosinophilic endarteritis in lung; similar lesions occur in small vessels of brain, kidney, and other organs.

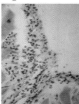 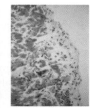

Acute eosinophilic and neutrophilic infiltration of subendocardium

Eosinophilic infiltration and early myocardial damage

Löffler endocarditis (eosinophilic endocarditis) likely a manifestation of same condition as Becker disease; both may be associated with eosinophilia and may be associated with a helminthic infestation.

Brain

Multiple embolic infarcts (lung, brain, spleen, kidney) and diffuse arteriolitis

Heart enlarged

Liver enlarged

Ascites

Edema

Leukocytosis, eosinophilia

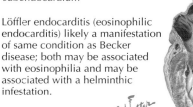

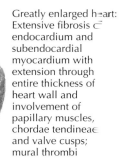

Greatly enlarged heart: Extensive fibrosis c̄ endocardium and subendocardial myocardium with extension through entire thickness of heart wall and involvement of papillary muscles, chordae tendineae and valve cusps; mural thrombi

FIG 31.2 Endomyocardial Causes of Restrictive Cardiomyopathy. *AV*, Atrioventricular.

feature that can become debilitating. Orthostasis is worsened by amyloid involvement in the adrenals and nephrotic syndrome due to renal involvement.

AL amyloidosis typically presents after the age of 40 years, wild-type TTR often occurs after the age of 60 to 70 years and mutant TTR presents at various ages from 30 to 70 years. AL cardiac amyloidosis carries the poorest prognosis and is generally harder to treat due to the associated orthostasis and frequent proteinuria.

Sarcoidosis is a granulomatous disease of unknown cause (Fig. 31.1C). Of the multiple organ systems commonly involved, including the heart, the most important is usually the lungs, where this involvement manifests as diffuse scarring and pulmonary hypertension that may lead to cor pulmonale. Myocardial involvement results in a restrictive or a dilated CM in <5% of systemic sarcoidosis patients. More commonly, focal cardiac involvement results in heart block, congestive failure, ventricular arrhythmias, or sudden cardiac death. The noncaseating granulomas have a propensity for involving the interventricular septum (hence, the high incidence of heart block) and the LV free wall. The scattered nature of granulomas contributes to the failure of right ventricular (RV) biopsies to detect the disease in approximately one-half the patients in which it is attempted. Cardiac MRI is sensitive for detection of cardiac involvement in patients with known sarcoidosis.

Clinically, patients with sarcoidosis generally present with syncope from conduction system disease or cor pulmonale from both the pulmonary manifestations and associated cardiac involvement. Myocardial sarcoidosis is usually gradually progressive, although it can be fulminant and lead rapidly to death.

Endomyocardial Causes

Endomyocardial fibrosis (sometimes called Becker disease) occurs primarily in Africa, especially in Uganda and Nigeria (Fig. 31.2A). In equatorial Africa, it is responsible for 10% to 20% of all deaths from heart disease. It is estimated that 12 million people worldwide may be affected by the disease. Pericardial effusions are common and may be quite large. Fibrous endocardial lesions are frequently noted in the ventricular inflow tracts and often involve the AV valves, which results in valvular regurgitation. The involved myocardium demonstrates a thick layer of collagen tissue overlying a layer of loosely arranged connective tissue. Fibrous and granulomatous tissue extend into the myocardium. Either or both ventricles may be involved and when the disease process is extensive. Papillary muscles and chordae may be matted with a mass of thrombus and endothelial tissue that will virtually fill the ventricular cavity. The clinical presentation depends on the extent of involvement of the RV, the LV, or both. Echocardiography and cardiac MRI can be diagnostic, with MRI having a greater sensitivity for detecting thrombus.

Eosinophilic endocarditis (Löffler endocarditis) is probably just an earlier manifestation of this same process (Fig. 31.2B). Both diseases are associated with eosinophilia. Some epidemiological evidence suggests that Löffler endocarditis is related to a worm (helminth) infestation. It is believed the myocardial damage occurs during the initial (necrotic) phase of hypereosinophilia. This is then followed a year or more by a thrombotic phase, and finally by a fibrotic, restrictive phase. Clinically, the initial phase is characterized by fever, weight loss, rash, and congestive heart failure. Localized thickening of the posterolateral LV wall and limited mitral valve movement may be noted. In some instances, the LV apex is virtually obliterated by thrombus. Later, a restrictive pattern with AV regurgitation dominates the hemodynamics, and pericardial effusions, sometimes quite large, are evident.

Patients with Churg-Strauss syndrome (asthma, eosinophilia, neuropathy, pulmonary infiltrates, paranasal sinus abnormalities, and/or extravascular eosinophils) may also develop endomyocardial fibrosis. The intracytoplasmic granular content of activated eosinophils may be toxic to the myocardial and endothelial cells, resulting in the damage observed.

Previous radiation therapy is an important cause of restrictive CM. It is believed that radiation may cause long-lasting injury to the capillary endothelial cells, leading to cell death, capillary rupture, and microthrombi. Cardiac complications usually occur many years after the initial insult and can vary widely, with constrictive pericarditis a more common manifestation than restrictive CM. Pericarditis with effusion, coronary artery fibrosis (especially ostial) and myocardial infarction, valvular stenosis or regurgitation, conduction system disease, and myocardial fibrosis may be the consequence of excessive previous radiation exposure. The severity of cardiac involvement is proportional to the radiation dose (more common at doses >45 Gy) and to the mass of myocardium exposed. Cardiac radiation exposure is most common after therapy for Hodgkin disease or breast cancer, and despite attempts to shield the heart from radiation and more focused radiation beam shaping, radiation heart disease remains a concern. In addition, damage to the myocardium may also occur from associated chemotherapy usage, with the ultimate result being either systolic or diastolic dysfunction, or both. Separating the effects of radiation from the consequences of chemotherapy is not always possible.

The most common cardiotoxic chemotherapeutic agents are the anthracyclines. After anthracycline exposure, cardiac toxicity usually is delayed and normally results in a dilated CM. However, early manifestations of primarily diastolic dysfunction may herald cardiotoxicity. There is a nonlinear increase in cardiotoxicity as the cumulative dose increases, with a 7% incidence with doxorubicin doses >550 mg/m^2. Cytotoxicity from anthracyclines seems to be due to the inhibition of an enzyme necessary for DNA repair and to the generation of free radicals that damage cell membranes, in part by lipid peroxidation. The heart may not be able to detoxify the free radicals because only a small amount of catalase needed to convert hydrogen peroxide to water is present. The anthracyclines also chelate iron and generate tissue-damaging hydroxyl radicals locally. For this reason, dexrazoxane, a drug that hydrolyzes to form a carboxylamine capable of removing the iron from the anthracycline-iron complex, is often used as a cardioprotectant in patients receiving anthracyclines. Other toxic drugs that have been implicated in the development of myocardial fibrosis include methysergide, ergotamine, mercurial agents, and busulfan. Endomyocardial biopsies with these drugs reveal considerable disruption of the normal muscle architecture. Valvular thickening and conduction abnormalities are also common.

Other Causes of Restrictive Cardiomyopathy

Less common causes of restrictive CM include certain inherited diseases. The most prominent is Fabry disease, an X-linked recessive disorder caused by deficiency of the lysosomal enzyme α-galactosidase. The accumulation of lysosomal glycolipids in cardiac tissue results in a severe, restrictive CM. Some patients with Fabry disease also have involvement of the cardiac valves, the skin, the kidneys, and the lungs.

HCM can present in a similar manner as a restrictive CM. Many mutations in sarcomeric proteins have been identified in the genetic profile of patients with HCM (see Chapter 30), and there is variability in the degree of diastolic dysfunction depending on both the genotype

as well as concomitant diseases (hypertension, diabetes). Generally, it is not difficult to distinguish HCM from other causes of restrictive CM. The law of Laplace defines wall tension as the product of the chamber pressure multiplied by the chamber radius divided by the wall thickness. In HCM, the thickened walls of the LV result in lowering wall tension, which results in a high LV ejection fraction (EF). In infiltrative myocardial diseases, the thickened LV walls reduce myocardial contraction and result in a small chamber with an abnormally low LVEF.

Other inherited diseases are rare, and hence, are a less common cause of restrictive CM. In Gaucher disease (characterized by a deficiency of the enzyme β-glucosidase, with accumulation of cerebrosides in various organs), there may be both myocardial dysfunction and hemorrhagic pericardial effusion. In Hurler syndrome, a deposition of mucopolysaccharide in the myocardium can cause a restrictive process. The cardiac valves and the coronary arteries may also be involved. Hemochromatosis, arising from inherited (autosomal-recessive) or acquired etiologies, is characterized by iron deposition in many organs, including the heart. Myocardial damage may result from direct tissue damage by the free-iron moiety, not from the infiltration of iron. Approximately 15% of patients have cardiac involvement that can be confirmed by cardiac MRI. Other rare systemic diseases include Danon disease (lysosome-associated membrane protein 2) and PRKAG2 (protein kinase adenosine monophosphate (AMP)–activated noncatalytic subunit γ-2) deficiencies, in which Wolff-Parkinson-White syndrome may be associated as well.

Many reports have described massive trabeculations in the LV toward the apex with large sinus recesses between the trabeculae, which is a pattern that defines ventricular noncompaction. Noncompaction is a genetic disorder that may present with any or all the features of a restrictive CM. Cardiac MRI is usually definitive.

Carcinoid heart disease primarily affects the right heart and is characterized by fibrous plaque that virtually coats the tricuspid and pulmonic valves and the RV endocardium. Valvular stenosis and regurgitation result, and RV dysfunction is common. The cardiac involvement in patients with carcinoid correlates with serotonin concentrations.

Friedreich ataxia is an autosomal recessive neurodegenerative disorder seen in Caucasians. It is caused by a mutation of the frataxin gene that results in diabetes, ataxia, and heart failure due to a restrictive CM in the second to third decade of life.

CLINICAL PRESENTATION

In addition to some of the unique clinical presentations described earlier, as a rule, patients with restrictive CM present with congestion and low-output symptoms. Dyspnea, paroxysmal nocturnal dyspnea, orthopnea, peripheral edema, ascites, and overall fatigue and weakness are common. Angina can be a presenting symptom if coronary arteries are involved. Atrial fibrillation is common, and heart block is a particularly common occurrence in patients with amyloidosis or sarcoidosis. Up to one-third of patients may present with thromboembolic complications.

DIFFERENTIAL DIAGNOSIS

Most patients present with right heart failure out of proportion to left heart failure and have normal or near-normal cardiac size on examination and chest x-ray. Although not specific for restrictive CM, this constellation of symptoms, signs, and findings should always raise the possibility of restrictive CM. The differential diagnosis of restrictive CM includes several cardiac causes: constrictive pericarditis, chronic RV infarction, RV dysfunction from RV pressure or (less likely) RV volume overload, intrinsic RV myocardial disease, or tricuspid valve disease. With evidence of right heart failure, ascites, and marked hepatic

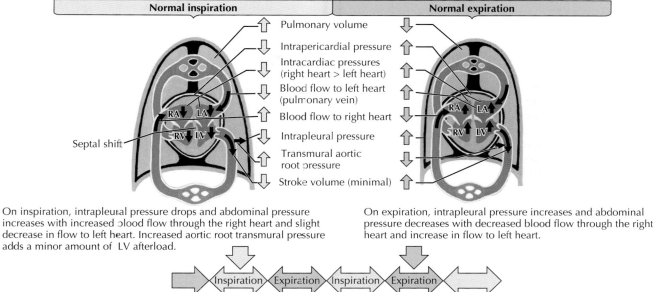

Normal inspiration	Normal expiration

Pulmonary volume ⇑ ⇓

Intrapericardial pressure ⇓ ⇑

Intracardiac pressures (right heart > left heart) ⇓ ⇑

Blood flow to left heart (pulmonary vein) ⇓ ⇑

Blood flow to right heart ⇑ ⇓

Intrapleural pressure ⇓ ⇑

Transmural aortic root pressure ⇑ ⇓

Stroke volume (minimal) ⇓ ⇑

Septal shift

On inspiration, intrapleural pressure drops and abdominal pressure increases with increased blood flow through the right heart and slight decrease in flow to left heart. Increased aortic root transmural pressure adds a minor amount of LV afterload.

On expiration, intrapleural pressure increases and abdominal pressure decreases with decreased blood flow through the right heart and increase in flow to left heart.

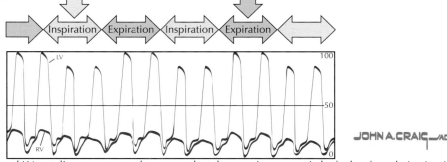

Inspiration Expiration Inspiration Expiration

JOHN A. CRAIG—AD

Simultaneous measurement of RV and LV systolic pressure reveals a concordant decrease in pressure in both chambers during inspiration, with a similar concordant increase in pressure in both ventricles during expiration. Pressure changes are exaggerated for emphasis.

FIG 31.3 Normal Cardiac Blood Flow During Inspiration and Expiration. *LA*, Left atrium; *LV*, left ventricle/ventricular; *RA*, right atrium; *RV*, right ventricle/ventricular.

dysfunction, separating primary from right heart-induced hepatic cirrhosis may be challenging at times. Distinguishing restrictive CM from constrictive pericarditis can generally be accomplished using noninvasive and invasive studies. These two entities affect hemodynamics in a subtly different manner, and distinguishing the two is important because of the difference in prognosis and treatment options.

Normal Hemodynamics

Intracardiac pressures reflect the contraction and relaxation of individual cardiac chambers and the changes imparted to them by the simultaneous pleural and pericardial pressures (Fig. 31.3). To help understand respiratory changes, one should picture inspiration as pulling venous blood through the RV to the pulmonary artery. This lowering of intrathoracic pressure results in increasing flow to the right side of the heart with simultaneous reduction in blood flow to the left heart. The fall in the intrapleural pressures with inspiration also slightly increases the transmural aortic root pressure, effectively increasing the impedance to LV ejection. The reverse occurs during expiration. In severe lung disease, such as asthma, the swings in blood flow in inspiration and expiration are exaggerated with a marked decrease in intrathoracic pressure with inspiration and a marked increase in intrathoracic pressure with expiration. These negative inspiratory intrapleural pressures and positive expiratory pressures result in magnified swings in LV filling, and a paradoxical pulse may result.

The normal atrial and ventricular waveforms are shown in upper Fig. 31.4. With atrial contraction, the atria becomes smaller and the atrial pressures rise (*a* wave). With the onset of ventricular contraction,

the AV valves bulge toward the atria, and a small *c* wave is typically detectable on hemodynamic tracings. As ventricular contraction continues, the AV annular ring is pulled into the ventricular cavity, and the atria go into their diastole, resulting in enlargement of the atria and a decrease in the atrial pressures (*x* descent). Passive filling of the atria during ventricular systole produces a slow rise in the atrial pressures (the *v* wave) until the AV valves reopen at the peak of the *v* wave, and the pressure then falls rapidly as the ventricles actively relax (the *y* descent), and blood runs from the atria to the ventricles. Passive filling of the ventricles continues while the AV valves are open through atrial contraction again, and the cycle repeats with the onset of the next ventricular contraction.

Ventricular diastole can be divided into an initial active phase (a brief period when the ventricle fills about halfway) and a passive filling phase. The nadir or lowest diastolic pressure during ventricular diastole occurs at the end of the early active relaxation phase (suction effect).

Constrictive Pericarditis Physiology

Constrictive pericarditis (Fig. 31.4B) and restrictive CM (Fig. 31.4C) alter the normal intracardiac pressures in several ways as described in these figures. Please refer to Chapter 57, which covers expected respiratory changes with their impact on ventricular flow in these two diseases.

Because the atrial and ventricular septi are normally unaffected by the pericardial process, in restrictive CM, both the RV systolic and LV systolic pressures should fall with inspiration. If constrictive pericarditis is present, with inspiration, the RV systolic pressure and area of the RV

A. Normal

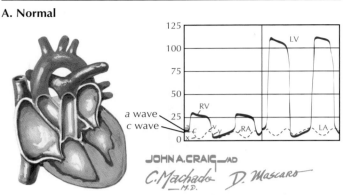

Atrial contraction reduces atrial volume and increases atrial pressure (a wave). Ventricular contraction closes the AV valve and creates the c wave. The AV ring is pulled into the atria, and atrial relaxation ensues with pressure decrease (x descent). Passive atrial filling causes v wave until AV valves open and pressure drops rapidly (y descent) while ventricles relax. Following ventricular systole, an active and passive diastolic filling phase follows, with ventricular pressure lowest in the active phase.

B. Constrictive pericarditis

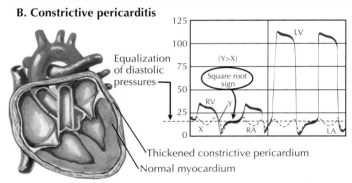

High atrial pressures when AV valves open result in rapid early filling (rapid y descent) until filling abruptly stops (square root sign). There is equalization of late diastolic pressures. The right ventricular diastolic is usually > one-third the right ventricular systolic.

C. Restrictive cardiomyopathy

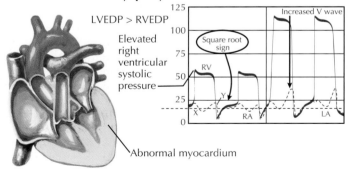

Restrictive cardiomyopathy exhibits high atrial pressures with early and rapid diastolic filling. Left heart diastolic pressures are higher than the right heart, and LVEDP is greater than RVEDP. A large v wave in left atrium reflects poor left atrial compliance. Pulmonary hypertension results, and the RV systolic pressure is elevated.

FIG 31.4 Comparisons of Normal and Pathological Intracardiac Pressures. *AV,* Atrioventricular; *LA,* left atrial; *LV,* left ventricular; *LVEDP,* left ventricular end-diastolic pressure; *RA,* right atrial; *RV,* right ventricular; *RVEDP,* right ventricular end-diastolic pressure.

pressure tracing will rise as the LV systolic pressure and area of the LV pressure tracing falls, which demonstrates ventricular interdependence. It is critical to demonstrate ventricular interdependence to diagnose constriction. In addition, in constrictive pericarditis, the RV and pulmonary arterial systolic pressures are usually normal, and there is equalization of the RV and LV end-diastolic pressures. The high RV end-diastolic pressure results in the RV end-diastolic pressure being greater than one-third of the RV systolic pressure.

Restrictive Cardiomyopathy Physiology

In restrictive CM, the atrial pressures are high, with the filling wave (*v* wave) at times markedly elevated due to the poor atrial compliance. When the AV valve opens, there is a high driving pressure from the prominent atrial *v* wave into the ventricle, and this results in rapid early ventricular filling. The stiff ventricle stops the rapid filling abruptly as diastole ensues. This sudden stoppage of inflow produces the "square root" sign in the diastolic filling pattern similar to that seen in constriction, although in this case, the myocardium provides the restraint. As opposed to constrictive pericarditis, the end-diastolic LV pressure is consistently higher (>5 mm Hg) than that of the end-diastolic RV pressure. The prominent left atrial (LA) *v* wave results in the mean LA pressure being quite high, and pulmonary hypertension results. This differs greatly from the expected normal pulmonary artery pressures in constrictive pericarditis and assists in separating the two syndromes (Fig. 31.4). In a patient with myocardial restriction but a normal pericardium, the normal inspiratory decrease in all intracardiac pressures is expected, and there are concordant changes in the RV and LV systolic pressures during the entire respiratory cycle. This lack of demonstrable ventricular interdependence helps define restrictive CM from constrictive pericarditis.

DIAGNOSTIC APPROACH

Procedures that will aid in the differential diagnosis of restrictive CM are outlined in Table 31.1.

Electrocardiography

The ECG in patients with restrictive CM is often abnormal but usually nonspecific. Low voltage may be a prominent feature, especially in amyloidosis. The QRS pattern often simulates myocardial infarction with poor R-wave progression in the precordial leads or a pseudoinfarction pattern in the inferior leads. If pulmonary hypertension is present, evidence of RV hypertrophy may be noted. Interatrial conduction delays (notched P waves) and evidence of atrial enlargement are also common. AV heart block is common in sarcoidosis. High-grade AV block is less commonly seen in amyloidosis, but first-degree AV block is often present. Atrial arrhythmias, especially fibrillation, are common, although these are rarely a presenting symptom; sick sinus syndrome is also frequent. Ventricular tachyarrhythmias increase because with disease progression and in amyloidosis, these may be a harbinger of sudden cardiac death.

Laboratory Testing

There are no specific blood markers for restrictive CM, and often blood tests are unrevealing. That being said, patients who present with a restrictive CM should be screened for any systemic disease that might be contributory. Serum troponin, brain natriuretic peptide (BNP), and proBNP have been found to be elevated in amyloidosis even without clinical heart failure, and are associated with poor prognosis. In one series, an N–terminal-proBNP >8500 was associated with a median survival in amyloidosis of 3 months. The presence of a serum or urine monoclonal paraprotein is important in the evaluation of amyloidosis. A complete blood count with differential can exclude anemia and

TABLE 31.1 Differential Diagnosis of Restrictive Cardiomyopathy Versus Constrictive Pericarditis

Examination Procedure	Restrictive Cardiomyopathy	Constrictive Pericarditis
Physical examination	Kussmaul sign is occasionally present. Paradoxical pulse is absent. Apical impulse is prominent. S_3 and S_4 are present. Regurgitant AV valve murmurs are common.	Kussmaul sign is common. Paradoxical pulse may be present. Apical impulse retracts or is absent. Pericardial knock may be present. Regurgitant AV valve murmurs are rare.
Chest x-ray	Enlarged atria Pulmonary edema at times	Normal heart size Occasional pericardial calcium
ECG	Low voltage Atrial hypertrophic P waves Conduction disease is common. Atrial fibrillation is common.	Occasional low voltage P waves reflect interatrial conduction delay. Conduction defects are rare. Atrial fibrillation is occasionally present.

Echocardiography	Small or normal LV cavity with large atria
	Increased wall thickness; sparkling texture
	Thickened cardiac valves at times
	Septal bounce rarely seen.
	Little septal movement with inspiration
	Thickened atrial septum
	<15% inspiratory decrease in MV velocity
	In PV: D>S (S/D ratio <1)
	
	TV inflow velocity with inspiration:
	  Mild decrease in E wave
	  No change in peak TR velocity
	Myocardial Ea <8.0 cm/s (reduced)
	M-mode slope of inflow color velocity edge <100 cm/s
		Mild or no atrial enlargement
		Normal wall thickness
		
		Abrupt septal bounce in early diastole
		Septal movement toward left ventricle with inspiration
		Normal atrial septum
		>25% inspiratory decrease in MV velocity
		In PV: S>D
		In PV: inspiratory decrease in S and D waves
		TV inflow velocity with inspiration:
		  Decreased inflow E wave
		  Increased peak TR velocity
		Myocardial Ea >8.0 cm/s (normal or increased)
		M-mode slope of inflow color velocity edge >100 cm/s

Cardiac catheterization	LVEDP – RVEDP >5 mm Hg Pulmonary hypertension Dip and plateau in RA and RV are common. RVEDP <⅓rd RV systolic Late inspiratory RV/LV systolic pressure in phase (concordant) Area of LV pressure tracing/area of RV pressure tracing ratio similar in both inspiration and expiration. Paradoxical pulse is rare.	Equalization of pressures LVEDP – RVEDP <5 mm Hg PA systolic rarely >40 mm Hg Dip and plateau in RA and RV are common. RVEDP >⅓rd RV systolic Inspiratory RV/LV systolic pressure discordant. Area of LV/area of RV pressure tracing ratio declines with inspiration as RV systolic pressure rises as LV systolic falls. Paradoxical pulse is more common.
CT/MRI	LA enlargement, LV hypertrophy, thickened atrial septum, hyperenhancement related to fibrosis, normal pericardium	Occasionally thickened pericardium or calcium

AV, Atrioventricular; *LA*, left atrial; *LV*, left ventricular; *LVEDP*, left ventricular end-diastolic pressure; *MV*, mitral valve; *PA*, pulmonary artery; *PV*, pulmonary vein; *RA*, right atrial; *RV*, right ventricular; *RVEDP*, right ventricular end-diastolic pressure; *TR*, tricuspid regurgitant; *TV*, tricuspid valve.

eosinophilia as causes or contributors to heart failure. The sedimentation rate may be reduced in patients with right heart failure due to lower serum proteins in liver congestion; therefore an elevated sedimentation rate is clearly abnormal and may suggest an inflammatory process such as sarcoidosis. Although insensitive, an elevated angiotensin-converting enzyme level may also be present in sarcoidosis. Renal failure should be excluded, because it may suggest Fabry disease or renal involvement from another systemic process. A 24-hour urine for total protein is indicated to exclude a nephrotic syndrome if the serum albumin is low. Hemochromatosis is characterized by an elevated plasma iron level, a normal or low total iron-binding capacity, elevated serum ferritin, high saturation of transferrin, and urinary iron. Carcinoid syndrome is associated with high levels of circulating serotonin and urinary 5-hydroxyindoleacetic acid. Endemic forms of endomyocardial

fibrosis have been related to high levels of cerium and low levels of magnesium.

Systemic amyloidosis may be demonstrated by abdominal fat biopsy (AL amyloid), and a bone marrow biopsy will demonstrate plasma cell dyscrasia in a high number of patients. A high plasma cell burden (>30% cellularity) suggests co-existent multiple myeloma.

Chest X-Ray

The chest x-ray in most restrictive CMs reveals a normal heart size with enlarged atria. If pulmonary hypertension is present, an enlarged RV and pulmonary arteries may be seen. Pericardial calcium is usually not present. Mediastinal nodes may be prominent if sarcoidosis is a consideration. Diastolic heart failure should always be considered in patients with a relatively normal heart size and pulmonary edema.

Echocardiography

Echocardiography is usually revealing and frequently diagnostic. Ventricular Doppler filling patterns can be assessed, and changes in the patterns with respiration recorded. Pulmonary venous and hepatic venous flow patterns in concert with mitral flow patterns provide additional information. Transesophageal echocardiography is unnecessary.

The classic restrictive CM two-dimensional echocardiographic image includes severe biatrial enlargement and thickened LV walls, often with a speckled or unusual myocardial texture if an infiltrative process is present. There is often thickening of the interatrial septum in amyloidosis.

The law of Laplace is defined by pressure multiplied by radius of a heart chamber divided by wall thickness. With increased wall thickness, wall tension is expected to be reduced and the EF increased. In patients with an infiltrative process, the walls are thick, but the LVEF is low, normal, or reduced. This is often a clue to an infiltrative process.

In restrictive CM, there is no ventricular septal bounce or septal shifting with inspiration as might be seen in constrictive pericarditis. Patients with endomyocardial fibrosis usually have involvement of the ventricular apices and the subvalvular apparatus with scar. In endomyocardial fibrosis, the ventricles may be virtually obliterated by the collagen tissue and thrombus. The echocardiogram in patients with ventricular noncompaction most often reveals massive trabeculations in the LV apical region, with large sinuses between.

The echocardiogram in HCM can be confused with a restrictive CM, but HCM results in segmental wall thickness and a minimal wall thickness of >1.5 cm. If the hypertrophy is subaortic, a dynamic outflow tract gradient may be demonstrated that is also not seen in a restrictive CM. The LVEF in HCM is also generally quite high in accordance with the law of Laplace, as discussed previously.

Echocardiography and/or Doppler Flow Velocity Patterns

Normal Doppler flow velocity patterns. Doppler filling patterns, especially during respiration, help differentiate constrictive pericarditis from restrictive CM (see Table 31.1). Normal Doppler echocardiographic patterns and definitions are shown in Fig. 31.5. Some definitions are useful to review. The time from aortic valve closure to mitral valve opening represents the isovolumic relaxation time. The E-wave acceleration time is the time from the opening of the mitral valve to the peak flow into the LV; the time from the peak flow (top of the E wave) to diastasis is the E-wave deceleration time. Normal atrial contraction results in an A wave, reflecting the acceleration of blood flow into the LV during atrial systole; the A-wave velocity may be increased in diastolic dysfunction because the atrial pressure is higher to push against a stiff LV myocardium. The tricuspid flow pattern reflects right-sided filling and usually mirrors the mitral flow pattern.

The Doppler pulmonary venous flow pattern characterizes filling of the left atrium from the pulmonary veins. The left atrium fills during both ventricular systole and diastole. It fills during ventricular systole in concert with the atrial diastole, and the mitral ring being pulled toward the LV both enlarge the left atrium. The left atrium fills again during ventricular diastole while the mitral valve is open to the ventricle. Normally, an equal amount of LA filling occurs during ventricular systole and ventricular diastole (so S = D). Also, under normal circumstances, when the atrial kick occurs, some reversal of flow is seen in the pulmonary vein because of the rapid rise in LA pressure. Hepatic flow can be interrogated as well, and it is similar to pulmonary venous flow with two phases of right atrial filling and reversal during atrial systole. Because of the low right atrial pressures, some reversal of flow also occurs during the *c* wave when the tricuspid valve bulges into the atrium at the onset of ventricular systole.

Doppler flow pattern in restrictive cardiomyopathy. Fig. 31.5 (bottom) shows the mitral inflow pattern of impaired early LV relaxation and contrasts the findings seen with impaired LV compliance that affects flow later in diastole. Compared with normal LV diastolic performance, if early relaxation is impaired, the rate of initial filling (E wave) is reduced, and there is reversal of the E/A ratio. The isovolumic relaxation time increases, and the mitral deceleration time is faster as the LV diastolic pressure rises quickly from the rapid filling. Because of impaired diastolic flow out of the left atrium, flow through the pulmonary vein is greater in systole than in diastole, and therefore, the S/D velocity ratio is >1.

In restrictive CM, the issue is not usually impaired early LV filling but abnormal LV compliance and restricted late filling. Most of the LV filling must occur early in diastole because little can occur in late diastole; this is manifested by a prominent E wave, and the time to fill the ventricle is reduced (a shortened isovolumic relaxation time). Because of the rapidly rising LV diastolic pressures, the deceleration time is shorter (faster), and the contribution from the atrial kick to the late flow velocities is reduced (the E is much more prominent than the A). The pulmonary venous pattern reflects this, with rapid flow during early ventricular diastole and little flow into the stiff left atrium during ventricular systole. Thus, the S/D flow ratio of the pulmonary venous flow pattern is much <1. Hepatic venous flow patterns again resemble the pulmonary venous flow pattern.

Tissue Doppler measures may contribute additional information. Tissue Doppler uses the same pulse wave sampling as flow velocity, but it is modified to filter the low-amplitude reflections. When the transducer is placed on the mitral annulus or at the myocardium near the mitral annulus, the velocities record the longitudinal movement of the heart in systole and diastole. Because the transducer is at the apex, movement toward the apex is recorded as a positive wave (Sa). When the ventricle goes into diastole, the movement away from the transducer is recorded as a negative wave (Ea). If Ea is reduced (<10 cm/s), it implies impaired early myocardial relaxation. If the E wave of the mitral flow pattern is prominent (rapid filling of the LV) while the Ea wave of the tissue Doppler is reduced, it means that there must be an elevated LA pressure. In other words, if there is more pressure pushing the blood into the LV than anticipated from the LV pulling blood into itself, then the LA pressure is presumed to be elevated. This ratio (E/Ea) has been used to provide an estimate of the LA pressure. In general, a ratio of ≥15 has a 90% predictive value of a mean pulmonary capillary wedge pressure being >15 mm Hg. The E/Ea ratio has the added advantage of being useful in atrial fibrillation and sinus tachycardia.

Color M-mode propagation velocity is another method for demonstrating the rapid early flow into the LV during restriction. As the LV relaxes, there are intracavitary pressure gradients that promote the propagation of flow from the mitral orifice to the LV apex. By placing an M-mode cursor on the edge of the color-flow envelope, a propagation velocity (first aliasing contour) can be recorded (Vp). A reduced Vp (<40 cm/s) implies impaired relaxation.

A schematic review of the various echo/Doppler patterns that might be observed in a patient with restrictive CM is shown in Fig. 31.6.

Because similar diastolic mitral inflow patterns may occur in constrictive pericarditis, patterns during respiration are the key to differentiating constriction from restriction. There is usually little respiratory change in the mitral and pulmonary venous flow patterns in restrictive CM, whereas a significant (>25%) inspiratory drop in the maximal velocity of these flow patterns has been seen in constriction. The increased inspiratory filling of the RV with constrictive pericarditis results in the previously described increased RV pressure, and that increased pressure can be recorded in the tricuspid regurgitant jet velocity with inspiration. In restriction, the RV systolic pressure falls normally with inspiration.

Normal mitral flow velocity studies

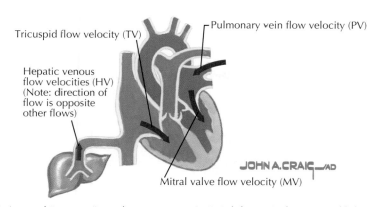

ECG provides cycle timing, and "pressure" panel represents aortic (Ao), left ventricular (LV), and left atrial (LA) pressures. Mitral valve flow pattern (MV) is contrasted with pulmonary vein (PV), tricuspid valve (TV), and hepatic venous (HV) flow velocities. The time from aortic valve closure (AVC) to opening of mitral valve (MVO) defines the isovolumetric relaxation time (IVRT) and reflects active myocardial relaxation. The MV Doppler pattern reflects early filling (E wave), with Doppler its acceleration time (AT) and deceleration time (DT). Following a diastasis period, atrial contraction creates the A-wave velocities. PV velocities reflect flow into the LA, with systolic flow (S) occurring during ventricular systole (atrial relaxation and mitral ring descent into LV) and again during ventricular diastole (D) while mitral valve is open. Reversal of flow (AR) occurs during atrial systole; tricuspid flows are similar to mitral. Hepatic flow velocities are similar to PV except direction is away from transducer (negative) and there is some flow reversal seen during early ventricular systole (C wave) and during atrial systole.

Mitral and pulmonary venous Doppler flow patterns in diastolic dysfunction and restrictive cardiomyopathy

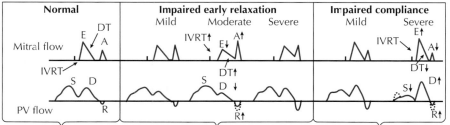

Normal	Impaired early relaxation	Impaired compliance
Note: Normal E > A and normal isovolumetric relaxation time (IVRT); DT = deceleration time of E wave; PV systolic velocity (S) about equal to diastolic (D); some flow reversal (R) during atrial systole	Note: Varying degrees of impaired relaxation with prolongation of IVRT and DT, reduced E wave and increased A wave and PV flow reversal; systolic is greater than diastolic pulmonary flow because of impaired early filling in diastole.	Note: Varying degrees of reduced LV compliance with E wave much greater than A wave. Reduced DT due to rapid rise in LV diastole pressure, increased PV flow reversal, and more PV flow in early diastole than in systole because the LV filling occurs primarily in early diastole.

FIG 31.5 Doppler Flow Studies: Comparison of Mitral and Pulmonary Vein Flow Velocities. MVC, Mitral valve closure; *VR*, ventricular relaxation. (Modified with permission from Klein AL, Scalia GM. Disease of the pericardium, restrictive cardiomyopathy and diastolic dysfunction. In: Topol EJ, ed. *Comprehensive Cardiovascular Medicine.* Philadelphia: Lippincott–Raven; 1998:669–716.)

Pericardial constriction and restrictive CM may occur together, and in this circumstance, the preceding findings do not clearly distinguish the two. The presence of atrial fibrillation makes Doppler flow patterns less complete (lacking an atrial component) and can complicate differentiating pericardial constriction and restrictive CM. Overall, it is estimated that equivocal echocardiographic patterns are present in up to one-third of the patients with possible constrictive pericarditis. The use of tissue Doppler adds some additional useful information in differentiating constriction from restriction, with a peak Ea >8.0 cm/s or an M-mode of the velocity color-flow pattern >100 cm/s, which suggests constriction rather than restriction.

Cardiac Nuclear Imaging

In patients with amyloidosis, technetium-99m (Tc) pyrophosphate myocardial imaging may be abnormally positive, and indium-labeled antimyosin antibody scans can also be positive, although these studies do not appear to be very sensitive. Imaging with ^{99m}Tc-DPD (3,3-diphosphono-1,2-propanodicarboxylic acid) has been shown to possibly distinguish between AL and TTR amyloidosis. Segmental perfusion defects are occasionally seen with perfusion imaging (thallium-201 or ^{99m}Tc sestamibi) in sarcoidosis; gallium-67 scans may also localize inflammation in this disorder.

Computed Tomography and Magnetic Resonance Imaging

Cardiac anatomic features and their relationship to the lungs are best defined by CT and MRI. Pericardial thickening is poorly detected by echocardiography, but both CT and MRI can detect pericardial thickening of ≥4 mm. However, a normal pericardium does not exclude constrictive pericarditis. A thickened interatrial septum suggests amyloidosis.

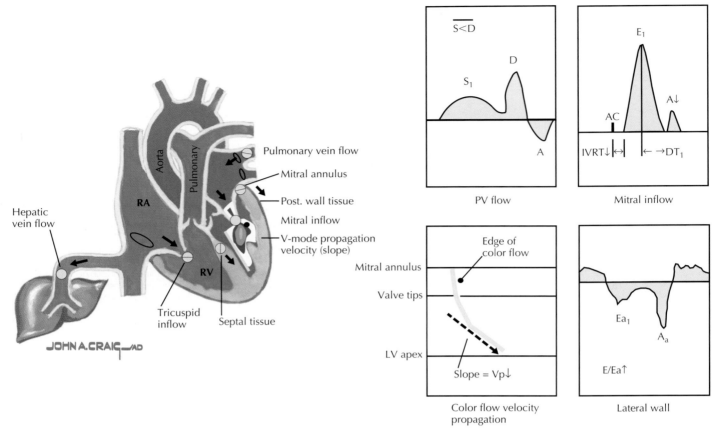

FIG 31.6 Diastolic Abnormalities in Restrictive Cardiomyopathy. There is more rapid filling in early diastole in the pulmonary venous (PV) flow (S<D) and in the mitral inflow (E>A). The high left atrial pressure results in the mitral valve opening earlier than after aortic closure (↓isovolumic relaxation time [IVRT]). Color flow velocity into the left ventricle (LV) is reduced (↓velocity propagation [Vp]), and the driving force pushing blood into the LV (E velocity) is greater than that pulling blood into the LV (Ea). Thus, the E/Ea ratio is increased. *AC,* Aortic closure; *D,* diastolic velocity; *DT,* deceleration time; *RA,* right atrium; *RV,* right ventricle; *S,* systolic velocity.

In addition, CT, and particularly, MRI may provide evidence of an infiltrative process (e.g., amyloid, sarcoid) in patients with restrictive CM. Cardiac MRI has emerged as a more sensitive test for cardiac amyloid than echocardiography. Up to 83% of amyloid patients have evidence of a pattern of global transmural or subendocardial late gadolinium enhancement. Both T1- and T2-weighted images can provide additional confirmatory data. Cardiac MRI is limited at times due to concerns about the rare occurrence of nephrogenic systemic fibrosis in patients with impaired renal function, and CT is limited because of the risk of contrast nephropathy.

Cardiac Catheterization and Endomyocardial Biopsy

Cardiac catheterization is often an important adjunct to noninvasive studies. The relationship between right and left heart filling pressures during inspiration is key to understanding the hemodynamics (see Table 31.1).

In restrictive CM, the LV end-diastolic pressure should be >5 mm Hg higher than the RV end-diastolic pressure at all phases of respiration, and pulmonary hypertension should be present (see Fig. 31.4). Hence, the RV end-diastolic pressure should be less than one-third of the RV systolic pressure despite an elevated RV end-diastolic pressure. This contrasts with constriction. Unfortunately, lung disease may also be present in the same patient, and other causes of pulmonary

hypertension may make this criterion less specific. The pulmonary vascular resistance is normal or near-normal in both constrictive pericarditis and restrictive CM unless there is associated lung disease. A prominent LA (or pulmonary capillary wedge) v wave is present in restriction CM because of abnormal LA compliance, and may be due to associated mitral valve regurgitation. An elevated v wave is unlikely in the pulmonary wedge tracing in constriction. The ventricular systolic pressures should be tracked together with inspiration, and both should decrease in restrictive CM, with discordance observed in constrictive pericarditis.

Endomyocardial biopsy is of limited value in dilated CM, but it may be helpful in restrictive CM. This is particularly true in cardiac amyloidosis, in which amorphous hyaline deposits are seen in the extracellular space. On electron microscopy, these are composed of nonbranching fibrils that bind Congo Red (leading to green birefringence under polarized light). Immunofluorescence microscopy and mass spectroscopy can distinguish the primary AL type (κ or λ immunoglobulin light chains) from the less common AA (nonimmunoglobulin protein A) or secondary amyloidosis. Sarcoidosis is spotty and may be missed by percutaneous biopsy. Fabry disease is distinctive, with deposition of glycolipid in the affected lysosomes; the diagnosis is confirmed by myocardial biopsy. Other diseases that result in a restrictive process cause myocardial fibrosis of a general nature, with interstitial fibrosis, loss of myofibrils, and vacuolation of cytoplasm. Myocardial biopsy is often not diagnostic in these latter circumstances.

MANAGEMENT AND THERAPY

Optimum Treatment

Diastolic Heart Failure

The treatment of diastolic heart failure centers on reducing symptoms and directing any therapy to the underlying process (Box 31.2). When diastolic pressures are elevated, diuretics are used to treat pulmonary and systemic congestion. However, the stiff ventricle is dependent on adequate preload, and the overzealous use of diuretics can result in hypotension, reduced renal blood flow, and renal dysfunction. Increased bowel edema may reduce the absorption of furosemide. Patients with restrictive CM usually present for hospitalization when oral diuretics are ineffective, and it is essential in this circumstance to give diuretics and other medications intravenously. Aquapheresis is occasionally helpful, but is currently rarely used. Oral torsemide or bumetamide are preferred loop diuretics when bowel edema is present. Spironolactone or eplerenone is a useful adjunct, especially if liver congestion and ascites are present. Metolazone can be used as an adjunct when loop diuretics and aldosterone antagonists are inadequate, although hypokalemia is common. Maintenance of slow heart rates improves diastolic time and allows for adequate diastolic filling. Beta-blockers or ivabradine can improve rate control in sinus rhythm. Calcium channel blockers are also used routinely under the assumption that they can both improve myocardial diastolic dysfunction and ventricular rate in patients with atrial fibrillation; however, worsening heart block at times limits their use. Sinus rhythm should be maintained if possible, because the atrial contribution to output may be significant in severe diastolic dysfunction. Angiotensin-converting enzyme inhibitors may also improve myocardial relaxation and are often useful despite relatively normal ventricular systolic function. Angiotensin receptor blockers have also been reported to provide symptomatic relief. Systemic blood pressure control is important to reduce the cardiac afterload and decrease any stimulus for further LV hypertrophy, although hypotension often limits its use. Hypotension can be a more difficult clinical problem than hypertension in restrictive CM due to associated autonomic dysfunction. Digoxin may result in increased arrhythmias, especially in patients with amyloidosis, and should not be used.

The use of the Doppler flow pattern has been suggested by some to help tailor therapy. For instance, fusion of the mitral inflow E and A waves implies inadequate diastolic time; therefore, heart rate reduction is needed. A pseudonormal or restrictive pattern (E>A) implies high diastolic filling pressures and the need for further therapy with angiotensin-converting enzyme inhibitors, calcium blockers, and diuretics. If the PR interval is prolonged, dual-chamber pacing may maximize the relationship of the atrial kick to ventricular contraction, thus improving LV filling. Anticoagulation with warfarin or novel anticoagulants are recommended to reduce the risk of atrial appendage thrombi in patients with continuous or paroxysmal atrial fibrillation or if there is evidence for LV thrombus.

Over time, medical therapy tends to be limited. Heart block should be treated with pacemaker therapy. Implantable cardioverter-defibrillators are controversial and may not prolong life. Because these need to be disabled at end of life, their use requires a thorough discussion with the patient and family. Cardiac transplantation in selected patients may be the only option, although significant pulmonary hypertension is often a complicating feature. Unfortunately, following cardiac transplantation, amyloidosis has been reported to recur in the transplanted heart, suggesting that cardiac transplantation should only be considered for those with isolated cardiac disease and not those with systemic involvement.

BOX 31.2 Therapy in Restrictive Cardiomyopathy

General

- Diuretics (furosemide, torsemide, bumetanide); rarely aquapharesis
  - Spironolactone or eplerenone
  - Metolazone
- Slow heart rate
  - In sinus rhythm: β-blockers, ivabradine
  - Antiarrhythmics to maintain sinus rhythm if possible
  - In atrial fibrillation: β-blockers, calcium channel blockers
- Improve diastolic relaxation
  - Calcium channel blockers
  - β-blockers
  - ACE inhibitors and ACE receptor blockers
- Control systemic blood pressure
- Avoid orthostatic hypotension
- Avoid digitalis preparations
- Pacemaker therapy when indications exist
  - ICD therapy controversial
- Anticoagulation with either warfarin or one of the novel anticoagulants
- Cardiac transplantation

Specific

- Amyloidosis: depends on type of amyloidosis
  - Alkylating agents, interferon, steroids, colchicine
  - For AL: other chemotherapy regimens (cyclophosphamide-thalidomide-dexamethasone, bortezomib, lenalidomide-dexamethasone), stem cell therapy
  - For ATTR, AApoA1: liver transplantation
  - For senile AA: treat underlying disorder
  - Under investigation for ATTR: drugs aimed at preventing misfolding of TTR (tafamidis), drugs aimed at stabilizing TTR (diflunisal), drugs that interfere with fibrillogenesis (doxycycline, TUDCA), drugs aimed at blocking transthyretin production
- Hypereosinophilic syndrome
  - Steroids
  - Hydroxyurea
  - Interferon
- Sarcoidosis
  - Steroids and other antiinflammatories
  - Pacemaker if heart block present
- Hemochromatosis
  - Phlebotomy
  - Desferrioxamine
  - Liver transplantation
- Fabry disease
  - α-galactosidase enzyme replacement
- Carcinoid syndrome
  - Somatostatin analogues
  - Serotonin antagonists
  - α-adrenergic blockers
  - Surgical valve replacement

AA, Secondary amyloidosis; *AApoA1,* A apolipoprotein-A1; *ACE,* angiotensin-converting enzyme; *AL,* primary amyloidosis; *ATTR,* familial or senile amyloidosis; *ICD,* implantable cardioverter-defibrillator; *TUDCA,* tauroursodeoxycholic acid.

Specific Therapy

Therapies directed at the underlying cause of the restrictive process are equally quite limited. The prognosis for primary amyloidosis is poor, with a median survival time of approximately 2 years, despite the use of alkylating agents and other approaches. Interferon has been tried, with little success, although the combination of steroids and interferon shows some promise. Combination therapy with melphalan, prednisone, and colchicine may relieve some of the noncardiac and renal aspects of the disease. The restrictive CM due to light chain deposition has been reported to be reversible, and this variant may have a better prognosis after remission of the plasma cell dyscrasia. A variety of treatment regimens are being investigated, including cyclophosphamide-thalidomide-dexamethasone, bortezomib, lenalidomide-dexamethasone, autologous stem cell transplants, and other novel chemotherapy combination agents. Liver transplantation (or combined liver-heart transplantation) may be an option in selected patients with hereditary ATTR, A-apolipoprotein-A1, and atrial fibrillation amyloidosis to remove or diminish the hepatic source of the protein. Treatment of senile AA amyloid usually focuses on treating the underlying problem (i.e., infectious, familial Mediterranean fever), interleukin-1 blockade with anakinra for those with auto-inflammatory disorders, and tumor necrosis factor inhibition for some rheumatologic disorders. Thus far, the experience in cardiac transplantation in these patients has been limited, but successes has been found in some with wild-type ATTR and V122I-related ATTR amyloidosis, especially in younger patients. Other therapies are aimed at preventing the misfolding of TTR in the plasma to maintain its normal soluble structure. Tafamidis has been developed for this purpose and to specifically to treat ATTR amyloidosis; early trials are encouraging. Diflunisal, a nonsteroid antiinflammatory drug, stabilizes transthyretin and is also undergoing trials. Doxycycline and tauroursodeoxycholic acid appear to interfere with TTR fibrillogenesis. Because transthyretin is manufactured in the liver, some novel RNA-inhibiting agents also hold promise. Finally, some immunotherapeutic targeting antibodies are being investigated that attack the amyloid deposits directly.

Corticosteroids and hydroxyurea are used in the early stages of the hypereosinophilic syndrome. There has also been some success with interferon in this disease. Surgery can debride the fibrous plaque, and valve replacement may be indicated if valvular dysfunction is a major part of the clinical presentation.

Corticosteroids and other inflammatory agents are used in sarcoidosis. Heart block can be treated with permanent pacing; implantable defibrillators help patients who are susceptible to severe ventricular tachyarrhythmias.

Enzyme replacement (β-glucosidase) and liver transplantation has improved some patients with Gaucher disease.

Hemochromatosis is generally managed by phlebotomy, chelating agents such as desferrioxamine, or both. Heart transplantation and combined heart-liver transplantation have also been used in patients whose hemochromatosis is refractory to standard therapy.

Fabry disease can now be treated with intermittent intravenous infusion of the enzyme α-galactosidase A, and early studies of its use to improve cardiac function are encouraging.

Carcinoid syndrome can be treated with somatostatin analogues, serotonin antagonists, and α-adrenergic blockers. Surgical tricuspid and/or pulmonary valve replacement is an option, especially in patients younger than 65 years of age, although the plaque deposition continues and will ultimately coat these valves.

Avoiding Treatment Errors

There are several important issues for patients with suspected or confirmed restrictive CM. First, it is critically important to be certain that the patient does have restrictive CM. Patients with pericardial constriction can benefit enormously from pericardiectomy. Patients with HCM have multiple other treatment options. Second, a diagnosis as to the cause of the restrictive CM should always be sought, because treatment options exist for some causes of restrictive CM. Third, optimal care requires close monitoring of patients to maintain intravascular volumes at a point that provides for patient comfort and ambulation but avoids hypotension and the downward spiral that occurs with worsening renal failure. Finally, in patients with severe restrictive CM, it is important for the physician to discuss treatment options and prognosis so that the patient and family can be involved in end-of-life decisions.

FUTURE DIRECTIONS

The definition of diastolic heart failure needs to be further standardized. Abnormalities of ventricular active relaxation and compliance are often dissociated from systolic dysfunction. Diastolic dysfunction may precede systolic dysfunction in many diseases, especially diseases with concentric hypertrophy, such as aortic stenosis and systemic hypertension. The prevalence of normal systolic and diastolic dysfunction in heart failure studies varies from 14% to 75%, emphasizing the nebulous nature for defining the role of diastolic disease. Abnormalities of early diastolic relaxation clearly differ from those of late diastolic compliance.

Clinically, older adults present with diastolic dysfunction more commonly than younger individuals. Despite this, the prognosis in patients with diastolic dysfunction is far better than that in systolic dysfunction, unless an infiltrative process is present. Diastolic dysfunction need not be present with even profound systolic dysfunction. Many patients who have a poor LVEF do not experience symptoms of congestion for many years because diastolic dysfunction only manifests when congestive symptoms emerge. A better basic understanding of the mechanisms that promulgate the diastolic dysfunction in various diseases is sorely needed.

Newer and more effective therapy for the various causes of restrictive CM could have a major effect in these diseases. This is particularly important for amyloidosis and for endocardial fibrosis in developing countries. A better understanding of the genetics of these diseases will go a long way to devising potential genetic interventions in familial causes. As noted previously, amyloidosis depositions are now being directly targeted, as are agents to minimize or prevent the production of abnormal proteins. These investigations hold great promise for the development of a more effective treatment in this devastating disease. The rarity of many of the restrictive CMs often places them in the orphan category for funding and research.

The treatment of diastolic heart failure in general remains a major challenge, and this is particularly true in restrictive CM. Although some advances have been made in symptomatic treatment, until satisfactory therapy is available for some of the underlying disease processes, therapies that improve ventricular diastolic performance are desperately needed for all patients with HFpEF and not only those with restrictive CM.

ADDITIONAL RESOURCES

Arbustini E, Narula N, Dec GW, et al. The MOGE(S) classification for phenotype-genotype nomenclature of cardiomyopathy: endorsed by the World Health Federation. *J Am Coll Cardiol.* 2013;62:2046.

A proposal to classify CM based on phenotype-genotype relationships. This scheme proposes a MOGE(S) classification, in which M = morphofunctional description, O = organ involvement, G = genetic or familial inheritance and transmission, E = etiology with specific gene mutation, and S = symptomatic status.

Elliott PM, Andersson B, Arbustini E, et al. Classification of the cardiomyopathies: a position statement from the European Society of Cardiology Working Group on Myocardial and Pericardial Disease. *Eur Heart J.* 2008;29:270.

Position paper from the European Society of Cardiology geared to everyday clinical practice. It emphasizes familial and/or genetic and nonfamilial and/or nongenetic causes, and excludes secondary causes and ion channelopathies. The paper attempts to put restrictive CM in prospective with other myocardial disease.

Maron BJ, Towbin JA, Theine G, et al. Contemporary definitions and classifications of the cardiomyopathies: an AHA Scientific Statement. *Circulation.* 2006;113:1807.

Position paper from the American Heart Association intended to provide methodologies for clinical diagnosis of CMs. Added to previous statements about those with ion channel CMs, even if there were no cardiac abnormalities detected.

EVIDENCE

Garcia MJ. Constrictive pericarditis versus restrictive cardiomyopathy. *J Am Coll Cardiol.* 2016;67:2061–2076.

Excellent overall review of both restrictive CM and constrictive pericarditis hemodynamics with contrasting tables and up-to-date discussion of current diagnostic and therapeutic options.

Gertz MA, Benson MD, Dyck PJ, et al. Diagnosis, prognosis and therapy of transthyretin amyloidosis. *J Am Coll Cardiol.* 2015;66:241–266.

Clinical review guide as to when to suspect the disease, the appropriate diagnostic evaluation and a literature review of treatment options for affected patients.

Gestke JB, Anaverkar NS, Nishamura RA, et al. Differentiation of constriction and restriction. Complex cardiovascular hemodynamics. *J Am Coll Cardiol.* 2016;68:2329–2347.

Good review of the similarities and differences between the hemodynamics of a restrictive myocardial process and a constrictive pericardial process. Contemporary view of diagnosis and treatment options.

Wechalekar AD, Gillmore JD, Hawkins PN. Seminar in systemic amyloidosis. *Lancet.* 2016;387:25641.

Excellent review of all the latest in the diagnosis and treatment of each form of amyloidosis. Provides literature review and comprehensive analysis of recent imaging and therapeutic options.

32

Hereditary Cardiomyopathies

Christopher Chien

The World Health Organization/International Society and Federation of Cardiology Task Force on the Definition and Classification of Cardiomyopathies define cardiomyopathies as a group of diseases of the myocardium that result in cardiac dysfunction. Although cardiomyopathy may be secondary to myocardial damage (e.g., myocardial infarction or hypertension), this chapter discusses the genetic basis of intrinsic cardiomyopathies without other identifiable causes.

Cardiomyopathies are classically divided into several categories based on anatomic and physiological properties: dilated cardiomyopathy (DCM), hypertrophic cardiomyopathy (HCM), restrictive cardiomyopathy (RCM), and arrhythmogenic right ventricular (RV) cardiomyopathy (ARVC). Each of these are associated with genetic mutations (Table 32.1 to Table 32.3).

Although genetic mutations can occur in familial or hereditary patterns, it is important to recognize that they can occur de novo, in the absence of family history of cardiomyopathy. In addition, familial cardiomyopathies can occur in the absence of an identifiable genetic mutation, because knowledge of genetics is expanding with newer technologies, such as next-generation sequencing. In this chapter, the term hereditary cardiomyopathy refers to all genetic cardiomyopathies, independent of familial history.

Genetic mutations may also be associated with multiple types of cardiomyopathies or arrhythmic disease. As examples, mutations of *MHY7* (β-myosin heavy chain) are associated with both HCM and DCM, and mutations in *SCN5A* (sodium ion channel) are associated with both DCM and arrhythmias. There is also increasing recognition of a genetic influence in cardiomyopathies that are not classically considered to be genetic or hereditary. For example, genetic testing of women with peripartum cardiomyopathy revealed that 15% of them had genetic mutations. Finally, genetic mutations can be associated with syndromes that involve extracardiac findings (see Table 32.1).

ETIOLOGY AND PATHOGENESIS

Dilated Cardiomyopathy

Patients with DCM develop eccentric cardiac remodeling, left and right ventricular dysfunction, heart failure, and arrhythmias. More than 50 mutations have been implicated in DCM, and approximately 35% of patients with familial DCM have an identifiable mutation. The most common affected genes are titin *(TTN)*, lamin A/C *(LMNA)*, β-myosin heavy chain *(MYH7)*, and cardiac troponin T *(TNNT)*. Mutations can be subcategorized by their histology and role in cardiac function (Fig. 32.1 and see Table 32.1)

Abnormalities of Force Production

Mutations in genes that code for sarcomeric proteins affect force production and transmission. Common mutations involve genes that code actin *(ACTC)*, β-myosin heavy chain *(MYH7)*, troponin *(TNNI3, TNNT2,*

TNNC1), and α-tropomyosin *(TPM1)*. Early-onset ventricular dilation and dysfunction are common. These are also associated with HCM. Inheritance is predominantly autosomal dominant, although incomplete penetrance is common.

Abnormalities of Force Transduction

Multiple mutations affect Z-disk interacting proteins that mediate detection and modulation of mechanical stress. Common mutations include desmin *(DES)*, dystrophin *(DMD)*, δ-sarcoglycan *(SGCD)*, and titin *(TTN)*. TTN is a giant protein that extends from the Z disk to the M-line of the sarcomere, acting as a spring that regulates passive tension and active contraction. Due to its immense size, its role in DCM was a technical barrier for years. However, with next-generation sequencing, *TTN* truncations can now be identified in 25% of cohorts of familial DCM. Extracardiac muscular dystrophies are also implicated in mutations of *DMD* (Duchenne and Becker muscular dystrophy) and *SGCD* (limb-girdle-muscular dystrophy).

Nuclear Proteins

Mutations that cause cardiomyopathy also occur in nuclear proteins, including *LMNA*, thymopoietin *(TMPO)*, and CARP *(ANKRD1)*. *LMNA* mutations result in a well-recognized genetic abnormality with several extracardiac phenotypes (muscular dystrophies, Charcot-Marie tooth disease) and a variety of cardiac phenotypes (including atrial fibrillation, DCM, RCM, and HCM). Notably, *LMNA* mutations are associated with progressive conduction abnormalities and high risk of sudden death and shocks from implantable cardiac-defibrillators (ICDs).

Hypertrophic Cardiomyopathy

HCM is characterized by myocardial hypertrophy (often involving the interventricular septum and left ventricular [LV] outflow obstruction), sudden cardiac death (SCD), and heart failure. Most mutations that cause familial HCM have autosomal dominant inherence and involve sarcomeric proteins (see Table 32.2). The most commonly affected genes are *MYH7* and myosin-binding protein C *(MYBPC3)*. Mutations of *MYH7*, *TNNT*, *TNNI*, and *TPM1* are also associated with a high risk of SCD, and ICD implantation may be warranted based on presence of these mutations. Wolff-Parkinson-White syndrome and HCM can be seen in mutations of *PRKAG2* and *LAMP2*. Danon disease is an X-linked dominant mutation in *LAMP2* that causes HCM, skeletal myopathies, intellectual impairment, and often requires consideration of cardiac transplantation.

Restrictive Cardiomyopathy

RCM is characterized by impaired diastolic function and relative preservation of the LV ejection fraction. RCM is most often secondary to a systemic or infiltrative disease, and some of these diseases have a hereditary pattern (such as familial transthyretin amyloidosis). However,

TABLE 32.1 Gene Defects Associated With Dilated Cardiomyopathy

Gene	Protein	Cardiac Features	Extracardiac Features	Inheritance
Abnormalities of Force Production				
MYH7	β-myosin heavy chain	Early-onset LV dilation Also causes HCM		AD
ACTC	Actin	Also causes HCM		AD
TNNI3	Troponin I	Also causes HCM		AD
TNNT2	Troponin T	Early onset LV dilation Also causes HCM		AD
TNNC1	Troponin C			AD
TPM1	α-tropomyosin	Also causes HCM		AD
Abnormalities of Force Transduction				
TTN	Titin	Also causes HCM Associated with peripartum cardiomyopathy		Mixed
DES	Desmin	Syncope	Skeletal myopathy	AD, AR
DMD	Dystrophin	Rapid progression to end-stage heart failure	Duchenne muscular dystrophy Becker muscular dystrophy	XR
SGCD	δ-sarcoglycan	Sudden death	Limb-girdle-muscular dystrophy (2F)	AR
Nuclear Proteins				
LMNA	Lamin A/C	Conduction abnormalities Sudden death Also associated with HCM, RCM, LVNC	Muscular dystrophy, Charcot-Marie tooth disease	AD
Other				
PLN	Phospholamban (reversible inhibitor of SERCA)	Progresses to end-stage HF in mid-life, requiring cardiac transplantation		AD
TAZ	Tafazzin	Endocardial fibroelastosis, associated with LVNC	Barth syndrome	XR
EYA4	EYA protein		Sensorineural hearing loss	AD

AD, Autosomal dominant; *AR,* autosomal recessive; *HCM,* hypertrophic cardiomyopathy; *HF,* heart failure; *LV,* left ventricle; *LVNC,* LV noncompaction cardiomyopathy; *RCM,* restrictive cardiomyopathy; *XR,* X-linked recessive.

mutations causing primary RCM have also been identified, including *TTNI3* and *DES*.

Arrhythmogenic Right Ventricular Cardiomyopathy

Patients with ARVC (also called arrhythmogenic RV dysplasia) have fibrofatty infiltration of their RV that causes arrhythmias and RV dysfunction. Notable arrhythmic findings include ventricular tachycardia with left bundle branch morphology and epsilon waves (terminal notch in the QRS complex). Most cases are familial, and it is commonly inherited in an autosomal-dominant pattern (Table 32.3). Most pathogenic mutations affect the desmosome, affecting the genes for desmocollin 2 *(DSC2)*, desmoglein 2 *(DSG2)*, junctional plakoglobin *(JUP)*, plakophilin 2 *(PKP2)*, and desmokplakin *(DSP)*. Many patients will carry more than one pathogenic variant. There is an association with *JUP* and *DSP* mutations and Naxos disease, which is characterized by palmoplantar keratoderma and wooly hair.

OTHER

There are several hereditary cardiomyopathies that do not fit one of the previous categories. LV noncompaction cardiomyopathy (LVNC) is characterized by a noncompacted myocardium. It has some overlap with DCM and HCM, but is associated with additional congenital defects (septal defects, patent ductus arteriosis), LV thrombus, and SCD. Sarcomeric genes and mutation of tafazzins *(TAZ)* have been implicated in LVNC. *TAZ*

mutation also causes Barth syndrome, an X-linked disorder of LVNC or DCM, and skeletal myopathy, neutropenia, and growth restriction.

Mitochondrial diseases can mimic HCM but often progress to DCM. They are associated with extracardiac syndromes, including MELAS (mitochondrial encephalomyopathy, lactic acidosis, and strokelike episodes) and MERRF (myoclonic epilepsy with ragged red fibers).

DIAGNOSTIC APPROACH

The American College of Cardiology/American Heart Association Guidelines recommend a two-generation family history in all patients with newly diagnosed heart failure. Family history should identify cases of cardiomyopathy, arrhythmia, and sudden (or unexplained) death. It is important to recognize that mutations of the same gene can cause different phenotypes, even in the same family. ECG should be performed to evaluate for conduction abnormalities. Physical examinations should include a full neuromuscular evaluation to identify any extracardiac muscular pathology.

Genetic Testing

Genetic testing is an increasingly used tool in patients with hereditary cardiomyopathies. The major purpose of genetic testing is to identify a pathogenic mutation to screen family members of affected patients. Genetic testing does not have a role in diagnosis of cardiomyopathy, and only has a limited role in prognostic or therapeutic implications.

TABLE 32.2   Gene Defects Associated With Hypertrophic Cardiomyopathy

Gene	Protein	Features	Inheritance
Thick-Filament Proteins			
MYH7	β-myosin heavy chain	High risk of sudden death	AD
MYL1	Myosin light chain-1	Papillary muscle thickening	AD
MYL2	Myosin light chain-2	Papillary muscle thickening	AD
Thin-Filament Proteins			
TNNT2	Troponin T	High risk of sudden death	AD
TNNI3	Troponin I	High risk of sudden death	AD
ACTC	Actin	Also causes DCM	AD
TPM1	α-tropomyosin	High risk of sudden death May progress from HCM to DCM	AD
MYBPC3	Myosin binding protein C	Mild presentation, later onset	AD
Lysosomal Protein			
LAMP2	Lysosome-associated membrane protein	Danon disease with skeletal, neurological, and hepatic involvement WPW Males often end-stage disease by second decade of life	XR
GLA	Lysosomal hydrolase α-galactosidase A protein	Cardiac Fabry disease Enzyme replacement therapy (α-galactosidase A)	XR
Glycogen Storage Cardiomyopathy			
PRKAG2	Gamma₂ regulatory subunit of AMP activated protein kinase	Atrioventricular block Atrial fibrillation WPW	AD

AD, Autosomal dominant; *AMP*, adenosine monophosphate; *AR*, autosomal recessive; *DCM*, dilated cardiomyopathy; *RCM*, restrictive cardiomyopathy; *WPW*, Wolff-Parkinson-White; *XR*, X-linked recessive.

TABLE 32.3   Gene Defects Associated With Arrhythmogenic Right Ventricular Cardiomyopathy

Gene	Protein	Features	Inheritance
PKP2	Plakophilin 2	Common mutation	AD
DSG2	Desmoglein 2	Common mutation	AD
JUP	Junctional plakoglobin	Associated with Naxos disease	AR
DSP	Desmoplakin	Associated with Naxos disease	AR
RYR2	Ryanodine receptor	Ryanodine receptor is also associated with catecholaminergic polymorphic VT	AD
DSC2	Desmocollin-2		AD

AD, Autosomal dominant; *AR*, autosomal recessive; *VT*, ventricular tachycardia.

Genetic testing should be performed in the appropriate population. It is most useful for diagnosing rare or specific cardiomyopathies, especially when there are specific phenotypic features (extracardiac features, conduction system disease, sudden death). Not surprisingly, the yield of genetic testing in the absence of family history of disease is low and is higher in patients with a family history of cardiomyopathy. However, genetic testing should be considered in all patients with phenotypic HCM.

Genetic testing should only be performed in conjunction with genetic counseling. This includes the following: (1) detailed family history and construction of a pedigree; (2) pretest counseling on the interpretation and implications of the result (with regards to patient care, family screening, and psychological impact); (3) decision-making and consent; and (4) disclosure of test results with posttest counseling. Genetic testing will demonstrate one of three outcomes: identification of a known disease-causing mutation, absence of any known disease-causing mutation, or the presence of mutations of unknown significance.

Screening of Family Members

Almost one-third of asymptomatic family members of patients with DCM will have echocardiographic abnormalities, such as LV enlargement or contractile abnormalities. Most of these family members will progress to develop overt DCM. Thus, the role of family screening should be considered. If a patient with cardiomyopathy has an identified pathological mutation, then screening for that specific mutation only can be offered to at-risk first-degree family members (depending on inheritance pattern). If there is no mutation, then no further cardiac screening is required. If the mutation is present in an asymptomatic family member, then they should undergo comprehensive cardiac evaluation and their offspring should also be offered screening (Fig. 32.2)

If a patient with hereditary cardiomyopathy (with a family history of similar disease) does not have an identifiable pathological mutation, then family screening can be considered every 3 to 5 years using ECG and echocardiography. More rigorous screening should be considered

In red, the defective proteins that are related to the cause of DCM, HCM, and ARVC

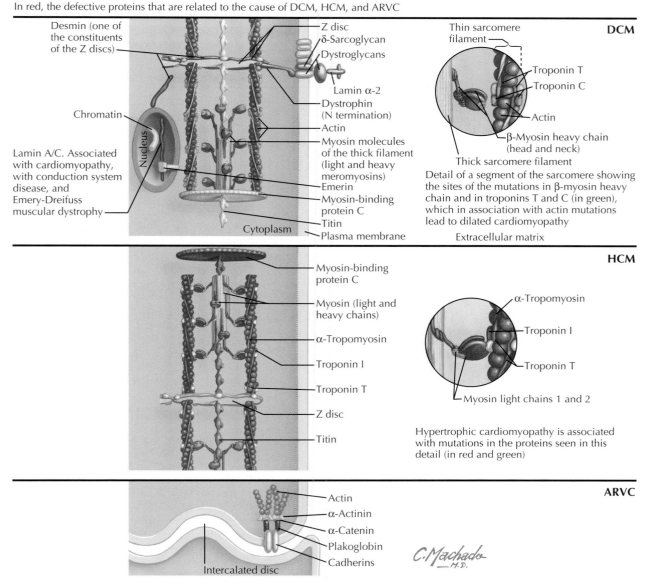

FIG 32.1 Interaction of Affected Proteins. Interaction of affected proteins in dilated cardiomyopathy (DCM), hypertrophic cardiomyopathy (HCM), and arrhythmogenic right ventricular cardiomyopathy (ARVC; cardiac muscle cell).

in adolescent family members of HCM patients when the family member is involved in competitive athletics because of the risk of SCD.

MANAGEMENT AND THERAPY

Treatment of DCM, HCM, and RCM are detailed in Chapters 29 to 31, respectively. The following discussion focuses on special management considerations in patients with identified pathogenic mutations.

There is limited evidence that genetic testing determines prognosis in DCM. However, sarcomeric mutations are most common in young patients, and their heart failure often progresses rapidly. Thus, advanced heart failure therapies such as transplantation or LV assist device placement can be indicated in these patients. In addition, mutations of *LMNA* or *SCN5A* are associated with a high risk of ventricular arrhythmias and heart block, but it is not clear that early implantation of ICDs is needed

before the usual guideline recommendations are met. In addition, there have been limited studies on the value of medical therapy in family members who are genotype positive, but phenotype negative.

Patients with HCM should undergo risk stratification for SCD as part of routine management. History of SCD in a first-degree relative is an established risk factor for which ICD implantation should be considered. Although some mutations carry increased risk of SCD, current guidelines do not recommend risk stratification based on genetic testing results alone. However, the presence of two or more mutations can be considered a risk factor in patients with borderline risk of SCD by other predictors.

The implications of mutations causing RCM are not known at this time, and do not affect management. ARVC is treated with ablation therapy, and sometimes, cardiac transplantation. Genetic testing does not alter the treatment strategy for patients.

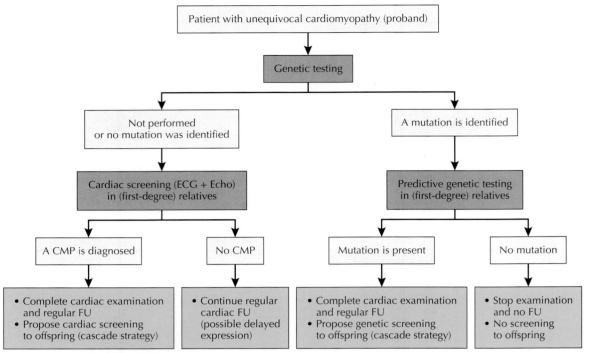

FIG 32.2 Family Screening Algorithm for Patients With Hereditary Cardiomyopathy (CMP). *FU,* Follow-up. (From Charron P, Arad M, Arbustini, E, et al. Genetic counselling and testing in cardiomyopathies: a position statement of the European Society of Cardiology Working Group on Myocardial and Pericardial Diseases. *Eur Heart J* 2010;31:2715–2728; Figure 2, p. 2720.)

FUTURE DIRECTIONS

Knowledge and identification of genetic pathways of cardiomyopathic disease continue to grow. With advances in screening techniques, increasing numbers of disease-causing mutations continue to be identified. Still, there are many unanswered questions, including the role of genotyping in prognosis and therapeutics, the relationship between genotype and phenotype over time, and the long-term implications of genetic testing. Finally, understanding of the genetic mechanisms that cause cardiac dysfunction may elucidate novel pathways of treatment.

ADDITIONAL RESOURCES

Ackerman MJ, Priori SG, Willems S, Berul C, Brugada R. HRS/EHRA expert consensus statement of the state of genetic testing for the channelopathies and cardiomyopathies. *Europace.* 2011;13:1077–1109.

Consensus statement from European and North American experts in inherited cardiomyopathies and channelopathies.

Ashley EA, Hershberger RE, Caleshu C, et al. Genetics and cardiovascular disease: a policy statement from the American Heart Association. *Circulation.* 2012;126:142–157.

This policy statement discusses some of the legal and financial considerations of genetic testing in cardiovascular disease, including a description of the Genetic Information Nondiscrimination Act (GINA).

Cahill TJ, Ashrafian H, Watkins H. Genetic cardiomyopathies causing heart failure. *Circ Res.* 2013;113:660–675.

This is a thorough review article on the contribution of genetics to DCM, HCM, ARVC, and RCM.

Charron P, Arad M, Arbustini E, et al. Genetic counselling and testing in cardiomyopathies: a position statement of the European Society of Cardiology Working Group on Myocardial and Pericardial Diseases. *Eur Heart J.* 2010;31:2715–2728.

This is a statement about the approach to genetic counseling, including principles, rationale, evidence, and recommendations for clinical practice.

Genetics home reference: your guide to understanding genetic conditions. https://ghr.nlm.nih.gov/.

This website from the National Institute of Health and the US National Library of Medicine provides easily searchable information about genes and genetic disorders.

EVIDENCE

Baig MK, Goldman JH, Caforio ALP, et al. Familial dilated cardiomyopathy: cardiac abnormalities are common in asymptomatic relatives and may represent early disease. *J Am Coll Cardiol.* 1998;31:195–201.

Approximately 30% of asymptomatic family members of patients with known familial DCM had echocardiographic abnormalities. Twenty-five percent of family members progressed to overt heart failure.

Herman DS, Lam L, Taylor MRG, et al. Truncations of titin causing dilated cardiomyopathy. *N Engl J Med.* 2012;366:619–628.

Seventy-two mutations of the TTN gene (which codes for titin) were identified, largely using next-generation sequencing. TTN was previously difficult to study due to its immense size.

McNair WP, Sinagra G, Taylor MRG. SCN5A mutations associate with arrhythmic dilated cardiomyopathy and commonly localize to the voltage-sensing mechanism. *J Am Coll Cardiol.* 2011;57:2160–2168.

Mutations of the SCN5A gene (voltage-gated sodium ion channel) have long been implicated in long QT syndrome, but it has been identified as a cause of DCM in this paper from the Familial Cardiomyopathy Registry Research Group.

Morita H, Rehm HL, Menesses A, et al. Shared genetic causes of cardiac hypertrophy in children and adults. *N Engl J Med.* 2008;358:1899–1908.

This paper from the Siedman laboratory showed that genetic mutations of sarcomeric proteins were identified in a high percentage of cases of cardiac hypertrophy in children, both with and without a previous family history of HCM.

Ware JS, Li J, Mazaika E, et al. Shared genetic predisposition in peripartum cardiomyopathies. *N Engl J Med.* 2016;374:233–241.

Women with peripartum cardiomyopathy have genetic mutations at a rate similar to patients with idiopathic DCM. The most common abnormality is a truncation of TTN.

33

Myocarditis

Daniel J. Lenihan

Myocarditis is an inflammatory process that can involve one or more components of the myocardium, including cardiomyocytes, the interstitium, and the coronary vasculature. This inflammatory process may result from infectious processes, responses to pharmacological or toxic agents, hypersensitivity reactions, or physical damage. Myocarditis may also be a cardiac manifestation of a systemic disease.

The clinical course of myocarditis is as diverse as its etiologies. Most patients have a subclinical, self-limited course, but myocarditis may also have fulminant, acute, or chronic presentations. The burden of myocarditis as a clinical entity is difficult to ascertain, at least in part because of its diversity and the elusiveness of diagnosis; for similar reasons, the ideal diagnostic and therapeutic approach to myocarditis has been an enigma. The future related to the diagnosis and treatment of myocarditis is encouraging, but this clinical problem will always remain challenging. Recent data have established a causal link between the long-term effects of viral myocarditis and dilated cardiomyopathy. New treatments for dilated cardiomyopathy and heart failure have focused on immunomodulating therapy partly based on this knowledge. It is clear that further elucidation of the pathogenesis of myocarditis will improve our collective treatment and management of left ventricular (LV) dysfunction and heart failure.

ETIOLOGY AND PATHOGENESIS

In North America and Europe, most cases of myocarditis probably result from viral infection. Many viruses have been associated with myocarditis (Box 33.1). Initial serological studies suggested that enteroviruses, such as coxsackie B, are common causes of viral myocarditis. However, the application of direct molecular techniques to endomyocardial biopsy specimens, and perhaps changing epidemiology, has led to increasing recognition of adenoviruses, parvovirus, and hepatitis C as etiologic agents. In HIV infection, there is often evidence of myocarditis when cardiac decompensation occurs, although it is unclear whether HIV or opportunistic infections are responsible.

The molecular mechanisms of myocardial injury in viral myocarditis remain incompletely understood. The initial phases of injury probably depend on viral attachment to myocytes and direct cell damage by the virus, resulting in myocyte necrosis. The finding of a common membrane receptor for adenoviruses and coxsackieviruses supports this hypothesis and the preponderance of these viruses as causative agents. Following the initial injury, host immune response to the virus most likely has an important role in myocardial injury. Animal models have shown that after the initial phase of entry and proliferation of the virus in the myocyte cytoplasm, inflammatory cells (including natural killer cells and macrophages) infiltrate with subsequent release of proinflammatory cytokines. T lymphocytes are activated through classic cell-mediated immunity. Cytotoxic T cells recognize viral protein fragments on the cell surface in a major histocompatibility complex–restricted

manner. Molecular mimicry can occur when antigens intrinsic to the myocyte cross react with viral peptides, inducing persistent T-cell activation. Cytokines, including tumor necrosis factor-α, interleukin (IL)-1, IL-2, and interferon-α have been identified as important mediators of chronic inflammatory disease. These cytokines can cause myocyte damage, which results in fewer contractile units with a resultant worsening of systolic function. Autoantibodies to myocyte components are often found in patients with myocarditis, although most studies that measured autoantibody levels were in patients with idiopathic-dilated cardiomyopathy. Even so, it seems apparent that cellular immunity has more of a role in the pathogenesis of myocarditis than does humoral immunity.

Rarely, bacterial infections, through spread from endogenous sources (Fig. 33.1), can produce focal or diffuse myopericarditis. One of the earliest recognized causes of myocarditis was diphtheria. Up to 20% of diphtheria patients have cardiac involvement, and myocarditis is the leading cause of death with this infection. The toxin produced by the diphtheria bacillus injures myocardial cells (Fig. 33.2). In South and Central America, the most common cause of infectious myocarditis is the protozoan *Trypanosoma cruzi*, which is the causative agent of Chagas disease.

Sarcoidosis, a systemic granulomatous disorder of unknown etiology, involves the myocardium in at least 20% of cases. Cardiac involvement ranges from a few scattered lesions to extensive involvement (Fig. 33.3). As a result, endomyocardial biopsy may be diagnostic, but it is frequently unreliable in confirming myocarditis. Giant cell myocarditis is a rare but highly lethal form of myocarditis of suspected immune or autoimmune etiology that may be associated with other inflammatory conditions (e.g., Crohn disease). Although the cumulative studies on immunosuppressive therapy for myocarditis are not positive (see the following), the previously mentioned causes of myocarditis do often respond to immunosuppression. Peripartum cardiomyopathy has been associated with myocarditis seen on endomyocardial biopsy, although the etiology or the frequency is still largely unknown.

Hypersensitivity reactions that result in myocarditis are characterized by eosinophilia and a perivascular infiltration of the myocardium by eosinophils and leukocytes. Any drug may cause hypersensitivity myocarditis, but clinically, this condition is rarely recognized. Therefore, a high index of suspicion should be maintained.

There are also a number of medications and toxins that can cause myocarditis. For example, cocaine use produces myocyte necrosis, mostly from profound sympathetic overstimulation. Anthracyclines (used as chemotherapeutic agents) are direct myocardial toxins with a dose-dependent toxic effect on the myocardium that can profoundly affect the function of the heart, even at low doses. A new breakthrough therapy for cancer, known as immunotherapy with checkpoint inhibitors, can activate the immune system, which results in improved cancer control in malignancies, such as melanoma and lung cancer, that were

BOX 33.1 Selected Etiologies of Myocarditis[a]

Infectious
Viral (coxsackievirus, adenovirus, HIV, hepatitis C, parvovirus)
Bacterial (meningococcus, *Corynebacterium diphtheria*)
Protozoal *(Trypanosoma cruzi)*
Spirochetal *(Borrelia burgdorferi)*
Rickettsial *(Rickettsia rickettsii)*
Parasitic *(Trichinella spiralis, Echinococcus granulosus)*
Fungal *(Aspergillus, Cryptococcus)*

Inflammatory Diseases
Sarcoidosis
Giant cell myocarditis
Scleroderma
Systemic lupus erythematosus
Hypersensitivity reactions
Serum sickness (antibiotics, tetanus toxoid, acetazolamide, phenytoin)

Toxic Exposures
Cocaine
Anthracyclines
Checkpoint inhibitors for the treatment of cancer (nivolumab, pembrolizumab)

[a]Examples are shown in each category, but this is not an all-inclusive list.

previously resistant to chemotherapy. These new agents have rarely been associated with myocarditis, but unfortunately, when this association occurs, the cardiac decompensation can be severe and even fatal.

CLINICAL PRESENTATION

The clinical course of a patient with myocarditis is variable. In up to 40% of patients, the disease is self-limited (Box 33.2). Some patients have a defined prodromal viral illness with fever and arthralgia. Cardiac symptoms are often nonspecific, and include fatigue, dyspnea, and chest pain with pleuritic features. Other patients present more acutely with progressive cardiac decompensation from heart failure and require intensive support. In some instances, the presentation of patients with focal myocarditis mimics that of acute myocardial infarction (MI), but with normal coronary arteries. Patients may present with symptoms of arrhythmias, including palpitations or syncope. Sudden death may also occur with myocarditis and is presumed to be secondary to arrhythmia, because even focal inflammation in the cardiac conduction system can be significant. Chronic immune-mediated myocardial injury or persistent myocyte viral gene expression may cause progressive dilatation and resultant LV dysfunction after the resolution of a clinically apparent or subclinical illness.

Physical findings in mild cases of infectious myocarditis may include low-grade fever, and a pericardial friction rub may be audible. Physical features of the underlying etiology, such as erythema nodosum

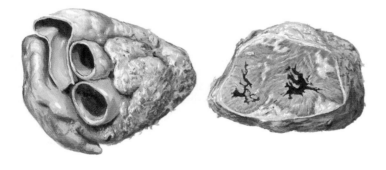

Heart serially sectioned, revealing multiple intramural and subepicardial abscesses with pericarditis

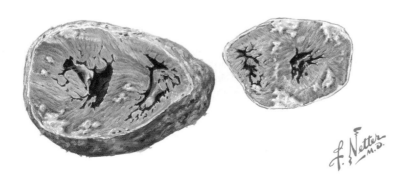

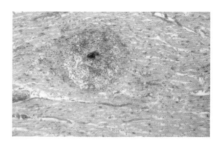

Abscess in heart muscle. Central mass of bacteria surrounded by leukocytes, destroyed muscle, and dilated blood vessels

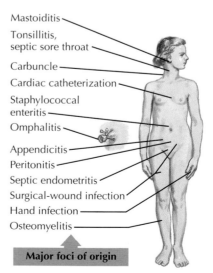

Mastoiditis
Tonsillitis, septic sore throat
Carbuncle
Cardiac catheterization
Staphylococcal enteritis
Omphalitis
Appendicitis
Peritonitis
Septic endometritis
Surgical-wound infection
Hand infection
Osteomyelitis

Major foci of origin

FIG 33.1 Septic Myocarditis and Myopericarditis.

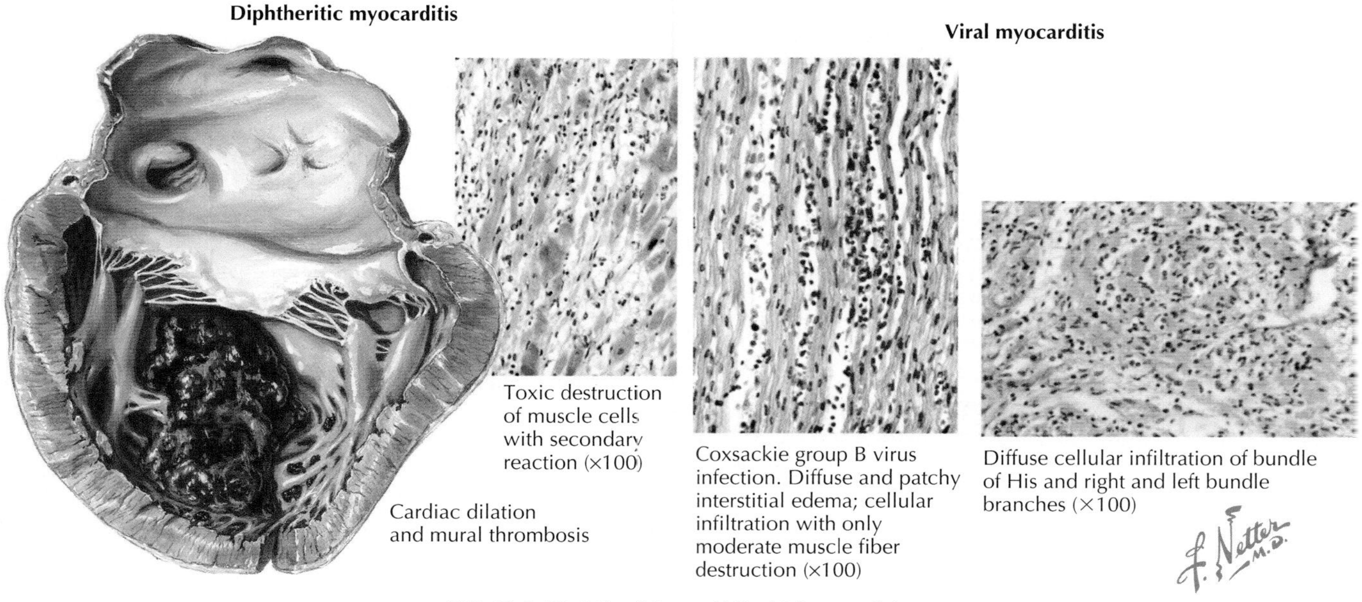

Diphtheritic myocarditis

Viral myocarditis

Toxic destruction
of muscle cells
with secondary
reaction (×100)

Cardiac dilation
and mural thrombosis

Coxsackie group B virus
infection. Diffuse and patchy
interstitial edema; cellular
infiltration with only
moderate muscle fiber
destruction (×100)

Diffuse cellular infiltration of bundle
of His and right and left bundle
branches (×100)

FIG 33.2 Diphtheritic and Viral Myocarditis.

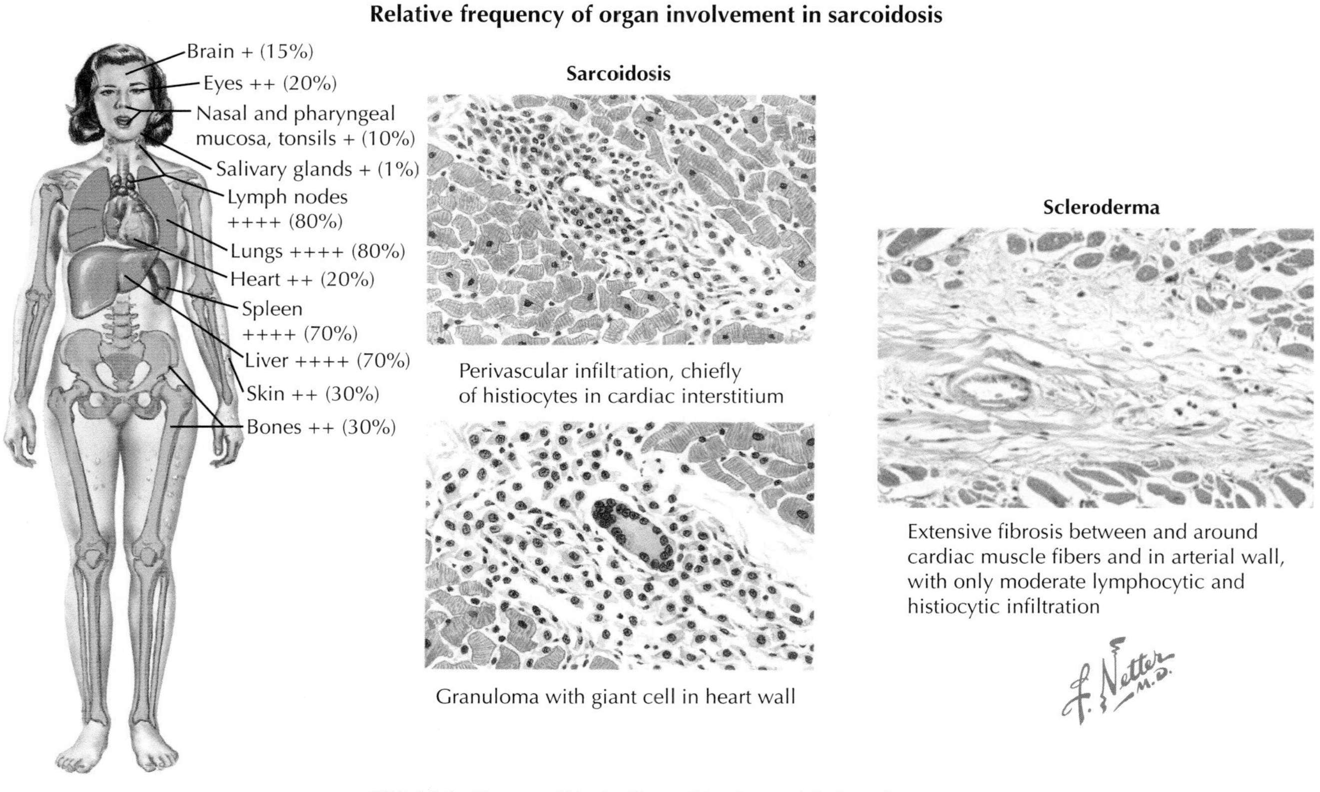

Relative frequency of organ involvement in sarcoidosis

Sarcoidosis

Brain + (15%)
Eyes ++ (20%)
Nasal and pharyngeal
mucosa, tonsils + (10%)
Salivary glands + (1%)
Lymph nodes
++++ (80%)
Lungs ++++ (80%)
Heart ++ (20%)
Spleen
++++ (70%)
Liver ++++ (70%)
Skin ++ (30%)
Bones ++ (30%)

Perivascular infiltration, chiefly
of histiocytes in cardiac interstitium

Scleroderma

Extensive fibrosis between and around
cardiac muscle fibers and in arterial wall,
with only moderate lymphocytic and
histiocytic infiltration

Granuloma with giant cell in heart wall

FIG 33.3 Myocarditis in Sarcoidosis and Scleroderma.

(sarcoidosis) and erythema chronica migrans (Lyme disease), can be
important clues in determining the cause of myocarditis and should
be elicited. If heart failure is evident, there may be a third heart sound,
jugular venous distention, or evidence of pulmonary edema. Sinus
tachycardia is usually prominent and out of proportion to temperature
elevation.

DIFFERENTIAL DIAGNOSIS

The differential diagnosis of myocarditis depends mainly on the presentation of the illness. Many illnesses are potentially implicated with
or are thought to be causal of myocarditis (see Boxes 33.1 and 33.2).
In terms of other causes of LV dysfunction or heart failure, the more

---

BOX 33.2   Clinical Presentations of Myocarditis

Unexplained fever or viral syndrome
Asymptomatic LV dysfunction
Symptomatic LV dysfunction
Acutely decompensated heart failure
Acute MI with normal coronaries
Sudden cardiac death
Arrhythmias
Troponin elevation without coronary artery disease

LV, Left ventricular; *MI,* myocardial infarction.

BOX 33.3   Diagnostic Testing Useful to Establish the Diagnosis of Myocarditis

Cardiac markers (CK-MB, natriuretic peptides, and troponins)
Serological tests for viral, spirochetal, or parasitic etiologies
Blood cultures (for infectious causes)
Markers of inflammation or underlying inflammatory disease (erythrocyte sedimentation rate, antinuclear antibodies, ACE level)
Electrocardiography
Echocardiography
Endomyocardial biopsy
Cardiac catheterization
Nuclear imaging
Magnetic resonance imaging

ACE, Angiotensin-converting enzyme; *CK-MB,* creatine kinase MB fraction.

---

common causes include long-standing hypertension, coronary artery disease, valvular heart disease, or inherited cardiomyopathy. Myocarditis, with evidence of LV dysfunction, is typically a diagnosis of exclusion after the other myriad causes that can result in LV dysfunction have been considered.

DIAGNOSTIC APPROACH

Few accurate and reliable diagnostic tests are available for myocarditis; therefore, clinical suspicion is vital (Box 33.3). Creatine kinase-MB fraction, natriuretic peptides (B-type natriuretic peptide or N-terminal pro–B-type natriuretic peptide), and cardiac troponins I and T concentrations are often increased, confirming the presence of cardiac dysfunction and myocardial cell injury. There may be evidence of a systemic infection with an increased white blood cell count and sedimentation rate. Blood cultures may confirm a bacterial etiology, but in viral infections, this is frequently not possible. Acute and convalescent titers for viruses (e.g., coxsackie B and Epstein-Barr) may provide some evidence of recent infection, especially if there is a twofold to fourfold increase in neutralizing antibody titers to a virus (or spirochetes in the case of Lyme disease). Other laboratory testing may confirm a systemic immunologic disease associated with myocarditis, such as sarcoidosis (angiotensin-converting enzyme level) or connective tissue diseases (antinuclear antibodies). Typical ECG findings include nonspecific ST-segment and T-wave abnormalities, atrial and ventricular arrhythmias, atrioventricular blocks, widened QRS complexes from intraventricular conduction delays, and rarely, Q waves. Intraventricular conduction abnormalities are associated with diffuse myocarditis and often predict a poor prognosis. As noted, some patients with myocarditis present with classic ECG findings of MI but have normal coronary arteries.

There are no specific radiographic findings in myocarditis; however, findings of cardiomegaly or pulmonary edema are often present. Echocardiography is useful to assess the global and regional LV functions, as well as diastolic filling abnormalities. Echocardiography can also demonstrate findings that result from myocarditis, including increased wall thickness, ventricular thrombi, valvular abnormalities, and pericardial involvement. Cardiac catheterization may exclude the presence of coronary disease or confirm the hemodynamic disturbances of heart failure. Nuclear imaging techniques, such as antimyosin antibody scanning, can identify myocardial inflammation but are not widely available. MRI may detect tissue alterations associated with myocarditis, and recent data suggest that contrast-enhanced imaging is the preferred test (Fig. 33.4).

The only gold standard to confirm myocarditis is endomyocardial biopsy. This method has a small defined risk to the patient, as well as disparities in interpretation. An expert panel of cardiac pathologists formulated the Dallas criteria to standardize the histological diagnosis of myocarditis on endomyocardial biopsy. They concluded that the histological hallmark of myocarditis is an inflammatory myocardial infiltrate with associated evidence of myocytolysis. Borderline myocarditis was defined as an inflammatory infiltrate without clear evidence of myocyte necrosis. The positive predictive value of endomyocardial biopsy using these criteria is low (10%); however, it can be marginally increased with more samples. These criteria probably underestimate the true incidence of myocarditis. Because there can be sampling errors due to nonuniformity of myocarditis throughout the myocardium or patchy infiltrates, as well as interobserver variability in interpretation, a negative result does not exclude the diagnosis of myocarditis. Confirming the presence of viral genomes by polymerase chain reaction or in situ hybridization is a relatively new development that has the potential for significant improvement of diagnosis of viral myocarditis and assessment of prognosis. Many recent studies on the use of MRI for the diagnosis of myocarditis from any cause have also recently been reported and highlight the usefulness of this as a diagnostic test.

MANAGEMENT AND THERAPY

Optimal Treatment

Nonpharmacological Therapy

The treatment of patients with myocarditis is largely supportive. Activity should be restricted to bed rest if acutely ill or modest nonstressful activity until active myocarditis is resolved. In animal models of myocarditis, exercise during an active period of cardiac inflammation resulted in increased myocardial damage. Athletes should refrain from sports for a 6-month period until heart size and function have returned to normal. Those with arrhythmias should refrain from athletic activities until the arrhythmias resolve. Salt restriction (typically emphasized in the management of heart failure) should be recommended for this population, especially in patients with LV systolic dysfunction. In the rare cases that progress to severe heart failure, supportive care may include an LV assist device or even cardiac transplantation. All unnecessary medications should be eliminated because of the potential that one drug may be responsible for a hypersensitivity reaction that results in myocarditis.

Pharmacological Therapy

The etiology established in a patient with myocarditis dictates the specific treatment plan. For example, in myocarditis caused by diphtheria, antitoxin should be administered immediately upon confirmation of the diagnosis. In the treatment of Lyme myocarditis, antibiotic therapy is used, although its efficacy has not been established. Efforts at treatment of Chagas disease focus on vector control and immunoprophylaxis.

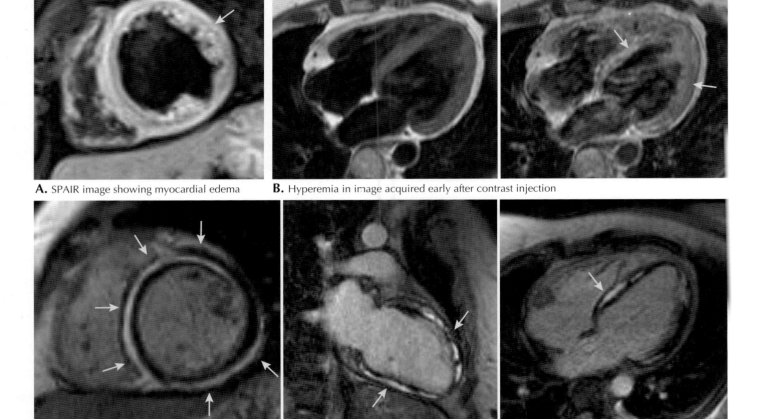

A. SPAIR image showing myocardial edema

B. Hyperemia in image acquired early after contrast injection

C. Epicardial Scar/Necrosis 15 minutes after contrast administration, inflammatory necrosis is noted with late gadolinium enhancement (LGE) along the epicardium

FIG 33.4 Acute Myocarditis. *SPAIR*, Spectral Attenuated Inversion Recovery. (Images courtesy Jai Singh, MD.)

Patients with dilated cardiomyopathy secondary to myocarditis are treated with conventional therapies for LV dysfunction, including renin-angiotensin system inhibitors, β-blockers, diuretics for volume overload, spironolactone for severe heart failure, and digoxin only if symptoms persist. During the acute phase of myocarditis, digoxin should be used with caution based on the notion that there is an increased sensitivity to digitalis in myocarditis, and hence, an increased likelihood of digitalis toxicity.

Immunosuppressive Therapy

Because the long-term effects of viral myocarditis are believed to be due in part to immune-mediated mechanisms, immunosuppressive therapy has been studied. The multicenter, U.S. National Institutes of Health–sponsored Myocarditis Treatment Trial evaluated the role of immunosuppressive therapy using prednisone with either cyclosporine or azathioprine in those with endomyocardial biopsy–proven myocarditis and an LV ejection fraction of <45%. There was no significant change in LV ejection fraction at 28 weeks and no survival difference between those treated with immunosuppression and control subjects in this prospectively randomized study. Smaller studies that evaluated the role of intravenous immunoglobulins (IVIGs) provided mixed results in myocarditis, but a large-scale randomized study failed to demonstrate a significant effect. Therefore, until evidence is presented with random-ized placebo-controlled studies of IVIGs in the treatment of acute

myocarditis, IVIG therapy should be considered only when the likeli-hood of benefit is greater, such as in systemic autoimmune disease, T-cell activation from an immune checkpoint inhibitor therapy for cancer, or biopsy-proven myocarditis with decompensation.

Avoiding Treatment Errors

If myocarditis is suspected, exercise should be minimized until the acute phase of illness is resolved, as has been shown by animal research. Efforts to uncover the underlying cause should be pursued, because treatments may differ depending on the etiology. The treatment of heart failure in any individual patient should be based on standard therapy for heart failure, but caution should be used when adding digoxin. Because a hypersensitivity reaction to most any medication is possible, elimination of all unnecessary medications is paramount.

FUTURE DIRECTIONS

Future therapy for myocarditis will probably be directed at the specific mechanisms of myocardial injury. The common pathway for many causes of myocarditis is the host immune response; therefore, antiviral drugs and virus-specific vaccines may well prove to be efficacious.

Immune-modulating therapy for heart failure is also under active investigation based on the hypothesis that these treatments may have a role in myocarditis or even idiopathic-dilated cardiomyopathy.

Proinflammatory cytokines may contribute to disease progression in heart failure by their direct toxic effects on the heart. Unfortunately, one example of this strategy using an inhibitor of tumor necrosis factor-α failed to produce a beneficial response in patients with LV dysfunction. Because of the large number of potential etiologies of myocarditis, it could well be the case that some etiologies of the disease respond to immunomodulation, whereas other etiologies do not. Further studies, with more accurate pre-enrollment characterization of the underlying etiology, should address this issue. Other forms of immunomodulating therapy, including plasma exchange and immunoabsorption, are also being investigated and perhaps may prove to be useful adjuncts to established therapy.

ADDITIONAL RESOURCES

Anzini M, Merlo M, Sabbadini G, et al. Long-term evolution and prognostic stratification of biopsy-proven active myocarditis. *Circulation.* 2013;128:2384–2394.
A nice review of outcomes of patients with biopsy-proven myocarditis.
Caforio AL, Pankuweit S, Arbustini E, et al. Current state of knowledge on aetiology, diagnosis, management, and therapy of myocarditis: a position statement of the European Society of Cardiology Working Group on Myocardial and Pericardial Diseases. *Eur Heart J.* 2013;34:2636–2648, 2648a–2648d.
A position statement from the European Society of Cardiology on myocarditis.
Cooper LT Jr. Myocarditis. *N Engl J Med.* 2009;360:1526–1538.
A beautiful review of the pathophysiology of myocarditis.
Francone M, Chimenti C, Galea N, et al. CMR sensitivity varies with clinical presentation and extent of cell necrosis in biopsy-proven acute myocarditis. *JACC Cardiovascular imaging.* 2014;7:254–263.
An important study indicating the utility of cardiac magnetic resonance in different types of myocarditis.

Fung G, Luo H, Qiu Y, Yang D, McManus B. Myocarditis. *Circ Res.* 2016;118:496–514.
A contemporary review of mechanisms of disease in myocarditis.
Johnson DB, Balko JM, Compton ML, et al. Fulminant myocarditis with combination immune checkpoint blockade. *N Engl J Med.* 2016;375:1749–1755.
An important report of two cases of myocarditis seen with combined checkpoint blockade. The myocarditis was confirmed unfortunately at autopsy.
Lurz P, Luecke C, Eitel I, et al. Comprehensive cardiac magnetic resonance imaging in patients with suspected myocarditis: the MyoRacer-Trial. *J Am Coll Cardiol.* 2016;67:1800–1811.
An important study examining the details of MRI for the diagnosis of myocarditis.

EVIDENCE

Gullastad L, Halfdan A, Fjeld J, et al. Immunomodulating therapy with intravenous immunoglobulin in patients with chronic heart failure. *Circulation.* 2001;103:220–225.
A smaller study that suggests the benefit of immunomodulation in the treatment of myocarditis. However, this is not a widely used method at present.
Mason JW, O'Connell JB, Herskowitz A, et al. A clinical trial of immunosuppressive therapy for myocarditis. *N Engl J Med.* 1995;335:269–275.
This is the initial large-scale study that failed to show a significant benefit of prednisone for the treatment of myocarditis.
McNamara D, Holubkov R, Starling RC, et al. Controlled trial of intravenous immune globulin in recent-onset dilated cardiomyopathy. *Circulation.* 2001;103:2254–2259.
An important study that described the lack of notable benefit for IVIG in a broad population of patients with possible myocarditis. Of note, the low percentage of patients who had biopsy-proven myocarditis might have influenced the results.

34

Cardiac Transplantation and Mechanical Circulatory Support Devices

Kristen A. Sell-Dottin, Benjamin Haithcock, Thomas G. Caranasos, Michael E. Bowdish, Michael R. Mill, Brett C. Sheridan

Cardiac transplantation developed in conjunction with research into myocardial protection and heart preservation, which facilitated safe open heart surgery. In 1961, Shumway and Lower published their seminal article describing the technique of orthotopic cardiac transplantation in a canine model, with successful functioning of the transplanted heart for several days. While Shumway was preparing to begin a human clinical trial of cardiac transplantation, Christiaan Barnard, a South African surgeon who had worked in the United States learning the techniques of immunosuppression and surgical transplantation, shocked the world in December 1967 by performing the first human-to-human heart transplantation in Capetown. His patient lived for 18 days before succumbing to infectious complications. Shumway performed the first successful cardiac transplantation in the United States in January 1968, beginning what has become the longest ongoing program of cardiac transplantation in the world.

Activity in cardiac transplantation exploded after these initial successes. However, a dismal initial 1-year survival rate of 22% led most programs to abandon the procedure. Early transplantation patients died of both immune rejection of the transplanted heart and infectious complications. Two major developments allowed surgeons and those caring for cardiac transplantation patients to more successfully balance the complications of graft rejection versus systemic infection. The development in 1971 of the cardiac bioptome by Caves, combined with the pathological grading system for rejection by Billingham, removed much of the treatment guesswork and permitted accurate diagnosis of rejection and rational strategies for maintenance immunosuppression and treatment of rejection. Cardiac transplantation improved rapidly again with the introduction of cyclosporine A in 1980. This calcineurin inhibitor dramatically reduced the incidence of rejection.

Recently, further investigation into basic mechanisms of transplantation rejection resulted in triple-drug immunosuppressive regimens that used smaller doses of prednisone, azathioprine, and cyclosporine, which allowed better rejection control with fewer infectious complications and adverse effects from these powerful immunosuppressive agents. Newer agents, such as tacrolimus, mycophenolate mofetil, and sirolimus, as well as the use of induction therapy, are now part of the antirejection armamentarium, and new drugs continue to be developed. With these advancements, >100,000 heart transplantations have been performed since December 1967. The International Society for Heart and Lung Transplantation (ISHLT) has a scientific registry that has followed outcomes of these patients since 1983. This registry allows for rigorous research and ongoing advancements in the field.

The development of durable mechanical support devices have dramatically increased the number of patients with heart failure who can be palliated. More than 5000 heart transplantations are performed worldwide each year, yet that leaves many heart failure patients untreated. In the United States in 2012, there were an estimated 6.6 million people with heart failure and a staggering 23 million people with heart failure worldwide. With only approximately 2000 donor hearts available in the United States each year, ventricular assist devices (VADs) have been increasingly used. These devices are used for three main indications: bridging to transplantation, bridging to recovery, and destination therapy.

INDICATIONS

Indications for cardiac transplantation include the presence of end-stage heart disease not amenable to standard medical or surgical therapy, New York Heart Association functional class IV heart failure on maximal medical therapy, and an estimated 1-year life expectancy of <50%. This includes patients in cardiogenic shock who require continuous inotropic support or circulatory support, patients with intractable life-threatening arrhythmias unresponsive to more conservative therapies, and patients with refractory angina symptoms from coronary artery disease (CAD) that is not amenable to percutaneous or surgical revascularization. Cardiopulmonary exercise testing, specifically peak oxygen consumption (VO_2) thresholds of <14 mL/kg per minute favors listing for transplantation. Alternatively, a predicted peak VO_2 <50% may be used as a threshold, especially for women and young patients (younger than 50 years old).

As other therapeutic approaches have improved—from coronary artery bypass grafting to percutaneous interventions to advances in medical therapy for congestive heart failure—patients who need transplantation are generally older and sicker, and have multiple comorbidities. In addition, the spectrum of individuals considered for cardiac transplantation today has been broadened to include older adult patients, children, and newborns. The most common indications for cardiac transplantations in the adult population are cardiomyopathies and end-stage CAD. A minority of transplantations are performed in patients with valvular heart disease, congenital heart disease, and as retransplantations (e.g., for graft vasculopathy). In children, the leading diagnoses are dilated cardiomyopathies and congenital heart disease.

Potential transplantation patients undergo an intensive screening process by a multidisciplinary team of cardiothoracic surgeons, cardiologists, transplantation coordinators, social workers, dietitians, physical therapists, psychologists/psychiatrists, and financial counselors. The screening ensures not only that the patient needs the transplantation but also that the patient is physically and mentally able to comply with the rigorous posttransplantation medical regimen and has the appropriate social support to undergo transplantation successfully.

DONORS

Transplantation donors are individuals who are brain dead but continue to have adequate cardiac function to temporarily support other organ function. Most die of catastrophic intracranial events or trauma. The hearts are carefully evaluated with respect to cause of death, need for cardiopulmonary resuscitation, and use of inotropic support; they undergo ECG and echocardiography to ensure adequate ventricular and valvular function. In men aged older than 45 years, women aged older than 55 years, and patients with other risk factors for CAD, cardiac catheterization and coronary angiography are frequently performed. Donors undergo thorough serological testing to rule out transmissible diseases, and their medical and social histories are evaluated. Donor heart exclusion criteria also include any malignancy with extracranial metastatic potential and systemic sepsis or endocarditis. Ideally, the cardiac donor has not sustained prolonged hypotension or hypoxemia and is younger than 55 years of age. There has been a trend toward more liberal donor selection criteria over the past 15 years, and hearts that have experienced cardiac arrest have successfully been used for transplantation.

DONOR–RECIPIENT MATCHING

Patients accepted for transplantation are placed on a national waiting list maintained by the United Network for Organ Sharing (UNOS). UNOS has a contract with the U.S. government to act as the organ procurement and transplantation network. Patients are evaluated on the waiting list by body size, ABO blood type, medical urgency status, and waiting time.

When a suitable donor is identified, UNOS generates a list that ranks potential recipients by distance from the donor hospital (to minimize the organ ischemic time during travel and implantation), size, ABO blood type, medical urgency, and waiting time. An organ is then offered to a transplantation center of a prospective recipient. If the transplantation physicians believe that the organ is suitable for their patient, arrangements are made to procure the organ and perform the transplantation. On occasion, a potential recipient is precluded from transplantation because of ongoing infection or another potentially reversible contraindication. If the initial center does not accept the organ, it is offered sequentially to all patients on the local list, followed by patients in ever-enlarging geographic circles until the nation is covered. Because of the number of patients actively awaiting transplantation, most hearts are placed within their local or regional areas. Other available organs are likewise matched with potential recipients.

DONOR PROCEDURE

After all the organs are allocated, procurement surgeons arrive at the donor hospital, and a coordinated procedure allows simultaneous procurement of all usable organs, often including the heart, lungs, liver, kidneys, and pancreas, and occasionally, the small intestine. The heart explantation procedure depends on whether only the heart will be used or whether the lungs will also be used separately or as a combined heart–lung transplantation. After initial dissection of the aorta and superior and inferior venae cavae, placement of a cardioplegia cannula in the ascending aorta, and completion of the other initial dissections by procurement teams, the donor is systemically heparinized. The superior vena cava is tied off, the left atrial (LA) appendage is amputated, and the inferior vena cava is partially transected to decompress the heart and prevent ventricular distention. The aorta is then cross-clamped, and cardioplegia is infused while the heart is lavaged with ice-cold saline (Fig. 34.1).

Simultaneously, the other organs are flushed with their own preservative solutions and lavaged with cold saline. After completing the cardioplegia infusion, the superior and inferior venae cavae are transected. If only the heart is to be used, the pulmonary veins and pulmonary arteries are divided at the pericardium, and the aorta is divided. If the lungs are to be used, the LA is divided at the midatrial level, leaving enough cuff of the LA for cardiac implantation and cuffs around the pulmonary veins for lung implantation. The pulmonary trunk is divided at its bifurcation to leave enough length on the pulmonary arteries for the lung implantation. If a combined heart–lung transplantation is planned, the two organs are resected en bloc by dividing the cavae, aorta, and trachea, and dissecting the heart–lung block from its mediastinal attachments. The organs are then stored in ice-cold saline in multiple layers of plastic bags to ensure sterility, and they are packed in an ice-filled cooler for transportation to the transplanting center.

RECIPIENT PROCEDURE

Two approaches to orthotopic cardiac transplantation are widely used. In the traditional Shumway and Lower technique, a biatrial anastomosis is performed, in which the donor and recipient atrial cuffs are sewn together. This technique does not require separate caval anastomoses, and therefore, saves time. An alternative technique, the bicaval technique, was developed in the 1990s and consists of sewing separate caval anastomoses. Purported advantages of this technique are related to improved atrial function, decreased risk of arrhythmia or need for permanent pacing, and decreased tricuspid regurgitation. However, in an outcomes analysis of the UNOS database between 1999 and 2005, no survival difference was identified between recipients of bicaval or biatrial orthotopic cardiac transplantation.

When a heart transplantation recipient is already on left ventricular assist device (LVAD) support, as is increasingly the case, chest reentry and recipient cardiectomy can be more complicated. Reentry via redo sternotomy and VAD explant typically requires additional time, which must be factored into the timing of donor cardiectomy to minimize ischemic time.

Biatrial Technique

The operation is performed through a standard median sternotomy using cardiopulmonary bypass with aortic and bicaval cannulation. The initial dissection and cannulation are performed while the heart is being transported to the recipient hospital. When the new heart arrives, cardiopulmonary bypass is instituted at moderate systemic hypothermia (~32°C), and caval tapes are secured around the caval cannulas. The aorta is cross-clamped and then divided just above the level of the aortic valve. The pulmonary trunk is divided above its respective valve, and the atria are divided at the midatrial level, with removal of the atrial appendages and preservation of the posterior atrial cuffs containing the pulmonary veins on the left and the cavae on the right. The donor heart is prepared by freeing the pulmonary artery from the aorta and the roof of the LA. The pulmonary venous orifices are interconnected to create a cuff for the LA anastomosis. Excess LA tissue can be removed to create a better size match for this anastomosis. The oval fossa of the donor heart is examined for a patent foramen ovale. If identified, it is closed primarily. The LA anastomosis is then fashioned with a suture in a continuous running fashion. The suture line is begun at the base of the donor LA appendage, just above the recipient left superior pulmonary vein (see Fig. 34.1). The donor right atrium is opened from the orifice of the inferior vena cava through the right atrial appendage and then sewn to the recipient atrial cuff. Next, the donor and recipient pulmonary trunks are cut to appropriate lengths. The pulmonary trunks are then anastomosed end to end with a running suture. Systemic rewarming is begun, and the donor and recipient aortas are trimmed and anastomosed with a running suture. The heart is de-aired, the suture line is secured, the patient is placed in a steep

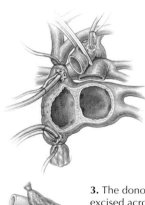

1. The recipient is placed on cardiopulmonary bypass support with venous drainage cannulas placed into the superior and inferior venae cavae. The cardiopulmonary bypass circuit returns oxygenated blood with controlled perfusion into the ascending aorta through a cannula placed distal to the aortic cross-clamp. Cardiopulmonary bypass provides systemic perfusion allowing excision of the recipient heart, retaining the posterior cuff of the right and left atria as well as the ascending aorta and main pulmonary artery.

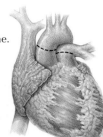

2. Dashed markings represent excision lines for removal of the donor heart.

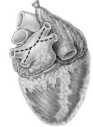

3. The donor heart is excised across the pulmonary veins, followed by preparation for transplantation by opening the posterior wall of the left atrium.

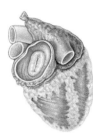

4. View of the donor mitral valve through the surgically opened left atrial posterior wall.

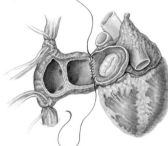

5. Initiation of cardiac implantation with anastomosis of left atrium of recipient to donor using a continuous monofilament suture line.

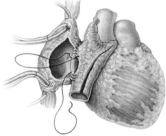

6. The left atrial anastomosis is completed, and the donor right atrium is opened from the inferior vena cava extending to the right atrial appendage.

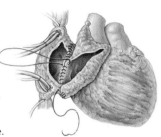

7. The right atrial cuff of the donor is anastomosed to the recipient right atrial cuff directly over the left atrial suture line reinforcing the edge of the interatrial septum.

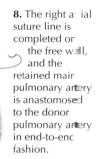

8. The right atrial suture line is completed on the free wall, and the retained main pulmonary artery is anastomosed to the donor pulmonary artery in end-to-end fashion.

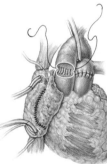

9. The fourth and final anastomosis aligns the ascending aorta of donor and recipient in end-to-end fashion.

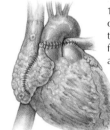

10. Completed biatrial orthotopic cardiac transplant with separation from cardiopulmonary bypass and removal of cannulas.

S. Moon, m.s.

FIG 34.1 Technique of Biatrial Cardiac Transplantation.

Trendelenburg position, and the cross-clamp is released, thus ending the donor heart ischemic time. During rewarming and reperfusion, the right side of the heart is de-aired, the caval tapes are removed, and the donor superior vena cava is oversewn. With rewarming and reperfusion, a spontaneous normal sinus rhythm usually develops. Regardless, temporary atrial and ventricular pacing wires are placed should temporary atrioventricular sequential pacing be needed postoperatively. After the onset of forceful ventricular contractions and completion of de-airing maneuvers, inotropic support is begun. Depending on the donor heart ischemic time and size, the pulmonary vascular resistance of the recipient, and the preoperative use of antiarrhythmic drugs (especially amiodarone), additional inotropic support or vasoconstrictive agents are sometimes necessary. The patient is then weaned from cardiopulmonary bypass. Heparin is reversed with protamine sulfate, and the heart is decannulated. After ensuring adequate hemostasis, chest drains are placed, and the sternotomy is closed.

Bicaval Technique

The operation is fundamentally the same as the biatrial technique. The differences in cardiectomy include developing the groove between the right and left atria to allow their separation. During excision of the heart, the superior vena cava is divided just above the level of the right atrium, and the inferior vena cava is divided just below the coronary sinus. After the aorta and pulmonary artery have been divided, an LA cuff is then created starting at the dome of the LA, carrying the incision inferiorly above the orifices of the right and left pulmonary veins (Fig. 34.2). During implantation, the LA cuff is sewn in a similar manner. Some surgeons place a vent through the right side of the LA

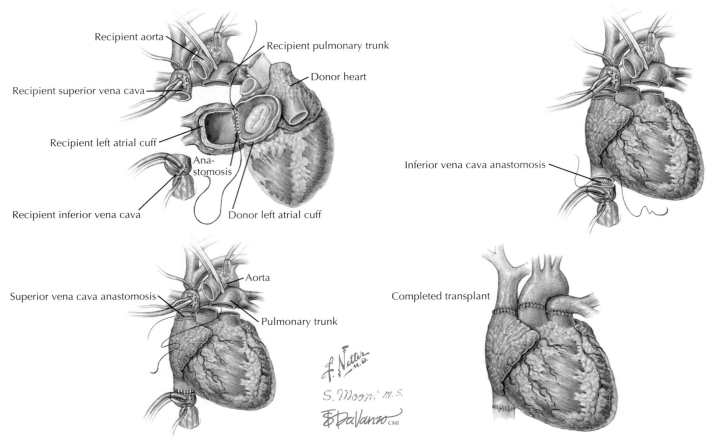

FIG 34.2 Technique of Bicaval Cardiac Transplantation.

suture line to assist in de-airing and to prevent warm blood from accumulating in the heart during the remainder of the implantation. Next, the recipient and donor inferior venae cavae are anastomosed, followed by the superior venae cavae. The pulmonary artery and aortic anastomosis are then completed similarly. An alternative is to complete the LA, inferior vena cava, and aortic anastomoses, and then release the cross-clamp, completing the remaining right-sided anastomoses with the heart beating and reperfused to decrease ischemic time. Weaning from cardiopulmonary bypass is the same as the biatrial technique.

POSTOPERATIVE MANAGEMENT

The initial postoperative treatment of cardiac transplantation recipients is similar to that of open heart surgery patients, especially in terms of fluid and electrolyte management, ventilator care and weaning, and pain control. The major differences include isolation precautions because of the increased infection risk and immunosuppression to prevent rejection. Multiple protocols for transplantation immunosuppression and rejection monitoring exist. Most rely on initial triple-drug immunosuppression with a calcineurin inhibitor (cyclosporine or tacrolimus), a purine synthesis inhibitor (azathioprine or mycophenolate mofetil), and prednisone. The doses of calcineurin inhibitors are monitored and adjusted based on daily serum concentrations, the standard doses of purine synthesis inhibitors are decreased if leukopenia or pancytopenia develops, and steroids are tapered by schedule in the absence of rejection. Most programs use a protocol of endomyocardial biopsies, supplemented when indicated by echocardiography, right-sided heart

catheterization, or both to diagnose rejection and monitor response to therapy. With significant rejection or hemodynamic compromise, patients are treated with bolus steroids. If this is ineffective or if a pattern of recurrent rejection develops in the patient, other treatment protocols are used. Because the donor heart is totally denervated, close monitoring of the heart rate is necessary in the early postoperative period. Denervation may lead to a slower intrinsic heart rate, necessitating the use of chronotropic medications, titrated to a goal heart rate of >90 beats/min.

During follow-up examinations, patients are monitored for the development of arrhythmias, immunosuppressive side effects, and signs and symptoms of infection. Routine ECGs often show two P waves when the biatrial technique is used: one from the recipient right atria and one from the donor right atria. This can be misdiagnosed as atrial fibrillation or premature atrial contractions. The correct diagnosis is established by confirming that one set of P waves (from the donor) is synchronous with the QRS complex. Routine chest radiography is vital to detect new infiltrates that most commonly represent preclinical pneumonias or early malignancies. Aggressive evaluation of these infiltrates is mandatory, because immunosuppressive agents increase infection risks and can accelerate growth of malignancies. Early detection and treatment can mean the difference between survival and death. Chronic renal insufficiency is a common adverse effect of long-term calcineurin inhibitor use and can be ameliorated by dose modulation. Likewise, chronic hypertension is a common result of the use of calcineurin inhibitors and steroids, and can necessitate treatment with multiple agents to control blood pressure. Hyperlipidemia also occurs with both agents, and evidence suggests all transplantation patients should be routinely treated with statins. Calcineurin inhibitors and steroids are also diabetogenic and usually necessitate aggressive therapy with insulin for adequate control. The frequency of endomyocardial biopsies gradually decreases in the absence of rejection; by 1 year, they are only performed with clinical suspicion of rejection or as part of the annual examination.

Results of Cardiac Transplantation

Data on >116,000 cardiac transplantation procedures from approximately 225 centers (all centers in the United States, which is mandatory for UNOS membership and voluntary for international centers), have been collected and analyzed by the ISHLT and UNOS since 1983. In 2014, the 31st "Official Adult Heart Transplant Report" was released by the ISHLT. The number of heart transplantation procedures reported to the registry declined annually from 1993 to 2004, and is now slowly increasing. In 2014, a total of 4196 heart transplantations were reported to the registry. More than 50% of the reporting centers perform >10 transplantations annually. The primary indications for adult heart transplantation are overwhelmingly CAD (36%) and nonischemic cardiomyopathy (55%). The remaining indications are adult congenital heart disease (3%), re-transplantation (2.5%), and valvular heart disease (2.8%). Recipients older than 60 years now include >25% of all recipients annually. In addition, a significant increase in the number of recipients on LVADs at the time of transplantation has occurred (41% currently vs. 24% during 2000–2008). Also, fewer recipients are now hospitalized immediately before transplantation (44% vs. 72%), which probably reflects the current practice of using an LVAD or inotropes in the outpatient setting as a bridge to transplantation. Donor use has become more liberal over the last decade, with an increase in the mean donor age from 23 years in 1983 to 35 years in 2014. In addition, although donors older than 50 years were rare before 1986, they now account for >12% of donors.

Postoperative immunosuppression has changed somewhat over the last decade, with increased use of perioperative antilymphocyte antibodies or interleukin-2 receptor antagonists. Tacrolimus is now the most commonly used calcineurin inhibitor, whereas mycophenolate mofetil remains the predominant antiproliferative agent. Sirolimus use remains low at <20%. Prednisone continues to be an important therapy because approximately 75% of patients are still on it 1 year posttransplantation; this decreases to >40% at 5 years posttransplantation.

Survival after cardiac transplantation remains excellent. The 1-, 5-, and 10-year survival rates are currently 84%, 70%, and 50%, respectively. After an initial drop in survival during the first 6 months, the survival curve then decreases at a linear rate of approximately 3.5% per year beyond 15 years after transplantation. However, it does not appear that there is a point where the slope of the survival curve decreases to reach that of the general population. Risk factors for 1-year mortality include the requirement of dialysis or prolonged mechanical ventilation at the time of transplantation, having an infection treated with intravenous antibiotics within 2 weeks of transplantation, requirement of short-term extracorporeal mechanical circulatory support, adults with congenital heart disease, preoperative use of a pulsatile VAD, recipient age, donor age, donor heart ischemic time, donor body mass index (inverse), transplantation center volume (inverse), recipient pulmonary artery diastolic pressure, and recipient pretransplantation bilirubin and creatinine levels.

At 7 years posttransplantation, approximately 90% of recipients have no functional limitations, and many have returned to full-time work. In the first year after transplantation, noncytomegalovirus infection, graft failure, and acute rejection are the most common causes of death. After 5 years, allograft vasculopathy accounts for 33% of deaths, followed by malignancies (23%) and noncytomegalovirus infections (11%). Posttransplantation morbidities remain significant. By 10 years

after transplantation, 99% of survivors have hypertension, 14% have severe renal insufficiency, 93% have hyperlipidemia, 37% have diabetes, and 53% have angiographic allograft vasculopathy.

Mechanical Circulatory Support Devices

Over the past 20 years, mechanical circulatory support devices (MCSDs) have been developed with the goal of supporting patients with advanced heart failure as a bridge to transplantation, bridge to recovery, and alternative to transplantation. MCSDs are defined as mechanical pumps that assist or replace the left, right, or both ventricles of the heart to pump blood. The current generation of devices allows a spectrum of support, ranging from short- to intermediate- to long-term duration. Depending on hemodynamic parameters, devices can be tailored for partial or complete LV support, right ventricular support, or biventricular support. Device positions range from paracorporeal pumps, to intracorporeal pumps with transcutaneous drive lines, to completely implantable systems. Device technology has also advanced, becoming progressively smaller, more reliable, less thrombogenic, and with lower infection risks. First-generation devices rely mostly on large pneumatic or electric drives, second-generation devices rely on axial flow technology, and third-generation rely primarily on magnetically levitated drives. Third-generation devices have now been approved for both as a bridge to transplantation therapy and as destination therapy.

Patient Selection and Indications

Patient selection remains paramount to success with MCSDs, and a multidisciplinary approach should be used. Indications for mechanical circulatory support are similar to heart transplantation. Clinical indications for MCSDs are both acute and chronic (Fig. 34.3). Acute indications include refractory cardiogenic shock after myocardial infarction, acute myocarditis, and failure to wean from cardiopulmonary bypass. The use of short-term MCSDs to treat acute heart failure falls outside the scope of this chapter and will not be discussed further, but it should be mentioned that MCSDs can be used with acceptable results in these patient populations at experienced centers.

Chronic indications are similar to those of heart transplantation and include ischemic cardiomyopathy, idiopathic cardiomyopathy, valvular cardiomyopathy, and congenital heart disease. Generally accepted hemodynamic criteria for MCSDs in these patients include New York Heart Association functional class IV heart failure refractory to medical therapy, a cardiac index of <2 L/min per meter², pulmonary capillary wedge pressure >25 mm Hg, systolic blood pressure <80 mm Hg, and an ejection fraction of >20%. Exclusion criteria for MCSDs in these patients remain a subject of debate but generally include evidence of fixed pulmonary hypertension (>6 Wood units), recent pulmonary infarction, active peptic ulcer disease, diabetes with end-organ damage, severe peripheral vascular disease, active infection, renal insufficiency (creatinine >2.5 mg/dL), significant liver or lung dysfunction, recent malignancy, excessive obesity (body mass index >35 kg/m²), active substance abuse, history of noncompliance, and severe psychosocial issues. Patients with chronic indications for MCSDs can be considered for a long-term or durable device. An endpoint for mechanical circulatory support should be identified preoperatively, with the caveat that the endpoint can change depending on patient status after device implantation. Possible endpoints include bridge to recovery, bridge to transplantation, and destination therapy (alternative to transplantation). For example, one may intend a device to be a bridge to recovery and find that cardiac function does not improve; these patients are then often candidates for consideration for either bridge-to-transplantation or destination therapy. We would caution against the use of durable devices in the acute setting before a full evaluation has been completed to avoid the dreaded endpoint of "bridge to nowhere."

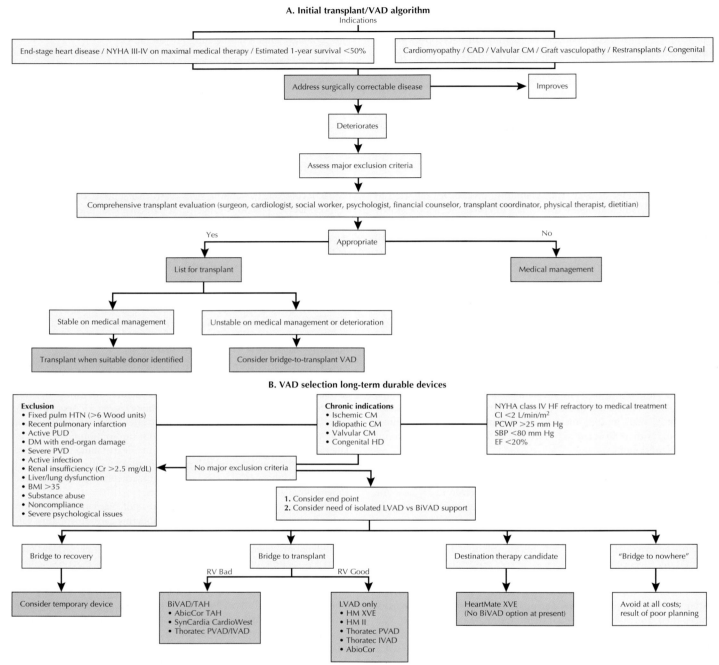

FIG 34.3 Ventricular Assist Device Selection. *BiVAD*, Biventricular assist device; *BMI*, body mass index; *CAD*, coronary artery disease; *CI*, cardiac index; *CM*, cardiomyopathy; *Cr*, creatinine; *DM*, diabetes mellitus; *EF*, ejection fraction; *HD*, heart disease; *HF*, heart failure; *HM*, HeartMate; *HTN*, hypertension; *IVAD*, implantable ventricular assist device; *LVAD*, lead ventricular assist device; *NYHA*, New York Heart Association functional class; *PCWP*, pulmonary capillary wedge pressure; *PUD*, peptic ulcer disease; *Pulm*, pulmonary; *PVAD*, paracorporeal ventricular assist device; *PVD*, peripheral vascular disease; *RV*, right ventricle; *SBP*, systolic blood pressure; *TAH*, total artificial heart; *VAD*, ventricular assist device; *XVE*, extended lead vented electric.

Long-Term Durable Mechanical Circulatory Support Devices

AbioCor Total Artificial Heart

The AbioCor (Abiomed, Inc., Danver, Massachusetts) is approved by the Food and Drug Administration (FDA) under a Humanitarian Device Exemption for use in patients who are not transplantation candidates and who are not candidates for LVAD destination therapy. It is implanted selectively at only a few centers in the United States. The device is a total artificial heart that uses transcutaneous energy transmission. Thromboembolic and bleeding complications have been high with this device, and its use is limited.

SynCardia Total Artificial Heart

The SynCardia CardioWest (SynCardia Systems, Inc., Tucson, Arizona) device is a temporary total artificial heart. It is approved for use as a bridge to transplantation for transplantation-eligible patients. This biventricular, pneumatic, pulsatile blood pump completely replaces the native ventricles of the patient and all four cardiac valves orthotopically. In a nonrandomized prospective study at 5 U.S. centers, 81 patients received the artificial heart device with a survival rate to transplantation of 79%, and overall 1-year survival of 70%. Bleeding events occurred in 62% of patients, infectious events in 77%, and neurological events in 27%.

Thoratec Paracorporeal Ventricular Assist Devices

The Thoratec Paracorporeal Ventricular Assist Device (Thoratec Corp., Pleasanton, California), which is based on designs from the 1970s, has been approved as a bridge to transplantation since 1995. It can be used in the right, left, or biventricular positions. It is relatively easy to implant, and it can be used in a wide range of patient sizes because of the paracorporeal location of the ventricles. Although patients can be ambulated with this device, its paracorporeal position limits its wide-ranging applicability and appeal.

HeartMate XVE

The HeartMate XVE (Thoratec Corp.) is a first-generation VAD that is an implantable, pulsatile, electrically driven device that can fully sustain circulation. The inflow cannula connects to the LV apex, and the outflow cannula connects to the aorta. The pump is implanted in an abdominal wall pocket, and a single transcutaneous cable exits the right epigastrium and connects to a wearable external driver. It has been approved as a bridge to transplantation since 1998, and it received FDA approval in 2003 for use as destination therapy. The use of this pump was limited by issues with durability and the size of the pump.

HeartMate II

The HeartMate II (Thoratec Corp.) was developed to overcome some of the limitations of pulsatile volume-displacement devices, such as the HeartMate XVE (including the large pump size and limited long-term mechanical durability). The HeartMate II device uses continuous-flow, rotary pump technology. The smaller pump size, compared with the HeartMate WVE, allows the extension of MCSD therapy to smaller patients (adolescents and some women). Another advantage is the potential for greater durability because this device has only a single moving part (the rotor). Implantation is similar to the HeartMate XVE; however, a much smaller abdominal wall pocket is needed due to the smaller device size. In a prospective multicenter trial without a concurrent control group, 133 patients underwent implantation of the HeartMate II device. The principal outcome (transplantation or alive at 6 months) was reached in 75% of patients, and the incidences of device failure and infection were lower than those in the HeartMate XVE destination therapy trial. Compared with newer, third-generation devices, HeartMate II LVADs have a higher rate of significant device thrombosis and thromboembolic events.

HeartMate III

The HeartMate III (Thoratec Corp.) is a third-generation device that uses a magnetically suspended centrifugal pump and has no bearings. It is fully implantable, and the small pump size allows for limited dissection and eliminates the need for an abdominal wall VAD pocket. The pump has been programmed with intrinsic pulsatility that is believed to decrease the risk of pump thrombosis, gastrointestinal bleeding, and stroke. The device has been FDA approved for both bridge-to-transplantation and destination therapy indications. Clinical trials with destination therapy patients are ongoing.

HeartWare

The HeartWare HVAD (Medtronic, Minneapolis, Minnesota) is a continuous-flow centrifugal pump that is fully implantable and small enough to be placed in an intrapericardial position. Magnetic and hydrostatic forces suspend the impeller within the pump, eliminating any physical contact between the impeller and pump. The Evaluation of the HeartWare Left Ventricular Assist Device for the Treatment of Advanced Heart Failure (ADVANCE) trial demonstrated comparable survival to other available devices for bridge-to-transplantation patients. The HeartWare Ventricular Assist System as Destination Therapy of Advanced Heart Failure (ENDURANCE) trial is a randomized, controlled trial that evaluated survival and outcomes for destination therapy HVAD implantations. Good survival and an acceptable complication profile led to approval for use of the HVAD in destination therapy patients in the fall of 2017.

Results From the Interagency Registry for Mechanically Assisted Circulatory Support

The Interagency Registry for Mechanically Assisted Circulatory Support (INTERMACS) database, funded by the U.S. National Heart, Lung, and Blood Institute (NHLBI), is a registry for patients who receive durable FDA-approved MCSDs for treatment of advanced heart failure. It was established to advance understanding and application of mechanical circulatory support to improve the duration and quality of life for individuals with advanced heart failure. It represents a unique collaboration of the NHLBI as the funding and scientific support agency, the FDA as the regulatory agency, and the Center for Medicaid and Medicare Services as the federal reimbursement agency, to establish a common language through which benefit and progress with respect to these devices can be expressed.

INTERMACS went live on June 23, 2006, and as of December 31, 2015, 158 centers were able to enroll patients into its database. From 2006 to 2015, >90% of patients received continuous-flow devices, and pulsatile devices continue to be phased out. An increase in VAD use for destination therapy was observed after 2008, but this plateaued in 2014 at nearly 46% of implantations being destination therapy. Approximately one-third of adult patients with VADs receive a heart transplantation by 1 year.

The actuarial survival for the entire cohort was 80% at 1 year and 70% at 2 years. One-year actuarial survival for destination therapy patients was almost 80%, whereas those who required biventricular VAD support had inferior survival, with only approximately 50% of patients surviving at 1 year. Preoperative risk factors for early death were critical cardiogenic shock, older age, ascites at the time of implantation, higher level of bilirubin, and placement of a biventricular assist device or a total artificial heart. Interestingly, the initial "strategy" at implantation had no discernible effect on survival (bridge to transplantation vs. bridge to recovery vs. bridge to candidacy). LVAD pump exchange became more prevalent and was associated with a significant decrease in 1-year survival compared with control subjects (patients who did not require exchange).

FUTURE DIRECTIONS

Cardiac transplantation is an established, safe, durable, and reliable therapy for patients with end-stage heart disease. Its application is limited only by an inadequate supply of donor organs, which mandates careful selection of recipients to ensure the best results in the use of this scarce resource. Initiatives for improvements in cardiac transplantation include development of a more scientific method to evaluate heart recipients and donors through development of a Heart Allocation Score and a Donor Risk Index. In addition, there are initiatives to standardize donor management among the regional Organ Procurement Organizations (OPOs), because donor selection and management varies widely geographically, with cardiac donation rates ranging from 4% to 60%, depending on the OPO. Advances in immunosuppression and immunomodulation will probably occur in the areas of co-stimulatory blockade and modification of antibody-mediated rejection. New research suggests that B-cell regulation, in addition to or as opposed to T-cell regulation, affects the development of chronic allograft vasculopathy. However, drugs to target these mechanisms remain in their infancy and require better understanding before they can be used clinically. Unfortunately, despite early enthusiasm, stem cell therapy for advanced heart failure remains far from a clinical reality.

MCSDs continue to evolve. The new, smaller rotary pumps seem to have increased durability, and they have lower infection and thromboembolic event rates than the pulsatile flow devices. In addition, these pumps have recently been approved for use in destination therapy. Future developments in MCSDs will undoubtedly continue, especially from the aspects of decreasing infections and thromboembolic events. Percutaneously placed or peripherally placed VADs that either fully or partially support the patient are also in development, perhaps moving the MCSD therapy to less sick patients before they progress to refractory heart failure. Because of the heart failure epidemic, research interest and clinical activity will continue, and it is likely that the future holds significant advances.

ADDITIONAL RESOURCES

Baumgartner WA, Reitz BA, Achuff SC, eds. *Heart and Heart-Lung Transplantation*. Philadelphia: W.B. Saunders; 1990.
A comprehensive review of heart transplantation from the leaders in the field.

Jatin A, Singh S, Antoun D, et al. Durable mechanical circulatory support versus organ transplantation: past, present, and future. *Biomed Res Int.* 2015;2015:849571.
Review article discussing the role of both mechanical circulatory support and transplantation in patient management.

EVIDENCE

International Society for Heart and Lung Transplantation. Available at: http://www.ishlt.org; The Scientific Registry of Transplant Recipients. Available at: https://www.srtr.org/; United Network for Organ Sharing. Available at: http://www.unos.org.
Useful web sites for information about U.S. organ donation, trends, and outcomes.
Kirklin JK, Naftel DC, Pagani FD, et al. Seventh INTERMACS annual report: 15,000 patients and counting. *J Heart Lung Transplant.* 2015;34:1495–1504.
Seventh annual report from the INTERMACS database, including device trends, morbidity and mortality data, and patient characteristics.
Lund LH, Edwards LB, Kucheryavaya AY, et al. Registry of the International Society for Heart and Lung Transplantation: Thirty-First Official Adult Heart Transplant Report—2014. *J Heart Lung Transplant.* 2014;33(10):996–1008.
Most recent registry report from the ISHLT.
Miller LW, Pagani FD, Russell SD, et al. Use of a continuous-flow device in patients awaiting heart transplantation. *N Engl J Med.* 2007;357:885–896.
Report showing that a continuous-flow LVAD can provide effective hemodynamic support for a at least 6 months in patients awaiting heart transplantation, with improved functional status and quality of life. This report led to FDA approval of the HeartMate II device as a bridge to transplantation in April 2008.
Rose EA, Gelijns AC, Moskowitz AJ, et al. Long-term use of a left ventricular assist device for end-stage heart disease. *N Engl J Med.* 2001;345:1435–1443.
Seminal article showing a survival benefit of LVADs in patients with advanced heart failure who are not candidates for heart transplantation compared with optimal medical management. This report led to FDA approval of the Heart Mate XVE device as destination therapy.

35

Stress-Induced Cardiomyopathy

Christopher D. Chiles, Rikin Patel, Charles Baggett

Stress-induced cardiomyopathy, also called Takotsubo cardiomyopathy, represents a syndrome of transient left ventricular (LV) dysfunction from a variety of psychological or physiological stressors. Patients in the critical care setting are particularly vulnerable, but ambulatory patients subject to severe emotional distress may also develop stress-induced cardiomyopathy. In the intensive care setting, sepsis, respiratory failure, intracranial hemorrhage, and pancreatitis are a few of the described precipitators. Despite its description more than 25 years ago and its increasing clinical recognition, the pathophysiology of stress cardiomyopathy remains speculative and the treatment empiric, but the prognosis is commonly favorable.

Takotsubo cardiomyopathy was originally described in the early 1990s in Japan, but is now recognized to occur worldwide. "Takotsubo" is a Japanese word for a narrow-necked fishing pot used for trapping octopi, and this pot resembles findings seen on the left ventriculogram in the most common pattern of stress cardiomyopathy (Fig. 35.1). Other names include transient LV apical ballooning and colloquially as "broken heart syndrome."

Stress-induced cardiomyopathy affects women much more often than men (>80% of cases are women), with a mean age of 66 years, and accounts for approximately 2% of suspected acute coronary syndromes. Treatment is primarily supportive.

ETIOLOGY AND PATHOGENESIS

Although numerous associations exist between putative etiologies and stress-induced cardiomyopathy, the pathogenesis of the disease is not well understood. Because a variety of clinical circumstances have been temporally associated with stress-induced cardiomyopathy, it has been proposed that mediators, such as excess catecholamines, histamines, and/or cytokines that result from a variety of stresses, could cause coronary artery spasm, microvascular dysfunction, or direct myocardial toxicity. Any combination of these could result in the transient ECG changes, depressed LV function, and elevated cardiac biomarkers that characterize stress-induced cardiomyopathy. In addition, multiple studies have associated a lack of estrogen with the predominance of this condition in postmenopausal women.

Observational studies indicate that most cases of Takotsubo cardiomyopathy are preceded by either emotional (14%–38%) or physiological (17%–77%) stress. However, in the International Takotsubo Registry, up to 28% of patients had no evident trigger. The association with stress would be consistent with the hypothesis that increased catecholamine levels could cause microvascular dysfunction or myocardial toxicity. Studies that evaluated plasma norepinephrine found elevated levels in most patients with Takotsubo cardiomyopathy. One report measured the magnitude of plasma catecholamine release in Takotsubo cardiomyopathy compared with patients with myocardial infarction (MI). In this study, concentrations of both epinephrine (1264 pg/mL

vs. 376 pg/mL) and norepinephrine (2284 pg/mL vs. 1100 pg/mL) were higher in patients with Takotsubo cardiomyopathy. Further support for a causative effect of catecholamines includes findings of transient myocardial perfusion abnormalities consistent with stunned myocardium or multivessel coronary artery vasospasm. In addition, endomyocardial biopsy specimens show histological signs of catecholamine toxicity in patients with stress cardiomyopathy.

CLINICAL PRESENTATION

Many patients with stress-induced cardiomyopathy present with severe LV dysfunction and are critically ill as a result. The most common chief complaint in Takotsubo cardiomyopathy is chest pain at rest (33%–71%), with shortness of breath, syncope, and shock also reported. It is important to note if there may be a history of severe emotional distress, such as death of a family member or other significant psychological stress, in the clinical presentation. Critical medical or surgical illness, panic attacks, arguments, and other emotionally charged situations have been reported as triggering scenarios. Cardiogenic pulmonary edema may develop in stress cardiomyopathy, particularly with fluid resuscitation in the setting of sepsis, pancreatitis, trauma, or the postoperative period.

ECG findings typically mimic those in ST-segment elevation MI (STEMI) or other forms of acute coronary syndrome. The presentation of stress-induced cardiomyopathy may also result in ECG changes similar to those seen in intracranial hemorrhage, stroke, or head trauma as well as deep symmetric T-wave inversions in the precordial leads with a prolonged QT interval. Acute systolic heart failure, cardiogenic shock, or dynamic LV outflow tract obstruction due to hyperdynamic basal segments (13%–18%) may also be part of the presentation.

DIFFERENTIAL DIAGNOSIS

Stress-induced cardiomyopathy typically presents with chest pain, respiratory distress, or pulmonary edema in conjunction with LV dysfunction, ECG abnormalities, and elevated cardiac biomarkers. The clinical presentation of Takotsubo cardiomyopathy often mimics MI.

Acute coronary syndromes are far more common than stress-induced cardiomyopathy. For this reason, the clinician who is evaluating a patient with suspected Takotsubo cardiomyopathy should still consider MI a high possibility in the differential. The diagnosis of stress-induced cardiomyopathy most often involves ruling out significant coronary artery disease (CAD) by angiography. Acute pulmonary embolism may also be considered in the differential diagnosis. The possibility of myocarditis may be more difficult to distinguish from Takotsubo cardiomyopathy at times. Either a characteristic pattern of wall motion abnormalities, findings at angiography, or a rapidly improving clinical course can help to distinguish stress-induced cardiomyopathy from an acute coronary syndrome or myocarditis.

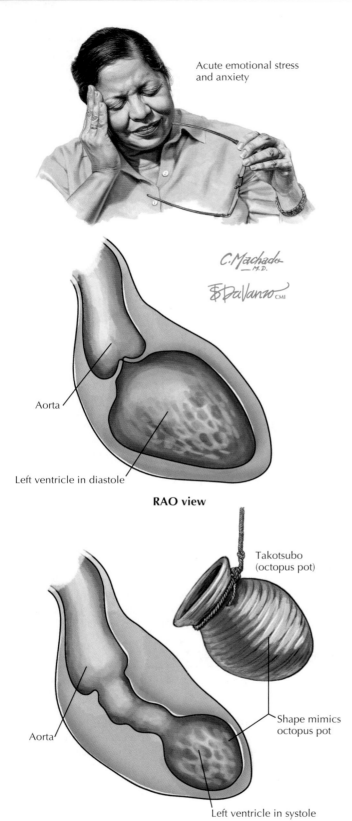

Acute emotional stress and anxiety

Aorta

Left ventricle in diastole

RAO view

Takotsubo (octopus pot)

Aorta

Shape mimics octopus pot

Left ventricle in systole

FIG 35.1 Octopus Pot. *RAO,* Right anterior oblique.

DIAGNOSTIC APPROACH

The diagnosis of stress-induced cardiomyopathy depends on an appropriate clinical history and the lack of evidence to support an alternative diagnosis. Clinical context, laboratory data, and the use of echocardiographic and angiographic imaging can help direct the clinician with the diagnosis.

Diagnostic criteria have been developed by a group at the Mayo Clinic. If all four of the following criteria are met, the diagnosis of stress cardiomyopathy can be confirmed:

1. Transient akinesis or dyskinesis of the LV apical and midventricular segments with regional wall motion abnormalities extending beyond a single epicardial vascular distribution. Exceptions are the focal and global variants.
2. Absence of obstructive coronary disease or angiographic evidence of acute plaque rupture. If CAD is present, the diagnosis of stress cardiomyopathy can still be made if the wall motion abnormalities are not in the distribution of the CAD.
3. New ECG abnormalities (either ST-segment elevation or T-wave inversion) or modest elevation in cardiac troponin.
4. Absence of pheochromocytoma or myocarditis.

Electrocardiography

As noted, the ECG is an important initial diagnostic tool in stress-induced cardiomyopathy. The most common ECG abnormalities are ST-segment and T-wave abnormalities. ST-segment elevation at presentation is reported in 43% of stress-induced cardiomyopathy cases. Anterior ST changes are more common than inferior or lateral ST abnormalities. Additional findings may include T-wave inversions, pathological Q waves, and prolonged corrected QT segments. Ogura et al. compared specific 12-lead ECG findings in Takotsubo cardiomyopathy and acute anterior MI. Q waves and inferior lead reciprocal changes were more common in acute anterior MI than in Takotsubo cardiomyopathy. T-wave inversion in precordial leads, a ratio of ST-segment elevation in leads V_4 to V_6 and leads V_1 to V_3 of >1.0, and QT dispersion were more common in Takotsubo cardiomyopathy. Absence of inferior lead reciprocal changes combined with the ratio of ST-segment elevation in leads V_4 to V_6 and leads V_1 to V_3 was the most powerful predictor of Takotsubo cardiomyopathy, with a specificity of 100% and an overall accuracy of 91%.

Cardiac Biomarkers

Most patients with stress-induced cardiomyopathy will have elevated serum cardiac troponin. In two case series, 100% of individuals with Takotsubo cardiomyopathy were found to be troponin-positive. The most common pattern of cardiac troponin elevation is a small, rapid increase with peak levels typically measured at presentation. Plasma B-type natriuretic peptide (BNP) or N-terminal pro-BNP are also commonly elevated in those with stress cardiomyopathy.

Cardiac Catheterization

Takotsubo cardiomyopathy commonly presents with chest pain and ST-segment elevation on ECG, necessitating emergent diagnostic coronary angiography. Even when the diagnosis of Takotsubo cardiomyopathy is suspected, initial management should proceed in accordance with current STEMI guidelines.

Although the absence of obstructive CAD at angiography is one of the typical diagnostic criteria, some patients may be found to have CAD. In the International Takotsubo Registry, 15% of patients had CAD. This incidence likely represents the background prevalence of CAD in older populations of patients at risk for stress-induced cardiomyopathy.

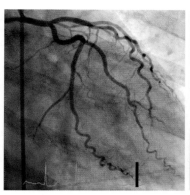
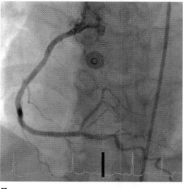
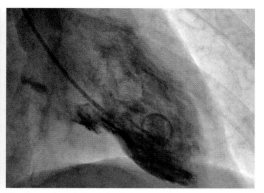

A. Coronary angiogram showing non-obstructive disease of the left coronary artery.

B. Coronary angiogram showing non-obstructive disease of the right coronary artery.

C. Normal end-diastolic left ventriculogram.

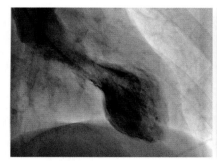
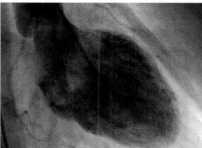
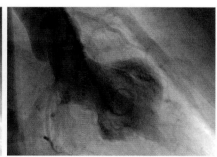

D. End-systolic left ventriculogram showing apical ballooning.

E. Normal end-diastolic left ventriculogram.

F. End-systolic left ventriculogram showing midventricular ballooning.

FIG 35.2 Takotsubo Cardiomyopathy.

The classic description of Takotsubo cardiomyopathy on left ventriculography is apical dyskinesis with depressed mid to apical segments and hyperdynamic basal segments in a distribution beyond that of a single coronary artery (Fig. 35.2A–D). However, there are additional subtypes of Takotsubo syndrome: midventricular (Fig. 35.2E and F), basal, focal, and global. These variants account for up to 20% of stress cardiomyopathy cases.

Intensive care unit patients with multiple co-morbidities and stress-induced cardiomyopathy may be unable to safely undergo coronary angiography. Patients with trauma, intracranial bleeding, pancreatitis, or acute kidney injury may be poor candidates for angiography or revascularization with concurrent use of iodinated contrast or anticoagulation. In these settings, the risk-to-benefit ratio of cardiac catheterization may preclude proceeding with an invasive evaluation.

Transthoracic Echocardiography

Transthoracic echocardiography is recommended for initial evaluation and serial follow-up of LV function with suspected stress-induced cardiomyopathy. The mean LV ejection fraction (EF) ranges between 39% and 49%, but may be as low as 20%. The EF rapidly increases over days to weeks to a mean follow-up LVEF of 60% to 76%. Although there is a focus on LV dysfunction in stress cardiomyopathy, both right and left ventricles may be involved. Many patients with Takotsubo syndrome have return of normal LV systolic function in as little as a week.

Cardiac Magnetic Resonance Imaging

Routine use of cardiac MRI is not generally required, although it has been recently examined in clinical studies. An important clinical use might be as a tool to help distinguish between myocarditis and atypical stress-induced cardiomyopathy. Absence of late gadolinium enhancement on MRI would support stress cardiomyopathy over the diagnosis of myocarditis or MI. One study of cardiac MRI in stress-induced cardiomyopathy showed that 26% of patients had right ventricular (RV) wall abnormalities. Those with RV dysfunction had an overall lower LVEF than did patients with normal RV function (40%–48%). Follow-up cardiac MRI showed typical improvement of LV function and resolution of RV function.

MANAGEMENT AND THERAPY

Optimal Treatment

There are limited data on optimal medical management for stress-induced cardiomyopathy. Current opinion suggests a medical regimen analogous to that recommended for treatment of patients with cardiomyopathy and systolic dysfunction. This includes initiation of a β-blocker (when the patient is euvolemic), an angiotensin-converting enzyme inhibitor, aspirin, and diuretics, as needed. Marked improvement in LV dysfunction over days to weeks is typical for patients with stress-induced cardiomyopathy. Anticoagulation to prevent thrombosis from significant LV dysfunction may be considered until LV function improves. Patients should be monitored for atrial and ventricular arrhythmias, heart failure, and mechanical complications while in the hospital. The long-term prognosis is probably similar to age- and disease-matched controls, and many patients can discontinue therapies for LV dysfunction over the ensuing months. However, there is a reported recurrence rate of between 2% and 10%.

Avoiding Treatment Errors

Severe hypotension and cardiogenic shock may develop in up to 10% of those with stress-induced cardiomyopathy. Cardiogenic shock may be due to LV or RV systolic dysfunction, but also can be caused by dynamic LV outflow tract (LVOT) obstruction. In the presence of cardiogenic shock, timely evaluation of an intraventricular pressure gradient by either left heart catheterization or transthoracic echocardiography is required. Such a gradient can occur if the LV base is hyperkinetic and obstructs LV outflow. Prompt diagnosis of this complication is important, because treatment differs from hypotension in the absence of intraventricular obstruction. With LVOT obstruction, treatment must focus on maintaining an adequate end-diastolic LV volume and decreasing the intraventricular pressure gradient. Maintenance of end-diastolic LV volume is achieved by avoiding excessive diuresis and fluid resuscitation if pulmonary congestion is absent. β-blocker therapy increases diastolic filling time and may decrease the magnitude of the LVOT gradient. β_1 agonists (particularly dobutamine) should be specifically avoided in the setting of hypotension with dynamic intraventricular obstruction. If hemodynamics do not improve with fluids and β-blockers, then phenylephrine or vasopressin can increase mean arterial pressure and reduce the gradient. Finally, placement of an intraaortic balloon pump can mechanically support the patient, although there is a small possibility that decreased afterload can worsen the intraventricular gradient.

FUTURE DIRECTIONS

Diagnosis of stress-induced cardiomyopathy depends on meeting criteria (in particular, biomarker positivity and LV dysfunction) in the presence of an appropriate clinical scenario and the absence of significant CAD. Advances in imaging may ultimately prove to be valuable tools in assessing stress-induced cardiomyopathy. Nuclear medicine techniques, including ^{123}I-metaiodobenzylguanidine myocardial scintigraphy, could help clarify regional adrenergic receptors in stress-induced cardiomyopathy. A rat model of Takotsubo cardiomyopathy may provide further insights into the pathogenesis. Studies of the potential role of the endocrine, central neural, and autonomic nervous systems may also be useful.

Although much remains to be understood regarding the pathophysiology of stress-induced cardiomyopathy, there are also unanswered questions about optimal therapy. Beta-blockers, which have been a cornerstone in treatment, did not seem to affect the development or recurrence in large registry data. The use of angiotensin-converting enzyme inhibitors or angiotensin receptor blockers were associated with the most favorable prognosis, raising additional questions about other neuroendocrine mechanisms in this interesting syndrome.

ADDITIONAL RESOURCES

"Uptodate" Online Medical Resource; 2008. Available at: <http://www.uptodate.com/home/index.html>. Accessed February 23, 2010.
An evidence-based, peer-reviewed medical information resource providing a synthesis of the literature, the latest evidence, and specific recommendations for patient care.

EVIDENCE

Akashi YJ, Goldstein DS, Barbaro G, Ueyama T. Takotsubo cardiomyopathy: a new form of acute, reversible heart failure. *Circulation.* 2008;118:2754–2762.
Provides details regarding the mouse model of disease and the potential for estrogen replacement as a therapy.
Bybee KA, Kara T, Prasad A, et al. Systematic review: transient left ventricular apical ballooning: a syndrome that mimics ST-segment elevation myocardial infarction. *Ann Intern Med.* 2004;141:858–865.
A review of a seven case series that proposed specific Mayo criteria for the clinical diagnosis of Takotsubo cardiomyopathy due to its characteristic presentation.
Ghadri JR, Cammann VL, et al. Differences in the clinical profile and outcomes of typical and atypical Takotsubo syndrome data from the International Takotsubo Registry. *JAMA Cardiol.* 2016;1(3):335–340.
This article helps to understand the clinical characteristics of the typical and atypical types of Takotsubo syndrome within the International Takotsubo Registry.
Kurowski V, Kaiser A, von Hof K, et al. Apical and midventricular transient left ventricular dysfunction syndrome (tako-tsubo cardiomyopathy): frequency, mechanism, and prognosis. *Chest.* 2007;132:809.
Reports demographic, clinical, and outcomes data on Takotsubo cardiomyopathy.
Ogura R, Hiasa Y, Yakahashi T, et al. Specific findings of the standard 12-lead ECG in patients with 'Takotsubo' cardiomyopathy: comparison with the findings of acute anterior myocardial infarction. *Circ J.* 2003;67:687–690.
Describes the 12-lead ECG findings in Takotsubo cardiomyopathy and acute anterior MI, and identifies which are most specific and most accurate for the diagnosis of Takotsubo cardiomyopathy.
Templin C, Ghadri JR, Diekmann J, et al. Clinical features and outcomes of Takotsubo (stress) cardiomyopathy. *N Engl J Med.* 2015;373:929–938.
Reviews clinical features, prognostic predictors, and outcomes of Takotsubo cardiomyopathy in the International Takotsubo Registry.

Cardiac Rhythm Abnormalities

36

Bradyarrhythmias

Fong T. Leong, Basil Abu-el-Haija, J. Paul Mounsey

In adults, bradycardia refers to a ventricular rate that is <60 beats/min. This figure is somewhat arbitrary and does not necessarily connote disease. For instance, it is common to find healthy athletes with resting heart rates of approximately 40 beats/min. In general, bradycardia becomes a clinical issue if it correlates with symptoms—syncope, dizziness, exercise intolerance, breathlessness, angina, fatigue, or mental confusion. These correlations can be difficult to establish. For example, fatigue is a common complaint and may be merely coincidental with, and not caused by, slow heart rates. In such circumstances, ambulatory cardiac monitors, and occasionally, invasive testing can determine whether bradycardia is truly pathological, and help to form the appropriate treatment plan.

ETIOLOGY AND PATHOGENESIS

It is simplest to regard bradycardia as a manifestation of quite a few non-cardiac and cardiac causes (Box 36.1). When due to cardiac causes, brady-cardia may be further categorized according to the site(s) of delay or block within the cardiac conduction system: the sinus node, the atrioventricular (AV) node, the bundle of His, and the bundle branches and/or Purkinje network. Conditions that alter the autonomic inputs to the sinus and AV nodes, diseases that interrupt the blood supply or the electrophysiology of these structures, or drugs that modify the ionic properties of conductive cardiomyocytes can all lead to bradycardia. By far, sinus node dysfunction (SND) and AV block (either nodal or infranodal) account for most clinically significant bradyarrhythmias. Reflex-mediated syncope (subtypes of which retard the heart to varying extents) is described in Chapter 43. In this chapter, we focus on the cardiac causes of bradyarrhythmias (Fig. 36.1).

Sinus Node Dysfunction

In SND, there is delay or loss of impulse propagation from the sinoatrial (SA) node to the atria. Although congenital forms of this condition do occur, SND is mainly a disease of older adults. The associated bradyarrhythmia is often progressive and also unpredictable in terms of how slow the heart rate may become. In addition, at the time of diagnosis, 17% of patients with SND have coexistent AV node dysfunction. In those with solitary sinus node disease, new AV conduction abnormalities develop at a rate of approximately 2.5% per year.

Four different clinical presentations of SND have been described. These subtypes of SND are not mutually exclusive and may overlap. The indications for pacing in SND are set out in Table 36.1.

Inappropriate Sinus Bradycardia

Persistent sinus bradycardia that does not improve with exercise is an early sign of SND. On the screening ECG, the PR interval is normal and the QRS complex is narrow, unless there is a bundle branch block (BBB) that is either concomitant with the bradycardia or dependent on it (deceleration-dependent BBB).

Sinus Arrest

In sinus arrest, the sinus node fails to depolarize, resulting in an atrial pause. The PP interval encompassing this pause is not an exact multiple of the basic PP interval (Fig. 36.2), indicating that the abnormality is not simply a blocked sinus impulse. Sinus pauses exceeding 3 seconds are highly suggestive of SND. Conversely, it is not uncommon to encounter asymptomatic sinus pauses of ≤2 seconds in the well-conditioned athlete or even in normal individuals, especially during sleep due to high vagal tone.

Sinoatrial Exit Block

In SA exit block, the SA node does fire automatically, but the impulse either fails to propagate into the atria (because of a conduction barrier within or around the SA node) or does so after a delay. In the former scenario, the atria are not depolarized, and the expected P wave fails to materialize. Like AV block, SA exit block can be graded as first, second, or third degree, with second-degree SA block further classified into Mobitz type I (Wenckebach) or Mobitz type II. Type II SA block is the most common. In this circumstance, the failure of the sinus impulse to exit the node is intermittent, and the atrial pause produced is an exact multiple of the prevailing PP interval (see Fig. 36.2). In Wenckebach SA block, the PP interval shortens progressively before the dropped beat. With third-degree SA block, the ECG only records the escape rhythm (see Fig. 36.2). If no P waves are present, it is impossible to distinguish (by ECG criteria alone) third-degree SA block from prolonged sinus arrest. Clinically, this distinction is not important; what matters is whether the patient is symptomatic. In first-degree SA block, there is an abnormally long interval between the sinus impulse and atrial capture. This condition also cannot be diagnosed from the surface ECG.

Tachy-Brady Syndrome

Also known as sick sinus syndrome, tachy-brady syndrome is a common manifestation of SND. The cardiac rhythm is interrupted by alternating periods of supraventricular tachyarrhythmias (most commonly, atrial fibrillation) and bradycardia. Typically, the bradycardia is seen immediately after spontaneous termination of the tachycardia, and it may take the form of a prolonged sinus arrest, SA block, or a junctional escape rhythm. Because bradycardia occurs suddenly, patients frequently experience dizziness or syncope. The highest incidence of syncope associated with SND probably occurs in this group. It is also possible for tachycardia to be initiated during spontaneous bradycardia or sinus arrest, perhaps because of the increased dispersion of refractoriness when the heart slows down. Some individuals with tachy-brady syndrome have periods of marked tachycardia and other unassociated periods of marked bradycardia. This condition can also be exacerbated by medications that slow AV node conduction.

BOX 36.1 Causes of Bradycardia

Noncardiac Causes

Drugs
Beta-blockers
Calcium channel blockers
Antiarrhythmic drugs (e.g., amiodarone, ibutilide, flecainide, lidocaine)
Digoxin
Adenosine
Opiate overdose
Lithium
Ivabradine
Clonidine
Fingolimod

Neurogenic
Reflex-mediated syncope
Raised intracranial pressure
Increased ocular pressure (e.g., during eye surgery)
Neuromuscular disorders (e.g., myotonic dystrophy, Friedreich ataxia)
Guillain-Barré syndrome
Dysautonomia (e.g., Shy-Drager syndrome)

Endocrine and Metabolic
Hypothyroidism
Acidosis
Electrolyte abnormalities
Anorexia nervosa
Porphyria

Environmental and Infection-Related
Hypothermia
Lyme disease
Chagas disease
Envenomation (e.g., snakebite)
Diphtheria
Acute rheumatic fever
Organophosphate insecticides

Others
Physiological
Iatrogenic (e.g., following aortic valve replacement or supraventricular tachycardia ablation)
Collagen vascular disease (e.g., rheumatoid arthritis, systemic lupus erythematosus, ankylosing spondylitis)
Congenital

Cardiac Causes
Sinus node dysfunction
Atrioventricular node dysfunction
Hisian and infra-Hisian block
Myocardial infarction (especially inferior)
Myocarditis
Myocardial infiltration: cardiac sarcoidosis, hemochromatosis, cardiac amyloidosis, Wegener granulomatosis

TABLE 36.1 Recommendations for Permanent Pacing in Sinus Node Dysfunction

Class	Recommendation	Level of Evidence[a]
I	Permanent pacemaker implantation is indicated for SND with documented symptomatic bradycardia, including frequent sinus pauses that produce symptoms.	C
	Permanent pacemaker implantation is indicated for symptomatic chronotropic incompetence.	C
	Permanent pacemaker implantation is indicated for symptomatic sinus bradycardia that results from required drug therapy for medical conditions.	C
IIa	Permanent pacemaker implantation is reasonable for SND with heart rate <40 beats/min when a clear association between significant symptoms consistent with bradycardia and the actual presence of bradycardia has not been documented.	C
	Permanent pacemaker implantation is reasonable for syncope of unexplained origin when clinically significant abnormalities of sinus node function are discovered or provoked in electrophysiological studies.	C
IIb	Permanent pacemaker implantation may be considered in minimally symptomatic patients with chronic heart rate <40 beats/min while awake.	C
III	Permanent pacemaker implantation is not indicated for SND in asymptomatic patients.	C
	Permanent pacemaker implantation is not indicated for SND in patients for whom the symptoms suggestive of bradycardia have been clearly documented to occur in the absence of bradycardia.	C
	Permanent pacemaker implantation is not indicated for SND with symptomatic bradycardia due to nonessential drug therapy.	C

[a]Evidence is ranked as: (1) level A, if the data were derived from multiple randomized clinical trials that involved a large number of individuals; (2) level B, if data were derived either from a limited number of trials that involved a comparatively small number of patients or from well-designed data analyses of nonrandomized studies or observational data registries; and (3) level C, if the consensus of experts was the primary source of the recommendation. See Evidence Section for more details.
SND, Sinus node dysfunction.

Atrioventricular Block

AV block occurs when there is a delay or nonconduction of an atrial impulse to the ventricles. It can result from normal or abnormal cardiac electrophysiology, can be transient (e.g., following inferior myocardial infarction [MI]) or permanent, and can occur at any or several levels of the AV node–His–Purkinje axis. Based on the ECG, AV block may be graded as first, second, or third degree, depending on whether AV conduction is merely delayed, intermittently blocked, or completely blocked. This classification has clinical implications, because the site of AV block (and hence, the prognosis of the patient) may be inferred with reasonable accuracy from the rhythm. It is important to note that when the atria and ventricles beat independently of each other, AV dissociation occurs (Fig. 36.3). In clinical parlance, this term is applied

P wave →	PR interval →	QRS complex and rhythm →	Diagnosis
Normal axis and rhythm. Each P wave followed by a QRS	Constant and ≤200 ms	QRS complex generally narrow but may be wide if there is BBB; each QRS preceded by a P wave.	Sinus bradycardia
Disappears intermittently and unpredictably	Constant, except for the pause(s)	QRS may be absent, narrow, or broad following the missing P wave, with variation reflecting escape rhythm.	Sinus arrest or exit block (+/− junctional or ventricular escape)
Absent. No fibrillatory waves evident	Not applicable	Narrow and regular	Junctional bradycardia
Normal axis and rhythm. Rate <60/min. Each P wave followed by a QRS	Constant and >200 ms	QRS complex generally narrow but may be wide if there is BBB; each QRS preceded by a P wave.	Sinus bradycardia with 1st degree heart block
Normal axis and rhythm. Rate may be < or ≥60/min. Not every P wave followed by a QRS	Lengthens progressively, until P wave fails to initiate QRS. Pattern then repeats.	QRS complex generally narrow but may be wide if there is BBB; fewer QRSs than Ps; irregular rhythm; QRS complexes 'dropped' in cyclical manner.	Sinus rhythm with Mobitz type I (Wenckebach) block
Normal axis and rhythm. Rate may be < or ≥60/min. Not every P wave followed by a QRS	Constant, except for the pause(s). PR after the dropped QRS is same as before.	QRS complex typically wide; fewer QRSs than Ps. QRS rhythm varies according to P/QRS ratio, but is generally regular.	Sinus rhythm with Mobitz type II block
Normal axis and rhythm. Rate may be < or ≥60/min. No relationship between Ps and QRSs	Not applicable as there is no relationship between Ps and QRSs.	QRS complex may be narrow or broad, depending on origin of escape rhythm. QRS < P wave rate. Rhythm is usually regular.	Sinus rhythm with complete heart block
Normal axis and rhythm. Rate <60/min. No relationship between Ps and QRSs	Not applicable as there is no relationship between Ps and QRSs.	QRS complex generally narrow. QRS rate = P wave rate. Regular rhythm.	Bradycardia with isorhythmic AV dissociation

FIG 36.1 Diagnostic Algorithm for Bradyarrhythmias (QRS rate <60 beats/min). *AV,* Atrioventricular; *BBB,* bundle branch block.

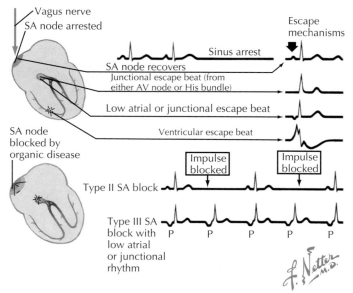

FIG 36.2 Sinus Arrest and Sinoatrial Exit Block. *AV,* Atrioventricular; *SA,* sinoatrial.

when the ventricular rate, driven by a subsidiary pacemaker, is the same or faster than the atrial rate. Because of this, the ventricles are functionally refractory to the slower atrial impulses.

First-Degree Atrioventricular Block

First-degree AV block is defined as a PR interval >0.2 second. Each P wave is followed, after a constant delay, by a QRS complex (see Fig. 36.3). In that sense, the label "AV block" is incorrect, because no P waves are actually blocked. Because the PR interval reflects the time between the earliest recorded atrial activity and the onset of ventricular depolarization, first-degree AV block can arise from conduction delay in the AV node (the most common mechanism), abnormally slow intraatrial conduction (less common), or even less often, His-Purkinje disease (in which case, the evoked QRS complex will be broad). In individuals with dual AV node physiology, transient, abrupt, first-degree AV block may be seen when antegrade conduction jumps from the fast pathway (used normally) to the slow pathway (see Chapter 37). In the presence of concomitant organic heart disease (e.g., cardiac involvement from myotonic dystrophy or aortic root abscess from endocarditis), first-degree AV block may evolve unpredictably into higher degrees of heart block. Serial ECGs over time will reveal if there is progression of the first-degree AV block. Isolated first-degree heart block is benign and is not associated with increased risk of mortality.

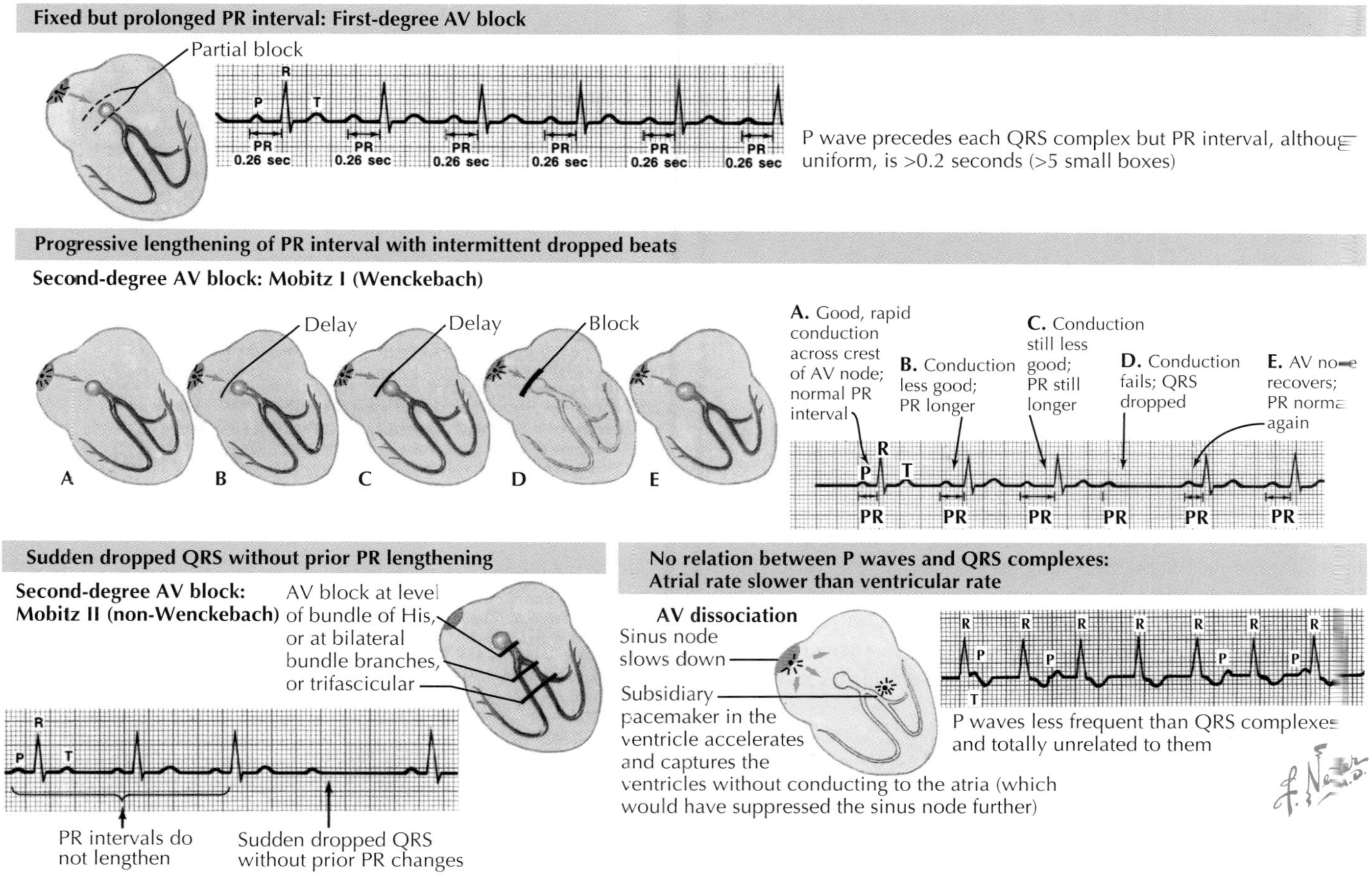

Fixed but prolonged PR interval: First-degree AV block

P wave precedes each QRS complex but PR interval, although uniform, is >0.2 seconds (>5 small boxes)

Progressive lengthening of PR interval with intermittent dropped beats

Second-degree AV block: Mobitz I (Wenckebach)

A. Good, rapid conduction across crest of AV node; normal PR interval

B. Conduction less good; PR longer

C. Conduction still less good; PR still longer

D. Conduction fails; QRS dropped

E. AV node recovers; PR normal again

Sudden dropped QRS without prior PR lengthening

Second-degree AV block: Mobitz II (non-Wenckebach)

AV block at level of bundle of His, or at bilateral bundle branches, or trifascicular

PR intervals do not lengthen

Sudden dropped QRS without prior PR changes

No relation between P waves and QRS complexes: Atrial rate slower than ventricular rate

AV dissociation

Sinus node slows down

Subsidiary pacemaker in the ventricle accelerates and captures the ventricles without conducting to the atria (which would have suppressed the sinus node further)

P waves less frequent than QRS complexes and totally unrelated to them

Features of two types of atrioventricular block

	"High"	"Low"
Site of block	AV node	Bundle of His, bilateral bundle branch, or trifascicular
Type of escape rhythm	Junctional escape rhythm Narrow QRS Adequate rate (40–55 beats/min)	Ventricular escape rhythm Wide QRS Inadequate rate (20–40 beats/min) Risk of asystole
Underlying pathology	Right coronary artery disease, inferior infarction, edema around AV node	Left anterior descending coronary artery disease, large anteroseptal infarction, or chronic degeneration of conduction system
Rhythm before complete block	Preceded by Mobitz I (Wenckebach) second-degree AV block	Preceded by Mobitz II second-degree AV block

FIG 36.3 Atrioventricular (AV) Conduction Abnormalities.

Second-Degree Atrioventricular Block

In second-degree AV block, there is intermittent interruption of AV conduction, so that some P waves are not followed by QRS complexes. Two types are recognized: Mobitz types I and II.

In Mobitz type I (Wenckebach) AV block, the delay in AV conduction increases with each successive impulse; in other words, the PR interval lengthens with each beat until a P wave is blocked (see Fig. 36.3). After the dropped ventricular beat, AV conduction recovers and the cycle repeats. Although the PR interval increases progressively, the magnitude of increment decreases during the Wenckebach cycle. Typically, the first P wave after the pause is associated with a normal PR interval, whereas the second P wave is associated with the greatest

PR increment. When the evoked QRS complex is narrow, the site of Wenckebach AV block is almost always nodal in location. Wenckebach block at the level of the His bundle is rare. Even if the QRS complex is broad, the block is still more likely to be within the AV node, but in this circumstance, it is also possible that the block is distal to the bifurcation of the His bundle. Mobitz type I block is often physiological and can be observed during sleep. Uncommonly, Mobitz I block can be incessant. In this case, symptoms of fatigue, or rarely, syncope, may require treatment.

In Mobitz type II AV block, the PR interval is constant and does not change until the block occurs (see Fig. 36.3). Typically, bifascicular block or BBB is also present—usually right (R) BBB with left anterior fascicular block (LAFB). In most of these cases, the site of block is at or below the level of the His bundle. When Mobitz type II block is seen with narrow QRS complexes (a rare combination), the block is generally within the bundle of His. Mobitz type II block can be differentiated from a nonconducted atrial ectopic beat by (1) its uniform P-wave configuration, (2) its constant PP interval, and (3) the observation that the PP interval encompassing the blocked P wave is twice as long as the prevailing PP duration. If two or more consecutive atrial beats are blocked but others conduct to the ventricles, then the term advanced type II AV block is used. The distinction between Mobitz type I and type II AV block is important because type II block often progresses to complete heart block (thus, compromising prognosis), whereas Wenckebach block rarely does so.

The question arises whether it is possible to designate fixed 2:1 AV block as either type I or type II if the basic pattern has only one conducted P wave in it. Although it is not always possible to distinguish the two, if the block worsens during exercise or with atropine and improves with vagal stimulation, it is likely to reside below the AV node, and therefore, to be indicative of the type II AV block. The converse observations will be true of type I AV block. In addition, if the PR interval is normal but the QRS complex is broad, type II block is again likely. Alternating BBB is also indicative of type II AV block. However, if the PR interval is prolonged and associated with a BBB, or if the PR interval and QRS complex are both normal (Fig. 36.4), then the site of block can only be defined using intracardiac electrode recordings.

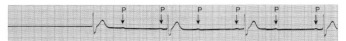

In the situation in which every other P wave is blocked, it is impossible to tell whether the PR interval is progressively increasing (since there is never more than one completed PR interval at a time). Thus, one cannot differentiate between Mobitz I and Mobitz II, and it is unclear whether the site of the block is at the AV node or in the His–Purkinje system. If this differentiation is clinically vital, intracardiac electrophysiological study is necessary.

FIG 36.4 Second-Degree Atrioventricular Block.

Complete or Third-Degree Atrioventricular Block

Third-degree AV block is characterized by the failure of all atrial impulses to reach the ventricles (Fig. 36.5). The site of block can be inferred from the features of the escape rhythm distal to the choke point. Complete block of the AV node unmasks an escape pacemaker in the His bundle. In the absence of antecedent BBB, the rhythm produced has (1) narrow QRS complexes, (2) a heart rate of 40 to 60 beats/min, and (3) a rate that increases with exercise or atropine. With block at or below the His bundle, the escape rhythm arises from a ventricular pacemaker, and (1) has a wide QRS complex, (2) a heart rate of 20 to 40 beats/min, and (3) a rate that fails to accelerate with atropine. The escape rate is not necessarily critical to the safety of the patient. Instead, it is the site of origin of the escape rhythm that matters. A subsidiary pacemaker distal to the bundle of His can stop at any time (resulting in ventricular standstill) and is vulnerable to overdrive suppression (e.g., from a spontaneous burst of pause-dependent ventricular tachycardia). In contrast, narrow complex escape rhythms are more stable.

Concealed His Extrasystoles

Rarely, premature junctional beats that do not conduct to the atria or the ventricles (and hence, remain "concealed" on the surface ECG) may penetrate the AV node retrogradely and cause conduction delay or even blockade of the subsequent atrial beat. This shows as first-degree or Mobitz type II AV block, respectively. Confirmation of this diagnosis requires His bundle recordings.

Chronic Multifascicular Blocks

A conduction disturbance of the right bundle branch or one of fascicles of the left (L) bundle branch is also known as a fascicular block (Box 36.2). By this definition, bifascicular block can be associated with any of the following: (1) RBBB + LAFB, (2) RBBB + left posterior fascicular block (LPFB), or (3) LBBB alone. Similarly, disease of all three ventricular fascicles can present as (1) alternating RBBB and LBBB, or (2) RBBB + LAFB alternating with RBBB + LPFB. Confusingly, the latter combinations are not generally referred to as "trifascicular block."

No relation between P waves and QRS complexes: QRS rate slower than P rate: Third-degree (complete) AV block

1. Atrial impulse blocked at AV node. Ventricles driven by an escape pacemaker in bundle of His (relatively fast, narrow complex escape rhythm)

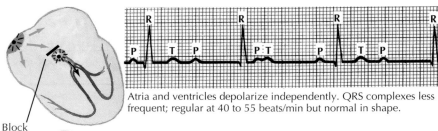

Atria and ventricles depolarize independently. QRS complexes less frequent; regular at 40 to 55 beats/min but normal in shape.

2. Atrial impulses blocked below the His bundle. Ventricles driven by a subsidiary ventricular pacemaker (slow broad complex escape rhythm)

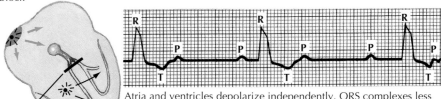

Atria and ventricles depolarize independently. QRS complexes less frequent; regular at 20 to 40 beats/min but wide and abnormal in shape.

FIG 36.5 Complete Atrioventricular (AV) Block.

TABLE 36.2 Recommendations for Permanent Pacing in Chronic Bifascicular Block

Class	Recommendation	Level of Evidence[a]
I	Permanent pacemaker implantation is indicated for advanced second-degree AV block or intermittent third-degree AV block.	B
	Permanent pacemaker implantation is indicated for type II second-degree AV block.	B
	Permanent pacemaker implantation is indicated for alternating bundle branch block.	B
IIa	Permanent pacemaker implantation is reasonable for syncope not demonstrated to be due to AV block when other likely causes have been excluded, specifically ventricular tachycardia	B
	Permanent pacemaker implantation is reasonable for an incidental finding at electrophysiological study of a markedly prolonged HV interval (≥100 ms) in asymptomatic patients.	B
	Permanent pacemaker implantation is reasonable for an incidental finding at electrophysiological study of pacing-induced infra-His block that is not physiological.	B
IIb	Permanent pacemaker implantation may be considered in the setting of neuromuscular diseases such as myotonic muscular dystrophy, Erb dystrophy (limb-girdle muscular dystrophy), and peroneal muscular atrophy with bifascicular block or any fascicular block, with or without symptoms.	C
III	Permanent pacemaker implantation is not indicated for fascicular block without AV block or symptoms.	B
	Permanent pacemaker implantation is not indicated for fascicular block with first-degree AV block without symptoms.	B

[a]Evidence is ranked as (1) level A, if the data were derived from multiple randomized clinical trials that involved a large number of individuals; (2) level B, if the data were derived either from a limited number of trials that involved a comparatively small number of patients or from well-designed data analyses of nonrandomized studies or observational data registries; and (3) level C, if the consensus of experts was the primary source of the recommendation. See Evidence Section for more details.

AV, Atrioventricular; *HV*, interval between the His bundle electrogram and the earliest recorded ventricular activation; 35–55 ms is considered normal

---

BOX 36.2 Fascicular Block

ECG Criteria for Left Anterior Fascicular Block
1. Left-axis deviation (−45 degrees or less[a])
2. RS pattern in leads II, III, aVF
3. QR pattern in lead aVL
4. Peak of R wave in lead aVL precedes peak of terminal R wave in lead aVR.
5. Peak of initial R wave in lead III precedes peak of initial R wave in lead II.

ECG Criteria for Left Posterior Fascicular Block
1. Right-axis deviation (≥120 degrees)
2. $S_I Q_{III}$ pattern, with RS in lead I and QR complexes in leads II, III, and aVF

[a]−45 degrees indicates a negative axis.

Instead, the term trifascicular block is commonly used to indicate abnormal PR prolongation with concurrent bifascicular block (the AV node and/or His bundle are regarded as an independent fascicle). Terminology aside, multifascicular blocks are clinically relevant because of the small but finite risk (~1% per year) of progression to complete heart block. This risk is lower in individuals who have the common RBBB + LAFB combination compared with those who have the rare RBBB + LPFB dyad. Indications for pacing in chronic fascicular block are listed in Table 36.2.

Atrioventricular Block After Myocardial Infarction

When AV or intraventricular conduction block complicates acute MI, the type of conduction disturbance, location of infarction, and relation of electrical disturbance to infarction must be considered if permanent pacing is contemplated.

Patients with acute MI who have intraventricular conduction defects, with the exception of isolated LAFB, have unfavorable short- and long-term prognoses and an increased risk of sudden death.

Regardless of whether the infarction is anterior or inferior, the development of an intraventricular conduction delay reflects extensive myocardial damage rather than an electrical problem in isolation.

AV block can complicate either inferior MI or anterior MI. AV block after acute inferior MI most often resolves spontaneously within 2–7 days, and pacing is therefore not recommended. This is unlike AV block that complicates an acute anterior MI, which is unlikely to improve. Most patients end up requiring permanent pacemaker implantation. Electrophysiological studies and observations in patients following acute MI suggest that the AV block in inferior MI is usually due to an ischemic lesion of the AV node, whereas AV block in anterior MI is due to extensive damage and necrosis involving both bundle branches (infra-Hisian block). The proximal AV conduction system usually has a dual arterial blood supply from both the right and left anterior descending coronary arteries, and may explain the transient behavior of AV block and lack of necrosis of the AV node seen in inferior MI as opposed to that seen in anterior MI patients. Patients with inferior MI may also be prone to bradycardia and AV block due to increased vagal tone associated with inferior injury, which has also been described after reperfusion as the Bezold-Jarisch reflex.

Recommendations for permanent pacing after the acute phase of MI are similar to the recommendations for pacing in AV block in general (Table 36.3). In other words, if the patient is symptomatic from the AV block (regardless of the location of block), if the AV block is high degree or third degree and is unlikely to resolve, then permanent pacemaker implantation is recommended.

Hypersensitive Carotid Sinus Syndrome

The hypersensitive carotid sinus syndrome is defined as syncope or presyncope resulting from an extreme reflex response to carotid sinus stimulation. There are two components of the reflex: (1) cardioinhibitory, which results from increased parasympathetic tone and is manifested by slowing of the sinus rate or prolongation of the PR interval and advanced AV block, alone or in combination; and (2) vasodepressor, which is secondary to a reduction in sympathetic activity that results in loss of vascular tone and hypotension. This effect is independent of heart rate changes. Permanent pacing is indicated for recurrent syncope caused by spontaneously occurring carotid sinus stimulation and carotid sinus pressure that induces ventricular asystole of >3 seconds. This topic is covered in detail in Chapter 43 on syncope.

TABLE 36.3   Recommendations for Permanent Pacing in Acquired Atrioventricular Block in Adults

Class	Recommendation	Level of Evidence[a]
I	Permanent pacemaker implantation is indicated for third-degree and advanced second-degree AV block at any anatomic level associated with bradycardia with symptoms (including heart failure) or ventricular arrhythmias presumed to be due to AV block.	C
	Permanent pacemaker implantation is indicated for third-degree and advanced second-degree AV block at any anatomic level associated with arrhythmias and other medical conditions that require drug therapy that results in symptomatic bradycardia.	C
	Permanent pacemaker implantation is indicated for third-degree and advanced second-degree AV block at any anatomic level in awake, symptom-free patients in sinus rhythm, with documented periods of asystole ≥3.0 s or any escape rate <40 beats/min, or with an escape rhythm that is below the AV node.	C
	Permanent pacemaker implantation is indicated for third-degree and advanced second-degree AV block at any anatomic level in awake, symptom-free patients with AF and bradycardia with ≥1 pauses of ≥5 s.	C
	Permanent pacemaker implantation is indicated for third-degree and advanced second-degree AV block at any anatomic level after catheter ablation of the AV junction.	C
	Permanent pacemaker implantation is indicated for third-degree and advanced second-degree AV block at any anatomic level associated with postoperative AV block that is not expected to resolve after cardiac surgery.	C
	Permanent pacemaker implantation is indicated for third-degree and advanced second-degree AV block at any anatomic level associated with neuromuscular diseases with AV block, such as myotonic muscular dystrophy, Kearns-Sayre syndrome, Erb dystrophy (limb-girdle muscular dystrophy), and peroneal muscular atrophy, with or without symptoms.	B
	Permanent pacemaker implantation is indicated for second-degree AV block with associated symptomatic bradycardia regardless of type or site of block.	B
	Permanent pacemaker implantation is indicated for asymptomatic persistent third-degree AV block at any anatomic site with average awake ventricular rates of ≥40 beats/min if cardiomegaly or LV dysfunction is present, or if the site of block is below the AV node.	B
	Permanent pacemaker implantation is indicated for second- or third-degree AV block during exercise in the absence of myocardial ischemia.	C
IIa	Permanent pacemaker implantation is reasonable for persistent third-degree AV block with an escape rate >40 beats/min in asymptomatic adult patients without cardiomegaly.	C
	Permanent pacemaker implantation is reasonable for asymptomatic second-degree AV block at intra- or infra-His levels found at electrophysiological study.	B
	Permanent pacemaker implantation is reasonable for first- or second-degree AV block with symptoms similar to those of pacemaker syndrome or hemodynamic compromise.	B
	Permanent pacemaker implantation is reasonable for asymptomatic type II second-degree AV block with a narrow QRS. When type II second-degree AV block occurs with a wide QRS, including isolated right bundle branch block, pacing becomes a class I recommendation.	B
IIb	Permanent pacemaker implantation may be considered for neuromuscular diseases such as myotonic muscular dystrophy, Erb dystrophy (limb-girdle muscular dystrophy), and peroneal muscular atrophy with any degree of AV block (including first-degree AV block), with or without symptoms, because there may be unpredictable progression of AV conduction disease.	B
	Permanent pacemaker implantation may be considered for AV block in the setting of drug use and/or drug toxicity when the block is expected to recur even after the drug is withdrawn.	B
III	Permanent pacemaker implantation is not indicated for asymptomatic first-degree AV block.	B
	Permanent pacemaker implantation is not indicated for asymptomatic type I second-degree AV block at the supra-His (AV node) level or that which is not known to be intra- or infra-Hisian.	C
	Permanent pacemaker implantation is not indicated for AV block that is expected to resolve and is unlikely to recur (e.g., drug toxicity, Lyme disease, or transient increases in vagal tone or during hypoxia in sleep apnea syndrome in the absence of symptoms).	B

[a]Evidence is ranked as: (1) level A, if the data were derived from multiple randomized clinical trials that involved a large number of individuals; (2) level B, if data were derived either from a limited number of trials that involved a comparatively small number of patients or from well-designed data analyses of nonrandomized studies or observational data registries; and (3) level C if the consensus of experts was the primary source of the recommendation. See Evidence Section for more details.
AF, Atrial fibrillation; *AV*, atrioventricular; *LV*, left ventricular.

DIAGNOSTIC APPROACH

The clinical evaluation of bradycardia focuses on (1) correlating the documented rhythm disturbance with symptoms and (2) ascertaining the site of the conduction block because of the importance of this in predicting the natural history, prognosis, and treatment of the bradyarrhythmia. To this end, a careful patient history and 12-lead ECG of the bradyarrhythmia are absolutely vital. Sometimes, it may be necessary to supplement the ECG with an atropine challenge or vagal stimulation to help differentiate nodal from infranodal conduction block. Exercise testing is also valuable because it can provide objective evidence of chronotropic incompetence and can also confirm the level of block in second-degree heart block. When the suspected bradyarrhythmia is intermittent or if symptom correlation is unclear, long-term rhythm recording is necessary. This can be done with an ambulatory Holter recorder (that documents the rhythm continuously for 24–72 hours), a patient-activated event monitor (typically kept by the patient for 1–3 months and activated at the time of symptoms), or an implantable loop recorder (inserted subcutaneously and capable of nonstop rhythm recording for up to 3 years). Rarely, invasive electrophysiology studies are required, usually because documentation of suspected high-grade AV block as the cause of dizziness or blackouts cannot be obtained noninvasively.

MANAGEMENT AND THERAPY

Optimum Treatment

In the absence of Torsades de pointes (see Chapter 43), documented asystole of ≥3 seconds, or a ventricular escape rhythm of <40 beats/min, asymptomatic bradycardia does not require medical intervention. Symptomatic bradycardia, however, is most often treated with implantation of a permanent pacemaker (see Tables 36.1–36.3). The role of drugs for chronotropic support is limited and is confined to emergency use. Atropine (used during acute resuscitation to abolish vagal slowing of the heart) and isoproterenol (sometimes used until pacing is established) are examples of drugs given for this purpose.

Avoiding Treatment Errors

With bradyarrhythmias, a careful assessment of the patient's symptoms, review of the drug history, and interpretation of the relevant ECG tracings are usually all that is necessary to avoid over- or undertreating the patient.

FUTURE DIRECTIONS

Important questions on the diagnosis, prognosis, and optimal treatment of bradyarrhythmias include (1) whether genetic abnormalities (yet to be defined) can be useful in assessing and establishing the timing of treatment in these patients, and (2) how best to determine the contribution of bradycardia to symptoms in patients with unclear presentation.

It seems unlikely that pharmacological approaches will be able to match the success of cardiac pacemakers in preventing symptoms, and mortality and morbidity in patients with bradyarrhythmias. In the last decade, significant advances have been made in pacemaker size and durability, and it is likely that advances in pacemaker design will continue.

ADDITIONAL RESOURCES

Fisher JD, Aronson RS. Rate-dependent bundle branch block: occurrence, causes and clinical correlations. *J Am Coll Cardiol.* 1990;16:240–243.
An excellent review of rate-dependent BBB.
Harrigan RA, Pollack ML, Chan TC. Electrocardiographic manifestations: bundle branch blocks and fascicular blocks. *J Emerg Med.* 2003;25:67–77.
Well-illustrated review of infranodal blocks.
Krahn AD, Klein GJ, Yee R, Skanes AC. The use of monitoring strategies in patients with unexplained syncope—role of the external and implantable loop recorder. *Clin Auton Res.* 2004;14(suppl 1):55–61.
Describes the use of loop recorders in unexplained syncope.

EVIDENCE

Epstein AE, DiMarco JP, Ellenbogen KA, et al. ACC/AHA/HRS 2008 Guidelines for Device-Based Therapy of Cardiac Rhythm Abnormalities: a report of the American College of Cardiology/American Heart Association Task Force on Practice Guidelines. *Circulation.* 2008;117:e350–e408.
Epstein AE, DiMarco JP, Ellenbogen KA, et al. 2012 ACCF/AHA/HRS focused update incorporated into the ACCF/AHA/HRS 2008 guidelines for device-based therapy of cardiac rhythm abnormalities. A report of the American College of Cardiology Foundation/American Heart Association Task Force on Practice Guidelines and the Heart Rhythm Society. *Circulation.* 2013;127(3):e283–e352.
Latest update of the guidelines on the management of bradyarrhythmias.

37

Supraventricular Tachycardia

Sunita Juliana Ferns, J. Paul Mounsey

Supraventricular tachycardia (SVT) is an abnormally rapid heart rhythm originating proximal to the bifurcation of the bundle of His. SVTs are relatively common clinical arrhythmias that present in people of all age groups. They are frequently symptomatic and often result in the patient seeking medical attention on an emergent or nonemergent basis. Vagal maneuvers may be useful to terminate SVTs that are atrioventricular (AV) node–dependent. In >80% of cases, a good history and a careful examination of the ECG allow for the diagnosis. Treatment decisions for SVT are usually based on whether the patient is stable or unstable when they present with the tachycardia. In most cases with SVT, patients are usually stable, and a nonemergent approach may be taken. Treatment often includes medications, catheter ablation procedures, or in some cases, surgery. Classification of SVTs are usually based on the site of origin, the nature of the arrhythmia, or the mechanism. In this chapter, we discuss classification, recognition, and treatment of the most common form of SVTs. Atrial flutter (AFl) and atrial fibrillation (AF), although both are forms of SVT, will be covered in a separate chapter.

ETIOLOGY AND PATHOGENESIS

Categorization of SVTs may be based on the site of origin, their mechanism, or their appearance on surface ECGs. Sites of origin include the sinus node, the atrium, the AV node, and the proximal His bundle. Some wide complex tachycardias are also supraventricular in origin and recognizing and differentiating them from ventricular tachycardias (VTs) are important. Fig. 37.1 details a stepwise algorithm to approaching a tachycardia based on the surface ECG appearance and response to clinical maneuvers.

Reentry is the most common mechanism of SVTs. Reentry requires two roughly parallel conducting pathways, shown as pathways A and B in Fig. 37.2, that must be connected proximally and distally by conducting tissue, thus forming a potential electrical circuit. Second, one of the pathways (pathway B in our example) must have a refractory period that is substantially longer than the refractory period of the other pathway. Third, the pathway with the shorter refractory period (pathway A) must conduct electrical impulses more slowly than the other pathway. If all these seemingly implausible prerequisites are met, reentry can be initiated when an appropriately timed premature impulse is introduced to the circuit. The premature impulse must enter the circuit at a time when pathway B (the one with the long refractory period) is still refractory from the previous depolarization and at a time when pathway A (the one with the shorter refractory period) has already recovered and is able to accept the premature impulse.

The other main mechanism is abnormal automaticity of tissue that may arise in any of the previously described sites for SVTs. Tachycardias due to abnormal automaticity may be unifocal or multifocal. The least common mechanism of tachycardia is triggered reentry.

HISTORY

Most SVTs present with palpitations as a common sign; however, more ominous presentations such as shortness of breath, obtunded consciousness, chest discomfort, or severe chest pain may also be presenting signs. Sudden cardiac death (SCD) is an extremely rare form of presentation and occurs in <0.3% of patients per year. SCD occurs almost exclusively in patients with Wolf-Parkinson-White (WPW) syndrome with rapid AF that degenerates to ventricular fibrillation (VF).

Abrupt onset and termination suggests a pathological tachycardia, and the response to vagal maneuvers indicates that the AV node may be an integral part of the circuit, such as AV reentrant tachycardia (AVRT) or AV nodal reentrant tachycardia (AVNRT). Statistically, these account for >90% of SVTs. However, abrupt termination with vagal maneuvers may also be seen more uncommonly in focal atrial tachycardia (FAT) and some types of VTs. A described irregularity could predict AF, AFl, or AT with variable block, although the awareness of regularity versus irregularity may vary widely.

Palpitations in patients with SVT are usually characterized by sudden onset and termination, which are hallmarks in differentiating them from sinus tachycardia. Episodes may last for seconds or minutes, but in rare cases, episodes can last several hours and sometimes for days. The frequency is also variable, and although some patients may present with several episodes per day, the usual presentation is more commonly a few a year. The frequency and duration of episodes, and severity of symptoms often help guide how aggressively a provider must pursue a diagnosis or treatment plan. However, patients may be instructed in how to count their pulse rate manually, and there are currently numerous smart phone applications that can reliably record a heart rate.

SVTs are usually triggered by ectopic beats in most people. Substances like asthma medications, cold supplements, herbal remedies, and dietary supplements, especially those containing sympathomimetic compounds, alcohol, caffeine, or tobacco may predispose people to increased ectopy and trigger an episode of SVT. Tiredness, emotional upheavals, or stress can also lead to an adrenergic surge, precipitating SVT.

A medical history such as hyperthyroidism or catecholamine-producing tumors may predispose patients to episodic palpitations.

EXAMINATION

Examination is an important and essential tool because it can differentiate the patient who needs an emergent treatment from one who does not.

A physical examination should include the general appearance of the patient, heart rate, blood pressure, and jugular venous pressure (JVP). Physical maneuvers, using methods such as ice to the face, a carotid sinus massage, Valsalva, or coughing may be both diagnostic and therapeutic if the AV node is an integral part of the circuit, as

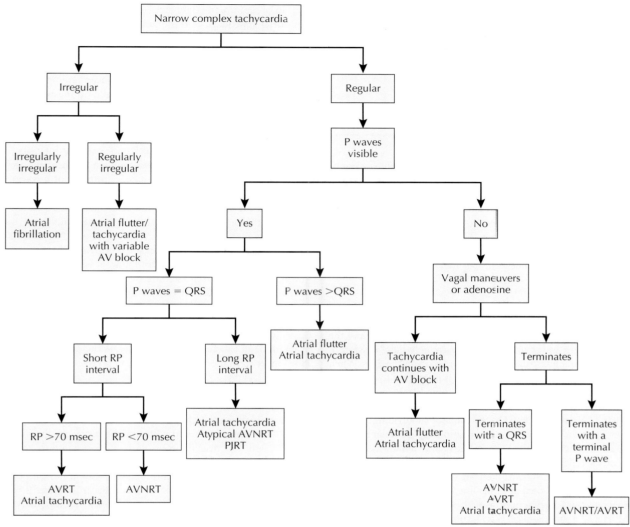

FIG 37.1 Approach to Narrow Complex Tachycardia. *AV*, Atrioventricular; *AVNRT*, AV nodal reentrant tachycardia; *AVRT*, AV reentrant tachycardia; *PJRT*, persistent junctional reciprocating tachycardia.

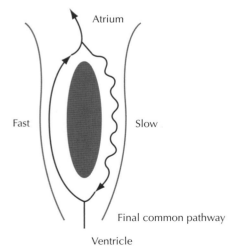

FIG 37.2 Reentry Mechanism.

described earlier. A slowing of the tachycardia with a vagal maneuver can uncover 1:1 AV conduction or help a bundle branch aberrancy recover and change a wide complex tachycardia to a narrow complex tachycardia. Presence of a murmur, displaced apical impulse, or a gallop can portend associated heart disease.

DIAGNOSTIC TOOLS

The ECG is the principal tool in diagnosis, especially during tachycardia. Many patients with SVTs may have normal resting ECGs, and longer term ECG monitoring may require a continuous ambulatory recorder, such as a 24-hour to 14-day Holter monitor. Event monitors may be useful in patients with infrequent symptoms. There are two types of event recording devices, one that has a capability of recording only when activated, and a second type, which is a looping recorder that continuously records the rhythm in addition to tracing several minutes before the recording and tracking the activation. Upper and lower rate parameters can also be programmed to record automatically on these devices. Again, these monitors are only useful if symptoms occur while the monitor is being worn; implantable loop recorders may be considered in patients with infrequent symptoms. These are especially useful for determining the presence or absence of an arrhythmia during symptoms of syncope or palpitations when conventional testing has proven inconclusive.

Other ambulatory tests such as an exercise stress to diagnose arrhythmias that occur during increased catecholamine surges may be useful.

Finally, an invasive electrophysiology (EP) study in which intracardiac catheters are used to record activity from several regions of the heart is useful for a definitive diagnosis and permanent treatment.

Electrocardiography

Most narrow complex tachycardias (QRS <120 ms) are SVTs, and wide complex tachycardias (QRS >120 ms) are VTs with some overlap (Box 37.1). Regardless of the QRS width, noting the P waves and the relationship of the P waves to the QRS is extremely helpful. More P waves than QRS complexes suggest a tachycardia of atrial origin. When there is a 1:1 relationship between the two, it is important to determine if the rates are identical and if not, if there is a predictable relationship between the PP and RR intervals. The P-wave axis is useful in determining the origin of atrial activation. One method for subdividing a narrow complex tachycardia is to examine the relationship between the QRS complex and the P wave on the ECG. A line is drawn halfway between two successive QRS complexes, and if the P waves are buried in the tail end of the QRS or before the line, these are considered short RP tachycardias. If the P wave is noted after the line, these are considered to be long RP tachycardias. A description of these tachycardias is listed in Table 37.1. Fig. 37.3 shows typical ECG recordings of the most common forms of SVT.

In some cases, P waves may not be discernable on the surface ECG and repeating an ECG at double standard or placing the arm leads in various chest positions to discern P waves (Lewis leads) may help. Esophageal recording, or intracavitary or epicardial recording may also be used. This is especially useful in postoperative patients who are often sedated and sometimes have temporary epicardial wires in place. Long rhythm strips and review of telemetry may be useful to look for perturbations and their resulting effects during the tachycardia.

DIFFERENTIAL DIAGNOSIS

Atrial Tachycardias

Atrial tachycardia (ATs) can be broadly classified as focal, macro-reentrant, micro-reentrant, or triggered. Oftentimes, it is clinically difficult to differentiate micro-reentrant and triggered reentry from automatic foci; therefore, for clinical purposes, ATs are more commonly classified as macro-reentrant or focal. Macro-reentrant tachycardias like AFl are usually precipitated by underlying structural heart disease or scars from cardiac surgery, and will be discussed separately.

Focal Atrial Tachycardia

FATs arise when an abnormal focus of atrial tissue spontaneously depolarizes faster than the underlying sinus node. They constitute approximately 5% of presenting SVTs. Common foci include the crista terminalis,

the atrial septum, the right atrial appendage, mitral valve annulus, the left atrial appendage, and the pulmonary veins. They may be seen in isolation or in the presence of structural heart disease. They are usually paroxysmal, but may be incessant, and atrial rates are generally between 120 and 250 beats/min. Incessant ATs usually occur at lower rates, and may, over time, produce a tachycardia-induced cardiomyopathy. Tachycardia rates may increase or decrease based on the sympathetic tone, and exercise or stress may precipitate these tachycardias. The atrial rate displays features of warming up and slowing down rather than the paroxysmal onset and termination noted in reentrant SVTs.

These may be regularly irregular, and a variable intensity of S_1 may be noted on the physical examination as a result of the varying AV block. The JVP may reveal an excessive number of *a* waves. Carotid sinus massage may uncover a flutter or multiple nonconducted P waves.

Adenosine is useful because it blocks the AV node usually without affecting the tachycardia focus, and may unmask multiple P waves that fail to conduct to the ventricle. Approximately 10% of FATs may be adenosine sensitive. Cardioversion and overdrive pacing may temporarily suppress FATs, but they usually resume again without an antiarrhythmic drug. Although FATs presenting in the first 6 months of life or the perioperative period after cardiac surgery may spontaneously resolve with time, those that persist beyond 3 years are unlikely to resolve and require medical or catheter ablation treatment. Medical treatment is usually with Vaughn Williams class IA, C, or III agents, such as procainamide in the acute setting, or flecainide, propafenone, or sotalol for longer term therapy. Treatment can reverse a tachycardia-induced cardiomyopathy.

Electrocardiographic Recognition

Distinct P waves are usually visible, and depending on the site of origin, the P-wave appearance and vector might vary from the sinus P wave. In ATs, with foci near the sinus node, P-wave contours are similar to those in sinus rhythm. Unlike in AFls, an isoelectric baseline may be seen in FATs. These are typically long RP tachycardias with the P waves occurring in the second half of the tachycardia cycle. P waves may conduct 1:1 at lower atrial rates or there may be a Mobitz type I block or higher degrees of heart block at faster rates. Analysis of P-wave configuration during tachycardia is useful to localize the focus of the tachycardia. Lead V_1 is the most useful lead because it is located to the right and anterior in relation to both atria. Positive P waves in lead V_1 suggest a left atrial focus, whereas right ATs, especially those from near the tricuspid annulus, have a negative or biphasic P wave in lead V_1. P waves in ATs originating near the septum are generally narrower than those arising in the right or left atrial free wall, and negative P waves in the inferior leads suggest a low atrial origin. Rhythm strips may show a gradual increase in the rate at the onset, with slowing down or speeding up, depending on the sympathetic tone.

Chaotic Atrial Tachycardia

In approximately a third of FATs, multiple atrial foci may be the source. Chaotic AT, also known as multifocal AT, is characterized by multiple foci that result in three or more P-wave morphologies and irregular PP intervals and varying PR intervals. Chaotic AT can occur in childhood in the setting of an acute viral bronchiolitis or advanced pulmonary disease. In adults, it usually occurs in the setting of chronic obstructive pulmonary disease and congestive heart failure, and may be a precursor to AF. Digitalis and theophylline toxicity can cause a chaotic AT. These tachycardias are usually difficult to treat and are frequently refractory to overdrive pacing, cardioversion, or catheter ablation. Antiarrhythmic agents such as class IA, C, or III agents have been used. Often correction of electrolyte or acid base imbalance and a treatment of the underlying disease is indicated.

TABLE 37.1 Characteristics of Narrow Complex Tachycardia

Type	Ventricular Rate	Rhythm	Presentation	Prevalence	P-wave Contour	RP Relationship	Ventricular Response to Vagal Maneuvers	Mechanism
FAT	75–200	Regular May be irregular	Paroxysmal May be incessant	Rare	Abnormal (depends on site of origin)	Long (May Wenckebach)	Abrupt slowing with return to normal rate	Automatic
Atrial flutter	75–175	Regular May be regularly irregular	Paroxysmal	Common	Saw tooth	Long (May Wenckebach)	Abrupt slowing with return to normal rate	Reentrant
AF	120–160	Grossly irregular	Paroxysmal May be incessant	Common	Baseline undulation	—	Slowing, irregularity remains	
AVNRT (typical)	120–250	Regular	Paroxysmal	Common	Retrograde Buried in terminal QRS	Short	Terminates	Reentrant
AVNRT (atypical)	100–250	Regular	Paroxysmal	Rare	Retrograde	Long	Terminates	Reentrant
ORT	130–280	Regular	Paroxysmal	Common	Retrograde	Short	Terminates	Reentrant
ART	130–280	Regular	Paroxysmal	Rare	Retrograde		Terminates	Reentrant
Preexcited AF	120–250	Irregular	Paroxysmal	Common	P waves difficult to see		May degenerate to VF	
PJRT	120–200	Regular May be irregular	Incessant	Rare	Retrograde	Long	Terminates	Reentrant
Mahaim	130–250	Regular	Paroxysmal	Rare	Retrograde	Short	Terminates	Reentrant
JET	120–280	Regular	Paroxysmal	Rare	Retrograde (may be AV dissociation)	Short	None or slowing down	Automatic

AF, Atrial fibrillation; ART, antidromic reentry tachycardia; AV, atrioventricular; AVNRT, AV nodal reentrant tachycardia; FAT, focal atrial tachycardia; JET, junctional ectopic tachycardia; ORT, orthodromic reentry tachycardia; PJRT, persistent junctional reciprocating tachycardia; VF, ventricular fibrillation.

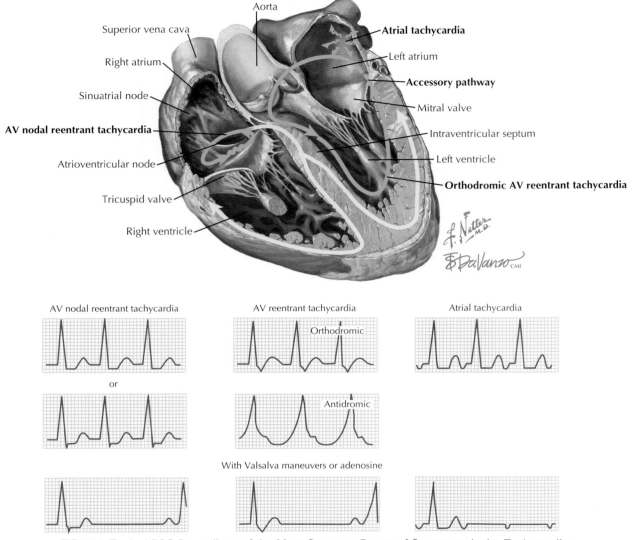

FIG 37.3 Typical ECG Recordings of the Most Common Forms of Supraventricular Tachycardia. *AV*, Atrioventricular.

Atrioventricular Node Reentry Tachycardia

AVNRT is one of the most common forms of SVT, accounting for 60% of all cases. It can present anytime, but typically presents between the second and fourth decade of life with another peak in the sixth and seventh decade.

AVNRT is characterized by the presence of two distinct pathways within the AV node referred to as the fast and slow pathways due to the difference in the conduction times in both. Typically, the pathway conducting faster has a longer refractory period, and the slower conducting pathway has the shorter refractory period. Under normal circumstances, sinus beats are initially conducted down both the fast and slow pathways. Tachycardia occurs when a critically timed atrial complex blocks in the fast pathway and conducts with a critical prolongation of AV nodal conduction time down the slow pathway. The delay in conduction down the slow pathway allows for fast pathway recovery, which is then available to take the impulse in the opposite direction from the ventricle to the atrium, thereby initiating AV nodal reentry. Variations in tachycardia rate usually reflect variation in the anterograde AV conduction time.

Typical AVNRT is the more common form (95%), in which antero-grade conduction to the ventricle occurs over the slow pathway and retrograde conduction occurs over the fast pathway. In atypical AV node reentry, the reentry occurs in the opposite direction. Other variations, such as with reentry over both slow pathways or a slow and intermediate pathway, may be noted. Spontaneous AV block can occur especially at the onset of the arrhythmia, and 2:1 AV conduction may be seen.

Electrocardiographic Recognition

AVNRTs are usually narrow QRS tachycardias, although the presence of a bundle branch aberrancy can rarely result in a wide complex appearance. Onset and offset is sudden with rates that may vary between 150 and 250 beats/min. Onset is usually after a premature atrial contraction (PAC) that is conducted with a long PR interval. Atrial activation is usually noted as a small disruption to the terminal QRS, with the P waves being buried in the distal QRS, resulting in a pseudo-S in lead II or pseudo R₁ I in lead V₁ (Fig. 37.4). Termination usually occurs in the slow pathway, and with typical AVNRT, this may be noted as a

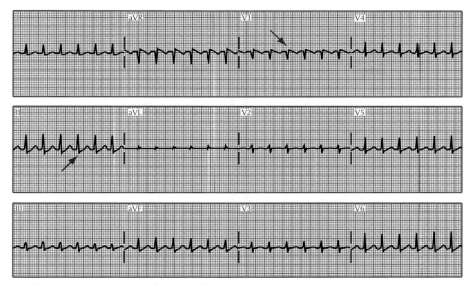

FIG 37.4 Atrioventricular Nodal Reentry Tachycardia. *Arrow* shows pseudo-S waves in II and pseudo R waves in lead V₁.

retrograde P wave before the tachycardia termination. The AV node is located inferiorly and posteriorly; therefore, the P-wave axis in the inferior leads is negative and positive in anterior leads, such as lead V_1.

Accessory Pathway–Mediated Tachycardia

Accessory pathway (AP)–mediated tachycardia accounts for approximately 30% of SVTs. In normal hearts, the atria and ventricle are isolated electrically from each other by the fibrous annulus of the AV valves, with the AV node being the only electric conduit between the atria and the ventricles. APs are fibers that connect the atrium or AV node to the ventricle outside the normal AV nodal–His-Purkinje conduction system. Most pathways are left-sided or posteroseptal. Right-sided pathways are less common. These pathways can conduct impulses anterograde or retrograde or in both directions, and are substrates for AV reentrant tachycardias. When the pathway is capable of anterograde conduction, the ventricle can be depolarized in part by the AP and produces a QRS complex that is preexcited (Fig. 37.5). Symptomatic patients with a preexcitation pattern on an ECG are said to have the WPW syndrome. Anterograde conduction of AF across these nondecremental APs can lead to VF and rarely result in SCD. The refractory period of the AP is the key determinant of the potential for these patients to have VF, and risk stratification by exercise testing, ambulatory monitoring, or an EP study may be performed. Unfortunately, noninvasive tests are limited in sensitivity and specificity, and the gold standard is ultimately invasive EP testing. In some cases, however, APs are only able to conduct retrograde and are said to be concealed. Initiation of SVT depends on a critical degree of AV delay that allows for the AP to recover excitability so that it can conduct retrograde, but unlike in AVNRT, this delay can occur in the node or in the His-Purkinje system and is not dependent on an AH interval prolongation. AVRT can be further classified into orthodromic reentry tachycardia (ORT) and antidromic reentry tachycardia, depending on whether the impulse travels anterograde down the node and retrograde up the AP or vice versa. ORT accounts for >95% of AVRTs.

Electrocardiographic Recognition

Localization of an AP is possible on a baseline ECG in the presence of ventricular preexcitation (Fig. 37.5). The preexcitation pattern is a short

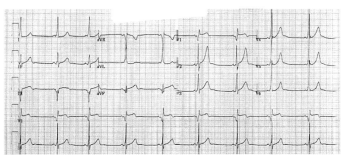

FIG 37.5 ECG of a Patient With Wolf-Parkinson-White Syndrome.

PR interval <120 ms and δ wave resulting in a wide QRS. In the absence of anterograde conduction, the baseline ECG is normal; however, during SVT with 1:1 AV conduction, if the retrograde P wave occurs after the terminal QRS, it suggests AVRT. Unlike in AVNRT, in which the atria and ventricles may be simultaneously depolarized, in AVRTs, ventricular depolarization must precede atrial activation. The P-wave vector may be useful because the atria are activated eccentrically in AVRT, and a negative P-wave vector will be seen in the lead closest to the site of pathway insertion. In addition, a bundle branch block on the site of pathway insertion results in a longer RP interval because the reentry circuit involves the ventricles. In ORT, termination with adenosine is due to a block in the AV node and seen as a retrograde P wave.

Atypical Pathways

Atypical pathways are variations in the standard AV connections and include Mahaim pathways, decrementally conducting APs, and fasciculoventricular or nodoventricular pathways (Table 37.2).

Mahaim fibers. Mahaim fibers are atriofascicular fibers that usually insert into the right bundle, thereby resulting in a preexcitation with a left bundle branch block pattern. These fibers are unique in the sense that they are almost like another AV node with decremental properties; however, unlike the AV node, they cannot conduct retrograde. SVTs due to Mahaim pathways are antidromic in nature with a left bundle branch block pattern similar to that seen during preexcitation. The

TABLE 37.2 Atypical Pathways

Pathway	PR Interval	Preexcitation	Tachycardia Type	Treatment
Mahaim	Normal	Present (LBBB, superior axis)	Antidromic	Drugs/ablation
Decremental pathway (PJRT)	Normal	Absent	Orthodromic	Ablation
Fasciculoventricular	Normal	Present	None	No treatment required
Nodoventricular/nodofascicular	Normal	May be present	Orthodromic/Antidromic	Slow pathway modification

LBBB, Left bundle branch block; *PJRT*, persistent junctional reciprocating tachycardia.

retrograde limb in SVT is over the right bundle branch–His bundle–AV node back to the atrium. The most common variant inserts into the right bundle; however some connect straight to the ventricle or other parts of the distal conduction system. They are often right-sided, usually right posterolateral or posteromedial.

Persistent junctional reciprocating tachycardia. Persistent junctional reciprocating tachycardia is an uncommon arrhythmia characterized by a long RP tachycardia with anterograde conduction over the AV node and by retrograde conduction via an AP. These decrementally conducting APs are usually located in the posteroseptal region and can cause an incessant tachycardia, resulting in a cardiomyopathy. The arrhythmias are usually refractory to drug treatment, and catheter ablation is the preferred choice of treatment. Because of the long ventriculoatrial (VA) time, these pathways are usually more difficult to map than the standard AP.

MANAGEMENT

Acute Management

Management often depends on the underlying heart disease, how well the tachycardia is tolerated, and the response to treatment in the past in an individual patient. For patients who are hemodynamically stable, the following sequential approach may be tried: vagal maneuvers, followed by IV adenosine, and lastly, IV β-blockers or calcium channel blockers. Although these maneuvers will usually not convert an AT, the transient AV nodal block may aid in the identification of the arrhythmia by exposing the underlying P-wave morphology.

For patients who are hemodynamically unstable, immediate direct current cardioversion (DCCV) under anesthetic is recommended, but this is seldom required. Vagal maneuvers may be used in the interim, as long as they do not delay cardioversion. In patients who have severe symptoms like angina, hypotension, or heart failure, but who are hemodynamically stable with IV access, adenosine may be preferred to DCCV.

Vagal maneuvers include a carotid sinus massage, the Valsalva and Müller maneuvers, gagging, coughing, and ice to the face. Vagal maneuvers work by increasing the parasympathetic tone and sympathetic withdrawal. Because most maneuvers depend on the AV node, slowing conduction in the AV node may terminate or slow the tachycardia. Carotid sinus massage should be performed with caution. Patients with a history of smoking, carotid sinus stenosis, or a bruit may not be good candidates.

Adenosine is the initial drug if vagal maneuvers do not work. It is preferred over other drugs because of its rapid onset and short half-life. Doses of 6 to 12 mg are usually successful at terminating the tachycardia in approximately 90% of cases. Lower doses may need to be used in heart transplantation patients or those on dipyridamole or carbamazepine. Side effects may include flushing, bronchospasm, chest discomfort, or transient heart block. Adenosine is contraindicated in patients with AF who have the WPW syndrome.

IV calcium channel blockers and β-blockers may be used if adenosine fails. These drugs rarely terminate an AT but may be used to provide symptomatic relief by slowing the ventricular rate. Disadvantages include their relatively longer half-life, and negative inotropic and hypotensive effects.

DCCV should be considered early in patients with hemodynamic compromise. It is important to sedate patients who are awake because the energy delivered is a painful stimulus. A synchronized direct current shock is delivered to avoid precipitation of VF. Most SVTs respond to energies in the range of 10 to 50 J. Antiarrhythmic medications can have an effect on defibrillation thresholds, and thresholds may be increased with drugs such as flecainide, propafenone, amiodarone, and lidocaine. When defibrillation fails, it is important to be able to differentiate an unsuccessful defibrillation due to inadequate energy or improper paddle placement from termination with immediate re-initiation of the arrhythmia.

Acute management of WPW with AF demands a DCCV if the patient is unstable. If stable, it is reasonable to administer a class IA or IC agent that prolongs the refractoriness of the pathway, such as procainamide, ibutilide, or flecainide. It cannot be overemphasized that adenosine, calcium channel blockers, or β-blockers should be avoided in this arrhythmia. Treatment with agents that block the AV node can lead to preferred conduction down the accessory pathway and precipitate ventricular fibrillation.

Pacing

If the patient has pacing wires in place, such as in the setting of a postoperative arrhythmia or in patient with a permanent pacemaker, overdrive atrial pacing may restore sinus rhythm. In certain situations, esophageal pacing may also be used.

Long-Term Treatment

The decision for long-term treatment largely depends on the frequency and severity of the episodes. If the attacks are infrequent, well tolerated, short, and easily terminated by the patient, they may not require therapy. In patients with infrequent episodes of prolonged, well-tolerated tachycardia, a pill in the pocket approach is reasonable in patients with AVNRT or AVRT without preexcitation. A single dose of flecainide, diltiazem, or propranolol may suffice in these patients.

Frequent recurrent episodes may require prophylactic options, including medical options or catheter ablation. In patients with AVNRT or orthodromic AVRT with a concealed pathway, a long-acting calcium antagonist, a long-acting β adrenoceptor blocker, and digitalis are reasonable initial choices that could be efficacious in preventing recurrences in up to 50% of patients. Class IC or III agents may also be used, but are generally associated with a broader side effect profile. Combination therapy may be attempted when monotherapy fails.

Catheter Ablation

For patients who are drug intolerant or in whom drugs are ineffective, radiofrequency (RF) catheter ablation is the preferred long-term choice of therapy. Catheter ablation is effective in more than 95% to 98% of cases, with a low incidence of complications, and over the long term is more cost effective. RF should be considered early in the management of patients with symptomatic recurrent episodes of tachycardia. Especially, in patients with WPW syndrome who are at risk for a rapidly conducting AF due to an AP, ablation should be considered as a firstline treatment. Ablation has replaced surgery in virtually all cases, and may be considered the initial treatment of choice in many symptomatic patients.

Catheter ablation allows for the targeting and selective destruction of areas of the heart that are strategically important for the genesis or propagation of arrhythmias by using a thin, flexible catheter inserted percutaneously and positioned under fluoroscopic guidance and electrophysiological mapping.

Several energy sources are available currently with RF energy, with cryoablation being the preferred choice with the best safety and efficacy profile. Over the past 15 years, three-dimensional electroanatomic mapping has been used extensively to facilitate mapping and reduce fluoroscopic exposure. The technology used is similar to a global positioning system to identify precise catheter tip position. These systems can provide three-dimensional localization of catheter electrodes using impedance or magnetic-based localization, and can catalogue catheter location and timing signals during mapping or ablation. These systems have contributed significantly to our understanding of arrhythmias and their mechanisms, enhanced success due to accurate localization, and made complete elimination of fluoroscopy during these procedures possible.

Catheter Ablation for Specific Tachycardias

Atrial tachycardia ablation. Almost all forms of FATs are amenable to catheter ablation. Catheter ablation is the first choice of treatment for this arrhythmia because of its high success rates and the morbidity of drug therapy. FATs are usually mapped during tachycardia, with attention initially directed at the anatomic location indicated by the P-wave morphology of the tachycardia. The means by which these arrhythmogenic foci are identified has evolved from single- or dual-catheter methods (probing different parts of the atria with multipolar electrodes) to the use of complex noncontact mapping systems. Regardless of technique, the aim remains the same: to pinpoint a site during tachycardia or atrial ectopy where local activation precedes the onset of the surface P wave by the greatest possible length of time (typically

30–100 ms). Overall, AT ablations are extremely low risk, and the rare complications that have been reported have occurred when an FAT focus was near or within a pulmonary vein, resulting in pulmonary vein stenosis in smaller patients, or when the focus was near the crista terminalis, with potential damage to the sinus node or phrenic nerve. Injury to the phrenic nerve is less likely in a patient who has never had heart surgery because the phrenic nerve continuously slides over the epicardial surface of the heart.

Atrioventricular nodal reentrant tachycardia ablations. AVNRT ablations are performed by modification of the slow pathway participating in AVNRT. The slow pathway is located in the posteromedial floor of the right atrium close to the os of the coronary sinus in a region known as the triangle of Koch. The ablation catheter is placed within the inferior aspect of the triangle of Koch and manipulated until a delayed, multicomponent atrial potential (believed to represent slow pathway depolarization) is recorded at the catheter tip. The goal of this overall strategy is to initiate RF ablation at the more distal points in the slow pathway, allowing for subsequent RF applications further superiorly and proximally if the initial therapy is unsuccessful. A single RF application suffices in most cases, and ablation at a successful site results in an accelerated junctional rhythm during RF energy application, suggesting damage to the slow pathway itself. Success rates are excellent and usually approach 98% to 100% with <1% risk of complete heart block. Cryoablation has been used as an alternative to RF ablation for treatment of AVNRT with excellent results.

Atrioventricular reentrant tachycardia ablations. The AP is targeted for ablation in AVRTs once it is determined that it is part of the tachycardia circuit or capable of rapid AV conduction during AF. Between 50% and 60% of APs are located in the free wall or nonseptal aspect of the mitral annulus. The remainder are distributed in the inferoseptal space (20%–30%), along the free wall of the tricuspid annulus (15%–20%), and in the superior and midseptal areas, close to the AV node (<10%) (Fig. 37.6). Multiple pathways are present in approximately 5% of patients. Occasionally, pathways may be located in an epicardial location and accessed with a catheter in the coronary sinus. Left-sided APs may be reached either retrograde (by extending the mapping-ablating catheter from a femoral artery up to the aorta and into the left ventricle), or with a transseptal puncture (crossing the fossa ovalis from the right

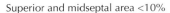

Superior and midseptal area <10%

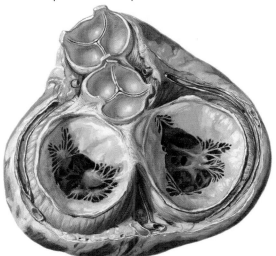

Mitral annular
free wall 50%–60%

Tricuspid annular
free wall 15%–20%

Inferoseptal space 20%–30%

FIG 37.6 Accessory Pathway Location.

atrium and then into the left ventricle). With manifest pathways, the ventricular insertion site can be determined by finding the site of the earliest onset of the ventricular electrogram in relation to the onset of the δ wave. Concealed pathways may be mapped during SVT or ventricular pacing if retrograde conduction is determined to be up the pathway as opposed to the AV node. Sometimes, a sharp AP potential may be recorded during sinus rhythm, indicating an appropriate site for ablation. During RF application, successful extirpation of the AP may be inferred from disappearance of the δ wave, termination of AVRT during RF energy delivery, or the sudden appearance of a crisp concentric-nodal conduction. Cryoablation may be used in mid or anterior septal APs with a high risk of heart block. Overall, APs have an excellent success rate, approaching 95% to 98% with minimal complications.

AVOIDING TREATMENT ERRORS

- As noted earlier, it is imperative that AV nodal blocking agents are not administered in patients with preexcited AF.
- Carotid sinus massage should only be attempted after bilateral carotid stenosis or a carotid bruit has been ruled out.
- Adenosine should be used with caution in patients with bronchospasm and in heart transplantation recipients.

FUTURE DIRECTIONS

Three-dimensional mapping has allowed for ablations to be performed routinely without fluoroscopy in most procedures. The evolution of contact force technology allows for more effective lesion delivery. Using stereotaxis and robotic navigation, operators can now manipulate catheters in a room remote from the patient. Newer technologies for energy delivery, such as ultrasound, microwave, and light amplification by stimulated emission of radiation technology are being explored. Future EP laboratories are likely to be portable, and hospitals will not require a traditional catheterization laboratory.

ADDITIONAL RESOURCES

Josephson ME. *Josephson's Clinical Cardiac Electrophysiology.* 5th ed. Philadelphia: Wolters Kluwer; 2016.
Provides a thorough understanding of the mechanisms of cardiac arrhythmias and therapeutic interventions.

Wellens HJ. 25 years of insights into the mechanisms of supraventricular arrhythmias. *Pacing Clin Electrophysiol.* 2003;26:1916–1922.
Summarizes developments that have contributed to accurate diagnosis and therapy for SVT.

Wellens HJ, Conover M. *The ECG in Emergency Decision Making.* 2nd ed. St Louis: Saunders; 2006.
Describes how to use 12-lead ECGs to make a rapid, informed decision in emergencies.

EVIDENCE

Al-Khatib SM, Arshad A, Balk EM, et al. Risk stratification for arrhythmic events in patients with asymptomatic pre-excitation: a systematic review for the 2015 ACC/AHA/HRS guideline for the management of adult patients with supraventricular tachycardia: A Report of the American College of Cardiology/American Heart Association Task Force on Clinical Practice Guidelines and the Heart Rhythm Society. *Heart Rhythm.* 2016;13(4):e222–e237.
Provides on overview for risk stratification in asymptomatic preexcitation.

Delacretaz E. Clinical practice. Supraventricular tachycardia. *N Engl J Med.* 2006;354:1039–1051.
Provides an excellent review on differential diagnosis, ECG recognition, and treatment of SVT.

Khairy P, Van Hare GF, Balaji S, et al. PACES/HRS expert consensus statement on the recognition and management of arrhythmias in adult congenital heart disease: developed in partnership between the Pediatric and Congenital Electrophysiology Society (PACES) and the Heart Rhythm Society (HRS). Endorsed by the governing bodies of PACES, HRS, the American College of Cardiology (ACC), the American Heart Association (AHA), the European Heart Rhythm Association (EHRA), the Canadian Heart Rhythm Society (CHRS), and the International Society for Adult Congenital Heart Disease (ISACHD). *Heart Rhythm.* 2014;11(10):e102–e165.
Provides an overview of recognition and treatment of tachycardias in the adult congenital population.

Page RL, Joglar JA, Caldwell MA, et al. 2015 ACC/AHA/HRS guideline for the management of adult patients with supraventricular tachycardia: executive summary: a report of the American College of Cardiology/American Heart Association Task Force on Clinical Practice Guidelines and the Heart Rhythm Society. *J Am Coll Cardiol.* 2016;67(13):1575–1623.
Provides recommendations for treatment of SVT.

38

Atrial Fibrillation: Rate Versus Rhythm

Matthew S. Baker, Anil K. Gehi, James P. Hummel, J. Paul Mounsey

Atrial fibrillation (AF) is the most common sustained cardiac rhythm abnormality. The prevalence of AF is increasing because of a combination of factors, including the aging of the population, a rising prevalence of chronic heart disease, and more frequent diagnosis by enhanced monitoring devices.

Because it is more common with advanced age, rates of AF in those older than 80 years have been reported to be 5% to 10%. It is more common in men and less common among African Americans. AF is often associated with structural heart disease, although a significant proportion of patients have no detectable heart disease.

DEFINITION AND CLASSIFICATION

AF is a supraventricular tachyarrhythmia characterized by uncoordinated atrial activity, which leads to ineffective atrial contraction. It is identified on ECG by irregular RR intervals (if atrioventricular [AV] conduction is intact) and the absence of repetitive, organized P waves.

The duration of AF episodes is used to divide the diagnosis into three categories. Paroxysmal AF (pAF) is AF that terminates spontaneously or with intervention within 7 days of onset. Persistent AF continues for >7 days. Permanent AF describes a shared decision by the patient and provider to cease attempts at restoration or maintenance of sinus rhythm.

Two other definitions are worth noting. Nonvalvular AF refers to AF in the absence of rheumatic mitral stenosis, a mechanical or bioprosthetic heart valve, or mitral valve repair. Lone AF generally refers to AF in a younger person without cardiac disease, hypertension, or diabetes. Because it has been used inconsistently, lone AF may be a confusing term, and as such, should not be used to guide clinical decision-making.

MECHANISM AND PATHOPHYSIOLOGY

The mechanisms underlying AF are numerous. AF can be looked at as a phenotype or common manifestation of a variety of pathologies, rather than as an isolated disease process of its own. The development of AF is promoted by disturbance of atrial architecture. Atrial fibrosis is most commonly due to those heart diseases that increase atrial pressure and wall stress (e.g., hypertension, coronary artery disease, valvular heart disease, and heart failure). The morbidity associated with AF is a reflection of the morbidity of those underlying maladies.

The initiation and maintenance of AF requires both a trigger and an appropriate atrial substrate. Ectopic foci often provide the trigger, and these commonly arise from left atrial tissue extending into the pulmonary veins. For this reason, pulmonary vein isolation remains fundamental to catheter ablation of AF. There are several theories to explain the maintenance of AF, including reentrant wavelets, spiral rotors, and multiple, rapidly firing foci. These are all potential therapeutic targets.

CLINICAL PRESENTATION

AF has been related to multiple risk factors (Box 38.1). Its onset can be associated with acute causes, such as binge alcohol intake, surgery, myocardial infarction, pericarditis, pulmonary disease, or hyperthyroidism (Fig. 38.1). Most often in these cases, treatment of the inciting conditions will lead to resolution of the AF. AF has also been associated with obesity and obstructive sleep apnea. Multiple cardiovascular conditions are linked to AF, including valvular heart disease, heart failure, coronary artery disease, hypertension (particularly with left ventricular hypertrophy), hypertrophic cardiomyopathy, restrictive cardiomyopathy, congenital heart disease, and pericardial disease. In these conditions, treatment of the underlying cause does not usually abolish AF. Familial AF has been increasingly recognized and is probably a result of genetic abnormalities, which lead to abnormal function of cardiac ion channels. Finally, approximately 30% to 45% of cases of pAF and 20% to 25% of persistent AF occur in patients without predisposing conditions.

The presentation of AF is diverse. Individual experiences of AF range from no symptoms to palpitations, dyspnea, or heart failure, with the most common symptom being fatigue. The hemodynamic or thromboembolic complications of AF are not infrequently the manner of its initial presentation (Fig. 38.2). Aside from the functional impairment associated with stroke, AF in and of itself can considerably impair quality of life.

EVALUATION

The initial evaluation of AF involves characterizing the pattern of episodes (i.e., pAF or persistent), determining its cause, investigating associated cardiac and noncardiac conditions, assessing its tolerability, and calculating the risk of the patient for thromboembolic complications. This can usually be accomplished with a thorough history and physical examination, ECG, echocardiogram, and basic tests of thyroid function. Consideration may be given to investigation of the patterns of arrhythmias by ambulatory cardiac monitoring. In particular, patients who are symptomatic with exercise should be assessed for adequacy of heart rate control during exercise.

MANAGEMENT

Optimal treatment of the patient with AF should be individualized to the needs of the patient, and include modification, when possible, of the underlying processes that lead to the arrhythmia, alleviation of symptoms, and prevention of tachycardia-mediated cardiomyopathy.

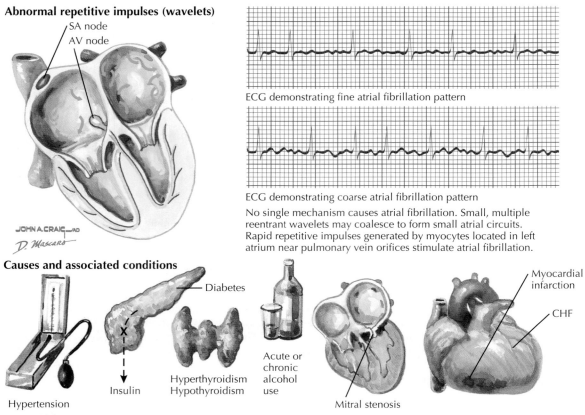

Abnormal repetitive impulses (wavelets)

SA node
AV node

JOHN A. CRAIG _MD
D. Mascaro

ECG demonstrating fine atrial fibrillation pattern

ECG demonstrating coarse atrial fibrillation pattern

No single mechanism causes atrial fibrillation. Small, multiple reentrant wavelets may coalesce to form small atrial circuits. Rapid repetitive impulses generated by myocytes located in left atrium near pulmonary vein orifices stimulate atrial fibrillation.

Causes and associated conditions

Diabetes

Insulin

Hyperthyroidism
Hypothyroidism

Acute or chronic alcohol use

Mitral stenosis

Myocardial infarction

CHF

Hypertension

FIG 38.1 Pathogenesis of Atrial Fibrillation. *AV,* Atrioventricular; *CHF,* congestive heart failure; *SA,* sinoatrial.

BOX 38.1 Clinical Risk Factors for Atrial Fibrillation

- Increasing age
- Hypertension
- Diabetes mellitus
- Myocardial infarction
- Valvular heart disease
- Heart failure
- Obesity
- Obstructive sleep apnea
- Cardiothoracic surgery
- Smoking
- Exercise
- Alcohol use
- Hyperthyroidism
- Increased pulse pressure

- European ancestry
- Family history
- Genetic variants
- ECG
  - Left ventricular hypertrophy
- Echocardiographic
  - Left atrial enlargement
  - Decreased LV fractional shortening
  - Increased LV wall thickness
- Biomarkers
  - Increased C-reactive protein
  - Increased B-type natriuretic peptide

LV, Left ventricular.

In principal, management of AF itself can be directed at controlling the ventricular rate (rate control), restoration of sinus rhythm (rhythm control), or both, along with prevention of thromboembolism. Strategies to prevent thromboembolism are discussed in Chapter 39.

Rate Control

The optimal heart rate target for patients in AF is not clear. In the randomized Rate Control Efficacy in Permanent Atrial Fibrillation (RACE II) trial, no benefit was seen for strict rate control (resting heart rate <80 beats/min) compared with lenient control (resting rate <110 beats/min). Optimal rate control thus depends on the extent of symptoms and individual patient characteristics. One approach would be to target a resting heart rate of <80 beats/min in those with rates <110 beats/min during moderate exercise in most symptomatic patients, although more lenient control may also be reasonable in asymptomatic patients with normal left ventricular function. Monitoring the heart rate over an extended period with a Holter monitor or another such telemetric device may be useful to evaluate the adequacy of rate control. Patients who are hemodynamically compromised as a result of rapid ventricular rates during AF require prompt attention. In addition, inadequacy of rate control may lead to tachycardia-induced cardiomyopathy and should be considered in any patient with idiopathic heart failure and rapid AF.

Drugs that prolong the refractory period of the AV node are generally effective agents for rate control. Beta-blockers and nondihydropyridine calcium channel blockers (verapamil or diltiazem) are considered the first-line agents for rate control. Multiple β-blockers have been studied and proven to be effective, including metoprolol, atenolol, nadolol, and carvedilol. Care should be taken when initiating β-blockers in patients with AF and heart failure who have a reduced ejection fraction. Verapamil and diltiazem are also effective agents. These agents should be avoided in patients with systolic heart failure (particularly if the left ventricular ejection fraction is <40%) because of their negative inotropic effects. However, these agents may be preferred over β-blockers in patients with bronchospastic pulmonary disease. Digoxin slows the heart rate predominantly by enhancing parasympathetic tone to the AV node. However, it is generally ineffective in the presence of

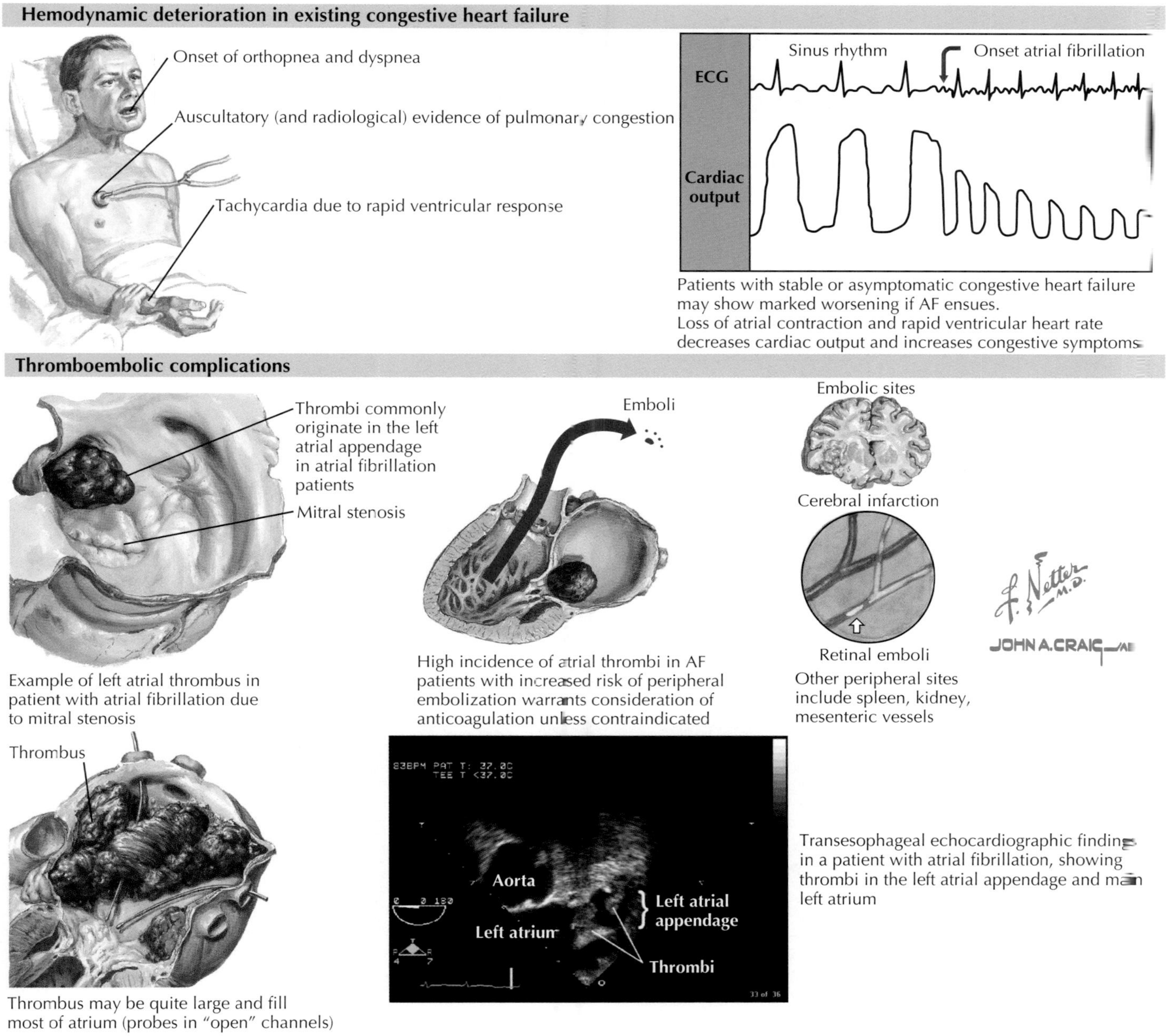

Hemodynamic deterioration in existing congestive heart failure

Onset of orthopnea and dyspnea

Auscultatory (and radiological) evidence of pulmonary congestion

Tachycardia due to rapid ventricular response

ECG

Sinus rhythm   Onset atrial fibrillation

Cardiac output

Patients with stable or asymptomatic congestive heart failure may show marked worsening if AF ensues.
Loss of atrial contraction and rapid ventricular heart rate decreases cardiac output and increases congestive symptoms

Thromboembolic complications

Thrombi commonly originate in the left atrial appendage in atrial fibrillation patients

Mitral stenosis

Example of left atrial thrombus in patient with atrial fibrillation due to mitral stenosis

Thrombus

Thrombus may be quite large and fill most of atrium (probes in "open" channels)

Emboli

High incidence of atrial thrombi in AF patients with increased risk of peripheral embolization warrants consideration of anticoagulation unless contraindicated

Embolic sites

Cerebral infarction

Retinal emboli

Other peripheral sites include spleen, kidney, mesenteric vessels

Aorta

Left atrium

Left atrial appendage

Thrombi

Transesophageal echocardiographic findings in a patient with atrial fibrillation, showing thrombi in the left atrial appendage and main left atrium

FIG 38.2 Clinical Presentation of Atrial Fibrillation.

increased sympathetic activity, such as during exercise. In addition, digoxin has a narrow therapeutic window with many potential side effects, with lower doses corresponding to serum levels of <0.9 ng/mL that are associated with better outcomes. Digoxin is thus most useful as an add-on agent in patients already on β-blockers or calcium channel blockers whose heart rates are not adequately controlled. Combination therapy in this manner may allow lower doses of each agent, thus limiting potential side effects. Amiodarone slows AV nodal conduction through sympatholytic and calcium channel–blocking mechanisms, and thus can also be used for rate control, such as in the critically ill patient. However, amiodarone is predominantly a rhythm control drug and is associated with many potential adverse extracardiac effects. It should only be used as a last resort for rate control, and replaced as soon as possible with a β-blocker and/or calcium channel blocker if no attempts to restore sinus rhythm are planned.

AV nodal ablation with permanent pacemaker implantation is a definitive option for long-term rate control management in medically refractory cases. However, it renders the patient permanently pacemaker-dependent, so it should only be used after all medical attempts at rate control (and potentially, rhythm control) have been exhausted.

Rhythm Control

Multiple randomized clinical trials have compared outcomes of a rate control and anticoagulation strategy versus a rhythm control (using pharmacological agents) and anticoagulation strategy in patients with AF. Although a rhythm control strategy may be expected to have theoretical advantages over rate control strategies through the addition of atrial contraction and the regularization of ventricular contraction, these studies did not demonstrate significant tangible benefits. Instead, there was no overall difference in mortality and an increase

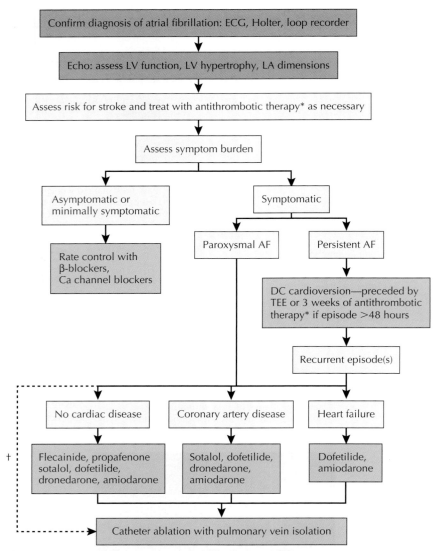

FIG 38.3 Management and Therapy for Atrial Fibrillation (AF). *, Options for antithrombotic therapy include warfarin (with target INR 2.0–3.0), apixaban, dabigatran, rivaroxaban, or edoxaban. *t*, Catheter ablation as an initial rhythm-control strategy is reasonable in paroxysmal AF and may also be considered in persistent AF. *Ca*, Calcium; *DC*, direct current; *INR*, international normalized ratio; *LA*, left atrium; *LV*, left ventricle/ ventricular; *TEE*, transesophageal echocardiography.

in hospitalization in the rhythm control group, mostly as a result of admissions for cardioversion. It might be that deleterious effects of antiarrhythmic drugs offset the benefits of sinus rhythm, or it might be that pharmacological agents were not effective enough at rhythm control to demonstrate a benefit. Nevertheless, the implication of these studies is that a rhythm control strategy should be an individualized decision based on the nature, intensity, and frequency of symptoms associated with AF, patient preferences, and response to treatment.

Should one make the decision to embark on a rhythm control strategy in the patient with symptomatic AF, there are many approaches (Fig. 38.3). In patients with recurrent pAF, several antiarrhythmic drugs may be effective. The choice of antiarrhythmic is largely dictated by safety considerations. For those with no or minimal heart disease, a wide range of choices is available, including flecainide, propafenone, sotalol, dronedarone, and dofetilide. Dofetilide has only shown efficacy in persistent AF, and therefore, is not used in patients with pAF.

Flecainide and propafenone are contraindicated in patients with coronary artery disease or significant left ventricular hypertrophy. Sotalol and dofetilide should be used with caution in those with renal insufficiency. For patients with significant systolic heart failure, the choice is generally limited to dofetilide or amiodarone, which have been shown to have a neutral mortality effect in this population. Amiodarone is generally a second-line agent. It is reserved for older adults or patients with significant cardiomyopathy because of its multiple potential toxicities. A decision for long-term amiodarone therapy should be based on discussions of the risk-to-benefit ratio with the patient. As an alternative or when first-line agents are ineffective, catheter or surgical ablation can be considered (see Fig. 38.3). Ablation is discussed in detail in Chapter 40, and is a highly effective method of rhythm control in AF, particularly in patients with pAF.

In a patient with persistent AF, a first attempt at rhythm control may be made with cardioversion alone, especially in the patient with no or minimal heart disease. Direct-current cardioversion under adequate anesthesia is a highly effective means to restore sinus rhythm acutely (see Fig. 38.1). However, pharmacological cardioversion with ibutilide is also a reasonable alternative. For patients with AF lasting ≥48 hours (or when the duration of AF is unknown), anticoagulation is recommended for at least 3 weeks before and 4 weeks after cardioversion, regardless of the method used for cardioversion. As an alternative to anticoagulation before cardioversion, a transesophageal echocardiogram can be performed to exclude the presence of left atrial thrombus. Even in those individuals with no evidence of a left atrial thrombus, anticoagulation after cardioversion is still necessary. If AF recurs in the patient with persistent AF, an antiarrhythmic drug may be effective in maintaining sinus rhythm following cardioversion.

Lifestyle Modifications

Modifiable risk factors such as obesity, hypertension, and diabetes contribute significantly to the development of AF. An aggressive risk factor modification program that included weight loss, regular exercise, smoking cessation, and abstinence from alcohol, as well as tight control of hypertension, diabetes, and sleep apnea, was shown to reduce AF burden after catheter ablation. In another study, regular aerobic training similarly reduced AF burden in a nonablation population with paroxysmal AF. Although long-term data are not available, if these lifestyle modifications can be sustained, they might have beneficial effects on the natural history of AF and overall cardiovascular risk.

Avoiding Treatment Errors

Management of AF should predominantly focus on the three principles of rate control, prevention of thromboembolism, and rhythm control. In addition, underlying factors contributing to the development of AF and increased cardiovascular risk should be modified when possible. Once rate control and prevention of thromboembolism are addressed, a rhythm control strategy should be adopted in patients with recurrent AF who continue to experience symptoms. Most common errors arise when one of these principles of management is not adequately addressed. In the case of failure to address stroke prophylaxis, a relatively common error, the consequences can be devastating.

FUTURE DIRECTIONS

Although rhythm control has potential theoretical advantages compared with rate control in terms of improved hemodynamics, it has failed to improve outcomes in multiple studies. It is possible that the benefits of maintaining sinus rhythm are offset by deleterious effects of antiarrhythmic drugs. The potential prognostic benefit of sinus rhythm compared with AF without the use of toxic drugs is currently being tested in several large randomized ablation trials. It is also possible that newer antiarrhythmic drugs such as those targeting more atrial specific channels (e.g., I_{Kur}) may be developed with less potential for ventricular proarrhythmia and lower systemic toxicity. In addition, studies are ongoing to investigate the effects of different agents in relation to patient clinical characteristics and biomarkers that could help tailor individual drug therapy to maximize benefit while minimizing adverse events.

ADDITIONAL RESOURCES

Haissaguerre M, Jais P, Shah DC, et al. Spontaneous initiation of atrial fibrillation by ectopic beats originating in the pulmonary veins. *N Engl J Med.* 1998;339:659–666.
Seminal description of the source of ectopic foci that initiate AF.

Klein AL, Grimm RA, Murray RD, et al. For the Assessment of Cardioversion Using Transesophageal Echocardiography Investigators. Use of transesophageal echocardiography to guide cardioversion in patients with atrial fibrillation. *N Engl J Med.* 2001;344:1411–1420.
Study describing the use of transesophageal echocardiography to obviate the need for anticoagulation before a cardioversion of AF.

Wyse DG, Waldo AL, DiMarco JP, et al. For the Atrial Fibrillation Follow-up Investigation of Rhythm Management (AFFIRM) Investigators. A comparison of rate control and rhythm control in patients with atrial fibrillation. *N Engl J Med.* 2002;347:1825–1833.
Largest study thus far comparing the alternative strategies of rate or rhythm control with anticoagulation in the management of AF.

EVIDENCE

Gage BF, Waterman AD, Shannon W, et al. Validation of clinical classification schemes for predicting stroke. Results from the National Registry of Atrial Fibrillation. *JAMA.* 2001;285:2864–2870.
Seminal study describing the use of a point scoring system to predict the risk for stroke in patients with AF.

January CT, Wann LS, et al. 2014 AHA/ACC/HRS Guideline for the management of patients with atrial fibrillation: a report of the American College of Cardiology/American Heart Association Task Force on Practice Guidelines and the Heart Rhythm Society. Developed in collaboration with the Society of Thoracic Surgeons. *J Am Coll Cardiol.* 2014;64(21):2305–2307.
Latest comprehensive guidelines for the management of AF developed by the major cardiology societies.

39

Atrial Fibrillation: Stroke Prevention

Joseph S. Rossi, J. Paul Mounsey

ETIOLOGY AND PATHOGENESIS

Approximately 800,000 strokes occur annually in the United States, and it is estimated that atrial fibrillation is the primary cause in approximately 15% of these events. The prevention of stroke remains a critical focus in the initial treatment of atrial fibrillation and should be carefully addressed at the time of presentation after symptoms are controlled, and the patient is able to engage in a complex decision-making process regarding the risks and benefits of oral anticoagulation (OAC). For some patients, the risk of stroke is outweighed by bleeding risk, and OAC therapy is deferred in lieu of strategies believed to be associated with a lower bleeding risk (aspirin alone or simple observation). However, there is considerable evidence that many patients and providers defer anticoagulation therapy despite low bleeding risk and elevated stroke risk, which results in undertreatment of this vulnerable population. It is estimated that of the older adult patients with atrial fibrillation in the United States with a CHADS score >3, <50% have ever filled a prescription for an anticoagulant.

Fortunately, there have been significant advances in stroke prevention therapies for atrial fibrillation in the last 5 years. Warfarin was the only OAC available until the approval of the first novel oral anticoagulant (NOAC) in 2009. Long-term warfarin therapy is associated with well-known limitations, including close regulation of vitamin K intake and regular blood testing to assure therapeutic levels. For patients who are not good candidates for warfarin therapy, there are now four NOAC agents widely available, all with favorable safety and efficacy profiles compared with warfarin in randomized clinical trials. In addition to widely available NOAC therapy, procedural options have progressed significantly, and there are now several catheter-based and open surgical techniques available to occlude the left atrial appendage (LAA), which is believed to be responsible for 90% of embolic strokes in patients with atrial fibrillation. In this chapter, we summarize the current strategies to determine stroke risk and bleeding risk in patients diagnosed with atrial fibrillation, and review the clinical usefulness of warfarin and newly available options for OAC and LAA occlusion.

STROKE RISK STRATIFICATION

The $CHADS_2$ score was initially described in 2001 and was validated to estimate stroke risk among a cohort of approximately 1800 patients aged older than 65 years with an average follow-up of approximately >1 year. The $CHADS_2$ score awards points for congestive heart failure, hypertension, age, diabetes, and history of embolic stroke. Stroke risk has generally been described as low ($CHADS_2$ score 0–1), intermediate ($CHADS_2$ score 1–2), and high ($CHADS_2$ score ≥3). Patients at intermediate or high risk for stroke are likely to benefit from OAC, and it is generally accepted that risk of stroke outweighs the risk of bleeding from OAC. This is more controversial among patients with borderline

stroke risk (score 1–2) and among patients at high bleeding risk. The $CHADS_2$ score provides an easy and accessible method to document stroke risk and became the mainstay of stroke risk stratification for a decade until the model was updated to account for additional risk factors.

A refined version of the $CHADS_2$ score was published in 2010 and sought to increase the predictive value by incorporating increased risk of stroke associated with advanced age, female sex, and known vascular disease and interventions (myocardial infarction, percutaneous coronary intervention and/or coronary artery bypass graft [CABG], and pulmonary vein disease). The CHA_2DS_2-VASc score is now a favored risk stratification tool and has been validated in several observational cohorts. It is viewed as a more complete risk stratification tool and has largely displaced the $CHADS_2$ score in clinical practice. Its main advantage is that it better separates, and therefore, risk stratifies low- and moderate-risk patients

It is important to emphasize that not all stroke events in patients with atrial fibrillation are due to left atrial and/or atrial appendage thrombus. Many patients with atrial fibrillation also have an increased risk of atherosclerotic and hypertensive stroke, which are the leading causes of stroke worldwide. Therefore, the CHA_2DS_2-VASc score can be considered an "inventory of comorbidities," and has also been shown to predict other acute cardiovascular events, including outcomes in patients with congestive heart failure. Because patients with elevated stroke risk also have an increased risk of bleeding events, significant efforts have been centered on bleeding risk prediction as well. Bleeding risk increases with age, and both the $CHADS_2$ and CHA_2DS_2-VASc scores have been shown to predict elevated bleeding risk. When the bleeding risk outweighs the risk of stroke, many patients choose to forego OAC regimens in favor of treatment associated with lower bleeding risk. In the current era, these choices include medical therapy with aspirin alone, or consideration of LAA occlusion procedures. The HAS-BLED (Hypertension, Abnormal renal/liver function, Stroke, Bleeding, Labile international normalized ratio, Elderly, Drugs or alcohol use) score has now been validated as the most predictive tool for estimating bleeding risk when counseling patients, and this is reflected in current guidelines.

HAS-BLED: BLEEDING RISK STRATIFICATION

Every patient who receives OAC should be appropriately counseled regarding the risk of bleeding associated with all OAC therapies. Bleeding risk increases significantly with age, and the interpretation of the risk/benefit ratio becomes extremely challenging among older adults and frail patients, and among patients with a clinical history of significant bleeding events. The HAS-BLED bleeding risk score incorporates most important comorbidities (hypertension, abnormal renal and/or liver function, stroke, bleeding history or predisposition, labile

TABLE 39.1 Summary of Risk Stratification Scores and Predicted Annual Event Risk

Score	CHADS$_2$ Annual Stroke Risk (%)	CHA$_2$DS$_2$-VASc Annual Stroke Risk	HAS-BLED Annual Bleeding Risk
0	1.9	0	1.1
1	2.8	1.3	1.0
2	4	2.2	1.9
3	5.9	3.2	3.7
4	8.5	4.0	8.7
5	12.5	6.7	12.5
6	18.2	9.8	N/A
7	N/A	9.6	N/A
8	N/A	6.7	N/A
9	N/A	15.2	N/A

HAS-BLED, Hypertension, Abnormal renal/liver function, Stroke, Bleeding, Labile international normalized ratio, Elderly, Drugs or alcohol use.

international normalized ratio, older adults, drugs and/or alcohol concomitantly) and is now recommended in the American College of Cardiology/American Heart Association/Heart Rhythm Society and European and Canadian Atrial Fibrillation guidelines to estimate major bleeding risk in atrial fibrillation patients on anticoagulation. HAS-BLED has been shown to be a better predictor of serious bleeding both in clinical trial cohorts and in observational studies. It is noteworthy that it has been validated only among patients taking warfarin, not those on NOAC drugs, and it is not clear that bleeding risk will interact with pathologies similarly among patients taking the different classes of drugs. The HAS-BLED score also remains the only prediction model that has been shown to correlate with risk of intracranial hemorrhage. The HAS-BLED score has been validated in both patients with and without atrial fibrillation, but is typically applied and cited as rationale to avoid anticoagulation therapy in atrial fibrillation patients believed to be at high risk for bleeding. Table 39.1 summarizes the annual event risk for both stroke and bleeding based on these risk stratification models.

ORAL ANTICOAGULATION WITH WARFARIN FOR STROKE PREVENTION

Warfarin therapy continues to be the most commonly prescribed regimen for OAC (although no longer for new prescriptions), and there is a large body of evidence from multiple randomized studies suggesting that the risk for stroke after initiation is reduced by >75%. Warfarin has been the standard of care for stroke prevention among atrial fibrillation patients for >30 years. However, maintenance of warfarin therapy has significant limitations. Although it is an effective antagonist of vitamin K–dependent clotting factors, determinants of hepatic metabolism can result in wide variability of effective doses among individuals. In addition, dietary intake of vitamin K can affect warfarin effectiveness, and patients must maintain significant discipline to avoid fluctuations in the international normalized ratio.

Genetic panels can be helpful to identify patients likely to require higher maintenance doses of warfarin. The *VKORCI* gene encodes the vitamin K epoxide reductase enzyme. A single nucleotide polymorphism G-A mutation in the promoter region of this gene results in less enzyme production, and therefore, decreased warfarin metabolism. In addition, several variant CYP2C9 alleles can also lower warfarin clearance due

to reduced enzymatic activity. The wild-type CYP2C9*1 allele is associated with normal warfarin metabolism, whereas the CYP2C9*2 and CYP2C9*3 alleles result in decreased warfarin clearance and therefore require lower maintenance doses. A testing algorithm has been proposed and added to the warfarin label that suggests starting doses of warfarin based on this genetic testing information.

NOVEL ORAL ANTICOAGULANTS FOR STROKE PREVENTION

The first NOAC therapy available in the United States was dabigatran, which was approved by the Food and Drug Administration (FDA) for stroke prevention in atrial fibrillation in 2009 based on the results of the Randomized Evaluation of Long-Term Anticoagulation Therapy (RE-LY) trial. Dabigratran was associated with a lower risk of intracranial hemorrhage and embolic events compared with warfarin. Although an effective anticoagulant, this medication, in particular, has been associated with higher rates of dyspepsia and gastrointestinal bleeding, especially among older adults, in both the randomized trial and observational studies. Although dabigatran is the only NOAC associated with a lower risk of embolic stroke than warfarin, its side effect profile has led to declining use recently with increased availability of oral factor Xa inhibitors.

Oral factor Xa inhibitors are rapidly becoming the standard of care for OAC for newly diagnosed atrial fibrillation. These agents are now widely available, and there have been multiple randomized trials that have suggested that apixaban, rivaroxaban, and edoxaban are noninferior to warfarin for the prevention of thromboembolic stroke, and are associated with a significant decrease in the risk of major bleeding, most importantly, intracranial hemorrhage. Because they have a rapid onset of action (<3 hours), they do not require bridging therapy with parenteral agents during initiation. In addition, all of these agents are well tolerated and have minimal side effects. However, NOAC therapies have not been compared to each other in randomized trials, making it difficult to choose one in favor of another. The randomized trials do provide some insight into their effectiveness and limitations, and these trials are summarized in Table 39.2. It is noteworthy that, although all NOACs were tested in patients at low, intermediate, and high risk of stroke, the edoxaban and rivaroxaban trials recruited, on average, patients with a higher vascular risk than the dabigatran and apixaban trials. It is not clear whether this difference should be used to guide therapy selection.

NOAC therapies have been approved for patients with nonvalvular atrial fibrillation. This has been a controversial stipulation because many patients with atrial fibrillation also have comorbid heart valve disease. Generally, nonvalvular atrial fibrillation has been defined as the absence of previous heart valve surgery or hemodynamically significant mitral valve stenosis. Patients with a history of heart valve surgery or mitral stenosis were excluded from all of the large randomized trials that compared NOAC therapy with warfarin. In practice, most physicians prescribe these agents for patients with treated and stable heart valve disease, with the exception of those with mechanical heart valve replacement. All patients with mechanical heart valves require anticoagulation therapy with warfarin, and there has been concern that NOAC therapies will be less effective in this population. Dabigatran, the only agent studied in a population with mechanical valves, was associated with increased risk of valve thrombosis compared with warfarin therapy.

INPATIENT ANTICOAGULATION FOR STROKE PREVENTION

There have been no randomized clinical trials to evaluate the effectiveness of immediate anticoagulation for stroke prevention among hospitalized patients with atrial fibrillation. For patients admitted with

TABLE 39.2	Comparison of Novel Oral Anticoagulation Therapies for Atrial Fibrillation						
	Clinical Trial (n)	Mean CHADS$_2$ Score	Prevention of Thromboembolic Stroke[a]	Intracranial Hemorrhage[a]	GI Bleeding[a]	Renal Clearance (%)	Notes
Dabigatran	RE-LY	2.1	Superior	Decreased	Increased	80	Efficacy for 150-mg but not 110-mg dose; higher risk of GI side effects increased dependence on renal clearance
Apixaban	ARISTOTLE	2.1	Noninferior	Decreased	Decreased	25	Studied in lower risk patients, decreased mortality compared with warfarin
Rivaroxaban	ROCKET-AF	3.5	Noninferior	Decreased	Increased	35	Poor INR management in warfarin arm of ROCKET-AF, no reduction in total bleeding events, once daily dosing
Edoxaban	ENGAGE-AF	2.8	Noninferior	Decreased	Decreased	50	Less effective in patients with GFR >90, once daily dosing

[a]Compared with warfarin.
GFR, Glomerular infiltration rate; *GI*, gastrointestinal; *INR*, international normalized ratio.

acute thromboembolic events, the choice of anticoagulation regimen is typically based on the underlying disease state, risk of bleeding, and renal function. Many patients with large embolic strokes have a significant risk of hemorrhagic transformation, and initiation of anticoagulation therapies should be considered in consultation with a neurologist when appropriate. For patients with normal renal function and a low risk of bleeding, enoxaparin provides effective, immediate anticoagulation. Heparin infusion is also immediately effective but requires monitoring and titration parameters. Vitamin K antagonists require several days to achieve therapeutic levels and typically require bridging therapy with heparin or enoxaparin. For patients with an elevated risk of stroke who are good candidates for initiation of a NOAC, these agents can be safely initiated in the hospital setting and provide prompt therapeutic anticoagulation within several hours.

ANTIPLATELET AGENTS FOR STROKE PREVENTION

It is important to note that no antiplatelet agent as monotherapy has been proven to reduce the risk of embolic stroke in patients with atrial fibrillation in a placebo-controlled clinical trial. Although aspirin is associated with a decreased risk of stroke and myocardial infarction in multiple trials, its efficacy in the setting of atrial fibrillation is largely untested. ACTIVE A (the 2009 Atrial Fibrillation Clopidogrel Trial with Irbesartan for Prevention of Vascular Events) compared aspirin and clopidogrel with aspirin alone in patients who could not tolerate warfarin therapy. Although combination antiplatelet therapy was slightly better than aspirin for prevention of the primary endpoint, this benefit was largely balanced by an increased risk of major bleeding. ACTIVE W (the 2006 Atrial Fibrillation Clopidogrel Trial with Irbesartan for prevention of Vascular Events) compared aspirin and clopidogrel with warfarin therapy. ACTIVE W was stopped early because of superiority of warfarin over dual antiplatelet therapy for the prevention of stroke. There was also a trend toward decreased bleeding in the warfarin arm. Dual antiplatelet therapy is associated with significant bleeding risk and cannot be recommended over OAC, particularly with available NOAC therapies.

When antiplatelet agents are compared with OAC, the results have generally suggested the superior efficacy of anticoagulation therapy, with similar or lower bleeding risk compared with antiplatelet therapies. The previously described ACTIVE W indicated superiority of warfarin compared with dual antiplatelet therapy. The 2011 Apixaban Versus Acetylsalicylic Acid to Prevent Stroke in Atrial Fibrillation Patients Who

Have Failed or Are Unsuitable for Vitamin K Antagonist Treatment (AVERROES) trial randomized 5599 patients with atrial fibrillation to apixaban or aspirin. With a mean follow-up of 1.1 years, the apixaban group had lower rates of stroke or systemic embolism than the aspirin group (1.6%/year vs. 3.7%/year) without any increase in rates of major bleeding (1.4%/year vs. 1.2%/year). The trial was stopped early because of early Data and Safety Monitoring Board (DSMB) analysis that suggested superiority of apixaban over aspirin alone for all clinically important endpoints.

BRIDGING THERAPY IN PATIENTS REQUIRING CESSATION OF ORAL ANTICOAGULATION

The management of anticoagulation for patients undergoing invasive or surgical procedures is a regular dilemma. It is clear that the cessation of OAC causes a marginal increase in stroke risk, and care must be taken to balance this risk against the bleeding risk of any invasive procedure. There are no specific guidelines to reference in making these decisions; however, a consensus statement was recently published that summarized some standard recommendations for cessation of NOAC therapy due to variability in half-life and renal clearance (Table 39.3). Interruption of NOAC therapy should be minimized, and care must be taken to account for renal function and the bleeding risk of any proposed procedure. Most physicians rely on clinical judgment and provide bridging therapy only in patients at highest risk for stroke. Generally, bridging therapy is recommended among atrial fibrillation patients with mechanical heart valves, especially valves in the mitral position. In this population, admission for heparin bridging within 48 hours of warfarin cessation is usually recommended, but enoxaparin can also be considered in many patients with normal renal function. Because of the short half-life of most NOAC therapies, bridging therapy with heparin or enoxaparin is generally not required.

PROCEDURES FOR STROKE PREVENTION: TARGETING THE LEFT ATRIAL APPENDAGE

Procedure-based therapies for stroke prevention provide an attractive alternative for patients unable to tolerate anticoagulation. The LAA has long been recognized as the predominant source for embolic events in the setting of atrial fibrillation; surgical resection was first reported in 1947. Unfortunately, randomized trials of surgical LAA ligation were never performed despite surgical excision becoming the standard of

TABLE 39.3 Cessation of Novel Oral Anticoagulation Therapy Before Invasive Procedures

Dabigatran						Apixaban, Edoxaban, or Rivaroxaban	
CrCl, mL/min	≥80	50–79	30–49	15–29	≥30	15–29	<15
Estimated drug half-life, h	13	15	18	27	6–15	Apixaban: 17	Apixaban: 17
						Edoxaban: 17	Edoxaban: 10–17
						Rivaroxaban: 9	Rivaroxaban: 13
Procedural bleed risk, recommendation for therapy cessation (h)							
Low	≥24	≥36	≥48	≥72	≥24	≥36	No data
Uncertain, intermediate, or high	≥48	≥72	≥96	≥120	≥48	No data	No data

CrCl, Creatinine clearance.
Adapted from Doherty JU, Glucksman TI, Hucker WJ, et al. 2017 ACC expert consensus decision pathway for periprocedural management of anticoagulation in patients with nonvalvular atrial fibrillation. *J Am Coll Cardiol.* 2017;doi:10.1016/j.jacc.2016.11.024.

care for patients with atrial fibrillation who underwent heart surgery. There is reasonable observational evidence that patients with surgical closure of the LAA have a mitigated stroke risk, possibly similar to that of an aged-matched population. Based on this observational data from early Cox-Maze patients, additional techniques and devices have been designed to exclude the LAA with a goal of mitigating stroke risk in the long term. The PLAATO (percutaneous left atrial appendage transcatheter occlusion) device was the first implantable LAA occluder tested in humans, but it was withdrawn for commercial reasons after a successful feasibility study.

The LAA represents vestigial tissue growth and does not have an important physiological function. However, the appendage has long been recognized not only as a site of stasis during atrial fibrillation and therefore as a source for thrombus and embolic events, but it is also a likely electrical trigger of atrial depolarization waveforms in many patients. It is possible that disruption of the tissue, either with surgical excision or device placement, could paradoxically increase the burden of atrial fibrillation. Ongoing randomized trials are currently attempting to address this issue, and one recently published randomized trial of cardiac surgery patients demonstrated that LAA excision was associated with an increased risk of paroxysmal atrial fibrillation before discharge.

Surgical Left Atrial Appendage Occlusion

The LAA is commonly oversewn during heart valve surgery in patients with atrial fibrillation. This is usually accomplished with the placement of a running suture line. Despite direct visualization of the appendage tissue, this portion of cardiac surgery is performed while the patient is on cardiopulmonary bypass. The LAA is therefore not expanded, and on occasion, this results in incomplete LAA closure. Retrospective studies have suggested a persistent LAA communication in 24% of patients who have undergone surgical LAA ligation, which has been associated with an increased risk of stroke and systemic embolism. As a result, there have also been several commercial products that have been marketed for direct LAA occlusion at the time of surgery. The most common is the AtriClip device (AtriCure, Mason, Ohio). Automated suture devices offer the advantage of quick deployment and consistent tissue approximation and may be more reliable than manual suturing techniques.

Pericardial Approach for Left Atrial Appendage Occlusion

The Lariat device (SentreHEART, Palo Alto, California) has been FDA approved for soft tissue ligation and was designed to facilitate LAA ligation with a surgical "lasso" from the pericardial space. The procedure uses a magnetic rail system, with one magnetic wire inserted through a transseptal puncture, and one magnetic wire inserted from the pericardial space (Fig. 39.1). The wires meet over the tip of the LAA, and a lasso is used to close the appendage. Although the device has been approved as a suture to close soft tissue, and published data have indicated that it is effective for LAA closure, it has not been proven in a clinical trial to be effective for the prevention of thromboembolic events. Despite this lack of FDA-approved indication, the pericardial approach offers a theoretical advantage over implantable devices because there is no foreign body left inside the heart. The Lariat system is therefore often used for LAA occlusion in patients who are unable to tolerate even short durations of anticoagulation therapy, which are currently mandated after Watchman (Boston Scientific, Marlborough, Massachusetts) implantation. Real-world application of the Lariat device has been described in multiple observational studies with success rates of >90%, and a relatively low risk of major complications. There was an increase in use of the pericardial approach before FDA approval of the Watchman device.

A recent adverse event report described 36 mortality events associated with the pericardial approach to LAA occlusion, with an unknown denominator. Several thousand procedures have now been performed in the United States despite the lack of FDA approval for this indication. Importantly, the LAA is a known trigger for some patients with atrial fibrillation, and the ongoing aMAZE trial (LAA Ligation Adjunctive to PVI for Persistent or Longstanding Persistent Atrial Fibrillation) will seek to determine whether a pericardial approach to left atrial appendage ligation is beneficial among patients undergoing percutaneous pulmonary vein isolation.

Watchman Device for Left Atrial Appendage Occlusion

There is currently only one implantable device available for stroke prevention in the United States. The Watchman device consists of a self-expanding nitinol frame covered with a permeable (160 μm) polyethylene terephthalate membrane and was approved in 2014 after a protracted process requiring two separate randomized controlled clinical trials. The device is inserted through a 14-Fr sheath delivered into the left atrium after a transseptal puncture (Fig. 39.2). The initial randomized PROTECT-AF trial now has follow-up data available up to 5 years and showed a statistically significant reduction in total mortality, cardiovascular mortality, and major bleeding events compared with warfarin therapy alone, with similar prevention of ischemic stroke. There was a procedural success rate of >90%. Because of concerns regarding early procedure-related complications, an additional randomized trial (PREVAIL) was required before FDA approval. Although the PREVAIL trial did not show a mortality benefit for Watchman and failed to meet the primary efficacy endpoint, it did demonstrate improved procedural success (95%), improved safety, and a significant reduction in major bleeding compared with warfarin. In total, the randomized

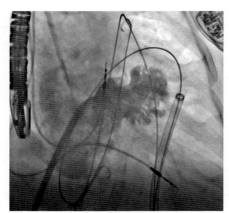

A. LAA angiogram with SL1 sheath

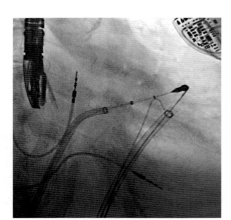

B. Magnetic rail system in place across LAA

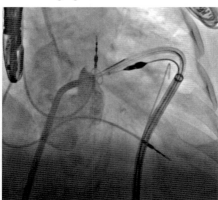

C. Snare advanced and secured around ostium of LAA

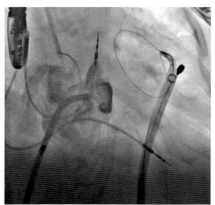

D. Completion angiogram with snare released

FIG 39.1 Stepwise Pericardial Approach to Left Atrial Appendage (LAA) Occlusion.

trials suggested that the Watchman device appeared to provide similar protection from stroke compared with warfarin therapy, and that cessation of warfarin associated with the successful Watchman procedure provided significant benefits to patients by decreasing bleeding risk associated with OAC. Table 39.4 summarizes the Watchman clinical trial results.

There were several consistent, and important criticisms of the randomized PROTECT and PREVAIL trials. Most importantly, the device arm was compared with warfarin only. This was an important limitation because most NOAC therapies are associated with a decreased bleeding risk compared with warfarin, and it is likely that the bleeding benefit of the Watchman device might be tempered compared with these newer agents. PROTECT and PREVAIL were also notable for the low stroke risk seen in both arms, and many have questioned whether the clinical trial populations could be generalized to contemporary clinical practice. A recent meta-analysis of clinical trial data suggested superiority of warfarin over Watchman for stroke prevention. However, many patients were unable to tolerate long-term anticoagulation with warfarin or NOAC therapy, and device occlusion of the LAA offers a promising alternative for selected patients with elevated bleeding risk. In current clinical practice, the Watchman device is approved for patients with "a rationale to seek alternatives to long term anticoagulation." The device is commonly offered to patients with recurrent severe bleeding events, medical and social conditions that predispose to bleeding and/or trauma, and an elevated HAS-BLED score in the setting of elevated stroke risk (CHA$_2$DS$_2$-VASc $\geq$2).

Atrial Fibrillation Ablation for Stroke Prevention

The techniques and evidence for atrial fibrillation ablation are described in detail in Chapter 40. In general, it seems logical that eliminating atrial fibrillation from a patient will have a positive effect on stroke risk. This remains controversial and has not been proven in properly designed randomized trials. We do know that continuation of anticoagulation is imperative in the period immediately after atrial fibrillation ablation when stroke risk is likely to be elevated because of inflammation of atrial tissue. Once a patient has a good response to ablation and maintains normal sinus rhythm, the decision to discontinue OAC therapy depends on stroke and bleeding risk. At this point, atrial fibrillation ablation should be viewed as a procedure to reduce the symptom burden of atrial fibrillation and not as a technique to attenuate stroke risk.

FUTURE DIRECTIONS

Recent analysis of prescribing habits suggest rapid uptake in the use of oral factor Xa inhibitors for stroke prevention in atrial fibrillation, with a corresponding decrease in warfarin use. This pattern is likely to improve safety outcomes and minimize bleeding risk. Real-world safety data on NOAC agents to this point have been reassuring, and as the agents become generic in the future, it is likely that warfarin prescriptions will continue to decline. Device-based therapies for stroke prevention are currently available and newer technologies are on the horizon. Use of procedural techniques for stroke prevention will be a focus of intense investigation in the coming years, and practicing cardiologists will be

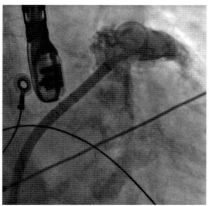

A. LAA angiogram with pigtail catheter in place

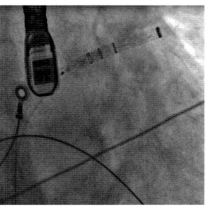

B. Watchman device advanced to tip of delivery sheath

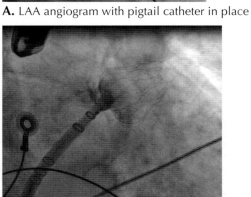

C. Watchman device unsheathed and deployed in LAA

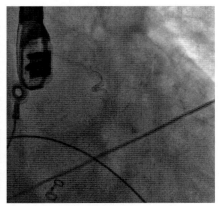

D. Device released and sheath retracted

FIG 39.2 Stepwise Watchman Implant. *LAA,* Left atrial appendage.

TABLE 39.4 Watchman Clinical Trial Results

Trial (n)	Design	Mean CHADS$_2$ Score	Procedural Success (%)	Frequency of Major Procedure-Related Safety Event	Overall Clinical Benefit
PROTECT-AF (707)	2:1 Watchman vs. warfarin	2.2	88	4.8% pericardial effusion in device group 1.1% procedure-related stroke 0.6% device embolization	Noninferior for prevention of ischemic stroke, significant reduction in hemorrhagic stroke, and major bleeding in the device group. Five-year follow-up suggests improved composite endpoint in device group
PREVAIL (407)	2:1 Watchman vs. warfarin	2.6	95	0.4% pericardial effusion with tamponade 0.7% device embolization 0.4% major bleeding	Improved procedural safety compared with PROTECT; noninferiority endpoint met for ischemic stroke but not for overall efficacy compared with warfarin; low event rates in both arms (18 total efficacy endpoints were met among 407 patients)
CAP registry (460)	Device-only registry	2.4	95	2.2% serous pericardial effusion No procedure-related stroke No device embolization	Continued improved procedural success, limited follow-up data published at this time with regard to late stroke and safety events

faced with complex treatment paradigms that require a multidisciplinary approach to optimize treatment outcomes.

ADDITIONAL RESOURCES

2016 ACC/AHA clinical performance and quality measures for adults with atrial fibrillation or atrial flutter. *Circ Cardiovasc Qual Outcomes.* 2016;9:443–488.
Summary of evidence-based recommendations for stroke prevention.
Doherty JU, Glucksman TI, Hucker WJ, et al. 2017 ACC expert consensus decision pathway for periprocedural management of anticoagulation in patients with nonvalvular atrial fibrillation. *J Am Coll Cardiol.* 2017;doi:10.1016/j.jacc.2016.11.024.
Contemporary review of strategies to minimize risk in the perioperative period.
http://www.strokeassociation.org/STROKEORG/LifeAfterStroke/ HealthyLivingAfterStroke/UnderstandingRiskyConditions/ When-the-Beat-is-Off---Atrial fibrillation_UCM_310782_Article.jsp#. WLIg2e8zVM -.
Excellent resource for updated stroke statistics from the American Heart Association.

EVIDENCE

Camm AJ, Lip GY, De Caterina R, et al; for the ESC Committee for Practice Guidelines. 2012 focused update of the ESC Guidelines for the management of atrial fibrillation: an update of the 2010 ESC Guidelines for the management of atrial fibrillation. *Eur Heart J.* 2012;33:2719–2747.
European guidelines including evidence for NOAC therapy in atrial fibrillation.
Connolly SJ, Ezekowitz MD, Yusuf S, et al. Dabigatran versus warfarin in patients with atrial fibrillation. *N Engl J Med.* 2009;361(12):1139–1151.
Pivotal dabigatran trial demonstrating efficacy for stroke prevention.
Giugliano RP, Ruff CT, Braunwald E, et al. Edoxaban versus warfarin in patients with atrial fibrillation. *N Engl J Med.* 2013;369(22):2093–2104.
Pivotal edoxaban trial demonstrating efficacy for stroke prevention.

Granger CB, Alexander JH, McMurray JJ, et al. Apixaban versus warfarin in patients with atrial fibrillation. *N Engl J Med.* 2011;365(11):981–992.
Pivotal apixaban study demonstrating efficacy for stroke prevention.
Holmes DR Jr, Doshi SK, Kar S, et al. Left atrial appendage closure as an alternative to warfarin for stroke prevention in atrial fibrillation: a patient-level meta-analysis. *J Am Coll Cardiol.* 2015;65(24):2614–2623.
Combined data from PROTECT and PREVAIL trials.
Holmes DR Jr, Kar S, Price MJ, et al. Prospective randomized evaluation of the WATCHMAN Left Atrial Appendage Closure device in patients with atrial fibrillation versus long-term warfarin therapy: the PREVAIL Trial. *J Am Coll Cardiol.* 2014;64(1):1–12.
Initial findings of the PREVAIL study, published 5 years after PROTECT-AF.
Holmes DR, Reddy VY, Turi ZG, et al. Percutaneous closure of the left atrial appendage versus warfarin therapy for prevention of stroke in patients with atrial fibrillation: a randomised non-inferiority trial. *Lancet.* 2009;374(9689):534–542.
Initial publication of the PROTECT-AF randomized trial.
Huisman MV, Rothman KJ, et al. Changing landscape for stroke prevention in AF: findings from the GLORIA-AF registry phase 2. *J Am Coll Cardiol.* 2017;69(7):doi:10.1016/j.jacc.2016.11.061.
Important real-world experience with available NOAC therapies.
January CT, Wann LS, Alpert JS. 2014 AHA/ACC/HRS guideline for the management of patients with atrial fibrillation: a report of the American College of Cardiology/American Heart Association Task Force on Practice Guidelines and the Heart Rhythm Society. *J Am Coll Cardiol.* 2014;64(21):e1–e76.
Most recent complete guideline recommendations for stroke prevention in atrial fibrillation.
Patel MR, Mahaffey KW, Garg J, et al. Rivaroxaban versus warfarin in nonvalvular atrial fibrillation. *N Engl J Med.* 2011;365(10):883–891.
Pivotal trial demonstrating efficacy of rivaroxaban for stroke prevention.

40

Invasive Management of Atrial Fibrillation and Atrial Tachycardias

Matthew S. Baker, Anil K. Gehi, J. Paul Mounsey

Although they were once considered investigational techniques, catheter and surgical ablation have evolved to become commonly performed procedures in major hospitals worldwide. Catheter ablation is the preferred therapy for typical atrial flutter, and it should be considered as a first-line therapy in select patients with atrial fibrillation (AF) when a rhythm control strategy is being pursued. A decision to pursue invasive management of atrial arrhythmias depends on a number of factors, including symptom burden, the type of arrhythmia, the presence of underlying cardiac structural abnormalities, the availability of noninvasive treatment alternatives, and patient preference. Current evidence is insufficient to demonstrate reduction of heart failure, stroke, or mortality after AF ablation, so the impetus to pursue ablation currently remains a reduction in symptoms and an improvement in quality of life. Symptomatic patients with paroxysmal AF have been best represented in clinical trials of catheter ablation and generally have the best chance of achieving a benefit from invasive therapies.

MAZE PROCEDURE

Ablation of AF is based on the concept that barriers to atrial conduction at critical locations would prevent maintenance of the abnormal rhythm (Fig. 40.1). Using cut-and-sew techniques to create atrial barriers has been termed the Maze procedure. The Maze procedure has gone through multiple iterations. Newer techniques use bipolar radiofrequency or cryoablation as alternatives to the cut-and-sew technique. The Maze procedure has a high reported success rate. However, because of its invasiveness and complexity, the Maze operation has not been widely adopted except in patients with AF who are undergoing cardiac surgery for another reason, such as valvular disease.

RADIOFREQUENCY CATHETER ABLATION

Catheter ablation initially emulated the surgical Maze procedure by using radiofrequency ablation to produce linear lines of electrical isolation in the atrial endocardium. After the observation that focal tachycardia from the pulmonary veins often provokes AF, there has been increasing enthusiasm for treatment of AF through ablation of these triggers. Electrical isolation of the pulmonary veins and their left atrial orifices has become the cornerstone of any AF ablation procedure.

Catheter ablation can be performed under general anesthesia or conscious sedation. Femoral venous access is used to introduce catheters into the right-sided cardiac chambers. From there, transseptal needle puncture provides a route to the primary chamber of interest in AF ablation, which is the left atrium. The procedure may be preceded by transesophageal echocardiography to exclude the presence of left atrial appendage thrombus. During the procedure, intravenous heparin is administered to prevent thrombus formation. Details of the complex anatomy of the left atrium are often evaluated by preprocedural CT or MRI. Fluoroscopy and three-dimensional electroanatomic mapping systems are used to reconstruct left atrial anatomy and to track catheter movement during AF ablation.

The delivery of radiofrequency energy via transvenous electrode catheter achieves myocardial ablation by conducting alternating electrical current through the resistive medium of myocardial tissue. After several seconds at a temperature >50° C, myocardial tissue necrosis occurs, resulting in nonconducting scar tissue.

In general terms, the number and configuration of radiofrequency lesions delivered to the atria vary according to the type of AF (see definition of types of AF in Chapter 38). In paroxysmal AF, complete electrical isolation of the pulmonary veins from the left atrium is usually sufficient to achieve clinical success. Current approaches to pulmonary vein isolation involve a wide ring of encircling lesions around the openings of the pulmonary veins into the left atrium (Fig. 40.2).

Compared with paroxysmal AF, the efficacy of pulmonary vein isolation in persistent AF has been more modest. For this reason, pulmonary vein isolation is sometimes combined with additional ablation in cases of persistent AF. Approaches vary, but may include (1) ablation at sites bearing complex fractionated atrial electrograms (CFAEs), (2) the application of additional atrial lesion lines, and/or (3) ablation of the ganglionated plexuses.

CFAEs are intracardiac atrial electrograms distinct from the normal electrical signals of atrial tissue. CFAEs may demonstrate fractionated and/or rapid signals. These are believed to represent areas of abnormal electrical conduction and possibly high-frequency "drivers" of persistent AF. CFAEs can be identified by visual assessment of intraatrial recordings or by automated computer analysis.

The creation of lines of lesions is an attempt to emulate the surgical Maze procedure. Originally intended to interrupt reentrant circuits in the atrium, other possible mechanisms by which linear ablation may improve AF ablation outcomes are the incidental elimination of CFAEs and/or autonomic ganglia along the course of the linear lesions. Lesion "sets" may include any combination of the following: a "roofline" between the two upper pulmonary veins, a mitral isthmus line from the left inferior pulmonary vein to the mitral annulus, linear lesions to isolate the other thoracic veins (namely, the coronary sinus and the superior vena cava) or the left atrial appendage, and a conventional cavotricuspid isthmus (CTI) line to eliminate typical atrial flutter.

The observation that changes in autonomic tone can be associated with the initiation of AF has led some operators to target autonomic ganglia during AF ablation. Vagal stimulation may lead to premature atrial depolarizations, changes in refractoriness of atrial myocardium, and the development of CFAEs. Ganglionated plexuses are part of the cardiac autonomic system and are located within epicardial fat pads. Destruction of ganglionated plexuses during endocardial catheter ablation is achieved by transmural radiofrequency heating.

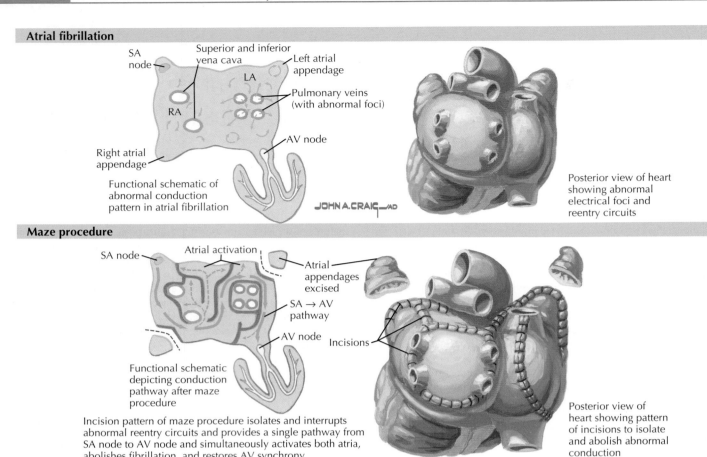

FIG 40.1 Surgical Management of Atrial Fibrillation. *AV,* Atrioventricular; *LA,* left atrium; *RA,* right atrium; *SA,* sinoatrial.

The optimal technique for ablation of persistent AF remains elusive. Recent studies have called into question the benefit of these strategies of ancillary ablation beyond the pulmonary veins.

CRYOBALLOON ABLATION

The use of cryothermal energy delivered via a balloon-based system to achieve pulmonary vein isolation as a substitute for radiofrequency pulmonary vein isolation has grown rapidly. A transvenous catheter is used to position a balloon sequentially in the antra of the pulmonary veins (Fig. 40.3). Liquid nitrous oxide is then delivered under pressure to the balloon, where it changes to gas, resulting in local tissue cooling. Freezing and ice crystal formation within tissue around the circumference of the balloon leads to disruption of cell membranes, changes in cellular metabolism, electrical activity, and microvascular blood flow. These changes ultimately lead to cell death and formation of a nonconductive scar.

SUCCESS AND COMPLICATIONS OF ATRIAL FIBRILLATION ABLATION

Recurrence of AF early (<3 months) after initial ablation is common and does not preclude long-term success. Antiarrhythmic medication and direct-current cardioversion may be used to maintain sinus rhythm during this period of atrial remodeling. Beyond 3 months, recurrence of AF may indicate reconnection of pulmonary veins and require long-term antiarrhythmic therapy or repeat catheter ablation to achieve desired outcomes.

Depending on the duration of follow-up, thoroughness of rhythm monitoring, and whether antiarrhythmic drugs are used during the postoperative period, success rates for radiofrequency or cryoablation of paroxysmal AF range from 65% to 95%. For persistent AF, the corresponding percentages are 40% to 80% (the results from the higher end of this range are usually obtained after multiple attempts at ablation). Robust data on the long-term outcomes of AF ablation are not available, and it remains uncertain if apparently "cured" AF may yet relapse years later.

Catheter ablation for AF is not without risk. The mortality rate associated with the procedure has been reported at 0.15%. Cardiac perforation with tamponade is the most common potentially life-threatening complication, with a reported incidence between 1.2% and 6%. Factors contributing to the risk of tamponade are extensive catheter manipulation and ablation within cardiac chambers, the common use of multiple transseptal punctures, and the need for systemic anticoagulation during the procedure.

Pulmonary vein stenosis can occur after radiofrequency or cryoballoon AF ablation. Significant pulmonary vein stenosis has been defined as >70% reduction in pulmonary vein luminal diameter. Symptoms include chest pain, dyspnea, cough, hemoptysis, and symptoms of pulmonary hypertension. The incidence of pulmonary vein stenosis has been reported to be <10%, but screening for asymptomatic stenoses is not routinely performed. Awareness of this potential complication has

ECG of atrial fibrillation demonstrating irregular R-R intervals and a lack of organized P waves

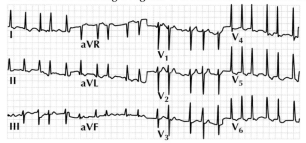

Catheter ablation of atrial fibrillation

Radiofrequency ablation lesion "sets"

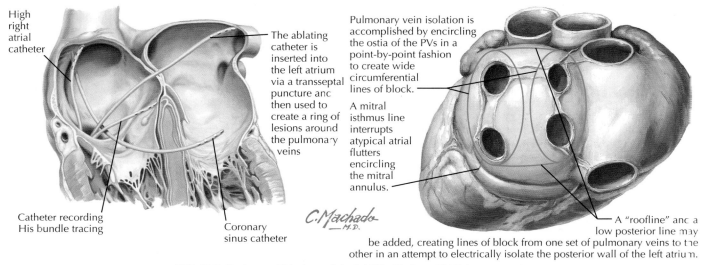

High right atrial catheter

The ablating catheter is inserted into the left atrium via a transseptal puncture and then used to create a ring of lesions around the pulmonary veins

Catheter recording His bundle tracing

Coronary sinus catheter

Pulmonary vein isolation is accomplished by encircling the ostia of the PVs in a point-by-point fashion to create wide circumferential lines of block.

A mitral isthmus line interrupts atypical atrial flutters encircling the mitral annulus.

A "roofline" and a low posterior line may be added, creating lines of block from one set of pulmonary veins to the other in an attempt to electrically isolate the posterior wall of the left atrium.

FIG 40.2 Catheter Ablation of Atrial Fibrillation. *PV,* Pulmonary vein.

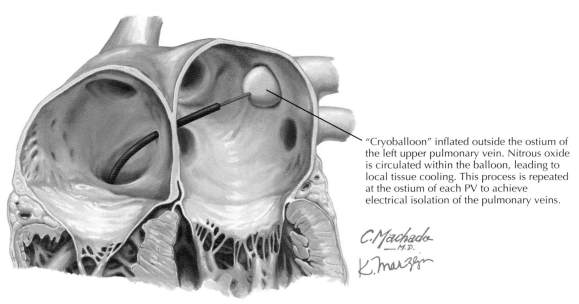

"Cryoballoon" inflated outside the ostium of the left upper pulmonary vein. Nitrous oxide is circulated within the balloon, leading to local tissue cooling. This process is repeated at the ostium of each PV to achieve electrical isolation of the pulmonary veins.

FIG 40.3 Cryoballoon Ablation of Atrial Fibrillation. *PV,* Pulmonary vein.

led most operators to avoid extensive ablation within the pulmonary veins.

Phrenic nerve injury can result from direct thermal injury, usually to the right phrenic nerve as it runs by the right superior pulmonary vein and superior vena cava. Patients can be asymptomatic or present with dyspnea, hiccups, cough, or thoracic pain. Phrenic nerve injury

is more common after cryoballoon ablation compared with radiofrequency ablation (up to 7.5% incidence vs. <1% incidence). Phrenic nerve function usually recovers fully by 12 months postablation.

Thromboembolic events (stroke and transient ischemic attack) are well-described complications of catheter ablation for AF, with an incidence reported between 0% and 7%. For this reason, anticoagulation is necessary during and for at least 2 months postoperatively, regardless of the long-term stroke risk of the patient. Even when catheter ablation is perceived to be successful, the long-term stroke risk of the patient should be managed after considering standard risk factors (i.e., CHADS-VASc score), bleeding risk, and patient preference.

The most feared complication of AF ablation is the development of an atrial–esophageal fistula, which has a reported incidence of 0.1% to 0.25%. The esophagus passes directly behind the left atrium, in close approximation to the posterior wall of the left atrium and one or more pulmonary veins. The precise mechanism of esophageal injury is not completely understood, but may involve direct thermal injury, acid reflux, infection from the esophageal lumen, and ischemia due to injury of microvasculature. Atrioesophageal fistula presents with fever and recurrent neurological events (from septic and/or air emboli) days to weeks after the procedure and carries a mortality rate of >70%. Prompt recognition and diagnosis by CT or MRI allows for successful treatment by urgent surgical intervention or esophageal stent placement.

CATHETER ABLATION OF ATRIAL TACHYCARDIAS

From a mechanistic standpoint, atrial tachycardias (ATs) may be segregated into those that are due to reentrant circuits ("atrial flutter") and those that are driven by one or more rapidly discharging foci ("focal atrial tachycardia"). Atrial flutters are, in turn, classified into those that require conduction via a narrow strip of right atrial tissue between the inferior vena cava and the tricuspid annulus (the CTI), as opposed to those "atypical" atrial flutters that do not.

Typical (CTI-dependent) atrial flutter usually activates the right atrium in a counterclockwise fashion, if the heart is viewed from its apex looking up at the tricuspid valve (Fig. 40.4). This is associated with a characteristic pattern of atrial activity on 12-lead ECG; an inverted sawtooth pattern is present in the inferior leads II, III, and aVF, with upright P waves in lead V_1. Although this arrhythmia is sensitive to external direct-current shocks, catheter ablation is considered a first-line treatment for this arrhythmia. Clockwise CTI-dependent atrial flutter (associated with a variable and less specific ECG pattern) is seen nine times less frequently than its counterclockwise cousin. However, it can

be ablated using the same method. Of patients with typical atrial flutter, approximately 30% have concomitant AF. Ablation of the atrial flutter does not cure AF.

Atypical atrial flutter is most frequently a reentrant circuit related to an atrial scar. A scar can be the result of previous cardiac surgery, previous ablation, or underlying fibrosis. The ECG in atypical atrial flutter can overlap with that of focal ATs and typical flutter. In general, P-wave durations are longer, isoelectric intervals shorter, and cycle length less variable compared with focal ATs. A sawtooth pattern, like that seen in typical atrial flutter, may or may not be present. The surface ECG has limited usefulness in localizing the circuit of atypical atrial flutter. Some atypical flutters are confined to the left atrium or interatrial septum, and some involve a complex figure-of-eight pattern.

Focal ATs can occur whether structural atrial abnormalities exist. Unlike atypical atrial flutter, the arrhythmogenic locus of a focal AT can be inferred with reasonable accuracy by analysis of the P wave on 12-lead ECG. Furthermore, these automatic foci have a predilection for particular regions. For example, in the right atrium, common sources are the crista terminalis, the tricuspid annulus, and the coronary sinus ostium; in the left atrium, the pulmonary veins are often the centers of electrical unrest.

Regardless of the underlying mechanism, all types of ATs are amenable to catheter ablation.

CATHETER ABLATION OF TYPICAL ATRIAL FLUTTER

Once confirmation of CTI–dependent atrial flutter is confirmed in the laboratory, the ablation strategy is to create a complete line of radiofrequency lesions across the CTI to achieve conduction block across that corridor of tissue. In experienced centers, catheter ablation of typical atrial flutter is associated with an acute success rate approaching 100%. During the first year after successful ablation, approximately 10% of patients experience recurrent atrial flutter, and a second ablation is successful in 95% of these patients. With a single procedure, 73% of patients will remain free of typical atrial flutter at 5 years. Procedure-related complications are rare.

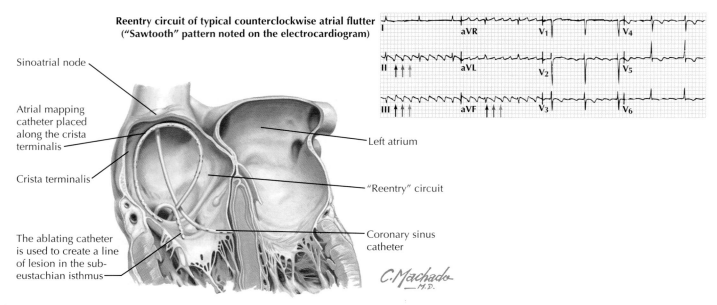

FIG 40.4 Catheter Ablation of Atrial Flutter.

TABLE 40.1	Outcomes of Catheter-Delivered Radiofrequency Ablation	
Type of Arrhythmia	**Success Rate (%)**	**Complications (Rate)**
AV node ablation	98–100	Sudden death (rare)
Atrial flutter	85–95 (typical flutter)	AV block (rare), stroke (rare)
	80–90 (atypical flutter)	
Focal atrial tachycardia	86	AV block, cardiac tamponade, stroke, phrenic nerve damage (collectively 1%–2%)
Atrial fibrillation	65–95 (for paroxysmal AF)[a]	Stroke (0.1%–7%), cardiac tamponade (1%–6%), LA flutter (up to 30%), phrenic nerve damage
	40–80 (for persistent AF)[a]	(<1%–7.5%),[b] PV stenosis (uncommon), atrioesophageal fistula (rare)

[a]Reported success rates vary widely, depending on definition of "success," number of repeat ablations, quality of postoperative surveillance, and so forth.
[b]The incidence of phrenic nerve damage is <1% with radiofrequency catheter ablation versus 4.7% to 7.5% with cryoballoon ablation.
AF, Atrial fibrillation; *AV*, atrioventricular; *LA*, left atrial; *PV*, pulmonary vein.

Atrial flutter and AF frequently coexist in the same hearts. For this reason, anticoagulation to prevent thromboembolic events is usually recommended in the same fashion as for patients with known AF (based upon their CHADS-VASc score). Even in patients without a history of AF, the rate of AF occurrence is 60% at 5 years after typical flutter ablation.

CATHETER ABLATION OF ATYPICAL ATRIAL FLUTTER

Targets for ablation in atypical atrial flutter were formerly identified using pacing maneuvers only. Although reliable, this method has the drawbacks of being time-consuming and prone to cause termination of tachycardia. Three-dimensional electroanatomic mapping systems now facilitate the study and treatment of these arrhythmias. These systems work equally well for focal ATs (see the following). Briefly, for an atypical atrial flutter, the aim is to create a "map" of the arrhythmia circuit and then confirm the importance of potential ablation targets through pacing maneuvers. These ablation targets are then destroyed by catheter ablation. It is often necessary to create a supplementary line of lesions to transect this and other parts of the atria that may be critical to tachycardia conduction. Such lines are usually extended from between electrically inert regions. Initial success rates with catheter ablation are high (Table 40.1), but recurrences have been observed in up to 20% of cases, mainly because these patients have extensive atrial disease with islands of scar tissue that can facilitate additional flutter circuits. Those who relapse are either palliated with antiarrhythmic drugs or treated with additional ablation.

FOCAL ATRIAL TACHYCARDIA ABLATION

Focal ATs are usually mapped during tachycardia, with attention initially directed to the anatomic location indicated by the abnormal P-wave morphology. The means by which these arrhythmogenic foci are identified has evolved from single- or dual-catheter methods (probing different parts of the atria with multipolar electrodes) to the use of three-dimensional mapping systems to create a virtual map of potential ablation targets. The aim of this technique is to pinpoint the earliest site of electrical activation during tachycardia or atrial ectopy. This spot is then destroyed by catheter ablation. As with atypical atrial flutter, success rates for catheter ablation of focal AT are high; potential complications are listed in Table 40.1.

ATRIOVENTRICULAR NODE ABLATION

An effective means of regulating and regularizing the ventricular rhythm is to perform ablation of the atrioventricular node. This can improve symptoms in select patients, such as those with tachycardia-mediated cardiomyopathy and high ventricular rates refractory to medical therapy. However, this procedure renders the patient dependent on a ventricular pacemaker. It is therefore generally reserved for older adult patients. After complete atrioventricular node ablation, the ventricular rate of the patient is independent of atrial activity and determined solely by the pacemaker; therefore, no rate-controlling medications are required. Because the upper chambers of the heart remain in AF, antithrombotic therapy must still be considered based on the risk of the patient, such as that assessed by the CHA_2DS_2-VASc score.

FUTURE DIRECTIONS

Remarkable advances have been made in the invasive management of atrial arrhythmias over the past two decades. Cardiac imaging and electrical mapping software capable of greater signal resolution, catheters with novel modes of energy delivery and the ability to record the force of catheter contact, and remotely operated robotic catheter steering systems are some developments in the evolution of ablation of cardiac arrhythmias. Technical advances such as these are anticipated to improve patient safety, and to increase procedure efficacy and efficiency for these often complex procedures.

ADDITIONAL RESOURCES

Huang SKS, Miller JM, eds. *Catheter Ablation of Cardiac Arrhythmias*. 3rd ed. Philadelphia: Saunders-Elsevier; 2015.
Well-illustrated reference for the mapping and ablation of arrhythmias.

EVIDENCE

Calkins H, Kuck KH, Cappato R, et al. 2012 HRS/EHRA/ECAS expert consensus statement on catheter and surgical ablation of atrial fibrillation: recommendations for patient selection, procedural techniques, patient management and follow-up, definitions, endpoints, and research trial design : a report of the Heart Rhythm Society (HRS) Task Force on Catheter and Surgical Ablation of Atrial Fibrillation. Developed in partnership with the European Heart Rhythm Association (EHRA), a registered branch of the European Society of Cardiology (ESC) and the European Cardiac Arrhythmia Society (ECAS); and in collaboration with the American College of Cardiology (ACC), American Heart Association (AHA), the Asia Pacific Heart Rhythm Society (APHRS), and the Society of Thoracic Surgeons (STS). Endorsed by the governing bodies of the American College of Cardiology Foundation, the American Heart Association, the European Cardiac Arrhythmia Society, the European Heart Rhythm Association, the Society of Thoracic Surgeons, the Asia Pacific Heart Rhythm Society, and the Heart Rhythm Society. *Heart Rhythm*. 2012;9(4):632–696.

Latest recommendations for catheter ablation of AF from major cardiology societies.

Haïssaguerre M, Jaïs P, Shah DC, et al. Spontaneous initiation of atrial fibrillation by ectopic beats originating in the pulmonary veins. *N Engl J Med.* 1998;10:659–666.

Original description of pulmonary vein isolation that is now the foundation of AF ablation.

January CT, Wann LS, et al. 2014 AHA/ACC/HRS guideline for the management of patients with atrial fibrillation: a report of the American College of Cardiology/American Heart Association Task Force on Practice Guidelines and the Heart Rhythm Society. Developed in collaboration with the Society of Thoracic Surgeons. *J Am Coll Cardiol.* 2014;64(21):2305–2307.

Comprehensive guidelines for the management of AF developed by the major cardiology societies.

41

Ventricular Arrhythmias

Khola S. Tahir, Eugene H. Chung, James P. Hummel, J. Paul Mounsey

Ventricular arrhythmias originate from the distal conduction system (distal to the His bundle) or ventricular myocardium, and with few exceptions, present with a wide QRS morphology on ECG. These may occur as isolated premature ventricular contractions (PVCs), couplets (2 consecutive PVCs), or as ventricular tachycardia (VT) (≥3 consecutive beats with a rate of >100 beats/min). Nonsustained VT refers to ≥3 self-terminating episodes that last between 3 beats and 30 seconds, whereas sustained VT refers to episodes that last >30 seconds or that require earlier termination due to hemodynamic instability. Ventricular fibrillation (VF) is a fast, irregular, and disorganized rhythm in the ventricles characterized by an undulating baseline without distinct QRS complexes on ECG. VF results in circulatory collapse, and if sustained, it usually results in death within 3 to 5 minutes if not corrected promptly.

Although wide QRS complex tachycardia is not synonymous with VT, 80% of patients with a wide complex tachycardia have VT as a diagnosis. VT is usually found in patients with underlying structural heart disease, predominantly coronary artery disease (CAD) and myocardial ischemia. It is often but not invariably associated with hemodynamic instability, and thus may cause symptoms such as chest pain, dyspnea, palpitations, or syncope, or lead to sudden cardiac death (SCD). The severity of symptoms determines the urgency of treatment. This chapter reviews the pathogenesis, diagnosis, and treatment of ventricular arrhythmias. SCD, a potential result of VT or VF, is addressed in greater detail in Chapter 42.

ETIOLOGY AND PATHOGENESIS

The type of VT, prognosis, and management of the arrhythmia are dependent on the presence of structural heart disease. The risk of sustained monomorphic VT is higher in patients with severe left ventricular (LV) dysfunction and extensive scarring. VT is also associated with myocardial ischemia, congestive heart failure, infiltrative cardiomyopathy, and high catecholamine states (Fig. 41.1). VT in patients with ischemic heart disease is most often due to a reentry circuit in a region of a previous myocardial infarction. In these areas, gap junctions are often disrupted, which leads to slow and disorderly conduction by surviving cardiomyocytes. This physiology can lead to initiation and maintenance of reentrant circuits. Intracardiac recordings in the electrophysiology laboratory from the VT site of origin during sinus rhythm demonstrate fractionated low-amplitude electrograms synonymous with slow electrical conduction. Fibrosis from nonischemic processes may also lead to reentry as the underlying cause of VT in patients without coronary disease.

DIFFERENTIAL AND ECG DIAGNOSIS

VT must be distinguished from other wide complex tachycardias: supraventricular tachycardia (SVT) with bundle branch block, preexcitation of the ventricle during SVT due to anterograde conduction over an accessory pathway (antidromic reciprocating tachycardia), or ventricular pacing. The decision that a wide complex tachycardia is VT is extremely important because misdiagnosis can delay life-saving treatment. Any wide complex tachycardia in a patient with ischemic or other structural heart disease should be managed as VT until proven otherwise. Many diagnostic algorithms exist for distinguishing VT from other wide complex tachycardias. These can be confusing and are often unhelpful. ECG clues that, if present, favor VT, are reviewed in the following. The two main groups of diagnostic criteria are related to abnormalities of QRS morphology and identification of independent P-wave activity.

QRS Morphology

If the QRS morphology changes during the tachycardia relative to baseline, then the diagnosis is probably VT. Intraventricular conduction is always abnormal in VT and results in broadening of the QRS. In general, the QRS duration is usually >120 ms in VT, with the caveat that VTs originating from the His-Purkinje system rarely have a normal QRS duration. The morphology of the QRS yields important information about the site of origin of the VT. Generally, a VT with right bundle branch block morphology (predominantly positive QRS complex in lead V_1) suggests an LV origin, whereas a VT with left bundle branch block morphology (predominantly negative QRS in lead V_1) suggests right ventricular (RV) or septal origin (Fig. 41.2A). A QRS with a superior axis during VT implies an inferior origin, whereas an inferior axis implies an origin on the anterior wall or near the outflow tracts. VT originating near the apex will result in dominant S waves in leads V_2 to V_5, whereas basal VTs will have dominant R waves in these leads. VT with a right bundle branch block pattern generally has an atypical appearance in lead V_1. The R wave is single or biphasic (QR or RS) or triphasic (with the initial R wave taller than the smaller r' and an S wave in between that crosses the baseline). Lead V_6 typically demonstrates small r and large S waves. Left bundle branch block patterns with initial R waves >30 ms or time to the nadir of the S wave of >60 ms in lead V_1 and time from QRS onset to the nadir of the S wave >100 ms in any precordial lead suggest VT rather than aberrancy. The S wave may be notched or slurred. Because SVT with aberration is due to a functional bundle branch block, the QRS should resemble a typical bundle branch block, and the S wave is neither notched nor slurred. If lead V_6 is used, a qS pattern suggests VT. Although sometimes useful, these findings have limited sensitivity and specificity. Change in the frontal plane QRS axis of >40 degrees, especially toward the "northwest quadrant" between −90 and −180 degrees (normal is −30 to 90 degrees), is highly suggestive of VT. Concordance refers to uniform direction of the QRS complexes in the precordial leads, which are either all positive or all negative; for example, in VT with a right bundle branch block pattern, the QRS is upright in all precordial leads (Fig. 41.2B).

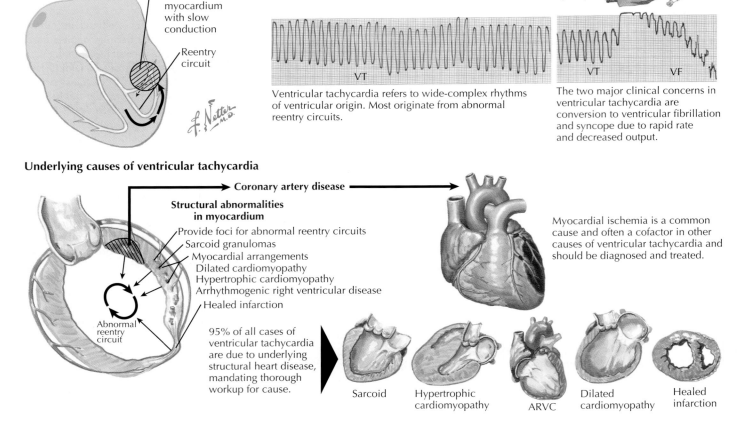

Ventricular tachycardia refers to wide-complex rhythms of ventricular origin. Most originate from abnormal reentry circuits.

The two major clinical concerns in ventricular tachycardia are conversion to ventricular fibrillation and syncope due to rapid rate and decreased output.

Underlying causes of ventricular tachycardia

Coronary artery disease

Structural abnormalities in myocardium
Provide foci for abnormal reentry circuits
Sarcoid granulomas
Myocardial arrangements
Dilated cardiomyopathy
Hypertrophic cardiomyopathy
Arrhythmogenic right ventricular disease
Healed infarction

Myocardial ischemia is a common cause and often a cofactor in other causes of ventricular tachycardia and should be diagnosed and treated.

95% of all cases of ventricular tachycardia are due to underlying structural heart disease, mandating thorough workup for cause.

Sarcoid   Hypertrophic cardiomyopathy   ARVC   Dilated cardiomyopathy   Healed infarction

FIG 41.1 Mechanisms of Ventricular Tachycardia (VT). *ARVC,* Arrhythmogenic right ventricular cardiomyopathy.

Independent P-Wave Activity

Atrioventricular (AV) dissociation indicates independent P-wave activity, and its presence is diagnostic of VT (Fig. 41.3A). The sinus rate is usually slower than the ventricular rate. The P waves should be upright in leads I and II if the origin is the sinus node. Variable deflections within the ST segment are suggestive of AV dissociation, and all 12 leads should be analyzed. AV dissociation can be difficult to discern, and its absence does not exclude VT because the patient may have underlying atrial fibrillation (in up to one-third of cases), or there may be retrograde ventricle-to-atrial conduction that results in AV association in VT. A fusion beat occurs when a sinus beat conducts to the ventricles via the AV node concurrent with a beat arising from the ventricles (Fig. 41.3B). The resulting QRS complex has an intermediate appearance between a normal beat and a VT beat.

A capture beat occurs when the ventricle is depolarized via the AV node, which results in a narrow (normal-appearing) QRS (Fig. 41.3C). The presence of capture and/or fusion beats indicates AV dissociation, and if present, this points to a diagnosis of VT. Their absence, however, does not exclude VT.

Additional Criteria

Two simpler alternative approaches have been reported. One looks for specific criteria for SVT and diagnoses VT by default if they are not present. Specifically, SVT is diagnosed only in the presence of typical left bundle branch block morphology (delay to the S-wave nadir in lead V_1 of <70 ms and no Q wave in lead V_6) or typical right bundle branch block morphology (rSR′ in lead V_1 and RS in lead V_6 with R height higher than S depth). Otherwise, VT is diagnosed. Another algorithm has been reported that restricted ECG analysis to a single lead, aVR, which is illustrated in Fig. 41.4. Initial R waves, or broad or notched initial downward deflections in aVR, support the diagnosis of VT.

CLINICAL PRESENTATION

There is a wide variation in the presentation of ventricular arrhythmias. PVCs are a common cause of palpitations, although these can also be asymptomatic and detected incidentally. When frequent, they can often result in nonspecific symptoms such as fatigue, dizziness, or dyspnea, especially when occurring in bigeminal (alternating normal and premature [and wide] QRS complexes) and trigeminal patterns (two normal beats for every PVC).

Most patients presenting with symptomatic monomorphic VT, especially those older than 40 years of age, have underlying ischemic heart disease. Acquired or inherited cardiomyopathies can also provide the substrate for monomorphic VT. Symptoms associated with VT depend on many factors, including the VT rate, presence of structural heart disease, and medications. Hemodynamic stability is not helpful in differentiating VT from SVT, because VT can often be well tolerated, and SVT can result in syncope. Exercise-induced VT in a normal heart may be better tolerated than even a slow VT in patients with a low ejection fraction. Anemia or preexisting orthostatic hypotension in a patient

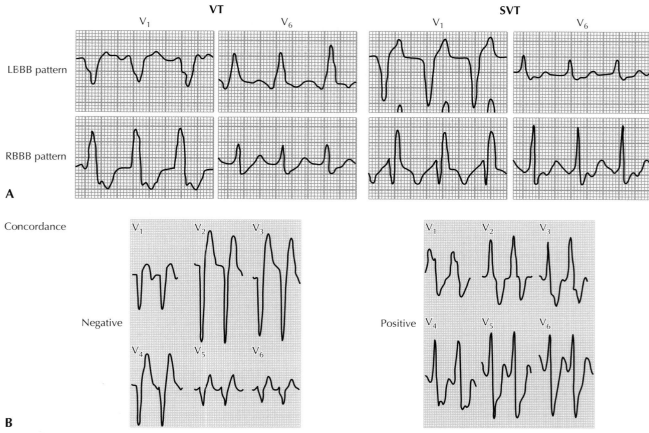

FIG 41.2 Changes in QRS Morphology in Ventricular Tachycardia *(VT)* and in Supraventricular Tachycardia *(SVT)*. (A) Typical patterns seen with left bundle branch block *(LBBB)* and in right bundle branch block *(RBBB)*. (B) Typical patterns of positive and negative concordance in QRS complexes. See text for details.

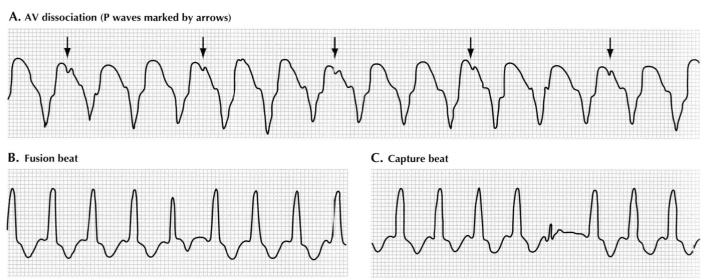

A. AV dissociation (P waves marked by arrows)

B. Fusion beat

C. Capture beat

FIG 41.3 Electrocardiographic Signs of Independent P-Wave Activity. *AV,* Atrioventricular.

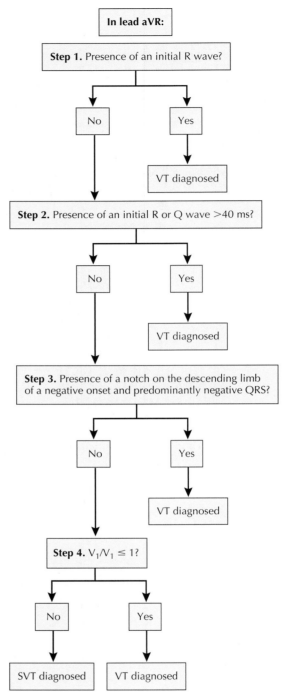

FIG 41.4 New aVR Algorithm for Diagnosing Wide Complex Tachycardia. *SVT*, Supraventricular tachycardia; *VT*, ventricular tachycardia. (Modified from Vereckei A, Duray G, Szénási G, et al. New algorithm using only lead aVR for differential diagnosis of wide QRS complex tachycardia. *Heart Rhythm.* 2008;5:89–98.)

with VT will usually result in early hemodynamic compromise. Patients may present with a range of symptoms: palpitations (regular or irregular), dizziness, shortness of breath, chest pain, presyncope, syncope, congestive heart failure, or SCD. Signs of AV dissociation, such as "cannon" A waves and varying intensity of S₁, can sometimes be elicited on physical examination and can help diagnose VT.

Polymorphic VT and VF generally result in rapid hemodynamic collapse if sustained and require prompt defibrillation.

DIAGNOSTIC APPROACH

Some maneuvers may aid in differentiating SVT from VT in the hemodynamically stable patient. During an episode of tachycardia, carotid massage or the Valsalva maneuver increases vagal stimulation and is most useful for tachyarrhythmias other than VT. Vagal stimulation can slow conduction over the AV node and thereby can terminate an AV nodal reentrant tachycardia or AV reentrant tachycardia, or unmask atrial flutter waves. Although the termination of a wide complex tachycardia with intravenous adenosine favors a diagnosis of SVT with aberrancy, adenosine-responsive VT has been reported in patients with normal LV function, and thus, responsiveness to adenosine does not rule out VT. However, the idea that the absence of a response to adenosine rules in a diagnosis of VT is also a fallacy. The most common reason adenosine fails to terminate an adenosine-sensitive arrhythmia is that an insufficient dose reaches the heart before the drug is inactivated in the circulation. Moreover, adenosine can precipitate hemodynamic compromise in a patient whose condition is already tenuous and promote VF; thus, it should only be used with caution in a patient in whom VT is the most likely diagnosis (see Chapter 37). If the diagnosis remains unclear, VT and aberrant SVT can be definitively differentiated by an electrophysiology study (EPS) if the arrhythmia can be re-induced.

EVALUATION OF THE PATIENT WITH VENTRICULAR ARRHYTHMIAS

Premature Ventricular Contractions

PVCs may be a marker for significant underlying conditions such as CAD, congestive heart failure, dilated cardiomyopathy (DCM), hypertrophic cardiomyopathy, infiltrative conditions, sarcoidosis, and arrhythmogenic RV cardiomyopathy. Thus, an echocardiogram to evaluate for the presence of structural heart disease is usually warranted. In the absence of CAD or structural heart disease, PVCs are generally benign, and most commonly arise from foci in the outflow tracts of the ventricles. Ambulatory ECG monitoring can document the PVC burden. Patients are at increased risk of a tachycardia-induced cardiomyopathy when ≥20% of recorded beats are ventricular ectopy. For patients whose symptoms persist and who have frequent PVCs (>5% of recorded beats), pharmacological therapy and/or radiofrequency ablation should be considered.

Ventricular Tachycardia

Much of the prognosis associated with VT is dependent on the presence or absence of underlying heart disease. Thus, a thorough investigation for structural heart disease is indicated. This usually starts with an echocardiogram but should also include ischemic evaluation, especially in patients with coronary risk factors and possibly a cardiac MRI in some patients. Patients with sustained VT and who are also found to have structural heart disease may be at risk of SCD and should be considered for defibrillator therapy.

The next sections review specific types of VT, associated conditions, and long-term management approaches. Fig. 41.5 shows examples of different types of VT.

VENTRICULAR TACHYCARDIA SYNDROMES

Monomorphic Ventricular Tachycardia

Monomorphic VT is the most common wide complex rhythm. Its prognosis depends on the presence or absence of underlying structural heart disease, and thus these conditions will be grouped separately.

Monomorphic VT

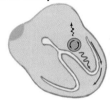

Most common wide complex rhythm. Monomorphic VT is usually a regular sustained rhythm. Reentry is usual mechanism, most commonly as a result of structural heart disease.

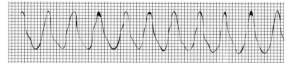

Monomorphic VT with RBBB

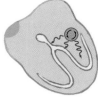

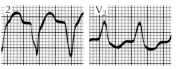

Usually arises from left ventricle focus

Monomorphic VT with LBBB

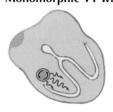

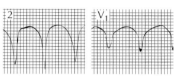

Usually arises in right ventricle or interventricular septum

Bundle branch reentry VT

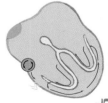

Usually seen in patients with dilated cardiomyopathy. Shows LBBB morphology.

JOHN A. CRAIG—AD

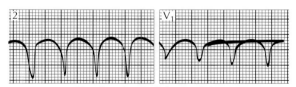

Usually arises in right ventricle

Accelerated idioventricular rhythm

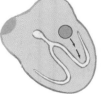

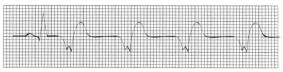

Wide complex rhythm with heart rate ranging between 50 and 120 bpm. Usually results after reperfusion as enhanced automaticity of ectopic ventricular focus.

Premature ventricular complexes

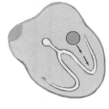

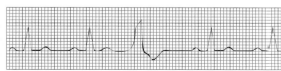

PVCs frequently asymptomatic. Some cause palpitations; are usually not significant, but increasing frequency may be marker of significant underlying condition.

Polymorphic VT

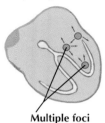

Wide complex tachycardia with two or more ventricular morphologies. Chaotic electrical activity due to multiple, simultaneous wave fronts.

Multiple foci

Normal QT interval

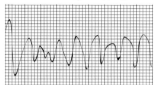

Polymorphic VT occurring with normal QT interval may be due to ischemia and is a cause of sudden cardiac death

Long QT interval

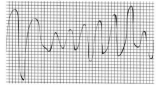

Torsades de pointes is VT with long QT interval. Many have family history of sudden cardiac death.

FIG 41.5 Types of Ventricular Tachycardia (VT). *bpm,* Beats per minute; *LBBB,* left bundle branch block; *PVCs,* premature ventricular complexes; *RBBB,* right bundle branch block.

Monomorphic Ventricular Tachycardia in the Structurally Normal Heart
Right Ventricular Outflow Tract Tachycardia

RV outflow tract VT tachycardia is a rare catecholamine-induced tachycardia that typically occurs in young patients with structurally normal hearts and is often induced by exercise. The ECG shows a left bundle branch block with an inferior axis. Ventricular arrhythmias can either occur as frequent ectopy and salvos of nonsustained VT or as sustained VT, and are due to triggered activity from catecholamine-mediated delayed afterdepolarizations. Sustained RV outflow tachycardia is often sensitive to adenosine and vagal maneuvers, and also responds well to treatment with β-blockers and flecainide. SCD rarely occurs in these patients, and for this reason, they may be treated pharmacologically. EPS with radiofrequency is an attractive option in patients in whom medical therapy fails. During EPS, isoproterenol is frequently required to initiate and/or maintain the tachycardia for mapping the VT origin, but the tachycardia can usually be cured.

Fascicular Tachycardia

Fascicular tachycardia typically occurs in young, predominantly male patients with structurally normal hearts. This VT is unique in that it is responsive to verapamil. The common type of fascicular tachycardia (90%–95%) originates from the region of the posterior fascicle and thus, the ECG usually shows almost classic right bundle branch block appearance similar to right bundle branch block with a left anterior fascicular block (left superior axis deviation). The mechanism involves a reentrant circuit that involves septal tissue and the left posterior fascicle. Less commonly, the arrhythmia can exit from the region of the anterior fascicle. If the patient remains symptomatic despite pharmacological therapy, the arrhythmia can be treated with catheter ablation. Although treatment with verapamil can be useful, it should only be considered in consultation with a cardiac electrophysiologist because verapamil is contraindicated for other forms of VTs.

Other common sites for ventricular arrhythmias, especially PVCs, to arise in the normal heart include the papillary muscles, coronary cusps, and areas around the mitral valve annulus.

Monomorphic Ventricular Tachycardia in Structural Heart Disease

Sustained VT is most common in patients with structural heart disease. Structural heart disease provides the substrate for disorderly conduction and reentrant VT. Patients with structural heart disease are at a higher risk of SCD from sustained VT because it can deteriorate further into VF. Therefore, it is extremely important to determine whether patients presenting with VT have structural heart disease due to a significant impact on management decisions. VT can occur in various forms of structural heart disease as described in this section.

Ischemic Heart Disease

Frequent ventricular ectopy and nonsustained VT may identify patients with ischemic heart disease at increased risk. The Multicenter Unsustained Tachycardia Trial (MUSTT; 1999) and the Multicenter Automatic Defibrillator Implantation Trial (MADIT I; 1996), which studied post–myocardial infarction patients with nonsustained VT, ejection fractions less than 35% to 40%, and inducible VT on EPS, showed a significant decrease in mortality from implantable cardioverter-defibrillator (ICD) placement versus antiarrhythmic therapy.

VT can present at various stages of ischemic heart disease. Sustained monomorphic VT rarely presents in the setting of an acute myocardial infarction. It is primarily seen in patients who have a healed previous myocardial infarction without ongoing ischemia. Viable myocardial tissue within the scar provides an area where the slowed conduction that is critical to the maintenance of a VT reentrant circuit may occur. Patients with large areas of myocardial injury and subsequently low ejection fractions are at a much higher risk of sustained monomorphic VT.

Patients with first-time presentation of sustained VT in which the etiology is likely CAD should undergo evaluation for ischemia. Coronary angiography with revascularization should be strongly considered in these patients. However, despite treatment for ischemia, these patients can have recurrent VT. In these situations, further structural evaluation using cardiac MRI or PET CT can be useful to assess for myocardial scar, which can serve as the substrate for monomorphic VT.

An ICD for secondary prevention is indicated in patients with ischemic heart disease and sustained VT. In patients who have recurrent VT, episode frequency can be reduced by antiarrhythmic agents such as amiodarone or sotalol. If patients have breakthrough VT on antiarrhythmic therapy, ablation can be pursued as well.

Dilated Nonischemic Cardiomyopathy

Up to 60% of the time, patients with DCM have multiple patchy areas of fibrosis in the left ventricle that are found at autopsy. DCM with these patchy areas can result in reentrant VT. These fibrotic areas and reentrant circuits are often located near the epicardium. Other mechanisms are possible in nonischemic cardiomyopathy, however, including enhanced automaticity or triggered activity, which can render these patients especially vulnerable to early or delayed after-depolarizations induced by QT interval–prolonging medications and/or metabolic abnormalities. Bundle branch reentry tachycardia, caused by a macro-reentrant circuit involving the His-Purkinje system is also a common cause of VT in DCM patients. Bundle branch reentrant VT usually presents as VT with a left bundle branch block morphology, often with

rapid rates (>200 beats/min). Bundle branch reentry occurs in patients with His-Purkinje disease, which usually manifests as QRS widening and a prolonged infrahisian conduction (measured as the HV interval, i.e., the time from the His bundle electrogram to the earliest recorded ventricular activation) in sinus rhythm. Retrograde conduction over the left bundle activates transseptal conduction, which then activates the right bundle branch, establishing the reentrant circuit. Although most patients with bundle branch reentrant VT do require ICD placement, radiofrequency ablation of the right bundle branch may completely or largely prevent VT recurrences, reducing the frequency of ICD discharges and prolonging device life.

Evidence-based heart failure therapy is essential in patients with DCM. They should be treated with maximum tolerated doses of β-blockers and angiotensin-converting enzyme inhibitors. Antiarrhythmics (e.g., amiodarone or sotalol) can be used in patients with recurrent VT or atrial arrhythmias who already have had an ICD implanted. It is also important to control concurrent atrial arrhythmias because they can lead to worsening LV function and dilatation.

Hypertrophic Cardiomyopathy

Myocyte disarray and interstitial fibrosis are pathological features of hypertrophic cardiomyopathy and can provide the substrate for reentrant VT. Patients with hypertrophic cardiomyopathy are at a higher risk of SCD from these ventricular arrhythmias. Risk factors for SCD in these patients are syncope, nonsustained VT, family history of SCD, insufficient blood pressure response with exercise, and interventricular septal thickness >30 mm found by echocardiography. Ambulatory ECG monitoring can be used to assess for occurrence of arrhythmias in these patients. ICD therapy should be considered for secondary prevention in patients with sustained VT or as primary prevention in those with risk factors for SCD. Amiodarone has not been shown to reduce mortality in patients with hypertrophic cardiomyopathy but may reduce recurrent tachyarrhythmias. Beta-blocker therapy should be used if possible because they also help decrease the LV outflow tract gradient.

Sarcoidosis

Symptomatic cardiac sarcoidosis occurs in 5% of patients with pulmonary or systemic sarcoidosis, although the rate of subclinical cardiac involvement may be much higher. Although abnormal automaticity and triggered activity can result from inflammation, macro-reentry around granulomatous scar, the hallmark of the disease, is the most common mechanism of ventricular arrhythmias. Patients with cardiac sarcoidosis and VT are at high risk of SCD and should be considered for an ICD. Due to the high prevalence of conduction disease and heart block in this population, consideration should be given to dual-chamber devices. Beta-blocker therapy is also generally required in these patients. Ablation can be considered for patients who have recurrent VT despite being on therapy and who have an ICD.

Arrhythmogenic Right Ventricular Cardiomyopathy

Arrhythmogenic RV cardiomyopathy is a genetic disorder inherited in an autosomal dominant fashion. It is a condition of segmental or diffuse replacement of the RV myocardium with fatty and fibrofatty tissue. Fatty tissue replacement is normally most severe in areas near the epicardium and mid-myocardium in the RV free wall, but the disease may also progress to the LV. These areas of fibrosis are sources of reentrant VT. ECG changes are present in approximately 95% of patients with arrhythmogenic RV cardiomyopathy. Classic findings include inverted T waves in leads V_1 to V_3, right bundle branch block, and a terminal notch in the QRS in leads V_1 to V_3 (referred to as the ε wave) (Fig. 41.6).

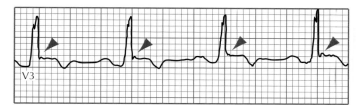

Epsilon waves (marked by the red arrowheads) are notches in the terminal portion of the QRS complex that reflect slowed intraventricular conduction.

FIG 41.6 Epsilon Wave in Arrhythmogenic Right Ventricular Dysplasia or Cardiomyopathy.

If the suspicion is high for arrhythmogenic RV cardiomyopathy based on ECG, an echocardiogram should be obtained. However, because RV visualization can be limited on echocardiography, cardiac MRI is normally used to establish the diagnosis. Patients with arrhythmogenic RV cardiomyopathy and VT are at high risk of SCD, and ICD therapy is recommended. In these patients, the RV ICD lead must be placed in the RV septum to avoid myocardial perforation because the RV free wall is usually abnormal in these patients. Antiarrhythmic therapy can be used in patients who have frequent ventricular arrhythmias. Patients who have refractory arrhythmias despite antiarrhythmic therapy can be referred for ablation.

Polymorphic Ventricular Tachycardia

Polymorphic VT is a wide complex tachycardia that has two or more ventricular morphologies. Polymorphic VT can be differentiated from VF based on the presence of clearly defined QRS complexes. It is also important to distinguish polymorphic VT from Torsades de pointes because the mechanisms are different and affect management. Specifically, Torsades de pointes is a polymorphic VT in the context of a prolonged QT, which is often initiated after a pause. It is characterized by twisting of the QRS complex along the isoelectric baseline. The VT is triggered by early afterdepolarizations during the prolonged refractory period. Normally, Torsades de pointes occurs in salvos and self-terminates; however, at times, it can deteriorate into VF. It is normally triggered by electrolyte derangements, particularly hypomagnesemia and hypokalemia, and QT-prolonging medications. Patients with Torsades de pointes respond well to magnesium sulfate infusion and removal of the inciting agents. Pacing can be used in patients with recurrent pause-dependent Torsades de pointes.

The various etiologies of polymorphic VT can be classified into three categories: structural heart disease, channelopathies, and reversible factors such as drug interactions and electrolyte derangements.

Structural Heart Disease

Structural heart disease, particularly myocardial ischemia, is the most common cause of polymorphic VT. In patients who have sustained polymorphic VT, it is essential to determine if they have an acute coronary syndrome. If an acute coronary syndrome is identified, these patients should undergo emergent coronary angiography and revascularization. Timely revascularization can lead to resolution of the arrhythmia. An echocardiogram should be obtained in patients presenting with polymorphic VT even if ischemia has been ruled out to assess cardiac function and to evaluate for structural abnormalities. In the absence of ischemia, polymorphic VT with DCM, hypertrophic cardiomyopathy, sarcoidosis, and arrhythmogenic RV cardiomyopathy is associated with a poor prognosis. Almost always, ICD implantation and subsequent therapy with a β-blocker or other antiarrhythmic therapy are indicated.

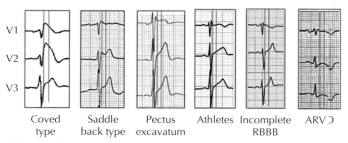

FIG 41.7 Classic Brugada ECG Patterns. Type 1 is considered diagnostic of Brugada syndrome. Types 2 and 3 were grouped together as Type 2 in a recent consensus report. (Reused with permission from Bayes LA, Brugada J, Baranchuk A, et al. Current electrocardiographic criteria for diagnosis of Brugada pattern: a consensus report. *J Electrocardiol* 2012;45:433–442.)

Channelopathies
Brugada Syndrome
Brugada syndrome is an autosomal dominant arrhythmogenic genetic disorder with increased risk of SCD due to ventricular arrhythmias. In 20% to 40% of the patients, there is a loss of function mutation involving the sodium channel SCN5A.

Brugada syndrome has been characterized by specific ECG patterns: types 1, 2, and 3 (Fig. 41.7). Only the type 1 cove-shaped pattern, with >2-mm ST elevations and T-wave inversions in leads V_1 to V_3, is now considered the diagnostic Brugada ECG pattern. Increased vagal tone, fever, sodium channel–blocking medications, and electrolyte abnormalities can bring out the ECG pattern. Manifestations of Brugada syndrome include syncope, nocturnal agonal breathing, documented VF or polymorphic VT, inducible VT, family history of SCD at age younger than 45 years, and coved type ECG in family members.

Because the type 1 Brugada ECG pattern can be intermittent, provocative drug challenge with intravenous sodium channel blockers (e.g., procainamide) may be of diagnostic benefit. Symptomatic patients with a type 1 Brugada ECG should undergo ICD placement. The management of the asymptomatic patient with a type 1 Brugada ECG remains the subject of debate, but the incidence of adverse events appears to be low. In these patients, avoidance of or aggressive treatment of conditions (e.g., fever) that can provoke the pattern and cardiac specialist referral seem reasonable measures.

Long QT Syndrome

Long QT syndrome (LQTS) is a genetic disorder in which repolarization is delayed, leading to a prolonged QT interval on ECG. In men, a QT interval >440 ms is considered prolonged. The threshold is higher in women, in whom a QT interval of 460 ms is prolonged. It is important to recognize that one-third of patients with LQTS can present with normal QT intervals.

Individuals with LQTS can present with syncope, seizures, ventricular arrhythmias, and SCD. Risk factors for arrhythmias in patients with LQTS include family history of LQTS, female sex, the length of the QT interval, and increasing age. Genetic testing can help determine the underlying mutation in 60% to 70% of patients.

The three most common forms of LQTS are LQT 1, 2, and 3. LQT 1 is associated with exercise (most often swimming), LQT 2 is associated with auditory or emotional stimuli (e.g., being awoken by an alarm clock), and LQT 3 often results in sudden death during sleep. LQT 1 and 2 are associated with loss of potassium channel function; LQT 3 is associated with gain of sodium channel (SCN5A) function.

Patients with LQTS should be educated to avoid medications that are known to prolong the QT interval. It is also important to maintain normal levels of potassium and magnesium in these patients. Beta blockers should be used because they decrease ventricular arrhythmias, particularly in LQT 1 patients. Patients with LQTS should be also instructed to avoid competitive sports. ICD implantation is recommended in patients with LQTS and a history of cardiac arrest. ICDs are also recommended in patients who have had syncope while on therapy with β-blockers and in individuals who have undergone genetic testing and have been determined to have high-risk LQTS, including LQT 2, LQT 3, and a QTc interval of >500 ms.

Catecholaminergic Polymorphic Ventricular Tachycardia

Catecholaminergic polymorphic VT (CPVT) is a genetic disorder that is characterized by polymorphic VT induced by release of catecholamines. These patients have normal heart rhythms at rest, but with exercise or when under stress, they can present with syncope, palpitations, and SCD.

Genetic testing may help identify individuals with CPVT. Approximately one-half of all cases are due to mutations in the ryanodine receptor that result in disruption of the normal handling of calcium within cardiac myocytes.

Pharmacological therapy including β-blockers and verapamil can help control the heart rate response to exercise. Antiarrhythmic therapy, specifically with flecainide, can be used to inhibit the release of calcium. ICDs can be used for secondary prevention in this patient population.

Reversible Factors

Electrolyte derangements such as hypokalemia and hypomagnesemia can lead to ventricular arrhythmias by prolonging ventricular repolarization.

QT-prolonging medications, such as antipsychotics, tricyclic antidepressants, macrolide antibiotics, and type 1A, 1C, and III antiarrhythmics, can also induce ventricular arrhythmias.

ACUTE MANAGEMENT AND THERAPY

Optimum Treatment

Acute management combines stabilizing the patient and terminating the VT, and takes priority over the diagnostic evaluation. If the patient is maintaining a pulse but is presyncopal, hypotensive, or in severe respiratory distress, the patient should, after appropriate sedation, receive a synchronized external direct-current cardioversion. If synchronization is difficult because of the width of the QRS complex, then unsynchronized defibrillation should be performed. Patients who are pulseless and/or unresponsive should be immediately treated according to the Advanced Cardiac Life Support guidelines with cardiopulmonary resuscitation and high-energy defibrillation.

If the VT is well tolerated, agents such as intravenous procainamide, lidocaine, amiodarone, and magnesium may be given. Procainamide is more effective than lidocaine unless the VT is in the context of acute myocardial ischemia or infarction. Amiodarone often requires 24 to 48 hours for effect and is less helpful acutely. Amiodarone may have to be administered concurrently with or after another drug (e.g., procainamide) has converted the rhythm. Intravenous magnesium is useful in Torsades de pointes. If the VT fails to terminate, a synchronized direct-current cardioversion should be performed, but only after the patient has received adequate and appropriate sedation. Potential precipitating causes such as myocardial ischemia, congestive heart failure, hypoxia, electrolyte disturbances, and/or drug toxicities should be addressed.

Subsequent management of the patient with VT depends on the etiology and the absence of reversible causes. Blood samples should be urgently obtained for complete blood count, electrolytes (including magnesium), blood urea nitrogen, creatinine, cardiac markers, blood glucose, and toxicology screen. When appropriate, an arterial blood gas measurement should also be obtained (Fig. 41.8).

For patients with an ICD, therapies should be delivered within the first 30 seconds to few minutes of arrhythmia onset, depending on individualized device programming. Therapy from a device can be a cardioversion (shock) or overdrive pacing. Interrogation of the device will usually provide sufficient information to determine whether the arrhythmia precipitated overdrive pacing or if the defibrillation was VT, as well as the frequency and treatment of similar (and other) tachyarrhythmias. A recurrent need for shocks requires exploration of precipitating triggers (most commonly, ischemia), programming of the ICD, and adjunctive antiarrhythmics if indicated. If a patient has presumed VT that has not triggered the ICD to initiate either overdrive pacing or cardioversion, there are several possible explanations. The VT rate could be slower than the programmed detection rate, or the arrhythmia could be mistaken for SVT by the ICD. If the ICD cannot be urgently reprogrammed by experienced personnel, the patient should be treated as if no ICD were present. The ICD should then be evaluated as soon as possible thereafter.

Avoiding Treatment Errors

In general, a patient with a new wide complex tachycardia should be presumed to have VT until proven otherwise, and intravenous verapamil or diltiazem should be avoided. Such drugs can precipitate hemodynamic compromise in a patient whose condition is already tenuous and can promote VF. AV nodal–blocking drugs of any kind are absolutely contraindicated unless there is a high index of suspicion that the diagnosis is SVT. Treatment of VT with AV nodal blockers can be disastrous. Treatment of SVT with antiarrhythmic drugs (as if it is VT) is not.

LONG-TERM MANAGEMENT AND THERAPY

Optimum Treatment

The long-term approach to preventing recurrent VT and SCD combines risk stratification, antiarrhythmic medications, and/or ICDs. Primary and secondary prevention of SCD is discussed in more detail in Chapter 42.

Patients with a history of sustained VT and depressed LV function or a history of a cardiac arrest clearly benefit from ICD implantation. If recurrent VT develops after the ICD is placed, which results in multiple shocks, amiodarone can be used to slow down the VT cycle length and possibly permit overdrive pacing to terminate subsequent episodes via the ICD.

If amiodarone is not effective, β-blockers, sotalol, procainamide, and mexiletine are options. However, these are usually not as effective as amiodarone. Medication-refractory hemodynamically stable VT can be studied in the electrophysiology laboratory. By using activation mapping and three-dimensional electroanatomic mapping techniques, the circuit can often be localized and transected with several radiofrequency ablation lesions. In patients with ischemic heart disease or DCM, multiple circuits may be present, making radiofrequency ablation difficult. In patients with complex recurring VT, which is hemodynamically poorly tolerated, scar mapping in sinus rhythm with linear ablations, which connect scar tissue, may be effective in decreasing the frequency of VT.

Future Directions

Patients with VT are at increased risk of SCD, and ICD implantation is recommended. For patients with medically refractory VT, catheter

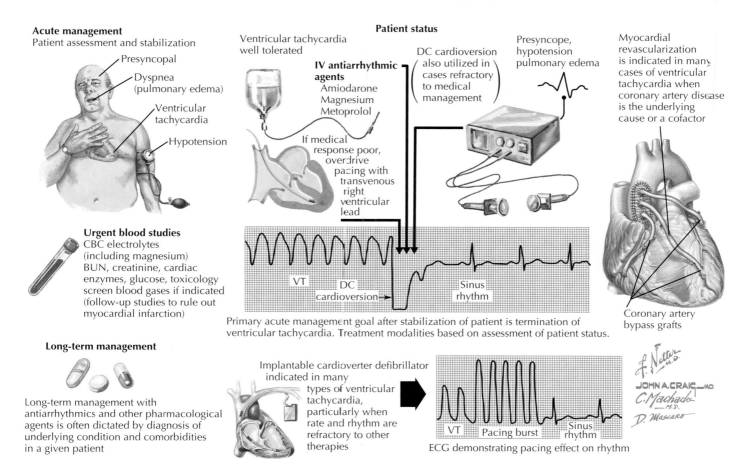

FIG 41.8 Management of Ventricular Tachycardia (VT). *BUN,* Blood urea nitrogen; *CBC,* complete blood count; *DC,* direct current; *IV,* intravenous.

ablation is an important option. Ablation catheter technologies continue to rapidly improve. High-density electroanatomic mapping has transformed identification of arrhythmogenic scar and critical isthmi for reentrant circuits. Techniques for pericardial access have become safer for those with nonischemic cardiomyopathies who need epicardial ablation.

ADDITIONAL RESOURCES

Bardy GH, Lee KL, Mark DB, et al. Amiodarone or an implantable cardioverter-defibrillator for congestive heart failure (SCD-HeFT). *N Engl J Med.* 2005;352:2022–2025.

The Sudden Cardiac Death in Heart Failure Trial (SCD-HeFT) included both ischemic and nonischemic cardiomyopathy patients. In these patients with ejection fractions ≤35% and New York Heart Association functional class II or III heart failure, overall mortality was significantly reduced in the ICD group (compared with amiodarone).

ECC Committee, Subcommittees and Task Forces of the American Heart Association. 2005 American Heart Association Guidelines for Cardiopulmonary Resuscitation and Emergency Cardiovascular Care. *Circulation.* 2005;112(suppl 1):IV-1–IV-203. Available at:: http://circ .ahajournals.org/content/vol112/24_suppl/#_AMERICAN_HEART _ASSOCIATION_ GUIDELINES_FOR_CARDIOPULMONARY _RESUSCITATION_ AND_EMERGENCY_CARDIOVASCULAR_CARE. Accessed February 23, 2010.

This report provides the latest guidelines from the American Heart Association.

Edhouse J, Morris F. ABC of clinical electrocardiography: broad complex tachycardia Part I. *Br Med J.* 2002;324:719–722.

The first of a series of reviews on the basics of ECG.

Griffith MJ, Garratt CJ, Mounsey JP, et al. Ventricular tachycardia as default diagnosis in broad complex tachycardia. *Lancet.* 1994;343 386–388.

This paper proposes using VT as the default diagnosis when evaluating a new broad complex tachycardia in contrast to most algorithms, which are based on a default diagnosis of SVT.

Wellens HJ, Bar FW, Lie K. The value of the electrocardiogram in the differential diagnosis of a tachycardia with widened QRS complex. *Am J Med.* 1978;64:27–33.

This was a retrospective case study that helped establish criteria to distinguish ventricular ectopy from aberrantly conducted SVT.

EVIDENCE

Brugada P, Brugada J, Mont L, et al. A new approach to the differential diagnosis of a regular tachycardia with a wide QRS complex. *Circulation.* 1991;83:1649–1659.

Reports the stepwise Brugada criteria for diagnosing VT.

Buxton AE, Lee KL, Fisher JD, et al. A randomized study of the prevention of sudden death in patients with coronary artery disease. Multicenter Unsustained Tachycardia Trial Investigators. *N Engl J Med.* 1999;341: 1882–1890.

The MUSTT Study, along with MADIT, examined post–myocardial infarction patients with nonsustained VT, ejection fractions less than 35% to 40%, and inducible VT on EPS, and showed a significant decrease in mortality from ICD placement as opposed to antiarrhythmic therapy.

Kadish A, Dyer A, Daubert JP, et al. Prophylactic defibrillator implantation in patients with nonischemic dilated cardiomyopathy. *N Engl J Med.* 2004;350:2151–2158.

In those with nonsustained VT and DCM (ejection fraction <36%), the Defibrillators in Non-Ischemic Cardiomyopathy Treatment Evaluation (DEFINITE) Study showed survival benefit for those receiving an ICD.

Moss AJ, Hall WJ, Cannom DS, et al. Improved survival with an implanted defibrillator in patients with coronary disease at high risk for ventricular arrhythmia. Multicenter Automatic Defibrillator Implantation Trial Investigators. *N Engl J Med.* 1996;335:1933–1940.

The MADIT Study, along with MUSTT, examined post-MI patients with NSVT, EF less than 35% to 40%, and inducible VT on EPS and showed a significant decrease in mortality from ICD placement as opposed to antiarrhythmic therapy.

Moss AJ, Zareba W, Hall WJ, et al. Prophylactic implantation of a defibrillator in patients with myocardial infarction and reduced ejection fraction. *N Engl J Med.* 2002;346:877–883.

The MADIT II Study showed that post–myocardial infarction patients with ejection fractions <30% and couplets or >10 PVCs per hour who did not undergo EPS also benefited from ICD therapy.

Vereckei A, Duray G, Szénási G, et al. New algorithm using only lead aVR for differential diagnosis of wide QRS complex tachycardia. *Heart Rhythm.* 2008;5:89–98.

Presents a new and simplified algorithm using aVR for differentiating VT from SVT and compares it with previously published approaches.

42

Sudden Cardiac Death

Basil Abu-el-Haija, Eugene H. Chung, J. Paul Mounsey

Sudden cardiac death (SCD) is defined as any death from a cardiac cause occurring within an hour of symptom onset. The term sudden cardiac arrest (SCA) refers to an event from which an individual is resuscitated or spontaneously recovers. Sudden unexpected death has many potential etiologies (Box 42.1). Patients with coronary artery disease (CAD) and previous myocardial infarction (MI) have an annual incidence of SCD of up to 30%, which is responsible for approximately 70% of fatal arrhythmias. Other high-risk groups include patients with previous cardiac arrest, congestive heart failure, cardiomyopathy (dilated, infiltrative, or hypertrophic), valvular heart disease, myocarditis, and congenital heart disease (CHD). Screening patients potentially at risk for SCD and addressing their risk factors is the crux of primary prevention. Secondary measures aim to prevent recurrent events in survivors of aborted SCA (Fig. 42.1).

EPIDEMIOLOGY

SCD occurs in 300,000 to 450,000 individuals in the United States annually. According to death certificates, SCD accounts for 15% of the total mortality in the United States. However, death certificates may overestimate the true prevalence of SCD as suggested by some investigators. In 1 study, the incidence of SCD according to death certificates in a particular year was 153 per 100,000, but when true causes of death were investigated by looking at findings in the medical records and autopsy results, the incidence of SCD (i.e., sudden unexpected death due to cardiac causes) was only 53 per 100,000 in the same population in that particular year. The causes of unexpected death due to noncardiac causes are many. Men are two to three times more likely to experience SCD than women (a few examples are shown in Box 42.1).

ETIOLOGY AND RISK FACTORS

The pathogenic electrical events leading to SCD are most commonly ventricular tachycardia (VT), ventricular fibrillation (VF), and eventually asystole (Fig. 42.2). Approximately 80% of SCDs involve VT, VF, or Torsades de pointes; the remaining 20% are due to bradyarrhythmias. SCD is most commonly associated with underlying structural heart disease. Less than 20% of out-of-hospital victims of SCA recover to hospital discharge. The likelihood of resuscitation diminishes 10% for every minute of delay. It has been estimated that 50% of those who survive a cardiac arrest will die within 3 years. This underscores the importance of primary and secondary prevention.

CAD accounts for 70% to 80% of SCD cases, especially in Western societies in patients aged older than 35 years. As such, two of the leading risk factors are previous heart attack and documented CAD. In those with chronic ischemic disease, the most powerful predictor is an ejection fraction (EF) <40%. Following CAD, patients with nonischemic cardiomyopathies (hypertrophic and dilated) and an EF <40% are at

the highest risk. Additional major risk factors for SCD include congestive heart failure of any etiology and a history of cardiac arrest. Channelopathies (e.g., long QT syndrome and Brugada syndrome) result in an increased risk for cardiac arrhythmias and SCD. CHDs are less common causes of SCD.

DIFFERENTIAL DIAGNOSIS

The most common etiologies are discussed in the sections that follow (see also Box 42.1).

Ischemic Heart Disease

Overwhelmingly, the most common cause of SCD is ischemic heart disease that results from coronary atherosclerosis. Arteritis, dissection, spasm, and congenital coronary anomalies are rare causes associated with myocardial ischemia. CAD has been attributed to 70% to 80% of all SCDs. In a study of 84 survivors of out-of-hospital cardiac arrest, immediate coronary angiography revealed significant disease of probable etiologic significance in 71% of patients; approximately one-half of these patients had complete occlusions. Acute occlusion of the left anterior descending or left circumflex coronary artery portends a higher risk of SCD. Patients with angina and previous MI are at much higher risk than those without any clinical manifestation of CAD. Unfortunately, SCD can be the first manifestation of CAD in one-third of CAD patients.

Causes of SCD in the CAD population include myocardial ischemia or MI, heart failure, electrolyte imbalance, drug toxicity, or primary (no precipitating cause identified). The probable mechanisms for VT or VF in patients with CAD are acute ischemia and reentry via myocardial scar, especially in those with a previous infarction. A meta-analysis of four non–ST-elevation MI trials found the risk of sustained or unstable ventricular arrhythmias (VT or VF) to be 2.1% (vs. 10% in ST-segment elevation MI [STEMI]) during the initial hospital admission. Patients with VT and VF had the highest mortality rate in the first 30 days (>60%) post-MI, followed by patients with VF only (>45%), followed by patients with VT only (>30%). This trend was consistent at 6 months, which correlated with a 5- to 15-fold increase in mortality within 6 months in patients with these arrhythmias. Patients in the Global Utilization of Streptokinase and Tissue Plasminogen Activator for Occluded Coronary Arteries (GUSTO I) Trial, which studied fibrinolytic therapies for STEMI, demonstrated higher overall incidences of sustained arrhythmias than in non-STEMI patients: specifically, 3.5% for VT only, 4.0% for VF only, and 2.6% for both VT and VF. Of these arrhythmias, 80% to 85% occurred within the first 48 hours ("early"). In-hospital mortality and 1-year mortality (for those who survived >30 days) after discharge of these patients were much higher among those with VT, VF, or VT and VF (18.6%, 24%, or 44% in-hospital, and 7.2%, 2.9%, or 7.1% at 1 year, respectively) than patients without these arrhythmias (4.2% in-hospital and 2.7% at 1-year). Patients with "late" (after the first

---

BOX 42.1 Major Etiologies of Sudden Cardiac Death

Ischemic Heart Disease
Coronary atherosclerosis (myocardial ischemia or infarction)
Congenital coronary anomalies
Arteritis
Dissection
Coronary spasm

Nonischemic Heart Disease
Dilated cardiomyopathy
Hypertrophic cardiomyopathy
Arrhythmogenic RV dysplasia or cardiomyopathy
Congenital heart disease (tetralogy of Fallot, Ebstein anomaly, transposition of great arteries)

Primary Electrophysiology Disorders
Long QT syndrome
Brugada syndrome

Idiopathic VF
Catecholaminergic polymorphic VT
Commotio cordis
Metabolic derangements

Sudden Expected Death Unrelated to Primary Heart Disease
Pulmonary embolism
Drug induced
Aortic rupture or other intravascular catastrophe
Intracranial hemorrhage
Airway obstruction

RV, Right ventricular; *VF,* ventricular fibrillation; *VT,* ventricular tachycardia.

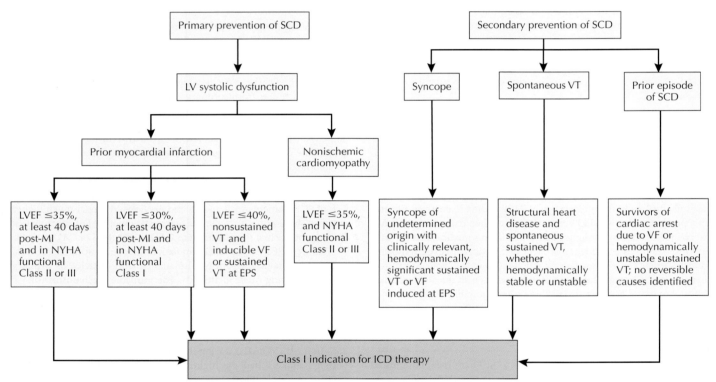

FIG 42.1 Treatment Algorithm for Implantable Cardioverter-Defibrillator (ICD)–Based Primary and Secondary Prevention of Sudden Cardiac Death (SCD). *EPS,* Electrophysiological study; *LV,* left ventricular; *LVEF,* left ventricular ejection fraction; *MI,* myocardial infarction; *NYHA,* New York Heart Association; *VF,* ventricular fibrillation; *VT,* ventricular tachycardia.

48 hours) ventricular arrhythmias had increased mortality at 1 year (24.7% for VT, 6.1% for VF, 4.7% for VT and VF) and were more likely to have had a previous MI, previous bypass surgery, and a longer time from the onset of MI and receiving treatment.

Nonischemic Cardiomyopathy
Idiopathic-Dilated Cardiomyopathy
Ten percent to 15% of SCD cases are attributable to cardiomyopathies not associated with CAD. In patients with dilated cardiomyopathies,

the presence of nonsustained VT, syncope, and/or advanced heart failure are high-risk predictors. SCD is the major cause (up to 72% in some studies) of death in patients with nonischemic cardiomyopathy. Most fatal arrhythmias are believed to be tachyarrhythmias, mainly polymorphic, and the less commonly monomorphic VTs. The primary mechanisms of polymorphic VT and VF are unknown, but subendocardial scarring, and interstitial and perivascular fibrosis are probably involved. A particular type of monomorphic VT (see Chapter 41) caused by bundle branch reentry is characteristic of

Potential etiologies

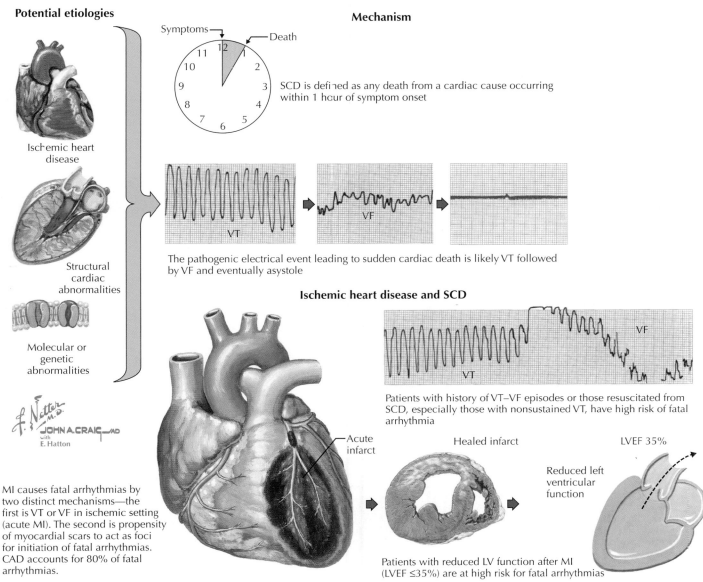

Ischemic heart disease

Structural cardiac abnormalities

Molecular or genetic abnormalities

Mechanism

Symptoms — Death

SCD is defined as any death from a cardiac cause occurring within 1 hour of symptom onset

VT

VF

The pathogenic electrical event leading to sudden cardiac death is likely VT followed by VF and eventually asystole

Ischemic heart disease and SCD

VT

VF

Patients with history of VT–VF episodes or those resuscitated from SCD, especially those with nonsustained VT, have high risk of fatal arrhythmia

MI causes fatal arrhythmias by two distinct mechanisms—the first is VT or VF in ischemic setting (acute MI). The second is propensity of myocardial scars to act as foci for initiation of fatal arrhythmias. CAD accounts for 80% of fatal arrhythmias.

Acute infarct

Healed infarct

LVEF 35%

Reduced left ventricular function

Patients with reduced LV function after MI (LVEF ≤35%) are at high risk for fatal arrhythmias

FIG 42.2 Mechanisms of Sudden Cardiac Death (SCD): Ischemic Heart Disease. *CAD,* Coronary artery disease; *LV,* left ventricular; *LVEF,* left ventricular ejection fraction; *MI,* myocardial infarction; *VF,* ventricular fibrillation; *VT,* ventricular tachycardia.

nonischemic cardiomyopathy. In bundle branch reentry, a macroreentrant circuit that involves both bundles, the Purkinje system, and the myocardium can be documented.

Hypertrophic Cardiomyopathy

Hypertrophic cardiomyopathy (HCM) is an autosomal-dominant inherited disorder estimated to affect 1 in 500 adults (see Chapter 30 and Fig. 42.3). The overall risk of SCD in patients with HCM is estimated at 1% to 4% per year, but within subgroups of patients with this disease the risk of SCD varies substantially. All first-degree relatives of a patient with HCM who had SCD must be screened. Generally, patients with HCM who are at highest risk for SCD are those with recurrent syncope, nonsustained VT on Holter monitoring, extreme left ventricular hypertrophy on an echocardiogram (>30 mm), abnormal blood pressure response to exercise, and a positive family history of SCD from HCM. Careful evaluation for HCM is of utmost importance in young

individuals because HCM is the most common cause of SCD in young athletes in the United States (Fig. 42.3). Genetic testing of first-degree relatives of an individual whose gene mutation has been identified may help establish risk but remains a controversial screening modality. Screening should include a detailed history and physical examination, ECG, and echocardiography.

Arrhythmogenic Right Ventricular Dysplasia and Cardiomyopathy

Arrhythmogenic right ventricular dysplasia and cardiomyopathy (ARVD/C) is an autosomal-dominant condition in which the right ventricular (RV) myocardium is replaced by fatty or fibro-fatty tissue. The left ventricle may be involved in later stages of the disease. SCD incidence in ARVD/C is 2% and usually presents before age 50 years.

The ECG may reveal left bundle branch morphology and left-axis deviation during VT, and ε waves and T-wave inversions in leads V_1

Structural congenital abnormalities

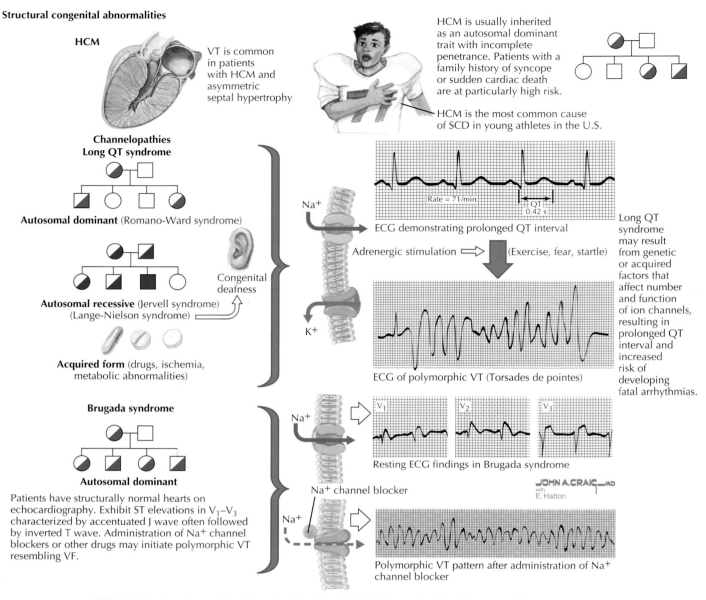

HCM

VT is common in patients with HCM and asymmetric septal hypertrophy

HCM is usually inherited as an autosomal dominant trait with incomplete penetrance. Patients with a family history of syncope or sudden cardiac death are at particularly high risk.

HCM is the most common cause of SCD in young athletes in the U.S.

Channelopathies
Long QT syndrome

Rate = 71/min   QT 0.42 s

ECG demonstrating prolonged QT interval

Autosomal dominant (Romano-Ward syndrome)

Na^+

Adrenergic stimulation ⇒ (Exercise, fear, startle)

K^+

Congenital deafness

Autosomal recessive (Jervell syndrome)
(Lange-Nielsen syndrome)

ECG of polymorphic VT (Torsades de pointes)

Acquired form (drugs, ischemia, metabolic abnormalities)

Long QT syndrome may result from genetic or acquired factors that affect number and function of ion channels, resulting in prolonged QT interval and increased risk of developing fatal arrhythmias.

Brugada syndrome

Na^+ V_1 V_2 V_3

Resting ECG findings in Brugada syndrome

JOHN A. CRAIG—AD
with E. Hatton

Autosomal dominant

Na^+ channel blocker

Patients have structurally normal hearts on echocardiography. Exhibit ST elevations in V_1–V_3 characterized by accentuated J wave often followed by inverted T wave. Administration of Na^+ channel blockers or other drugs may initiate polymorphic VT resembling VF.

Na^+

Polymorphic VT pattern after administration of Na^+ channel blocker

FIG 42.3 Mechanisms of Sudden Cardiac Death (SCD): Inherited Cardiomyopathies. *HCM,* Hypertrophic cardiomyopathy; *K⁺,* potassium; *Na⁺,* sodium; *VF,* ventricular fibrillation; *VT,* ventricular tachycardia.

through V_3 during sinus rhythm (Fig. 42.4). The most useful imaging study to confirm the diagnosis of ARVD/C is MRI, which classically shows fatty infiltration of the myocardium, RV dilatation or dyskinesia, or both, but if the MRI is nondiagnostic, additional confirmatory tests may be required.

Other Congenital Anomalies

Coronary artery anomalies are uncommon but account for a disproportionate percentage of deaths in young athletes. The mechanism of SCD is believed to be ischemia from coronary spasm or abnormal tension placed on the ectopic coronary artery by the ascending aorta and the pulmonary trunk (Fig. 42.5). The most consistent fatal anomaly occurs when the left coronary artery originates from the right coronary sinus and courses between the aorta and the pulmonary artery.

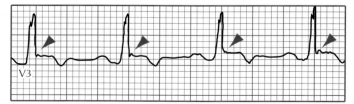

V3

Epsilon waves (marked by the red arrowheads) are notches in the terminal portion of the QRS complex that reflect slowed intraventricular conduction.

FIG 42.4 Epsilon Wave in Arrhythmogenic Right Ventricular Dysplasia or Cardiomyopathy.

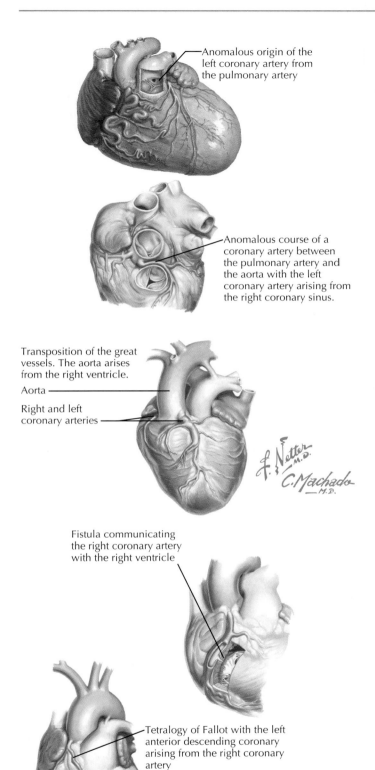

Anomalous origin of the left coronary artery from the pulmonary artery

Anomalous course of a coronary artery between the pulmonary artery and the aorta with the left coronary artery arising from the right coronary sinus.

Transposition of the great vessels. The aorta arises from the right ventricle.

Aorta

Right and left coronary arteries

Fistula communicating the right coronary artery with the right ventricle

Tetralogy of Fallot with the left anterior descending coronary arising from the right coronary artery

FIG 42.5 Congenital Coronary Artery Anomalies.

Other infrequent congenital diseases associated with an increased risk of SCD are mitral valve prolapse, aortic stenosis, Ebstein anomaly, coarctation of the aorta, tetralogy of Fallot, transposition of the great arteries, and Eisenmenger physiology. When surgical correction is possible, the risk of SCD decreases but is not eliminated.

Sudden Cardiac Death in the Absence of Structural Heart Disease or Congenital Heart Disease

Approximately 10% of cases of SCD in patients younger than 40 years occur in the absence of CHD or structural heart disease. These deaths can be due to a variety of causes. Primary electrical disorders of the conduction system constitute most of these causes.

Primary Electrophysiology Disorders
Long QT Syndrome

Channelopathies account for up to 5% to 10% of SCDs annually but generate considerable interest because patients with channelopathies have structurally normal hearts. The most recognized of the channelopathies are manifested by prolongation of the QT interval with a concomitant increased risk of VT and SCD. Patients with long QT syndrome (LQTS) have QTc intervals >440 ms (see Fig. 42.3); LQTS can be congenital or acquired. The annual incidence of SCD is between 1% and 2%, and approximately 9% in affected individuals with syncope. Life-threatening arrhythmia presents as Torsades de pointes. Torsades de pointes, or "twisting of the point," is a polymorphic VT associated with a prolonged QT interval, R-on-T premature ventricular contractions, and long–short coupled RR intervals.

Multiple forms of LQTS have been recognized and associated with at least 12 different genes. LQTS 1 and 2 are due to potassium channel defects. Potassium channels are responsible for cardiac repolarization; loss of function results in prolongation of repolarization and thus lengthening of the QT interval. SCD can occur with exercise stress or unexpected auditory stimulation (sudden loud sounds or a phone ringing in the middle of the night have been reported to cause SCD in LQTS). LQTS 3 results from a gain of function in the cardiac sodium channel gene *SCN5A*, which is associated with rapid cardiac depolarizations. Too much depolarization upsets the balance between depolarization and repolarization, and results in QT prolongation. SCD occurs during sleep. Beta-blockers are a mainstay of treatment in all patients with congenital LQTS, regardless of symptoms, because they mitigate the effect of enhanced sympathetic activity. Animal studies and registry data have shown β-blockers to be most efficacious in LQTS 1 and least efficacious in LQTS 3. This finding is probably due to the differing roles of sympathetic stimulation by genotype. Beta-blockers also shorten the QT interval; however, the exact mechanism is unknown. Implantable cardioverter-defibrillators (ICDs) are recommended for patients with a diagnosis of LQTS who are survivors of a cardiac arrest (class I) and can be useful in patients with a diagnosis of LQTS who experience recurrent syncopal events while on beta-blocker therapy (class IIa).

Acquired LQTS is reversible QT prolongation due to secondary causes (medications, electrolyte abnormalities, or ischemia). It is unclear whether there is always a genetic predisposition to the acquired form of LQTS, but cases have been described in which patients with apparent acquired LQTS have a subtle genetic abnormality.

Brugada Syndrome

Brugada syndrome, an autosomal-dominant disease, causes 20% of SCD in young people with structurally normal hearts. The most common recognized cause is a loss-of-function mutation in the cardiac sodium channel *SCN5A* that results in early repolarization of the RV myocardium. However, the genetic abnormality has not been recognized in most patients. SCD is associated with rest or nocturnal settings, as well as elevated temperatures (e.g., febrile illness or hot tubs). Diagnosis is based on symptoms and 12-lead ECG showing ST elevations of >2 mm in leads V₁ through V₃, characterized by an accentuated J wave (often followed by a negative T wave) (see Fig. 42.3). The type 1 pattern (a coved ST-segment elevation >2 mm in >1 of leads V₁ to V₃, followed by a negative T wave; see Fig. 42.3) is diagnostic of Brugada syndrome. The type 2 pattern has a "saddleback" ST elevation in the right precordial leads. The type 3 pattern can have the morphology of either type 1 or type 2 (coved or saddleback), but with <2 mm of ST-segment elevation, and can be mistaken as a normal variant of early repolarization. Sodium channel blockade with flecainide or procainamide can unmask Brugada ECG patterns when the diagnosis is in doubt, because the main problem is loss of function of sodium channel. Sodium channel blockers can augment the abnormality. Electrophysiology study (EPS) should be considered in patients with the spontaneous type 1 pattern regardless of symptoms, and if positive for inducible VT, an ICD should be considered. In patients with type 1 pattern provoked by a sodium channel blocker, EPS is recommended in those with a family history of SCD. Any patient with a history of syncope or cardiac arrest and a type 1 pattern should be considered for an ICD.

Other Electrical Disorders

In Wolff-Parkinson-White syndrome, rapid conduction of atrial fibrillation or flutter down an accessory pathway can lead to rapid ventricular rates and degenerate to VF. Patients with Wolff-Parkinson-White syndrome are at higher risk of SCD if multiple pathways are present, and if the RR interval during preexcited atrial fibrillation is <250 ms (or 240 beats/min). Short QT syndrome, characterized by a QT interval of <300 ms, is caused by gain-of-function mutations in genes encoding potassium channels. It presents with syncope, atrial fibrillation, or VT, and typically affects young healthy patients with structurally normal hearts. Bradyarrhythmias can result in SCD and are discussed in Chapter 36. Other potential but rare causes of SCD include catecholaminergic polymorphic VT, idiopathic VF, and congenital heart block (which results in VF).

Commotio Cordis

Commotio cordis is SCD from blunt, nonpenetrating chest blows, which occur in an individual without structural anomalies in the heart and without traumatic injury to the sternum, the ribs, or the heart. Chest impact during the 15 to 30 ms preceding the peak of the T wave can induce VF. The harder the projectile, the more reliably VF was induced in swine model experiments. The overall survival rate is <25%, and when cardiopulmonary resuscitation was initiated after 3 minutes (38 patients) in 1 study, only 3% survived. Prevention with protective sporting equipment, softer baseballs, and rapid bystander cardiopulmonary resuscitation (including immediate access to automated external defibrillators) represent the best strategies. Teenaged boys are particularly at risk because of the sports they play and the underdevelopment of their chest walls.

SUDDEN CARDIAC DEATH IN YOUNG ATHLETES

SCD in young (age younger than 35 years) athletes is rare, with U.S. incidence at approximately 1 in 200,000. The three most common etiologies in the United States are HCM, commotio cordis, and coronary anomalies. In athletes older than 35 years, CAD remains the most common cause of SCD. Screening focuses on the history and physical examination; any athlete who reports previous exertional syncope or near syncope must undergo further cardiac evaluation. Routine use of ECG and echocardiography remains controversial. The 36th Bethesda Conference provided recommendations for athletic participation in patients at risk of SCD (see the discussion elsewhere in this book for additional information).

DIAGNOSTIC APPROACH

Early response is critical, and patients are far more likely to survive to hospital discharge if bystander cardiopulmonary resuscitation and early defibrillation are available. Thus, advanced cardiac life support and the rapid response system must be activated as soon as possible. The evaluation of survivors of SCD should include a detailed history and physical examination, including the circumstances of the SCD, medication and drug history, a family history of SCD, and potential risk factors. Diagnostic testing may include any combination of ECG, echocardiography, cardiac catheterization, CT, MRI, telemetry monitoring, stress testing (exercise or pharmacological), and EPS. Unless a clearly reversible cause is found, most SCD survivors will require ICD implantation to prevent further events. Attempts to reduce SCD must be centered on prevention, because mortality is so high.

RISK FACTORS FOR SUDDEN CARDIAC DEATH WITHOUT A HISTORY OF HEART DISEASE

Many risk factors have been identified and associated with an increased risk of SCD among people without a history of CHD or structural heart disease. In summary, any risk factor for CHD is a risk factor for SCD. These risk factors include cigarette smoking; in a large prospective study that consisted of a cohort of women without CHD, a strong dose–response relationship between cigarette smoking and SCD risk was observed. Smoking cessation significantly reduced and eventually eliminated excess SCD risk. Hypertension, hyperlipidemia, diabetes, excessive alcohol intake, physical inactivity, and a family history of SCD or premature CHD are also among the risk factors recognized of having SCD.

SUMMARY OF IMPLANTABLE CARDIOVERTER-DEFIBRILLATOR TRIALS

Results of multiple clinical trials have helped define the role of ICDs in primary and secondary prevention of SCD. EF is the most potent predictor of SCD, and ICDs are superior to antiarrhythmic drug therapy in most cases. Recent important trials are briefly reviewed in the following (Tables 42.1 and 42.2).

Primary Prevention

Several trials sought to identify patients at risk of SCD and to assess the role of ICD or antiarrhythmic therapy as primary prevention measures. The broad categories of patients consisted of (1) history of myocardial ischemia or infarction, or both, and (2) congestive heart failure of any etiology. The first of these studies, the Multicenter Automatic Defibrillator Implantation Trial (MADIT I 1996), directly compared ICDs versus antiarrhythmic therapy, with amiodarone in patients with a previous MI, EFs of ≤35%, and an abnormal EPS. It was stopped early because the ICD group had a 55% reduction in total mortality. The Multicenter Unsustained Tachycardia Trial (MUSTT 1999) enrolled a patient population similar to that of MADIT I but which had EFs of ≤40%. The goal of this study was to compare medical therapy with EPS-guided therapy (antiarrhythmic drug or ICD). The incidence of arrhythmic death was significantly lowered, but only in those who received an ICD. MADIT II (2002) evaluated patients whose MI had occurred at least 30 days before the trial began, whose bypass surgery or percutaneous coronary intervention had taken place at least 3 months before, or both, and who had EFs ≤30%. No other risk stratification was undertaken. This trial was also stopped early because the ICD group showed a marked 29% reduction in all-cause mortality compared with the conventional medical therapy group. The Defibrillator in Acute Myocardial Infarction Trial (DINAMIT 2004) evaluated whether early ICD implantation in an immediate (6–40 days, average 18 days) post-MI population conferred benefit. Although arrhythmic deaths were more frequent in the non-ICD arm of the study, no significant benefit in all-cause mortality was noted. The Coronary Artery Bypass Graft Patch

TABLE 42.1 Summary of Major Implantable Cardioverter-Defibrillator Trials—Primary Prevention

Trial	Inclusion Criteria	Key Findings
MADIT I (1996)	Previous MI, EF ≤35%, nonsustained VT, abnormal EPS (VT induced)	ICDs reduced overall mortality by 54% compared with medical therapy.
MUSTT (1999)	Previous MI, EF ≤40%, nonsustained VT	Cardiac arrest or death from arrhythmia was significantly lower in those receiving an ICD compared with those receiving no therapy or those with EPS-guided antiarrhythmic drug therapy.
MADIT II (2002)	Previous MI, EF ≤30%	These patients have a high risk of SCD regardless of the presence of nonsustained VT or the results of EPS.
DINAMIT (2004)	MI within preceding 6–40 days, EF ≤35%	ICD did not reduce overall mortality in patients with recent MI. ICD was associated with reduced arrhythmic death, but that was offset by increased rate of nonarrhythmic death.
CABG Patch (1997)	Planned CABG, EF <36%, abnormal SAECG	ICD at time of revascularization did not improve overall therapy compared with medical therapy.
DEFINITE (2004)	Nonischemic dilated cardiomyopathy, EF ≤35%, nonsustained VT	Significant reduction in all-cause mortality in NYHA class III heart failure patients, trend toward significance in all study patients receiving ICD.
SCD-HeFT (2005)	Ischemic or nonischemic cardiomyopathy, class II and III heart failure, EF ≤35%	ICD group had 23% reduction in overall mortality. Amiodarone without ICD did not confer survival benefit.
DANISH trial (2016)	Nonischemic cardiomyopathy, NYHA II or higher, EF ≤35%	SCD was significantly lower in the ICD group

CABG, Coronary bypass grafting; EF, ejection fraction; EPS, electrophysiological study; ICD, implantable cardioverter-defibrillator; MI, myocardial infarction; NYHA, New York Heart Association; SAECG, signal-averaged ECG; SCD, sudden cardiac death; VT, ventricular tachycardia.

TABLE 42.2 Summary of Major Implantable Cardioverter-Defibrillator Trials—Secondary Prevention

Trial	Inclusion Criteria	Key Findings
CASH (1994)	Survivors of SCD	ICDs reduced overall mortality by 23% compared with either amiodarone or metoprolol and 63% reduction compared with propafenone.
CIDS (2000)	Cardiac arrest survivors due to VT or VF or syncope thought due to arrhythmia	Patients at highest risk of death benefited most from ICD. Age, poor ventricular function, and poor functional status predict risk.
AVID (1997)	Resuscitated VF or sustained VT with syncope or sustained VT with chest pain and EF ≤40%	ICD therapy was associated with 39%, 27%, and 31% reductions in mortality at 1, 2, and 3 years, respectively, compared with antiarrhythmic drug therapy.

EF, Ejection fraction; ICD, implantable cardioverter-defibrillator; SCD, sudden cardiac death; VF, ventricular fibrillation; VT, ventricular tachycardia.

(CABG Patch 1997) trial also examined the potential benefit of an early (epicardial) ICD system implantation at the time of bypass surgery. Patients had EFs <36% and a positive signal-averaged ECG (a more detailed ECG that averages recordings taken over a period of 20 minutes). There was no significant benefit in overall mortality, which emphasized the powerful effect of coronary revascularization in SCD prevention. The ICD group did have a relative 45% reduction in arrhythmia-associated death.

Based on the results of these primary prevention trials, current guidelines recommend ICD implantation for primary prevention in patients with ischemic cardiomyopathy (EF ≤35%) whose MI occurred at least 40 days before implantation or whose revascularization occurred at least 3 months before.

To examine the role of ICD in patients with nonischemic cardiomyopathy, the Defibrillators in Non-ischemic Cardiomyopathy Treatment Evaluation (DEFINITE 2004) Trial enrolled patients with EFs <35% and nonsustained VT. Patients who received an ICD demonstrated a strong but not quite significant trend in reduction of all-cause mortality. The Sudden Cardiac Death Heart Failure Trial (SCD-HeFT 2005) included both ischemic and nonischemic cardiomyopathy patients. In these

patients with EFs ≤35% and New York Heart Association (NYHA) functional class II or III heart failure, overall mortality was significantly reduced in the ICD group (compared with amiodarone or a placebo). In the latest guidelines, any patient meeting SCD-HeFT criteria qualifies for an ICD.

In patients who are candidates for cardiac resynchronization therapy, the Comparison of Medical Therapy, Pacing, and Defibrillation in Chronic Heart Failure (COMPANION) trial demonstrated significant reduction in all-cause mortality. Cardiac resynchronization therapy is reviewed in Chapter 44.

A more recent study, the Defibrillator Implantation in Patients with Nonischemic Systolic Heart Failure (DANISH) trial, brought some controversy about the role of ICDs in primary prevention of SCD in patients with nonischemic cardiomyopathy. In this randomized controlled trial, patients with symptomatic systolic left ventricular dysfunction (EF ≤35%) not caused by CHD were randomized between ICD and usual care. After a median follow-up of >5 years, there was no significant mortality difference between the two groups, although SCD was significantly lower in the ICD group versus that in the control group (4.3% vs. 8.2%). The effect of this trial on the guidelines for ICD implantation in nonischemic cardiomyopathy has not yet been determined.

Secondary Prevention

For survivors of SCD without a reversible cause, ICD implantation is extremely beneficial in preventing death from VT or VF. Three randomized controlled trials have assessed the role of ICDs in secondary prevention. Two meta-analyses confirmed a significant reduction (25%–28%) in overall mortality with an ICD compared with amiodarone, especially in patients with an EF of ≤35%.

The Cardiac Arrest Survival in Hamburg (CASH 2000) trial compared an ICD with metoprolol, propafenone, or amiodarone. A 23% reduction in mortality ($P = 0.08$) was seen in the ICD group compared with those taking metoprolol or amiodarone. Propafenone was stopped prematurely in the study because of increased mortality rates. The Canadian Implantable Defibrillator Study (CIDS 2000) did not show significant reduction in total mortality with an ICD compared with amiodarone after 5-year follow-up. Further analysis showed that the highest risk patients (with two of the following: EF ≤35%, NYHA failure class III or IV heart failure, aged older than 70 years) did derive a significant survival benefit with an ICD. Both CASH and CIDS might have lacked the statistical power to demonstrate significant mortality benefit. In the Antiarrhythmic Drug Versus Defibrillator (AVID 1997) trial, >1000 patients who survived cardiac arrest and who had an EF ≤40% were randomized to ICDs or medical therapy with amiodarone or sotalol. Survival was significantly higher in the ICD group, and there was >50% reduction in arrhythmic death. In addition, improved survival was seen most in patients with EFs of 20% to 35%.

MANAGEMENT AND THERAPY

Optimum Treatment

A summary of the current guidelines is shown in Box 42.2. Patients with ischemic cardiomyopathy and an EF <35% should receive an ICD after optimization of antiischemia therapy and after at least 40 days have passed since MI or 3 months after revascularization, or both. For patients with a previous MI and an EF between 35% and 40%, but who have a history of nonsustained VT or syncope, an EPS should be performed. If the patient has inducible VT, an ICD should be implanted. Medical therapy, including angiotensin-converting enzyme inhibitors, β-blockers, antiplatelet agents, and lipid-lowering therapy, should be optimized.

For patients with persistent nonischemic cardiomyopathy, NYHA functional class II heart failure, and an EF ≤35%, an ICD should be placed. In the case of bundle branch reentry VT, radiofrequency ablation may be beneficial, although patients in this group will still require ICD placement if the EF is ≤35%. Other specific diseases require more aggressive approaches. In patients with Wolff-Parkinson-White syndrome and aborted SCA, radiofrequency ablation is necessary. Patients with a family history of SCD who have HCM, arrhythmogenic RV dysplasia, LQTS, or Brugada syndrome should undergo ICD placement, and any agent known to precipitate acquired LQTS should be discontinued immediately. Finally, patients without a demonstrable cause for documented VF or VT are still at risk for SCD and should be offered ICD therapy.

Beta-blockers have a favorable effect on prevention of SCD and other benefits in patients with congestive heart failure. The Metoprolol Controlled-Release Randomized Intervention Trial in Heart Failure showed a 41% decrease in SCD in heart failure patients with an EF of <40% (mean ~28%) with β-blocker therapy. A β-blocker may be added to amiodarone in most cases without causing worrisome bradycardia. The combined post hoc analysis of the European Myocardial Infarction

---

BOX 42.2 Summary of Indications for Implantable Cardioverter-Defibrillator (ICD)

ICD Implantation for Secondary Prevention

- Documented cardiac arrest due to VF and not due to a reversible cause.
- Documented sustained VT, spontaneous or induced during EPS, not associated with acute MI or reversible cause.
- ICD therapy is indicated before discharge in patients who develop sustained VT/VF >48 hours after STEMI, provided the arrhythmia is not due to transient or reversible ischemia, reinfarction, or metabolic abnormalities.

ICD Implantation for Primary Prevention

- ICD therapy is recommended for primary prevention of SCD to reduce total mortality in selected patients with nonischemic cardiomyopathy, or ischemic heart disease at least 40 days post-MI with LVEF of ≥35% and NYHA functional class II or III symptoms on long-term GDMT, who have reasonable expectation of meaningful survival for >1 year.
- Documented previous MI and EF ≤30% (MADIT II criteria) and NYHA functional class I symptoms on long-term GDMT, who have reasonable expectation of meaningful survival for >1 year.
- ICD therapy is indicated in patients with nonsustained VT due to previous MI, LVEF <40%, and inducible sustained VT at electrophysiological study.

The Following Conditions Must Be Met Before ICD Implantation for Primary Prevention:

- At least 40 days have passed since the most recent MI
- At least 3 months have passed since revascularization (CABG or PCI)
- Optimization of cardiomyopathy medical therapy (β-blockers, ACE-i/ARB) for 3 months
- Expected survival with a good functional status of at least 1 year
- Exclusions include:
  - Previous MI within the past 40 days (DINAMIT criteria)
  - Hypotension or cardiogenic shock while in a stable baseline rhythm
  - CABG or PCI within the past 3 months
  - Symptoms or findings that would make the patient a candidate for revascularization
  - Noncardiac disease associated with expected survival of <1 year or irreversible brain damage

ACE-i, Angiotensin-converting enzyme inhibitors; *ARB*, angiotensin receptor blockers, *CABG*, coronary bypass grafting; *EF*, ejection fraction; *EPS*, electrophysiological study; *GDMT*, guideline-directed medical therapy; *LVEF*, left ventricular ejection fraction; *MI*, myocardial infarction; *NYHA*, New York Heart Association; *PCI*, percutaneous coronary intervention; *SCD*, sudden cardiac death; *STEMI*, ST-segment elevation myocardial infarction; *VF*, ventricular fibrillation; *VT*, ventricular tachycardia.

Amiodarone Trial and the Canadian Amiodarone Myocardial Infarction Arrhythmia Trial revealed a 61% decrease in SCD in post-MI patients treated with both β-blockers and amiodarone, although no change in overall mortality was noted.

Avoiding Treatment Errors

Implantation of ICDs has become a routine procedure for cardiac electrophysiologists, but they should be implanted by experienced operators. Rare procedural complications include pneumothorax, cardiac tamponade, bleeding, or infection.

Compared with antiarrhythmic therapy, ICDs are clearly superior in the prevention of SCD. Individualization of medical treatment must be balanced with adherence to the latest guidelines to identify and treat patients who are most likely to benefit from ICD therapy.

Primary prevention of SCD in the general population has been an area of active research and investigation. There is no evidence that routine screening effectively identifies populations at increased risk of SCD. Even in young athletes, there is controversy regarding the use of routine ECGs, echocardiograms, or stress testing. However, obvious interventions to reduce the risk of SCD are the same interventions that reduce the risk of CHD because most SCD cases are due to CHD. In other words, smoking cessation, lipid control, active lifestyle and exercise, good diabetes and blood pressure control, and moderation in alcohol consumption have all been shown to decrease the risk of SCD.

FUTURE DIRECTIONS

Ongoing research involves finding genetic, electrical, and biochemical markers for increased risk of SCD. Although the EF is a powerful predictor of those at risk of SCD, its measurement can be variable depending on the testing modality used and the physiological state of the patient. Follow-up data from SCD-HeFT showed that >80% of patients did not require therapy from their prophylactic ICD. Development of an SCD "risk score," much like the $CHADS_2$ index that guides oral anticoagulation in atrial fibrillation patients or the Thrombolysis In Myocardial Infarction risk score for guiding management of non-STEMI, may be the best means of stratifying risk and controlling costs. Such a score could incorporate a combination of invasive and noninvasive studies such as the EPS, signal-averaged ECG, microvolt T-wave alternans, heart rate variability, maximum oxygen consumption, and serum B-type natriuretic peptide. To enhance survival of out-of-hospital cardiac arrests, the rapid response system must be expanded as much as possible by teaching basic life support in schools and increasing the availability of automated external defibrillators.

ADDITIONAL RESOURCES

Al-Khatib SM, Granger CB, Huang Y, et al. Sustained ventricular arrhythmias among patients with acute coronary syndromes with no ST-segment elevation: incidence, predictors, and outcomes. *Circulation.* 2002;106:309–312.

This study pooled data from multiple trials on patients with NSTEMI and showed that ventricular arrhythmias are associated with increased 30-day and 6-month mortality.

Arizona Center for Education and Research on Therapeutics. QT Drug Lists by Risk Groups. Available at: https://crediblemeds.org/index.php/login/dlcheck. Accessed February 23, 2010.

Connolly SJ, Hallstrom AP, Cappato R, et al. Meta-analysis of the implantable cardioverter defibrillator secondary prevention trials. AVID, CASH and CIDS Studies. *Eur Heart J.* 2000;21(24):2071–2078.

Meta-analysis of second prevention trials.

Epstein AE, DiMarco JP, Ellenbogen KA, et al. ACC/AHA/HRS 2008 Guidelines for Device-Based Therapy of Cardiac Rhythm Abnormalities: a report of the American College of Cardiology/American Health Association Task Force on Practice Guidelines (Writing Committee to Revise the ACC/AHA/NASPE 2002 Guideline Update for Implantation of Cardiac Pacemakers and Antiarrhythmia Devices) developed in collaboration with the American Association for Thoracic Surgery and Society of Thoracic Surgeons. *J Am Coll Cardiol.* 2008;51:e1–e62.

The latest guidelines update from the American College of Cardiology/American Heart Association/Heart Rhythm Society.

Gehi A, Haas D, Fuster V. Primary prophylaxis with the implantable cardioverter-defibrillator. *JAMA.* 2005;294(8):958–960.

Review highlighting the need for a better means of stratifying patients at risk for SCD.

Huikuri HV, Castellanos A, Myerburg RJ. Sudden cardiac death due to cardiac arrhythmias. *N Engl J Med.* 2001;345:1473–1482.

Review on the pathogenesis of SCD.

Lee DS, Green LD, Liu PP, et al. Effectiveness of implantable defibrillators for preventing arrhythmic events and death: a meta-analysis. *J Am Coll Cardiol.* 2003;41(9):1573–1582.

Meta-analysis of first and second prevention trials.

Maron BJ, Doerer JJ, Haas TS, et al. Sudden deaths in young competitive athletes. *Circulation.* 2009;119:1085–1092.

An analysis of the 27-year-old registry of cardiovascular deaths in young athletes in the United States.

Maron BJ, Gohman TE, Kyle SB, et al. Clinical profile and spectrum of commotio cordis. *JAMA.* 2002;287:1142–1146.

Describes the presentation, management, and outcome of cases from the U.S. Commotio Cordis Registry.

Maron BJ, Zipes DP. Task Force 12: Legal aspects of the 36th Bethesda Conference. *J Am Coll Cardiol.* 2005;45:1313–1375.

Newby KH, Thompson T, Stebbins A, et al. Sustained ventricular arrhythmias in patients receiving thrombolytic therapy: incidence and outcomes. *Circulation.* 1998;98:2567–2573.

Data analysis from the GUSTO I Study showed the negative impact of ventricular arrhythmias despite thrombolytic therapy at the time of acute MI.

Spaulding CM, Joly L, Rosenberg A, et al. Immediate coronary angiography in survivors of out-of-hospital arrest. *N Engl J Med.* 1997;336:1629–1633.

Early study that demonstrated the high prevalence of significant CAD in out-of-hospital survivors of SCA.

EVIDENCE

The Antiarrhythmics versus Implantable Defibrillators (AVID) Investigators. A comparison of antiarrhythmic-drug therapy with implantable defibrillators in patients resuscitated from near-fatal ventricular arrhythmias. *N Engl J Med.* 1997;337:1576–1583.

Report from the AVID Trial.

Bardy GH, Lee KL, Mark DB, et al. Amiodarone or an implantable cardioverter-defibrillator for congestive heart failure. Sudden Cardiac Death in the Heart Failure Trial (SCD-HeFT). *N Engl J Med.* 2005;352:225–237.

Report of SCD-HeFT.

Bigger JT Jr. Prophylactic use of implanted cardiac defibrillators in patients at high risk for ventricular arrhythmias after coronary-artery bypass graft surgery. Coronary Artery Bypass Graft (CABG) Patch Trial Investigators. *N Engl J Med.* 1997;337:1569–1575.

Report from the CABG Patch Trial.

Buxton AE, Lee KL, Fisher JD, et al. A randomized study of the prevention of sudden death in patients with coronary artery disease. Multicenter Unsustained Tachycardia Trial Investigators. *N Engl J Med.* 1999;341:1882–1890.

Report from the MUSTT.

Connolly SJ, Gent M, Roberts RS, et al. Canadian implantable defibrillator study (CIDS): a randomized trial of the implantable cardioverter defibrillator against amiodarone. *Circulation.* 2000;101:1297–1302.

Report from CIDS.

Hohnloser SH, Kuck KH, Dorian P, et al. Prophylactic use of an implantable cardioverter-defibrillator after acute myocardial infarction. *N Engl J Med.* 2004;351:2481–2488.

Report from the DINAMIT.

Kadish A, Dyer A, Daubert JP, et al. Prophylactic defibrillator implantation in patients with nonischemic dilated cardiomyopathy. *N Engl J Med.* 2004;350:2151–2158.

Report from the DEFINITE Trial.

Køber L, Thune JJ, Nielsen JC, et al. Defibrillator implantation in patients with nonischemic systolic heart failure. *N Engl J Med.* 2016;375(13):1221–1230.

Report of the DANISH Trial.

Kuck KH, Cappato R, Siebels J, et al. Randomized comparison of antiarrhythmic drug therapy with implantable defibrillators in patients resuscitated from cardiac arrest: the Cardiac Arrest Study Hamburg (CASH). *Circulation.* 2000;102:748–754.

Report from CASH.

Moss AJ, Hall WJ, Cannom DS, et al. Improved survival with an implanted defibrillator in patients with coronary disease at high risk for ventricular arrhythmia. Multicenter Automatic Defibrillator Implantation Trial Investigators. *N Engl J Med*. 1996;335:1933–1940.
Report from MADIT I.

Moss AJ, Zareba W, Hall WJ, et al. Prophylactic implantation of a defibrillator in patients with myocardial infarction and reduced ejection fraction. *N Engl J Med*. 2002;346:877–883.
Report from MADIT II.

43

Syncope

Pamela S. Ro, J. Paul Mounsey

Syncope is a transient, self-limited loss of consciousness and voluntary muscle tone. It is typically followed quickly by spontaneous recovery of consciousness. The incidence rate of syncope varies between 0.80 and 0.93 per 1000 person-years. Syncope accounts for 3% to 5% of emergency department visits and 1% to 3% of hospital admissions. There is an increased association with acute illness and noxious stimuli. There is also a familial tendency. Normal cerebral blood flow is 60 mL/min per 100 g tissue (11.4 mL oxygen/min per 100 g). Syncope occurs when <3.5 mL oxygen/min per 100 g tissue is delivered for >8 seconds. This can occur due to sudden cerebrovascular tone dysregulation, drop in perfusion pressure, change in heart rate, drop in cardiac preload, or drop in arteriolar resistance.

ETIOLOGY AND PATHOGENESIS

The various etiologies of syncope can be divided into four categories: orthostatic hypotension, cardiac anatomic abnormalities, cardiac arrhythmias, and neurally-mediated syncope (NMS).

Orthostatic Hypotension

Orthostatic hypotension is a common cause of syncope (Fig. 43.1). This is especially true for older adults and individuals with certain medical conditions. Some primary disorders of the autonomic nervous system can cause orthostatic hypotension, such as Parkinson disease and Shy-Drager syndrome. There are also disorders that secondarily affect the autonomic nervous system, such as diabetes mellitus or a paraneoplastic process. Pregnancy and medications that can cause or exacerbate orthostatic hypotension should be considered as causes. The American Autonomic Society defines orthostatic hypotension as a drop in systolic blood pressure of ≤20 mm Hg or a drop of diastolic blood pressure of ≤10 mm Hg within 3 minutes of standing.

Cardiac Anatomic Abnormalities

Various cardiac anatomic abnormalities can cause syncope. This can be related to ventricular outflow tract obstruction or decreased cardiac output. Mechanical outflow tract obstruction of the left ventricle can be due to hypertrophic cardiomyopathy, aortic valve stenosis, and myocardial tumors (including myxomas, rhabdomyomas, and fibromas). Right-sided outflow tract obstruction can be due to pulmonary valve stenosis and unrepaired tetralogy of Fallot. Diagnoses that can lead to decreased cardiac output include dilated cardiomyopathy, restrictive cardiomyopathy, and pulmonary hypertension (either primary or secondary). Diagnosis of these etiologies requires a careful physical examination with confirmation by echocardiography.

Cardiac Arrhythmias

Both bradyarrhythmias and tachyarrhythmias can cause syncope. Bradycardia or asystole due to sinus node dysfunction is often abrupt in onset. Atrioventricular block also tends to be sudden in onset. These etiologies must be especially considered in postoperative cardiac surgical patients. Although it is most commonly idiopathic, atrioventricular block can also be seen in the setting of rheumatic fever, Lyme disease, sarcoidosis, electrolyte abnormalities, viral myocarditis, and Duchenne muscular dystrophy.

Both supraventricular and ventricular tachycardia can cause symptoms of palpitations, shortness of breath, and lightheadedness, as well as syncope. Supraventricular tachycardia can include atrioventricular reciprocating tachycardia, as well as atrial flutter and atrial fibrillation. The rate of tachycardia is probably most predictive of syncope. However, tachycardia in the setting of elevated activity level and its association with increased metabolic demands, as well as tachycardia in the setting of relative dehydration, can also increase the risk of syncope. Patients with atrial fibrillation and patients with Wolff-Parkinson-White syndrome should be monitored. Those patients with Wolff-Parkinson-White syndrome and a fast anterograde conduction pathway may be at risk for life-threatening arrhythmias (see Chapter 37).

Structural abnormalities such as ischemic and nonischemic cardiomyopathies, hypertrophic cardiomyopathy, arrhythmogenic right ventricular cardiomyopathy, and coronary artery abnormalities can predispose individuals to ventricular arrhythmias. An inherited ion channel disorder should also be considered, especially if syncope occurs in the setting of exercise or stress. These disorders include long QT syndrome, catecholaminergic polymorphic ventricular tachycardia Brugada syndrome, and short QT syndrome.

In general, syncope associated with anatomic cardiac abnormalities, cardiomyopathies, and inherited ion channel disorders carries an adverse prognosis. The same is true for atrioventricular block but not for supraventricular tachycardia or sinus node dysfunction.

Neurally-Mediated Syncope

NMS, also referred to as vasovagal syncope, vasodepressor syncope, and neurocardiogenic syncope, is the most common cause of syncope. The "typical faint" is not a pathological cardiac condition. It most likely represents a remnant defense mechanism in response to stress. The pathophysiology of NMS remains to be fully elucidated. It is mostly believed to be a disturbance in the autonomic control of heart rate and blood pressure. Several theories involve baroreceptor reflex abnormalities that lead to a disconnection between the autonomic nervous system and the cardiovascular system. Another theory proposes that venous pooling, which occurs in an upright position, leads to reduced cardiac filling, which then activates mechanoreceptors that cause a paradoxical withdrawal of sympathetic tone. The triad of apnea, bradycardia, and hypotension was first termed the Bezold-Jarisch Reflex in the 1940s, when it was appreciated that afferent and efferent pathways in the vagus nerve control both heart rate and vasomotor tone by increasing or decreasing parasympathetic discharge to the heart (Fig. 43.2). In general,

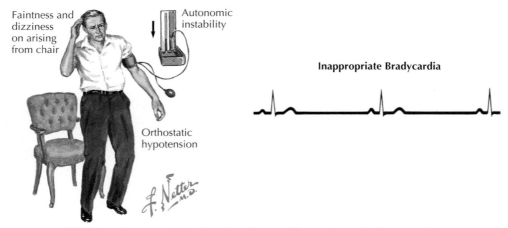

FIG 43.1 Autonomic Dysfunction Causes Hemodynamic Abnormalities.

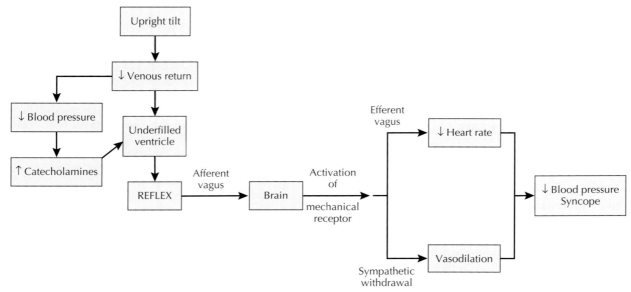

FIG 43.2 The Bezold-Jarisch Reflex.

an initial trigger leads to a pronounced sympathetic surge followed by a paradoxical parasympathetic input. Several types of situational syncope are also neurally mediated, such as coughing, micturition, defecation, postprandially, by hair grooming, and postexercise.

CLINICAL PRESENTATION

Determining the etiology of a syncopal episode can be difficult and confusing. It is essential to obtain a careful and detailed history, perform a complete physical examination, and obtain directed laboratory studies (Fig. 43.3).

When asking a patient regarding the event, it is important to ask specific details (Box 43.1). Prompt evaluation is essential. The further a patient is from the event, the less the patient will remember regarding the details. The symptoms that surround a syncopal event can often aid in determining the underlying etiology. The quality and duration of symptoms preceding the loss of consciousness can vary considerably, depending on the cause. Observations made by witnesses are also important and can help recreate the events that led from prodromal symptoms to duration of unconsciousness and mental status upon arousal. Typical

prodromal symptoms may consist of lightheadedness, weakness, headache, vision or hearing changes, palpitations, nausea, diaphoresis, yawning, or anxiety. A longer prodrome is more often seen with NMS, whereas a sudden onset or lack of prodrome can be associated with an arrhythmic etiology. A patient with an arrhythmia may be more likely to complain of palpitations beforehand. Tonic-clonic movements are associated with a seizure disorder, whereas posturing can be seen both with seizure disorders and NMS. Loss of consciousness typically is brief (usually <1 minute) for patients with NMS, whereas patients with a seizure disorder may have a post-ictal period for up to half an hour. Following the event, the NMS patient may feel fatigued but should be alert and oriented. NMS generally occurs when the patient is in an upright position. Cardiac structural abnormalities must be considered if syncope occurs during exertion. Chest pain suggests coronary disease as an etiology.

Other aspects of the history of the patient are important. A detailed medical history and family history can help determine if a patient is at increased risk for syncope related to arrhythmias. Recent changes in medication should be investigated. A syncopal event associated with a family history of sudden death warrants immediate attention. Obtaining a fluid history can also help elucidate the etiology.

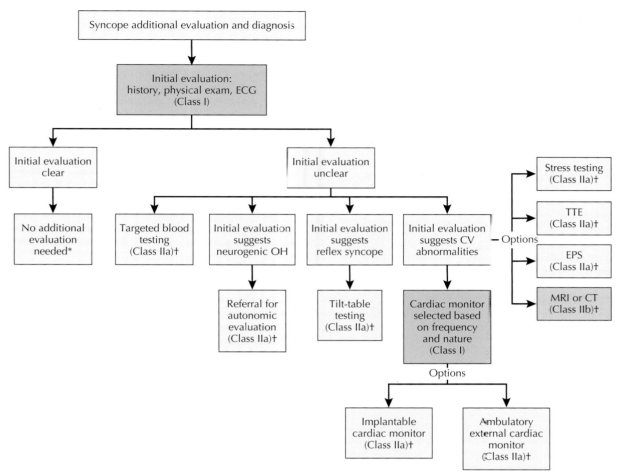

FIG 43.3 Flowchart for the Evaluation and Diagnosis of Syncope. *Green*, Class (strong); *yellow*, class IIa (moderate); *orange*, class IIb (weak). *, Applies to patients after a normal initial evaluation without significant injury or cardiovascular morbidities; patients followed up by primary care physician as needed.†, In selected patients. *CV,* Cardiovascular; *EPS,* electrophysiological study; *OH,* orthostatic hypotension; *TTE,* transthoracic echocardiography. (From Shen WK, Sheldon RS, Benditt DG, et al. 2017 ACC/AHA/HRS guideline for the evaluation and management of patients with syncope. A report of the American College of Cardiology, American Heart Association Task Force on Clinical Practice Guidelines, and the Heart Rhythm Society. *J Am Coll Cardiol* 2017;70:620–663.)

DIFFERENTIAL DIAGNOSIS

Differentiating syncope from other conditions of altered consciousness can be challenging. Neurological etiologies can include seizure disorders, basilar migraines, and increased intracranial pressure. Metabolic etiologies include hypoglycemia and hypercalcemia. Behavioral and psychiatric etiologies include panic attacks, conversion reactions, and malingering. Most syncope is benign and not fatal. However, patients with rare life-threatening disease must be identified. A careful history, thorough physical examination, and directed diagnostic tests are necessary to determine the underlying cause.

DIAGNOSTIC APPROACH

A careful physical examination is essential. Vital signs should be noted, including orthostatic vital signs with blood pressure and pulse measured in the supine, sitting, and standing positions for 5 minutes in each position. Often the results of the examination are normal. A loud systolic ejection murmur at the left or right upper sternal border can indicate right or left outflow tract obstruction. Changes in the quality of the

murmur in different positions can indicate hypertrophic cardiomyopathy. In a patient with hypertrophic cardiomyopathy, performing a Valsalva maneuver will increase the intensity of the murmur, and squatting will decrease the intensity of the murmur. Patients with ischemic or dilated cardiomyopathies may exhibit signs of left ventricular enlargement and dysfunction, with a displaced maximal precordial impulse and evidence of hepatomegaly and edema if in cardiac failure. Carotid sinus massage can be performed to elicit carotid sinus hypersensitivity. Baroreceptor stimulation may cause a drop in blood pressure or even development of profound asystole. This can be especially true for older adult men in whom baroreceptor function declines with advancing age. Therefore, it is not recommended to perform carotid massage on older patients with carotid bruits or suspected carotid vascular disease. When the history, physical examination, and ECG are insufficient, further testing may be required (Fig. 43.4).

Electrocardiogram

An ECG should be obtained for any patient who presents with syncope (Fig. 43.5). The ECG will often be normal. However, evidence of various degrees of atrioventricular block, bundle branch block, or pacemaker

BOX 43.1 Pertinent Questions to Ask a Patient With a History of Syncope

- Activity Associated With Syncopal Event
  Positional changes
  Exercise
  Micturition
  Defecation
  Coughing
  Hair styling
  Phlebotomy
  Looking upward
- Prodromal Symptoms
  Palpitations
  Lightheadedness
  Vision changes
  Diaphoresis
  Pale appearance
  Abdominal pain
- Syncopal Event
  Time of the day
  Location
  Length of time for loss of consciousness
  Incontinence
  Tonic-clonic movements
- Symptoms Upon Return to Consciousness
  Palpitations
  Nausea
  Vomiting
  Chest pain
  Shortness of breath
- Historical Information
  Previous illness with fever, vomiting, diarrhea
  Recent travel
  Recent trauma
- Medications
  Antihypertensives
  Insulin
  Other prescription medications
  Over-the-counter medications
  Illicit drug use
  Alcohol
  New medications
  Change in dose of previous medications
- Family History of Sudden Unexplained Death

Blood and Urine Tests

Hematocrit and urinalysis can be helpful to determine volume status. Blood glucose can be checked acutely if hypoglycemia is suspected. A urine human chorionic gonadotropin (hCG) should be obtained if pregnancy is suspected. Electrolyte abnormalities such as hypokalemia and hypomagnesemia can also predispose to both ventricular and supraventricular arrhythmias. Blood and urine toxicology screening is useful when illicit drug use is suspected.

Echocardiography

Echocardiograms are not necessary in all patients who present with syncope. However, most adults will undergo echocardiography. If left ventricular dysfunction is suspected or abnormal cardiac findings are present on physical examination or an ECG, then an echocardiogram may be helpful. Echocardiograms can evaluate for any evidence of ventricular dysfunction, hypertrophy, or structural abnormalities.

Exercise Stress Test

Exercise stress tests can be helpful in making a diagnosis, especially in patients who have syncope with exertion and a normal echocardiogram. Normally, the corrected QT interval should shorten with an increased heart rate. Prolongation of the corrected QT interval at peak exercise and early recovery can be seen in patients with long QT syndrome. Patients with catecholaminergic polymorphic ventricular tachycardia may have completely normal ECGs at baseline, but they may develop evidence of ventricular ectopy, such as multifocal premature ventricular contractions and bidirectional ventricular tachycardia, with exercise. Some ventricular outflow tract tachycardias may only become evident with exercise. Ischemic changes may be seen during exercise in patients with coronary abnormalities.

ECG Monitors

Continuous rhythm assessment with ambulatory monitors are useful in correlating symptoms with an arrhythmia. However, the monitors are only useful if the patient is symptomatic during the monitoring period. A Holter monitor is typically worn for 24 to 48 hours, and a patch monitor can be worn for up to 2 weeks. Both monitors continuously record the cardiac rhythm. This is an effective method for symptoms that occur frequently or can be reproducibly recreated. External loop recorders and transtelephonic event monitors are worn for up to a couple months. They can aid in recording the heart rhythm of a patient during symptoms; however, their usefulness may be limited by the ability of the patient to activate the device before cessation of symptoms, the physical size of the device, or the ability of the patient to sleep comfortably or participate in activities with the device. Implantable loop recorders provide long-term monitoring of infrequent symptoms without external electrodes. The device is implanted under the skin and can remain in place for up to 3 years. The smallest device weighs 2.5 g.

Head-Up Tilt Table Test

A head-up tilt table test is used to attempt to reproduce symptoms in a controlled setting while documenting vital signs and rhythm. It is performed with a controlled passive upright posture to 60 to 80 degrees. Tilt table testing can improve the diagnostic evaluation of syncope. A positive result is defined as a drop in heart rate (cardioinhibitory), blood pressure (vasodepressor), or both (mixed). The sensitivity of the head-up tilt table test is variable. Isoproterenol or nitroglycerin can be administered to help reproduce symptoms and increase sensitivity by increasing heart rate and myocardial contractility, thus triggering ventricular mechanoreceptors. Symptoms can also be induced in asymptomatic patients, decreasing the specificity of the study. The procedure

malfunction that indicates bradycardia as a cause of syncope must be evaluated. Evidence of left or right ventricular hypertrophy can indicate a cardiac structural abnormality. Delta waves (a short PR interval with a slurred upstroke of the QRS complex) are the classic ECG finding of a patient with Wolff-Parkinson-White syndrome. The corrected QT interval is often prolonged in patients with long QT syndrome. The QT interval must be calculated; the automated ECG computer interpretation algorithm will often miscalculate the actual QT interval. Brugada syndrome typically demonstrates a coved ST-segment elevation in association with an incomplete right bundle branch block pattern in leads V_1 to V_3. Arrhythmogenic right ventricular cardiomyopathy may demonstrate an ε wave at the terminal portion of the QRS complex or evidence of T-wave inversion in leads V_1 to V_3.

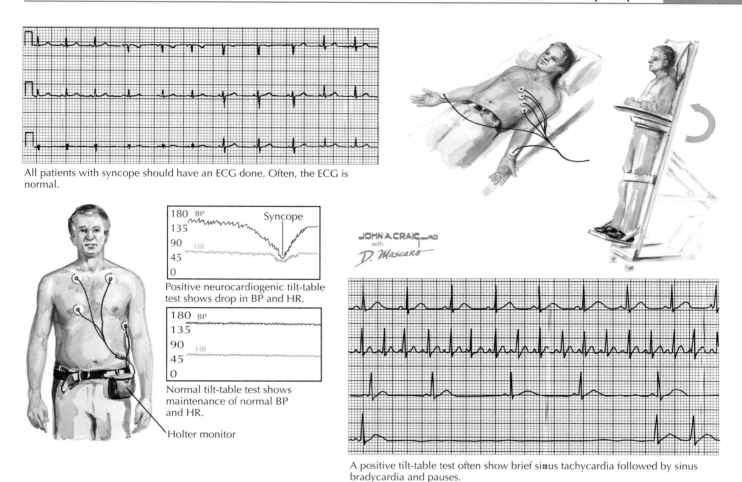

All patients with syncope should have an ECG done. Often, the ECG is normal.

180 BP
135
90 HR
45
0
Syncope

Positive neurocardiogenic tilt-table test shows drop in BP and HR.

180 BP
135
90 HR
45
0

Normal tilt-table test shows maintenance of normal BP and HR.

Holter monitor

JOHN A. CRAIG__AD
with
D. Mascaro

A positive tilt-table test often show brief sinus tachycardia followed by sinus bradycardia and pauses.

FIG 43.4 Syncope: Diagnostic Evaluation. *BP*, Blood pressure; *HR*, heart rate.

can be useful in confirming the diagnosis in a patient suspected of having NMS. However, most patients with NMS do not require a tilt test if the history and physical examination suggest a diagnosis of NMS.

Intracardiac Electrophysiology Study

An intracardiac electrophysiology study involves placement of transvenous catheters within the heart. The procedure can assess the function of the sinus node and atrioventricular node as well as susceptibility to supraventricular and ventricular arrhythmias. The yield of an electrophysiology study is low in someone with a normal physical examination and negative cardiac evaluation. In addition, the sensitivity of an electrophysiology study is low for detecting bradyarrhythmias such as sinus node dysfunction or atrioventricular block. Therefore, electrophysiology studies are not routinely performed in patients presenting with syncope unless other risk factors are identified. In patients with a history of myocardial infarction, an electrophysiology study can help risk stratify those who may be at higher risk for ventricular arrhythmias. However, if ischemia is suspected, ischemia evaluation with a stress test or heart catheterization should be performed before the electrophysiology study. The electrophysiology study is less useful in patients with nonischemic cardiomyopathy. Patients with an ejection fraction of <35% may qualify for an implantable cardioverter-defibrillator regardless of electrophysiology results. A procainamide challenge may be helpful if Brugada syndrome is suspected. Brugada syndrome is a sodium channelopathy. Procainamide is a sodium channel blocking agent. Compared with the standard electrophysiology study that evaluates for inducible ventricular

arrhythmias, a procainamide challenge test may provoke morphological changes in the ECG typically seen in patients with Brugada syndrome, particularly ST-segment changes in leads V_1 to V_3. For patients suspected of having catecholaminergic polymorphic ventricular tachycardia, an epinephrine infusion can be considered to evaluate for bidirectional ventricular tachycardia.

Optimum Evaluation

The laboratory examination is guided by the history and physical examination. There should be a thoughtful application of tests obtained. Not all patients with syncope require an admission to the hospital or a brain magnetic resonance imaging study. If a patient has a classic history for NMS with a normal cardiovascular and neurological examination, as well as a normal ECG, no further study may be needed. Furthermore, it sometimes may not be possible to determine the cause of syncope. Therefore, it is important to remember that the purpose of evaluation is not only to determine a cause but also to risk stratify the patient. If the patient has been thoroughly evaluated and risk stratified for dangerous arrhythmias or other life-threatening conditions, then the evaluation has been worthwhile even if a definitive diagnosis was not obtained.

MANAGEMENT AND THERAPY

Optimum Treatment

Prescribing the appropriate treatment for a patient is dependent on making the correct diagnosis. If a bradyarrhythmia is the cause, then

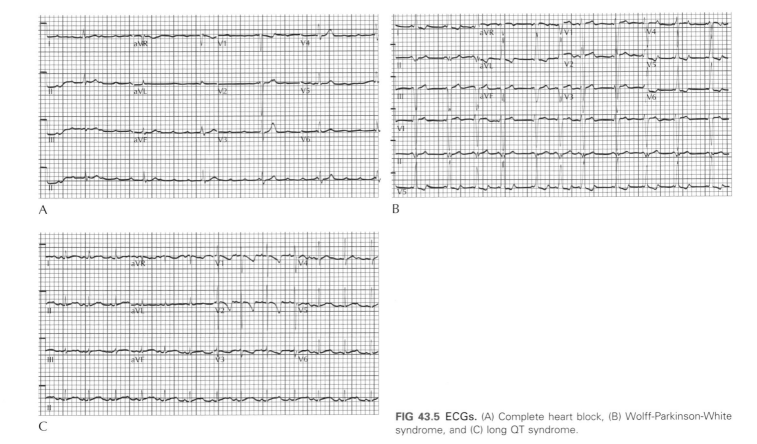

FIG 43.5 ECGs. (A) Complete heart block, (B) Wolff-Parkinson-White syndrome, and (C) long QT syndrome.

the patient may benefit from placement of a pacemaker for rate support. If a tachyarrhythmia has been detected, then the patient may require medications, radiofrequency or cryoablation, or placement of an internal cardiac defibrillator. Cardiac structural abnormalities may require interventional cardiac catheterization or surgical intervention. Treatment for NMS has evolved considerably and includes nonpharmacological and pharmacological aspects.

Nonpharmacological Treatment for Neurally-Mediated Syncope

Most patients respond well to behavioral and lifestyle modification alone. It is essential to educate patients about NMS, its physiology, and its excellent prognosis. Education about prodromal symptoms will allow patients to lay down rather than try to "walk it off," thus preventing a syncopal episode that may ultimately lead to physical harm from the fall. For those who cannot lay down, various isometric counterpressure maneuvers, such as leg crossing, hand-grip exercises, and tensing the arm and leg muscles, have been found to be effective. These exercises increase systemic blood pressure and decrease venous pooling, aborting an impending syncopal event. Squatting is also effective in increasing venous pressure and preventing syncope.

Volume expansion is the baseline treatment for these patients. Patients must increase fluid intake to 2 to 3 L/day taken throughout the day. Liberalizing salt intake can also be beneficial in patients who do not have other medical conditions that would make this contraindicated. Caffeine should be limited because it is a diuretic and may counteract any attempts to expand volume with fluids. These maneuvers are easy to accomplish and well tolerated. Compression stockings can help avoid venous pooling in the lower extremities. These may be especially useful

for those patients who stand for long periods of time. Tilt training is another safe and easy tool. Patients are instructed to stand against a wall for 30 minutes or until symptoms appear on a routine, daily basis. Unfortunately, tilt training is not well accepted by patients, and results of tilt training have been inconsistent. Physical therapy and core exercise may be beneficial in a portion of patients who are debilitated by NMS.

The benefits of pacing have not yet been established. It had been thought that pacing would be beneficial to treat the bradycardia and asystole that are associated with vasovagal episodes. There have been mixed results for the use of pacemaker therapy in this population. Exceptions have been made for patients with a marked cardioinhibitory response. However, in general, pacemaker therapy is not considered an established treatment option for these patients.

Pharmacological Treatment for Neurally-Mediated Syncope

Pharmacotherapy should be reserved for patients with NMS who do not respond to conservative measures. Studies on drug therapy have had conflicting results, making definitive treatment guidelines difficult. Fludrocortisone is frequently used. It is a synthetic corticosteroid with mineralocorticoid activity that increases blood pressure. Adverse side effects include elevated blood pressure, edema, and decreased potassium levels. Midodrine is another frequently used drug. It acts as a central α agonist to increase blood pressure, but it has adverse side effects, including headache, facial flushing, goosebumps, and supine hypertension. Droxidopa is a prodrug of norepinephrine. It acts by increasing blood pressure, but it also has a side effect of supine hypertension. If this medication is being contemplated, referral to a specialist may be in order. Once considered the mainstay of treatment, β-blocker therapy has been ineffective in randomized studies and is no longer the treatment of choice. Paroxetine and other serotonin reuptake inhibitors have been found to significantly reduce syncopal episodes in randomized studies. Although the mechanism is not fully elucidated, activated serotonin receptors are known to directly affect vagal tone, blood pressure, and heart rate in animal models. Ivabradine, a cardiotonic agent, blocks the sinus node pacemaker channel. This slows the sinus node and thus may be a treatment option for those with postural orthostatic tachycardia syndrome and marked sinus tachycardia. Ultimately, medication treatment should be tailored on an individual patient basis. Some patients may find effective treatment with a multidrug regimen in small doses rather than a large dose of a single agent.

Special Patient Populations
Pediatric Patients

The frequency of vasovagal episodes in this age group often leads to dismissal of symptoms. Obtaining a careful personal and family history, as well as reviewing an ECG, are essential elements that can help distinguish benign vasovagal syncope from a potentially life-threatening etiology. Concerning elements in the history include syncope that occurs while supine, during exercise, in response to a loud noise or fright, and a family history of sudden death in a young person. Whenever these elements are elicited in a patient, further evaluation is warranted.

Older Adult Patients

Falls in the older adults are a common occurrence. Many falls may be due to syncope; however, many are not. The ability to make the diagnosis is complicated by poor patient recall of the event and the clinical overlap among mechanical falls, orthostatic intolerance, generalized dizziness, and vasovagal syncope. Syncope can be the first manifestation of an autonomic disorder or central nervous system problem. Older adult patients are more prone to vasovagal syncope due to reduced fluid intake and an age-related decline in baroreceptor and autonomic functions. It is particularly important to be cognizant of polypharmacy in this at-risk age group. Consideration should be given to restricting driving privileges, particularly if the syncopal events are profound and without much warning.

FUTURE DIRECTIONS

Treatment strategies for cardiac structural abnormalities and cardiac arrhythmias continue to improve. However, our understanding of the pathophysiology of NMS and autonomic function in general is still incomplete. Further study will lead the way for more effective treatment strategies. Future modification of guidelines and protocols, as well as increased use of specialized syncope units, will further promote a cohesive structured-care pathway that can be efficient and cost-effective.

ADDITIONAL RESOURCES

Grubb BP. Clinical practice. Neurocardiogenic syncope. *N Engl J Med.* 2005;352:1004–1010.
A complete review of the evaluation and treatment of patients with neurocardiogenic syncope.

Hogan TM, Constantine ST, Crain AD. Evaluation of syncope in older adults. *Emerg Med Clin North Am.* 2016;34:501–627.
A review of the management of syncope, specifically in the older adult population.

Kanter RJ. *Syncope. Clinical Pediatric Arrhythmias.* 2nd ed. Philadelphia, PA: Saunders; 1999.
A thorough resource for the differential diagnosis of syncope in pediatric patients; however, most of the chapter is applicable to the adult population as well.

Moya A, Sutton R, Ammirati F, et al. Guidelines for the diagnosis and management of syncope (version 2009). Task Force for the Diagnosis and Management of Syncope. *Eur Heart J.* 2009;20:2631–2671.
An update on the European Task Force guidelines, with new guidelines for evaluation and treatment of syncope.

Shen WK, Sheldon RS, Benditt DG, et al. 2017 ACC/AHA/HRS guideline for the evaluation and management of patients with syncope. A report of the American College of Cardiology/American Heart Association Task Force on Clinical Practice Guidelines, and the Heart Rhythm Society. *J Am Coll Cardiol.* 2017;03.003.
An update to the guidelines for treatment of all patients with various forms of syncope.

EVIDENCE

D'Angelo RN, Pickett CC. Diagnostic yield of device interrogation in the evaluation of syncope in an elderly population. *Int J Cardiol.* 2017;236:164–167.
The study demonstrated that device interrogation is rarely useful in elucidating a cause of syncope in the older adult population.

Health Quality Ontario. Long-term continuous ambulatory ECG monitors and external cardiac loop recorders for cardiac arrhythmia: a health technology assessment. *Ont Health Technol Assess Ser.* 2017;17:1–56.
This study demonstrated that although both long-term continuous ambulatory ECG monitors and external loop recorders were more effective than 24-hour Holter monitors in detecting symptoms, there was no evidence to suggest that the devices differed in effectiveness.

Solbiati M, Casazza G, Dipaola F, et al. The diagnostic yield of implantable loop recorders in unexplained syncope: a systematic review and meta-analysis.
A review of the literature with a meta-analysis that demonstrates that implantable loop recorders diagnosed a large percentage of patients with unexplained syncope.

Varosy PD, Chen LY, Miller AL, et al. Pacing as a treatment for reflex-mediated (vasovagal, situational, or carotid sinus hypersensitivity) syncope: a systematic review for the 2017 ACC/AHA/HRS guideline for the evaluation and management of patients with syncope: a report of the American College of Cardiology. American Heart Association Task Force on Clinical Practice Guidelines and the Heart Rhythm Society. *Heart Rhythm.* 2017;1547–1571.
A systematic review of literature that demonstrates that evidence does not support the use of pacing for reflex-mediated syncope beyond those used for recurrent vasovagal syncope and asystole documented by implantable loop recorder.

Wenzke KE, Walsh KE, Kalscheur M, et al. Clinical characteristics and outcome of patients with situational syncope compared to patients with vasovagal syncope. *Pacing Clin Electrophysiol.* 2017;10.1111.
Study of a large cohort of patients with syncope found that situational syncope consists of a low percentage of patients with reflex syncope.

44

Cardiac Pacemakers and Defibrillators

Anil K. Gehi, J. Paul Mounsey

Technological advances have improved the versatility and function of implantable devices used to treat bradyarrhythmias and tachyarrhythmias. Surgical placement of pacemakers and implantable cardioverter-defibrillators (ICDs) can be performed on an outpatient basis, with low risk and minimal morbidity, which allows most patients to return to full functional capacity quickly.

INDICATIONS FOR IMPLANTATION OF CARDIAC RHYTHM DEVICES

Pacemakers

Pacemakers are indicated primarily for patients with symptomatic bradycardia or impressive bradycardia without symptom correlation but which is associated with a high risk of progression to a symptomatic bradycardia. Precise indications are published in the American College of Cardiology/American Heart Association Guidelines for Pacemaker and ICD Implantation. Symptoms of bradycardia may be subtle (lightheadedness, fatigue) or dramatic (syncope or cardiac arrest). Bradycardia may be the result of dysfunction of the sinus node (referred to as sick sinus syndrome), the atrioventricular node, or the infranodal conduction system. Damage to the conduction system results most commonly from fibrosis or infarction, but may be the result of numerous other etiologies, including infection, pharmacological agents, electrolyte imbalance, or thyroid disease. It is imperative to rule out potentially reversible causes before committing a patient to device-based therapy (Fig. 44.1).

Biventricular Pacemakers

Based on the concept that "dyssynchronous" electrical activation of the left ventricle—as with bundle branch block or right ventricular pacing—translates to inefficient cardiac function, biventricular pacing has been developed as a therapeutic approach for patients with impaired cardiac function who would not otherwise have an indication for pacemaker therapy (Fig. 44.2). For instance, in patients with left bundle branch block, delayed electrical activation of the lateral wall of the left ventricle leads to delayed contraction of this same wall. In an individual with normal systolic function, delayed contraction of the lateral wall of the left ventricle may not result in any significant decrement in function. However, in an individual with markedly impaired left ventricular function, the disorganized ventricular contraction resulting from left bundle branch block can result in decreased pumping efficiency and increased mitral regurgitation. By positioning pacemaker leads in the right ventricle and in a lateral branch of the coronary sinus on the epicardium of the left ventricle, simultaneous pacing of both walls of the left ventricle improves ventricular synchrony. Biventricular pacing is indicated for treatment of patients with symptomatic heart failure (New York Heart Association functional class III or IV) despite optimal medical therapy, reduced left ventricular ejection fraction, and a widened QRS duration (either intrinsically or due to a long-term need for pacing).

Implantable Cardioverter-Defibrillators

ICDs are indicated for patients with structural heart disease at risk for malignant ventricular tachyarrhythmias (i.e., ventricular tachycardia or ventricular fibrillation). These indications include patients with a history of resuscitated cardiac arrest or ventricular tachycardia, as well as patients at high risk for future cardiac arrest or ventricular tachyarrhythmia (e.g., a patient with ischemic or nonischemic cardiomyopathy or hypertrophic cardiomyopathy). ICDs are also often indicated in patients with structurally normal hearts who are at high risk for ventricular tachyarrhythmias, such as those with inherited disorders of cardiac rhythm: long QT syndrome, Brugada syndrome, or catecholaminergic polymorphic ventricular tachycardia. The indications for ICD implantation, particularly in patients with tachyarrhythmias, are discussed in detail in this chapter and summarized in Fig. 44.3.

PACEMAKER TECHNOLOGY

A pacemaker consists of a pulse generator and endocardial leads capable of sensing and pacing. The pulse generator contains a microprocessor to control the analysis of sensed activity and a battery. Pacemakers can be configured as single-chamber, dual-chamber, or biventricular devices. To clarify pacemaker characteristics, a four-letter code describes features specific to each pacemaker. The first letter or category of the code indicates the chamber(s) paced, and the second describes the chamber(s) sensed. Options for these positions include O (none), A (atrium), V (ventricle), and D (dual = A + V). The third position of the code indicates the response of the device to a sensed event; options include O (none), T (triggered), I (inhibited), and D (dual = triggered or inhibited). The fourth position indicates programmability of rate modulation. The letter R in this position indicates that the device has an active responsive sensor. For example, a pacemaker programmed to VOO mode paces the ventricle at a specified rate and will ignore any signal sensed by the ventricular lead. A pacemaker programmed to VVI paces the ventricle at a specified rate but will inhibit pacing in the ventricle if an appropriate signal is sensed by the ventricular lead. A pacemaker programmed to DDD mode paces both the atrium and ventricle, unless it is inhibited by an appropriate signal in the atrium or ventricle. Ventricular pacing can also be triggered after atrial sensing or pacing. Turning on the rate sensor with any mode of pacing allows the specified rate to increase in response to exercise that is detected by a sensor contained in the pacemaker (most commonly an accelerometer or a respiration sensor). In a patient with chronotropic incompetence, the pacing rate can adjust as necessary to correspond with and compensate for the activity of the patient.

DEFIBRILLATOR TECHNOLOGY

As with a pacemaker, an ICD consists of a pulse generator and endocardial leads. In addition, an ICD requires high-voltage defibrillator

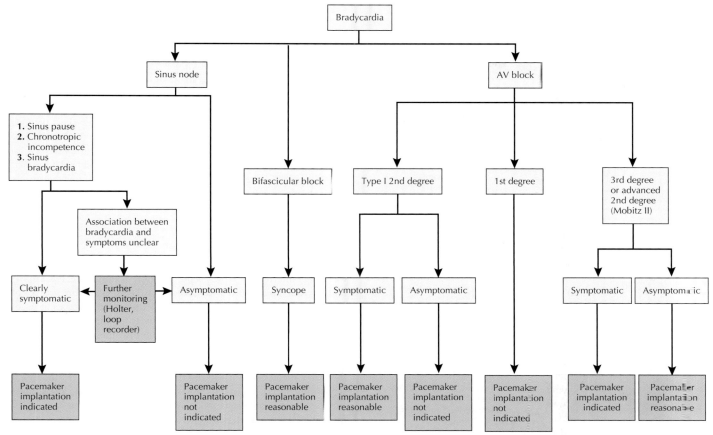

FIG 44.1 Algorithm Detailing Evaluation of Patients With Bradycardia and Indications for Pacemaker Implantation. In general, pacemaker implantation is indicated for significant bracycardia associated with symptoms. *AV,* Atrioventricular.

coils, which are integrated into the right ventricular endocardial lead. An ICD pulse generator contains not only a microprocessor and a battery but also a high-voltage capacitor. Besides being capable of pacing for bradycardia when necessary, ICDs use therapies for detected ventricular tachyarrhythmias. An ICD considers an episode of tachycardia as a potential malignant ventricular arrhythmia first, based on a preprogrammed rate cutoff. Beyond this, an ICD can distinguish a tachyarrhythmia as ventricular in origin based on the associated activity in the atrium, the rapidity of onset (to distinguish it from sinus tachycardia), the regularity of ventricular activity (to distinguish it from atrial fibrillation with a rapid ventricular response), and the morphology of the ventricular signal. If diagnosed as a ventricular tachyarrhythmia, the ICD may use therapies such as antitachyarrhythmic pacing, low-energy cardioversion, or high-energy defibrillation (Fig. 44.4). These therapies can be tailored to tachycardias in multiple rate tiers, allowing for different treatments for different types of tachycardia. This multitiered therapy helps reduce the need for high-energy defibrillation without compromising ICD efficacy.

DEVICE IMPLANTATION

Endocardial leads are introduced via access through the subclavian, axillary, or cephalic vein, typically on the left side. Epicardial lead placement may be required (if endocardial implantation is not feasible). Epicardial lead placement requires a more invasive surgical approach and is therefore used only when percutaneous endocardial lead

placement is not possible or if a patient needing a pacemaker o- ICD placement is undergoing an open cardiac surgical procedure.

Endocardial leads are positioned and secured in the right atrium, right ventricle, and in the case of biventricular pacing devices, a branch of the coronary sinus, using fluoroscopy. A pacemaker lead typically has two electrodes (bipolar) in contact with the atrial or ventricular myocardium (Fig. 44.5A). A biventricular pacemaker has an additional lead on the epicardium of the lateral left ventricle via the coronary sinus (Fig. 44.5B). Impulses delivered by the pulse generator through these electrodes pace the heart. The additional high-voltage coils of an ICD lead act as shocking electrodes in conjunction with the ICD pulse generator itself (Fig. 44.6). Once positioned, the leads are inserted into the header of the pulse generator, which is implanted into the subcutaneous or submuscular region below the clavicle. The entire procedure can generally be accomplished within 1 to 2 hours, depending on the complexity of the device, under conscious sedation or general anesthesia.

POSTPROCEDURE CARE AND LONG-TERM FOLLOW-UP

Postoperatively, patients are instructed to keep the surgical incision clean and dry for approximately 10 days and to notify their provider of any evidence of infection. They are asked to limit ipsilateral arm use to below shoulder level and to avoid heavy lifting for a few weeks to prevent lead dislodgment and promote wound healing. Driving

Delayed ventricular activation

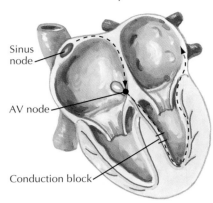

Sinus node

AV node

Conduction block

- Delayed lateral wall contraction
- Disorganized ventricular contraction
- Decreased pumping efficiency
- Increased mitral regurgitation

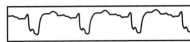

Ventricular resynchronization

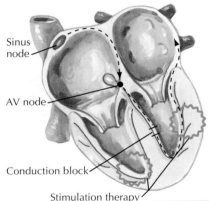

Sinus node

AV node

Conduction block

Stimulation therapy

JOHN A.CRAIG_AD
D. Mascaro

- Organized ventricular activation sequence
- Coordinated septal and free-wall contraction
- Improved pumping efficiency
- Less mitral regurgitation

In patients with conduction block (e.g., left bundle branch block), there is delayed lateral wall electrical activation and mechanical contraction leading to decreased pumping efficiency. By simultaneously pacing the septal and lateral walls of the left ventricle with right ventricular and left ventricular leads (via the coronary sinus), the ventricular walls are "resynchronized," thereby improving pumping efficiency.

FIG 44.2 Benefit of Biventricular Pacing. *AV,* Atrioventricular.

restrictions are typically imposed for approximately 6 months in patients who have had an ICD placed for documented sustained ventricular tachycardia or ventricular fibrillation. Occasionally, it may be reasonable to shorten the driving restrictions. Patients who undergo ICD implantation for primary prevention are generally not restricted from driving. It is recommended that commercial driving be permanently prohibited. Pacemaker and defibrillator patients are ideally monitored remotely through wireless technology over the internet by a central device clinic. Remote monitoring allows for near continuous monitoring for adverse events, including malignant arrhythmias and device malfunction. More extensive evaluation including battery voltage, lead integrity testing, and electrographic evaluation of arrhythmic events can be done remotely on a quarterly basis or for urgent evaluation of patient symptoms.

Remote monitoring has been demonstrated to reduce both morbidity and mortality in long-term follow-up.

The management of a single ICD shock does not necessarily require an emergent office or emergency department visit. Although an ICD shock can be an anxiety-provoking experience, occasional shocks are to be expected. In the event of a single shock, a patient who is otherwise well should be reassured and referred for evaluation within the week. However, if the shock is associated with worrisome symptoms such as syncope, shortness of breath, persistent palpitations, or chest pain, or if a patient experiences multiple ICD shocks over a short period of time, an emergency department visit is required. In the event of an ICD shock, the appropriateness of ICD therapy should be determined by evaluation of stored recordings in the ICD. Any potentially reversible cause should be treated. Otherwise, management often requires optimization of ICD programming, the use of antiarrhythmic agents, or catheter ablation.

Electromagnetic Interference

Electromagnetic interference occurs when a source emits electromagnetic waves that interfere with the proper function of the device. It is important for individuals with pacemakers or ICDs to avoid any sources of electromagnetic interference. That said, with recent advances in pacemaker and ICD technology there are relatively few devices that interfere with their function. There is no restriction on the use of household items such as microwaves, televisions, radios, or electric blankets because these are not sources of electromagnetic interference. Although passage through a metal detector will not harm ICD or pacemaker function, it is recommended that patients with these devices not be in close contact with handheld metal detectors or scanning wands that contain magnets. Instead, patients are advised to present their device identification card to security personnel and request a hand search. Cellular telephone use is not prohibited, although patients are advised to use the phone on the contralateral ear (>10 cm from the device) and not to carry the phone in the breast pocket on top of the implanted device. Electronic article surveillance systems are not likely to cause a negative interaction with an implanted device as long as the patient is not standing close to the scanning system for a prolonged period of time. Patients are instructed to walk normally through such devices.

Medical sources of potential electromagnetic interference include MRI scanners, radiation therapy, transthoracic cardioversion, and electrocautery. The effect of a strong magnetic field differs for pacemakers and ICDs: pacemaker exposure to an electromagnetic field usually results in asynchronous pacing (i.e., VOO); and exposure of an ICD can result in "blinding" of the device, which potentially results in inappropriate withholding of therapy for tachyarrhythmias. MRI scans are generally contraindicated in patients with implanted devices. Direct radiation (i.e., radiation therapy) that focuses on the area where an implanted pacemaker or ICD is present is not recommended; if necessary, the device should be moved to the opposite side and shielded from the direct beam. Implanted ICDs and pacemakers should be evaluated before and after electrical cardioversion, and the external electrodes used for cardioversion (anterior–posterior position) should be positioned as far as possible (>5 cm) from the implanted device. Surgical electrocautery presents unique concerns for the ICD patient, because electrical output from the cautery can be mistakenly detected by the ICD, resulting in inappropriate delivery of therapy during a normal rhythm. Hence, the detection function of the ICD should be inactivated before any surgery or procedure during which electrocautery may be used. Electrocautery may also interfere with pacemaker sensing and inhibit output. In the pacemaker-dependent patient, the pacemaker should be programmed to asynchronous mode; otherwise, the anesthesiologist may need to apply a magnet to the pacemaker to provide asynchronous pacing. In

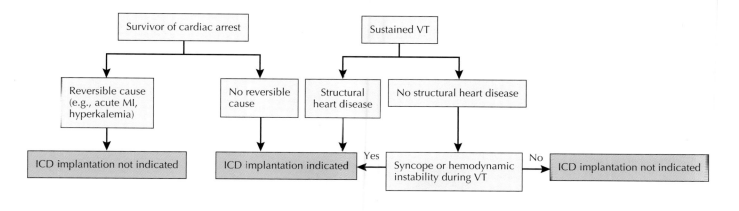

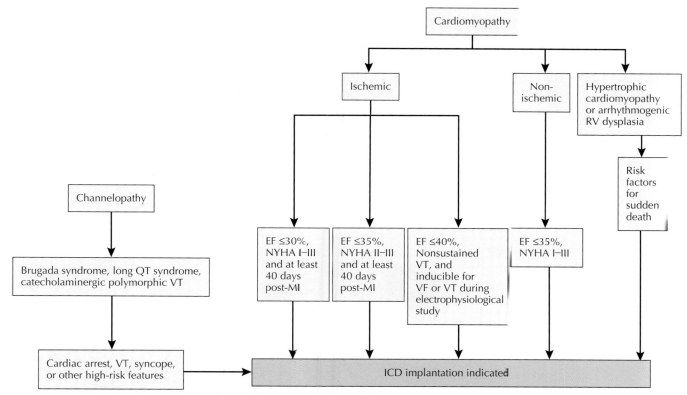

FIG 44.3 Algorithm Detailing Evaluation of Patients With Sudden Cardiac Death and/or Tachyarrhythmias and Indications for Implantable Cardiac Defibrillator (ICD) Implantation. In general, ICD implantation is indicated for secondary prophylaxis in survivors of cardiac arrest or hemodynamically significant sustained ventricular tachycardia (VT). ICDs are indicated for primary prophylaxis in patients with cardiomyopathy or channelopathies of various etiologies and risk factors for sudden death. *EF*, Ejection fraction; *MI*, myocardial infarction; *NYHA*, New York Heart Association (functional class); *RV*, right ventricular; *VF*, ventricular fibrillation.

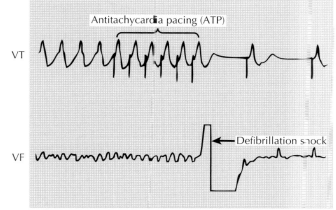

FIG 44.4 Therapy for Ventricular Tachycardia (VT). *VF*, Ventricular fibrillation.

In the situation of VT, burst rapid ventricular pacing at a rate faster than the rate of the VT (known as antitachycardia pacing) will often terminate VT. In the situation of VF, a high-voltage defibrillation shock is delivered through defibrillation coils positioned on the right ventricular lead to terminate the arrhythmia.

A. Dual-chamber pacing

The endocardial leads are usually introduced via the subclavian or the cephalic vein (left or right side), then positioned and tested

A pocket for the pulse generator is commonly made below the midclavicle adjacent to the venous access for the pacing leads. The incision is parallel to the inferior clavicular border, approximately 1 inch below it.

The pulse generator is placed either into the deep subcutaneous tissue just above the prepectoralis fascia, or into the submuscular region of the muscle pectoralis major

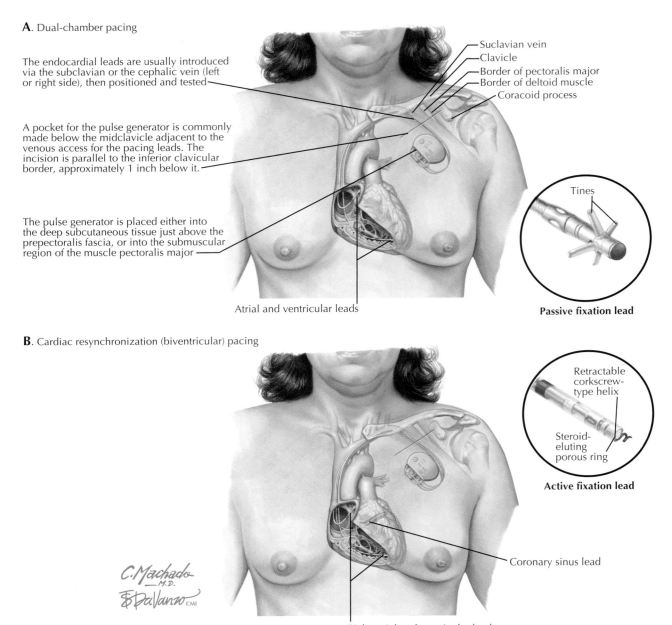

Suclavian vein
Clavicle
Border of pectoralis major
Border of deltoid muscle
Coracoid process

Tines

Passive fixation lead

Atrial and ventricular leads

B. Cardiac resynchronization (biventricular) pacing

Retractable corkscrew-type helix

Steroid-eluting porous ring

Active fixation lead

C.Machado
— M.D.
BDaVanzo CMI

Coronary sinus lead

Right atrial and ventricular leads

The leads connecting the pulse generator to the endocardium can be different types: unipolar or bipolar and of active fixation or passive fixation. The unipolar system has a single electrode (cathode, negative pole) in contact with the endocardium, and the anode is the pulse generator itself. The bipolar system lead has both a cathode and an anode at the tip of the same lead. Passive fixation leads have tines, barbs that anchor the lead to the endocardial trabecular muscle of the chamber in which it is implanted. Active fixation leads have a corkscrew-type device or helix that is placed into the myocardium. Both types irritate the myocardium, causing inflammatory reaction and cellular growth around the lead. To minimize the inflammatory reaction, most leads have steroid-eluting tips. The coronary sinus lead allows for "resynchronization" of disorganized ventricular contraction in selected patients with impaired cardiac function and conduction block.

FIG 44.5 Implantable Cardiac Pacemaker.

In all aspects, the surgical procedure for ICD implantation is very similar to that of cardiac pacemaker implantation. The venous access and the "pocket" for the pulse generator in the subcutaneous region above the prepectoralis fascia or in the submuscular region below the midclavicle are the same as those used for pacemaker implants.

Due to the number of functions the ICD can perform (cardioverter, defibrillator, and pacemaker), the ICD is usually slightly larger than a pacemaker. The surface of the ICD functions as one of the electrodes of the defibrillation system.

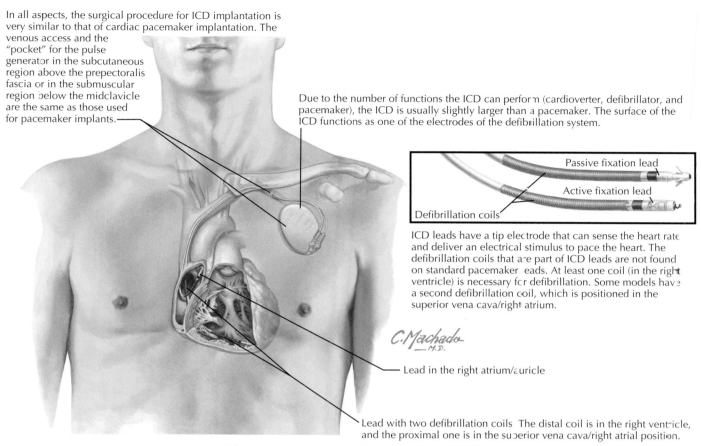

Passive fixation lead

Active fixation lead

Defibrillation coils

ICD leads have a tip electrode that can sense the heart rate and deliver an electrical stimulus to pace the heart. The defibrillation coils that are part of ICD leads are not found on standard pacemaker leads. At least one coil (in the right ventricle) is necessary for defibrillation. Some models have a second defibrillation coil, which is positioned in the superior vena cava/right atrium.

C.Machado
_M.D.

Lead in the right atrium/auricle

Lead with two defibrillation coils The distal coil is in the right ventricle, and the proximal one is in the superior vena cava/right atrial position.

FIG 44.6 Implantable Cardiac Defibrillator (ICD).

addition, it is recommended that the rate-responsive feature be disabled. In a patient who is not pacemaker-dependent, no reprogramming aside from disabling the rate-responsive feature is necessary. Electrocautery in close proximity to an older pacemaker may render it nonoperational. It is recommended that postoperative ECGs, with and without magnet application, be performed after the use of electrocautery to confirm proper pacemaker function.

"LEADLESS" TECHNOLOGY

Recent innovations in device technology allow for "leadless" management of both tachyarrhythmias and bradyarrhythmias. A completely subcutaneous defibrillator has recently been approved for management of patients at risk for malignant ventricular arrhythmias. However, this subcutaneous device is not capable of long-term pacing. A "bullet-like" device with a self-contained pulse generator can be implanted in the right ventricular apex to allow for leadless pacing. These subcutaneous or leadless pacing devices preclude the need for transvenous leads. Because transvenous leads may deteriorate over time or lead to venous occlusion, necessitating lead extraction, leadless technology has distinct advantages. Future advances may incorporate both leadless pacing and defibrillation, potentially with multichamber pacing capabilities, allowing for fully leadless systems for all bradyarrhythmia or tachyarrhythmia indications.

FUTURE DIRECTIONS

Advances in pacemaker and ICD technology have substantially improved survival and quality of life for patients with cardiac arrhythmias. In the future, indications for ICD therapy will probably expand as proper identification of patients at risk for future ventricular tachyarrhythmic events improves (see Fig. 44.3). In addition, enhanced functionality is continuously being added to modern devices.

EVIDENCE

Abraham WT, Fisher WG, Smith AL, et al. Cardiac resynchronization in chronic heart failure. *N Engl J Med.* 2002;346:1845–1853.
One of the early seminal studies of cardiac resynchronization therapy that demonstrated clinical improvement in patients with moderate-to-severe heart failure and intraventricular conduction delay.
AVID Investigators. A comparison of antiarrhythmic-drug therapy with implantable defibrillators in patients resuscitated from near-fatal ventricular arrhythmias. *N Engl J Med.* 1997;337:1576–1583.
This article demonstrates the clear benefit of implantable defibrillators in patients who were successfully resuscitated from near-fatal ventricular arrhythmias.
Epstein AE, DiMarco JP, Ellenbogen KA, et al. ACC/AHA/HRS 2008 guidelines for device-based therapy of cardiac rhythm abnormalities. *J Am Coll Cardiol.* 2008;51:1–62.

A consensus statement of guidelines for device-based management of cardiac rhythm disturbances.

Gehi AK, Mehta D, Gomes JA. Evaluation and management of patients after implantable cardioverter-defibrillator shock. *JAMA.* 2006;296:2839–2847.

A review article discussing the evaluation and management of patients who receive a shock from their implantable defibrillator.

Kusumoto FM, Goldschlager N. Cardiac pacing. *N Engl J Med.* 1996;334:89–97.

A review article discussing indications, function, and management of cardiac pacemakers.

Mangrum JM, DiMarco JP. The evaluation and management of bradycardia. *N Engl J Med.* 2000;342:703–709.

Review article describing the anatomy and pathology of the conduction system of the heart.

Moss AJ, Zareba W, Hall WJ, et al. Prophylactic implantation of a defibrillator in patients with myocardial infarction and reduced ejection fraction. *N Engl J Med.* 2002;346:877–883.

Seminal article demonstrating the benefit of implantable defibrillators for primary prophylaxis in patients with previous myocardial infarction who have a severely reduced ejection fraction.

Valvular Heart Disease

45

Aortic Valve Disease

Timothy A. Mixon, Gregory J. Dehmer

The aortic valve is a semilunar valve that includes three pocket-like cusps of approximately equal size. The normal aortic valve opens completely during systole, allowing ejection of blood from the left ventricle (LV), whereas closure during diastole prevents retrograde blood flow from the aorta into the LV. Dysfunction of the valve can lead to either impairment of LV outflow or valvular incompetence with regurgitation, either of which reduce effective forward cardiac output.

AORTIC STENOSIS

Etiology and Pathogenesis

LV outflow may be limited due to abnormalities of the aortic valve or narrowing of the outflow tract either above or below the aortic valve. The most common cause of LV outflow obstruction is valvular aortic stenosis (AS). However, nonvalvular obstruction of LV outflow may result from a congenital abnormality, such as a membrane either above or below the valve, or hypertrophic obstructive cardiomyopathy (HOCM) (see Chapter 30).

The etiology of valvular AS varies with the age of the patient at presentation. In childhood, congenital abnormalities predominate, including valves that are unicuspid, bicuspid, or rarely, even quadricuspid (Fig. 45.1). Unicuspid valves usually are severely narrowed at birth and produce symptoms in infancy. Bicuspid valves rarely cause symptoms during childhood but may undergo progressive calcification, which leads to detectable stenosis between 40 and 70 years of age. One study found two-thirds of aortic valve replacements (AVRs) for AS in patients aged younger than 70 years were due to a bicuspid valve. Calcific degeneration of a previously normal tricuspid valve predominates in patients diagnosed after age 70 years, with a prevalence of 3% to 5% in patients older than 75 years old (Fig. 45.2).

Rheumatic involvement of the aortic valve is currently rare in the United States and typically results in a combination of stenosis and regurgitation, usually with concomitant mitral valve disease. The rheumatic valve is characterized by commissural fusion and calcification, whereas the more common degenerative AS shows calcification progressing from the base of the cusps toward the leaflets and sparing the commissures (see Fig. 45.2). Rheumatic AS generally presents between ages 30 and 50 years. Less common causes of AS include obstructive vegetations from endocarditis, radiation therapy, rheumatoid involvement with severe nodular thickening of the leaflets, and systemic diseases, including Paget disease, Fabry disease, ochronosis, and end-stage renal disease.

Bicuspid aortic valve disease merits special consideration because of its prevalence (~1.3%) in the general population and the association of bicuspid aortic valve disease with ascending aortic dilatation (range: 20%–80% in various studies). Aortopathy is believed to develop based on both genetic and hemodynamic factors. Due to the propensity for aortic dilatation, imaging of the aorta is indicated in patients with a bicuspid aortic valve, and consultation with a specialized surgical center is recommended if the aorta measures >4.5 cm.

Clinical Presentation

AS is asymptomatic for years. Progressive pressure overload imposed by the valve stenosis results in concentric LV hypertrophy (LVH). This compensatory adaptation lowers wall stress and maintains forward flow but also leads to detrimental effects, including an abnormal diastolic filling pattern and subendocardial ischemia.

Classic symptoms of AS are angina, syncope, and dyspnea, with the latter being a manifestation of congestive heart failure (CHF). Based on natural history studies, the average survival without valve replacement is 5 and 3 years in patients who present with angina or syncope, respectively. The most concerning presentation is CHF, because those patients have an average survival without valve replacement of <2 years. In contemporary trials, survival is even worse among patients with AS who also have other co-morbidities.

Angina occurs in two-thirds of patients with severe AS, and approximately one-half of these have significant coronary artery disease (CAD). In the absence of significant CAD, angina is caused by subendocardial ischemia due to increased wall thickness, prolonged ejection time, and increased LV end-diastolic pressure.

Syncope may arise from various mechanisms. During physical exertion, systemic vascular resistance declines, whereas the necessary increase in cardiac output is blunted by the fixed valvular obstruction, which results in systemic hypoperfusion. Common arrhythmias such as atrial fibrillation may result in syncope due to a decline in cardiac output because the atrial contribution to cardiac output is more important in the presence of LVH. Finally, life-threatening arrhythmias, such as ventricular tachycardia or fibrillation, although uncommon, may occur at rest or with exertion, leading to the potential for sudden cardiac death.

Initially, CHF symptoms are mostly from diastolic dysfunction (heart failure with preserved ejection fraction). Later, systolic dysfunction with progressive ventricular dilatation may occur, with a rapid worsening of symptoms. To compensate for the LV pressure load, the left atrium (LA) hypertrophies and develops vigorous contractions that support LV filling by elevating LV end-diastolic pressure without necessarily increasing mean LA pressure. However, as the disease progresses, or with physical activity, LA pressure increases further, leading to higher pulmonary venous pressures and eventually to pulmonary congestion and edema. Pulmonary edema may develop abruptly during activity or with the loss of atrial function, as in atrial fibrillation.

Other clinical manifestations of AS include gastrointestinal bleeding from angiodysplasia (so-called Heyde syndrome), which is associated with a mild form of acquired von Willebrand disease, embolic events (including stroke) from detachment of small calcium deposits, or infective endocarditis (see Chapter 49) with its associated complications.

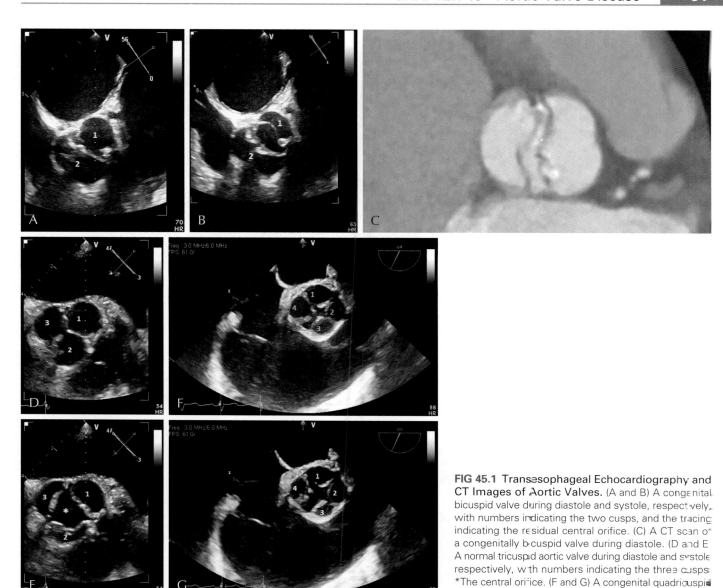

FIG 45.1 Transesophageal Echocardiography and CT Images of Aortic Valves. (A and B) A congenital bicuspid valve during diastole and systole, respectively, with numbers indicating the two cusps, and the tracing indicating the residual central orifice. (C) A CT scan of a congenitally bicuspid valve during diastole. (D and E) A normal tricuspid aortic valve during diastole and systole respectively, with numbers indicating the three cusps. *The central orifice. (F and G) A congenital quadricuspid valve during diastole and systole respectively.

Physical Examination

There are three key focus areas in the physical examination: evaluation of the carotid artery, auscultation of the murmur and second heart sound, and evaluation for signs of CHF. With severe AS, the carotid artery has a diminished pulsation and slowed upstroke (pulsus parvus et tardus), with the maximum carotid upstroke noticeably delayed after the apical impulse (Fig. 45.3). A marked vibration or "thrill" may also be felt. These abnormal carotid findings are fairly specific for severe AS, but are not seen in all patients.

The first heart sound is usually normal, but the second heart sound has a reduced aortic closure sound or may be single because the pulmonic closure sound is unaffected; in severe cases, it may be paradoxically split from the marked delay of LV ejection. The murmur of AS may be preceded by an early systolic ejection click, heard more frequently with a bicuspid valve or a congenital form of AS in which the leaflets have preserved pliability. The murmur is characteristically crescendo–decrescendo, harsh in quality, located at the upper sternal border, with transmission into the carotids. High-frequency resonation

may be heard at the apex (Gallavardin phenomenon) and can be mistaken for mitral regurgitation (MR). With worsening AS, the murmur peaks later during systole, which is consistent with delayed LV ejection. There is often a fourth heart sound (S_4), which reflects the reduced LV compliance during atrial contraction, and a third heart sound (S_3) if LV dysfunction has developed.

The jugular venous pressure is not elevated unless CHF is present. Late in the disease, a prominent "v" wave may occur from tricuspid insufficiency caused by pulmonary hypertension and bulging of the hypertrophied septum into the right ventricle. As the stenosis severity progresses, the LV apical impulse is displaced inferiorly and laterally, with a palpable presystolic pulsation (palpable S_4).

With aging, the aortic valve leaflets can become thickened and calcified with slightly reduced mobility but without hemodynamically significant stenosis, which is a condition termed aortic sclerosis. The murmur of aortic sclerosis is similar to that in AS but tends to be an early peaking murmur with normal carotid pulsations. Aortic sclerosis, while not directly leading to serious sequelae, has been associated with a significantly higher prevalence of CAD and cardiovascular mortality.

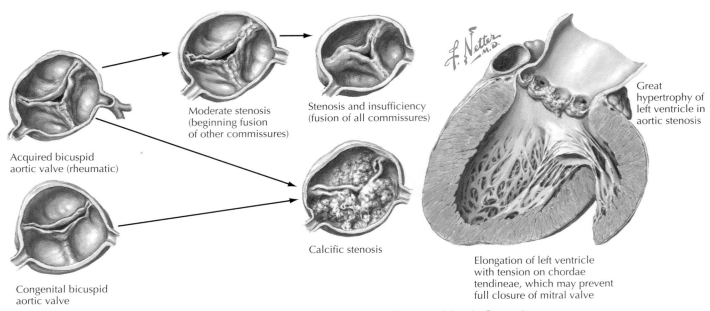

FIG 45.2 Rheumatic and Nonrheumatic Causes of Aortic Stenosis.

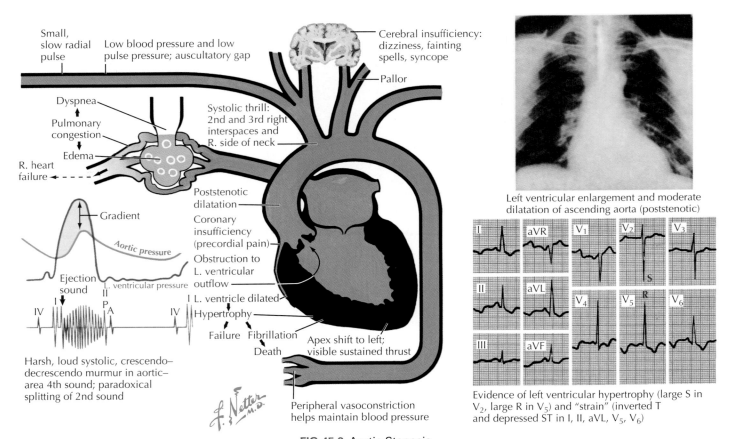

FIG 45.3 Aortic Stenosis.

Differential Diagnosis

Differentiation of valvular AS from other causes of LV outflow tract obstruction is important, because treatment and prognosis differ. Subvalvular and supravalvular outflow tract obstruction may be due to a discrete fibrous membrane. It is important to distinguish the murmur of MR and HOCM from that of AS. The MR murmur is holosystolic, with a more musical quality and constant intensity despite variations in cardiac cycle length. In contrast, the murmur of AS is accentuated after pauses, such as after a premature ventricular contraction or long cycles in atrial fibrillation. The outflow murmur associated with HOCM

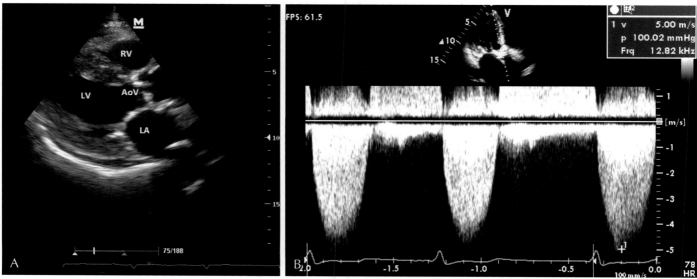

FIG 45.4 Two-Dimensional Echocardiography and Doppler Analysis in a Patient With Aortic Stenosis. (A) A parasternal long-axis view of the heart including the left ventricle *(LV)*, left atrium *(LA)*, right ventricle *(RV)*, and aortic valve *(AoV)*. (B) A continuous-wave Doppler signal across the valve in an apical long axis image, showing a peak velocity of 5 m/s, representing a peak transvalvular gradient of 100 mm Hg.

TABLE 45.1 Echocardiographic Assessment of the Severity of Aortic Valve Stenosis

Degree of Stenosis[a]	Aortic Valve Area (cm^2)	Mean Pressure Gradient (mm Hg)	Aortic Jet Velocity (m/s)
Mild	≥1.5	<20	<3.0
Moderate	1.0–1.5	20–39	3.0–3.9
Severe	<1.0	≥40	>4.0

[a]Instead of relying on one single value, assessment of aortic stenosis is best viewed as a continuum, with integration of multiple measurements necessary to accurately characterize severity.

often sounds similar to that of AS and increases in intensity after premature ventricular contractions, but responds uniquely to provocative maneuvers. In contrast to valvular AS, the murmur of HOCM becomes more prominent with decreasing preload, such as the straining phase of the Valsalva maneuver or standing upright. Furthermore, the carotid upstroke in HOCM is rapid and may have a bisferious (double peak) quality.

Diagnostic Approach

Two-dimensional echocardiography with Doppler is the most useful and common test for evaluating suspected AS. A complete transthoracic echocardiogram can identify the location of the aortic outflow obstruction, estimate the severity of valvular obstruction, and provide information about LV function, the degree of LVH, LA size, and the presence or absence of associated valvular abnormalities (Fig. 45.4). Doppler interrogation across the aortic valve reliably provides the transvalvular mean and peak pressure gradients (Table 45.1). The transvalvular gradient depends on the severity of the stenosis and the flow volume across the valve, which may vary depending on factors such as exercise, anxiety, anemia, hypovolemia, concomitant aortic regurgitation, and LV systolic function. Transvalvular gradients are reported as a mean or a peak

instantaneous gradient. In general, a peak transvalvular gradient >64 mm Hg (4.0 m/s) or a mean transvalvular gradient >40 mm Hg is consistent with severe AS. Aortic valve area (AVA) is estimated by the continuity equation or measured directly by planimetry. Because the pressure gradient can vary considerably under different conditions, the calculated AVA is generally believed to be a more reliable measure of severity than the pressure gradient alone. An AVA <1.0 cm^2 or an index of <0.6 cm^2/m^2 suggest severe AS. One pitfall is relying solely on Doppler-derived AVA without visualization of the valve for calcification and altered mobility. An increased outflow tract gradient due to HOCM can be mistaken for valvular AS and lead to an inappropriate referral for AVR. In patients with poor acoustic windows, transesophageal echocardiography may provide better visualization to corroborate Doppler findings; some centers have expertise in using cardiac CT and cardiac magnetic resonance imaging to confirm the diagnosis.

Because of the relationship of flow and pressure across the valve, some patients with low cardiac output have a low mean transvalvular pressure gradient (20–40 mm Hg) despite having significant AS. Valve area calculations appear mismatched, with a small AVA but an unexpectedly low gradient. This may be observed in a few clinical situations that are important to differentiate, so the correct treatment is chosen. Repeat measurements during a low-dose dobutamine infusion is often helpful. If severe AS exists, but the cause of the low gradient is significant LV systolic dysfunction, dobutamine will often increase the cardiac output by producing a peak velocity of >4.0 m/s, whereas the AVA remains at <1.0 cm^2 (low-flow, low-gradient AS). If the increase in cardiac output causes a substantial increase in the calculated AVA with no change in transvalvular gradient, the clinical problem is likely a cardiomyopathy, rather than AS (pseudo-AS). In some cases, no augmentation of LV function, and hence, cardiac output is observed, indicating a lack of contractile reserve, making the assessment of AS severity more problematic (this variant of low-flow, low-gradient AS is likely to have a worse prognosis due to the lack of contractile reserve after AVR). Finally, it has now been recognized that low-flow, low-gradient AS can occur without LV systolic dysfunction, which is often caused by LVH with small LV cavity size, severe diastolic dysfunction, and even significant MR. In these cases, dobutamine testing is not helpful; CT assessment of aortic valve calcification, demonstration of an AVA indexed to body surface area (<0.6 cm^2/m^2), and a reduced stroke volume index (<35 mL/m^2) help confirm the diagnosis.

Other Diagnostic Modalities

The ECG most commonly shows sinus rhythm until late in the disease course. The most common ECG findings are LVH ($>80\%$) and LA hypertrophy. Less common findings are ST-segment depression in leads V$_4$ through V$_6$ (strain pattern) and conduction system disease.

A chest x-ray usually shows a normal-sized cardiac silhouette, because the LV may be hypertrophied, but it is usually not grossly dilated unless end-stage CHF is present. Other findings could include LA enlargement, signs of pulmonary venous congestion, and poststenotic dilatation of the ascending aorta.

Coronary angiography is necessary to identify CAD and is indicated for all patients aged older than 35 years who require AVR or who have two or more risk factors for CAD. Invasive hemodynamic measurements are no longer necessary if a good quality echocardiogram is available and historical, physical examination, and echocardiographic findings are in agreement. However, when there is discordant or inconclusive information, right- and left-sided heart catheterizations are indicated to obtain pressure gradients and to measure cardiac output.

If echocardiography is nondiagnostic, cardiac CT or MRI may serve as alternatives for diagnosing AS severity. Cardiac CT or MRI also accurately and reproducibly assess the aortic root, if enlargement is suspected; serial examinations are indicated if enlargement is identified, with aortic root replacement considered when the diameter is >5.1 to 5.5 cm or is >4.5 cm if AVR is independently indicated. MRI is also useful for assessing LV volume, function, and mass.

Management and Therapy
Optimum Treatment

AVR is indicated in adults with severe and symptomatic AS. Medical therapy for valvular AS is limited to treatment of complications, such as CHF, rhythm disturbances, and infective endocarditis. Heart failure from LV systolic dysfunction is treated in the usual fashion (see Chapter 29). Systemic hypertension should be controlled. Investigations have failed to show a role for specific drugs to slow the progression of AS.

Atrial fibrillation may occur late in the disease course and can lead to significant hemodynamic deterioration. It is treated in the usual manner, with emphasis on the maintenance of sinus rhythm, if symptomatic, and anticoagulation as indicated, based on usual assessment tools for the risk of stroke. In patients presenting with atrial fibrillation and hemodynamic compromise, urgent electrical cardioversion is indicated.

Volume depletion should be avoided, because it reduces LV filling pressures and may lead to severe hypotension. Volume depletion can develop with aggressive diuresis but can also occur during or after noncardiac surgery from the effects of anesthesia or bleeding. Aggressive volume and blood replacement may be necessary to reverse the clinical deterioration. Caution is needed if arterial vasodilators or venodilators such as nitroglycerin are used because they can easily cause hypotension.

Infective endocarditis occurs more frequently with congenital valvular abnormalities and prosthetic valves, and is less common with senile, calcific AS. Endocarditis prophylaxis is no longer recommended in native AS unless other risk factors are present. Patients with moderate to severe degrees of outflow tract obstruction should not engage in vigorous, unsupervised exercise.

Aortic Valve Replacement

AVR is indicated for the treatment of symptomatic AS, and is covered in Chapter 54. In general, AVR can be delayed until symptoms develop, although some centers advocate for earlier valve replacement. Asymptomatic patients with severe AS generally have an acceptable course and prognosis without valve replacement, with a rate of sudden death of $<1\%$ per year, which is lower than formerly feared. However, close clinical follow-up is needed, because less than one-half are free of cardiac symptoms at 5 years without AVR.

Future Directions

Ongoing studies are exploring potential causes of AS in an attempt to find therapies that can alter the natural history. Multidisciplinary valve teams have brought transcatheter AVR (TAVR) into the mainstream for inoperable, high risk, and intermediate surgical risk patients. Current studies are comparing surgical AVR to TAVR in low-risk patients, and additional trials are planned. Innovative surgical techniques are also being explored to minimize incisions and improve patient recovery after surgical AVR.

AORTIC REGURGITATION

Aortic valve regurgitation (AR) results in impaired cardiac output and volume overload of the LV. The distinction between acute and chronic forms of AR is important because this informs etiologies, associated diseases, prognosis, and treatment.

Etiology and Pathogenesis

Etiologies of chronic AR may be broadly categorized based on one of two structural defects—those involving the valve cusps or those involving the aortic root.

Common causes of acute AR include ascending aortic dissection with distortion of the normal valve architecture, infective endocarditis, traumatic disruption, and spontaneous rupture or prolapse of a valve cusp secondary to degenerative diseases of the valve. Acute AR also may occur with sudden dehiscence of the sewing ring of a prosthetic valve and after balloon valvuloplasty.

Aortic Valve and/or Leaflet Pathology

The most common cause of valve or leaflet disease is infective endocarditis; other causes include rheumatic heart disease, congenital abnormalities of the aortic valve (especially bicuspid valves), calcific or myxomatous degenerative disease, traumatic leaflet disruption, or perivalvular leak. Infective endocarditis may cause AR by several mechanisms, including (1) perforation of a single leaflet or a flail leaflet, and (2) weakening of the cusp and valve annulus as a result of an expanding aortic root abscess. Rheumatic disease is characterized by shortening and scarring of the cusps and is frequently accompanied by mitral valve involvement.

Aortic Root Diseases

Aortic root disease is responsible for approximately 50% of cases of AR. Common aortic root problems include connective tissue disorders (such as Marfan syndrome, Loeys-Dietz syndrome, and type IV Ehler-Danlos) that may lead to annuloaortic ectasia or ascending aortic dissection, and resulting distortion of valve structure and/or weakened support of the aortic valve leaflets (Fig. 45.5). In long-standing systemic hypertension, AR may occur from dilatation of the ascending aorta.

Less common causes of AR include syphilitic aortitis, ankylosing spondylitis, osteogenesis imperfecta, systemic lupus erythematosus, rheumatoid arthritis, psoriatic arthritis, Behçet syndrome, ulcerative

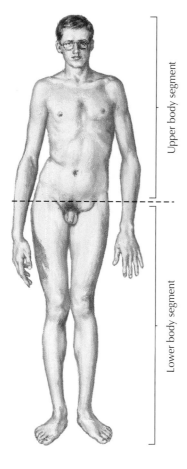

Tall, thin person with skeletal disproportion. Upper body segment (top of head to pubis) shorter than lower body segment (pubis to soles of feet). Fingertips reach almost to knees (arm span-to-height ratio greater than 1.05). Long, thin fingers (arachnodactyly). Scoliosis, chest deformity, inguinal hernia, flatfoot

Upper body segment

Lower body segment

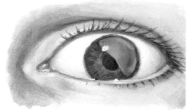

Ectopia lentis (upward and temporal displacement of eye lens). Retinal detachment, myopia, and other ocular complications may occur

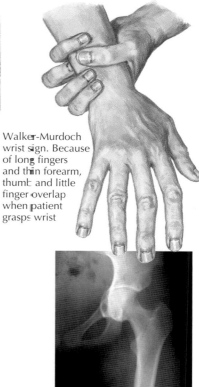

Walker-Murdoch wrist sign. Because of long fingers and thin forearm, thumb and little finger overlap when patient grasps wrist

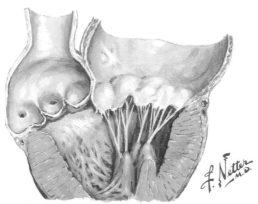

Dilatation of aortic ring and aneurysm of ascending aorta due to cystic medial necrosis cause aortic regurgitation. Mitral valve prolapse causes regurgitation. Heart failure is common.

Radiograph shows acetabular protrusion (unilateral or bilateral)

FIG 45.5 Aortic Regurgitation in Marfan Syndrome.

colitis, discrete subaortic stenosis, and ventricular septal defect with prolapse of an aortic cusp (Fig. 45.6).

Natural History

The natural history of chronic AR is incompletely known. Data from the presurgical era indicate that patients with chronic severe AR who had angina or heart failure had a prognosis similar to those with severe AS, with mortality rates of at least 10% to 20% per year. Asymptomatic patients with normal LV function developed symptoms of LV dysfunction at a rate of approximately 4% annually, but the occurrence of sudden death was rare (<0.2% per year). However, 25% of patients who died or progressed to LV dysfunction did so before manifesting symptoms, emphasizing the importance of serial quantitative assessments of LV function. Asymptomatic patients who developed LV dysfunction had higher event rates, with >25% developing symptoms annually.

In contrast, the natural history of acute AR—especially if severe—is dire, with morbid complications such as pulmonary edema and cardiogenic shock that may be refractory to intensive medical therapy. In such cases, early mortality is high even with urgent surgical repair.

Clinical Presentation

Clinical presentation of AR varies with the onset (acute or chronic) and the degree to which compensatory changes have occurred within the LV in response to volume overload (Table 45.2). In acute AR, the presentation is usually dramatic. Compensatory LV dilatation has not yet developed, so LV compliance is normal and remains so despite the

sudden regurgitation. The acute volume overload is poorly tolerated, because the LV is abruptly and markedly distended, resulting in impaired systolic function and severely increased LV diastolic pressure, which, in turn, causes severely increased LA and pulmonary capillary wedge pressures, with resultant pulmonary edema. Forward cardiac output is reduced, and sinus tachycardia develops in an attempt to augment cardiac output. Because of these changes, the patient with acute AR usually appears severely ill, manifesting tachycardia, hypotension, peripheral vasoconstriction, and pulmonary edema, but lacks many of the classic signs seen with chronic regurgitation.

Chronic AR may be asymptomatic for years. When symptoms develop, they are usually indolent, reflecting the slow, progressive nature of the disease. Frequent complaints include exertional dyspnea, orthopnea, paroxysmal nocturnal dyspnea, angina pectoris, and palpitations. As AR develops, the LV slowly dilates, with an increase in end-diastolic volume and chamber compliance plus hypertrophy (Fig. 45.7). In the early phases of chronic AR, the increased end-diastolic volume is not associated with major increases in end-diastolic pressure. The resulting increased stroke volume maintains a normal forward cardiac output, usually without substantial increases in heart rate despite the regurgitation. The augmented aortic systolic pressure from the increased stroke volume plus the lower aortic diastolic pressure from regurgitation into the LV results in a wide pulse pressure, leading to many of the classic findings of chronic AR (Table 45.3; see Fig. 45.7). During exercise, the systemic vascular resistance and diastolic filling period decrease, resulting in less regurgitation per beat, which leads to increased forward cardiac output without substantial increases in LV end-diastolic pressure.

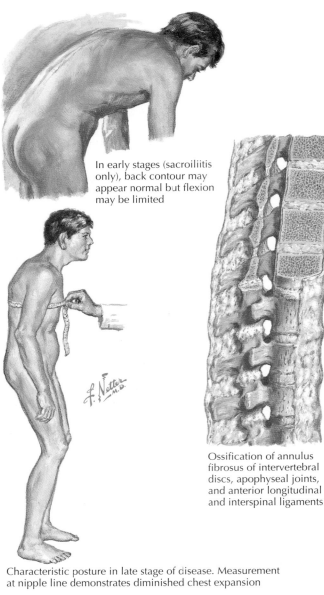

In early stages (sacroiliitis only), back contour may appear normal but flexion may be limited

Ossification of annulus fibrosus of intervertebral discs, apophyseal joints, and anterior longitudinal and interspinal ligaments

Characteristic posture in late stage of disease. Measurement at nipple line demonstrates diminished chest expansion

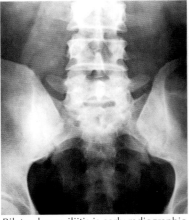

Bilateral sacroiliitis is early radiographic sign. Thinning of cartilage and bone condensation on both sides of sacroiliac joints

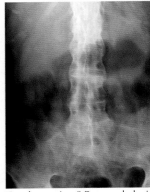

"Bamboo spine." Bony ankylosis of joints of lumbar spine. Ossification exaggerates bulges of intervertebral disks

Complications

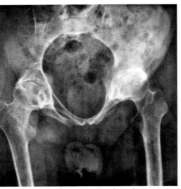

Radiograph shows complete bony ankylosis of both sacroiliac joints in late stage of disease

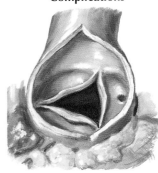

Dilatation of aortic ring with valvular regurgitation

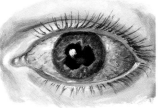

Iridocyclitis with irregular pupil due to synechiae

FIG 45.6 Aortic Regurgitation in Ankylosing Spondylitis.

With time and worsening regurgitation, the ability of the LV to compensate for the chronic volume overload is exceeded, and LV systolic failure develops. As the LV ejection fraction decreases, the ventricle dilates further, initiating a vicious cycle that eventually leads to the typical symptoms of CHF, which may become irreversible.

Physical Examination
Acute Aortic Regurgitation

In acute severe AR, systolic blood pressure is normal or decreased, and diastolic blood pressure is slightly elevated, which results in a pulse pressure that is normal or slightly narrowed. Although tachycardia is usually present, the precordium is relatively quiet. The first heart sound is soft because of premature closure of the mitral valve and may be absent in severe AR. The second heart sound is also soft, and a third heart sound is frequently present due to rapid early diastolic filling of the LV. In contrast to chronic AR, the diastolic murmur of acute regurgitation is often short, only heard in early diastole, and is soft in intensity

or even absent in severe cases. This occurs because diastolic flow across the valve stops when the aortic diastolic pressure equalizes with the rapidly rising LV diastolic pressure. A systolic murmur may also be present but is usually not particularly loud because of the reduced forward output.

Chronic Aortic Regurgitation

In chronic compensated AR, increased carotid pulse volumes may be accompanied by a bruit or transmitted systolic murmur. Peripheral pulses are bounding as a result of the high stroke volume and wide pulse pressure, with systolic hypertension and a low diastolic blood pressure. The LV apical impulse is enlarged, forceful, and displaced inferiorly and laterally. The first heart sound is normal or soft, and the second heart sound may be normal, single, or paradoxically split. Ejection clicks may be heard, especially in patients with a dilated aortic root. A fourth heart sound can be detected as LV hypertrophy develops, and a third heart sound occurs later in the clinical course of AR when

TABLE 45.2   Hemodynamic Features of the Stages of Severe Aortic Regurgitation

	Acute Severe Regurgitation	Chronic, Severe Regurgitation (compensated)	Chronic, Severe Regurgitation (late decompensation)
LV compliance[a]	Not increased	Increased	No longer increased
LVEDP	↑↑↑	Normal	↑↑↑
LV dimensions	Normal	↑↑	↑↑
Aortic SBP	Normal or low	↑	Normal or low
Aortic DBP	Normal	↓↓	Normal
Pulse pressure	Normal to ↓	↑↑↑	Normal
LVEF	Normal	Normal to ↑	↓ to ↓↓↓
Total stroke volume	↑	↑↑↑	↑
Heart rate	↑↑↑	Normal	↑↑
Regurgitant volume	Large	Very large	Large
Effective cardiac output	↓↓	Normal	↓
Arterial pulse volume	Normal to ↑	↑↑↑	Normal

↑, Slight increase; ↑↑, moderate increase; ↑↑↑, severe increase; ↓, slight decrease; ↓↓, moderate decrease; ↓↓↓, severe decrease; *DBP*, diastolic blood pressure; *LV*, left ventricular; *LVEDP*, left ventricular end-diastolic pressure; *LVEF*, left ventricular ejection fraction; *SBP*, systolic blood pressure.

[a]Arrows are not used in the first row, because the changes in LV compliance are complex. In acute severe regurgitation, compliance is not really normal but is not increased. In the right-hand column, compliance is not really normal but is reduced compared with the state described in the middle column.

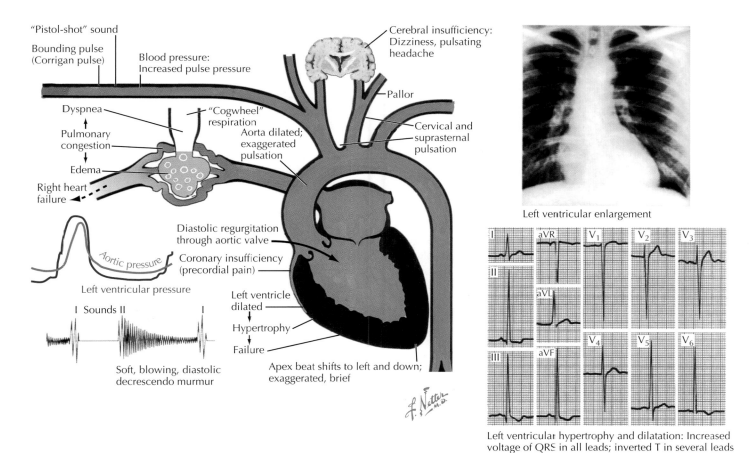

Left ventricular enlargement

Left ventricular hypertrophy and dilatation: Increased voltage of QRS in all leads; inverted T in several leads

FIG 45.7 Manifestations of Aortic Regurgitation.

TABLE 45.3   Physical Examination Findings With Severe Aortic Regurgitation

Finding	Description
De Musset sign	Head bob with each systolic pulsation
Corrigan pulse	Bounding pulse, alternatively named "water-hammer pulse"
Traube sign	Booming systolic and diastolic sounds ("pistol shots") over the femoral arteries
Müller sign	Systolic pulsation of the uvula
Duroziez sign	Systolic murmur over the femoral artery when compressed proximally, diastolic murmur when compressed distally
Quincke sign	Capillary pulsations noted in the nail beds or fingertips with each cardiac cycle
Hill sign	Popliteal systolic pressure exceeding brachial pressure by 30–60 mm Hg

the LV decompensates. The diastolic murmur of chronic AR is best heard at the base of the heart along the left sternal edge or in the second right intercostal space. It is best detected with the diaphragm of the stethoscope while the patient is leaning forward during held expiration. The etiology of the regurgitation is more likely to be valvular if the murmur is louder to the left of the sternum, whereas aortic root disease may be the cause if the murmur is louder to the right of the sternum. The diastolic murmur begins at the second heart sound and continues for a variable portion of diastole. Severity of the regurgitation is better correlated with the length of the murmur than with its intensity. However, when the LV begins to fail and end-diastolic pressure increases, the murmur begins to shorten again. A systolic murmur may be present from increased forward flow across the aortic valve or concomitant AS. A low-pitched rumbling mid-diastolic murmur best heard at the cardiac apex (Austin Flint murmur) may be present in severe AR and mistaken for the murmur of mitral stenosis.

Differential Diagnosis

Several conditions can mimic AR and should be considered in the differential diagnosis. First, patients with pulmonic regurgitation have a blowing diastolic decrescendo murmur but would not usually have a wide pulse pressure or bounding carotid pulse. The murmur of pulmonic regurgitation should increase with inspiration; the pulmonic valve closure sound is often increased in intensity, and a right ventricular (RV) heave may be present. The ECG would show signs of RV strain or hypertrophy rather than left-sided abnormalities, and chest radiography would show signs of RV enlargement. Second, in those presenting at a younger age, the diagnosis of patent ductus arteriosus should be considered. It causes a wide pulse pressure, as seen in chronic AR, but the murmur is continuous, with a low-pitched diastolic component. The ECG in this condition would be normal or show signs of LV hypertrophy, and chest radiography would show increased flow in the pulmonary vasculature. Third, if symptoms of dyspnea and chest pain begin suddenly, a ruptured sinus of Valsalva aneurysm into the RV should be considered. The pulse pressure is usually increased, but the murmur is continuous instead of only diastolic. Chest radiography would show signs of increased flow in the pulmonary vasculature. Finally, and rarely, a coronary arteriovenous fistula may present with a murmur that can be confused with AR. The murmur should be continuous, but occasionally the diastolic component can dominate, mimicking AR. Echocardiography, and, if necessary, cardiac catheterization, can be performed to distinguish all of these conditions from AR.

Diagnostic Approach

Echocardiography is valuable for the initial assessment of acute and chronic AR and for serial follow-up examinations. Echocardiography provides information about the etiology and severity of AR (assessed accurately and quantitatively), the presence of concomitant valve disorders, and the state of LV compensation as assessed by chamber size, function, and wall thickness. Additional information from echocardiography, notably, LV ejection fraction and chamber dimensions, can be followed serially to determine the timing of surgical intervention. For patients in whom echocardiography is inadequate or inconclusive, cardiac MRI is an accurate method to assess AR severity, LV volumes, and LV function.

With chronic AR, the ECG frequently shows left-axis deviation and LV hypertrophy. Other findings are nonspecific, including interventricular conduction defects, nonspecific ST-segment and T-wave changes, and PR interval prolongation, especially if the etiology is inflammatory. None of these findings correlate with regurgitation severity.

Chest radiography in chronic AR shows LV dilatation that may be massive (cor bovinum). An enlarged aortic root size suggests this as the etiology of the regurgitation. Pulmonary vasculature may be engorged during a decompensated state. With acute severe AR, there is minimal cardiac enlargement, with florid pulmonary edema the only finding.

AR can also be evaluated by cardiac catheterization. Hemodynamic tracings in severe AR show a wide pulse pressure and an elevated LV end-diastolic pressure. Aortic root angiography provides a semiquantitative assessment of severity, whereas quantitative calculations can also be performed. Catheterization is not routinely necessary, but may be useful when clinical assessment and noninvasive evaluation are discordant.

Management and Therapy
Acute Aortic Regurgitation

Regardless of the etiology, acute AR requires rapid diagnosis with aggressive medical therapy followed by urgent definitive surgical therapy, if feasible. Definitive therapy is surgical repair or (more commonly) valve replacement. Occasionally, a brief period of medical stabilization is possible and desirable. Medical stabilization includes afterload-reducing agents to augment forward cardiac output if hypotension does not preclude this therapy, and antimicrobials if the etiology is acute endocarditis. Intraaortic balloon counterpulsation is contraindicated because it increases regurgitation. Slowing the heart rate with β-blockers is not recommended, because it lengthens the time during which regurgitation can occur and blunts the compensatory tachycardia. However, if acute aortic dissection is the etiology, β-blockers reduce the force of LV ejection and should be coupled with aggressive lowering of the blood pressure. With endocarditis, surgery occasionally can be delayed a few days to allow further antibiotic therapy but should not be postponed if there is significant hemodynamic instability or heart failure. Recent studies have favored early surgical therapy and reported lower in-hospital mortality, and reduced risk of stroke in the setting of large vegetations.

With acute aortic dissection, the clinical picture may be dominated by other sequelae, including myocardial infarction from compromise of a coronary artery, hemopericardium with tamponade, hemorrhagic shock, or stroke due to involvement of a great vessel; all of these can alter treatment and the outcome.

Chronic Aortic Regurgitation

Medical therapy. Vasodilator therapy using a dihydropyridine calcium channel blocker, angiotensin-converting enzyme inhibitor, or angiotensin II receptor blocker is indicated for treatment of hypertension in patients with any degree of AR, or in patients with severe, symptomatic AR who are not surgical candidates. Data are inconclusive as to the role of these medications in patients with chronic, severe, asymptomatic AR who have normal LV systolic function. Specifically, in patients with Marfan syndrome, long-term administration of β-blockers, angiotensin-converting enzyme inhibitors, and angiotensin receptor blockers slows the rate of aortic dilatation and progression to aortic complications.

Surgical therapy. Valve replacement should be considered for most patients with symptomatic severe AR, unless comorbid conditions preclude surgery. However, the timing of surgery in asymptomatic patients with severe AR is controversial. If the routine activity level of a patient is low, exercise testing may be considered with reclassification of patients as "symptomatic" if: (1) functional capacity is low; (2) symptoms are elicited; or (3) an abnormal hemodynamic response develops.

Surgery is strongly recommended in asymptomatic patients with severe AR who have a depressed LV ejection fraction (<50%) and may be considered in asymptomatic patients with normal LV ejection fraction but severe ventricular dilatation (LV end-systolic dimension >50 mm or end-diastolic dimension >65 mm, by echocardiography) or in patients who are undergoing cardiac surgery for another indication.

Future Directions

Minimally invasive AVR, most commonly with a small thoracotomy to the right of the sternum, is becoming more common as surgical techniques improve. This approach seems to shorten length of stay and recovery periods before returning to normal activity, but it is unclear whether there are long-term advantages or hazards. AR has generally been an exclusion criteria in TAVR studies, so data are limited, but percutaneous approaches are being investigated with alternatives to the current valves used for TAVR in AS.

ADDITIONAL RESOURCES

Carabello BA. Aortic stenosis. *N Engl J Med.* 2002;346:677–682.
General, timeless overview of AS.
Clavel MA, Magne J, Pibarot P. Low-gradient aortic stenosis. *Eur Heart J.* 2016;37:2645–2657.
Review of the various causes of low gradient AS, how to evaluate, and treat.
Dal-Bianco JP, Khandheria BK, Mookadam F, et al. Management of asymptomatic severe aortic stenosis. *J Am Coll Cardiol.* 2008;52:1279–1292.
Review of the management of asymptomatic severe AS with emphasis on identifying patients at high risk of complications.
Enriquez-Sarano M, Tajik AJ. Clinical practice. Aortic regurgitation. *N Engl J Med.* 2004;351:1539–1546.
Concise review of the diagnosis and management of AR.
Otto CM. Valvular aortic stenosis: disease severity and timing of intervention. *J Am Coll Cardiol.* 2006;47:2141–2151.
Review article on the pathogenesis, clinical spectrum, and treatment of calcific AS in adults.

Ross J Jr. Afterload mismatch in aortic and mitral valve disease: implications for surgical therapy. *J Am Coll Cardiol.* 1985;5:811–826.
Classic article explaining the changes in LV function occurring in aortic and mitral regurgitation in terms of afterload mismatch.
Verma S, Siu SC. Aortic dilatation in patients with bicuspid aortic valve. *N Engl J Med.* 2014;370:1920–1929.
Review of the aortopathy associated with bicuspid aortic valves.

EVIDENCE

Evangelista A, Tornos P, Sambola A, et al. Long-term vasodilator therapy in patients with severe aortic regurgitation. *N Engl J Med.* 2005;353:1342–1349.
Long-term vasodilator therapy with nifedipine or enalapril did not reduce or delay the need for AVR in patients with asymptomatic severe AR and normal LV systolic function.
Hiratzka LF, Creager MA, Isselbacher EM, et al. Surgery for aortic dilatation in patients with bicuspid aortic valves. A statement of clarification from the American College of Cardiology/American Heart Association Task Force on Clinical Practice Guidelines. *J Am Coll Cardiol.* 2016;67:724–73.
Brief update considering the optimal timing for surgical treatment of aortic dilatation in patients with bicuspid aortic valves.
Nishimura RA, Grantham JA, Connolly HM, et al. Low-output, low-gradient aortic stenosis in patients with depressed left ventricular systolic function. The clinical utility of the dobutamine challenge in the catheterization laboratory. *Circulation.* 2002;106:809–813.
Dobutamine challenge aids in the identification of patients with AS who can benefit from valve replacement.
Nishimura RA, Otto CM, Bonow RO, et al. 2014 AHA/ACC guideline for the management of patients with valvular heart disease. *J Am Coll Cardiol.* 2014;63:e57–e185.
Outlines the evaluation and management of patients with AS, AR, and other valve diseases as defined by an expert committee assembled by the American College of Cardiology and the American Heart Association.
Pellikka PA, Sarano ME, Nishimura RA, et al. Outcome of 622 adults with asymptomatic hemodynamically significant aortic stenosis during prolonged follow-up. *Circulation.* 2005;111:3290–3295.
Describes long-term outcome of hemodynamically significant asymptomatic AS in adults.
Shores J, Berger KR, Murphy EA, Pyeritz RE. Progression of aortic dilatation and the benefit of long term beta-adrenergic blockade in Marfan's syndrome. *N Engl J Med.* 1994;330:1335–1341.
Prophylactic β-adrenergic blockade slowed the rate of aortic dilatation and reduced development of aortic complications in some patients with Marfan syndrome.
Tornos P, Sambola A, Permanyer-Miralda G, et al. Long-term outcome of surgically treated aortic regurgitation: influence of guideline adherence toward early surgery. *J Am Coll Cardiol.* 2006;47:1012–1017.
Provides further support for the recommendations of the American College of Cardiology/American Heart Association guidelines on the timing of AVR.

46

Mitral Valve Disease

Michael Yeung, Thomas R. Griggs

The origin of the word mitral comes from the Latin *mitre*, which means "bishop or Pope's hat" due to the physical resemblance between them. The mitral valve is a bicuspid valve, that is, it consists of two leaflets that separate and coordinate the flow of blood between the left atrium (LA) and the left ventricle (LV). During diastole, LA pressure surpasses LV pressure, which allows the anterior and posterior mitral valve leaflets to open to permit passive flow of blood from the LA to the LV. At the end of diastole, atrial contraction or the "atrial kick" occurs, which allows the final 20% of blood to be forcefully pushed into the LV. At the end of diastole, the mitral valve closes to prevent back flow of blood into the LA.

The mitral valve opening is enclosed by a fibrous ring termed the mitral valve annulus. The mitral valve leaflets are further attached to the chordae tendineae, which are tendon-like projections that prevent prolapse of the leaflets and regurgitation of blood into the LA. The chordae tendineae are further attached to the papillary muscles from the wall of the LV. For example, ischemia to the papillary muscles can cause dysfunction of the mitral valve apparatus, which leads to significant valvular regurgitation.

ETIOLOGY AND PATHOGENESIS

Mitral Stenosis

Most cases of mitral stenosis are due to rheumatic fever, and at present, this is seen predominantly in developing countries where there is still a lack of widespread use of antibiotics and access to care. The estimated prevalence of rheumatic disease worldwide is between 15 and 20 million people, whereas there are approximately 200,000 deaths every year from acute or chronic sequelae of rheumatic fever. Rheumatic fever occurs as an immune response to repeated episodes of untreated group A β-hemolytic streptococcal pharyngitis, whereby immune antibodies attack the valve tissue due to the molecular mimicry seen between the streptococcal antigens and the valve. This immune attack leads to leaflet thickening and calcification, as well as commissural fusion of the mitral valve and chordae shortening, all of which contribute to further narrowing of the mitral valve orifice and decreased mobility of the mitral valve leaflets. Approximately 40% of all patients with rheumatic fever have mitral stenosis, with the rest having a mixture of mitral regurgitation (MR) and/or aortic valve disease. Other causes of mitral stenosis involve calcific mitral stenosis and congenital mitral stenosis, both of which are rare.

The normal mitral valve cross-sectional area in diastole is 4 to 6 cm^2. Blood flow is impaired when the valve orifice is narrowed to <2 cm^2, creating a pressure gradient with exertion. A valve area <1 cm^2 is considered critical mitral stenosis and results in a significant pressure gradient across the valve at rest with chronically increased LA pressures (Fig. 46.1).

Chronically increased LA pressures associated with mitral stenosis result in LA enlargement and predisposition for atrial fibrillation. Valves affected by mitral stenosis are also vulnerable to recurrent thrombus formation due to blood stasis in the LA and implantation of bacteria in a diseased valve, which leads to infective endocarditis.

The hemodynamic effects of chronic mitral stenosis include pulmonary venous and arterial hypertension; right ventricular (RV) hypertrophy, dilation, and failure; peripheral edema; tricuspid regurgitation; ascites; and hepatic injury with cirrhosis (Fig. 46.2).

Mitral Regurgitation

Numerous etiologies contribute to MR, including mitral valve prolapse, coronary artery disease (ischemic MR), rheumatic heart disease, bacterial or fungal endocarditis, certain collagen vascular diseases, and heart failure (functional MR). In general, it is important to differentiate the etiology of MR between primary and secondary causes. Primary MR refers to abnormal valve function due to degenerative changes seen at the valve level itself, either due to myxomatous mitral valve prolapse, rheumatic leaflet changes, or ischemic heart disease that results in a dysfunctional papillary muscle apparatus. Secondary MR, or functional MR, is a result of progressive enlargement of the LV that leads to mitral annular dilatation and further displacement of the papillary muscle structures. Secondary MR is due to worsened heart failure due to nonischemic cardiomyopathy.

With MR, blood leaks back into the LA in addition to traveling its usual forward route through the aortic valve and into the aorta. If the regurgitant volume is significant, LA remodeling occurs with dilation to accommodate increased volumes without intolerable LA hypertension (Fig. 46.3). Over time, as an increasing fraction of ventricular volume is regurgitant, the forward ventricular output is reduced, and symptoms and other findings of MR become obvious (Fig. 46.4). Patients are generally clinically well if the regurgitant fraction (regurgitant volume/total ejection volume) is <0.4. Patients with regurgitant fractions >0.5 predictably develop LV failure and have high morbidity and mortality. Any evidence of LV failure (LV ejection fraction <60%) is a critical marker of poor prognosis and an indication to proceed to mitral valve surgery.

Infectious endocarditis, spontaneous rupture of chordae tendineae, or ischemic injury of a papillary muscle may cause acute MR. In these cases of abruptly increased regurgitant flow, because there is no adaptation of the LA or pulmonary vasculature to the increased regurgitant volumes, acute pulmonary edema suddenly occurs. Aggressive use of vasodilators is the medical treatment of choice, but this is often a temporary measure because survival often depends on emergency repair or replacement of the valve.

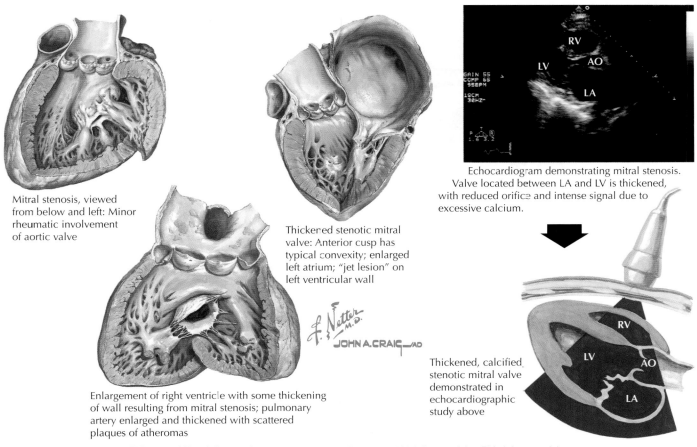

Mitral stenosis, viewed from below and left: Minor rheumatic involvement of aortic valve

Thickened stenotic mitral valve: Anterior cusp has typical convexity; enlarged left atrium; "jet lesion" on left ventricular wall

Echocardiogram demonstrating mitral stenosis. Valve located between LA and LV is thickened, with reduced orifice and intense signal due to excessive calcium.

Enlargement of right ventricle with some thickening of wall resulting from mitral stenosis; pulmonary artery enlarged and thickened with scattered plaques of atheromas

Thickened, calcified stenotic mitral valve demonstrated in echocardiographic study above

FIG 46.1 Mitral Stenosis. *AO*, Aorta; *LA*, left atrium; *LV*, left ventricle; *RV*, right ventricle.

CLINICAL PRESENTATION

Mitral Stenosis

Patients notice the effects of moderate (valve area = 1–2 cm^2) mitral stenosis with activity. However, in severe mitral stenosis, dyspnea with minimal exertion and paroxysmal nocturnal dyspnea may occur. In some cases a sudden, dramatic onset of atrial fibrillation produces the first symptoms, occasionally resulting in acute episodes of pulmonary edema. When the development of atrial fibrillation is clinically silent, the initial event may be a stroke or other thromboembolic event. The classic presentation of severe cor pulmonale with ascites and edema is rarely seen today except in medically underserved populations. Mitral valve disease increases the risk for bacterial seeding into the diseased valve tissue, which results in infective endocarditis.

Auscultatory findings in a patient with mitral stenosis include a loud first heart sound, an opening snap after the second heart sound, and a low-pitched diastolic murmur with presystolic accentuation if the patient is in sinus rhythm. The opening snap is the sound generated by sudden full opening of the mitral valve. It reflects the severity of the pressure gradient across the mitral valve, because greater LA pressures generate earlier opening than lesser pressures. Therefore, the shorter the interval from the second heart sound to the opening snap, the greater the pressure gradient, and the more severe the stenosis.

The characteristic diastolic, low-frequency "rumble" or murmur associated with mitral stenosis is best heard at the apex with the patient in the left lateral decubitus position and the bell over the point of maximal ventricular intensity. The rumble occurs throughout diastole, with accentuation in late diastole (presystole) in patients who have preserved normal sinus rhythm. This murmur can be difficult to hear, and is soft and brief when the stenosis is minor. Therefore, heightened awareness of possible mitral stenosis is necessary. If the murmur is inaudible, it can be accentuated by having the patient exercise before auscultation or perform maneuvers such as isometric handgrip. This murmur sequence—loud first sound, opening snap, and diastolic rumble—is specific for mitral stenosis. Murmurs that mimic mitral stenosis include the Austin Flint murmur with aortic regurgitation, mitral diastolic murmurs in patients with large intracardiac shunts, and occasionally murmurs that are caused by an LA myxoma. However, none have all three components of classic mitral stenosis.

ECG changes in mitral stenosis may range from minor ST-segment and T-wave abnormalities to ECG evidence of severe pulmonary hypertension and RV enlargement. The ECG pattern of LA and RV enlargement is a classic indicator. Atrial fibrillation is common.

Mitral Regurgitation

Acute MR following sudden failure of the valve apparatus is almost always immediately and severely symptomatic. In this situation, the regurgitant volume competes for forward systemic blood flow and is simultaneously leaking back considerably into a small, noncompliant LA. This results in an acute increase in LA pressures and acute pulmonary edema, and is often coupled with hypotension or shock. The physical examination will reflect the respiratory distress and evidence of poor

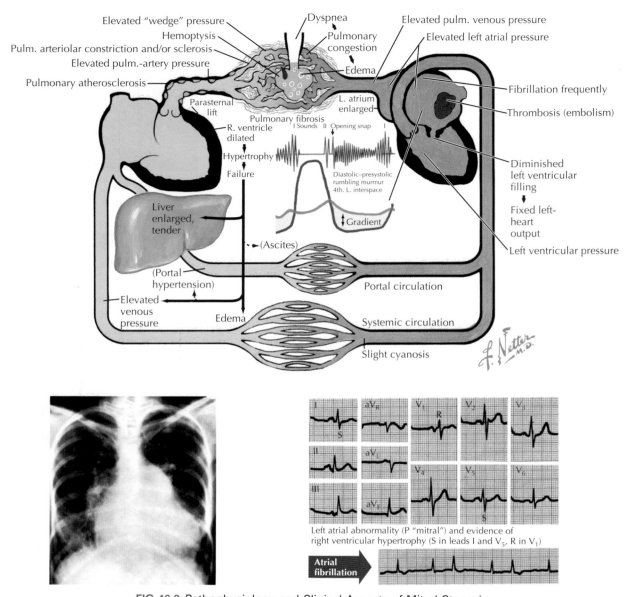

FIG 46.2 Pathophysiology and Clinical Aspects of Mitral Stenosis.

systemic perfusion, such as tachycardia, cool extremities, and diaphoresis. However, at times, the cardiac examination may not be helpful because acute MR may not be well appreciated, and a systolic murmur is often difficult to hear or may be absent. Emergent diagnosis usually requires echocardiography.

In contrast to acute MR, severe chronic mitral insufficiency may be tolerated without symptoms for years. Many cases of chronic MR are discovered during routine examinations when the characteristic holosystolic murmur is noticed. Symptoms usually begin as dyspnea on exertion and fatigue. Patients may also present with slowly progressive pulmonary edema or evidence of RV failure. Sudden decompensation can occur with the onset of atrial fibrillation due to further loss of atrial contraction and emptying into the LV.

With chronic MR, the precordial cardiac impulse may be normal or may show a displaced, sustained LV impulse with a rapid filling wave. On auscultation, the most prominent feature is a holosystolic murmur that classically radiates to the axilla. The intensity may not correlate with the severity of the MR; even severe MR can be associated with virtually no murmur. ECG changes in MR are nonspecific and are primarily changes of LV hypertrophy and strain; atrial fibrillation is common.

DIFFERENTIAL DIAGNOSIS

Primary pulmonary diseases (pneumonia, tuberculosis, chronic obstructive lung disease, and pulmonary thromboembolism) may present similarly to mitral valve disease, with dyspnea on exertion or pulmonary edema. Dyspnea may also be present in chronic interstitial pulmonary diseases, pulmonary hypertension, and malignancies that involve the chest. Other cardiovascular conditions that present similarly include ischemic heart disease, congenital heart disease, dilated cardiomyopathy, and hypertrophic cardiomyopathy. Chronic pericardial disease with restriction can cause RV failure that mimics the pulmonary hypertension associated with mitral valve disease.

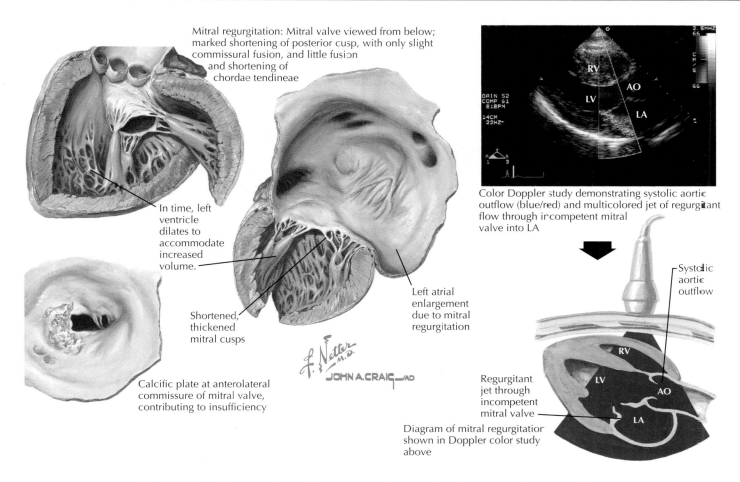

Mitral regurgitation: Mitral valve viewed from below; marked shortening of posterior cusp, with only slight commissural fusion, and little fusion and shortening of chordae tendineae

In time, left ventricle dilates to accommodate increased volume.

Shortened, thickened mitral cusps

Calcific plate at anterolateral commissure of mitral valve, contributing to insufficiency

Left atrial enlargement due to mitral regurgitation

Color Doppler study demonstrating systolic aortic outflow (blue/red) and multicolored jet of regurgitant flow through incompetent mitral valve into LA

Systolic aortic outflow

Regurgitant jet through incompetent mitral valve

Diagram of mitral regurgitation shown in Doppler color study above

FIG 46.3 Mitral Regurgitation. *AO*, Aorta; *LA*, left atrium; *LV*, left ventricle; *RV*, right ventricle.

DIAGNOSTIC APPROACH

Many pulmonary diseases can be differentiated from mitral valve disease by chest imaging, including both radiography and CT scanning. When an initial evaluation has focused the differential diagnosis on mitral valve disease, the most helpful clinical tool is echocardiography (see also Chapter 9).

In rheumatic mitral valve disease, echocardiography can demonstrate thickening, calcification, poor valve mobility, and thickening of sub-valvular structures. The degree of valvular stenosis or regurgitation can be estimated using Doppler ultrasonography. When necessary, the anatomy of the valve and subvalvular apparatus can be further defined by transesophageal echocardiography. The goals of echocardiography are to evaluate the severity of the stenosis or regurgitation, the mobility of the valve, the involvement of subvalvular structures, and the degree of calcification, as well as to detect intracardiac thrombi. Echocardiography provides information about LV contractile function and an accurate estimation of pulmonary artery pressure and RV function. It can also identify bacterial and fungal vegetations, intracardiac masses (especially LA myxoma), and intraventricular septal defects, which are conditions that can complicate the diagnosis of mitral valve disease.

Cardiac catheterization is indicated when there is a questionable diagnosis, when clinical and echocardiographic findings are inconsistent, and in many patients for whom surgical treatment is contemplated. Catheterization is performed to quantify the mitral valve area, to document key elements of hemodynamics such as cardiac output and systemic resistance, to define the degree of pulmonary hypertension, and to determine whether coronary artery disease is also present.

MANAGEMENT AND THERAPY

Mitral Stenosis

Asymptomatic patients in normal sinus rhythm with mild, uncomplicated mitral stenosis require only periodic monitoring for symptoms and prophylaxis against rheumatic fever. In symptomatic patients, diuretics can help reduce pulmonary congestion. With mitral stenosis, ventricular filling time is critically important; the heart rate should be maintained as low as is practical with a β-blocker or a rate-affecting calcium channel blocker. Patients with atrial fibrillation must be treated with warfarin anticoagulation, unless it is contraindicated.

Optimum Treatment

Symptomatic mitral stenosis can be treated by percutaneous mitral balloon valvotomy (PMBV), surgical valvotomy, or surgical replacement of the mitral valve. On the basis of recent guidelines, intervention should be considered for symptomatic patients with an MVA <1.5 cm^2 (see Table 46.2). PMBV is the treatment of choice in selected patients in whom there is mild valvular calcification, little involvement of the sub-valvular apparatus, and minimal or no mitral valve regurgitation. It is essential to exclude LA thrombi by transesophageal echocardiography

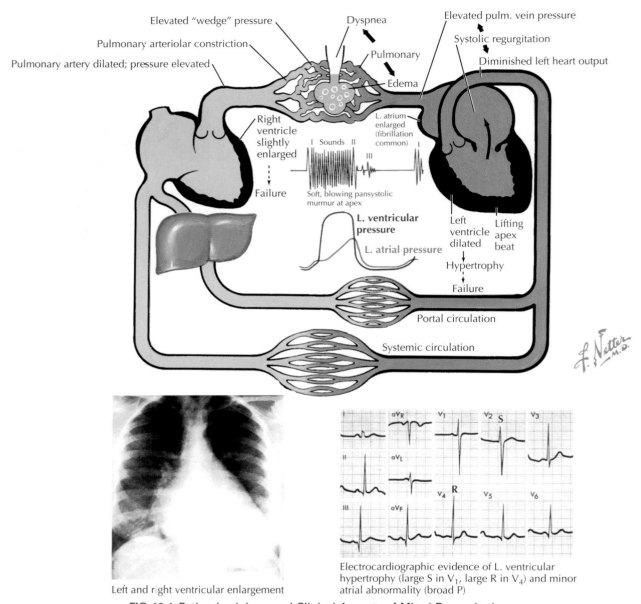

Elevated "wedge" pressure

Pulmonary arteriolar constriction

Pulmonary artery dilated; pressure elevated

Dyspnea

Pulmonary

Edema

Elevated pulm. vein pressure

Systolic regurgitation

Diminished left heart output

Right ventricle slightly enlarged

Failure

L. atrium enlarged (fibrillation common)

Sounds

Soft, blowing pansystolic murmur at apex

L. ventricular pressure

L. atrial pressure

Left ventricle dilated

Lifting apex beat

Hypertrophy

Failure

Portal circulation

Systemic circulation

Left and right ventricular enlargement

Electrocardiographic evidence of L. ventricular hypertrophy (large S in V_1, large R in V_4) and minor atrial abnormality (broad P)

FIG 46.4 Pathophysiology and Clinical Aspects of Mitral Regurgitation.

in patients being considered for PMBV. The results of PMBV depend on operator experience. Longitudinal studies in expert centers have documented event-free survival to be >70% at 7 years.

Open valvotomy is a repair procedure that involves direct visualization of the valve by the surgeon and facilitates debridement of the valve structure and reconstruction of the subvalvular apparatus. This approach also permits valve replacement per the judgment of the surgeon. Mitral valve replacement is indicated for patients with severe mitral stenosis who are not candidates for percutaneous commissurotomy or surgical repair (Tables 46.1 to 46.3) (see Chapter 50).

Avoiding Treatment Errors

Many patients unknowingly minimize mitral stenosis symptoms by adopting a sedentary lifestyle. This situation may be suspected following a careful history and documented with exercise testing. These patients may benefit greatly from PMBV. Alternatively, patients may report severe

symptoms despite echocardiographic data that suggest mild mitral stenosis. Exercise testing with simultaneous echocardiography or catheterization is indicated in this situation and may disclose dramatic worsening of atrial and pulmonary hypertension, and the need for intervention.

Rheumatic fever can affect all heart valves. Therefore, multiple valve disease must be considered in all patients. Special attention should be given to the possibility that echocardiography can underestimate the degree of aortic regurgitation in patients with severe mitral stenosis. Tricuspid stenosis may be similarly underestimated or even undetected, and may complicate the immediate postoperative recovery after mitral valve repair or replacement.

Atrial fibrillation is a frequent cause of decompensation in patients with mitral stenosis, and must be anticipated and managed aggressively. Similarly, pregnancy increases requirements for cardiac output and requires special planning and management. In women with rheumatic or congenital mitral stenosis, initial symptoms often manifest with

TABLE 46.1	Management Approach for Patients With Asymptomatic Mitral Stenosis	
	Yearly Follow-Up	**Consider Percutaneous Mitral Balloon Valvotomy**
Asymptomatic	Mild stenosis (MVA >1.5 cm²) or MVA <1.5 cm² but valve morphology not favorable for PMBV	Moderate or severe stenosis (MVA <1.5 cm²) and Pulmonary artery systolic pressure >50 mm Hg or Exercise test results: Pulmonary artery pressure >60 mm Hg Pulmonary artery wedge pressure >25 mm Hg or New-onset atrial fibrillation and No LA thrombus or significant mitral regurgitation (3+ or 4+)

LA, Left atrial; *MVA*, mitral valve area; *PMBV*, percutaneous mitral balloon valvotomy.

TABLE 46.2	Management Approach for Patients With Symptomatic Mitral Stenosis		
	Periodic Follow-Up	Consider PMBV	Consider Open Valvotomy or Mitral Valve Replacement
Mildly symptomatic (NYHA functional class II)	Mild stenosis (MVA >1.5 cm²) and Exercise test results: PASP <60 mm Hg PAWP <25 mm Hg MVG <15 mm Hg or Valve morphology not favorable for PMBV	Progressive mitral stenosis (MVA >1.5 cm²) and Exercise test results: PASP >60 mm Hg PAWP >25 mm Hg MVG >15 mm Hg and Valve morphology favorable for PMBV and No LA thrombus or significant mitral regurgitation (3+ to 4+)	Moderate or severe stenosis (MVA <1.5 cm²) and Valve morphology not favorable for PMBV and Pulmonary pressure >60–80 mm Hg
	Moderate or severe stenosis (MVA <1.5 cm²) and Valve morphology not favorable for PMBV and Pulmonary pressure <60 mm Hg	Moderate or severe stenosis (MVA <1.5 cm²) and Valve morphology favorable for PMBV and No LA thrombus or significant mitral regurgitation (3+ to 4+)	
Moderately to severely symptomatic (NYHA functional class III–IV)	Mild stenosis (MVA >1.5 cm²) and Exercise test results: PASP <60 mm Hg PAWP <25 mm Hg MVG <15 mm Hg	Moderate or severe stenosis (MVA <1.5 cm²) and Valve morphology favorable for PMBV or High-risk surgical candidate with less than favorable morphology for PMBV and No LA thrombus or significant mitral regurgitation (3+ to 4+)	Moderate or severe stenosis (MVA <1.5 cm²) and Valve morphology not favorable for PMBV and Acceptable surgical risk

LA, Left atrial; *MVA*, mitral valve area; *MVG*, mitral valve gradient; *NYHA*, New York Heart Association; *PASP*, pulmonary artery systolic pressure; *PAWP*, pulmonary artery wedge pressure; *PMBV*, percutaneous mitral balloon valvotomy.

TABLE 46.3	Management Approach for Patients With Chronic Severe Mitral Regurgitation		
	Follow-Up With Echo Every 6 Months or Medical Therapy	Mitral Valve Repair	Mitral Valve Replacement
No subjective symptoms and no suggestion of symptoms by exercise testing	Normal LV function (EF >60% and ESD <40 mm) and No new-onset atrial fibrillation and No pulmonary hypertension and Mitral valve repair unlikely[a]	LV dysfunction (EF <60%, ESD >40 mm) or Pulmonary hypertension or New-onset atrial fibrillation	LV dysfunction (EF <60%, ESD >40 mm) and Mitral valve repair not possible
Symptoms	Severe LV dysfunction[b] (EF <30% and/or ESD >55 mm) and Chordal preservation not likely	EF >30% ESD <55 mm	Intervention indicated but mitral valve repair not possible

EF, Ejection fraction; *ESD*, end-systolic dimension of the left ventricular chamber; *LV*, left ventricular.
[a]Mitral valve repair may be an option for asymptomatic patients with normal LV function in an experienced center.
[b]Transcatheter MV repair may be considered for severely symptomatic patients (NYHA class III/IV) with chronic severe primary MR (stage D) who have a reasonable life expectancy but a prohibitive surgical risk because of severe comorbidities.

pregnancy. Bacterial endocarditis should be considered whenever symptoms worsen in patients with mitral stenosis.

Mitral Regurgitation

Primary MR is a degenerative structural problem that causes valve incompetency that can only be corrected adequately by valve repair or replacement, and recently, by a percutaneous mitral clip procedure. Therefore, the primary role of the physician is to monitor patients with MR for development of symptoms and evidence of LV dysfunction, which are events that portend the need for intervention. A mitral clip is a minimally invasive transfemoral percutaneous procedure that mimics the surgical Alfieri stitch repair by placing the mitral clip device preferentially at the A2P2 portions of the mitral valve leaflets. Current use of the mitral clip procedure is limited to patients who are at high risk for open heart surgery. Although the mitral clip cannot match the reduction of MR compared with the open surgical approach, the clinical symptomatic improvement is comparable to the surgical cohorts, and the lack of morbidity makes this an attractive approach for patients who are poor candidates for surgery.

Secondary or functional MR is more challenging to treat because the main problem lies not with the valve itself, but with the progressive cardiac dysfunction and subsequent LV and mitral annular dilatation. Although mitral valve intervention, either surgical or percutaneous, may ameliorate the mitral insufficiency, it does not halt or reverse the natural course of LV dysfunction.

Medical therapy for chronic MR, including vasodilators and β-blockers, have not been adequately documented to delay the need for intervention. Aggressive treatment of hypertension is useful in patients with chronic MR.

Optimum Treatment

The timing of surgical intervention for patients with chronic MR is critical. In most cases, MR is well tolerated, and patients are asymptomatic for many years. Delaying surgery as long as possible avoids the trauma, expense, and risk of surgery. However, every effort must be made to proceed with surgery before ventricular function worsens. Close echocardiographic follow-up is necessary, and there is current discussion

that earlier intervention before the development of LV dysfunction may be beneficial because most of these patients present with irreversible heart failure. In general, mitral valve surgery should be considered in patients with known moderate to severe MR when they are symptomatic or there is objective evidence of decreased LV function (LV ejection fraction <60%).

Valve repair for severe MR lessens mortality and decreases the frequency of complications. Valves must be relatively free of calcification and have pliable leaflets with chordae tendineae that can be separated, reinforced, or reattached as needed. Placement of a reinforcing mitral ring is frequently included in the mitral valve repair due to secondary causes. Valve repair, as opposed to replacement, preserves the mitral apparatus and significantly improves postoperative LV function, and is the surgical option of choice when feasible. In addition, as opposed to mitral valve replacement, surgical repair does not require long-term anticoagulation that significantly reduces the life-long risk of bleeding.

Avoiding Treatment Errors

MR that results from dilated cardiomyopathy is caused by dilation of the mitral ring and ventricles with anatomic deformity of the spatial and functional relationship of the papillary muscles and chordae tendineae to the mitral valve leaflets. In severe LV dysfunction, mitral valve repair or replacement may fail to improve symptoms and is associated with a high risk of operative death. New surgical and percutaneous approaches for correction of MR in this circumstance are being studied in clinical trials to determine safety and efficacy.

Coronary heart disease can cause MR by several mechanisms. The mitral valve is tethered to papillary muscles that depend on myocardial blood flow. Acute ischemia of the papillary muscles can cause temporary MR and can be corrected with coronary revascularization, either surgically or percutaneously. Acute myocardial infarction that involves a papillary muscle frequently causes acute life-threatening MR, with mortality rates near 30%. These are often managed surgically, with both repair of the valve and the subvalvular apparatus, as well as simultaneous revascularization.

Any structural abnormality of the valve can result in flow aberrations that promote deposition of microthrombi. These can be the nidus

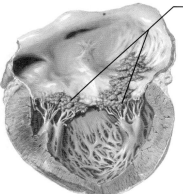

Bacterial vegetations first appear along "contact line" of mitral valve but spread to involve atria and chordae tendineae with subsequent rupture and shrinkage of the latter.

Perforation of aortic valve cusp   Bacterial perforation of anterior mitral cusp

Left ventricular hypertrophy

Late sequelae of bacterial endocarditis may result in mitral regurgitation via destruction of mitral valve cusps or by widening of annular valve ring due to left ventricular enlargement due to aortic insufficiency

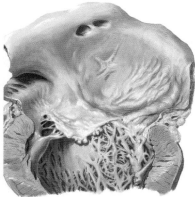

Thickening and erosion of mitral valve with stumps of ruptured chordae tendineae resulting in valvular incompetence, regurgitation, and atrial enlargement

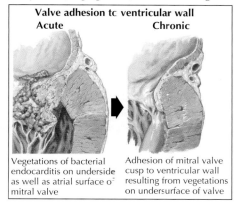

Valve adhesion to ventricular wall

Acute   **Chronic**

Vegetations of bacterial endocarditis on underside as well as atrial surface of mitral valve

Adhesion of mitral valve cusp to ventricular wall resulting from vegetations on undersurface of valve

FIG 46.5 Bacterial Endocarditis in Mitral Valvular Disease.

for a bacterial or fungal infection that results in further damage from endocarditis (Fig. 46.5). Endocarditis can affect valve competency because of interference in valve function by vegetations or by destruction or fenestration of the valve leaflets. Although endocarditis is usually managed with antibiotics, the damage caused by the bacteria is permanent, as is the resultant MR. Indications for surgery after cured bacterial endocarditis are identical to those for other causes for MR. In addition, acute surgical care is indicated for extremely large vegetations, when heart failure is otherwise unmanageable, when a myocardial abscess is documented, and for patients with persistent bacteremia.

FUTURE DIRECTIONS

Improving worldwide morbidity and mortality associated with rheumatic heart disease necessitates better systems of hygiene and improved prophylactic treatment of streptococcal infection. The prevalence of MR has increased as the population ages, spurring improvements in several areas: imaging with more accurate estimates of ventricular reserve; surgical technology with early repair of severely regurgitant valves; balloon valvotomy with improved patient selection and equipment; and minimally invasive percutaneous techniques with reduced recovery time and morbidity, such as the mitral clip or percutaneous mitral valve replacement.

ADDITIONAL RESOURCES

Carabello BA. Modern management of mitral stenosis. *Circulation.* 2005;112:432–437.

Carabello BA. The current therapy for mitral regurgitation. *J Am Coll Cardiol.* 2008;52:319–326.

State-of-the-art reviews by a noted expert.

EVIDENCE

Nishimura RA, Otto CM, Bonow RO, et al. 2014 AHA/ACC guideline for the management of patients with valvular heart disease: a report of the American College of Cardiology/American Heart Association Task Force on Practice Guidelines. *Circulation.* 2014;129:e521–e643.

In this recently updated report from a panel of experts assembled by the American College of Cardiology and American Heart Association, the authors cite 1000 articles and provide a comprehensive review of the diagnosis and management of valvular heart disease. Tables and algorithms provide easy access to the practical aspects of patient care.

47

Cardiovascular Manifestations of Rheumatic Fever

Lucius Howell, Sidney C. Smith, Jr.

ETIOLOGY AND PATHOGENESIS

Acute rheumatic fever (ARF), also known as scarlet fever, is caused by an autoimmune reaction to group A β-hemolytic streptococcal pharyngitis, which is caused by the common childhood infection of bacterial streptococcal pharyngitis, also known as "strep throat." It typically affects children between the ages of 5 and 15 years. Group A streptococcus is a bacteria that lives in oral flora and is spread through contact with droplets from infected persons with cough, sneeze, or touch. ARF is caused by an autoimmune response after exposure to group A streptococcal throat infection. Although not completely understood, the pathogenesis of the autoimmune response appears to be linked to the host's immune reaction to bacterial surface proteins. Streptococcal bacteria have surface proteins, M, T, and R, which are recognized by the host human leukocyte antigen (HLA) class II molecules. The HLA molecules produce antibodies that bind to the bacterial surface proteins, but the antibodies also bind to host proteins through molecular mimicry, which causes an autoimmune reaction. These autoantibodies cause a systemic autoimmune reaction that can interact with the joints, skin, brain, and heart. The autoimmune antigenic mimicry leads to destruction of human heart cardiac proteins that involve the cardiac valvular endocardium. During ARF, carditis and valvulitis can be present but are typically self-limiting. Recurrent or severe bouts of ARF then cause permanent cardiac valve damage, which leads to chronic rheumatic heart disease (RHD). This chapter outlines the evaluation and management of both ARF and chronic RHD.

CLINICAL PRESENTATION OF ACUTE RHEUMATIC FEVER

According to the Centers for Disease Control and Prevention, ARF predominantly affects children between 5 and 15 years old. It begins as a streptococcal throat infection and is characterized by a sore throat with fever and absence of cough (Fig. 47.1). This may also be associated with a red rash that appears on the neck, arm, and groin that then spreads all over the body. The rash is characterized by fine red bumps and feels like sandpaper. The rash lasts for about a week, and then it fades. At that time, the skin around the finger tips and toes may peel. Other common symptoms include an erythematous sore throat, a whitish coating of the tongue, and/or a red and bumpy tongue (strawberry tongue), headaches, swollen glands, nausea, and vomiting.

The earliest symptoms of ARF develop 2 to 3 weeks after the group A strep pharyngitis. These are typically fever and a painful migratory arthritis. Severe cases can manifest as the following: myocarditis, pericarditis, or valvulitis, or combination of the three; erythema marginatum, which are enlarged macular rings or crescent shaped with clear centers; subcutaneous nodules, which are firm nontender nodules over tendons;

and Sydenham chorea, an involuntary and irregular movement disorder of the tongue, face, and upper extremities.

Approximately 50% of patients with ARF will develop an autoimmune inflammatory carditis. Acute cardiac manifestations typically occur within 2 to 3 weeks of exposure. Acute rheumatic valvulitis or carditis develops after a few weeks, presenting as persistent sinus tachycardia predominantly at night, a prolonged PR interval, and a pansystolic murmur characteristic of rheumatic valvulitis. Valvulitis occurs in approximately 10% of patients with ARF and is characterized by inflammation and edema of the valve leaflets secondary to autoimmune destruction. Pericarditis is also common in ARF and is characterized by chest pain and a pericardial friction rub.

DIFFERENTIAL DIAGNOSIS FOR ACUTE RHEUMATIC FEVER

ARF has a variable presentation that can make diagnosis difficult based on symptoms alone. In patients with arthritis, carditis, and chorea, the differential diagnosis is extensive and includes diseases like Lyme disease, infective endocarditis, Henoch-Schönlein purpura, Kawasaki disease, drug intoxication, Wilson disease, encephalitis, systemic lupus erythematosus, systemic vasculitis, sarcoidosis, and hyperthyroidism. Obtaining a good clinical history, using the Jones criteria, and if possible, a rapid strep titer or transthoracic echocardiogram, can all help differentiate between ARF and other causes of acute systemic illness.

DIAGNOSTIC APPROACH TO ACUTE RHEUMATIC FEVER

History and Laboratory Evaluation

To make a diagnosis of acute ARF, there must be evidence of a preceding streptococcal infection by history or laboratory evidence, whenever possible, including rising antistreptolysin O titers, positive throat culture for group A β-hemolytic streptococci, or a positive rapid group A streptococcal carbohydrate antigen test.

Other laboratory investigations should include a complete blood count, C-reactive protein levels, and erythrocyte sedimentation rate.

Echocardiography

Echocardiographic and valvular findings of carditis and/or valvulitis include mitral regurgitation (MR), mitral annular dilation, and elongation of the chordae tendons and nodular leaflet tips. More severe findings include coaptation defects, restricted leaflet motion with prolapse, and in rare cases, chordal rupture.

An echocardiogram is now recommended in all cases of ARF and in cases of possible rheumatic fever. In cases in which ARF meets some of the criteria but not all, an echocardiogram is recommended to look

Cardiac Manifestations of Acute Rheumatic Fever

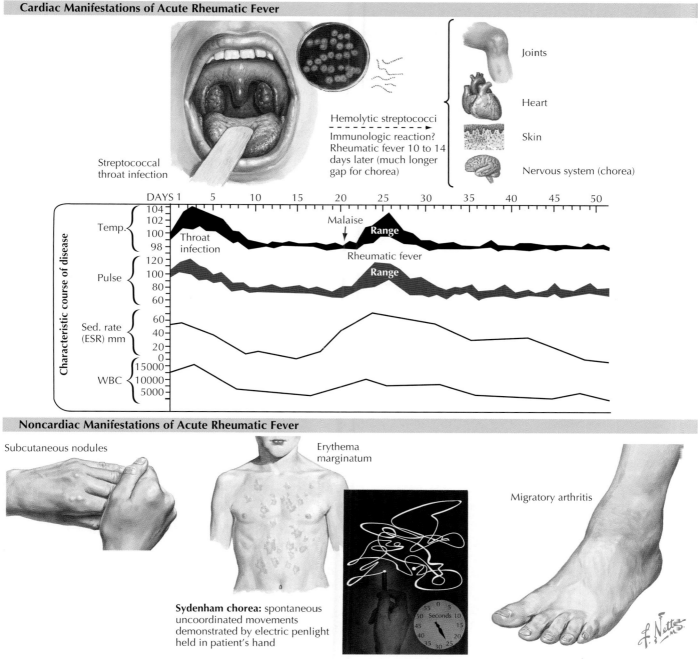

FIG 47.1 Cardiac and Noncardiac Manifestations of Acute Rheumatic Fever. *ESR*. Erythrocyte sedimentation rate; *WBC*, white blood count.

for evidence of subclinical carditis. During the early courses of ARF, the mitral and aortic valves may be normal on echocardiography. Serial echocardiograms should be performed in patients who develop chorea and/or clinical evidence of carditis.

Electrocardiogram

The most common finding on an ECG is sinus tachycardia. In carditis, there may be a prolonged PR interval and occasionally a first-degree heart block.

Jones Criteria for Diagnosis of Rheumatic Fever

The initial description of ARF and its symptoms were published in 1944, known as the Jones criteria. These criteria were updated by the American Heart Association in 2015. The diagnosis of ARF primarily falls into the history, physical examination findings, and echocardiographic findings. It includes two sets of criteria: one for low-risk populations, and one for moderate- to high-risk populations. The criteria have also been updated to account for recent evidence to support the use of echocardiography in addition to presentation and examination in making the diagnosis.

BOX 47.1 Revised Jones Criteria for Diagnosis of Acute Rheumatic Fever

Low Risk Populations (ARF incidence <2 per 100,000 school age children, <1/1000 general population)
Major Criteria
- Carditis: clinical and/or subclinical
- Polyarthritis
- Chorea
- Erythema marginatum
- Subcutaneous nodules

Minor Criteria
- Polyarthralgia
- Fever >38.5°C
- ESR >60 mm/h or CRP >3 mg/dL
- Prolonged PR interval

Moderate and High-Risk Population (not clearly from a low risk population)
Major Criteria
- Carditis: clinical and/or subclinical
- Monoarthritis or polyarthritis
- Chorea
- Erythema marginatum
- Subcutaneous nodules

Minor Criteria
- Monoarthralgia
- Fever >38.5°C
- ESR >30 mm/h or CRP >3 mg/dL
- Prolonged PR interval

Initial Diagnosis of Acute Rheumatic Fever
- Two major criteria or one major plus two minor criteria
- Evidence of preceding group A streptococcal infection (elevated or rising antistreptolysin O or other streptococcal antibody, or positive throat culture, or positive rapid antigen test)

Recurrent Diagnosis of Acute Rheumatic Fever
- Two minor criteria
- Evidence of preceding group A streptococcal infection (elevated or rising antistreptolysin O or other streptococcal antibody, or positive throat culture, or positive rapid antigen test)

CRP, C-reactive protein; *ESR,* erythrocyte sedimentation rate.

Revised Jones Criteria for Diagnosis of Acute Rheumatic Fever

See Box 47.1.

MANAGEMENT AND THERAPY

Due to the prevalence of the disease being located in underdeveloped and low-income areas, the biggest barriers to treatment and prevention of ARF are related to lack of infrastructure, geography, and biopsychosocial issues.

Acute Rheumatic Fever and Rheumatic Carditis and/or Valvulitis

Penicillin and penicillin derivatives are the treatment for ARF. Urgent surgery is recommended for patients with severe carditis and evidence of uncontrolled heart failure due to acute rheumatic MR, but surgery can be typically avoided with medical therapy alone. Acute rheumatic valvulitis with valvular insufficiency can be typically managed medically with antibiotics, diuretics, and afterload reducers.

Primary and Secondary Prevention

There are many factors that influence the incidence of rheumatic fever and RHD, including streptococcal group strains, overcrowding, and access to medical care. Primary prevention includes treating group A strep pharyngitis early and eradicating group A strep with penicillin, which then prevents ARF. This is done through active sore throat screenings and treatment of pharyngitis by oral antibiotics; typically, penicillin is given intramuscularly and/or orally, and amoxicillin is administered orally. Vaccine development is also another possibility for rheumatic fever prevention. There are several multivalent vaccines that have been developed and have completed phase II trials, but unfortunately, there are currently no vaccines available.

Secondary prevention programs focus on patients with previous ARF or echocardiographic evidence of RHD; these programs then concentrate on preventing recurrent ARF episodes with prophylactic antibiotics. For ARF, the World Health Organization recommends 5 years of secondary prophylaxis after the initial attack or until 18 years of age, whichever is longer. For mild RHD, prophylaxis is recommended for 10 years or until the age of 25 years. For moderate, severe cases or after valve surgery, secondary prophylaxis is recommended to be lifelong. Some institutions in places with high endemic areas of rheumatic fever recommend long-term and/or lifelong prophylaxis in patients with evidence of RHD or previous valvular surgery. The biggest issue with secondary prevention is poor compliance due to lack of community-based networks and medicine.

In addition, active echocardiographic screening in asymptomatic children and adolescents has been proposed in areas with a high prevalence, but such screening is rarely performed due to lack of availability. For each country with moderate to high and different populations of RHD, focus must be placed on raising awareness, surveillance, and prevention.

CLINICAL PRESENTATION OF RHEUMATIC HEART DISEASE

RHD is often diagnosed in patients who have experienced one or more ARF episodes, but as many as one-half will never have been diagnosed with ARF. Patients will typically present with shortness of breath, heart failure symptoms, stroke, and/or new atrial arrhythmias in their third, fourth, and fifth decades, with or without a history of ARF.

RHD typically affects the left-sided mitral and aortic valves. Isolated mitral valve involvement occurs in 70%, mitral and aortic involvement in 20%, and isolated aortic, tricuspid, or pulmonic involvement are rare. As discussed previously, the endothelium of these valves is permanently damaged due to the autoimmune antigenic mimicry.

The right-sided valves, which are the tricuspid and pulmonic valves, are typically unaffected. Tricuspid regurgitation can be seen in patients with RHD, but it is often functional because of high pulmonary pressures and right ventricular modification due to severe left-sided valvular disease. Severe mitral and aortic valve disease can lead to elevated left ventricular and/or left atrial pressures that cause left atrial dilation and to high pulmonary pressures that lead to complications such as atrial arrhythmias (e.g., atrial fibrillation), hemoptysis, stroke, pulmonary edema, and right-sided heart failure.

Major complications from RHD present as acute heart failure, atrial fibrillation, stroke, and/or infective endocarditis. Unfortunately, RHD can remain undetected for many years until the disease has progressed into the late stages. Clinical diagnosis is based on pathological valvular defects detected on both auscultation and echocardiography, as described in the following.

Mitral Valve Disease in Rheumatic Heart Disease

RHD is the most common cause of mitral stenosis worldwide. Early stages of RHD manifest primarily as MR. In the second and third decades of life, the disease progresses to a mixed MR and mitral stenosis. In the second, third, and fourth decades of life, the mitral valve thickens further, and mitral stenosis becomes the predominant disease pattern.

Rheumatic MR is typically characterized by elongation of the chordae and thickening of the leaflet tips, which creates an incompetent coaptation of the valve that allows blood to flow retrogradely into the left atrium during systole. Echocardiographically, rheumatic MR typically shows leaflet thickening, a prolapsing anterior valve leaflet, and elongation of the chordae, with an eccentric posterior-directed MR jet (Figs. 47.2 and 47.3). On examination, the peripheral pulses are typically normal, but in severe MR, the arterial pulse drops rapidly due to a decreased ejection time. Auscultation will reveal a loud holosystolic murmur best heard over the apex. There is typically a diminished S_1 heart sound and wide splitting of the S_2 heart sound due to early closure of the aortic valve. The pulmonic component of S_2 can be loud when pulmonary hypertension is present.

Rheumatic mitral stenosis is characterized by fusion of the anterior and posterior leaflet commissures and valvular thickening that leads to a narrowing of the orifice of the mitral valve, thus restricting blood flow

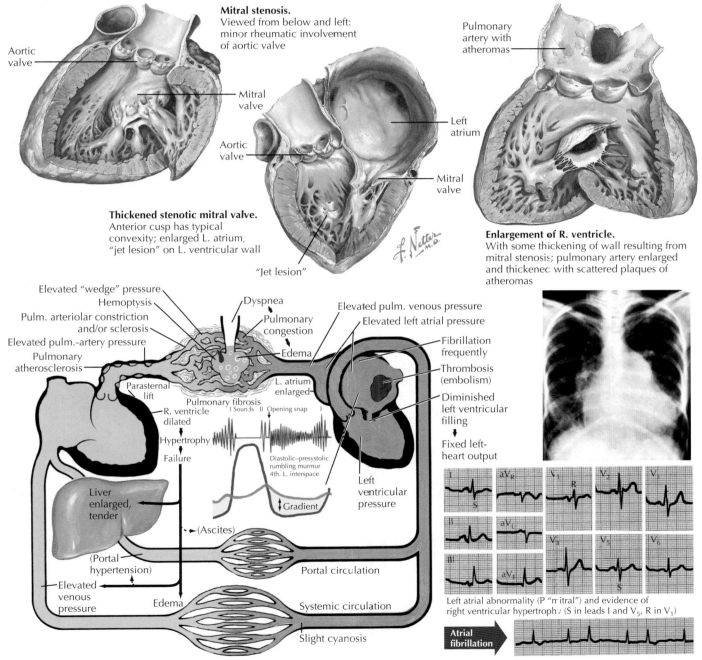

Mitral stenosis.
Viewed from below and left: minor rheumatic involvement of aortic valve

Aortic valve

Mitral valve

Aortic valve

Pulmonary artery with atheromas

Left atrium

Mitral valve

Thickened stenotic mitral valve.
Anterior cusp has typical convexity; enlarged L. atrium; "jet lesion" on L. ventricular wall

"Jet lesion"

Enlargement of R. ventricle.
With some thickening of wall resulting from mitral stenosis; pulmonary artery enlarged and thickened with scattered plaques of atheromas

Elevated "wedge" pressure
Hemoptysis
Pulm. arteriolar constriction and/or sclerosis
Elevated pulm.-artery pressure
Pulmonary atherosclerosis
Parasternal lift
R. ventricle dilated
Hypertrophy
Failure

Dyspnea
Pulmonary congestion
Edema
L. atrium enlarged
Pulmonary fibrosis
I Sounds II Opening snap I
Diastolic–presystolic rumbling murmur 4th. L. interspace
Gradient

Elevated pulm. venous pressure
Elevated left atrial pressure
Fibrillation frequently
Thrombosis (embolism)
Diminished left ventricular filling
Fixed left-heart output

Left ventricular pressure

Liver enlarged, tender
(Portal hypertension)
Elevated venous pressure
Edema
(Ascites)
Portal circulation
Systemic circulation
Slight cyanosis

Left atrial abnormality (P "mitral") and evidence of right ventricular hypertrophy (S in leads I and V_5, R in V_1)

Atrial fibrillation

FIG 47.2 Pathophysiology and Clinical Aspects of Mitral Stenosis.

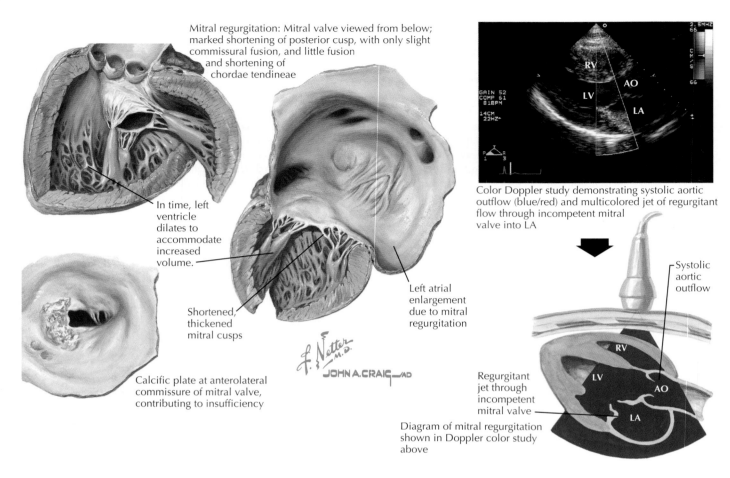

Mitral regurgitation: Mitral valve viewed from below; marked shortening of posterior cusp, with only slight commissural fusion, and little fusion and shortening of chordae tendineae

In time, left ventricle dilates to accommodate increased volume.

Shortened, thickened mitral cusps

Calcific plate at anterolateral commissure of mitral valve, contributing to insufficiency

Left atrial enlargement due to mitral regurgitation

Color Doppler study demonstrating systolic aortic outflow (blue/red) and multicolored jet of regurgitant flow through incompetent mitral valve into LA

Systolic aortic outflow

Regurgitant jet through incompetent mitral valve

Diagram of mitral regurgitation shown in Doppler color study above

FIG 47.3 Mitral Regurgitation. *AO*, Aorta; *LA*, left atrium; *LV*, left ventricular, *RV*, right ventricle.

from the left atrium to the left ventricle, which causes severe stenosis. Patients typically do not have symptoms until the valve area become severe and measures <1.5 cm². On examination, the peripheral pulses will be decreased. There is a loud S_1 heart sound due to closure of stiff leaflets, and the pulmonic component of S_2 can be increased when pulmonary hypertension is present. In diastole, there is an opening snap followed by a diastolic murmur (rumble) best heard with the bell of the stethoscope. As mitral stenosis worsens, the opening snap occurs earlier in diastole.

Aortic and Mixed Valve Disease in Rheumatic Heart Disease

Aortic valve disease caused by RHD typically involves both aortic and mitral valves. Similar pathophysiology of the mitral valve causes valve leaflet damage that involves the leaflet tips, which can cause fibrosis, thickening, cusp retraction, and calcification, leading to both aortic insufficiency and aortic stenosis. The presentation and examination depends on the relative severity of each lesion that cause serial altered flow dynamics. The examination may reveal multiple varying systolic and diastolic flow murmurs. Patients with aortic disease or mixed aortic and mitral valve disease will present with symptoms of heart failure, angina, or syncope when aortic stenosis is present. To properly diagnose aortic stenosis, attention must be focused on the hemodynamic assessment of each individual valve and the features and morphology of each valve using transthoracic or transesophageal echocardiographic modalities.

Tricuspid Valve Disease

Tricuspid valve disease typically is secondary to left-sided valvular disease, which leads to pulmonary hypertension and right ventricular strain dilation that leads to functional tricuspid regurgitation. However, some studies have suggested that the tricuspid valve can be involved, which leads to stenosis regurgitation or mixed disease. Surgical correction of tricuspid regurgitation or stenosis could be completed at the time of left-sided heart surgery.

COMPLICATIONS OF RHEUMATIC HEART DISEASE

Advanced single or multivalvular dysfunction leads to single ventricle or biventricular heart failure in RHD. In addition to the previously discussed cardiac auscultative valve findings, an S_3 or S_4 heart sound, and a laterally and apically displaced point of maximal impulse (PMI) can be present. Typical presentation is progressive shortness of breath, paroxysmal nocturnal dyspnea, orthopnea, elevated jugular vein pressure, and lower extremity swelling. An Australian study published in 2013 estimated that 27% of patients would develop heart failure within 5 years after a diagnosis of RHD.

Stroke

Stroke due to RHD is typically caused by a thromboembolic event that is the result of thrombus collecting on the valvular apparatus or by thrombus attached to the left atrial wall or left atrial appendage in patients with atrial fibrillation. Currently, the annual rate of stroke in patients with atrial fibrillation and RHD is approximately 6%.

Atrial Fibrillation

Atrial fibrillation is a common presentation of RHD. It is typically caused by fibrosis, high pressures, and severe dilation of the left atrium due to severe valvular disease, typically mitral stenosis or regurgitation. This leads to initially subclinical atrial fibrillation, followed by persistent, and then chronic atrial fibrillation. Atrial fibrillation then leads to serious potential combinations, including stroke from systemic embolism and worsening of heart failure symptoms.

DIFFERENTIAL DIAGNOSIS OF RHEUMATIC HEART DISEASE

Primary pulmonary diseases such as pneumonia, tuberculosis, and chronic obstructive pulmonary disease may present similarly to mitral valve disease. Other cardiac conditions, including congestive heart failure, advanced congenital heart disease, and pericardial disease, can also present with similar symptoms.

DIAGNOSTIC APPROACH IN CHRONIC RHEUMATIC HEART DISEASE

History and Laboratory Evaluation

Chronic RHD typically presents as heart failure symptoms, new-onset arrhythmias, or stroke. Baseline laboratory investigation includes blood count, renal function, and measurement of B-type natriuretic peptides (BNP).

Electrocardiogram

In chronic RHD, the ECG may show evidence of atrial or ventricular chamber enlargement and/or complicating arrhythmias like atrial fibrillation.

Echocardiography

Typical morphological echocardiographic changes of the mitral valve include leaflet thickening, subvalvular apparatus thickening, shortened chordae tendon, commissural fusion, calcification, and restricted leaflet motion. The fixed leaflet tips during diastole resemble a hockey stick. The degree of valvular stenosis or regurgitation can be estimated using Doppler ultrasonography. When necessary, the anatomy of the valve and subvalvular apparatus can be further defined by transesophageal echocardiography. Echocardiography provides information about left and/or right ventricular contractile function and pulmonary artery pressure. It can also identify evidence of infective endocarditis. The aortic valve may have thickened cusps, incomplete coaptation, and restricted movement.

Cardiac Catheterization

Cardiac catheterization is indicated when there is a questionable diagnosis, multivalvular disease, and in patients undergoing surgical treatment. Catheterization allows documentation of hemodynamics (e.g., cardiac output and systemic resistance) to define the degree of pulmonary hypertension and to determine whether coronary artery disease is also present.

MANAGEMENT OF CHRONIC RHEUMATIC HEART DISEASE

The main focus in treatment of RHD is to slow the progression of further valve damage, medically manage the valvular disease, and to use surgery or minimally invasive procedures when available (Fig. 47.4). All patients with chronic RHD should be placed on secondary antibiotic prophylaxis.

Asymptomatic patients in normal sinus rhythm with mild, uncomplicated valvular disease require only periodic monitoring with echocardiography, evaluation of symptoms, and prophylaxis against rheumatic fever.

Therapy is difficult for MR, but consists of afterload reduction that reduces the outflow resistance, which increases cardiac output, and thus reduces workload of the heart. There is little evidence that angiotensin-converting enzyme inhibitors or dihydropyridines are beneficial in MR. In patients with severe symptomatic MR, mitral valve repair or replacement is the only definitive therapy.

There are no medications that change the natural progression of mitral stenosis. However, diuretic therapy for pulmonary congestion and reduction of heart rate to increase the diastolic filling time can

Second generation of synthetic prosthetic valves and biological valves

Second-generation synthetic prosthetic valves were hingeless pivoting disk valves and hinged bileaflet valves.

Tissue valves made of porcine aortic valves, pericardium, or cadaver homografts are also important in valve replacement surgical therapy.

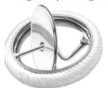

Medtronic-Hall pivoting disk valve

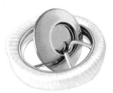

Björk-Shiley valve

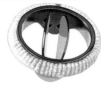

St. Jude bileaflet valve

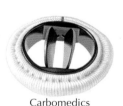

Carbomedics bileaflet valve

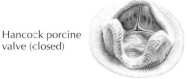

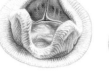

Hancock porcine valve (closed)

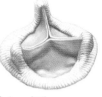

Edwards-Carpentier valve (closed)

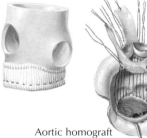

A Medtronic freestyle valve

Aortic homograft being settled

Aorta artery wall

Anterior mitral leaflet

FIG 47.4 Management and Treatment of Chronic Rheumatic Heart Disease.

improve symptoms. Optimization of ventricular filling time is critically important; the heart rate should be maintained as low as practical with a β-blocker or a rate-affecting calcium channel blocker. In symptomatic patients with rapid response to atrial fibrillation, cardioversion to normal sinus rhythm can be an important adjunct to medical therapy.

When the mitral valve area is severe, and the patient is symptomatic, mitral stenosis can be improved by percutaneous mitral balloon valvotomy (PMBV), surgical valvotomy, or surgical replacement of the mitral valve. PMBV is the treatment of choice in selected patients in whom there is little valvular calcification, little involvement of the subvalvular apparatus, and minimal or no mitral valve regurgitation (Fig. 47.5). It is essential to exclude left atrial thrombus by transesophageal echocardiography in patients being considered for PMBV. Mitral valve replacement is indicated for patients with advanced RHD and severe mitral stenosis who are not candidates for percutaneous commissurotomy or surgical repair.

MR or mixed mitral valve pathology with greater than mild MR will likely require surgical intervention with either mitral valve repair or replacement with a prosthetic or metal valve. Aortic valve and/or mixed valvular pathologies require surgical intervention. Mixed valve disease has a much higher operative risk, with no minimally invasive options. Multivalvular surgery has a higher operative risk and decreased long-term durability compared with that for single valve surgery. This makes the timing and postsurgical management challenging.

Treating heart failure or arrhythmias can help improve symptoms but does not change the natural course of the disease. In patients who develop heart failure, the mainstay therapies include a combination of β-blockers, angiotensin-converting enzyme inhibitors, afterload reducing agents, and digoxin if indicated. In addition, loop diuretics are used for symptoms of shortness of breath associated with pulmonary edema and swelling. Individuals with heart failure require cardiac surgery or percutaneous valve interventions to improve long-term survival.

Anticoagulation with warfarin is recommended for all patients with atrial fibrillation or a history of stroke. Treatment of atrial fibrillation with rate control or rhythm control is also recommended to maximize diastolic filling of the left ventricle.

Many women present with heart failure symptoms during pregnancy. Pregnancy in patients with RHD is associated with a higher mortality, especially when pulmonary hypertension is present due to mitral stenosis or left ventricular failure. Heart failure associated with moderately severe MR is also associated with higher mortality in pregnancy. Symptoms and associated heart failure generally occur in the second and third trimester when the cardiac output and volume overload associated with pregnancy occur.

RHD is a risk factor for infective endocarditis; therefore, it is important to teach such patients good dental hygiene. Endocarditis prophylaxis before any dental or surgical procedure is recommended for patients who have prosthetic valves or a history of endocarditis.

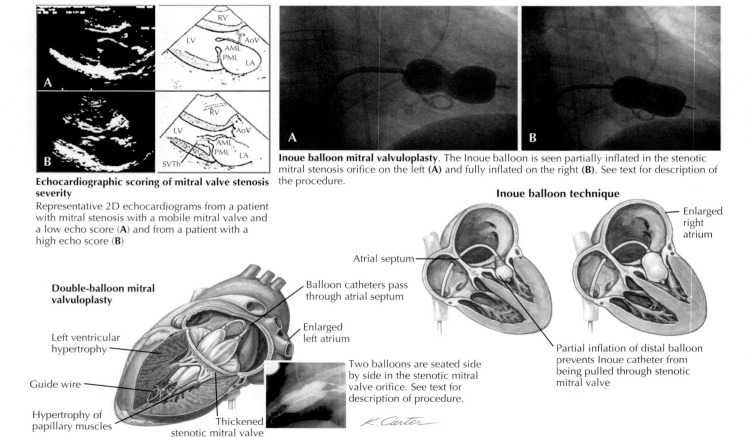

Echocardiographic scoring of mitral valve stenosis severity
Representative 2D echocardiograms from a patient with mitral stenosis with a mobile mitral valve and a low echo score (**A**) and from a patient with a high echo score (**B**)

Inoue balloon mitral valvuloplasty. The Inoue balloon is seen partially inflated in the stenotic mitral stenosis orifice on the left (**A**) and fully inflated on the right (**B**). See text for description of the procedure.

Inoue balloon technique

Enlarged right atrium

Atrial septum

Partial inflation of distal balloon prevents Inoue catheter from being pulled through stenotic mitral valve

Double-balloon mitral valvuloplasty

Left ventricular hypertrophy

Guide wire

Hypertrophy of papillary muscles

Balloon catheters pass through atrial septum

Enlarged left atrium

Two balloons are seated side by side in the stenotic mitral valve orifice. See text for description of procedure.

Thickened stenotic mitral valve

K. Carter

FIG 47.5 Mitral Balloon Valvuloplasty. *AML,* Anterior mitral leaflet; *AoV,* aortic valve; *LA,* left atrium; *LV,* left ventricular; *PML,* posterior mitral valve; *RV,* right ventricle; *SVTh,* subvalvular leaflet thickening.

FUTURE DIRECTIONS

ARF and RHD continue to be global problems in underdeveloped and low-income countries. Both prevention and surgical or percutaneous interventions are major humanitarian challenges throughout the underdeveloped world. Because there is currently no vaccine to prevent streptococcal pharyngitis, creating regional centers of expertise for treatment are key to reducing the overall global burden of RHD.

ADDITIONAL RESOURCES

Dougherty S, Khorsandi M, Herbst P. Rheumatic heart disease screening: current concepts and challenges. *Ann Pediatr Cardiol.* 2017;10:39–49.
Contemporary review of screening for rheumatic heart disease in children.
Hugenholtz PG, Ryan TJ, Stein SW, et al. The spectrum of pure mitral stenosis. Hemodynamic studies in relation to clinical disability. *Am J Cardiol.* 1962;10:773–784.
Important summary of hemodynamic findings related to functional status in patients with mitral stenosis.
Nishimura RA, Otto CM, Bonow RO, et al. 2014 AHA/ACC guideline for the management of patients with valvular heart disease: a report of the American College of Cardiology/American Heart Association Task Force on Practice Guidelines. *Circulation.* 2014;129:e521–e643.
Most recent heart valve disease guidelines provide therapeutic recommendations based on accumulated evidence and expert opinion.

Schlosshan D, Aggarwal G, Mathur G, et al. Real-time 3D transesophageal echocardiography for the evaluation of rheumatic mitral stenosis. *JACC Cardiovasc Imaging.* 2011;4:580–588.
Important resource summarizing 3D echo strategies in the evaluation of rheumatic mitral stenosis.

EVIDENCE

Gerber MA, Baltimore RS, Eaton CB, et al. Prevention of rheumatic fever and diagnosis and treatment of acute Streptococcal pharyngitis: a scientific statement from the American Heart Association Rheumatic Fever, Endocarditis, and Kawasaki Disease Committee of the Council on Cardiovascular Disease in the Young, the Interdisciplinary Council on Functional Genomics and Translational Biology, and the Interdisciplinary Council on Quality of Care and Outcomes Research: endorsed by the American Academy of Pediatrics. *Circulation.* 2009;119:1541–1551.
Comprehensive summary of evidence regarding the prevention and treatment of acute rheumatic fever.
Patel JJ, Shama D, Mitha AS, et al. Balloon valvuloplasty versus closed commissurotomy for pliable mitral stenosis: a prospective hemodynamic study. *J Am Coll Cardiol.* 1991;18:1318–1322.
Early clinical trial demonstrating the efficacy of mitral balloon valvuloplasty for rheumatic mitral stenosis.

48

Tricuspid and Pulmonic Valve Disease

Allie E. Goins, David A. Tate, George A. Stouffer

Acquired disease of the right-sided cardiac valves is much less common than disease of the left-sided valves, possibly because of the relatively lower pressures and hemodynamic stress to which the right-sided valves are subjected. Indeed, right-sided valvular dysfunction most commonly occurs when morphologically normal valves are subjected to abnormal hemodynamic stresses (e.g., pulmonary hypertension) but can also be seen with congenitally malformed valves (tricuspid and pulmonic valvular abnormalities are part of numerous congenital syndromes; discussed in Section VIII) or with infective endocarditis (discussed in Chapter 49). Tricuspid and pulmonic valvular abnormalities are also part of numerous congenital syndromes (discussed in Section VIII).

TRICUSPID STENOSIS

Etiology, Pathogenesis, and Differential Diagnosis

The normal tricuspid valve has a valve area of 4 to 6 cm^2. Tricuspid stenosis is uncommon, and most cases are due to rheumatic heart disease. When rheumatic tricuspid stenosis is present, it is generally associated with mitral stenosis, which usually accounts for most of the presenting signs and symptoms. Carcinoid heart disease may also cause tricuspid stenosis, and the signs and symptoms may be mimicked by tumors (myxoma or metastasis), or vegetations that obstruct right ventricular (RV) inflow, particularly those associated with pacemaker leads (Box 48.1).

Clinical Presentation

The symptoms of tricuspid stenosis are mainly due to increased systemic venous pressure that results from a hemodynamically significant tricuspid valve lesion (Fig. 48.1). Peripheral edema, ascites, hepatic enlargement, and right upper quadrant discomfort may develop with chronic tricuspid stenosis or regurgitation. Decreased cardiac output may cause pronounced fatigue, and patients will occasionally complain of the appearance or sensation of the prominent *a* wave in the jugular veins, which results from increased jugular venous pressure due to impaired RV filling during atrial systole. The murmur of tricuspid stenosis is a low-pitched diastolic murmur at the lower left sternal edge. However, this can be difficult to differentiate from the murmur of mitral stenosis if it is also present. The physical examination may demonstrate the presence of tricuspid stenosis in patients with mitral stenosis, including when there is accentuation of the diastolic murmur during inspiration (as is the case for most right-sided murmurs), a prominent *a* wave in the jugular venous pulse, or both. An opening snap is occasionally appreciated but may be difficult to distinguish from that of coexistent mitral stenosis. When appreciated, it is usually heard following and more medial to the mitral opening snap.

Diagnostic Approach

Useful diagnostic studies include chest radiography, ECG, and echocardiography with Doppler evaluation. Right atrial (RA) enlargement is frequently evident on radiographs and manifests on the ECG as a large peaked P wave in lead II (Fig. 48.2). Because of the increased RA pressure, atrial fibrillation is often present.

Echocardiography typically reveals thickened tricuspid leaflets, decreased mobility, scarred chordae, and sometimes doming, if the tricuspid valve leaflets remain pliable. Carcinoid heart disease is associated with a distinctive morphology of a thickened tricuspid valve that is narrowed and fixed in the open position. Doppler evaluation allows estimation of the diastolic pressure gradient by the modified Bernoulli equation. Cardiac catheterization is generally not necessary for the diagnosis of tricuspid stenosis, but when performed, it calls for separate, simultaneous catheters in the RA and the RV. If cardiac output is low, tricuspid gradients may also be low and are not adequately evaluated using a catheter pullback. Clinically significant tricuspid stenosis is usually associated with a valve area of <1.0 to 1.5 cm^2.

Management and Therapy

Initial treatment of tricuspid stenosis includes diuretics and nitrates to relieve venous congestion. Refractory cases have traditionally required open tricuspid valve repair or replacement, and the concomitant mitral valve disease has primarily determined the indication and timing for surgery. A surgical approach may also be indicated for debulking of obstructive tumors or myxoma. However, although no randomized trials are available because of the relatively low prevalence of this condition, published studies suggest that percutaneous techniques are effective and safe, either as therapy for isolated tricuspid stenosis or for combined mitral and tricuspid disease; referral to experienced centers should be considered. The most recent American Heart Association/American College of Cardiology guidelines on the management of valvular heart disease state that percutaneous balloon valvotomy may be considered as a treatment option for patients with severe, symptomatic tricuspid stenosis who are inoperable or at an increased surgical risk. However, because percutaneous balloon valvotomy may worsen tricuspid regurgitation, this therapy should not be undertaken if there is more than mild associated tricuspid regurgitation, as is often the case.

TRICUSPID REGURGITATION

Etiology and Pathogenesis

Tricuspid regurgitation may be due to primary disease of the valve apparatus or diseases that cause pulmonary hypertension with RV pressure overload and secondary annular dilatation. Annual dilation is the predominant cause of tricuspid regurgitation and can be seen with any condition that causes pulmonary hypertension, including left ventricular failure, mitral regurgitation, mitral stenosis, primary pulmonary disease, and primary pulmonary hypertension. The rare causes of primary tricuspid regurgitation include rheumatic heart disease, myxomatous disease (prolapse), infective or marantic endocarditis, carcinoid heart

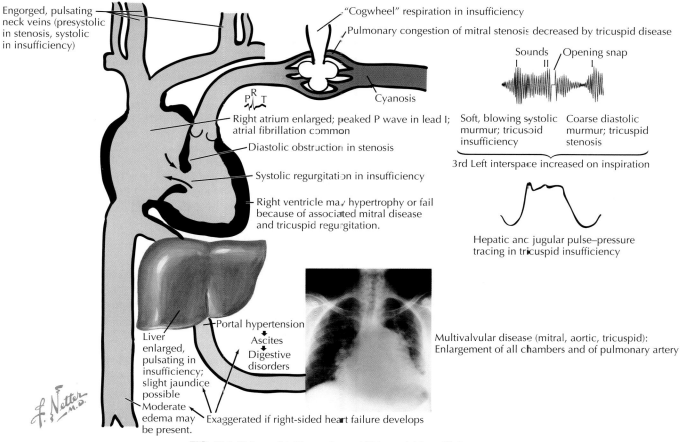

FIG 48.1 Tricuspid Stenosis and Tricuspid Insufficiency.

BOX 48.1 Differential Diagnosis of Tricuspid Stenosis

Rheumatic disease
Right atrial myxoma causing right ventricular inflow obstruction
Metastatic disease causing right ventricular inflow obstruction
Vegetations resulting from endocarditis of pacemaker leads or prosthetic valves
Congenital stenosis or atresia
Carcinoid disease

disease, iatrogenic injury during endomyocardial biopsy or placement of pacemaker or defibrillator leads, and trauma.

Clinical Presentation

Symptoms are often due to associated left-sided heart disease or pulmonary disease. Prominent signs and symptoms of right-sided heart failure suggest tricuspid regurgitation as a component. A patient will occasionally present with a pulsatile sensation in the neck. Endocarditis or carcinoid syndrome may be associated with characteristic systemic symptoms.

Jugular venous pressure is usually increased, and there is a prominent *cv* wave produced by regurgitant flow into the RA. The typical murmur is holosystolic and located at the left sternal edge or the subxiphoid area. The murmur is generally of low intensity and may be absent even in the presence of severe regurgitation. Augmentation of the murmur with inspiration (due to increased venous return) helps distinguish

tricuspid regurgitation from mitral regurgitation. When severe RV enlargement is present, a right-sided S_3 may be appreciated, which is also accentuated with inspiration.

Diagnostic Approach

Chest radiography often reveals RV enlargement manifested as filling of the retrosternal space. Dilation of the RV often causes incomplete or complete right bundle branch block, which is seen on the ECG.

Two-dimensional echocardiography evaluates the structure of the valvular apparatus and size of the RA and RV. Pulse-wave or color flow Doppler reveals the presence, direction, and magnitude of the regurgitant jet. Severe regurgitation is generally associated with systolic flow reversal in the hepatic veins and a vena contracta width (the narrowest portion of the regurgitant jet) of >0.7 cm. Finally, continuous-wave Doppler and the modified Bernoulli equation can be used to estimate the RV and pulmonary artery systolic pressures. In tricuspid regurgitation, the gradient between the RV and the RA during systole equals four times the square of the velocity. This gradient is then added to the estimated RA pressure (the jugular venous pressure) to estimate RV systolic pressure. In the absence of pulmonic stenosis, this also equals pulmonary systolic pressure. It is important to recognize that this calculation estimates the pulmonary systolic pressure, not the volumetric severity of the tricuspid regurgitation itself.

Management and Therapy

The mainstay of therapy for tricuspid regurgitation caused by RV pressure overload is the treatment of the condition that is causing pulmonary hypertension. Diuretics may be useful for refractory fluid retention.

Arrows indicate major atrial electrical vectors.

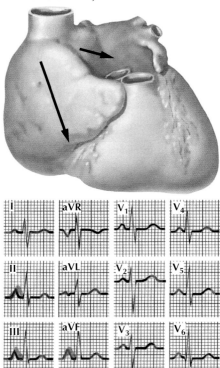

Tall P waves in leads II, III, and aVF ≥2.5 mm

Causes

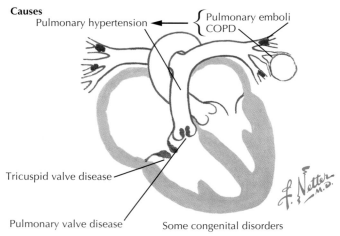

Pulmonary hypertension ← { Pulmonary emboli / COPD

Tricuspid valve disease

Pulmonary valve disease   Some congenital disorders

FIG 48.2 Causes of Right Atrial Enlargement. *COPD*, Chronic obstructive pulmonary disease.

Surgical tricuspid annuloplasty, which generally involves placement of a semi-rigid prosthetic valvuloplasty ring, is occasionally necessary for patients whose condition is refractory to medical therapy. It is commonly performed at the time of operation for concurrent left-sided valvular disease. In this circumstance, tricuspid annuloplasty should be performed in patients with severe tricuspid regurgitation. If the left-sided disease is mitral valve prolapse, even mild tricuspid regurgitation should be repaired, because myxomatous involvement often leads to progressive regurgitation. Surgical tricuspid valve replacement is rarely necessary. Bioprostheses are favored in surgical tricuspid valve replacement because the tricuspid valve may be relatively prone to thrombosis.

Percutaneous techniques to treat patients with severe tricuspid regurgitation, who are deemed to be inoperable or at high-risk of developing complications from traditional surgery, are being developed. The proximity of the tricuspid valve to the right coronary artery, atrioventricular node, and the trabeculated RV make the development of percutaneous techniques for the treatment of tricuspid valve disease difficult. The tricuspid valve annulus is also typically more fragile compared with the mitral valve annulus. Percutaneous devices that focus on improving coaptation of the tricuspid leaflets are currently being developed and studied. Other transcatheter annuloplasty devices that aim to reduce dilatation of the annulus are being developed for the treatment of tricuspid regurgitation, as well as transcatheter valves positioned at the junction of the RA and the vena cava. The goal of these valves will be to help reduce the symptoms caused by venous congestion rather than actually altering the grade of tricuspid regurgitation itself.

PULMONIC STENOSIS

Etiology and Pathogenesis

RV outflow obstruction may be subvalvular, valvular, or supravalvular (Fig. 48.3). Both the subvalvular and the supravalvular forms of RV outflow obstruction are usually associated with other congenital heart disease, as discussed in Section VIII. However, true valvular pulmonic stenosis usually occurs as an isolated congenital defect. In addition, it may occur as the sole cardiac abnormality in patients with Noonan syndrome. Rarely, pulmonic stenosis is due to rheumatic disease, endocarditis, or carcinoid syndrome.

Clinical Presentation

Patients with pulmonic stenosis are often asymptomatic. Patients may reach the fourth through sixth decades of life with significant pressure gradients across the pulmonic valve but with no symptoms and no evidence of right-sided heart failure. If right-sided heart failure does develop, abdominal swelling, peripheral edema, abdominal discomfort, and fatigue may be present. Patients seldom present with chest pain or exertional syncope.

The physical examination typically reveals a mid-systolic crescendo–decrescendo murmur at the left sternal edge. An associated ejection click, which usually decreases with inspiration, is often present. P_2 is soft and delayed, producing a widely split S_2, but one that narrows with appropriate physiological changes (unlike the fixed, widely split S_2 present in patients with an atrial septal defect). Occasionally, a right-sided S_4 is appreciated at the left sternal border. An RV lift may also be present. If RV failure is present, there may be peripheral edema, hepatomegaly, abdominal swelling, and jugular venous distention with a prominent *a* wave.

Diagnostic Approach

ECG may be normal with mild-to-moderate stenosis, but in more severe cases, it will often reveal right-axis deviation, RA enlargement, and RV hypertrophy. A complete or incomplete right bundle branch block is sometimes present, although patients with Noonan syndrome characteristically have a left bundle branch block. Chest radiography reveals poststenotic dilatation of the pulmonary artery but diminished peripheral pulmonary vascular markings. RV hypertrophy and enlargement are highly variable.

Echocardiography with Doppler evaluation is useful for establishing the diagnosis and assessing therapy. Morphological assessment is best performed with the parasternal short-axis and subcostal views, and will generally reveal thickened but pliable leaflets with restricted motion and doming. Occasionally, patients will have more severe thickening with severely dysplastic valves. This is important to recognize, because

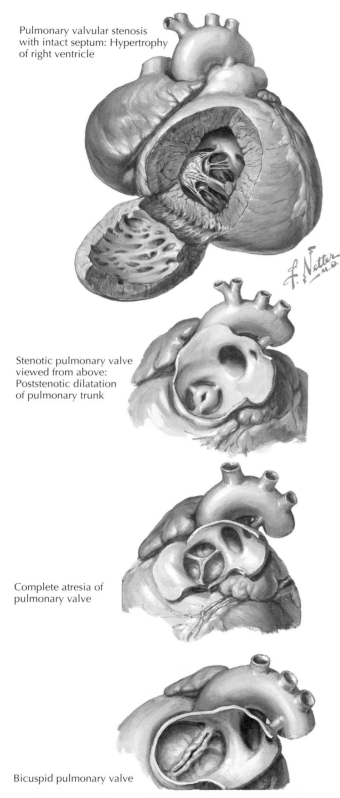

Pulmonary valvular stenosis with intact septum: Hypertrophy of right ventricle

Stenotic pulmonary valve viewed from above: Poststenotic dilatation of pulmonary trunk

Complete atresia of pulmonary valve

Bicuspid pulmonary valve

FIG 48.3 Pulmonary Valvular Stenosis and Atresia.

such patients are not well-suited to percutaneous valvuloplasty. Transesophageal echocardiography is not usually necessary but can be performed if a transthoracic study fails to provide an adequate assessment. The RV may be normal, particularly in childhood, but stenosis of long duration, greater severity, or both is usually associated with RV hypertrophy and enlargement. Paradoxical motion of the interventricular septum is often present. Continuous-wave Doppler evaluation is highly reliable in establishing the gradient across the pulmonic valve. Cardiac catheterization is usually not necessary but may be performed if Doppler studies are suboptimal or immediately before (and after) planned balloon valvuloplasty.

Management and Therapy

Adult patients with mild pulmonic stenosis generally do well and require no intervention. More severe disease is appropriately treated with percutaneous balloon valvotomy, which is highly effective and generally well-tolerated. The 2008 American College of Cardiology/American Heart Association guidelines recommend percutaneous balloon valvotomy in symptomatic adults with a peak instantaneous Doppler gradient >50 mm Hg or a mean Doppler gradient >30 mm Hg (in association with less than moderate pulmonic regurgitation) and in asymptomatic patients with a peak instantaneous Doppler gradient >60 mm Hg or a mean Doppler gradient >40 mm Hg (in association with less than moderate pulmonic regurgitation).

PULMONIC REGURGITATION

Etiology and Pathogenesis

A minor degree of pulmonic valve regurgitation evident by Doppler echocardiography is an essentially normal finding present in many healthy individuals. Moderate or severe regurgitation is usually secondary to severe pulmonary hypertension (either primary or secondary), pulmonary artery dilatation, or both. Rarely, it is secondary to endocarditis, carcinoid syndrome, rheumatic heart disease, trauma, Marfan syndrome, previous pulmonary valve surgery, or congenital valvular abnormalities.

Clinical Presentation

Accordingly, the dominant symptoms in pulmonic regurgitation are usually those of the underlying disease process. Patients without severe underlying disease are often asymptomatic. However, patients with severe pulmonic regurgitation may ultimately have typical symptoms and signs of right-sided heart failure.

The characteristic physical finding is a decrescendo diastolic murmur, loudest at the left third and fourth intercostal spaces, which increases with inspiration. S_2 is usually widely split with an accentuated pulmonic component if there is significant pulmonary hypertension. In the absence of pulmonary hypertension, the murmur is low-pitched. The more common high-pitched murmur associated with a prominent P_2 in the presence of severe pulmonary hypertension is the classic Graham Steell murmur. There is occasionally an associated crescendo–decrescendo systolic murmur from increased flow across the valve, or a holosystolic murmur due to coincident tricuspid regurgitation. Jugular venous distention and signs of right-sided heart failure may be apparent.

Diagnostic Approach

The findings on ECG and chest radiography are generally those of the underlying disease and of RV hypertrophy and dilatation. Echocardiography with Doppler can identify and grossly quantitate pulmonic regurgitation, and assess the size and contractility of the RV. Regurgitation is considered severe when the color Doppler jet fills the RV outflow tract, and there is a dense continuous-wave Doppler signal associated with rapid deceleration.

Management and Therapy

Treatment is generally directed at the underlying disease process. Valve surgery will rarely be necessary for severe regurgitation and progressive right heart failure. Occasionally, valve surgery will be necessary when the valve is damaged at the time of other surgery on the RV outflow tract, as in tetralogy of Fallot. In the absence of other indications, pulmonic regurgitation does not require endocarditis prophylaxis for dental procedures.

FUTURE DIRECTIONS

The treatment of pulmonic and tricuspid valve disease will continue to benefit from the steady evolution of percutaneous techniques. Pulmonic valvuloplasty was introduced in the early 1980s. It reduces the pressure gradient across the valve, and many patients have a subsequent further decrease in the RV outflow gradient due in part to resolution of infundibular hypertrophy. This success has led to a generally lower threshold for intervention with each iteration of guidelines. Follow-up studies confirm the continued long-term effectiveness of a percutaneous approach. With respect to tricuspid stenosis, valvuloplasty techniques that use multiple balloons or the Inoue balloon appear promising.

ADDITIONAL RESOURCES

American Society of Echocardiography [home page on the Internet]. http://www.asecho.org. Accessed April 5, 2018.
Because of the importance of echocardiographic and Doppler techniques in the assessment of valvular disease, this site is helpful in providing expert consensus guidelines on the optimal evaluation of lesion severity.
European Society of Cardiology [home page on the Internet]. http://escardio.org. Accessed April 5, 2018.
Provides the latest guidelines from a consensus of European authorities.

EVIDENCE

Baumgartner H, Falk V, Bax JJ, et al. 2017 ESC/EACTS Guidelines for the management of valvular heart disease. *Eur Heart J.* 2017;38:2739–2791.
European guidelines for the management of patients with valvular heart disease.

Nishimura RA, et al. AHA/ACC 2014 guidelines for the management of patients with valvular heart disease. A report of the American College of Cardiology/American Heart Association Task Force on Practice Guidelines. *Circulation.* 2014;129:e521–e643.
This joint American College of Cardiology/American Heart Association report outlines the appropriate diagnosis and management of valvular heart disease according to a panel of experts. It is thoroughly referenced, and the level of evidence is cited for the recommendations.
Rao PS. Percutaneous balloon pulmonary valvuloplasty: state of the art. *Catheter Cardiovasc Interv.* 2007;69:747–763.
This review article illustrates the ongoing technical advances in balloon valvuloplasty that have led to recommendations for lower thresholds for intervention.
Rodes-Cabau J, et al. Transcatheter therapies for treating tricuspid regurgitation. *J Am Coll Cardiol.* 2016;67(15):1829–1845.
A review article that illustrates the technical advances in transcatheter therapies used to treat tricuspid regurgitation.
Rodes-Cabau I, Taramasso M, O'Gara PT. Diagnosis and treatment of tricuspid valve disease: current and future perspectives. *Lancet.* 2016;388:2431–2442.
This review article focuses on the treatment of both tricuspid regurgitation and tricuspid stenosis, and the new advances in percutaneous therapy options for tricuspid regurgitation.
Warnes CA, et al. AHA/ACC 2008 guidelines for the management of adults with congenital heart disease. *Circulation.* 2008;118:2395–2451.
This joint American Heart Association/American College of Cardiology report outlines the appropriate diagnosis and management of congenital heart disease and valvular heart disease as a result of congenital heart disease. The recommendations are made according to a panel of experts.
Zoghbi WA, Enriquez-Sarano M, Foster E, et al. Recommendations for evaluation of the severity of native valvular regurgitation with two-dimensional and Doppler echocardiography. *J Am Soc Echocardiogr.* 2003;16:777–802.
Provides a critical review of echocardiographic and Doppler techniques used to evaluate the severity of regurgitant valvular lesions.

49

Infective Endocarditis

Thelsa Thomas Weickert, Kristine B. Patterson, Cam Patterson

Infective endocarditis (IE) is an infection caused by organisms that enter the bloodstream and that typically infect one or more of the cardiac valves, the endocardial surface of the heart, or an intracardiac device. Despite advances in medical and surgical interventions, IE continues to be associated with high morbidity and mortality, especially because of worsening antimicrobial resistance. Early diagnosis, prompt and appropriate antimicrobial therapy, echocardiographic evaluation, and timely surgical intervention are cornerstones of successful management.

ETIOLOGY AND PATHOGENESIS

The two main bacterial causes of IE are streptococci (community acquired) and staphylococci (healthcare associated and community acquired). *Staphylococcus aureus* has now replaced viridans group streptococci as the leading cause as a result of the increased frequency of oxacillin-resistant *S. aureus* in tertiary care centers and community-acquired infections.

IE most often occurs in the setting of an already damaged endothelial surface or on artificial valves. This provides a suitable site for bacterial colonization and adherence, which allows replication to a critical mass and a mature infected vegetation to form.

RISK FACTORS

See Box 49.1.

CLINICAL PRESENTATION

Any organ system can be involved in patients with IE, and thus the clinical presentation is highly variable. Four processes contribute to the clinical manifestations of IE: (1) the infectious process on the valve that causes local intracardiac complications (e.g., perivalvular abscess, valvular regurgitation, conduction disturbances, congestive heart failure [CHF]) (Fig. 49.1); (2) vascular phenomena (e.g., septic embolic lungs, brain, kidneys, spleen, and so forth; mycotic aneurysm, intracranial hemorrhage); (3) bacteremic seeding of remote sites (e.g., vertebral osteomyelitis, psoas or perirenal abscess, septic arthritis) (Fig. 49.2); and (4) immunologic phenomena (e.g., glomerulonephritis, Osler nodes, Roth spots, positive rheumatoid factor, and antinuclear antibodies).

The presentation of IE is straightforward when the classic signs and symptoms are present: fever; bacteremia or fungemia; valvular incompetence with evidence of vegetation on echocardiography; peripheral emboli; and immune-mediated vasculitis as seen in subacute IE. However, acute IE may evolve too quickly for immunologic phenomena to develop, and patients may present only with fever or severe manifestations such as those related to valve incompetency. In both acute and subacute IE, fever is the most common presenting symptom (up to 90% of patients).

Frequently, the diagnosis can be made clinically if a careful physical examination is performed. Attention should be given to the conjunctiva (hemorrhages), dilated fundoscopic examination (Roth spots), complete cardiovascular examination (new or changing murmur, especially aortic, mitral, or tricuspid regurgitation, and signs of CHF), splenomegaly, and extremities (splinter hemorrhages, septic emboli, Janeway lesions, or Osler nodes) (Fig. 49.3). The comprehensive physical examination can be complemented by several nonspecific, yet suggestive laboratory studies. Findings in IE include (but are not limited to) anemia, thrombocytopenia, leukocytosis, elevated inflammatory markers (erythrocyte sedimentation rate and/or C-reactive protein), active urinary sediment, hypergammaglobulinemia, positive rheumatoid factor, antinuclear antibodies, hypocomplementemia, and false-positive VDRL and Lyme disease serology.

DIAGNOSTIC APPROACH

Since 1994, the Duke criteria have been the most consistently used diagnostic strategy in stratifying patients suspected of having IE into definite, possible, or rejected categories. These criteria have been modified to include newer diagnostic methods. Although the modified Duke criteria can provide a primary diagnostic schema, they should not replace clinical judgment (Box 49.2).

Microbiology

The first definitive test should be at least three sets of blood cultures drawn from separate venipuncture sites in the first 24 hours of observation. More cultures may be necessary if the patient received antibiotics in the preceding weeks. Almost 50% of culture-negative IE can be attributed to antibiotic use before obtaining cultures. Organisms such as the *Haemophilus* species, *Actinobacillus actinomycetemcomitans*, *Cardiobacterium hominis*, *Eikenella corrodens*, and *Kingella* species (HACEK) group and *Brucella* are slow growing and require extended incubation of cultures (4 weeks). Special culture techniques or media may be required for some organisms (e.g., *Legionella*). Genetic sequencing is being used more frequently for organisms that have been difficult to identify through traditional microbiological methods. Blood culture results are negative in >50% of fungal endocarditis cases. Serological studies are frequently necessary to diagnose Q fever, brucellosis, legionellosis, and psittacosis, and are now included as surrogate markers in lieu of positive blood cultures for diagnosis.

Specific Pathogens
Staphylococcal Endocarditis

Staphylococci are now the most common cause of IE, especially *S. aureus* native valve IE. Increasing rates of infection with methicillin-resistant *S. aureus* are being reported. The course of *S. aureus* infection is typically fulminant with myocardial and valve ring abscesses, with

Early lesions

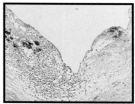

Deposit of platelets and organisms (stained dark), edema, and leukocytic infiltration in very early infective endocarditis of aortic valve

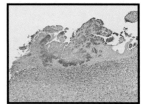

Development of vegetations containing clumps of bacteria on tricuspid valve

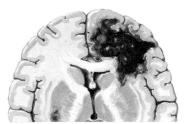

Infarct of brain with secondary hemorrhage from embolism to right anterior cerebral artery; also small infarct in left basal ganglia

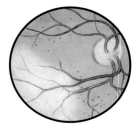

Embolus in vessel of ocular fundus with retinal infarction; petechiae

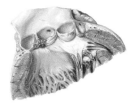

Early vegetations of infective endocarditis on bicuspid aortic valve

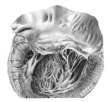

Early vegetations of infective endocarditis at contact line of mitral valve

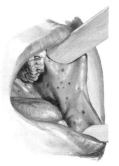

Petechiae of mucous membranes

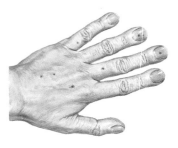

Multiple petechiae of skin and clubbing of fingers

Advanced lesions

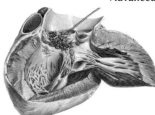

Advanced infective endocarditis of aortic valve: perforation of cusp; extension to anterior cusp of mitral valve and chordae tendineae: "jet lesion" on septal wall

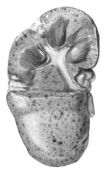

Petechiae and gross infarcts of kidney

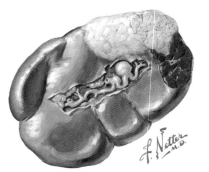

Mycotic aneurysms of splenic arteries and infarct of spleen; splenomegaly

FIG 49.2 Infective Endocarditis: Remote Embolic Effects.

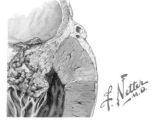

Vegetations of infective endocarditis on under-aspect as well as on atrial surface of mitral valve

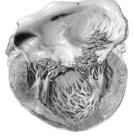

Advanced lesion of mitral valve: vegetations extending onto chordae tendineae with rupture of two chordae; also extension to atrial wall and contact lesion on opposite cusp

FIG 49.1 Infective Endocarditis.

BOX 49.1 **Risk Factors of Infective Endocarditis**

Patient Factors
- Older age (usually >60 years)
- Male gender
- History of IV drug use
- Poor dentition
- Immunosuppression/HIV
- Chronic hemodialysis

Cardiac Factors
- Valvular heart disease
- Congenital heart disease
- Prosthetic heart valves
- Intracardiac devices
- History of IE

IE, Infective endocarditis; *IV,* intravenous.

widespread metastatic infection being common. IE caused by oxacillin-resistant *S. aureus* is particularly common in injection drug users or patients with nosocomial infection. Coagulase-negative staphylococci are an important cause of prosthetic valve endocarditis (PVE). Right-sided IE is more commonly seen in injection drug users and may be either sensitive or resistant to oxacillin.

Streptococcal Endocarditis

Streptococci are now the second most common causative agents of IE, with the viridans group streptococci the most common subgroup. The cure rate exceeds 90%, but complications occur in approximately 30% of cases.

Streptococcus pneumoniae IE is rare and usually involves the aortic valve. It frequently has a fulminant course and is often associated with perivalvular abscess, pericarditis, and concurrent meningitis. *S. anginosus* has a predilection to disseminate and form abscesses, and may require

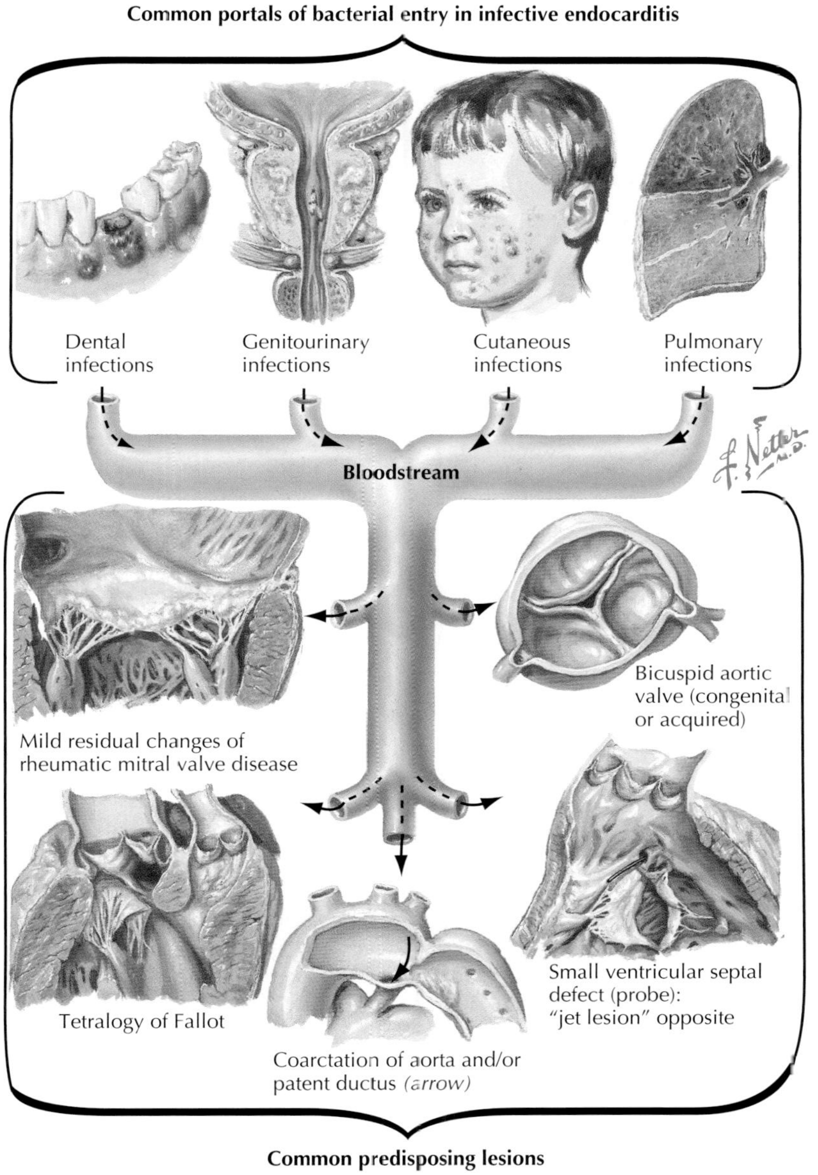

Common portals of bacterial entry in infective endocarditis

Dental infections

Genitourinary infections

Cutaneous infections

Pulmonary infections

Bloodstream

Mild residual changes of rheumatic mitral valve disease

Bicuspid aortic valve (congenital or acquired)

Tetralogy of Fallot

Small ventricular septal defect (probe): "jet lesion" opposite

Coarctation of aorta and/or patent ductus (*arrow*)

Common predisposing lesions

FIG 49.3 Frequent Origins of Infective Endocarditis in Nonimmunocompromised Individuals.

BOX 49.2 Diagnostic Approach to Infective Endocarditis

Definite IE Is Established in the Presence of Any of the Following:

Pathological Criteria

- Microorganisms demonstrated by culture or histological examination of a vegetation, a vegetation that has embolized or an intracardiac abscess specimen
- Vegetation or intracardiac abscess showing active endocarditis

Clinical Criteria

- Two major clinical criteria, one major, and three minor clinical criteria or five minor clinical criteria

Major Clinical Criteria

Positive Blood Cultures

- Typical microorganisms from two separate blood cultures: *Staphylococcus aureus*, streptococci (viridans and bovis), HACEK, or community acquired enterococci
- Persistently positive blood cultures
- Single positive blood culture for *Coxiella burnetii* or single phase I IgG antibody titer >1:800

Evidence of Endocardial Involvement

- Echocardiographic evidence of IE: vegetation, abscess, new partial dehiscence of prosthetic heart valve or new valvular regurgitation

---

HACEK, *Haemophilus species*, *Actinobacillus actinomycetemcomitans*, *Cardiobacterium hominis*, *Eikenella corrodens*, and *Kingella* species; *IE*, infective endocarditis; *IgG*, immunoglobulin G.

a longer course of therapy compared with other α-hemolytic strepto-cocci. *S. bovis* IE should prompt a colon malignancy evaluation.

Enterococcal Endocarditis

Enterococcus faecalis and *E. faecium* IE usually affects older men after genitourinary tract manipulation or younger women after an obstetric procedure. Classic peripheral manifestations are uncommon. The rate of penicillin-resistant enterococcal infection in tertiary care centers is rapidly increasing.

Gram-negative endocarditis. Individuals who use injection drugs, prosthetic valve recipients, and patients with cirrhosis are at increased risk for gram-negative endocarditis.

Salmonella IE usually involves preexisting valvular disease and is associated with significant valvular destruction, atrial thrombi, myo-carditis, and pericarditis. Valve replacement after 7 to 10 days of anti-microbial therapy is typically required.

Pseudomonas IE is almost exclusively seen in injection drug users and often affects normal valves. Embolic phenomena, inability to ster-ilize valves, neurological complications, ring and annular abscesses, splenic abscesses, bacteremic relapses, and progressive heart failure are common.

Neisseria gonorrhoeae rarely causes IE and typically follows an indo-lent course, with aortic valve involvement, large vegetations, valve ring abscesses, CHF, and nephritis.

HACEK Endocarditis

The gram-negative bacilli of the HACEK group account for 5% to 10% of cases of native valve IE. All are fastidious and may require ≥3 weeks for primary isolation. HACEK endocarditis is more common in patients who have dental infections or in injection drug users who contaminate the injection with saliva.

Fungal Endocarditis

Candida and *Aspergillus* species are the most common cause of fungal IE. *Candida* species are more common in persons with central venous catheters or in patients who are receiving parenteral nutrition. Both can be seen following prosthetic valve insertion. Other *Candida* species, *C. parapsilosis* and *C. tropicalis*, predominate in injection drug users. Blood culture results are usually negative in *Aspergillus* IE. Surgical intervention is almost always required, especially with the large vegeta-tions, after a course of antifungal agents. Lifelong antifungal suppressive therapy is frequently considered.

Culture-Negative Endocarditis

Culture-negative IE is common. Causes include recent administration of antimicrobial agents; slow growth of fastidious organisms, such as the HACEK group; fungal endocarditis; *Coxiella* species; intracellular parasites such as the *Bartonella* or *Chlamydia* species; and noninfectious endocarditis.

Prosthetic Valve Endocarditis

PVE occurs in up to 10% of patients during the lifetime of the pros-thesis. Early PVE (within 60 days after implantation) usually results from valve contamination during the perioperative period. Late PVE (after 60 days) results from transient bacteremia. Clinical manifestations are similar to those of native valve IE; however, new or changing murmurs are more common. Persistently positive blood culture results and val-vular dysfunction by echocardiography are the hallmarks. Transesophageal echocardiography (TEE) is recommended for diagnosis and assessment of complications (e.g., perivalvular abscess and regurgitation). Coagulase-negative staphylococci are the dominant cause of PVE in the first year. After 1 year, the causative organisms are similar to those of native valve

IE. Rifampin and gentamicin can be added to nafcillin or oxacillin for methicillin-sensitive *S. aureus* or to vancomycin for methicillin-resistant *S. aureus*. For culture-negative PVE, vancomycin and gentamicin should be used to provide broad bactericidal coverage.

Mycobacterium chimaera Endocarditis

Mycobacterium chimaera is a slow growing nontuberculosis mycobac-terium distinguished as a species within the *M. avium* complex. Recently, investigators in Switzerland identified *M. chimaera* contamination in heating–cooling units that were used to regulate the temperature of blood during extracorporeal membrane oxygenation as the potential source of invasive *M. chimaera* infections after open heart surgery. All patients identified underwent open heart surgery involving implanta-tions (prosthetic valves and aortic grafts), which resulted in bacteremia and endocarditis. Other accompanying symptoms included fatigue, fever, hepatitis, renal insufficiency, splenomegaly, and pancytopenia.

Healthcare providers involved in caring for patients who have under-gone open-heart surgery should be vigilant for cases of endocarditis and consider testing for slow-growing nontuberculosis mycobacteria, such as *M. chimaera*.

Echocardiography

Echocardiography is an essential tool in the diagnosis and management of patients with IE and should be performed in all patients with sus-pected and confirmed IE (Fig. 49.4). An oscillating vegetation or mass, annular abscess, prosthetic valve dehiscence, and new regurgitation are all major Duke criteria, and as such, confirm IE. Transthoracic echo-cardiography (TTE) is rapid, noninvasive, and has excellent specificity for vegetations (98%); however, sensitivity is <60%. TEE allows imaging of very small vegetations, prosthetic valves, and perivalvular areas for abscesses. TEE has a substantially higher sensitivity (76%–100%) and specificity (94%) than TTE for perivalvular extension of infection. If clinical sus-picion of IE persists after an initially negative TEE, a repeat study is warranted within 7 to 10 days. The combination of a negative TEE and a negative TTE confers a 95% negative predictive value.

MANAGEMENT AND THERAPY

Optimum Treatment

Antimicrobial Therapy

After initial broad spectrum empiric therapy, antimicrobial agents should be tapered based on susceptibility testing of the isolated causative microbe (Table 49.1). Prolonged administration of antimicrobial agents is required, almost always via the parenteral route. Bactericidal agents or antibiotic combinations that produce synergistic, rapidly bactericidal effects are the agents of choice. Although serum antibiotic levels are broadly useful, in particular, if aminoglycosides are part of the therapeutic regimen, it is important to monitor serum concentrations carefully to avoid toxicity. Blood culture specimens should be obtained early in therapy to ensure eradication of the bacteremia, and throughout therapy when persistent or recurrent fever is present. Patients with IE complicated by cardiac arrhythmias and CHF require close observation in an intensive care unit. Anticoagulation is contraindicated in patients with native valve IE.

Many of the newer antimicrobial agents may not have been specifi-cally evaluated in IE patients. Daptomycin, a cyclic lipopeptide antibiotic, is bactericidal in vitro against most gram-positive bacteria, especially oxacillin-sensitive and -resistant *S. aureus*. Daptomycin was shown to be equivalent to standard therapy for bacteremia and right-sided IE.

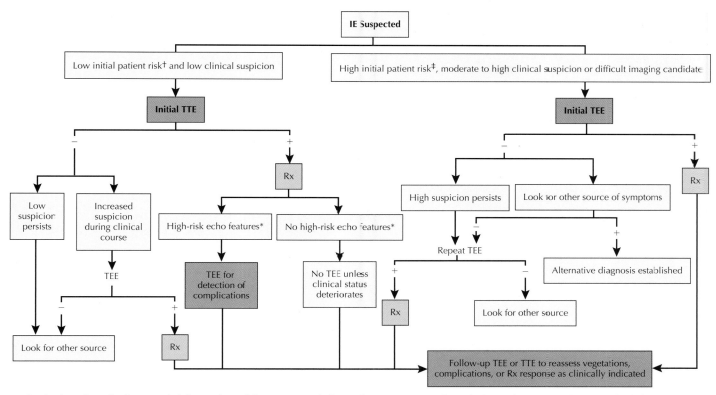

*High-risk echocardiographic features include large and/or mobile vegetations, valvular insufficiency, suggestion of perivalvular extension, or secondary ventricular dysfunction.
†For example, a patient with fever and a previously known heart murmur and no other stigmata of IE.
‡High initial patient risks include prosthetic heart valves, many congenital heart diseases, previous endocarditis, new murmur, heart failure, or other stigmata of endocarditis.

FIG 49.4 Echocardiography in the Diagnosis and Management of Infective Endocarditis (IE). *Rx*, Antibiotic treatment for endocarditis; *TEE*, transesophageal echocardiography; *TTE*, transthoracic echocardiography. (From Bayer AS, Bolger AF, Taubert KA, et al. Diagnosis and management of infective endocarditis and its complications. *Circulation* 1998; 98:2936–2948.)

Indications for Surgical Intervention

Appropriate, timely surgical intervention can reduce morbidity and mortality substantially. Relatively substantiated indications for surgical intervention include:

- Refractory CHF;
- More than one serious systemic embolic episode;
- Fungal IE, especially involving a prosthetic valve;
- IE with antibiotic-resistant bacteria or ineffective antimicrobial therapy;
- Persistent positive blood cultures following 1 week of antibiotic therapy;
- Left-sided IE with *Pseudomonas* or *Salmonella* species;
- Prosthetic valve IE ≤12 months after initial replacement; and
- Echocardiographic findings:
  - Vegetations >10 mm, especially those on the anterior mitral leaflet (greater risk for embolization) or vegetations that increase in size while on therapy;
  - Acute severe aortic or mitral insufficiency or valve perforation or rupture;
  - Large abscess or abscess unresponsive to therapy;
  - New heart block; and
  - Prosthetic valve dehiscence.

Avoiding Treatment Errors

Effective treatment of IE requires a multidisciplinary approach with input from infectious disease specialists, cardiologists, and cardiothoracic surgeons. Although guidelines and criteria such as the Duke criteria have been established, treatment should be individualized based on clinical judgment.

After a person is put on appropriate antimicrobial therapy, it is imperative to ensure that repeat blood cultures are negative. Blood cultures should be repeated near the end of antimicrobial therapy and shortly after completing therapy to ensure resolution, and a new baseline echocardiogram should be obtained. It is imperative to educate patients regarding signs or symptoms of IE. The need for thorough dental evaluation and treatment for substance abuse are often overlooked.

Prophylaxis

In 2007, the American Heart Association simplified its recommendations regarding antibiotic prophylaxis, and they currently recommend prophylaxis only for patients with the highest risk for IE, which include patients with:

1. A prosthetic heart valve or who have had a heart valve repaired with prosthetic material;
2. A history of endocarditis;
3. A history of heart transplantation with abnormal heart valve function; and
4. Certain congenital heart defects, including:
   a. Cyanotic congenital heart disease that has not been fully repaired, including children who have had surgical shunts and conduits;
   b. A congenital heart defect that has been completely repaired with prosthetic material or a device for the first 6 months after the repair procedure; and
   c. Repaired congenital heart disease with residual defects.

TABLE 49.1 Antimicrobial Therapy for Infective Endocarditis

Etiology	Antimicrobial Therapy[a]
Viridans streptococci and *S. bovis* penicillin-susceptible (MIC <0.1 µg/mL)	Penicillin G 12–18 million U/24 hrs IV either continuously or q4h for 4 wks or Ceftriaxone 2 g IV once daily for 4 wks, or Penicillin G 12–18 million U/24 hrs IV either continuously or in 6 doses for 2 wks with gentamicin 3 mg/kg per 24 hrs IV or IM in 1 dose for 2 wks, or Vancomycin 30 mg/kg/24 hrs IV in two divided doses for 4 wks (recommended only for patients allergic to β-lactams)
Viridans streptococci and *S. bovis* relatively resistant to penicillin (MIC 0.1–0.5 µg/mL)	Penicillin G 24 million U/24 hrs IV either continuously or q4h for 4 wks with gentamicin 3 mg/kg daily for 2 wks (ceftriaxone 2 g IV once daily may be substituted for penicillin in patients with penicillin hypersensitivity not of the immediate type), or Vancomycin 30 mg/kg/24 hrs IV in 2 divided doses for 4 wks (only recommended for patients allergic to β-lactams)
Enterococci (penicillin-susceptible)	Penicillin G 18–30 million U/24 hrs either continuously or q4h with gentamicin 3 mg/kg IV in 2–3 equally divided doses for 4–6 wks, or Ampicillin 2 g every 4 hrs with gentamicin 3 mg/kg IV in 2–3 equally divided doses for 4–6 wks, or Vancomycin 30 mg/kg/24 hrs IV in 2 divided doses for 4–6 wks with gentamicin 3 mg/kg IV in 2–3 equally divided doses for 4–6 wks (only recommended for patients allergic to β-lactams; cephalosporins are not acceptable alternatives for patients allergic to penicillins)
Enterococci (penicillin-resistant)	Vancomycin 30 mg/kg/24 hrs IV in 2 divided doses for 6 wks plus gentamicin 3 mg/kg per 24 hrs IV or IM in 3 divided doses or Linezolid 600 mg IV orally every 12 hrs for >6 wks or Daptomycin 10–12 mg/kg/dose for >6 wks
Staphylococci (oxacillin-susceptible strains)	Nafcillin or oxacillin 12 g IV q24 hrs in 4–6 equally divided doses for 6 wks or Cefazolin (or other first-generation cephalosporin) 6 g IV q 24h in 3 equally divided doses for 6 wks (for allergic to penicillin)
Staphylococci (oxacillin-resistant strains)	Vancomycin 30 mg/kg/24 hrs IV in 2 divided doses for 6 wks or daptomycin >8 mg/kg/dose for 6 wks
HACEK microorganisms	Ceftriaxone 2 g IV or IM once daily for 4 wks or Ampicillin 2 g/24 hrs IV q 4 hrs for 4 wks or Ciprofloxacin 1000 mg/24 hrs orally or 800 mg/24 hrs IV in 2 equally divided doses
Culture-negative (native valve)	Ampicillin-sulbactam 12 g/24 hrs IV in 4 doses for 4–6 wks plus gentamicin 1 mg/kg q8h for 4–6 wks or Vancomycin 30 mg/kg IV in 2 doses for 4–6 wks plus gentamicin 1 mg/kg IV in 3 doses for 4–6 wks plus Ciprofloxacin 1000 mg/24 hrs PO in 2 divided doses or 800 mg/24 hrs in 2 doses IV for 4–6 wks
Prosthetic valve endocarditis	Refer to 2015 American Heart Association endocarditis guidelines
Mycobacterium chimaera endocarditis (macrolide sensitive)	Daily azithromycin + rifampin + ethambutol for 12–18 months +/– IV amikacin for 3 months
Mycobacterium chimaera endocarditis (macrolide insensitive)	Daily rifampin + ethambutol + (other drug[b]) for 12–18 months +/– IV amikacin for 3 months

HACEK, Haemophilus species, Actinobacillus actinomycetemcomitans, Cardiobacterium hominis, Eikenella corrodens, and *Kingella* species; *IV,* Intravenous; *IM,* intramuscularly; *MIC,* minimum inhibitory concentration; *PO,* per os.

[a]Antimicrobial doses are for adult patients with normal renal and hepatic function. Aminoglycosides are used for synergy for gram-positive infections. When gentamicin is administered in multiple daily doses, the dose should be adjusted according to the renal function of the patient to achieve a peak concentration of approximately 3 mg/L and a trough concentration of <1 mg/L. Vancomycin doses should be adjusted according to the renal function of the patient to achieve a peak concentration of 30 to 45 mg/L and a trough concentration of 10 to 15 mg/L. Dosing of penicillin, nafcillin, and oxacillin is frequent and often problematic for home therapy patients. Because these drugs are stable for 24 hours at room temperature, they may be given via a pump that remains with the patient, requiring adjustment only once every 24 hours. Test infecting strain of *Enterococcus* for resistance to aminoglycosides. High-level resistance means loss of synergy, and thus aminoglycosides should not be used in these instances. Therapy should be prolonged to 8 to 12 weeks.

[b]Other drug options: clofazimine, moxifloxacin, ciprofloxacin or bedaquiline.

Adapted from Baddour LM, Wilson WR, Bayer AS, et al. Infective endocarditis in adults: diagnosis, antimicrobial therapy, and management of complications. *Circulation* 2015;132:1435–1486.

FUTURE DIRECTIONS

Some clinicians believe that the size of the vegetation and other echocardiographic characteristics predict which patients are at risk for poor outcome and need early surgery. However, specific echocardiographic criteria have not been demonstrated. Future studies will help to determine whether echocardiographic findings other than perivalvular or myocardial abscesses are added to the current list of indications for surgery.

ADDITIONAL RESOURCES

American Heart Association [home page on the Internet]. http://www .americanheart.org. Accessed February 16, 2010.
Provides guidance in the management of other cardiac-related diseases.
Bayer AS, Bolger AF, Taubert KA, et al. Diagnosis and management of infective endocarditis and its complications. *Circulation.* 1998;98:2936–2948.
This article clearly outlines the global management of IE.

European Society of Cardiology. European Society for Cardiologist guidelines for infective endocarditis; 2004. http://www.escardio.org/knowledge/guidelines/Guidelines_list.htm. Accessed February 16, 2010.

Reviews European guidelines, which differ from the Infectious Disease Society of America and American Heart Association guidelines.

Schlant RC, Alexander RW, O'Rourke RA, et al, eds. *Hurst's the Heart.* 10th ed. New York: McGraw-Hill Inc; 2001.

Comprehensively reviews the management of IE from the perspective of a cardiologist.

EVIDENCE

Baddour LM, Wilson WR, Bayer AS, et al. Infective endocarditis in adults: diagnosis, antimicrobial therapy, and management of complications. *Circulation.* 2015;CIR.0000000000000296, originally published September 15, 2015.

American Heart Association scientific statement on IE in adults.

Fowler VG Jr, Boucher HW, Corey GR, et al. Daptomycin versus standard therapy for bacteremia and endocarditis caused by *Staphylococcus aureus. N Engl J Med.* 2006;355:653–665.

Describes use of a newer generation antibiotics in resistant bacterial infections.

Infectious Diseases Society of America. American Heart Association infective endocarditis guidelines. http://www.idsociety.org/Content.aspx?id=9088. Accessed February 16, 2010.

Publishes updated guidelines for the management of IE, an essential tool in managing these complicated patients.

Li JS, Sexton DJ, Mick N, et al. *Clin Infect Dis.* 2000;30:633.

Modified Duke criteria for diagnosis of IE.

Mandell GL, Bennett JE, Dolin R, eds. *Mandell, Douglas, and Bennett's Principles and Practice of Infectious Diseases.* 6th ed. New York: Churchill Livingstone; 2005.

Provides more specific guidance in the diagnosis and treatment of suspected and/or confirmed IE. Less common pathogens and complicated IE are comprehensively reviewed.

Sax H, et al. Prolonged outbreak of Mycobacterium chimaera infection after open-chest heart surgery. *Clin Infect Dis.* 2015;61:67–75.

Mycobacterium chimaera *outbreak information.*

50

Surgical Treatment of Valvular Heart Disease

Timothy Brand, Thomas G. Caranasos, Michael E. Bowdish, Michael R. Mill, Brett C. Sheridan

Competency of the atrioventricular valves allows blood to enter the ventricles, where pressure is generated. When adequate systolic blood pressure is generated, the aortic and pulmonary valves open, allowing blood to enter the arterial system. The atrioventricular valves close, preventing the flow of blood into the atria. During diastole, the aortic and pulmonary valves close, the atrioventricular valves open, the ventricles fill, and ultimately begin the cycle of pulsatile blood flow through the systemic and pulmonary vascular tree.

Malfunction of any of the cardiac valves results in a less efficient circulatory system. Valvular dysfunction causes work overload in one or both ventricles. In extreme cases, this results in heart failure.

Valvular heart disease treatment is evolving with the addition of new technologies. Valve replacement technology has changed with the development of more durable tissue valves and new mechanical valves. The addition of transcatheter therapies has led to a paradigm in the treatment of valvular heart disease.

FIRST-GENERATION PROSTHETIC VALVES

Initial attempts to duplicate valve leaflets with flexible, nonbiological materials failed. The leaflets of these valves were too stiff in comparison with normal valve leaflets. Efforts at using nonflexible leaflets by constructing hinged-valve leaflets resulted in hinge thrombosis and malfunction. Design engineers then focused on free-floating occluders, such as disks or balls retained in a cagelike housing. This general valve design produced the first clinically useful valves. In 1958, the Starr-Edwards valve was used in the first clinically successful valve replacement.

Although these early designs functioned as intended, the first caged-ball valves had major shortcomings: (1) they were bulky in design and did not fit well into a small ventricle or aorta; (2) they had a small internal orifice, making them relatively stenotic; and (3) they stimulated thrombus formation, which precipitated thromboembolic events, which then necessitated long-term anticoagulation therapy.

Second-Generation Prosthetic Valves

The disadvantages of early prosthetic valves led to the development of two divergent lines of valve design using synthetic materials (mechanical valves) or biological tissue (bioprosthetic valves). The caged-ball valves were modified, and pivoting hingeless disk valves, such as the Lillehei-Kaster, Medtronic-Hall, and Björk-Shiley valves, were developed. The St. Jude and Carbomedics valves were the first successful hinged-leaflet valves (Fig. 50.1, top).

Homograft valves harvested at autopsy and preserved in antibiotic solution or frozen were the first nonsynthetic valves to be implanted successfully. Their limited availability prompted the use of porcine valves procured from slaughterhouses. Porcine valves were preserved with glutaraldehyde and mounted on modified nylon-covered plastic or metal stents. Valves made of pericardium were also developed and used successfully (Fig. 50.1, bottom). Porcine and bovine pericardial valves are commonly used bioprosthetic valves today, whereas the hinged leaflet valves are the commonly used mechanical valves. No valve has proven to be the perfect replacement, but durability has dramatically improved over the years.

ETIOLOGY AND PATHOGENESIS

Cardiac valve pathology consists of two broad categories: congenital valve deformity and acquired valvular dysfunction. Congenital deformity can occur in one or more cardiac valves (see Section VIII). Patients with severe congenital valvular dysfunction can die if prompt surgical intervention is not undertaken. In patients with normally developed hearts, infection can cause valvular dysfunction at any age. Rheumatic heart disease secondary to untreated streptococcal infection and bacterial endocarditis can destroy a normal heart valve. Generalized inflammatory illnesses, such as lupus erythematosus, rheumatoid arthritis, and eosinophilic endocarditis, as well as carcinoid disease, similarly can cause valvular dysfunction. Connective tissue diseases, such as Ehlers-Danlos syndrome and myxomatous degeneration, can cause valve deformity and dysfunction. Severe myocardial ischemia and injury can cause papillary muscle dysfunction, which can result in mitral valve insufficiency. Finally, aging often results in atherosclerotic changes and calcium deposition in arterial walls, and aging can also affect the aortic valves, sometimes with severe calcification of the leaflets. The mitral valve annulus can also be severely calcified, with or without valvular dysfunction.

Clinical Presentation

The presenting symptoms in patients with dysfunctional valves vary considerably, depending on the type and severity of dysfunction and the location of the affected valves. Diseased valves can become incompetent, stenotic, or both. Young patients with moderate aortic valve stenosis are often asymptomatic. Likewise, many patients with moderate mitral valve stenosis or insufficiency may be asymptomatic. In general, patients whose valve dysfunction progresses eventually experience dyspnea on exertion. Syncope or angina pectoris, alone or in association with dyspnea, can develop in patients with aortic stenosis.

DIFFERENTIAL DIAGNOSIS

In patients presenting with dyspnea and fatigue, noncardiac causes, such as anemia, hypertension, pulmonary pathology, and hypothyroidism, should be excluded. Primary cardiac myopathy should be considered. Coronary artery disease must be ruled out if angina pectoris is a symptom.

Second-generation synthetic prosthetic valves were hingeless pivoting disk valves and hinged bileaflet valves.

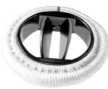

Medtronic-Hall
pivoting disk valve

St. Jude bileaflet valve

Björk-Shiley valve

Carbomedics
bileaflet valve

Tissue valves made of porcine aortic valves, pericardium, or cadaver homografts are also important in valve replacement surgical therapy.

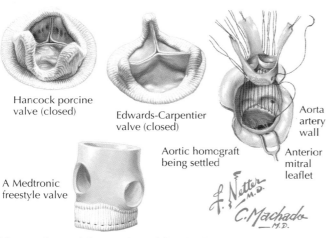

Hancock porcine
valve (closed)

Edwards-Carpentier
valve (closed)

Aortic homograft
being settled

A Medtronic
freestyle valve

Aorta
artery
wall

Anterior
mitral
leaflet

FIG 50.1 Second Generation of Synthetic Prosthetic Valves and Biological Valves.

DIAGNOSTIC APPROACH

Physical findings such as cardiac murmurs, wide pulse pressure, cardiomegaly, hepatomegaly, ascites, or pedal edema help to confirm abnormal circulatory conditions. Chest radiography and ECG offer supportive evidence of cardiac pathology. The most descriptive and definitive tests pinpointing cardiac valve anomalies are echocardiography in association with hemodynamic data from cardiac catheterization.

MANAGEMENT AND THERAPY

Optimum Treatment
Surgical Therapy
A variety of procedures are available to treat cardiac valvular disease. Replacing diseased valves with prosthetic valves has become a routine procedure, and valve repair—particularly mitral and tricuspid valve repair—has evolved considerably. Techniques routinely used in the repair of mitral and tricuspid insufficiencies include ring annuloplasty, resection of prolapsing portions of leaflets not supported by chordae, shortening or using artificial chordae, and increasing or decreasing the leaflet area by sliding annuloplasty. In patients who need aortic valve

replacement, some surgeons advocate aortic valve repair and resuspension, if possible, to preserve the native valve. An alternative to replacement is the Ross procedure, which entails transplanting the pulmonary valve of the patient into the aortic position. This provides the patient with a living, durable, nonthrombogenic, and hemodynamically superior valve. The pulmonary valve is then reconstructed using a tissue homograft valve. The choice of procedure depends on many factors, including the valve pathology, age, and ability of the patient to tolerate and comply with long-term anticoagulation.

Mitral and Tricuspid Valves
Patients with mitral and tricuspid valve pathology should be considered for valve repair rather than replacement, because the operative mortality associated with repair of these valves is lower than that associated with their replacement.

Conditions precluding satisfactory repair of the mitral and tricuspid valves include severe scarring and deformation by a disease process such as advanced rheumatic heart disease or advanced lupus, or another inflammatory process involving the valve leaflets and destruction of valve leaflets and annuli by endocarditis. Under these circumstances, the valve should be replaced (Fig. 50.2). Mitral valve replacement should include preservation of a portion of the subvalvular chordae and papillary muscles to aid in preserving normal ventricular contractility.

Aortic Valves
Adult patients with aortic valve pathology are seldom candidates for valve repair, and thus valve replacement is usually the preferred treatment for significant aortic stenosis or regurgitation. The age, lifestyle, and preferences of the patient, as well as the preferences of the surgeon dictate the type of prosthetic valve replacement (see Fig. 50.2B and Fig. 50.3).

Avoiding Treatment Errors
Issues With Prosthetic Valve Replacement
Patients with bioprosthetic valves have a lower incidence of bleeding, because long-term anticoagulation is not required in patients in sinus rhythm. Unfortunately, all bioprosthetic tissue valves eventually deteriorate and become insufficient. Deterioration of tissue valves occurs at an accelerated rate in younger patients and in patients with end-stage renal disease on hemodialysis. For older patients, particularly those with a risk of falling, a bioprosthetic valve may be the most appropriate choice, because long-term anticoagulation is not required for bioprosthetic aortic valves. Younger patients, with a natural life expectancy exceeding 15 to 20 years, should have prosthetic valves made of durable synthetic materials, such as pyrolytic carbon, titanium, stainless steel, or a combination of these. Use of mechanical valves necessitates indefinite anticoagulation.

Mechanical valves must have an appropriate sewing ring sutured to the annulus of the valve of the patient after the leaflets are excised. Sewing rings are usually circular and rigid, and vary in thickness. The rigid sewing rings change the natural shape of the valve annulus, and depending on thickness, decrease the size of the internal orifice of the prosthetic valve. Implanting a valve with a circular sewing ring into a noncircular annulus can generate unnatural tension between the valve annulus and sewing ring, which can lead to paravalvular leaks; the surgical approach in these instances must take this possibility into account.

The use of rigid circular sewing rings is unnecessary in bioprosthetic valves implanted in the aortic position. Freehand suturing is used to insert autograft pulmonary valves into the aortic position (the Ross procedure). It is also used in homograft cadaver valve implantation and with nonstented freestyle porcine valves.

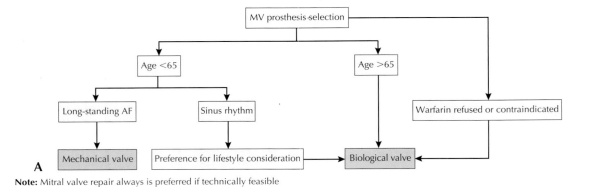

A

Note: Mitral valve repair always is preferred if technically feasible

B

FIG 50.2 **Algorithm for Prosthesis Selection in Valvular Heart Disease.** (A) Mitral valve (MV) prosthesis selection. (B) Aortic valve prosthesis selection. *AF*, Atrial fibrillation. (Adapted from Bonow RO, Carabello BA, Chatterjee K, et al. ACC/AHA 2006 guidelines for the management of patients with valvular heart disease: a report of the American College of Cardiology/American Heart Association Task Force on Practice Guidelines [Writing Committee to Develop Guidelines for the Management of Patients with Valvular Heart Disease]. *Circulation* 2006;114:e84–e213.)

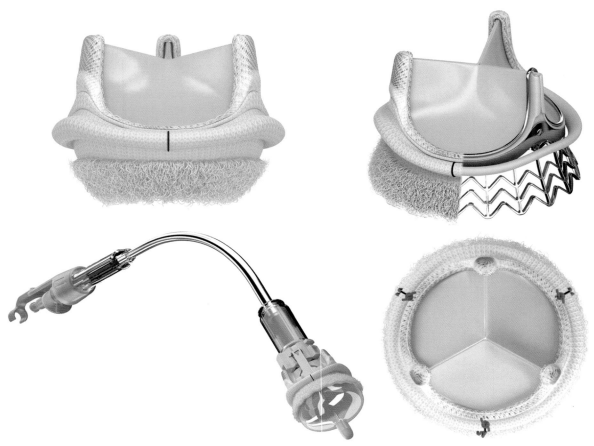

FIG 50.3 **Edwards Intuity Elite Valve System.** (Used with permission from Edwards Lifesciences LLC, Irvine, California.)

Exposing the mitral valve through the interatrial septum and an extension of the incision through the roof of the left atrium is common. This surgical exposure allows excellent visualization of the mitral and tricuspid valves and can be performed through a standard sternotomy, as well as through a variety of partial sternotomy and right thoracotomy incisions.

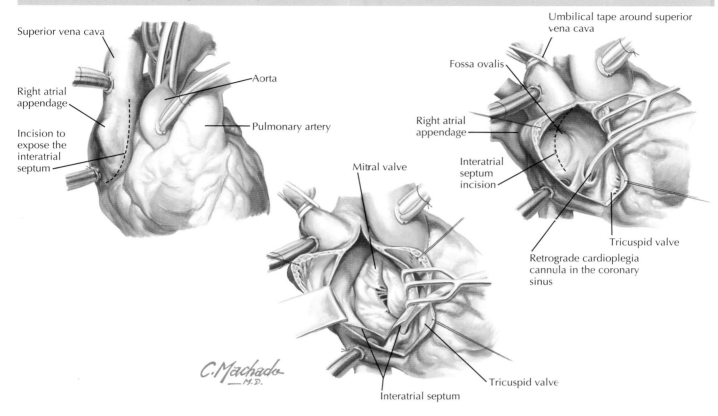

FIG 50.4 Exposing the Mitral Valve Through the Interatrial Septum.

Minimally Invasive Techniques

Minimally invasive coronary artery revascularization surgery uses small incisions and therefore is performed on a beating heart, obviating the use of cardiopulmonary bypass. In valve repair and replacement procedures, the use of smaller incisions is possible, but eliminating cardiopulmonary bypass is not feasible with current techniques and prosthetic valves.

Good visualization of the operative field is a prerequisite for proper valve repair or replacement. Smaller incisions limit visualization, although the use of miniature video cameras improves the view of the operative field. The mitral valve is generally the most difficult to visualize, so many surgeons approach it through the interatrial septum, sometimes extending the incision to the roof of the left atrium (Fig. 50.4).

FUTURE DIRECTIONS

Refinements in manufacturing mechanical prosthetic valves and their sewing rings will continue to decrease thromboembolic complications while improving their hemodynamic characteristics. Better chemical preservation of bioprosthetic valves will improve their longevity and resistance to deterioration, and make bioprosthetic valves a more attractive choice for younger patients.

The teaching of valve repair techniques to surgical trainees is already becoming more standardized. The appropriate surgical repair technique will be more predictable from the preoperative evaluation, including echocardiographic and hemodynamic data. Freehand valve implantation techniques will find increased use in selected patients, particularly for patients in whom the annulus is small and in which the valve sewing rings make the prosthetic valves too stenotic. Finally, with clinical acceptance of genetic engineering, farms of genetically altered pigs and baboons might provide viable biological leaflets, valves, and entire hearts for implantation.

Newer "sutureless" valves have come to market that are mounted on balloon expandable frames that can be inserted in a similar way as transcatheter valves, which can be placed with a standard sternotomy or facilitate easier placement with a minimally invasive approach.

ADDITIONAL RESOURCES

Bonow RO, Carabello BA, Chatterjee K, et al. ACC/AHA 2006 guidelines for the management of patients with valvular heart disease: a report of the American College of Cardiology/American Heart Association Task Force on Practice Guidelines (Writing Committee to Develop Guidelines for the Management of Patients with Valvular Heart Disease). *Circulation.* 2006;114:e84–e213.

American College of Cardiology/American Heart Association guidelines regarding the management of patients with valvular heart disease. Essential reading for clinicians caring for patients with valvular heart disease.

David TE, Feindel CM, Webb GD, et al. Long-term results of aortic valve-sparing operations for aortic root aneurysm. *J Thorac Cardiovasc Surg.* 2006;132:347–354.
Important contribution regarding aortic valve repair.
David TE, Ivanov J, Armstrong S, Rakowski H. Late outcomes of mitral valve repair for floppy valves: implications for asymptomatic patients. *J Thorac Cardiovasc Surg.* 2003;125:1143–1152.
Outcomes for mitral valve repair from a leading center for patients with myxomatous disease.

EVIDENCE

Carpentier A. Cardiac valve surgery: the "French connection." *J Thorac Cardiovasc Surg.* 1983;86:323–337.
Important contribution to mitral valve repair surgery.

Moon MR, Pasque MK, Munfakh NA, et al. Prosthesis-patient mismatch after aortic valve replacement: impact of age and body size on late survival. *Ann Thorac Surg.* 2006;81:481–489.
Important contribution regarding patient size and valve size in aortic valve replacement.

Structural Heart Disease

51

Clinical Presentation of Adults With Congenital Heart Disease

Joseph S. Rossi, Elman G. Frantz

ETIOLOGY AND PATHOGENESIS

Congenital heart disease refers to any heart defect present at birth. The etiology of such defects is multifactorial, with environmental and genetic factors playing important roles. In utero development can be affected by metabolic stress from toxins, hypoxemia, and medications. Chromosomal abnormalities, such as trisomy 21, or inherited single gene disorders can also play important roles. Congenital heart disease therefore can present along a spectrum from very mild to life threatening depending on the severity of structural involvement. Many cases have no identifiable cause and are generally assumed to be due to complex multifactorial genetic influences.

Among adult patients with congenital heart disease, symptoms and clinical trajectory can vary dramatically on the basis of type and severity of the underlying condition. Because of improved imaging techniques and widely available screening tests, most life-threatening congenital heart disease is diagnosed in utero in the United States. In patients who have congenital heart disease in adulthood, many have been appropriately treated (often surgically corrected), followed by a pediatric/congenital cardiologist, and remain on a stable trajectory. For patients who present for the first time with congenital heart disease in adulthood, there is typically a reason that the presentation was delayed. Among patients with severe congenital heart disease (cyanotic heart disease, large ventricular septal defect, or atrial septal defect), this is often due to lack of proper medical care and surveillance, but many patients can also present with progression of a clinical condition that was not previously detected despite adequate medical attention. Many patients also present after being lost to follow-up years after initial surgical treatment. It is helpful to group these patients on the basis of underlying pathophysiology and the presence or absence of previous surgical correction.

UNCORRECTED CYANOTIC HEART CONDITIONS

It is rare for cyanotic heart conditions to be diagnosed in adulthood, and when this occurs, it is typically due to lack of access to medical care. Cyanosis associated with congenital heart disease typically is the result of a significant amount of poorly oxygenated blood being shunted into the systemic circulation. This can occur due to improper mixing of blood at the atrial or ventricular level, with increased pulmonary outflow resistance that results in a right-to-left shunt. Examples of this type of cyanotic defect include pulmonary atresia with ventricular septal defect (VSD), tetralogy of Fallot (TOF), and Eisenmenger syndrome. Cyanosis can also result from the mixture of pulmonary and systemic venous returns despite normal or increased pulmonary blood flow. In most cardiac malformations classified in this group, a single chamber receives the total systemic and pulmonary venous returns. The mixing of oxygenated and desaturated blood can occur at any level: venous (e.g., total anomalous pulmonary venous connection [TAPVC]), atrial (e.g., single atrium), ventricular (e.g., single ventricle), and great vessel (e.g., persistent truncus arteriosus). In all these circumstances, near-uniform mixing of the venous returns usually occurs. Complete transposition of the great arteries (TGA) (Fig. 51.1) can be included in this group, although only partial admixture of the two venous returns occurs, leading to severe hypoxemia.

Most of these patients require surgical correction in childhood. In the rare patient in whom presentation with cyanosis occurs in adulthood, careful evaluation of the pulmonary vascular resistance is required, and surgical correction is the treatment of choice in most cases when there is a viable pulmonary vascular tree, and systemic and pulmonic ventricular function remains preserved. Consultation with a congenital heart specialist and a surgeon specializing in the treatment of adults with congenital heart disease is essential. A summary of surgical techniques involved in the correction of cyanotic congenital heart defects can be found in Chapter 53.

Eisenmenger Syndrome

Chronic overload of the pulmonary circulation due to acyanotic congenital heart defects, including VSD, atrial septal defect (ASD), and patent ductus arteriosus (PDA), can result in arterial remodeling and a gradual increase in the pulmonary vascular resistance, which results in severe pulmonary hypertension. Eventually, resistance across the pulmonary circuit becomes elevated to the point where the shunt reverses, which results in cyanosis and right ventricular (RV) failure. The condition was first described by Dr. Victor Eisenmenger in 1897 and is relatively uncommon today in the developed world. However, in cases of lack of access to appropriate medical care, large ASDs, VSDs, or PDAs can present with gradual overload of the pulmonary vascular circulation and result in Eisenmenger syndrome.

This condition is difficult to treat with surgical correction of the underlying defect because severe and chronic pulmonary hypertension is often a contraindication to corrective surgery. For patients with severe elevation of pulmonary vascular resistance, closing the source of intracardiac shunt can lead to increased afterload and failure of the RV. Therefore, Eisenmenger syndrome is generally considered inoperable, and quality of life and survival are likely better with medical management only. In some patients, it has been reported that Eisenmenger syndrome can be successfully treated with pulmonary vasodilator therapy, and eventual successful closure of the primary defect. For patients in whom complete ASD or VSD closure is believed to be contraindicated, a fenestrated repair that leaves a small residual shunt can also be considered, with complete repair occurring at a later date.

Balloon Atrial Septostomy (Technique)

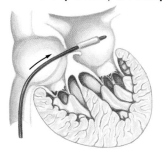

1. Balloon-tipped catheter introduced into left atrium through patent foramen ovale

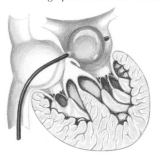

2. Balloon inflated

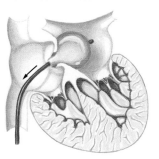

3. Balloon withdrawn producing large septal defect

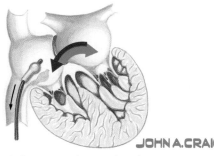

JOHN A.CRAIG—AD

4. Common atrium produced by septostomy allows mixing of oxygenated and deoxygenated blood

FIG 51.1 Transposition of the Great Arteries. The technique shown is used to promote venous mixing while awaiting surgical repair.

UNCORRECTED ACYANOTIC CONDITIONS

Atrial Septal Defect

Congenital heart defects that result in left-to-right shunting in the absence of hypoxemia are much more likely to allow survival into adulthood without clinical detection. The most common cause of acyanotic heart disease in the adult is ASD. Defects of the ostium secundum are the most common and often present later in life with dyspnea and RV enlargement and/or arrhythmias. Rarely, undiagnosed secundum ASD can result in severe pulmonary hypertension and even Eisenmenger syndrome, if left untreated. For patients with evidence of severe RV enlargement or with significant left-to-right shunt (>2:1) in the setting of secundum ASD, closure of the defect is recommended, and this can often be performed with catheter-based techniques (see Chapter 52). However, for patients with complex ASDs that involve abnormal venous return (sinus venosus ASD) or the septum primum (primum ASD), surgical closure is the treatment of choice due to the involvement of other cardiac structures. Primum ASD is often associated with abnormalities of the mitral valve and endocardial cushions, and superior sinus venosus ASD is commonly associated with anomalous pulmonary venous return. These defects do not occur with a complete tissue rim, making device-based closure impractical (Fig. 51.2).

Ventricular Septal Defect

VSD is typically diagnosed early in life due to the significant amount of turbulence causing an audible murmur on auscultation (the classic murmur of a VSD is a loud pansystolic murmur with an early diastolic component). However, in patients with lack of access to medical care, VSD can be well tolerated and allow survival into adulthood with relatively good functional status. This depends on the size of the degree of shunting associated with the defect. For "restrictive" VSD (<10 mm), patients will often present with a loud murmur without signs or symptoms of congenital heart failure. These small defects can often be observed without clinical consequence and are associated with normal pulmonary artery pressure and lack of left heart volume overload. Nonrestrictive VSD can progress to severe overload of the pulmonary vascular circuit, which results in severe pulmonary hypertension and Eisenmenger syndrome.

Anatomically, VSDs can be classified into four separate groups. Perimembranous VSD is the most common and accounts for 80% of clinically diagnosed defects (small muscular VSDs may be more common but these typically close spontaneously and remain undiagnosed). These defects are adjacent to the left ventricular outflow tract, and can be associated with aneurysmal deformation of the septal leaflet of the tricuspid valve and possibly left ventricular to right atrial shunting. The defect is often restrictive and can be followed conservatively. The second most common anatomic grouping is muscular VSD, which accounts for 5% to 10% of all cases. Muscular VSDs can often be multiple, and sometimes are amenable to percutaneous closure. Less common types of VSDs include supracristal (subpulmonic) and posterior (canal type). Supracristal VSD is usually associated with abnormalities of the right coronary cusp that causes aortic regurgitation, and when symptomatic, requires surgical VSD repair and repair and/or replacement of the aortic valve. Posterior or canal-type VSD is usually not associated with abnormalities of the atrioventricular valve and is typically isolated in the posterior portion of the ventricular septum. Together, supracristal and posterior VSDs account for <10% of all clinical presentations (Fig. 51.3).

Patent Ductus Arteriosus

PDA is a third form of acyanotic heart defect that can lead to persistent left-to-right shunting and overload of the pulmonary circulation. Although PDA closure usually occurs spontaneously at the time of birth due to the lack of exposure to maternal prostaglandins and increases in neonatal blood oxygen content, the presence of stressors at the time of birth can lead to persistent patency. The degree of shunting through the defect is dependent on the length and width of the PDA and the

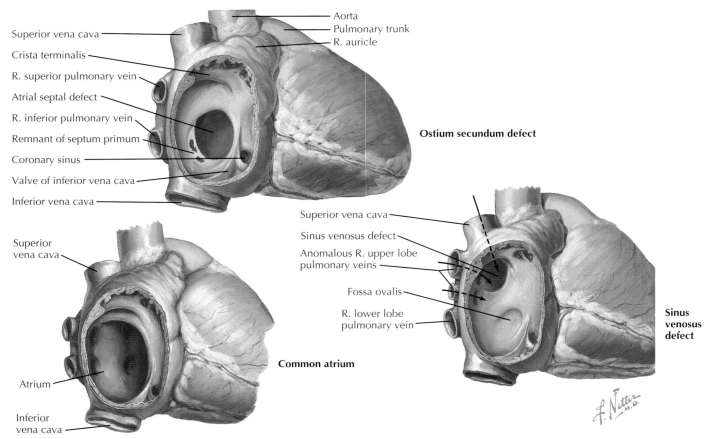

Superior vena cava

Crista terminalis

R. superior pulmonary vein

Atrial septal defect

R. inferior pulmonary vein

Remnant of septum primum

Coronary sinus

Valve of inferior vena cava

Inferior vena cava

Aorta
Pulmonary trunk
R. auricle

Ostium secundum defect

Superior vena cava

Atrium

Inferior vena cava

Common atrium

Superior vena cava

Sinus venosus defect

Anomalous R. upper lobe pulmonary veins

Fossa ovalis

R. lower lobe pulmonary vein

Sinus venosus defect

FIG 51.2 Defects of the Atrial Septum.

underlying resistance to pulmonary blood flow. Patients with low pulmonary vascular resistance can develop a persistent shunt into adulthood. Persistent shunting can lead to pulmonary hypertension and left ventricular overload. Fortunately, most PDA shunts can now be effectively closed with percutaneous techniques in most patients. In addition, medical treatment of PDA with nonsteroidal antiinflammatory agents can also be an effective measure to initiate physiological closure.

SURGICALLY CORRECTED CONDITIONS LIKELY TO PRESENT TO THE ADULT CARDIOLOGY CLINIC

Tetralogy of Fallot

TOF is a congenital heart disease present in approximately 1 in 2000 live births. It is characterized by an overriding aorta, VSD, pulmonary stenosis, and RV hypertrophy. The cause of TOF is largely unknown but is associated with advanced maternal age, maternal comorbid conditions (e.g., diabetes and hypertension), and alcohol abuse during pregnancy. Patients with TOF can usually survive early in life if adequate blood supply can be provided to the pulmonary circulation. A palliative and/or corrective shunt (Blalock-Taussig procedure) can be performed to shunt blood into the pulmonary circulation while definitive corrective surgery is planned. The first surgery to correct TOF was reported in 1954, and patients with surgical correction can now be expected to have a normal life span, with increased risk of morbidity due to RV failure and arrhythmias. Due to increased safety and standardization of techniques, TOF repair is now performed at most pediatric surgery centers, usually within the first year of life. Most patients survive with a good prognosis, and female patients can have uncomplicated

pregnancies. Because most patients require reconstruction of the RV outflow tract, there is often residual pulmonary valve disease that can progress into adulthood. In general, the goals of therapy for adult patients with previous TOF repair include: (1) monitoring of the pulmonic valve and RV outflow for both regurgitation and stenosis; (2) monitoring of RV function; (3) monitoring for ventricular and atrial arrhythmias; and (4) monitoring of previous VSD repair.

Most patients with TOF will have residual pulmonic valve disease. In some cases, this can result in pulmonic stenosis into adulthood if there is incomplete growth of the main pulmonary artery after surgical repair. More commonly, however, there is progressive pulmonic insufficiency that can lead to progressive RV failure if left untreated. Percutaneous valve replacement with the Melody Transcatheter Pulmonary Valve System (Melody TPV) (Medtronic, Minneapolis, Minnesota) has now been approved by the Food and Drug Administration and is commonly used in treatment of prosthetic RV-to-pulmonary artery conduits and rarely for native conduit disease. Specifically, the Melody TPV is approved for existence of a full (circumferential) RV outflow tract conduit that was ≥16 mm in diameter when originally implanted, with at least moderate regurgitation, and/or stenosis with a mean gradient of ≥35 mm Hg. This population represents a small number of patients, and it is likely that the Melody TPV will largely be used in native RV-to-pulmonary artery conduits in the future (Fig. 51.4).

D-Transposition of the Great Arteries

In patients with simple D-TGA, survival after birth is dependent on the presence of a large ASD and a PDA that allows a supply of oxygenated blood to the systemic circulation. Some patients require balloon

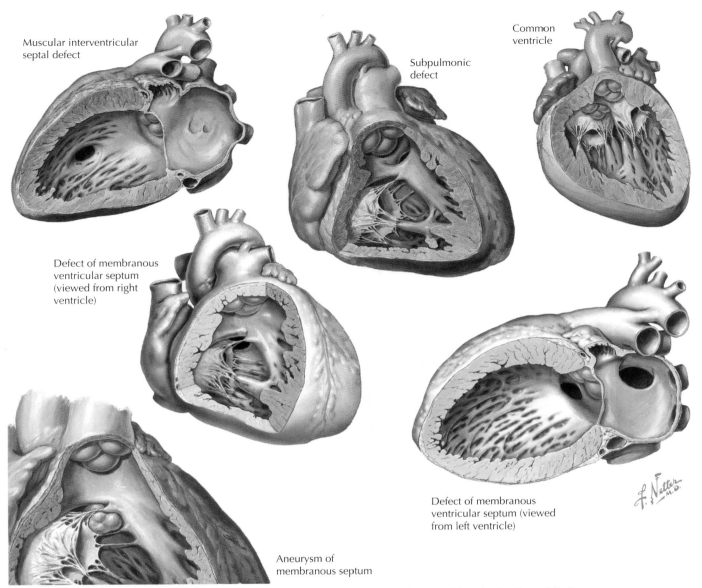

Muscular interventricular septal defect

Subpulmonic defect

Common ventricle

Defect of membranous ventricular septum (viewed from right ventricle)

Defect of membranous ventricular septum (viewed from left ventricle)

Aneurysm of membranous septum

FIG 51.3 Anatomic Features of Perimembranous and Muscular Ventricular Septal Defects.

atrial septostomy (Rashkind procedure) to increase the amount of oxygenated blood available in the systemic circulation. When uncorrected, this condition is generally not compatible with life past the neonatal period, and definitive correction with an atrial switch or arterial switch procedure is required. There are several subtypes of D-TGAs that are described based on the presence of outflow tract obstruction and VSDs. Patients with successful atrial switch have a baffle placed to divert deoxygenated blood into the subpulmonic left ventricle and are left with a systemic RV that receives baffled and oxygenated venous blood from the pulmonary veins. These patients will have increased risk of systemic ventricle failure. In patients with arterial switch procedures, there is an increased risk of acquired valvular heart disease. Long-term survival with both operations is now >90%.

In the adult population, previous atrial switch procedure requires regular clinical follow-up to follow baffle patency and evaluate for atrial and ventricular arrhythmias associated with this condition. It is not uncommon for the patients to require catheter ablation of electrical

disturbance later in life, and intracardiac navigation to ablate reentrant tachycardia can be challenging due to the presence of atrial baffles.

Tricuspid Atresia/Hypoplastic Right Heart

Most patient with tricuspid atresia and hypoplasia of the RV can survive in the presence of a VSD and an ASD that allows shunting of blood into the pulmonary circulation. However, the absence of a right-sided atrioventricular connection requires definitive surgical repair. Initial therapy includes prostaglandin E1 (PGE1) to maintain a PDA. Eventually, a modified Blalock-Taussig shunt can be performed to maintain pulmonary blood flow by placing a conduit between the subclavian artery and the pulmonary artery. In patients with normal pulmonary artery outflow, banding can be required to prevent overcirculation in the presence of a large VSD. A more definitive staged repair (Fontan operation) usually involves superior cavopulmonary anastomosis (hemi-Fontan or bidirectional Glenn) followed by a Fontan completion to redirect venous blood from the inferior vena cava and hepatic vein.

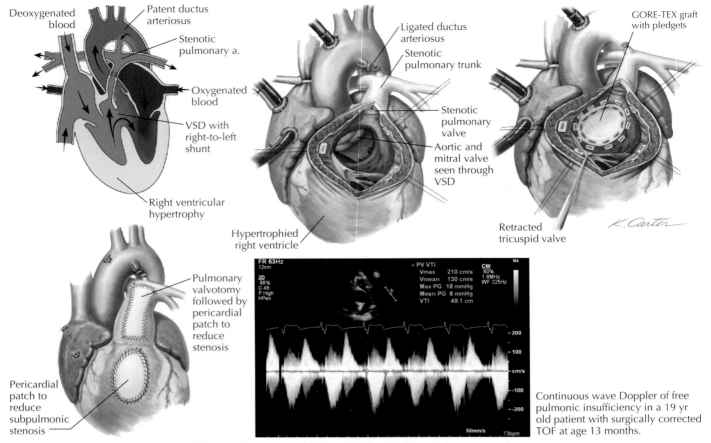

FIG 51.4 Tetralogy of Fallot (TOF). *VSD*, Ventricular septal defect.

These procedures are described in more detail in Chapter 53. Patients with a history of venous diversion surgery and a single functioning ventricle have been demonstrated to have a 76% survival at 25 years, and patients with hypoplastic right heart disorders are much more likely to survive into adulthood compared with patients with a hypoplastic left heart.

Total Anomalous Pulmonary Venous Connection

TAPVC is a rare congenital heart condition in which all of the pulmonary venous connections are made into the right atrium. This defect is not compatible with life unless corrected surgically shortly after birth. For patients with surgically corrected TAPVC who survive into adulthood, pulmonary venous stenosis can arise as the heart grows, and there is an increased incidence of supraventricular arrhythmias, including atrial fibrillation. Cardiac MRI is useful to evaluate the patency of the pulmonary venous connections, and ambulatory monitoring should be pursued aggressively for all patients complaining of palpitations and/or syncope.

UNCORRECTED CONDITIONS LIKELY TO PRESENT IN THE ADULT CARDIOLOGY CLINIC

Levo-Transposition of the Great Arteries

Levo-TGA (L-TGA) is an acyanotic congenital heart condition also known as a congenitally corrected transposition. L-TGA is usually diagnosed in the neonatal period by ultrasound, but because there is no need for immediate corrective surgery (unless it is associated with a VSD or pulmonic stenosis), these patients are usually followed conservatively during childhood. Adult patients with L-TGA are at increased risk of systemic ventricle failure and must be monitored closely for these sequelae. Afterload reduction of the systemic ventricle is likely to provide long-term benefit, and close monitoring of ambulatory blood pressures is essential. Early referral to an advanced heart failure clinic should be considered for patients with clinical evidence of systemic ventricular failure.

Coarctation of the Aorta

Although many severe forms of aortic coarctation are diagnosed in utero, milder phenotypes can present in adolescents with exercise-induced claudication, and occasionally, severe hypertension. Rarely, patients with milder phenotypes and mild pressure gradients can present in adulthood, but most patients presenting to the adult clinic will be those followed for recurrent coarctation after surgical repair earlier in life. Physical examination often reveals a systolic murmur with radiation to the back, and advanced imaging with CT or MRI can characterize the extent and severity of aortic pathology. For patients in whom the aortic narrowing is mild or moderate, invasive hemodynamic assessment can be beneficial to determine if surgical correction is necessary. Percutaneous intervention is also a reasonable option for some patients with focal stenosis amenable to placement of aortic stents or stent grafts.

Bicuspid Aortic Valve

Bicuspid aortic valve is the most common adult congenital heart condition, present in approximately 1 in 100 live births. Cases can be sporadic, but there is heritable component in many cases, and a gene mutation in *NOTCH1* has been strongly linked to the condition. Most patients with bicuspid aortic valve remain asymptomatic well into adulthood and are usually diagnosed after auscultation of a systolic ejection murmur.

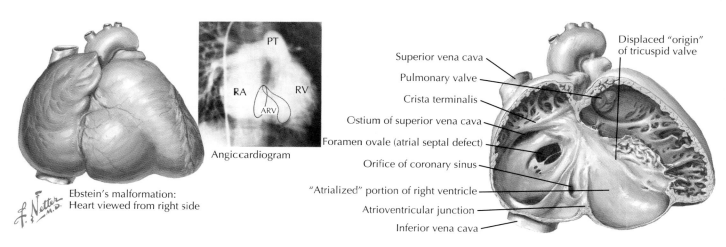

FIG 51.5 Ebstein Malformation. *ARV,* "Atrialized" right ventricle; *PT,* pulmonary trunk; *RA,* right atrium; *RV,* right ventricle.

The murmur is often present in the aortic area despite a lack of significant stenosis or even aortic sclerosis, and can be attributed to increased turbulence across the abnormal valve. There can also be a mid-systolic click associated with maximal expansion of a bicuspid valve immediately after S_1. Bicuspid aortic valve can also be associated with other syndromes of congenital heart disease. There is an increased risk of bicuspid aortic valve in patients with coarctation of the aorta, Turner syndrome, and dextrocardia.

It is imperative that patients with a bicuspid valve be evaluated for aortic pathology as well. There is an increased risk of aortic root enlargement and dissection. Many patients will initially present with aortic root enlargement and aortic insufficiency, which require surgical repair. The timing of aortic valve surgery is somewhat controversial, with most surgeons recommending early aortic valve replacement in the setting of aortic insufficiency when the aortic root measures >45 mm in diameter. This threshold is supported by surgical recommendations of the American College of Cardiology/American Heart Association/Society of Thoracic Surgery guidelines. It is now common practice to obtain a baseline MRI in most patients with a bicuspid aortic valve after the age of 40 years, with serial examinations every 6 months to 1 year when the aortic root measures >40 mm in diameter.

Dextrocardia

In approximately 1 in 1000 patients, the heart is located on the right side of the chest. In some patients, this is simply due to incomplete rotation of the heart during development and is also known as isolated dextrocardia or dextrocardia of embryonic arrest. Patients with isolated dextrocardia are more likely to have other conditions associated with arrested embryonic development, including pulmonary hypoplasia. When dextrocardia occurs in the setting of reversal of the internal organs (situs inversus), there is a higher risk of ciliary immotility due to a genetic mutation that leads to Kartagener syndrome, which is a multisystem disease characterized by recurrent infections of the upper and lower respiratory tract and sinuses, as well as infertility in men. Patients with dextrocardia and situs inversus are also more likely to experience additional congenital heart defects, including pulmonary atresia and endocardial cushion abnormalities.

Ebstein Anomaly

Apical malposition of the tricuspid annulus is the hallmark of the Ebstein anomaly. Many patients with this condition present with rhythm disturbance, and there is a high incidence of Wolf-Parkinson-White syndrome. More commonly, Ebstein anomaly is detected due to the presence of a systolic murmur due to tricuspid regurgitation, or as an incidental finding on an echocardiogram obtained for another indication. The incidence of Ebstein anomaly is <1 in 100,000 live births. Affected patients typically have significant right atrial enlargement on echocardiography as well, and ECG will typically reveal RV conduction delay. The incidence of accessory pathway–mediated supraventricular tachycardia is believed to be >20%, and evaluation by an electrophysiologist to consider catheter ablation should be considered in all patients with symptomatic tachycardia and/or syncope. Many patients will have multiple accessory pathways; therefore, there is an increased risk of recurrence compared with normal adults and other patients with Wolf-Parkinson-White syndrome (Fig. 51.5).

DIAGNOSTIC TESTING IN ADULTS WITH CONGENITAL HEART DISEASE

Electrocardiography and Ambulatory Monitoring

ECG plays an important role in monitoring the baseline rhythm of patients with congenital heart disease. In addition, patients with ventricular hypertrophy should be followed regularly with ECG to monitor for voltage changes and axis shift, which can be a precursor to the development of clinical heart failure. Ambulatory event monitors and Holter monitors can be useful in patients with congenital heart disease and unexplained syncope. All patients with congenital heart disease are at increased risk of both tachyarrhythmias and bradyarrhythmias, and monitors can indicate the need for electrophysiological study with or without ablation, and on occasion may confirm the need for permanent pacemaker placement.

Echocardiography

Transthoracic echocardiography remains the gold standard imaging technique for screening and evaluation of known congenital heart defects. Chest wall echocardiography typically allows adequate visualization of the anterior chambers of the heart, including the aortic valve and proximal ascending aorta, pulmonary outflow tract and the RV, and is very useful to evaluate the size and significance of ventricular and outflow tract abnormalities. Doppler analysis can typically provide useful quantification of shunt fraction and reliable measurement of the proximal great vessels.

Chest wall echocardiography provides limited visualization of the more posterior cardiac structures, including pulmonary venous inflow,

ASDs, and some endocardial cushion abnormalities. In these cases, transesophageal echocardiography can greatly improve anatomical definition of the major cardiac structures. Transesophageal echocardiography typically allows for adequate visualization of the pulmonary veins, coronary sinus, atrial septum, and the distal inferior vena cava and superior vena cava, and can adequately differentiate most common types of ASDs and VSDs. However, the intrathoracic course of aberrant anatomy is often poorly defined, necessitating advanced imaging techniques such as cardiac CT and MRI.

Advanced Cardiac Imaging Techniques

Among adults presenting with a first diagnosis of congenital heart disease, there has been significant improvement in the resolution and availability of advanced imaging techniques, such as cardiac MRI and CT to carefully evaluate conditions that are poorly differentiated by echocardiography. Gated imaging now allows for high-resolution, contrast-enhanced imaging of complex congenital heart defects such as ASD, anomalous venous return, and atrioventricular canal defects. Cardiac MRI allows for radiation-free surveillance of ventricular and atrial dimensions, and flow mapping can provide accurate quantification of the shunt fraction, the regurgitant fraction, and great vessel dimension in patients who require serial imaging. Advanced MRI imaging is now available at virtually all congenital heart centers, and has dramatically improved preprocedure planning for adult patients contemplating corrective surgery.

Cardiopulmonary Exercise Testing

Properly performed cardiopulmonary exercise testing (CPET) evaluation can provide accurate measurements of total oxygen consumption (VO_2), gas exchange, and aerobic capacity. The testing is versatile, because in addition to standard treadmill exercise, it is commonly performed with both a bicycle and upper arm exercise. CPET can now be used routinely in general cardiology practice and has gained particular relevance in the monitoring of patients with chronic heart failure. In adult patients with congenital heart disease, particularly those with a systemic RV, VO_2 monitoring can be an important physiological measure of systemic ventricle function in patients being considered for ventricular assist devices or transplantation.

Peak VO_2 is the most important measure reported during CPET. As workload increases, VO_2 increases as well in a linear fashion up to a peak value. When work demand on the muscles surpasses the delivery of oxygen, anaerobic metabolism begins. This is known as the anaerobic threshold. At peak VO_2, anaerobic metabolism begins, and patients experience rapid muscle fatigue as ventilator efficiency declines. Declining VO_2 and low VO_2 in general have been associated with an increased risk of mortality in adult patients with congenital heart disease. Several scoring systems have been derived to predict mortality in heart failure patients, with the most common system incorporating Ve/VCO_2 slope, heart rate recovery, oxygen uptake efficiency slope, and peak VO_2. These variables have all been associated with decreased survival among adult patients with congenital heart disease.

Cardiac Catheterization

Invasive evaluation plays an important role in defining the anatomy and treatment plan of adults with congenital heart disease. Hemodynamic assessment allows for quantification of pulmonary hypertension, QP/QS, and filling pressures. Coronary angiograms are useful for surgical planning to evaluate for coronary anomalies, and ventriculograms offer additional evaluation of atrioventricular valve regurgitation and outflow tract morphology. Exercise testing in the catheterization laboratory can assess cardiac output in response to stress, and pulmonary vasoreactivity studies are often performed to assess response to vasodilatory challenge among patients with longstanding pulmonary hypertension.

HEART TRANSPLANTATION FOR ADULTS WITH CONGENITAL HEART DISEASE

Among adults with severe congenital heart disease who survive to adulthood, the use of advanced heart failure therapies remains a controversial topic. For patients with severe pulmonary hypertension or Eisenmenger syndrome who present as adults, heart–lung transplantation can be required and is associated with a significantly increased risk compared with heart transplantation alone. For patients with L-TGA, hypoplastic left heart, or other conditions that exist with a system RV, clinical congestive heart failure is often inevitable, and close surveillance and monitoring with a specialist in advanced heart failure techniques is essential. Because patients with congenital heart disease are more likely to have syndromes involving other organ systems, mortality after transplantation has been shown to be higher, and the risk of death while on the heart transplantation waiting list is increased. Patients with adult congenital heart disease require careful screening for psychosocial risk factors before organ transplantation due to increased risk of mental health disorders associated with chronic illness.

FUTURE DIRECTIONS

Increased prevalence of intrauterine screening for cardiac defects, primarily with ultrasound and routine newborn pulse oximetry, is likely to result in improved rates of childhood surgical correction of severe congenital heart disease and improved long-term survival. However, increased use of fertility treatments and advanced maternal age in addition to the increasing prevalence of maternal diabetes and hypertension will continue to be public health challenges that increase the risk of the entire spectrum of associated birth defects. Appropriate recognition of congenital heart disease in the adult will remain an important focus of primary care and hospital medicine. Appropriate use of advanced imaging techniques and risk stratification studies will lead to guideline-based surveillance of identified patients, and referral to specialized centers will be required in a minority of patients with complex conditions.

ADDITIONAL RESOURCES

ACC/AHA 2008 Guidelines for the management of adults with congenital heart disease. *Circulation.* 2008;118:e714–e833. https://www.achaheart.org.
Important resource for physicians and patients.
Alshawabkeh LI, Hu N, Carter KD, et al. Wait-list outcomes for adults with congenital heart disease listed for heart transplantation in the U.S. *J Am Coll Cardiol.* 2016;68:908–917.
Resource for physicians considering heart transplant for patients with congenital heart disease.
Inuzuka R, Diller GP, Borgia F, et al. Comprehensive use of cardiopulmonary exercise testing identifies adults with congenital heart disease at increased mortality risk in the medium term. *Circulation.* 2012;125:250–259.
Important prognostic information regarding CPET results among patients with ACHD.
Olsen M, Soresnson HT, Hjortdal VE, et al. Congenital heart defects and developmental and other psychiatric disorders. *Circulation.* 2011;124:1706–1712.
Observational data demonstrating the prevalence of psychiatric disorders in patients with congenital heart disease.

Catheter-Based Therapies for Adult Congenital Heart Disease

Elman G. Frantz

Sometime at the turn of the millennium, due to improved treatment and outcomes, the prevalence of congenital heart disease in adults surpassed that of children. With longer term survival, this disproportionate share of adult patients will continue to grow. Many of these patients will have stable mild disease with a favorable natural history. However, a substantial number of patients will require close surveillance and specialized treatment in adult life due to late presentation, the cumulative effects of chronically altered hemodynamics, postoperative residual abnormalities, or the additional burden of acquired disease. In many cases, these patients are amenable to catheter-based therapies that may replace or minimize the need for open chest surgical interventions and associated morbidity. The techniques for these procedures are similar or identical to those used in children with congenital heart disease but with different frequencies of application. The training and experience essential to performing these procedures are generally in the province of pediatric interventional cardiologists, and with a few exceptions, rarely in the practice of adult interventionalists.

BALLOON ATRIAL SEPTOSTOMY

Although this procedure is common in the adult population, it is included here for several reasons. The cyanotic newborn with transposition of the great arteries is perhaps the best example of dramatically improved survival that results in a growing population of adult congenital heart patients. Survival to 1 year of age improved from <20% to >90% with the introduction of the Rashkind procedure; subsequent surgical correction and long-term survival are currently the norm. Also, the daring procedure introduced by William J. Rashkind in 1968, ushered in the era of interventional cardiac catheterization and remains an important adjunct today. A large balloon is passed transvenously across the foramen ovale and pulled forcefully across the atrial septum, tearing the thin tissue in the floor of the oval fossa, thereby creating a larger atrial septal defect (ASD), thus improving intracardiac mixing and systemic oxygen delivery. Balloon atrial septostomy is safely performed at the bedside under echocardiographic guidance (Fig. 52.1 and Video 52.1).

CATHETER INTERVENTIONS FOR CONGENITAL VALVULAR DISEASE

Balloon Valvuloplasty

Percutaneous balloon valvuloplasty is a commonly performed procedure for congenital semilunar valve stenosis early in life, but in adults, the disease is usually mild or has been successfully treated. Occasionally, adults may require intervention due to hemodynamic changes secondary to calcific degeneration or long-standing burden of disease.

Balloon pulmonary valvuloplasty is performed using a balloon diameter 20% to 30% greater than the diameter of the valve annulus, or if the annulus is large, two balloons may be used simultaneously (Fig. 52.2). Unless there is severe valve dysplasia, calcification, or annular hypoplasia, this technique is highly successful, durable, and has replaced surgical intervention in most cases. Residual gradients are typically <20 mm Hg, with mild nonprogressive pulmonary regurgitation. In selected neonates, the procedure is used to treat pulmonary atresia with an intact ventricular septum after initial radiofrequency perforation of the atretic valve membrane.

Bicuspid aortic valve is the most common congenital heart malformation. When significant commissural fusion and leaflet thickening are associated, the severity of stenosis often justifies intervention early in life, and balloon valvuloplasty can delay valve replacement surgery for decades. Avoidance of a prosthetic valve and associated anticoagulation is particularly appealing during the years of athletic participation and childbearing. When significant calcific degeneration is associated late in life, surgical valve replacement or transcatheter aortic valve replacement is preferred therapy. Balloon aortic valvuloplasty is performed with a balloon to valve annulus diameter ratio of 0.9 to 1.0. In teenagers and young adults, the large valve annulus often requires the double balloon technique (sum of balloon diameters/annulus ratio ~ 1.3) assisted by rapid pacing (Fig. 52.3). Gradient reductions of 50% to 70% are typical, usually with a well-tolerated degree of aortic regurgitation. Less than one-half of patients will require surgical aortic valve replacement within 10 years of follow-up.

Transcatheter Pulmonary Valve Implantation

Many surgical repairs (e.g., for pulmonary atresia, truncus arteriosus, the Rastelli repair for complex transposition of the great arteries, and the Ross pulmonary autograft procedure for aortic valve disease) require placement of a right ventricular to pulmonary artery conduit. Tetralogy of Fallot repair results in residual pulmonary valve dysfunction. Long-standing residual pulmonary valve or conduit dysfunction leads to late complications, namely, right ventricular failure and life-threatening arrhythmias. Repeated surgical replacement of conduits carries morbidity, has limited durability, and confers a cumulative risk of late arrhythmogenic death. Transcatheter implantation of a pulmonary valve produces an excellent hemodynamic result in most cases, allows a delay in surgical intervention, and minimizes the number of surgical procedures in the lifetime of a patient. Two transcatheter valves have received Food and Drug Administration approval in the United States, the Medtronic Melody valve (Medtronic, St. Paul, Minnesota) and the Edwards Sapien valve (Edwards Lifesciences, Irvington, California) (Video 52.2). Because the routine practice of prestenting has been adopted, the early problems of stent fracture and restenosis are now rare, and freedom from reintervention for the Melody valve is 89% at 7 years of follow-up. These valves are indicated for patients with a preexisting surgically implanted dysfunctional conduit (>16 mm) or bioprosthetic valve, but occasional

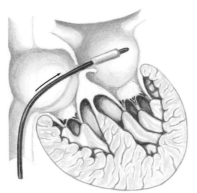

1. Balloon-tipped catheter introduced into left atrium through patent foramen ovale

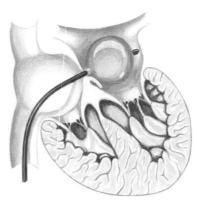

2. Balloon inflated

JOHN A. CRAIG—AD

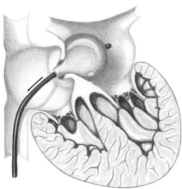

3. Balloon withdrawn producing large septal defect

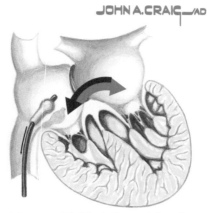

4. Large septal defect allows mixing of oxygenated and deoxygenated blood

FIG 52.1 Balloon Atrial Septostomy for Transposition of the Great Arteries (see Video 52.1**).**

patients with repaired tetralogy of Fallot and an intact pulmonary annulus (<24 mm) may be considered.

CATHETER INTERVENTIONS FOR VASCULAR STENOSES

Pulmonary Artery Stenosis

Pulmonary artery stenosis is a common residuum of congenital heart surgery and is difficult to manage by reoperation; therefore, catheter interventions are often preferred. In smaller growing patients, balloon angioplasty is favored over stent implantation, but relief of stenosis is usually incomplete. In adults, stent therapy produces better outcomes. A variety of stents designed for iliac or biliary applications are used off label and delivered through a long sheath after hand crimping onto the selected balloon (Fig. 52.4).

Coarctation of the Aorta

Native coarctation of the aorta may not produce symptoms and may be diagnosed in adolescents or adults during the evaluation of hypertension. Recurrent postoperative aortic coarctation may develop with somatic growth, particularly after neonatal repair, and may be associated with transverse aortic arch hypoplasia. Balloon angioplasty is well accepted and effective for growing children with discrete recurrent coarctation, but transcatheter stent implantation provides excellent relief of stenosis and the pressure gradient, and is typically used in older children and adults who often have more diffuse stenoses and more accommodative femoral arteries. Residual pressure gradients

are often zero, but occasionally may be up to 20 mm Hg in patients with complex or unusually resistant stenoses. Bare-metal stents have been successfully used for decades but more recently, covered stents have been available and have provided a margin of safety in controlling aortic wall injury. Bare-metal stents are hand-crimped onto the balloon of choice, and covered stents are premounted. Rapid pacing during stent deployment aids precise stent positioning, which may be especially important when the stenosis is adjacent to a carotid artery (Fig. 52.5).

TRANSCATHETER CLOSURE OF CONGENITAL SHUNTS

Persistent Ductus Arteriosus

Although the ductus arteriosus is a necessary vascular channel in fetal life, the postnatally persistent arterial duct can cause congestive heart failure, pulmonary hypertension, or endarteritis. A patent ductus may be diagnosed in adults due to poor access to care or sometimes subtle physical findings. In adults, the patent ductus is often calcified or is associated with pulmonary hypertension, thus increasing surgical risk. In the current era, percutaneous endovascular closure has become routine. A variety of closure devices are available (Gianturco coils [Cook Medical LLC, Bloomington, Indiana], Nit-Occlud coils [PFM Medical, Carlsbad, California], vascular plugs), but the St. Jude Amplatzer Duct Occluder (Abbott, Abbott Park, Illinois) is specifically designed for the typical ductal anatomy. It is a mushroom-shaped plug of nitinol wire mesh with polyester fabric patches sewn into the framework. The device

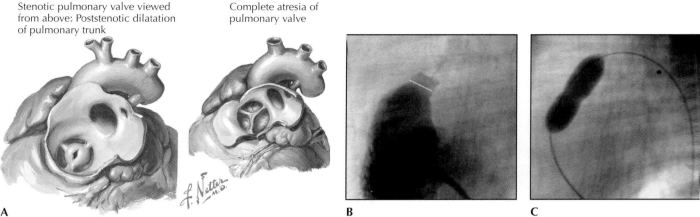

Stenotic pulmonary valve viewed from above: Poststenotic dilatation of pulmonary trunk

Complete atresia of pulmonary valve

A **B** **C**

(A) The anatomic features of congenital pulmonary stenosis and atresia are illustrated. (B) A lateral-view right ventricular angiogram in a neonate with critical pulmonary valve stenosis shows the doming valve with an annulus diameter of 5.9 mm and a tiny poststenotic jet. (C) A lateral view of an 8-mm-diameter balloon dilation catheter fully inflated across the annulus. The balloon has been passed over a guide wire that had been placed across the ductus to the descending aorta.

FIG 52.2 Congenital Pulmonary Valve Stenosis and Balloon Valvuloplasty.

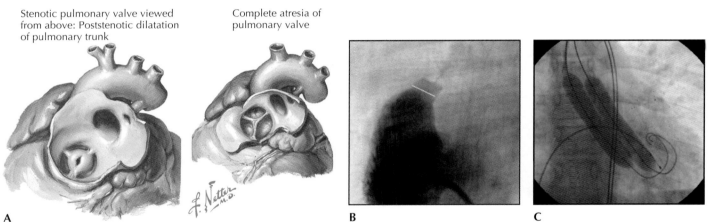

Stenotic pulmonary valve viewed from above: Poststenotic dilatation of pulmonary trunk

Complete atresia of pulmonary valve

A **B** **C**

(A) The anatomic features of congenital pulmonary stenosis and atresia are illustrated. (B) A lateral-view right ventricular angiogram in a neonate with critical pulmonary valve stenosis shows the doming valve with an annulus diameter of 5.9 mm and a tiny poststenotic jet. (C) A lateral view of an 8-mm-diameter balloon dilation catheter fully inflated across the annulus. The balloon has been passed over a guide wire that had been placed across the ductus to the descending aorta.

FIG 52.3 Congenital Aortic Valve Stenosis and Double-Balloon Valvuloplasty (see Video 52.2).

is attached to a delivery cable, advanced through a long sheath placed transvenously through the ductus, positioned, and then released in a controlled fashion. After deployment, the outer walls of the expanded plug "stent" the lumen of the vessel, securing the device in position and achieving complete closure (Fig. 52.6 and Video 52.3).

Atrial Septal Defect

ASDs are often incidentally diagnosed in adult life during evaluation of unrelated symptoms. Many patients are asymptomatic with minimal physical findings early in life. Unrepaired ASDs can lead to pulmonary hypertension, atrial arrhythmias, or right heart failure. Defects large enough to produce right heart enlargement should be closed to preempt these morbidities. Anatomic subtypes other than secundum defects require surgical correction (Fig. 52.7). Transcatheter closure of ASDs has become one of the most widely accepted catheter-based procedures, with excellent outcomes and avoidance of cardiopulmonary bypass.

In the United States, two septal occluders are approved by the Food and Drug Administration. The Amplatzer Septal Occluder (Abbott, Abbott Park, Illinois) is the first implantable device approved specifically for this indication, and it has been widely used since the late 1990s. It is a self-expanding, double-disk nitinol frame with a central waist sized to stent the atrial septal rims, and polyester patches are sewn into the frame to aid endothelialization and closure (Fig. 52.8). With transesophageal or intracardiac echocardiographic monitoring, a balloon-sizing catheter is used to obtain the stop-flow diameter of the defect. An occluder with a central waist equal to the stop-flow diameter is selected, attached to the delivery cable, loaded, and then delivered through a long 7- to 12-Fr femoral venous delivery sheath previously placed across the ASD into the left atrium. After deployment, the occluder position and rim capture are evaluated echocardiographically, and if the results are not ideal, the occluder can be recaptured, repositioned, or completely removed. After proper positioning is confirmed, the device

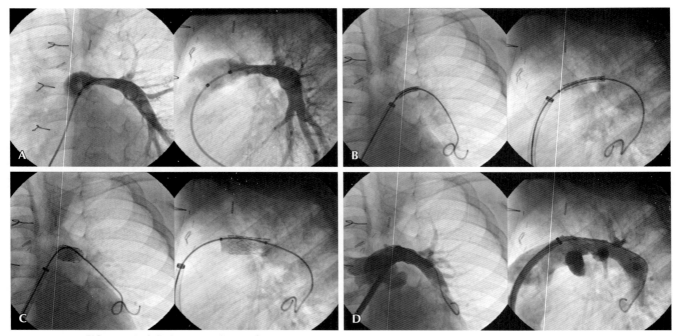

FIG 52.4 Left Pulmonary Artery Stenosis Stepwise Stent Implantation. (A) Initial angiogram. (B) Stent positioning. (C) Stent expansion. (D) Final angiogram.

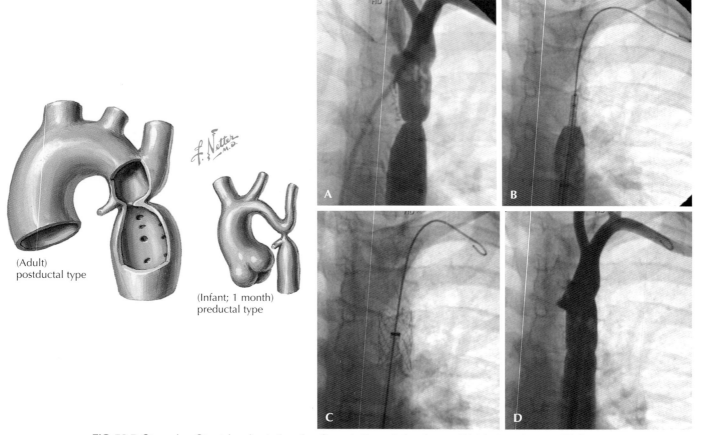

FIG 52.5 Stepwise Stent Implantation for Coarctation of the Aorta. (A) Initial angiogram. (B) Stent positioning. (C) Expanded stent. (D) Final angiogram.

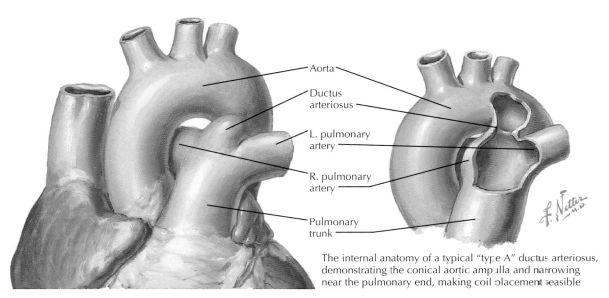

The internal anatomy of a typical "type A" ductus arteriosus, demonstrating the conical aortic ampulla and narrowing near the pulmonary end, making coil placement feasible

FIG 52.6 Patent Ductus Arteriosus (see Video 52.3).

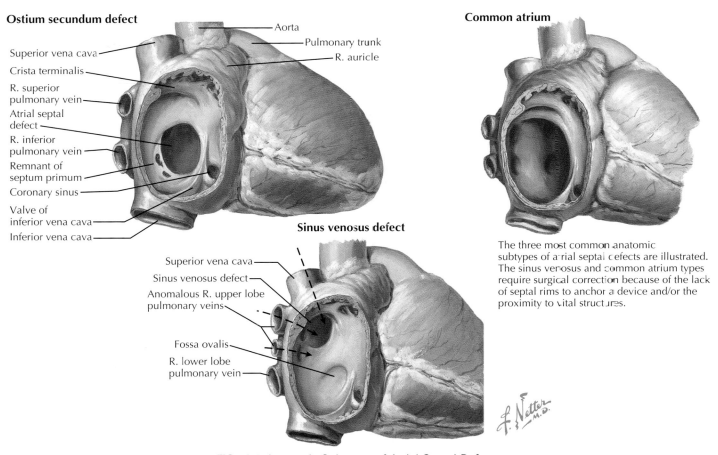

The three most common anatomic subtypes of atrial septal defects are illustrated. The sinus venosus and common atrium types require surgical correction because of the lack of septal rims to anchor a device and/or the proximity to vital structures.

FIG 52.7 Anatomic Subtypes of Atrial Septal Defects.

The Amplatzer Septal Occluder is deployed from its delivery sheath forming two disks, one for either side of the septum, and a central waist available in varying diameters to seat on the rims of the atrial septal defect.

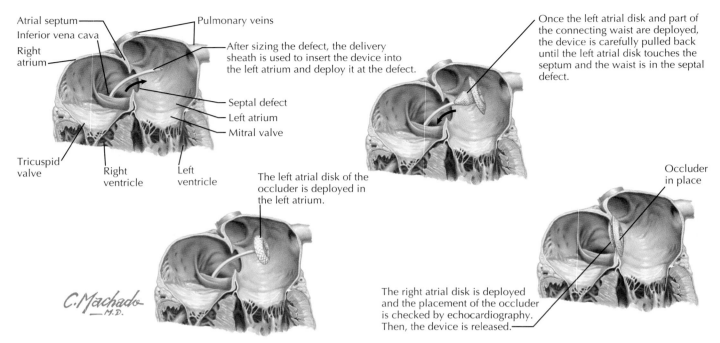

FIG 52.8 Amplatzer Septal Occluder (see Video 52.4).

is released by unscrewing the delivery cable (Video 52.4). In carefully selected patients, complete closure is achieved with a low rate of complications. The rare serious complication of late erosion of the atrial free wall or aortic root appears to be mostly avoidable with attention to case selection and judicious sizing methods.

The Gore Cardioform occluder (W. L. Gore & Associates, Inc., Flagstaff, Arizona) has been more recently approved and is being more widely adopted. It is a preassembled, single-wire nitinol frame upon which a thin polytetrafluoroethylene patch is suspended. It is delivered through a 10-Fr short venous sheath (Fig. 52.9). This occluder has the theoretical advantages of being lower profile, softer, and more compliant, but it is not self-centering and is only applicable to defects <17 mm in diameter.

Patent Foramen Ovale

The foramen ovale is a necessary vascular channel in the fetus, but it usually closes spontaneously in the first months of life. With provocative imaging, a potential right-to-left shunt at the patent foramen ovale (PFO) can be seen to persist in perhaps 15% of adults. Most of these patients have no adverse health outcomes, and the finding is often incidental. However, a PFO may rarely be the source of paradoxical embolism and cryptogenic stroke. Although controversial, some patients with no other identifiable stroke etiology may benefit from transcatheter closure of the PFO. Young patients (aged <55 years) with embolism documented by neuroimaging and who have a PFO, and a strongly positive contrast echocardiogram, atrial septal aneurysm, or thrombophilia, are most likely to benefit. The technique and applicable occluders are similar to those described for ASD closure (Video 52.5).

Ventricular Septal Defect

Most ventricular septal defects (VSDs) are not amenable to transcatheter closure, and surgical closure is routine. The precise anatomy of a VSD determines whether transcatheter closure is feasible. The proximity of perimembranous defects to the aortic valve and atrioventricular node (Fig. 52.10) makes device closure challenging and usually contraindicated. When the defect has undergone partial aneurysmal closure, it is more remote from these vital structures and may allow placement of an occluder in selected patients. Muscular VSDs in adults are generally small and do not require closure. Large muscular VSDs in infants are difficult to approach surgically because of their remote location; the transcatheter "hybrid" periventricular approach is often preferred. Although not congenital, selected postinfarction VSDs may be successfully closed percutaneously, and the morbidity and mortality of surgical closure in these patients is high. Transcatheter closure is most successful in patients who have survived for several weeks postinfarction when the viable myocardial margins of the VSD are better defined. A specially designed Amplatzer postinfarction septal occluder (Abbott) is available for this indication (Fig. 52.10A and 52.10B).

FUTURE DIRECTIONS

With improved survival, the number of adult patients with congenital heart disease is rising and now exceeds 1.2 million. A small minority of these patients will be candidates for catheter-based therapy to replace the need for surgical intervention or to treat postoperative residual disease. In general, the techniques and specialized equipment required for these interventions are the same as those used to treat infants and children with congenital heart disease. Because of their orphan status and limited market, the obstacles to innovation and regulatory approval by industry are daunting, and off-label use of equipment designed for other applications is common. Continued advances in catheter-based therapy for congenital heart disease are certain, but surgical intervention will remain the primary treatment method for many patients. A spirit of collaboration and mutual support between interventional cardiologists and surgeons is essential.

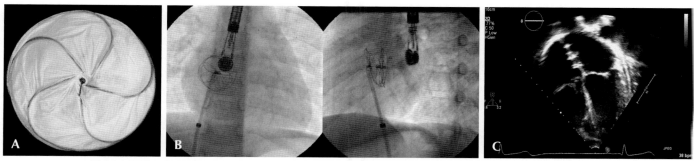

FIG 52.9 The Gore Cardioform Septal Occluder for Catheter-Based Closure of Selected Secundum Atrial Septal Defects. (A) Occluder en face. (B) Fluoroscopy of occlude pre-release. (C) Echocardiogram showing low profile of occlucer. (Courtesy W. L. Gore & Associates.)

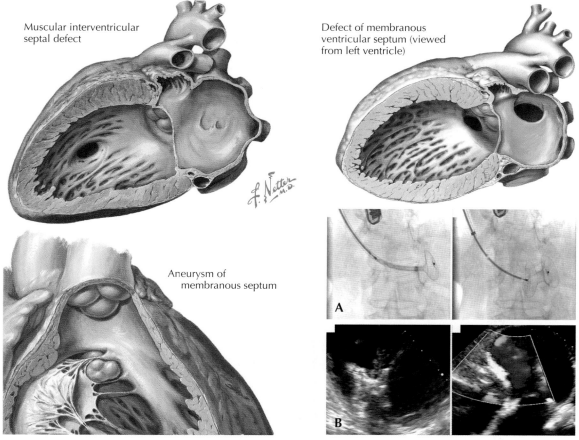

Muscular interventricular septal defect

Defect of membranous ventricular septum (viewed from left ventricle)

Aneurysm of membranous septum

FIG 52.10 Anatomic features of perimembranous versus muscular ventricular septal defects and depiction of (A) postinfarction ventricular septal defect occluder implant and (B) follow-up echocardiogram.

ADDITIONAL RESOURCES

Arzamendi D, Miró J. Percutaneous intervention in adult congenital heart disease. *Rev Esp Cardiol (English edition)*. 2012;65:690–699.

An authoritative and comprehensive review of catheter-based therapies for adults with congenital heart disease.

Pediatric and Adult Interventional Cardiac Symposium [home page on the Internet]. Available at: http://www.picsymposium.com/2015-livecases .html. Accessed March 31, 2017.

This state-of-the-art conference convenes internationally recognized experts and provides video tutorials of live cases for many of the catheter-based procedures discussed in this chapter.

EVIDENCE

Cheatham JP, et al. Clinical and hemodynamic outcomes up to 7 years after transcatheter pulmonary valve replacement in the US melody valve investigational device exemption trial. *Circulation*. 2015;131:1960–1970.

The longest available follow-up from the multicenter Investigational Device Exemption (IDE) trial showing durable results for the Melody transcatheter pulmonary valve replacement.

Humenberger M, et al. Benefit of atrial septal defect closure in adults: impact of age. *Eur Heart J*. 2011;32:553–560.

An important study demonstrating the therapeutic benefit of ASD closure in adults of all ages, including older adults.

Khan AR, et al. Device closure of patent foramen ovale versus medical therapy in cryptogenic stroke: a systematic review and meta-analysis. *JACC Cardiovasc Interv.* 2013;6:1316–1323.

A careful review of this controversial topic showing benefit of transcatheter closure.

Petit CJ. Pediatric transcatheter valve replacement. Guests at our own table? *Circulation.* 2015;131:1943–1945.

An excellent editorial contrasting the therapeutic goals, outcomes, and device development pathways for catheter-based treatments of pediatric and adult patients.

Rashkind WJ, Miller WW. Transposition of the great arteries. Results of palliation by balloon atrioseptostomy in thirty-one infants. *Circulation.* 1968;38:453–462.

The landmark report describing the first interventional catheter-based treatment for the formerly lethal transposition of the great arteries.

53

Surgical Interventions for Congenital Heart Disease

Robert D. Stewart, Anirudh Vinnakota, Michael R. Mill

Our understanding of the complexities of congenital heart disease, which is a deviation from normal cardiac anatomic development that affects 8 in 1000 births, has progressed immensely since the establishment of the Board of Pediatric Cardiology in 1961. Improvements in diagnostic imaging (including echocardiography, cardiac angiography, and MRI) and innovations in surgical repair techniques have resulted in greatly improved outcomes for children with congenital heart disease. This chapter provides a broad overview of the most common congenital heart lesions and the role of surgical interventions.

Embryological development of the heart begins with the fusion of angiogenic cell clusters within the splanchnic mesoderm layer of the primitive embryo to form the heart tube at 18 to 21 days of gestation. The heart begins to rhythmically contract as early as day 17, once functional units of the myocytes begin to form. Myocardial growth proceeds with segmentation and looping of the heart tube, as well as cellular differentiation and migration along the embryological axes, with the establishment of laterality, and with the organization of the primitive cells into a sophisticated organ. Deviations from this complex process of cardiac development lead to congenital cardiac anomalies, with clinical presentations that in some cases occur in the immediate postnatal period and in other cases in young adulthood.

Therapy for congenital heart disease has evolved with surgical and nonsurgical innovations. The development of pediatric cardiac surgery has led to the survival of many children with complex congenital heart disease. These successes have depended on improved diagnoses, advances in surgical technique, and the development of extracorporeal circulation—cardiopulmonary bypass (CPB). Complex repairs for previously fatal lesions such as transposition of the great arteries (TGA) and hypoplastic left-sided heart syndrome (HLHS) have become routine, with declining mortality rates and improved long-term outcomes. The development of transcatheter procedures has made therapeutic cardiac catheterization a viable alternative to surgery for specific congenital cardiac lesions.

SURGICAL TREATMENT

Many congenital heart lesions can be surgically repaired, meaning that approximately normal anatomy and physiology are established. The closure of atrial septal defects (ASDs) and ventricular septal defects (VSDs) can, when successfully accomplished in a young patient, eliminate the long-term consequences of the defect. Other lesions, most notably, the single-ventricle defects, cannot be repaired but can be successfully palliated with operative modifications that provide a viable alternative for cardiopulmonary physiology. These palliative operations can also be useful as a bridge to complete repair after a period of growth and development.

Palliative Surgical Procedures

The Blalock-Taussig (BT) shunt was first performed in 1944 at the Johns Hopkins Hospital (Baltimore, Maryland) to supply blood to the branch pulmonary arteries (PAs) of a severely cyanotic patient with tetralogy of Fallot (TOF). The shunt was created by dividing the right subclavian artery and directly anastomosing it to the right PA. Since that time, the creation of a systemic-to-PA shunt (a BT shunt) has been used for a variety of congenital heart defects with severe PA stenosis or atresia as a bridge to more definitive surgical correction. The technique of creating a BT shunt has been modified significantly by using an interposition graft, most commonly made of expanded polytetrafluoroethylene(ePTFE) (Gore-Tex; W. L. Gore & Associates, Newark, Delaware), between the systemic and pulmonary vessels. The modified BT shunt operation can be performed through a lateral thoracotomy or a median sternotomy, and can be performed on either the right or the left. A significant development in congenital heart surgery has been the increasing trend toward definitive repair at an earlier age, including the neonatal period. For this reason, the use of BT shunts is decreasing, but remains an important tool for the palliation of cyanotic heart lesions.

The PA band is an important palliative procedure for congenital heart lesions in which there is excessive pulmonary blood flow. The PA band is simply a Teflon (DuPont, Wilmington, Delaware) tape looped around the main pulmonary trunk and tightened to restrict pulmonary blood flow. The PA band was originally developed to treat large VSDs by decreasing the left-to-right shunt. Currently, the PA band is most commonly used for single-ventricle lesions with nonrestrictive pulmonary blood flow. The band is used to balance the systemic and pulmonary circulations, and to protect the pulmonary vasculature from prolonged exposure to high pressure, which could lead to a fixed increase in pulmonary vascular resistance and irreversible pulmonary hypertension. The PA band in these patients with single ventricles is a bridge to eventual Fontan physiology, or total cavopulmonary blood flow. There are still some instances in which a PA band is useful for the treatment of a VSD, most commonly in patients with multiple VSDs, which are also known as a "Swiss cheese septum."

The superior bidirectional cavopulmonary anastomosis, often referred to as the Glenn shunt, is the second stage in the palliation of all or most defects of the single-ventricle type. This shunt involves the disconnection of the superior vena cava (SVC) from the right atrium and a direct anastomosis of the SVC to the right PA (Fig. 53.1). This allows all of the systemic venous return from the upper body to flow directly to the lungs. The Glenn shunt is typically performed between 4 and 9 months of age, allowing for enough lung maturity to permit this passive blood flow. Patients will not be fully saturated following the Glenn shunt, because the venous return from the lower body still returns to the heart to mix with the fully oxygenated pulmonary venous blood

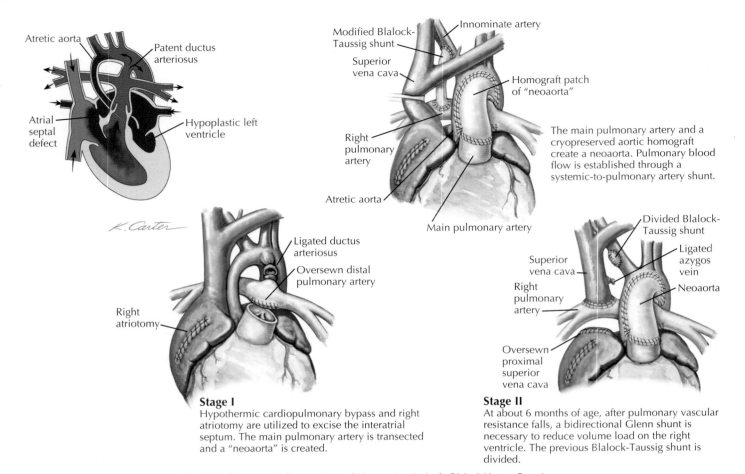

Stage I
Hypothermic cardiopulmonary bypass and right atriotomy are utilized to excise the interatrial septum. The main pulmonary artery is transected and a "neoaorta" is created.

Stage II
At about 6 months of age, after pulmonary vascular resistance falls, a bidirectional Glenn shunt is necessary to reduce volume load on the right ventricle. The previous Blalock-Taussig shunt is divided.

FIG 53.1 Norwood Correction of Hypoplastic Left-Sided Heart Syndrome.

Depending on the particular cardiac defect, the procedure may be combined with the removal of a BT shunt or removal of a PA band, with division of the main pulmonary trunk from the heart. In either instance, the attendant decrease in the volume load on the heart is beneficial to the function of the single ventricle and its long-term durability.

The ability of the pulmonary circulation to accept the entire cardiac output passively is limited, and thus, this is the rationale for creating total cavopulmonary circulation in two stages. The Glenn shunt is performed in the first year of life, and the completion of the Fontan is done in the second or third year of life. There are two distinct techniques for completing the Fontan: the lateral tunnel and the extracardiac conduit. The lateral tunnel involves creating a tunnel inside of the right atrium that extends from the opening of the inferior vena cava (IVC) to the opening of the SVC, which is, in turn, connected to the right PA, thus baffling all of the systemic venous return to the lungs. The extracardiac Fontan is created by disconnecting the IVC from the right atrium and sewing a graft of ePTFE from the open end of the IVC to the PAs (Fig. 53.2). Using either strategy, a direct connection of the IVC flow to the lungs establishes total cavopulmonary circulation, with the result being that after repair, the patient should have nearly normal oxygen saturation. Postsurgical outcomes with the Fontan, with either technique, have improved, with most recent data showing 95% 10-year survival.

Special Considerations for Specific Single-Ventricle Lesions

Tricuspid atresia is a rare congenital lesion with an absent right-sided arteriovenous connection and occurs only in <1% of patients with congenital heart disease. Left ventricular preload is dependent on interatrial blood flow via an ASD. This lesion is commonly associated with transposed great vessels, and the PA can range anywhere from atretic to enlarged. The physiology of the lesion varies by the amount of pulmonary blood flow. The original surgical repair, the classic Fontan procedure, involved constructing a direct connection between the right atrium and the main PA. Present-day conversion to the Fontan circulation usually requires a two-stage surgical approach after early palliation. The initial palliation may involve a BT shunt for lesions that include pulmonary stenosis or a PA band for those with a normal PA and excessive blood flow. A Glenn shunt is then created between 4 and 9 months of life, followed by the Fontan procedure, which is performed between 12 months and 3 years of age. In the Fontan era, mortality for tricuspid atresia decreased significantly, with 81% 1-year survival and 70% 10-year survival.

HLHS is a congenital lesion with univentricular physiology. HLHS generally involves a diminutive nonfunctional left ventricle that results from stenosis or atresia in both the mitral and aortic valves, as well as hypoplasia of the ascending aorta. Systemic blood flow is ductal-dependent, and the appearance of symptoms in the neonatal period usually correlates with spontaneous closure of the ductus arteriosus. Early management with prostaglandin E_1 to maintain ductal patency is life sustaining. The appropriate balance between pulmonary and systemic blood flow (Qp/Qs) is critical. The most common neonatal palliative approach is the Norwood procedure, in which a "neoaorta" is created by performing an aortopulmonary connection, then augmenting the hypoplastic ascending aorta with a homograft patch. A

Stage III

A modified Fontan procedure is completed 6–12 months after stage II utilizing an extracardiac Gore-Tex conduit to connect inferior vena cava blood flow to the pulmonary artery.

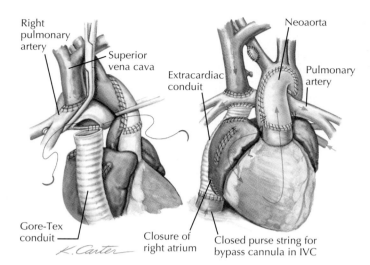

Systemic venous blood bypasses the right heart directly to the pulmonary arteries and lungs. Oxygenated blood is pumped from the left to right atrium through a septotomy. The "neoaorta" directs oxygenated systemic blood flow from the right ventricle.

FIG 53.2 Norwood Correction of Hypoplastic Left-Sided Heart Syndrome: Fontan Circulation. *IVC,* Inferior vena cava.

systemic-to-pulmonary shunt is required for pulmonary blood flow, and an atrial septectomy is always performed to permit unobstructed flow of left atrial blood through the tricuspid valve to the right ventricle (see Figs. 53.1 and 53.2). The surgery is usually performed during the neonatal period and carries a 20% to 30% risk of mortality. The Norwood procedure is followed by a bidirectional Glenn shunt at 4 to 6 months of age and a Fontan procedure at 2 to 3 years of age.

SURGICALLY CORRECTABLE LESIONS

Patent Ductus Arteriosus

Patent ductus arteriosus describes postnatal persistence of a normal fetal vascular connection between the main pulmonary trunk or proximal left PA and the descending thoracic aorta. This anomaly accounts for 10% of congenital heart lesions. In full-term infants, the ductus arteriosus is usually functionally closed by 10 to 15 hours after birth. Persistent blood flow through the ductus arteriosus is often associated with other congenital anomalies, and depending on the vascular connections, pulmonary blood flow may be dependent on patency of the ductus, as in lesions with right ventricular (RV) outflow tract obstruction. In this case, the vessel may be kept open with prostaglandin E_1 therapy until a BT shunt is surgically created. When no other associated anomalies exist, and ductus closure has not occurred after medical therapy with indomethacin for 48 to 72 hours, direct surgical ligation or division via a left posterolateral thoracotomy, or alternatively, catheter-based device closure, is indicated. Surgical closure before 10 days of age reduces the duration of ventilatory support, the length of hospital stay, and overall morbidity.

Ventricular Septal Defects

VSD is the most common congenital cardiac anomaly, occurring in 10% to 20% of patients with congenital heart disease. An interventricular communication occurs with the failure of the tissue ridges to fuse during formation of the septum. VSDs are traditionally classified by their location, and there are four types. Perimembranous defects form in the area around the membranous septum, and are by far the most common, consisting of approximately 80% to 85% of lesions. Inlet, or atrioventricular septal defect (AVSDs) form under the AV valves and are relatively rare as an isolated defect, but include approximately 10% of VSDs when included in the family of AVSDs. Conal VSDs form beneath the pulmonic and aortic valves in the conal septum and are referred to by various names, including supracristal VSD and double committed subarterial VSD. Muscular VSDs can form anywhere within the muscular septum in the trabeculations. The incidence of muscular VSDs is highly variable because they may occur more commonly in young infants but have a tendency to close spontaneously. Therefore, the incidence drops by age. Muscular VSDs are the only type that have a relatively high rate of spontaneous closure.

The hemodynamic significance of a VSD is related to the degree of left-to-right shunting. This produces overcirculation, which if severe enough, results in congestive heart failure in the infants. They fail to grow significantly despite adequate nutrition, are frequently tachypneic, and often sweat during feeding. This is an indication for early surgical repair. Smaller VSDs may not produce symptoms, but the excess shunting can produce enlargement of the left atrium and ventricle. This is also an indication for surgical closure, along with less common indications, including endocarditis or aortic valve prolapse and/or regurgitation caused by flow through the VSD. The closure of all VSDs involves a patch closure. Most of these defects are approached through the right atrium and tricuspid valve (Fig. 53.3), although the conal defects are frequently repaired through the PA and pulmonary valve. The most worrisome complication after VSD repair is complete heart block that requires a pacemaker, which occurs in approximately 1% of perimembranous and inlet VSDs. Efforts to close VSDs with catheter-delivered devices has been successfully accomplished in muscular and perimembranous VSDs, although current devices have limited usefulness with perimembranous VSDs due to a higher rate of complete heart block (see Chapter 52). Untreated large VSDs can cause reactive thickening of the PAs, which results in fixed pulmonary hypertension. When pulmonary hypertension becomes severe, shunting through the VSD shifts to right-to-left, and is known as Eisenmenger physiology. At this point, the VSD is not closable without causing RV failure.

Atrial Septal Defects

An interatrial communication accounts for 10% to 15% of congenital cardiac anomalies. ASDs refers to a spectrum of anomalies that are broadly classified into three categories: oval fossa or secundum defects; defects of the ostium primum, which are also known as partial AVSDs; and sinus venosus defects. Each type of ASD is unique. The oval fossa defect is by far the most common (80%–85%), and the indication for closure is excessive left-to-right shunting with a Qp/Qs >1.5:1 or significant enlargement of the right heart. Most oval fossa defects can be closed using a transcatheter device (see Chapter 52). If the defect cannot be closed with a device, it can be closed surgically either with a patch or by direct suture (Fig. 53.4, upper panel). Sinus venosus ASDs result from an overriding SVC that causes an atrial communication superior to the true atrial septum. Most sinus venosus ASDs are associated with anomalous pulmonary venous drainage (95%) and so cannot be closed by a device. A transatrial repair must include baffling of the anomalous

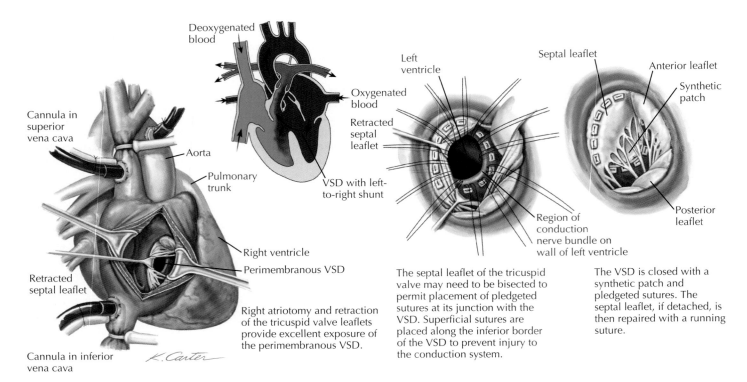

Deoxygenated blood

Oxygenated blood

Left ventricle

Septal leaflet

Anterior leaflet

Synthetic patch

Cannula in superior vena cava

Aorta

Pulmonary trunk

Retracted septal leaflet

VSD with left-to-right shunt

Right ventricle

Perimembranous VSD

Retracted septal leaflet

Cannula in inferior vena cava

K. Carter

Region of conduction nerve bundle on wall of left ventricle

Posterior leaflet

Right atriotomy and retraction of the tricuspid valve leaflets provide excellent exposure of the perimembranous VSD.

The septal leaflet of the tricuspid valve may need to be bisected to permit placement of pledgeted sutures at its junction with the VSD. Superficial sutures are placed along the inferior border of the VSD to prevent injury to the conduction system.

The VSD is closed with a synthetic patch and pledgeted sutures. The septal leaflet, if detached, is then repaired with a running suture.

FIG 53.3 Transatrial Repair of a Ventricular Septal Defect (VSD).

pulmonary venous drainage into the left atrium (Fig. 53.4, lower panel). The partial AVSD must also be closed surgically, because the inferior edge of these defects is the AV valve, and currently available devices would cause valvular dysfunction. In addition, nearly all partial AVSDs involve a cleft in the anterior leaflet of the mitral valve, which requires simultaneous repair (Fig. 53.5). ASD closure has excellent long-term outcomes, with surgery performed in childhood having a long-term survival similar to that of age-matched controls.

Atrioventricular Septal Defects

AVSDs are defects that involve deficiencies in the AV septum and abnormalities of the AV valves (mitral and tricuspid), which are also referred to commonly as AV canal defects. AVSDs account for 4% to 5% of cases of congenital heart disease. There is a wide spectrum of lesions, with a partial AVSD being limited to a deficiency in the atrial portion of the AV septum and a common AV valve (ostium primum ASD), and a complete AVSD referring to a deficiency of the entire AV septum and a common AV valve. Down syndrome is present in approximately 80% of patients with complete AVSDs. Complete AVSD is also seen in conjunction with TOF. The mortality rate for unrepaired complete AVSDs at 2 years of age is as high as 80% because of progressive congestive heart failure and pulmonary vascular disease. Because of the high risk of developing pulmonary vascular disease, surgical repair is performed at 3 to 6 months of age. Repair is performed via a median sternotomy with CPB with exposure through a right atriotomy. The complete AVSD is repaired by either closing both the ventricular and atrial components of the septal defect with a single patch or closing each component with separate patches. The common AV valve is divided into left and right components by the septal closure. The cleft in the left AV valve is then closed in a manner similar to that used in the repair of the partial AVSD (see Fig. 53.5). Late insufficiency of the left

AV valve following complete AVSD repair requires reoperation in 15% to 25% of patients.

Tetralogy of Fallot

Classically, TOF refers to four major congenital defects: VSD, infundibular pulmonary stenosis, dextroposition of the aorta, and RV hypertrophy (Fig. 53.6). The common anatomic abnormality responsible for all features is anterior malalignment of the outlet septum. TOF can present with a range of clinical findings: from cyanosis at birth to mild oxygen desaturation without cyanosis ("pink tetralogy"). The degree of compromise is determined by the severity of the RV outflow obstruction and the size and location of the VSD. Infants with severe forms of TOF who are profoundly cyanotic at birth are often maintained on prostaglandin E_1 to maintain a patent ductus arteriosus that provides adequate pulmonary blood flow until they undergo either a BT shunt or a complete repair. Acyanotic infants typically undergo complete repair between 3 and 6 months of age. Some infants who are initially acyanotic will have hypercyanotic episodes known as "Tet spells," which is when they have a dynamic increase in their RV outflow tract obstruction, thus shunting deoxygenated blood to their systemic circulation through the VSD. This is an indication for early repair. Total correction is accomplished by closure of the VSD and relief of subvalvular, valvular, and supravalvular pulmonary stenosis. The operation can often be performed through the right atrium and pulmonary trunk, but in cases of severe outflow tract stenosis, an RV incision is required. In many cases, a diminutive pulmonary valve annulus must be sacrificed to prevent obstruction, and the outflow tract obstruction is relieved by a transannular patch. The pulmonary regurgitation that results is generally well tolerated for many years, but most of these individuals will require late pulmonary valve insertion to avoid the development of arrhythmias, RV dysfunction, and sudden cardiac death.

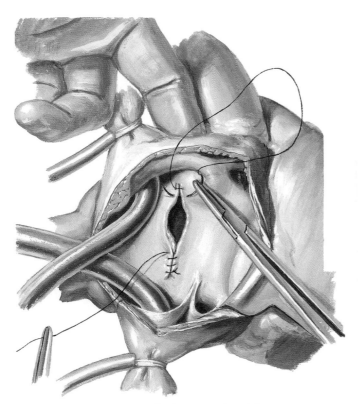

Direct suture of ostium secundum defect

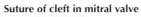

Suture of cleft in mitral valve

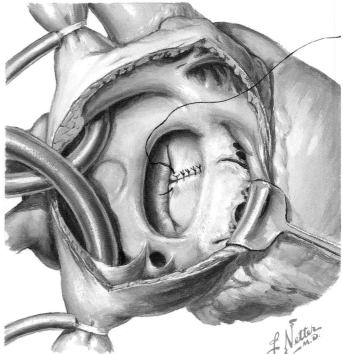

Partial atrioventricular septal defect

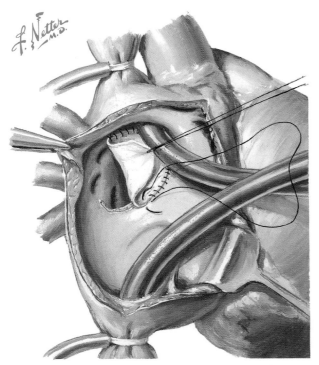

Application of patch for closure of sinus venous defect

FIG 53.4 Defects of the Atrial Septum.

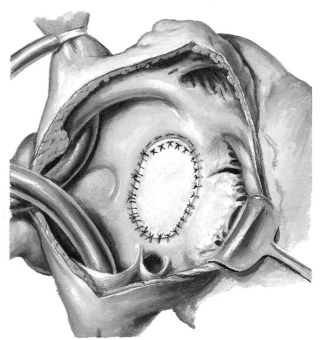

Patch applied to ostium primum defect

FIG 53.5 Endocardial Cushion Defects.

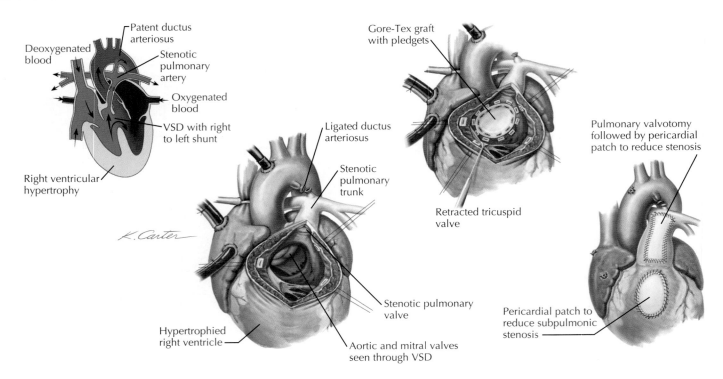

FIG 53.6 Tetralogy of Fallot. *VSD,* Ventricular septal defect.

Total Anomalous Pulmonary Venous Return

There are three types of total anomalous pulmonary venous return (TAPVR): supracardiac (most common, 50%), with pulmonary venous drainage into the innominate vein through a vertical vein; intracardiac, with drainage into the coronary sinus or the right atrium (least common, 10%–20%); and infracardiac, with drainage through a descending vertical vein into the IVC (30%–40%). All types of TAPVR are typically repaired in infancy by direct anastomosis of the common pulmonary venous confluence to the left atrium, which can be accomplished emergently under circulatory arrest or low-flow continuous CPB. Total anomalous pulmonary venous return may present with pulmonary venous obstruction and pulmonary edema. This is one of the few true congenital heart surgical emergencies. Even emergent repair has a mortality rate as high as 30% to 50%. The most concerning complication that occurs in up to 10% to 15% of patients after initial repair of TAPVR is stenosis of the individual pulmonary veins. Repair of this pulmonary vein stenosis is sometimes accomplished with a procedure in which the pericardial wall is sewn directly to the atrium with large fenestrations through the stenotic vessels. This procedure is referred to as the "sutureless" technique or marsupialization.

Transposition of the Great Arteries

The neonate with discordant ventriculoarterial connections is dependent on intracardiac mixing for survival and typically presents with cyanosis at birth. The initial management of TGA with prostaglandin E_1 and balloon atrial septostomy (see Chapter 52) to increase atrial mixing is life sustaining, but the mortality rate without surgical repair is very high. Historically, the surgical correction involved an intraatrial baffle to create AV discordance, which was then corrected by the ventriculoarterial discordance. Late right (systemic) ventricular failure and ventricular arrhythmias have led to widespread acceptance of the arterial switch as the optimal repair (Fig. 53.7). For this procedure, the great

vessels are first transected at the sinotubular junction, and the coronary arteries are mobilized and then transferred. The ascending aorta is then anastomosed to the original pulmonary valve, which becomes the neo-aorta. The PA is then connected to the original aorta, thus correcting the discordance. Of patients with TGA, approximately 50% have a VSD that must be addressed at the initial operation. Surgical outcomes with the arterial switch have been excellent, with 25-year survival ranging from 96% to 97%.

TRUNCUS ARTERIOSUS

Truncus arteriosus, a relatively uncommon defect, consists of a single semilunar valve (the truncal valve) that regulates outflow from the single arterial trunk to the aorta, PAs, and coronary circulation. The disease is frequently associated with microdeletion 22q.11 (DiGeorge syndrome) and velocardiofacial syndrome, with 33% of patients with truncus having DiGeorge syndrome. The single arterial trunk overrides the interventricular septum. Patients are occasionally cyanotic at birth but most often develop symptoms of congestive heart failure within the first weeks of life. The mortality rate for untreated truncus arteriosus is as high as 65% at 6 months. Surgical repair can be accomplished safely in the neonatal period by detachment of the PAs from the truncus, patch closure of the VSD committed to the left ventricle, and placement of a conduit from the RV to the PA (Fig. 53.8).

AVOIDING TREATMENT ERRORS

Surgical treatment errors can result from incorrect diagnosis, inappropriate timing of treatment, and poor surgical technique. The use of a multidisciplinary team that includes pediatric cardiologists, congenital heart surgeons, pediatric intensive care specialists, and pediatric cardiac anesthesiologists has become the standard of care for patients undergoing surgery for congenital heart defects. Review of preoperative studies

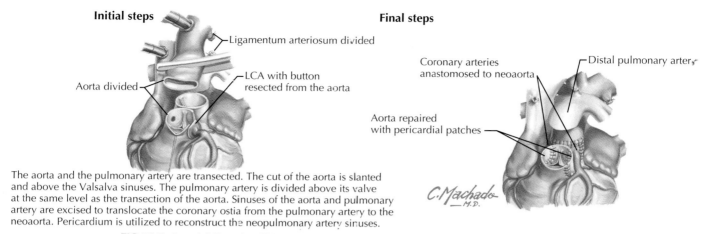

Initial steps

Ligamentum arteriosum divided

Aorta divided

LCA with button
resected from the aorta

Final steps

Coronary arteries
anastomosed to neoaorta

Distal pulmonary artery

Aorta repaired
with pericardial patches

C. Machado
—M.D.

The aorta and the pulmonary artery are transected. The cut of the aorta is slanted
and above the Valsalva sinuses. The pulmonary artery is divided above its valve
at the same level as the transection of the aorta. Sinuses of the aorta and pulmonary
artery are excised to translocate the coronary ostia from the pulmonary artery to the
neoaorta. Pericardium is utilized to reconstruct the neopulmonary artery sinuses.

FIG 53.7 Arterial Repair of Transposition of the Great Arteries. *LCA,* Left coronary artery.

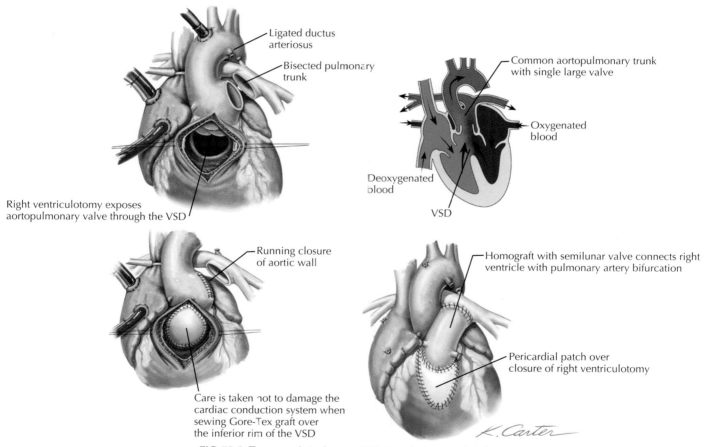

Ligated ductus
arteriosus

Bisected pulmonary
trunk

Common aortopulmonary trunk
with single large valve

Oxygenated
blood

Deoxygenated
blood

VSD

Right ventriculotomy exposes
aortopulmonary valve through the VSD

Running closure
of aortic wall

Homograft with semilunar valve connects right
ventricle with pulmonary artery bifurcation

Pericardial patch over
closure of right ventriculotomy

Care is taken not to damage the
cardiac conduction system when
sewing Gore-Tex graft over
the inferior rim of the VSD

K. Carter

FIG 53.8 Truncus Arteriosus. *VSD,* Ventricular septal defect.

and a comprehensive management strategy must be created for each child, with attention to the particular lesion and any comorbidities. This dedicated team approach minimizes the potential complications related to anesthesia, surgery, and postoperative care.

FUTURE DIRECTIONS

The technical excellence in transcatheter techniques achieved by interventional cardiologists in parallel with ongoing efforts by surgeons to find less invasive means to correct congenital heart defects has led to an emerging field that combines the tools of both disciplines, referred to as hybrid surgery. Important examples of hybrid surgery include intraoperative angioplasty and stenting of distal vascular stenoses as part of an open operative repair, periventricular echocardiography-guided device closure of muscular VSDs through a median sternotomy, and bilateral branch pulmonary banding in conjunction with stent placement in the ductus arteriosus as an alternative to the Norwood procedure for stage 1 palliation of HLHS. The primary theoretical benefits of these combined efforts include less invasive or less extensive operations, and the avoidance or reduction in the need for CPB. Although some early reports are encouraging, mid- and long-term results are still pending.

ADDITIONAL RESOURCES

Jonas RA, DiNardo J, Laussen PC, Howe R. *Comprehensive Surgical Management of Congenital Heart Disease.* London: Hodder Arnold Publication; 2004.

An outstanding textbook of congenital heart surgery primarily from the scope of a single author, Richard Jonas.

Mavroudis C, Backer CL. *Pediatric Cardiac Surgery.* 3rd ed. Philadelphia: Mosby; 2003.

The collective work of numerous outstanding surgeons, which is beautifully illustrated.

Nichols DG, Ungerleider RM, Spevak PJ, et al. *Critical Heart Disease in Infants and Children.* 2nd ed. St. Louis: Mosby; 2006.

This textbook has a greater scope than congenital heart surgery alone, with significantly more background in the medical aspects of congenital heart lesions.

Wilcox BR, Anderson RH, Cook AC. *Surgical Anatomy of the Heart.* 3rd ed. Cambridge, UK: Cambridge University Press; 2006.

Contains perhaps the most beautiful operative and anatomic photographs of congenital heart lesions ever published.

EVIDENCE

Bacha EA, Cao QL, Galantowicz ME, et al. Multicenter experience with perventricular device closure of muscular ventricular septal defects. *Pediatr Cardiol.* 2005;26:169–175.

Describes the state-of-the-art of hybrid VSD closure, including the lessons learned in developing this technique. The authors are the leading experts in the United States on hybrid congenital heart surgery.

Hjortdal VE, Redington AN, de Leval MR, Tsang VT. Hybrid approaches to complex congenital cardiac surgery. *Eur J Cardiothorac Surg.* 2002;22:885–890.

This article from Great Ormond Street Hospital describes the scope of procedures that have been modified with hybrid techniques for the treatment of congenital heart defects.

54

Transcatheter Aortic Valve Replacement

Sameer Arora, John P. Vavalle

PATHOPHYSIOLOGY

Age-related degeneration of the valve leaflet is the most common cause of aortic stenosis (AS). Degeneration of the aortic valve involves lipid accumulation, inflammation, and ultimately, calcification. In patients with a bicuspid or a unicuspid aortic valve, abnormal architecture makes the leaflet more susceptible to hemodynamic stress. This, in turn, leads to valve thickening, calcification, and stenosis of the valve orifice (Fig. 54.1).

DIAGNOSIS AND TREATMENT

History and physical examination are essential in diagnosing AS. Although the presentation among patients with AS may vary, it is recognized by the classic triad of dyspnea, angina, and syncope. The classic physical examination finding is largely characterized by a late-peaking harsh systolic murmur in the second right intercostal area with a diminished aortic valve closure sound and delayed carotid upstroke. Echocardiography or invasive hemodynamics are the confirmatory tests to confirm the presence of AS and to determine its severity.

Aortic valve replacement is the only definitive therapy for treatment of severe symptomatic aortic valve stenosis. Medical therapy proved ineffective in the treatment of aortic valve stenosis, except in a palliative role to alleviate symptoms. For decades, surgical aortic valve replacement was the only treatment option before the advent of transcatheter aortic valve replacement (TAVR). Unfortunately, many patients with degenerative AS were at an increased risk of complications with surgical valve replacement due to older age, frailty, and comorbidities. As a result, many patients who would have benefited from aortic valve replacement did not undergo surgical valve replacement. TAVR now fills the need for treatment. Since its first use in humans almost two decades ago, TAVR has emerged as one of the most revolutionary technologies in cardiovascular medicine and has transformed the treatment of aortic valve stenosis.

TRANSCATHETER AORTIC VALVE REPLACEMENT

Cribier and colleagues first described TAVR in humans in 2002. TAVR is currently the standard of care for the treatment of many patients with aortic valve stenosis. Two types of prostheses are approved in the United States for commercial use for TAVR. The self-expandable Medtronic CoreValve system (Medtronic, Minneapolis, Minnesota) and the balloon-expandable Edwards Sapien 3 system (Edwards Sapien Lifesciences, Irvine, California) are both approved for the treatment of severe symptomatic AS in patients who are deemed to be at least at intermediate risk for surgical aortic valve replacement (Fig. 54.2).

The Edwards S3 aortic valve is a balloon-expandable, trileaflet, bovine pericardial valve attached to a cobalt chromium framework, and is available in 20-, 23-, 26-, and 29-mm sizes. They are designed for transfemoral, transapical, or direct aortic access delivery. The Sapien 3 system, with a lower device profile, improved delivery catheter, and the additional feature of a polyethylene terephthalate outer skirt, has shown reduced rates of vascular complications and paravalvular regurgitation.

The Medtronic CoreValve Evolut Pro, which has a self-expanding nitinol frame, contains a trileaflet porcine pericardial tissue valve and a pericardial outer skirt; it is self-expanding, fully recapturable, and repositionable. It is available in four sizes (23, 26, 29, and 34 mm) and is designed to be delivered via a transfemoral, subclavian, or direct aortic approach. It is the only repositionable and recapturable device currently commercially available in the United States.

Both valves carry a Food and Drug Administration label for the treatment of severe symptomatic calcific aortic valve stenosis in those who are at intermediate, high, or extreme surgical risk, and for valve-in-valve TAVR, for the treatment of failed surgical bioprosthetic aortic valves.

INDICATIONS

Aortic valve replacement (surgical or TAVR) is indicated in patients with severe symptomatic AS. Severe AS is defined as an aortic valve area <1.0 cm^2, a mean gradient of >40 mm Hg, or an aortic jet velocity >4 m/s. Although studies are now underway that are studying patients with symptomatic moderate AS, the treatment of such patients currently remains an off-label procedure. The decision to use TAVR versus surgical valve replacement largely depends on surgical risk assessment before valve replacement. The Society of Thoracic Surgery (STS) score and the EuroSCORE are the two most commonly, currently used scores for risk stratification of patients with severe symptomatic AS. Although these surgical risk scores are available to assist physicians in quantifying the risk, the ultimate decision depends on the clinical judgment of a multidisciplinary heart team that consists of interventional cardiologists, cardiac surgeons, imaging specialists, geriatricians, and neurologists, as needed. Currently, the American Heart Association/American College of Cardiology recommends TAVR as a class I indication for patients who are considered inoperable and who are at high risk for surgery, and as a class IIa indication for patients at intermediate risk for surgery (Table 54.1).

When contemplating TAVR as a treatment option, many factors must be considered in addition to the surgical risk of the patient. A detailed preoperative assessment is needed. This includes high-resolution gated CT imaging to determine valve size, the risk for complications (e.g., ostial coronary occlusion), and route of access (Fig. 54.3). A multidisciplinary team approach is used to determine functional status, cognitive ability, frailty, and likelihood of survival and symptom benefit after TAVR. Coronary angiography is often performed before TAVR to evaluate for obstructive coronary artery disease.

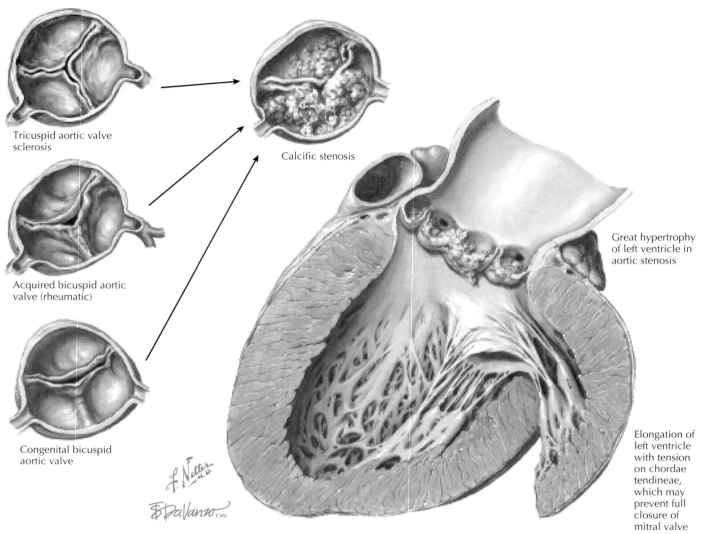

Tricuspid aortic valve sclerosis

Calcific stenosis

Acquired bicuspid aortic valve (rheumatic)

Congenital bicuspid aortic valve

Great hypertrophy of left ventricle in aortic stenosis

Elongation of left ventricle with tension on chordae tendineae, which may prevent full closure of mitral valve

FIG 54.1 Degenerative Calcific Aortic Valve Stenosis May Originate From Slow Calcification of a Trileaflet Aortic Valve, or Be Hastened by Bicuspid or Rheumatic Pathology.

Certain factors uncovered in this preoperative assessment may help sway the treatment decision toward an open approach, such as a heavily calcified bicuspid aortic valve at high risk for paravalvular leak after TAVR or multivessel coronary artery disease that would benefit from concomitant coronary artery bypass grafting at the time of surgical aortic valve replacement.

ROUTE OF ACCESS

If TAVR is selected as the treatment modality, the route of access for TAVR must be determined, usually from CT angiography of the peripheral vessels. The transfemoral route has been associated with the best outcomes and is generally considered the least invasive method of performing TAVR. If transfemoral TAVR is not an option due to severe peripheral vascular disease, other routes, such as transapical, direct aortic, subclavian, suprasternal, or transcaval TAVR, can be used (Fig. 54.4).

In the transapical approach, a minithoracotomy incision is made near the apex of the heart, and the valve is inserted anterograde through a sheath placed in the left ventricular apex. When the direct aortic approach is used, a small sternotomy incision is used to directly visualize the ascending aorta, and the valve is inserted through a sheath that is inserted into the ascending aorta. With subclavian access, a surgical cut-down is used to access the subclavian artery, and the valve is inserted via that approach. Suprasternal access is a method of performing direct aortic TAVR that allows for direct visualization of the aortic arch or innominate artery via a small incision above the manubrium without a sternotomy or thoracotomy. Finally, transcaval access has recently been developed as a way to perform TAVR via a femoral vein and a percutaneously created arteriovenous fistula from the inferior vena cava into the abdominal aorta. Once access is obtained into the abdominal aorta, the procedure is performed similarly to any other transfemoral TAVR. At the conclusion of the procedure, the arteriovenous fistula is closed with an Amplatzer occluder device (Abbott Laboratories, Abbott Park, Illinois).

EVIDENCE FOR CURRENT INDICATIONS

The Placement of AoRTic TraNscathetER Valve Trial (PARTNER) was a randomized prospective trial that divided patients into two cohorts: PARTNER A and PARTNER B. The PARTNER A cohort compared

Edwards Sapien Valve

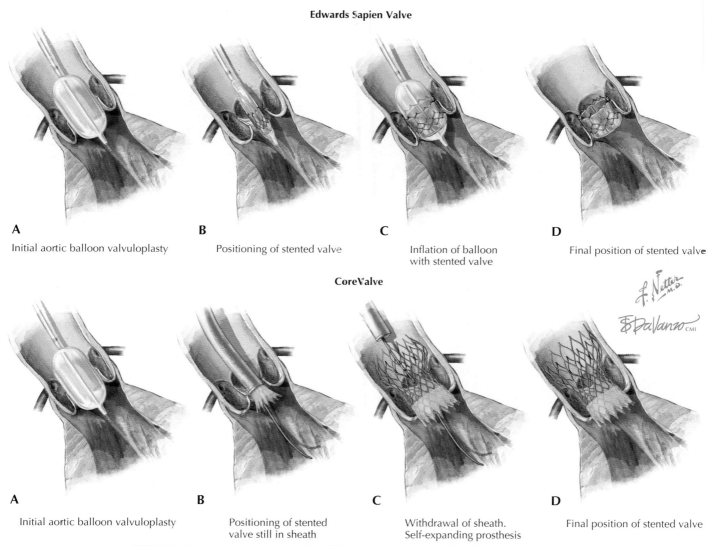

A	B	C	D
Initial aortic balloon valvuloplasty	Positioning of stented valve	Inflation of balloon with stented valve	Final position of stented valve

CoreValve

A	B	C	D
Initial aortic balloon valvuloplasty	Positioning of stented valve still in sheath	Withdrawal of sheath. Self-expanding prosthesis	Final position of stented valve

FIG 54.2 Percutaneous Aortic Valve (Edwards Sapien and CoreValve) Replacement.

TABLE 54.1   2017 American Heart Association/American College of Cardiology Focused Update on Valvular Heart Disease Guidelines

Class I	TAVR is recommended for symptomatic patients with severe AS (Stage D) and a prohibitive risk for surgical AVR who have a predicted post-TAVR survival >12 months.
Class I	The recommendation for either surgical AVR or TAVR among high-risk patients with severe, symptomatic AS (stage D), after consideration by a heart valve team.
Class IIa	After consideration by a heart valve team, TAVR is a reasonable alternative to surgical AVR for patients with severe, symptomatic AS (stage D) and intermediate surgical risk.

AS, Aortic stenosis; *AVR*, aortic valve replacement; *TAVR*, transcatheter aortic valve replacement.
From Nishimura RA, Otto CM, Bonow RO, et al. 2017 AHA/ACC focused update of the 2014 AHA/ACC guideline for the management of patients with valvular heart disease: a report of the American College of Cardiology/American Heart Association Task Force on Clinical Practice Guidelines. *Circulation.* 2017;135:e1159–e1195. https://doi.org/10.1161/CIR.0000000000000503.

TAVR against surgery in high-risk surgical patients, and PARTNER B compared TAVR against medical therapy in patients who were at prohibitive risk for open surgery. The PARTNER A trial included 351 patients who underwent surgery and 348 patients who underwent TAVR. The 30-day mortality rate for TAVR was 3.4%, and the rate was 6.5% for surgery. The 1-year mortality rate was 24.2% and 26.8% for TAVR and surgery, respectively ($P = 0.001$ for noninferiority). The PARTNER B trial compared TAVR versus medical therapy, with the results significantly favoring the TAVR group. The 1-year mortality rate for TAVR was 30.7% versus 50.7% for conventional medical therapy ($P < 0.001$). The benefits of TAVR were sustained at 5 years, with a significantly lower mortality rate than medical treatment (71.8% vs. 93.6%; $P < 0.0001$).

The CoreValve US Pivotal Trial was a multicenter noninferiority trial performed at 45 clinical sites in the United States that compared TAVR using a CoreValve with open surgery in patients who had severe symptomatic AS and an increased risk of death from surgery. The primary endpoint was all-cause death at 1 year, and 795 patients underwent randomization in the United States. All-cause death at 1 year in the TAVR group was 14.2% versus 19.1% in the surgical group ($P < 0.001$ for noninferiority and $P = 0.04$ for superiority). The 2-year mortality results were congruent with the 1-year results: an all-cause mortality

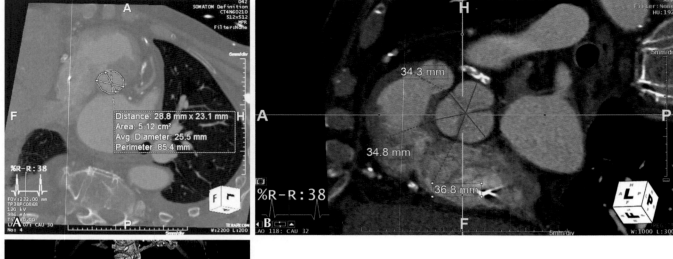

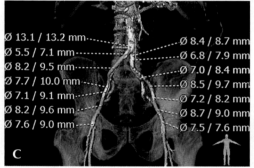

FIG 54.3 (A) Assessing the size of the aortic annulus to determine appropriate valve selection. (B) Measurements of the sinuses of Valsalva to ensure adequate coronary filling after transcatheter aortic valve replacement. (C) Assessing the diameters of the peripheral arteries to determine appropriate vascular access.

rate of 22.2% in the TAVR group and of 28.6% in the surgery group. Hemodynamic performance was superior in the TAVR group at all times. This study, for the first time, showed superiority for TAVR versus surgery in a high-risk surgical cohort.

These trials paved the way for the intermediate-risk trials, PARTNER 2 for the balloon-expandable valve, and the SURTAVI (SUrgical Replacement and Transcatheter Aortic Valve Implantation) trial for the self-expanding valve. The PARTNER 2 Trial, sponsored by Edwards Sapien Lifesciences, was conducted as a multicenter, randomized control trial across 57 centers in the United States and Canada. Patients with STS scores between 4% and 8% fell into the intermediate-risk category and were included for randomization. The prosthesis used for TAVR was the second-generation Sapient XT valve (Edwards Sapien Lifesciences). A total of 2032 patients were randomized into the TAVR group (n = 1011) and surgery group (n = 1021). The primary endpoint of the trial was death from any cause or disabling stroke at 2 years. A statistical difference was not found between TAVR and surgery with respect to this outcome both in the intention-to-treat analysis (19.3% vs. 21.1%, $P = 0.25$) or in the as-treated analysis (18.9% vs. 21.0%; $P = 0.16$) at 2 years. However, when the transfemoral TAVR cohort was compared with surgery, mortality was found to be lower for the transfemoral TAVR group both in the intention-to-treat (16.8% vs. 20.4%; $P = 0.05$) and as-treated analyses (16.3% vs. 20.0%; $P = 0.04$).

The SURTAVI trial, sponsored by Medtronic, was conducted across 87 centers across the United States, Canada, and Europe, and included 1746 intermediate-risk patients; it compared TAVR with its self-expandable prosthesis with surgery. The primary endpoint was a composite of death from any cause or disabling stroke at 24 months in patients who underwent attempted aortic valve replacement. At 24 months, the estimated incidence of the primary endpoint was similar in the two groups (12.6% in the TAVR group and 14.0% in the surgery group). The investigators concluded that TAVR was a noninferior alternative to surgery in patients with severe AS who were at intermediate surgical risk.

COMPLICATIONS

The Valve Academic Research Consortium has proposed standard endpoints for the TAVR clinical trials. The purpose was to standardize definitions for postoperative complications of TAVR, such as cerebral embolism causing stroke, myocardial infarction, bleeding sequelae, acute kidney injury, vascular compromise, prosthetic valve performance, and other sequelae related to prosthetic valve placement, including death.

The risk of stroke has been a major concern since the results of the original PARTNER trial, in which higher rates of cerebrovascular events were noted for TAVR compared with surgery, both at 30 days (5.5% vs. 2.4%) and 1 year (8.3% vs. 4.3%). Studies detected cerebral microembolism via ultrasound and MRI in earlier TAVR studies. However, data from recent studies showed a declining rate of neurological complications after TAVR, which was attributed to increased operator experiences, advancements in valve technology, and improvement in patient selection. Recent data suggested a lower rate of stroke with TAVR than with open surgical valve replacement. The S3 intermediate-risk observational study of patients who underwent TAVR or surgical valve replacement found a 1.0% disabling stroke rate for TAVR compared with 4.4% for surgery.

Another limitation to TAVR is the higher rates of permanent pacemaker following TAVR compared with surgical valve replacement. High rates of pacemaker implantation have traditionally been associated with the self-expandable TAVR valve rather than the balloon-expandable

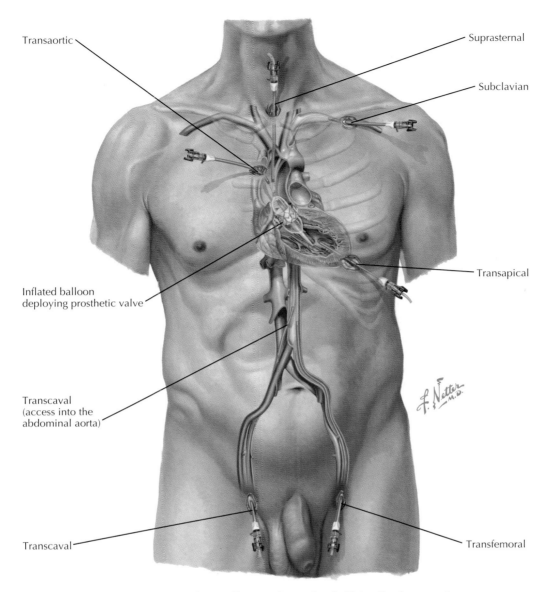

FIG 54.4 Approaches to Transcatheter Aortic Valve Replacement.

valve. This has been attributed to valve design and the potential for deeper implantation into the left ventricular outflow tract, which can cause more damage to the atrioventricular node and left bundle branches. However, with improved operator experience, and higher (more aortic) implantations, pacemaker rates have decreased, but generally remain around 10%.

Vascular complications remain prevalent among patients undergoing TAVR. These are largely due to the large-bore vascular access sheaths used for valve delivery in a generally frail and older population with significant vascular disease. As the delivery systems have improved and have become smaller with a lower profile, and patient selection has improved, so too have the rates of major vascular complications.

Lastly, one of the initial limitations of TAVR was the high rate of paravalvular leak compared with surgical valve replacement. With refinements in the valve technology, this has largely been mitigated. The polytetrafluoroethylene skirt in the S3 valve has resulted in lowering of the rates of paravalvular regurgitation by providing a seal around the valve. Similarly, the pericardial skirt now available for the Evolut Pro valve has resulted in a reduction of paravalvular leak rates for that valve.

FUTURE OF TRANSCATHETER AORTIC VALVE REPLACEMENT

Formal clinical trials are currently underway in the United States and Canada to investigate TAVR in low surgical risk patients, using the Sapien 3 valve (PARTNER 3, NCT02675114) and the Evolut R valve (NCT02701283). This is a major step toward approval of TAVR in patients at all levels of surgical risk. Other TAVR valves, such as the PORTICO valve (Abbott, Chicago, Illinois) and the Lotus Edge Valve (Boston Scientific Corporation; Natick, Massachusetts) are currently under investigation in the United States with anticipated Food and Drug Administration approval forthcoming. With more treatment options, improved technological advances, broader indications for use, and improved patient selection, TAVR is poised to become the primary modality for aortic valve replacement in those with aortic valve stenosis across the surgical risk spectrum.

ADDITIONAL RESOURCES

Grover FL, Vemulapalli S, Carroll JD, et al. STS/ACC TVT Registry. 2016 Annual Report of The Society of Thoracic Surgeons/American College of Cardiology Transcatheter Valve Therapy Registry. *Ann Thorac Surg.* 2017;103(3):1021–1035.

Society of Thoracic Surgery/American College of Cardiology Transcatheter Valve Therapy annual report of outcomes from commercial TAVR across the United States.

Kappetein AP, Head SJ, Généreux P, et al. Updated standardized endpoint definitions for transcatheter aortic valve implantation: the Valve Academic Research Consortium-2 consensus document. *J Am Coll Cardiol.* 2012;60(15):1438–1454.

Valvular Academic Research Consortium standardized endpoint definitions for TAVR.

Nishimura RA, Otto CM, Bonow RO, et al. 2017 AHA/ACC focused update of the 2014 AHA/ACC guideline for the management of patients with valvular heart disease: a report of the American College of Cardiology/American Heart Association Task Force on Clinical Practice Guidelines. *J Am Coll Cardiol.* 2017;70(2):252–289.

Updated valvular heart disease guidelines now including recommendations for TAVR in intermediate-risk patients, in addition to those at high and extreme risk.

EVIDENCE

Adams DH, Popma JJ, Reardon MJ, et al; for the U.S. CoreValve Clinical Investigators. Transcatheter aortic-valve replacement with a self-expanding prosthesis. *N Engl J Med.* 2014;370:1790–1798.

Randomized controlled trial comparing CoreValve TAVR with surgery in those at high risk for surgical valve replacement. For the first time, TAVR beat open surgical valve replacement on the outcome of mortality in a high-risk population.

Leon MB, Smith CR, Mack MJ, et al; for the PARTNER Trial Investigators. Transcatheter aortic-valve implantation for aortic stenosis in patients who cannot undergo surgery. *N Engl J Med.* 2010;363:1597–1607.

First randomized trial of TAVR, comparing the Sapien TAVR valve with medical therapy in those who were at too high risk for surgery. It demonstrated a significant mortality benefit for TAVR over medical therapy and established TAVR as the standard of care for patients with severe symptomatic AS who could not undergo surgical aortic valve replacement.

Reardon MJ, Van Mieghem NM, Popma JP, et al; for the SURTAVI Investigators. Surgical or transcatheter aortic-valve replacement in intermediate-risk patients. *N Engl J Med.* 2017;376:1321–1331.

Another randomized trial comparing CoreValve TAVR with surgery in patients at intermediate risk for surgery. This provided further evidence to support the use of TAVR in an intermediate-risk population.

Smith CR, Leon MB, Mack MJ, et al; for the PARTNER Trial Investigators. Transcatheter versus surgical aortic-valve replacement in high-risk patients. *N Engl J Med.* 2011;364:2187–2198.

Randomized controlled trial comparing the Sapien TAVR with surgical valve replacement. This study demonstrated that TAVR was an acceptable alternative to surgery in those at high risk for surgical valve replacement.

Smith CR, Leon MB, Mack MJ, et al; for the PARTNER 2 Investigators. Transcatheter or surgical aortic-valve replacement in intermediate-risk patients. *N Engl J Med.* 2016;374:1609–1620.

A randomized comparison of SAPIEN TAVR with surgery in patients at intermediate risk for surgery. This paved the way for approval for TAVR in intermediate-risk patients.

55

Transcatheter Mitral Valve Repair

Sameer Arora, John P. Vavalle

Mitral regurgitation (MR) is one of the most commonly encountered valvular diseases, and incidence rises precipitously with age. Severe symptomatic MR leads to heart failure, arrhythmias, pulmonary hypertension, and left ventricular failure. Mitral valve regurgitation is generally categorized based on its etiology as either primary degenerative MR or secondary functional MR. Degenerative mitral valve regurgitation is due to an anatomical defect of the valve apparatus itself, such as chordal rupture or mitral valve prolapse. Myxomatous degeneration, fibroelastic deficiency, connective tissue disorders, infective endocarditis, or even rheumatic heart disease may lead to degenerative mitral valve regurgitation. Functional, or secondary, mitral valve regurgitation is due to underlying left ventricular dilation that results in leaflet tethering and annular dilation that prevents leaflet coaptation.

Surgical correction with mitral valve repair or replacement is the mainstay of therapy in severe degenerative MR that requires intervention. Surgical intervention for secondary MR is more controversial, and its benefits are less well proven because the underlying problem is ventricular dysfunction more than true valvular pathology. However, many patients with chronic severe degenerative MR are not considered candidates for surgery due to advanced age, pulmonary hypertension, poor ventricular function, frailty, or other comorbidities. In these patients, transcatheter mitral valve repair, using the MitraClip system (Abbott Vascular, Menlo Park, California), is considered a reasonable alternative.

MITRACLIP

The MitraClip system, first described by St. Goar and colleagues, uses a catheter-based percutaneously delivered clip via a transseptal approach to accomplish an edge-to-edge repair of the mitral valve, similar to the Alfieri stitch first introduced by Alfieri in the early 1990s. The MitraClip, much like the Alfieri stitch, results in a double orifice mitral valve by approximating the anterior and posterior leaflets of the mitral valve (Fig. 55.1). This results in a reduction in the degree of mitral valve regurgitation, especially when the regurgitant jet is centrally located and the clips can be successfully placed at the location of the regurgitant orifice. The MitraClip is currently the only percutaneous transcatheter mitral repair device approved by the U.S Food and Drug Administration (FDA) for commercial use, and is approved for use in patients with primary MR.

TECHNIQUE

The current MitraClip device consists of a steerable guide catheter and a clip delivery system. The clip is a polyester-covered cobalt chromium device with two gripping arms to capture both the anterior and posterior mitral valve leaflets. A transseptal puncture from the femoral vein allows the delivery of a steerable catheter into the left atrium. The guide catheter is equipped with a steering knob at the back end to allow precise orientation and positioning. The clip delivery system, with an attached clip, is advanced into the left atrium through the guide catheter. From the left atrium, it is passed across the mitral valve while being centered over the origin of the regurgitant mitral jet. Transesophageal echocardiography (TEE) is used to aid in the positioning of the clip. The clip has two arms that are opened and closed by control mechanisms on the clip delivery system. On the inner portion of the clip are two "grippers" that match up to each arm and help to secure the leaflets from the atrial aspect as they are captured during closure of the clip. Leaflet tissue is secured between the arm and corresponding grippers simultaneously for the anterior and posterior leaflets under TEE guidance (Fig. 55.2). After satisfactory reduction in MR, the clip is closed and locked to effectively achieve a double orifice repair. Once satisfied with clip position and MR reduction, the clip is released. If further MR reduction is needed, additional clips can be placed, so long as severe mitral valve stenosis, as assessed by mean mitral valve gradient, is not created with the placement of additional clips.

EVIDENCE

The Endovascular Valve Edge-to-Edge Repair Study (EVEREST II) was designed as a multicenter, prospective, randomized control trial across 37 centers in the United States and Canada to evaluate the efficacy and safety of percutaneous mitral valve repair compared with conventional mitral valve surgical repair or replacement. Eligible patients had 3+ or 4+ chronic MR, and symptomatic patients were required to have a left ventricular ejection fraction of >25% and a left ventricular end-systolic diameter of ≤55 mm. If patients were asymptomatic, one of the following was required for eligibility: an ejection fraction of 25% to 60%, left ventricular end-systolic diameter of 40 to 55 mm, new atrial fibrillation, or pulmonary hypertension. A total of 279 patients were assigned in a 2:1 ratio to the percutaneous arm versus the surgical arm. Freedom from death, from surgery for mitral valve dysfunction, and from an MR grade 3+ or 4+ at 12 months was the primary composite endpoint to determine efficacy. The composite of major adverse events at 30 days was the primary safety endpoint. At 12 months, the primary efficacy endpoint was reached in 53% of the percutaneous repair group and in 73% of the surgical group ($P = 0.007$). The difference was largely governed by the higher rates of mitral valve surgery for mitral valve dysfunction in the percutaneous repair group compared with the surgical group (20% vs. 2%). However, the rate of major adverse events was lower in the percutaneous repair group compared with the surgical group (15% vs. 48%). This was largely due to higher rates of >2 U of blood transfusion that was required in the surgical group (45% vs. 13%). Despite the MitraClip being less effective in reducing MR compared with open surgery, the improvements in New York Heart Association (NYHA) functional class were superior with the MitraClip over

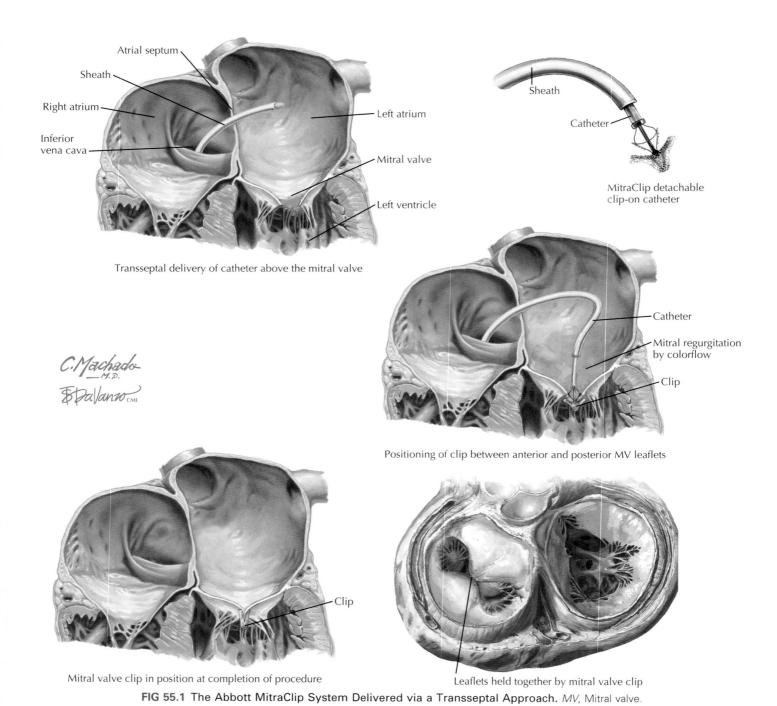

Transseptal delivery of catheter above the mitral valve

MitraClip detachable clip-on catheter

Positioning of clip between anterior and posterior MV leaflets

Mitral valve clip in position at completion of procedure

Leaflets held together by mitral valve clip

FIG 55.1 The Abbott MitraClip System Delivered via a Transseptal Approach. *MV,* Mitral valve.

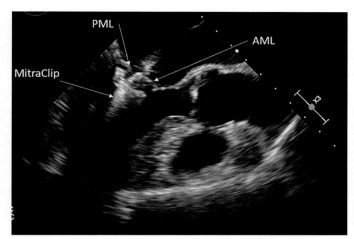

FIG 55.2 Transesophageal Guidance for Capturing the Anterior and Posterior Mitral Valve Leaflets With the MitraClip. *AML,* Anterior mitral leaflet; *PML,* posterior mitral leaflet.

surgery, which suggested that complete elimination of MR might not be necessary for symptom improvement and that the morbidity associated with open mitral valve surgery might outweigh the benefits in many patients.

The EVEREST II High-Risk registry and REALISM (Real World Expanded Multicenter Study of the MitraClip System) Continued Access Study High-Risk Arm were prospective registries designed to evaluate the efficacy of the MitraClip in a high surgical risk population. The 12-month outcomes in these high-risk patients were favorable, showing an 84% reduction in MR to ≤2+, low rates of adverse events, improvements in left ventricular remodeling, reductions in heart failure hospitalizations, and improved functional class. Furthermore, a propensity-matched comparison of medically managed patients with 3+/4+ MR with high-risk MitraClip patients showed a reduction in mortality at 30 days and 1 year for the MitraClip arm, which remained significant even after adjustment for baseline differences.

A prohibitive risk group was formed by retrospective evaluation of prohibitive risk patients from the high-risk arms of the EVEREST II high-risk and the EVEREST II REALISM registries. A total of 127 patients were identified. They underwent successful clip implantation in 95% of the cases. There were 30 deaths (23.6%) at 1 year. Most surviving patients (82.9%) sustained a reduction of MR of ≤2+, and 86.9% were in NYHA functional class I or II at 1 year. The study also saw an improvement in left ventricular parameters, quality of life indexes, and a reduction in heart failure hospitalizations in patients with reduced MR. These data led to the FDA approval of the MitraClip for high-risk and inoperable patients who have degenerative symptomatic 3+/4+ mitral valve regurgitation.

REAL-WORLD EXPERIENCE

Since its approval, there have been >35,000 implantations world-wide. In the United States, data from the Transcatheter Valve Therapies (TVT) national registry has demonstrated a >92% success rate, which is defined as a reduction of the MR to ≤2+, with an in-hospital mortality rate of <3% and a median hospital length of stay of 3 days. As expected, because of the FDA approval only for degenerative MR, >90% of the cases performed in the United States are for degenerative MR. However, globally, most MitraClip cases are being performed for functional mitral valve regurgitation. The Cardiovascular Outcomes Assessment of the MitraClip Percutaneous Therapy for Heart Failure Patients with

Functional Mitral Regurgitation Trial (COAPT) in the United States and Canada is specifically designed to test the MitraClip against medical therapy for the treatment of functional mitral valve regurgitation. Until the results of this study are known, it is unlikely that the FDA will expand its indication to include functional MR.

OTHER TECHNIQUES FOR TRANSCATHETER MITRAL VALVE REPAIR

Carillon Mitral Contour System

The Carillon Mitral Contour System (Cardiac Dimensions Inc., Kirkland, Washington) is a curved nitinol bridge that is delivered via the right internal jugular vein. After anchoring in the great cardiac vein, tension is applied by pulling on the system, which results in reshaping of the mitral annulus (Fig. 55.3). After animal studies suggested a significant reduction in mitral valve regurgitation, the European trial Carillon Mitral Annuloplasty Device European Union Study (AMADEUS I) was subsequently conducted. The trial demonstrated a successful deployment of the device in 30 of 43 (70%) patients, with 80% of the patients noted to have at least one grade reduction in MR. The major adverse event rate was 13% at 30 days. A subsequent trial called TITAN (Transcatheter Implantation of Carillon Mitral Annuloplasty Device) studied a modified device. In this study, 36 of 53 (68%) patients had the device successfully implanted, and the 30-day adverse event rate was 1.9%. In comparison with the control group, those who had the device implanted had significant reductions in MR, left ventricular volumes, and improved symptoms. The TITAN II trial studied another modification to the device in 36 patients; the device was successfully implanted in 30 (83%) patients. As in previous studies, there were reductions in MR, reduced annular diameters, and improved NYHA functional classifications. The device has CE Mark approval in Europe to treat functional MR, and a Phase III US trial is forthcoming.

Mitralign System

The Mitralign system (Mitralign, Inc., Boston, Massachusetts) is an attempt to replicate a surgical suture annuloplasty via transcatheter methods (Fig. 55.4). Via the femoral artery, a 14-Fr catheter is inserted across the aortic valve, and using a deflector tip, the catheter is pointed toward the mitral annulus. Pledgets are then anchored across the mitral annulus from the left ventricle to the left atrium in several positions along the mitral annulus. These anchors are then tethered, and the tension between them decreases the septal-lateral annulus diameter. European studies of the device have demonstrated safety and efficacy of the device, with improved 6-minute walk test results, as well as improved left ventricular dimensions and remodeling. The device currently has CE mark approval for use in the European Union for treatment of functional MR.

TRANSCATHETER MITRAL VALVE REPLACEMENT

Much of the interest and investment in transcatheter therapies for mitral valve regurgitation has now pivoted toward the development of transcatheter mitral valve replacement (TMVR) technology. Over the last several years, there has been significant investment to expedite the development of this technology. The development of TMVR valves has been more challenging than the development of transcatheter aortic valve replacement valves, primarily due to the D-shaped annulus, subvalvular structures, noncalcified annulus, transseptal approach, and the large-bore delivery systems.

Although there are several different prototypes in development, they all share similar features in that they have a nitinol self-expanding frame, three bovine or porcine pericardial leaflets, and an anchoring mechanism.

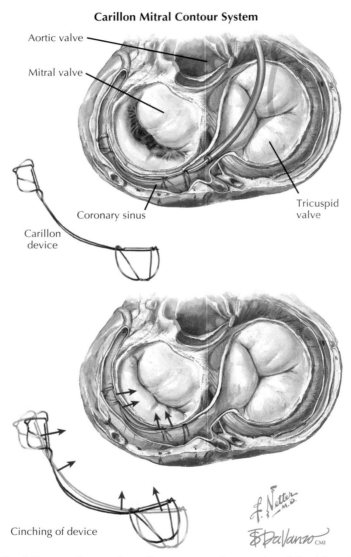

Carillon Mitral Contour System

Aortic valve

Mitral valve

Coronary sinus

Carillon device

Tricuspid valve

Cinching of device

FIG 55.3 The Carillon Mitral Contour System for a Percutaneous Approach to Mitral Annuloplasty.

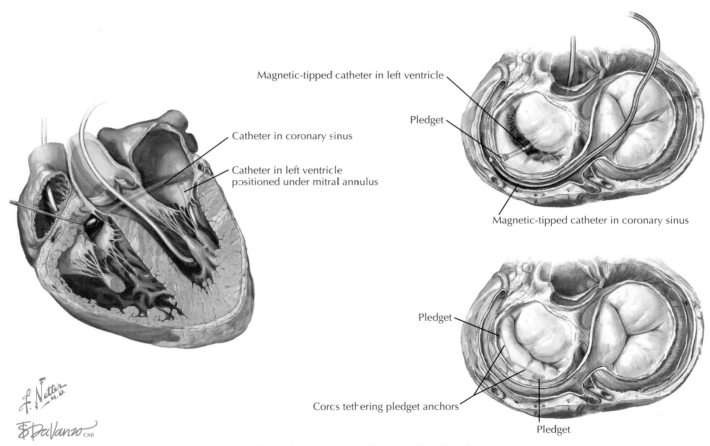

Magnetic-tipped catheter in left ventricle

Catheter in coronary sinus

Catheter in left ventricle
positioned under mitral annulus

Pledget

Magnetic-tipped catheter in coronary sinus

Pledget

Cords tethering pledget anchors

Pledget

FIG 55.4 Mitral Annuloplasty With the Mitralign System.

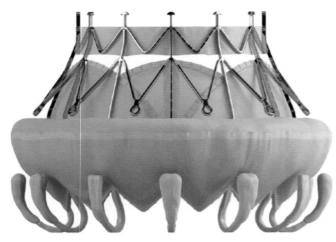

A CardiAQ-Edwards™ Transcatheter Mitral Valve

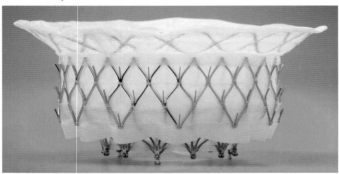

B Metronic Intrepid™ transcatheter heart valve

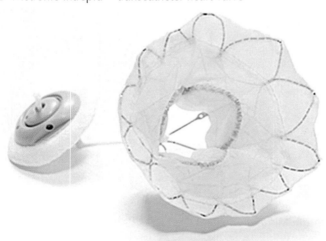

C Tendyne™ Mitral Valve System

FIG 55.5 Transcatheter Mitral Valve Replacement Prototypes. (A), CardiAQ-Edwards Transcatheter Mitral Valve. (B), Metronic Intrepid transcatheter heart valve. (C), Abbott Tendyne Mitral Valve System. (A, reused courtesy Edwards Lifesciences, Irvine, California; B, reused with permission from ©Medtronic 2017, Minneapolis, Minnesota; C, reused with permission from Tendyne Holdings, LLC, a subsidiary of Abbott Vascular, Roseville, Minnesota.)

Some designs have a sealing skirt to minimize paravalvular leak, and some are repositionable and recapturable. The valves that are furthest along in their development are the Edwards CardiAQ valve (Edwards Lifesciences, Irvine, California), which is the only design with a transseptal delivery system, the Medtronic Intrepid valve (Medtronic, Minneapolis, Minneapolis), and the Abbott Tendyne Valve (Abbott Vascular) (Fig. 55.5), which are all currently transapical only.

ADDITIONAL RESOURCES

Mitraclip.com.
Website for the manufacturer of the MitraClip device that provides general information on the device.
Nishimura RA, Otto CM, Bonow RO, et al. 2017 AHA/ACC focused update of the 2014 AHA/ACC guideline for the management of patients with valvular heart disease: a report of the American College of Cardiology/American Heart Association Task Force on Clinical Practice Guidelines. *J Am Coll Cardiol.* 2017;70(2):252–289.
Updated valvular heart disease guidelines that provide guidance for transcatheter mitral valve repair.
Nkomo VT, Gardin JM, Skelton TN, Gottdiener JS, Scott CG, Enriquez-Sarano M. Burden of valvular heart diseases: a population-based study. *Lancet.* 2006;368:1005–1011.
A population-based study describing the burden of valvular heart disease.
Rogers JH, Franzen O. Percutaneous edge-to-edge MitraClip therapy in the management of mitral regurgitation. *Eur Heart J.* 2011;32:2350–2357.
A summary of MitraClip therapy.

EVIDENCE

Feldman T, Foster E, Glower DD, et al; EVEREST II Investigators. Percutaneous repair or surgery for mitral regurgitation. *N Engl J Med.* 2011;364(15):1395–1406.
Randomized trial comparing MitraClip with surgery in the treatment of mitral valve regurgitation.
Glower DD, Kar S, Trento A, Lim DS, et al. Percutaneous mitral valve repair for mitral regurgitation in high-risk patients: results of the EVEREST II study. *J Am Coll Cardiol.* 2014;64(2):172–181.
High-risk registry of patients who underwent MitraClip therapy.
Lipiecki J, Siminiak T, Sievert H, et al. Coronary sinus-based percutaneous annuloplasty as treatment for functional mitral regurgitation: the TITAN II trial. *Open Heart.* 2016 Jul 8;3(2).
Results of the Carillon percutaneous mitral annuloplasty trial.
Regueiro A, Granada JF, Dagenais F, Rodés-Cabau J. Transcatheter mitral valve replacement: insights from early clinical experience and future challenges. *J Am Coll Cardiol.* 2017;69(17):2175–2192.
A state-of-the-art review of TMVR technologies.
Sorajja P, Mack M, Vemulapalli S, et al. Initial experience with commercial transcatheter mitral valve repair in the United States. *J Am Coll Cardiol.* 2016;67(10):1129–1140.
Results from real-word use of the MitraClip in the United States.
Velazquez EJ, Samad Z, Al-Khalidi HR, et al. The MitraClip and survival in patients with mitral regurgitation at high risk for surgery: a propensity-matched comparison. *Am Heart J.* 2015;170(5):1050–1059.
A propensity-matched comparison of patients who underwent MitraClip therapy versus medical therapy. This study suggested a mortality benefit with MitraClip over medical therapy alone.

Pericardial Diseases

56

Pericardial Disease: Clinical Features and Treatment

Allie E. Goins, Christopher D. Chiles, George A. Stouffer

The pericardium is a two-layered sac that encircles the heart (Fig. 56.1). The visceral pericardium is a mesothelial monolayer that adheres to the epicardium. It is reflected back on itself at the level of the great vessels, where it joins the parietal pericardium, which is the tough fibrous outer layer. Under normal conditions, a small amount of fluid (~5–50 mL) separates the two layers and decreases friction between them.

The normal pericardium serves three primary functions: fixing the heart within the mediastinum; limiting cardiac distention during sudden increases in intracardiac volume; and limiting the spread of infection from the adjacent lungs. However, the importance of these functions has been questioned because of the benign prognosis associated with congenital absence of the pericardium.

This chapter discusses the clinical features and treatment of four pathological conditions that involve the pericardium: acute pericarditis, chronic pericarditis, constrictive pericarditis, and pericardial effusions. The hemodynamic effects of pericardial pathology are discussed in Chapter 57.

ACUTE PERICARDITIS

Etiology and Pathogenesis

The most common presentation of a pericardial abnormality is acute pericarditis, which is inflammation of the pericardium (Fig. 56.2). In general, this is a self-limited disease that is responsive to oral antiinflammatory medication. Acute pericarditis infrequently necessitates hospital admission. It is more common in men than in women and more common in adults than in children. The two most common causes of acute pericarditis in the United States are viral and idiopathic. Viruses that have been implicated in causing pericarditis include coxsackie virus B; echovirus; adenoviruses; influenza A and B viruses; enterovirus; mumps virus; Epstein-Barr virus; HIV; herpes simplex virus type 1; varicella-zoster virus; measles virus; parainfluenza virus type 2; respiratory syncytial virus; cytomegalovirus; and hepatitis viruses A, B, and C. Other causes include uremia, pericardiectomy associated with cardiac surgery, pulmonary embolism, collagen-vascular diseases, Dressler syndrome, malignancy, tuberculosis, fungus (e.g., histoplasmosis), parasites (e.g., amoeba), myxedema, radiation, acute rheumatic fever, and trauma (Fig. 56.3).

Clinical Presentation

The clinical presentation of pericarditis is most often dominated by chest pain, which is generally sharp, pleuritic, and positional in nature, increased by lying supine and improved by leaning forward. Symptoms may include dyspnea, palpitations, coughing, and fever, and the patient may have a history of a viral prodrome. On physical examination, a pericardial friction rub is generally the most remarkable finding. The classic description is of a scratchy sound heard best along the lower left sternal border. It typically has three components (when the patient

is in sinus rhythm), which correspond to atrial systole, ventricular systole, and rapid ventricular filling during early diastole. The component corresponding to rapid ventricular filling (atrial systole) may be absent, resulting in a two-component friction rub. In one series of 100 patients with acute pericarditis, a three-component friction rub was detected in approximately 50% of the patients, whereas any friction rub (one, two, or three components) was present in almost all cases.

Differential Diagnosis

The differential diagnosis of acute pericarditis includes other pathologies involving the chest and heart, with two of the most common being myocardial ischemia and pulmonary embolus. Features that distinguish the discomfort of myocardial ischemia from acute pericarditis include previous exertional symptoms, lack of variation with respiration or position, associated symptoms of nausea or diaphoresis, and/or dyspnea. In addition, the discomfort of pericarditis is often described as "sharp" or "stabbing," whereas the pain of myocardial infarction is pressure-like. ECG changes of ST elevation can be seen in both pericarditis and myocardial ischemia or infarction; however, the ST elevation present with myocardial infarction is generally localized to a vascular bed and is accompanied by reciprocal ST depression. PR depression is common in acute pericarditis and exceedingly rare in myocardial infarction (it would imply atrial infarction in this setting). Cardiac biomarkers can be elevated in both conditions. Other conditions that can mimic acute pericarditis include disease states that involve inflammation of structures in close proximity to the pericardium, including cholecystitis, pancreatitis, and pneumonia.

Diagnostic Approach

According to the European Society of Cardiology (ESC) 2015 guidelines, the diagnosis of acute pericarditis requires at least two of the following: (1) the presence of chest pain typical of pericarditis (sharp, pleuritic, positional in nature); (2) pericardial friction rub on cardiac auscultation; (3) diffuse ST-segment elevation or PR depression on ECG, and (4) new or worsening pericardial effusion noted on echocardiography. Laboratory studies are nondiagnostic in acute pericarditis. Nonspecific markers of inflammation, such as white blood cell count or C-reactive protein, may be elevated. If concurrent myocarditis is present, cardiac biomarkers (creatine kinase and troponin) may be elevated.

As mentioned previously, ECG changes can help diagnose acute pericarditis, but a lack of ECG changes does not exclude the diagnosis of pericarditis. ECG abnormalities are present in approximately 90% of patients with acute pericarditis, with approximately 50% of patients showing all four stages of ECG changes commonly associated with the evolution of acute pericarditis (see Fig. 56.2 [ECG]; Fig. 56.4). Stage I changes accompany the onset of chest pain and include the classic ECG changes associated with acute pericarditis, which are diffuse concave ST elevation with PR depression (see Chapter 7). Stage II occurs several

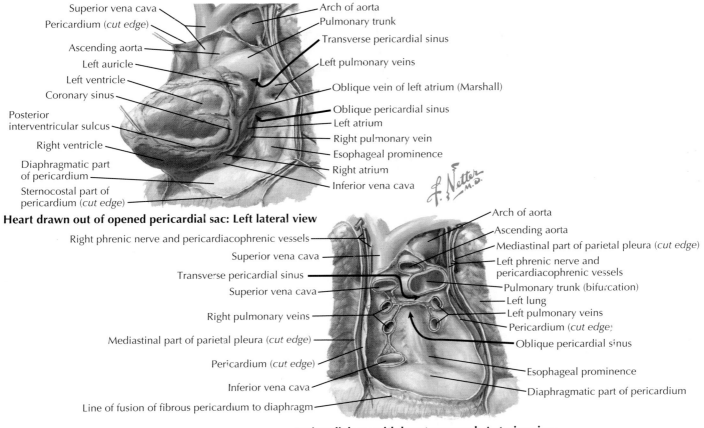

Heart drawn out of opened pericardial sac: Left lateral view

Superior vena cava
Pericardium (*cut edge*)
Ascending aorta
Left auricle
Left ventricle
Coronary sinus
Posterior interventricular sulcus
Right ventricle
Diaphragmatic part of pericardium
Sternocostal part of pericardium (*cut edge*)

Arch of aorta
Pulmonary trunk
Transverse pericardial sinus
Left pulmonary veins
Oblique vein of left atrium (Marshall)
Oblique pericardial sinus
Left atrium
Right pulmonary vein
Esophageal prominence
Right atrium
Inferior vena cava

Pericardial sac with heart removed: Anterior view

Right phrenic nerve and pericardiacophrenic vessels
Superior vena cava
Transverse pericardial sinus
Superior vena cava
Right pulmonary veins
Mediastinal part of parietal pleura (*cut edge*)
Pericardium (*cut edge*)
Inferior vena cava
Line of fusion of fibrous pericardium to diaphragm

Arch of aorta
Ascending aorta
Mediastinal part of parietal pleura (*cut edge*)
Left phrenic nerve and pericardiacophrenic vessels
Pulmonary trunk (bifurcation)
Left lung
Left pulmonary veins
Pericardium (*cut edge*)
Oblique pericardial sinus
Esophageal prominence
Diaphragmatic part of pericardium

FIG 56.1 Anatomy of the Pericardium.

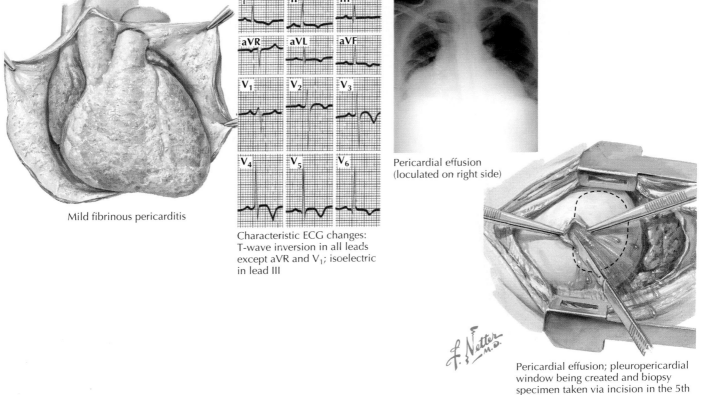

Mild fibrinous pericarditis

Characteristic ECG changes: T-wave inversion in all leads except aVR and V_1; isoelectric in lead III

Pericardial effusion (loculated on right side)

Pericardial effusion; pleuropericardial window being created and biopsy specimen taken via incision in the 5th left intercostal space

FIG 56.2 Diseases of the Pericardium: Presentation and Treatment of Pericarditis.

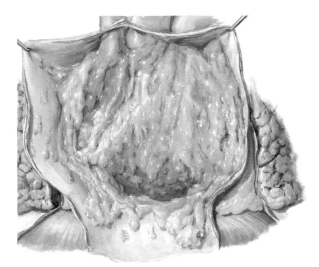

Purulent pericarditis

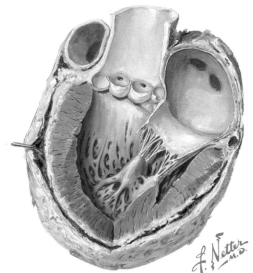

Tuberculous pericarditis

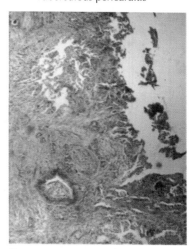

Biopsy specimen revealing
carcinomatous infiltration
of pericardium

FIG 56.3 Diseases of the Pericardium: Etiologies.

days later and is represented by the return of ST segments to baseline and T-wave flattening. In stage III, T-wave inversion is seen in most leads. The ECG in stage IV shows the return of T waves to an upright position. The approximate time frame for passage through all four stages of ECG changes in most cases of acute pericarditis is 2 weeks. Other ECG presentations include isolated PR depression, absence of one or more stages, and persistence of T-wave inversion. Atrial arrhythmias are seen in 5% to 10% of cases.

Echocardiography can be used to evaluate for the presence of pericardial effusion. It can also be used to evaluate for ventricular dysfunction, which might occur if the myocardium is involved in addition to the pericardium. However, a normal echocardiogram does not exclude the diagnosis of acute pericarditis.

Management and Therapy
Optimum Treatment

Most cases of acute pericarditis are self-limited, although symptoms can persist for weeks. The goals of acute pericarditis management include pain relief, identification, and treatment of the underlying cause, as well as observation for evidence that a pericardial effusion is developing with or without pericardial tamponade. Nonsteroidal antiinflammatory drugs (NSAIDs), such as aspirin, ibuprofen, and indomethacin, are generally first-line therapy for pain relief in acute pericarditis. Therapy with colchicine has been shown to provide more rapid relief of symptoms than NSAIDs and reduces the rate of recurrent symptoms.

Studies have shown that patients with acute pericarditis, due to viral or idiopathic etiology, are at risk of experiencing recurrent symptoms following discontinuation of steroid treatment. As a result, steroids are not recommended as first-line therapy for acute, viral, or idiopathic pericarditis unless the patient is unable to take NSAIDs or does not improve with NSAIDs and colchicine. If steroids are used, low to moderate doses with a slow taper are preferred over high doses to help prevent the return of symptoms at the end of treatment.

It is important to identify patients with pericarditis who are more likely to develop complications and experience an adverse outcome. Some of the risk factors found to be associated with a poor prognosis in multiple studies include fever >38°C, subacute onset of symptoms, presence of a large pericardial effusion or cardiac tamponade, lack of response to NSAID treatment, myocardial involvement as suggested by elevated cardiac biomarkers and/or ventricular dysfunction, recent trauma, current oral anticoagulant therapy, and long-term immunosuppression.

In general, patients with acute pericarditis have a favorable long-term prognosis, especially in cases of viral and idiopathic pericarditis. Tamponade has been reported in up to 15% of patients with acute pericarditis. Transient constrictive physiology within the first 30 days after an acute episode of pericarditis has been found in some patients—9% of patients with pericarditis in one study—but generally, it is self-limiting and abates within 3 months. Constrictive pericarditis develops in a small number of patients with acute pericarditis but generally is not clinically evident for many years (discussed in more detail later).

Avoiding Treatment Errors

Acute pericarditis can be confused with several life-threatening disorders, including myocardial ischemia and pulmonary embolus. A careful history and physical examination in combination with accurate ECG interpretation will often establish the diagnosis of acute pericarditis. It is also important to consider the pretest probability of various disorders in a specific patient: the risk of myocardial infarction will be higher in older patients with coronary artery disease risk factors; the risk of pulmonary embolus is increased in individuals with prothrombotic disorders or recent immobilization; and the likelihood of acute pericarditis is increased in younger patients with an antecedent viral illness.

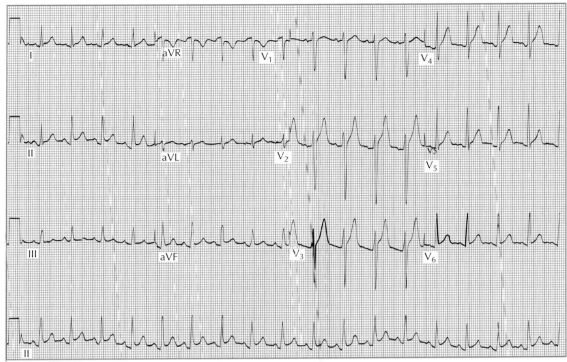

FIG 56.4 Typical Stage I Electrocardiographic Findings in a Patient With Acute Pericarditis. Note the diffuse ST elevation.

CHRONIC OR RECURRENT PERICARDITIS

Recurrent pericarditis is defined as pericarditis that reoccurs after a patient has been symptom free for at least 4 to 6 weeks, whereas chronic pericarditis (also referred to as "incessant pericarditis") is defined as symptoms lasting for at least ≥3 months. Recurrent or chronic symptoms develop in approximately 25% of patients with acute pericarditis. The mechanism is unknown, although there is evidence that recurrent infection or autoimmune processes may have a contributory role in individual patients. Most cases of recurrent pericarditis are treated with NSAIDs or colchicine, and steroids if no improvement is seen with these drugs. There are data that colchicine reduces recurrent symptoms in comparison to NSAID use alone. In severe cases, more potent immunosuppressive therapy and even pericardiectomy are occasionally necessary.

CONSTRICTIVE PERICARDITIS

Etiology and Pathogenesis

Constrictive pericarditis is characterized by a dense, fibrous thickening of the pericardium that adheres to and encases the myocardium, resulting in impaired diastolic ventricular filling (Fig. 56.5). The general paradigm is that constrictive pericarditis occurs over a period of years as a result of an acute injury (e.g., a viral infection) that elicits a chronic fibrosing reaction or as a result of a chronic injury that stimulates a persistent reaction (e.g., renal failure). Clinically, constrictive pericarditis generally is a chronic disease with symptom progression over a period of years. The presentation is that of right-sided heart failure, and it may resemble restrictive cardiomyopathy, cirrhosis, cor pulmonale, or other conditions. Because pericardial constriction is uncommon, patients occasionally are treated for an incorrect diagnosis (left- or right-sided heart failure, hepatic failure, or others) for years. Newer diagnostic technologies and a change in the predominant etiologies of constriction

have increased the recognition of subacute presentations that occur over a period of months.

The most common causes of constriction in industrialized countries are cardiac surgery, mediastinal radiation, pericarditis, and idiopathic etiologies (Table 56.1). Other causes include infection (e.g., fungal or tuberculosis), malignancies such as breast cancer or lymphoma, connective tissue disease (e.g., systemic lupus erythematosus or rheumatoid arthritis), trauma, and drugs.

Clinical Presentation

History

The symptoms and signs of constrictive pericarditis result from reduced cardiac output (CO), elevated systemic venous pressure, and pulmonary venous congestion. The typical history is progressively worsening dyspnea, edema, or other volume overload symptoms. Patients generally have features of right-sided heart failure with ascites and edema, but other features may include anorexia; nausea; fatigue; orthopnea; and sometimes, cardiac tamponade, atrial arrhythmia, and frank liver disease. Chest pain typical of angina may be related to underperfusion of the coronary arteries or compression of an epicardial coronary artery by the thickened pericardium.

Physical Examination

The physical examination in constrictive pericarditis generally reveals increased jugular venous pressure, a prominent y descent in the jugular pulse, and an increase of jugular venous pressure on inspiration (Kussmaul sign), which results from the thickened pericardium's impairment of venous return to the right side of the heart. The pulse pressure may be reduced, and a pulsus paradoxus may be present in up to one-third of patients. Tachycardia may develop to compensate for the diminished stroke volume. The apical impulse is reduced, and it is rarely displaced because the heart size is generally normal. The heart sounds may be

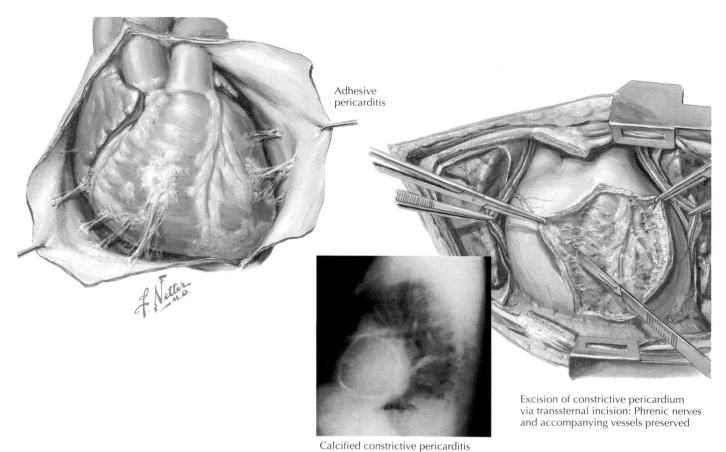

Adhesive pericarditis

Calcified constrictive pericarditis

Excision of constrictive pericardium via transsternal incision: Phrenic nerves and accompanying vessels preserved

FIG 56.5 Diseases of the Pericardium: Constrictive Pericarditis.

TABLE 56.1   Mayo Clinic Experience: Causes of Constrictive Pericarditis and Pericardial Effusions Requiring Pericardiocentesis in Different Cohorts

	CONSTRICTIVE PERICARDITIS		PERICARDIAL EFFUSION (REQUIRING PERICARDIOCENTESIS)		
	1936–1982 (n = 231; %)	1985–1995 (n = 135; %)	1979–1986 (n = 182; %)	1986–1993 (n = 354; %)	1993–2000 (n = 441; %)
Idiopathic	73	33	9	8	8
Infectious	6	3	7	4	7
After cardiac surgery	2	18	21	22	28
Connective tissue disease	2	7	6	3	4
Exposure to radiation	5	13	—	—	—
Acute pericarditis	10	16	—	—	—
Invasive procedure	—	—	4	9	14
Neoplastic	—	—	41	39	25

Adapted from Ling LH, Oh JK, Schaff HV, et al. Constrictive pericarditis in the modern era: evolving clinical spectrum and impact on outcome after pericardiectomy. *Circulation* 1999;100:1380–1386; and Tsang TS, Enriquez-Sarano M, Freeman WK, et al. Consecutive 1127 therapeutic echocardiographically guided pericardiocenteses: clinical profile, practice patterns, and outcomes spanning 21 years. *Mayo Clin Proc* 2002:77:429–436.

distant, and the first heart sound is typically soft because the mitral and tricuspid valves are nearly closed at end-diastole (because almost all ventricular filling occurs early in diastole). A pericardial knock (heard best along the left sternal border) often occurs shortly after the second heart sound as a result of a sudden deceleration of ventricular filling. A pericardial knock may be confused with an S_3 gallop, but knocks usually occur earlier in the cardiac cycle and have a higher acoustic frequency. Pericardial knocks can also be confused with the opening snap of mitral stenosis. Murmurs found at diagnosis are generally unrelated to pericarditis. Ascites, pleural effusions, and peripheral edema may be found. In addition, hepatosplenomegaly and its clinical sequelae, such as protein-losing enteropathy from impaired lymphatic drainage from the gut, may occur. Because the most impressive physical findings are often the insidious development of hepatomegaly and ascites, patients with constrictive pericarditis may initially be mistakenly thought to have hepatic cirrhosis or an intraabdominal tumor.

Differential Diagnosis

Constrictive pericarditis and restrictive cardiomyopathy are different diseases sharing a similar hemodynamic profile. The primary hemodynamic abnormality in both conditions is impaired diastolic filling of the ventricles. In constrictive pericarditis, the impediment to filling is caused by the thickened, unyielding pericardium. In restrictive cardiomyopathy, the abnormality is a result of a poorly compliant myocardium that limits the ability of the ventricles to expand and accept the filling volume of the atria. There is rarely overlap, and both entities can coexist (e.g., radiation-induced myopericardial disease). The heart failure that develops is insidious in onset and predominantly right-sided. These syndromes may mimic many other disease entities, and it is common for both conditions to go undiagnosed for years.

The differentiation of these two entities can be challenging to the clinician. Although various hemodynamic factors are helpful in differentiating constrictive pericarditis from restrictive cardiomyopathy, it is usually not possible to arrive at a firm diagnosis of either condition based on hemodynamics alone. Plain chest x-ray has some value in chronic pericardial constriction because calcification of the pericardium can be seen in up to 25% of cases. Pericardial thickening can sometimes be visualized by echocardiography, but a lack of pericardial thickening on echocardiography does not rule out constrictive pericarditis. Pericardial effusions can be seen but are generally small. CT scanning and cardiac MRI are now widely used to visualize the pericardium in patients with suspected constrictive pericarditis. A pericardial thickness of >3 mm suggests pericardial constriction, but it is important to note that pericardial thickening was absent in 20% of cases of surgically proven constrictive pericarditis in one series. Similarly, not all patients with a thickened pericardium will have constrictive pericarditis; however, a thickness of >6 mm adds considerable specificity to the diagnosis.

Diagnostic Approach

Laboratory evaluation might show the result of congestive hepatopathy with an elevated bilirubin concentration, mild elevation of hepatic transaminase concentrations, a low albumin concentration, and an elevated prothrombin time.

Electrocardiographic results are rarely normal in constriction. They may reveal low-voltage QRS and diffuse flattening of the T waves. Low voltage can result from effusive constrictive disease or myocardial atrophy. Conduction abnormalities and other nonspecific abnormalities may be present. Atrial fibrillation occurs in approximately one-third of patients.

When tuberculous pericarditis was common, chest radiography showed classic pericardial calcification in up to one-third of chronic cases, but this finding is less common today (see Fig. 56.5). The lack of pericardial calcification in constrictive pericarditis is now the rule rather than the exception. Cardiac size is generally normal.

The two-dimensional echocardiographic features of constriction include a thickened pericardium, abnormal ventricular septal motion, flattening of the left ventricular (LV) posterior wall during diastole, respiratory variation in ventricular size, and a dilated inferior vena cava. Doppler echocardiographic features include impaired diastolic filling and dissociation of intracardiac and intrathoracic pressures. The thickened pericardium acts as a buffer to the transmission of the usual intrathoracic pressure changes on the intrapericardial structures. This dissociation between the respiratory (intrathoracic) pressure variations is one feature of constriction but may also occur in tamponade. This

may be seen as an inspiratory decrease in the mitral inflow velocity of >25%. A decrease in LV filling during inspiration allows more room for right ventricular (RV) filling as the interventricular septum moves to the left, and hepatic diastolic flow velocities increase. During expiration, LV filling increases, with a concomitant decrease in right-sided heart filling and a decrease in hepatic diastolic forward-flow velocity. In constriction, diastolic forward flow is usually greater than systolic forward flow. In addition, hepatic diastolic flow reversal is increased because the inflow across the tricuspid valve is interrupted by the pericardium and movement of the septum toward the RV with expiration.

CT and MRI of the heart can be important in determining pericardial thickness. These modalities directly visualize the pericardium and can detect thickness >2 mm. The finding of normal pericardial thickness does not exclude constrictive pericarditis, because up to 20% of patients with surgically confirmed disease have normal pericardial thickness on these imaging modalities. Recall that not all patients with a thickened pericardium have constrictive pericarditis, but a thickness >6 mm adds considerable specificity to the diagnosis.

Left- and right-sided heart catheterization provides important information in evaluating potential constrictive pericarditis. There are three key features: elevation and equalization of the diastolic pressures in each cardiac chamber, an early diastolic "dip-and-plateau" configuration in the RV and LV tracings, and a prominent y descent on right atrial (RA) pressure tracings (for a more detailed discussion of hemodynamics, see Chapter 57).

Management and Therapy
Optimum Treatment

Chronic constrictive pericarditis is a progressive disease without spontaneous reversal of pericardial abnormalities, symptoms, or hemodynamics. A minority of patients survive for years with modest jugular venous distention and peripheral edema controlled by the judicious use of diuretics and dietary restriction of sodium intake. Drugs that slow the heart rate (e.g., β-blockers and calcium channel blockers) should be avoided, because mild sinus tachycardia is a compensatory mechanism. Most patients become progressively more disabled, with some developing severe cardiac cachexia.

The mainstay of therapy is surgical removal of the pericardium. In cases with a firmly adherent pericardium, scoring of the pericardium may "loosen" it, but results are less than optimal in many cases. Pericardiectomy is associated with significant risk for morbidity and mortality, especially in older adult patients or those with significant preoperative symptoms, organ dysfunction, or coexisting coronary artery disease. Mortality with pericardiectomy has also been reported to range from 5.6% to 19% and to correlate with RA pressure. In one series, survival of individuals after pericardiectomy at 5 and 10 years was 78 ± 5% and 57 ± 8%, respectively, and was inferior to that of an age- and sex-matched US population. In another single-center series, long-term survival after pericardiectomy was related to the etiology of the constrictive pericarditis, LV systolic function, renal function, serum sodium, and pulmonary artery systolic pressure. Idiopathic constrictive pericarditis had the best prognosis, followed by constrictive pericarditis that occurred after surgery or radiation treatment. Pericardial calcification had no impact on survival.

Of patients who survive pericardiectomy, 90% report symptomatic improvement, and approximately 50% become asymptomatic. Symptom resolution may be immediate but can take weeks to months. In some patients, symptoms may recur.

Avoiding Treatment Errors

A major difficulty in treating patients with constrictive pericarditis is that the diagnosis is often made many years after symptoms develop.

As noted, pericardiectomy is associated with significant morbidity and mortality, and, in general, outcomes are better in patients with better functional status before the operation.

PERICARDIAL EFFUSION

Etiology and Pathogenesis

Pericardial effusions are generally exudative and a response to pericardial injury. Exudative effusions occur secondary to inflammatory, infectious, malignant, or autoimmune processes within the pericardium. Transudative effusions can result from obstructed fluid drainage, which occurs through lymphatic channels. The hemodynamic effects of pericardial effusions occur on a spectrum with increasing pericardial pressure, which results in increased intracardiac diastolic pressures. Cardiac tamponade is a clinical syndrome caused by increased intrapericardial pressure due to the accumulation of exudative fluid, blood, pus, other fluid, or gas in the pericardial space. Cardiac tamponade can cause hemodynamic collapse by impairing venous return, which impairs diastolic ventricular filling and CO.

There are few data regarding etiologies of pericardial effusions in a community setting or in patients who do not require drainage. The most common etiologies that require pericardiocentesis include malignancy, previous cardiac surgery, a complication during a percutaneous procedure (e.g., RV perforation during pacemaker lead placement), idiopathic etiologies, connective tissue disorder, and infection (Table 56.1). Other causes include acute pericarditis, renal failure, coagulopathy, hypothyroidism, trauma, previous radiation, HIV, and myocardial infarction. Transudative effusions can be seen in congestive heart failure, cirrhosis, nephrosis, and pregnancy.

Pericardial effusions are common after cardiac surgery, occurring in >80% of cases. The maximal size is apparent by 10 days, and the effusions usually resolve spontaneously within 1 month after surgery.

Malignancy is one of the most common causes of pericardial effusions, reported in up to 20% of patients with cancer in autopsy series. The primary tumors most often associated with pericardial effusions are lung (40%), breast (23%), lymphoma (11%), and leukemia (5%). Pericardial effusions in patients with cancer are malignant approximately 50% of the time. Nonmalignant causes of pericardial effusions in patients with cancer include radiation-induced pericarditis and infections.

Clinical Presentation

Clinical manifestations of pericardial effusion depend on the intrapericardial pressure, which, in turn, depends on the amount and rate of fluid accumulation in the pericardial sac. As intrapericardial pressure increases, ventricular diastolic pressure increases. Atrial pressures increase to maintain forward flow across the tricuspid and mitral valves. Further increases in intrapericardial pressure cause ventricular filling to decrease, leading to impaired CO and hypotension. Rapid accumulation of pericardial fluid may elevate intrapericardial pressures with as little as 80 mL of fluid, whereas slowly progressing effusions can grow to 2 L without symptoms. When pericardial fluid accumulation is rapid or sustained, pericardial tamponade may result, the hemodynamics of which are discussed in detail in Chapter 57.

History and Physical Examination

Most pericardial effusions are asymptomatic. If symptoms occur, the most common complaints include dyspnea (85%), coughing (30%), orthopnea (25%), and chest pain (20%). The common signs of pericardial effusion are a paradoxic pulse (45%), tachypnea (45%), tachycardia (40%), hypotension (25%), and peripheral edema (20%), all of which raise the possibility that pericardial tamponade is present.

Small pericardial effusions are generally not detectable by physical examination. Large effusions result in muffled heart sounds and occasionally in Ewart sign, which is a dullness to percussion beneath the angle of the left scapula from compression of the left lung by pericardial fluid.

Patients with pericardial tamponade generally are tachycardic and tachypneic, and appear ill (Fig. 56.6). Pericardial tamponade is a medical emergency that necessitates intervention to remove fluid to reduce pericardial pressure and thus relieve the associated hemodynamic abnormalities. The description by Beck of pericardial tamponade included the classic triad of hypotension, muffled heart sounds, and jugular venous distention. Tamponade is generally associated with a pulsus paradoxus, and a decrease in systolic blood pressure of >10 mm Hg with inspiration. Systolic blood pressure normally decreases during inspiration, but cardiac tamponade causes an exaggeration of physiological respiratory variation in systemic blood pressure from decreasing CO during inspiration. However, pulsus paradoxus is neither sensitive nor specific for cardiac tamponade. It can also occur in constrictive pericarditis, obstructive lung disease, RV infarction, pulmonary embolus, or large pleural effusions.

Differential Diagnosis

The differential diagnosis of tachycardia and hypotension is broad and includes hypovolemia, cardiogenic shock (from either LV failure or RV infarction), neurogenic shock, anaphylactic shock, adrenal insufficiency, massive pulmonary embolus, pneumothorax, and pericardial tamponade. Of these conditions, elevated RA pressure (jugular venous distention on examination) is seen in pericardial tamponade, cardiogenic shock, pulmonary embolus, or pneumothorax. The etiology of shock will often be suggested by the clinical presentation, physical examination, ECG findings, and chest x-ray. Echocardiography can be useful in these patients and is the best modality for determining whether a pericardial effusion is present (Fig. 56.7). In some patients, right heart catheterization may also be helpful.

Diagnostic Approach
Electrocardiography

Typical findings include sinus tachycardia and low voltage. If associated pericarditis is present, PR-segment depression, diffuse ST elevation, and possibly, atrial tachyarrhythmias may be apparent. Electrical alternans, in which R-wave voltage varies from beat to beat, is the most specific ECG finding, but it is rarely found and only in association with large pericardial effusions.

Chest Radiography

An enlarged cardiac silhouette is seen after the accumulation of at least 200 mL of fluid. A large pericardial effusion results in a so-called water bottle appearance. One-third to one-half of patients have a coexisting pleural effusion, with the left side being more common than the right. Separation of the epicardial fat pad from the outer border of the cardiac silhouette can occasionally be observed, especially in the lateral view.

Echocardiography

Echocardiography is the gold standard test for evaluating pericardial effusions. Pericardial fluid appears as an echo-free space between the visceral and parietal pericardia. Effusions can be circumferential (completely surrounding the heart) or loculated. In cardiac tamponade, echocardiographic findings include diastolic collapse of the right atrium and/or ventricle. Doppler interrogation demonstrates marked respiratory variation in flow across the tricuspid and mitral valves. Echocardiography is a sensitive and specific test for pericardial effusions; however, false-positive results can occur in pleural effusions, pericardial thickening, increased pericardial fat (especially the anterior epicardial fat pad),

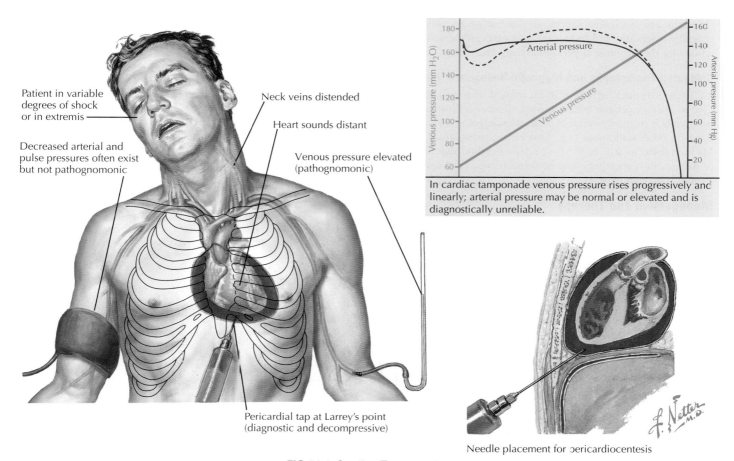

In cardiac tamponade venous pressure rises progressively and linearly; arterial pressure may be normal or elevated and is diagnostically unreliable.

Patient in variable degrees of shock or in extremis

Decreased arterial and pulse pressures often exist but not pathognomonic

Neck veins distended

Heart sounds distant

Venous pressure elevated (pathognomonic)

Pericardial tap at Larrey's point (diagnostic and decompressive)

Needle placement for pericardiocentesis

FIG 56.6 Cardiac Tamponade.

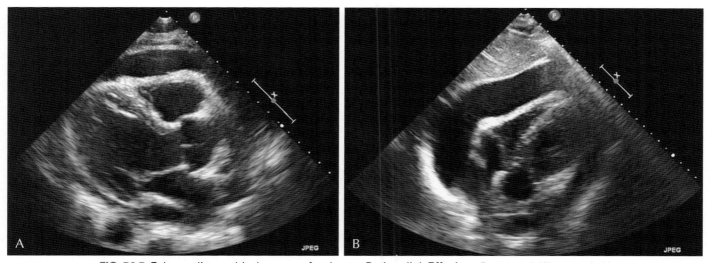

FIG 56.7 Echocardiographic Images of a Large Pericardial Effusion. Parasternal (A) suoxyphoid (B) views.

atelectasis, and mediastinal lesions. Transthoracic echocardiography is generally diagnostic, and transesophageal echocardiography is rarely needed for the diagnosis of pericardial tamponade.

Computed Tomography and Magnetic Resonance Imaging

A CT scan may detect as little as 50 mL of fluid. This modality is rarely used to evaluate patients with suspected effusions; effusions are more commonly incidentally found in patients undergoing chest CT evaluation for other indications (e.g., lung cancer, unexplained dyspnea). MRI can detect as little as 30 mL of pericardial fluid and may be used to distinguish hemorrhagic and nonhemorrhagic effusions based on T_1 and T_2 signal intensities.

Management and Therapy
Optimum Treatment

Most pericardial effusions resolve without drainage. However, in some patients, pericardiocentesis is needed as emergent treatment for tamponade (see Fig. 52.6) or for diagnostic purposes, including to evaluate the possibility of an infectious or malignant etiology. Pericardiocentesis can be performed percutaneously or surgically. Surgical procedures can enable drainage of loculated effusions and access to pericardial tissue for biopsy. However, percutaneous pericardiocentesis is simpler, more rapid, and associated with a quicker recovery.

A subxyphoid approach is generally used for percutaneous pericardiocentesis, although echocardiographically guided approaches via the chest wall are widely used. Needle insertion can be performed under ECG, echocardiographic, or radiographic guidance. Although pericardiocentesis usually leads to clinical improvement, pulmonary edema, hypotension, and acute ventricular dysfunction have been reported after the procedure. The safety and efficacy of this procedure is dependent on the skill of the operator and the size of the effusion. Recurrence rates of 12% to 40% have been reported after successful drainage.

Malignant pericardial effusions tend to recur, and several approaches have been advocated to prevent the need for repeated pericardiocentesis. The literature consists of small prospective or larger retrospective studies, and no consensus on the best approach has been formed. Balloon pericardiotomy, which forms a hole in the pericardium with a balloon, allows pericardial fluid to drain into the pleural space. Pericardial sclerosis involves application of a sclerosing agent (e.g., tetracycline, doxycycline, cisplatin, 5-fluorouracil, bleomycin) to scar the visceral and parietal pericardia with elimination of the pericardial space. Success rates of as high as 91% have been reported at 30 days, but potential complications include intense pain, atrial arrhythmias, fever, and infection. Another viable approach, surgical creation of a subxyphoid pericardial window, is associated with low morbidity, mortality, and recurrence rates, and can be performed under local anesthesia. However, this approach is not effective with loculated pericardial effusion. In some cases, a pleuropericardial window can be created via thoracotomy under general anesthesia.

Avoiding Treatment Errors

Cardiac tamponade is a medical emergency and may lead to hypotension and death if untreated. The diagnosis is occasionally missed because the patient does not have any clues in the history to point to the presence of pericardial disease. Because the initial presentation of malignancy and other disorders can be pericardial effusion, the lack of a history of pericardial disease or predisposing factors (e.g., chest radiation or cardiac surgery) does not exclude the diagnosis. In general, any patient with unexplained hypotension should undergo echocardiographic evaluation.

FUTURE DIRECTIONS

Diagnosis of pericardial diseases continues to become more accurate, resulting in improved therapies. Future challenges include development of more effective therapies for the more serious pericardial diseases, including refractory pericarditis, pericardial constriction, and pericardial tamponade. Little improvement in this area has occurred in the past decade, perhaps because of diagnostic inaccuracies. A renewed focus on a better understanding of pericardial response to injury and inflammation, combined with advances in diagnostic modalities and therapeutic options, provides a blueprint for development of improved treatments for pericardial disease.

ADDITIONAL RESOURCES

Little WC, Freeman GL. Pericardial disease. *Circulation*. 2006;113:1622–1632.
Reviews pericardial disease, including acute pericarditis, effusive constrictive pericarditis, cardiac tamponade, and constrictive pericarditis.
Spodick DH. Diagnostic electrocardiographic sequences in acute pericarditis: significance of PR segment and PR vector changes. *Circulation*. 1973;48:575–580.
A detailed study of the ECG changes seen in acute pericarditis.
Spodick DH. Pericardial rub: prospective, multiple observer investigation of pericardial friction rub in 100 patients. *Am J Cardiol*. 1975;35:357–362.
In this series of 100 patients with acute pericarditis, a three-component friction rub was detected in approximately 50% of the patients, whereas any friction rub (one, two, or three components) was present in almost all cases.

EVIDENCE

Adler Y, et al. 2015 ESC Guidelines for the diagnosis and management of pericardial diseases: The Task Force for the Diagnosis and Management of Pericardial Diseases of the European Society of Cardiology. *Eur Heart J*. 2015;36(42):2921-2964.
The 2015 European Society of Cardiology guidelines on the diagnosis and treatment of pericardial disease.
Bilchick KC, Wise RA. Paradoxical physical findings described by Kussmaul: pulsus paradoxus and Kussmaul's sign. *Lancet*. 2002;359:1940–1942.
A brief description of the history and significance of Kussmaul sign.
Imazio M, Bobbio M, Cecchi E, et al. Colchicine as first-choice therapy for recurrent pericarditis results of the CORE (COlchicine for REcurrent pericarditis) Trial. *Arch Intern Med*. 2005;165:1987–1991.
A prospective, randomized study of colchicine plus aspirin versus aspirin for the first episode of recurrent pericarditis in 84 patients. Treatment with colchicine significantly decreased the recurrence rate and symptom persistence at 72 hours.
Imazio M, Gaita F, LeWinter M. Evaluation and treatment of pericarditis: a systematic review. *JAMA* 2015; 314(14):1498–1506.
A review of the diagnostic approach and treatment of pericarditis.
Imazio M, Lazaros G, Brucato A, Gaita F. Recurrent pericarditis: new and emerging therapeutic options. *Nat Rev Cardiol*. 2016;13(2):99–105.
A review of the expanding knowledge base on recurrent pericarditis.
Lilly LS. Treatment of acute and recurrent idiopathic pericarditis. *Circulation* 2013; 127:1723–1726.
A review of the treatment options available for acute and recurrent idiopathic pericarditis.
Lotrionte M, Biondi-Zoccai G, et al. International collaborative systematic review of controlled clinical trials on pharmacologic treatments for acute pericarditis and its recurrences. *Am Heart J*. 2010; 160:662–670.
A review of the pharmacological treatments for acute pericarditis.
Nishimura RA. Constrictive pericarditis in the modern era: a diagnostic dilemma. *Heart*. 2001;86:619–623.
A review of the challenges in making the diagnosis of constrictive pericarditis.
Sagristà-Sauleda J, Angel J, Sánchez A, et al. Effusive constrictive pericarditis. *N Engl J Med*. 2004;350:469–475.
The largest study of patients with effusive-constrictive pericarditis.

57

Pericardial Disease: Diagnosis and Hemodynamics

Thomas M. Bashore

NORMAL PERICARDIAL PATHOLOGY AND PHYSIOLOGY

The pericardium can be conceptualized as a "balloon" with the heart being a fist pushed into it. The visceral pericardium adheres to the heart itself and is separated from the parietal pericardium by a space, the pericardial cavity. The entire structure is housed in the fibrous pericardium. The serosal space normally holds a small collection of approximately 50 mL of fluid that is transudative with low protein content. It also contains prostaglandins that modulate cardiac reflexes and coronary tone. The fluid within the pericardial space is in dynamic equilibrium with the blood serum. Because there are many smaller sinuses and recesses in the pericardial space (around the atria, the superior vena cava [SVC], the great vessels, the pulmonary veins [PVs], and the inferior vena cava [IVC]), 250 mL is the approximate limit of fluid; the normal pericardial reserve volume is exceeded with more than this amount, and the intrapericardial pressure rises.

The fibrous pericardium is essentially made of collagen and short elastic fibrils. Superiorly, it is continuous with the adventitia of the great vessels and attaches to the central tendon of the diaphragm inferiorly. Anteriorly, it attaches to the sternum via ligaments. Laterally, it is contiguous with the parietal lung pleura, and posteriorly, it is contiguous with the bronchi, esophagus, and descending aorta. The phrenic nerves and pericardiophrenic vessels track between the fibrous pericardium and mediastinal pleura anteriorly. Arterial supply is via branches of the internal mammary arteries and descending aorta. Venous drainage is into the superior intercostal veins and internal thoracic veins to the innominate vein.

The serosal pericardium is characterized by the surfaces of the "balloon" and is made of a single layer of mesothelium that covers the heart as epicardium and that lines the fibrous pericardium to form the parietal pericardial structure. Beneath the visceral pericardium and the myocardium are variable amounts of adipose tissue that are particularly prominent in the atrioventricular (AV) and interventricular grooves, and the acute border of the right ventricle (RV). The normal thickness of the pericardium is approximately 1.5 mm, depending upon the imaging method used to assess it.

The pericardium provides a thin tissue barrier between the heart and the surrounding structures; it exerts constant pressure on the heart, which affects the thin structures (the atria and the RV) more than the thicker walled left ventricle (LV). Resting diastolic pressures within the heart are directly affected by this pericardial constraint, and the restraint differs among the chambers. For instance, pericardial removal results in greater dilatation of the RV than of the LV. Pericardial influence on the thinner walled RV and right atrium (RA) accounts for approximately 50% of their normal diastolic pressures.

Normal intrapericardial pressures range from −6 to −3 mm Hg, which directly reflects the intrapleural pressures. The pressure differential between the pericardium and the cardiac chambers (transmural pressure) is approximately 3 mm Hg. The pericardium is much stiffer than cardiac muscle, and once the pericardial reserve volume is exceeded, the pressure–volume curve of the normal pericardium rises steeply. The pericardium has little effect on ventricular systole; however, interactions between the right- and left-sided cardiac chambers are enhanced by the pericardium because atrial and ventricular septal movements are independent of pericardial constraint.

Intracardiac pressures reflect the contraction and relaxation of individual cardiac structures and the changes imparted to them by the pleural and pericardial pressures (Fig. 57.1). Changes in pleural or pericardial pressure primarily affect the intracardiac diastolic pressure. With inspiration, the intrapleural pressures drop and the abdominal cavity pressure increases. Blood flow to the right side of the heart increases, whereas blood return to the left side of the heart decreases slightly. The fall in the intrapleural pressures also causes an increase in the transmural aortic root pressure, which slightly increases impedance to the LV ejection. The reverse occurs during expiration. In the normal setting, the respiratory changes are reflected in the intrapericardial and intracardiac pressures, with inspiration lowering the measured RA pressures and the systolic RV pressure more than the left-sided heart pressures.

The slight reduction in LV filling and the slightly increased impedance to LV ejection with inspiration normally produce a modest decline in the LV stroke volume and slightly lower systolic aortic pulse pressures with inspiration. Marked swings in the intrapleural pressures from negative during inspiration to positive during expiration (which occur in asthma or severe chronic obstructive lung disease) exaggerate these changes in LV filling and may produce a paradoxical pulse (>10 mm Hg decline in the aortic systolic pressure with inspiration) purely from the associated pleural pressure swings. Such a paradoxical pulse related to marked swings in the intrapleural pressure must be differentiated from a similar phenomenon due to pericardial tamponade.

The normal atrial and ventricular waveforms are shown in Fig. 57.2. With atrial contraction, the atrial pressures rise (a wave). With the onset of ventricular contraction, the AV valves bulge toward the atria, and a small c wave results (the c wave is evident on hemodynamic tracings but usually is not visible to the examiner observing the jugular venous pulsations). As ventricular contraction continues, the AV annulus is pulled into the ventricular cavity, and the atria undergo diastole, enlarging the atria and decreasing the atrial pressure (represented by the x descent). Passive filling of the atria during ventricular systole produces a slow rise in the atrial pressure (the v wave) until the AV valves reopen at the peak of the v wave; the pressure then abruptly falls

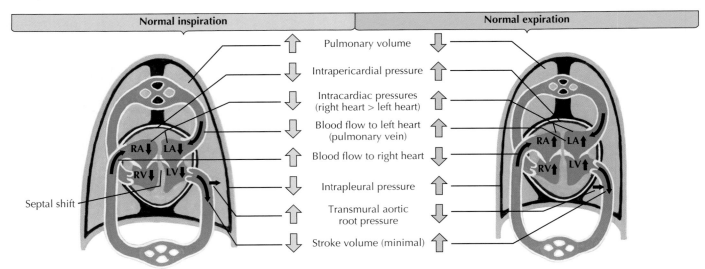

On inspiration, intrapleural pressures drop conceptually pulling blood from the periphery into the lungs through the right heart. The reduced intrathoracic pressures result in an increase in pulmonary venous blood volume and a slight increase in transmural aortic root transmural pressure (impedance). The result is increased right heart filling and decreased left heart filling.

On expiration, the reverse occurs and the pooled blood is returned to left heart while there is decreased flow through the right heart.

JOHN A. CRAIG—MD

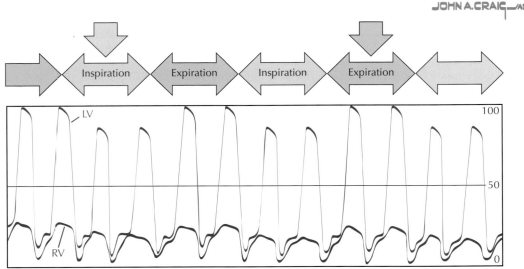

Simultaneous measurement of RV and LV intracardiac pressures reveals a concordance pattern between the two chambers in both inspiration and expiration.

FIG 57.1 Normal Cardiac Blood Flow During Inspiration and Expiration. *LA,* Left atrial; *LV,* left ventricular; *RA,* right atrial; *RV,* right ventricular.

as the ventricles begin active relaxation. Passive filling of the ventricles then follows until atrial contraction recurs, and the cycle repeats. Ventricular diastole can be conceptually divided into an initial active phase (a brief period when the ventricle fills about halfway) and a later, passive filling phase. The nadir, or lowest, diastolic pressure during ventricular diastole occurs during the early active relaxation phase (suction effect).

Hemodynamics of Pericardial Constriction and Pericardial Tamponade

Constrictive pericarditis and pericardial tamponade alter the normal intracardiac pressures in distinctive ways. Some of the hemodynamic abnormalities, such as ventricular interdependence, are seen in both processes, whereas other findings, such as the magnitude of the *y* descent, are unique to each (see Fig. 57.2).

PERICARDIAL CONSTRICTION

Constrictive pericarditis was recognized at autopsy in the 19th century and was described as a "chronic fibrous callous thickening of the wall of the pericardial sac that is so contracted that the normal diastolic filling of the heart is prevented" (Fig. 57.3). The variable severity of the constrictive process results in a spectrum of hemodynamic changes. Recent guidelines suggest that three separate syndromes should be identified: transient constriction, effusive–constrictive pericarditis, and chronic constrictive pericarditis. Transient constriction occurs at times during the acute phase of pericarditis and resolves within weeks after antiinflammatory therapy. Effusive–constrictive pericarditis is uncommon in developed countries, with tuberculosis being the most common cause. The epicardial layer results in the constriction and is usually not

Normal

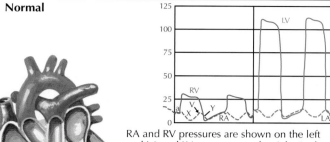

RA and RV pressures are shown on the left and LA and LV pressures on the right. In the atrial tracings, atrial contraction produces an "a" wave followed by the "x" descent due to atrial relaxation and the AV ring being pulled into the ventricle during ventricular systole. Passive filling of the atrium occurs creating the "v" wave that then falls with the opening of the AV valve. In ventricular diastole the atrial ventricular tracings track each other for the most part.

Constrictive pericarditis

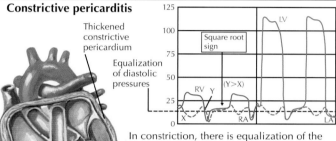

In constriction, there is equalization of the end-diastolic pressures in all chambers. Filling of the ventricles occurs primarily early in diastole then stops creating a "square-root sign." LV filling is rapid due to the high atrial pressures. The Y descent is greater than the X descent therefore. Because pulmonary pressures are normal, the RVEDP is generally >1/3 of the RV systolic pressures.

Cardiac tamponade

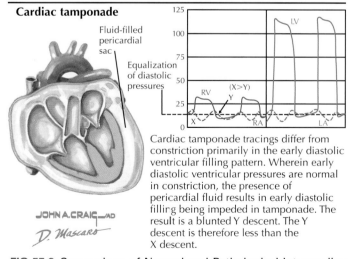

Cardiac tamponade tracings differ from constriction primarily in the early diastolic ventricular filling pattern. Wherein early diastolic ventricular pressures are normal in constriction, the presence of pericardial fluid results in early diastolic filling being impeded in tamponade. The result is a blunted Y descent. The Y descent is therefore less than the X descent.

FIG 57.2 Comparison of Normal and Pathological Intracardiac Pressures. See text for more details. *AV,* Atrioventricular; *LA,* left atrial; *LV,* left ventricular; *RA,* right atrial; *RV,* right ventricular; *RVEDP,* right ventricular end-diastolic pressure.

thickened. Effusive–constrictive pericarditis is confirmed when there is remaining evidence of constrictive pericarditis after the associated pericardial effusion is drained. Surgically, it requires sharp dissection of small visceral pericardial fragments until ventricular motion is improved. In chronic constrictive pericarditis, both the visceral and parietal pericardial layers are typically fused.

Hemodynamics of Pericardial Constriction

In constrictive pericarditis, the diastolic pressures in the atria are elevated due to the restriction of ventricular diastolic inflow. As opposed to a restrictive myocardial process, myocardial relaxation is typically normal. In constriction, the elevated atrial pressures and the normal early LV filling result in a rapid decrease in atrial pressure after the AV valves open and are responsible for the rapid *y* descent (see Fig. 57.2). However, the constraint imposed by the pericardium as the ventricle rapidly fills results in the sudden halting of this rapid early flow and an abrupt rise in diastolic pressure, which produces the "square root sign" or "dip and plateau" in the pressure tracings. The *x* descent is generally minimally affected; thus, the atrial *y* descent is greater than the *x* descent in constrictive pericardial disease. RV systolic and pulmonary systolic pressures are usually normal or only mildly elevated, with the result that the RV end-diastolic pressure (EDP) tends to be greater than one-third of the RV systolic pressure. Because the ventricles are confined by the pericardium at the end of ventricular diastole, the RV and LV EDPs equalize.

The normal respiratory changes in cardiac flow are also altered in constriction. With inspiration, the lower intrathoracic pressure is transmitted to the PVs but not to the left atrium (LA) due to the rigid pericardium; this reduces the gradient between the two and reduces the inflow into the LA and the LV. However, the normal increased flow to the right heart with inspiration still occurs from the IVC to the RA because the abdomen is not exposed to the lower intrathoracic pressures. However, flow in the exposed SVC to the RA fails to increase for the same reason as flow to the LA. Therefore the normal inspiratory fall in the RA pressures may not occur, and the pressure in the RA may not fall or may even rise (Kussmaul sign). This is thought of as the inspiratory "pulling" of blood into the lung through a stiff rigid vessel (the RA and the RV). Kussmaul sign is not specific for pericardial constriction because it can also be observed in acute or chronic RV failure, RV infarction, RV volume overload, and restrictive cardiomyopathy. In these latter conditions, the constrictive physiology is due more to RV volume overload (reaching the limit of RV chamber capacity) than to constriction from the pericardium.

Because the atrial and ventricular septa are unaffected by the pericardial process, changes in atrial and ventricular filling on the right side of the heart can affect left-sided filling (ventricular interdependence). Demonstration of ventricular interdependence is generally accepted as a fundamental requirement for diagnosing constrictive pericarditis. In constriction, as the negative intrapleural pressure draws blood through the RV with inspiration, the increase in RV filling into the confined RV results in an increase in RV systolic pressure, whereas a normal decrease in LV systolic pressure occurs. This phenomenon is illustrated in Fig. 57.4 and is referred to ventricular discordance. For further quantification, normally with inspiration, the area within the RV pressure tracing should fall in a compensatory manner compared with that of the simultaneous LV pressure tracing area. During inspiration in constriction, the RV receives more flow than the LV, and the RV pressure tracing area increases, whereas the LV pressure tracing area decreases. The simultaneous LV/RV pressure tracing area ratio thus becomes smaller with inspiration compared with the LV/RV ratio with expiration. When this inspiratory ratio is divided into the expiratory ratio, a number >1 would therefore be expected if constriction is present. When the Mayo

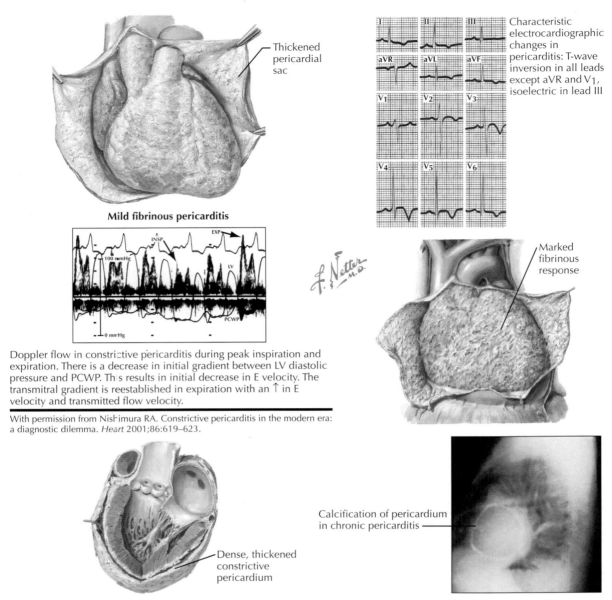

Thickened pericardial sac

Mild fibrinous pericarditis

Doppler flow in constrictive pericarditis during peak inspiration and expiration. There is a decrease in initial gradient between LV diastolic pressure and PCWP. This results in initial decrease in E velocity. The transmitral gradient is reestablished in expiration with an ↑ in E velocity and transmitted flow velocity.

With permission from Nishimura RA. Constrictive pericarditis in the modern era: a diagnostic dilemma. *Heart* 2001;86:619–623.

Characteristic electrocardiographic changes in pericarditis: T-wave inversion in all leads except aVR and V₁, isoelectric in lead III

Marked fibrinous response

Calcification of pericardium in chronic pericarditis

Dense, thickened constrictive pericardium

FIG 57.3 Constrictive Pericarditis. Mitral inflow Doppler reveals an inspiratory (INSP) decrease in gradient between the pulmonary wedge pressure and the left ventricular end-diastolic pressure and an increase in this gradient with expiration (EXP). *LV*, Left ventricular; *PCWP*, pulmonary capillary wedge pressure.

Clinic found this expiratory ratio/inspiratory ratio (index) to be >1.1, their report revealed that the sensitivity was 97%, with a specificity of 100%, a positive predictive value of 100%, and a negative predictive value of 95% for constrictive pericarditis.

Another hemodynamic observation considered reduced LA filling with inspiration in a patient with constriction by noting a lower pulmonary capillary wedge pressure to LV diastolic gradient in inspiration and a greater pulmonary capillary wedge pressure/LV diastolic gradient in expiration (see Fig. 57.3).

Clinical Examination, Chest X-Ray, and Electrocardiography

Pericardial constriction may be subtle, whereas significant constriction presents as primarily right-sided heart failure with normal LV systolic function and clear lungs. A history of antecedent pericarditis, pericarditis induced by drug use, uremia, cardiac surgery, or thoracic radiation

(which may also be a contributing factor in restriction) may be a clue. There is usually evidence of venous congestion, pedal edema, ascites (often out of proportion to peripheral edema), fatigue, dyspnea, and low cardiac output. Tachycardia occurs to compensate. Atrial arrhythmias are common. Jugular venous distention is universal, and a positive Kussmaul response is expected. Sharp, rapid x and y descents can be seen in the jugular venous pulsations at bedside by careful observation. Because the jugular veins may be so distended that they are invisible when the patient is reclining, patients should be examined in an upright position. To time the pulse waveforms, the opposite carotid pulse should be felt—the x descent in the jugular venous pulse (JVP) occurs during ventricular systole (the positive carotid impulse). The rapid y descent should then be observed immediately after the carotid impulse. The JVP thus looks like two prominent positive waves at the beginning of the carotid impulse and at the end of the carotid impulse. This is

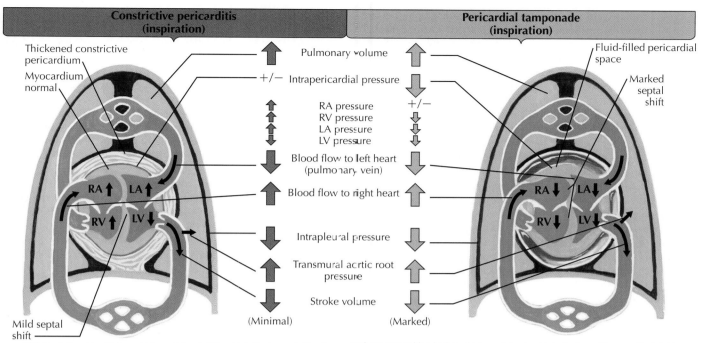

With inspiration blood is brought through the right heart into the lungs. Pulling the blood through the encased right atrium results in a failure of the JVP to drop (Kussmaul sign) as blood flow from the abdomen is outside the lung fields. The LA is within the lung fields and a drop in intrapleural pressures results in pooling of the incoming blood and a reduction in flow to the left heart similar to that normally seen. Some interventricular septal shift to the LV occurs resulting in a further reduction in LV inflow.

With inspiration blood is brought through the heart into the lungs. The compliant right heart receives the blood and no Kussmaul occurs. The heart is in a fixed space though and the increased blood flow to the RV forces a significant shift of the interventricular septum toward the LV and markedly reduces the LV inflow creating the pulsus alternans.

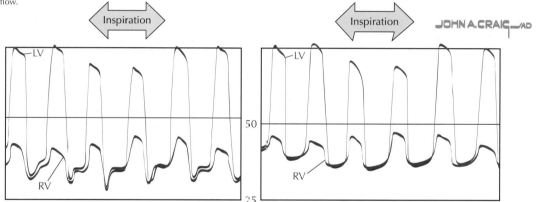

Simultaneous measures of LV and RV ventricular pressures with inspiration and expiration. On the left panel is an example of constriction and on the right panel tamponade. In both instances, there is evidence for ventricular interdependence with a rise in the RV systolic pressure associated with a fall in the LV systolic pressure with inspiration (ventricular discordance). In constrictive pericarditis, though, there is evidence for rapid early diastolic filling that does not occur in pericardial tamponade.

FIG 57.4 Comparison of Blood Flow in Constrictive Pericarditis and Pericardial Tamponade. *JVP*, Jugular vein pulse; *LA*, left atrial; *LV*, left ventricular; *RA*, right atrial; *RV*, right ventricular.

sometimes described as a "W" in the JVP. Precordial palpation may be normal, or the apex may even retract with systole. The rapid filling of the ventricles may produce a loud filling sound (pericardial knock) on auscultation, although this is less common now than in the past. The liver is often enlarged, and ascites is often the prominent examination feature. A paradoxical pulse is not usually demonstrated unless associated lung disease or concurrent pericardial tamponade exists.

As discussed in Chapter 56, although they are often helpful, the ECG and chest radiograph should not be relied on to diagnose either pericardial constriction or pericardial tamponade, or to distinguish the two. In pericardial constriction, the ECG is frequently abnormal, with occasional low voltage and abnormal T waves being common (see Fig. 57.3). Interatrial block demonstrated by a wide P wave is common.

An RV strain pattern may present, together with right-axis deviation. In chronic pericardial constriction, myocardial calcification and fibrosis can affect coronary perfusion and the conduction system. Stress tests in patients with pericardial constriction can produce a false-positive result, with ECG changes due to ischemia caused by myocardial calcification and fibrosis rather than typical coronary artery disease. Atrial arrhythmias, especially fibrillation, are common. The chest x-ray reveals a normal size heart with clear lung fields. Pericardial calcification (that spares the LV apex) may be present (see Fig. 57.3).

Echo-Doppler Measurements

Distinguishing features between constrictive pericarditis and restrictive cardiomyopathy can be found in Chapter 31. Increased pericardial thickness and calcium may be noted on echocardiography but are often difficult to discern. Some correlates of constrictive hemodynamics include diastolic flattening of the LV posterior wall and abrupt posterior motion of the interventricular septum (septal bounce) in early diastole. LV systolic function is generally normal or near-normal. Wall motion abnormalities are seen at times, especially if there is myocardial involvement.

Doppler flow is important in establishing the diagnosis. Because the ventricle fills almost entirely during the first third of diastole, the early filling (E wave) is usually high and has a shortened deceleration time (<160 ms). The atrial filling wave is usually reduced. Normally, with inspiration, the LV minimal pressure and the LA pressures fall equally, and no change is noted in the Doppler mitral inflow velocities. Reflecting the hemodynamics in constriction, the reduced inspiratory LV flow is highlighted by observing a >25% decrease in the peak mitral E-wave inflow velocity in the first beat of inspiration (see Fig. 57.3). At the same time, the tricuspid velocity usually increases >40%. The ventricular interdependence can be further documented by examining the hepatic vein (or SVC), the tricuspid and mitral inflows, and the PV inflow patterns with expiration and inspiration (Fig. 57.5). With inspiration, the hepatic systolic (S) and diastolic (D) waves, together with the tricuspid inflow E and A waves, increase, whereas the mitral E and A waves decrease, together with the pulmonary S and D waves. A "w" pattern is seen in the hepatic flow. Up to one in five patients with constriction may not reveal classic interdependence on echo-Doppler due to high LA pressures, and maneuvers to decrease preload (e.g., sitting or head-up tilt) may unmask the changes. Rapid inflow during

early diastole is also responsible for the commonly observed septal bounce.

Tissue Doppler echocardiography measures myocardial motion. Because myocardial relaxation is preserved in constrictive pericarditis, the early relaxation observed on tissue Doppler velocity patterns (Ea) is normal. If it is abnormal, then a primary myocardial problem is more likely to be present. For example, if the Ea is >7 cm/s, then that is consistent with constriction, whereas an Ea of <7 cm/s is more indicative of myocardial restriction. With severe constriction, although there is tethering of the lateral mitral annulus to the thickened pericardium, "annulus reversus" may occur when the lateral annular e′ velocity (normally less than the medial annulus e′) becomes greater. This observation has been shown to normalize after pericardiectomy.

A method of speckle tracking of B-mode echoes allows for global assessment of stress and strain (deformation) of the myocardium. When speckle tracking has been performed, constrictive pericarditis appears to have constrained circumferential deformation, whereas restrictive cardiomyopathy exhibits attenuation in the longitudinal direction.

Computed Tomography

CT can identify pericardial thickness when it is >4 mm. It is important to note that 20% to 28% of surgically proven constrictive pericarditis cases have normal pericardial thickness on imaging studies. CT can detect pericardial calcium, usually in the regions of pericardial fat; up to 50% of patients with constriction have some pericardial calcium present. CT may also reveal straightening of the interventricular septum, impaired diastolic filling and associated pleural effusion, and ascites

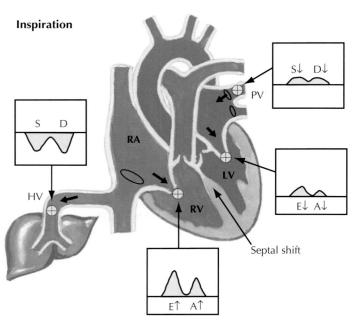

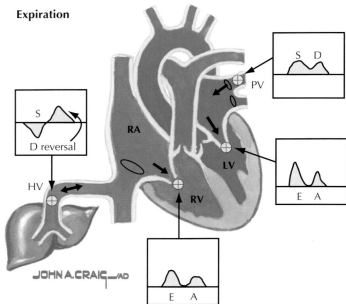

With inspiration, blood is "pulled" through the right heart and there is reduced filling of the left heart (reduced flow in the PV and mitral inflow) while there is increased right heart filling (increased systolic and diastolic flow in the hepatic veins and tricuspid inflow).

With expiration, there is a reduction in flow through the right heart and increased flow to the left heart. This is demonstrated by flow that is only systolic in the hepatic veins (reversed in diastole) and reduced flow through the tricuspid valve on the right side. On the left side there is increased flow in the PV and through the mitral valve. This pattern is seen in both constriction and tamponade except the early filling (E wave) is prominent in constriction and of short duration while the E wave is blunted in tamponade. *D*, Diastolic; *HV*, hepatic vein; *LA*, left atrial; *LV*, left ventricular; *PV*, pulmonary vein; *RA*, right atrial; *RV*, right ventricular; *S*, systolic.

FIG 57.5 Respiratory Echo-Doppler Flow Patterns in Pericardial Disease.

and/or hepatosplenomegaly. Observations that the immediate pulmonary structures are "frozen" during cardiac motion is a telltale sign of constriction. Evidence for pleural effusions and ascites may also be present.

Gated-Cardiac Magnetic Resonance Imaging

Although echo/Doppler remains the noninvasive gold standard modality, cardiac MRI (CMR) provides both similar and additional information at times. It can provide information on pericardial thickening, small pericardial effusions, dilated right-sided structures, the presence of a septal bounce, and evidence of pericardial inflammation (via late gadolinium enhancement). It can help differentiate pericardial constriction from myocardial restriction. Ventricular interaction can be demonstrated by phase-encoding velocimetry, in which similar transmitral and transtricuspid flow variations can be derived, similar to echo/Doppler. Extracardiac findings can also be observed, similar to CT, as described previously.

CARDIAC CATHETERIZATION

The hemodynamics of constrictive pericarditis were described earlier; catheterization allows their documentation (see Figs. 57.2 and 57.4). It is important to track all right-sided heart pressures in relation to the left-sided heart pressures and to note any respiratory changes in systolic and diastolic pressures. Right-sided heart catheterization by itself is usually inadequate for diagnosing pericardial disease. Observations to be made at cardiac catheterization include nearly equal levels of EDPs in all chambers, relatively normal or only slightly elevated pulmonary pressures with a normal pulmonary vascular resistance, a discrepancy of <5 mm Hg between the LVEDP and the RVEDP, a positive Kussmaul sign in the RA, and the classic square root (dip and plateau) pattern in the atrial and diastolic ventricular waveforms.

The crucial role of cardiac catheterization should be to demonstrate ventricular interdependence. The demonstration of discordant peak systolic RV and LV pressures or an increased RV/LV pressure time-to-area ratio >1.1 with inspiration and expiration, as noted earlier, is critical to confirming ventricular interdependence. The RVEDP is usually more than one-third the RV systolic pressure because the pulmonary pressure is normal and the RVEDP is elevated. A paradoxical pulse is unusual. In significant constriction, the nadir of the ventricular pressures usually approaches zero. At times, rapid fluid loading is required to reveal the constrictive physiology in patients with hypovolemia. If the patient is in atrial fibrillation, it may be impossible to sort out the subtle changes between the LV and RV pressures without using a temporary RV pacemaker to pace at a higher than baseline rate to establish a regular rhythm. In addition, an RA angiogram in the anteroposterior view may reveal a cardiac "peel" or thickening at the interface of the RA free wall and the lung fields. Similarly, contrast angiography of the coronary arteries may reveal a peel or a radiographic shadow between the coronary arteries and the lung fields, and segments of the coronaries on angiography may appear frozen in the pericardium during cardiac motion.

PERICARDIAL TAMPONADE

Pericardial tamponade occurs when pericardial fluid exceeds pericardial reserve volume. The result is cardiac compression and restricted diastolic filling of all the cardiac chambers (see Figs. 57.2, 57.4, and 57.6). The amount of pericardial fluid required for tamponade to manifest depends on the parietal pericardial compliance and the rate of fluid accumulation. Acute tamponade can result with even a small rapid increase in pericardial fluid because of the normally steep pericardial pressure–volume relationship. When fluid accumulates slowly, as in patients with

metastatic cancer or chronic uremia, the parietal pericardium adapts and stretches. Tamponade in a chronic situation occurs only after the accumulation of a large amount (sometimes >1 L) of fluid. When pericardial effusion follows acute pericarditis, the therapy focuses on treatment of the acute inflammatory process, with colchicine and aspirin as the cornerstones of therapy. Chronic pericardial effusions require a careful assessment of the etiology and may not require pericardial drainage unless hemodynamic compromise is evident.

Hemodynamics of Tamponade

As fluid accumulates in the pericardium, the thinnest walled chambers (the RA and the RV) are affected first. Right-sided diastolic pressures are normally lower than left-sided diastolic pressures, and collapse of the RA and the RV in diastole is observed early in tamponade (e.g., often before a paradoxical pulse). With cardiac contraction, the heart is also less full, and there is literally more room in the pericardial space for the left and right ventricles. With the onset of diastole, the high intrapericardial pressures are transmitted to the early diastolic atrial and ventricular pressures. When the AV valves open, the diastolic pressures in each chamber are already elevated, and this is reflected in the reduced y descent and loss of rapid ventricular filling in early ventricular diastole (see Fig. 57.2). The high diastolic pressures may also cause premature closure of the AV valves even before ventricular systole initiates. As the ventricles contract and eject blood, they become smaller, and the pericardial space increases; the atria can then still fill in atrial diastole (preserving the x descent). Therefore, the x descent is greater than the y descent in pericardial tamponade, which is the opposite of that observed in constrictive pericarditis. Increasing intrapericardial pressures progressively affect the RA diastolic pressure, then the RV diastolic pressure (especially in the thinner RV outflow tract), and eventually the left-sided heart diastolic pressure. This eventually restricts filling of all the cardiac chambers and finally results in the equalization of EDPs throughout the heart.

As in constriction, the increased filling of the right side of the heart, mandated by the negative intrathoracic pressure during inspiration, increases the early filling of the right heart structures and reduces filling of the left. Ventricular interdependence is present (see Fig. 57.4). Because there is a fixed space in which the heart can reside, it cannot expand in tamponade, but a leftward shift in the atrial and ventricular septa takes place as the right heart fills to the detriment of LV filling. Importantly, atrial reservoir function increases during pericardial tamponade; the left atrium may fill only during expiration, with subsequent emptying only during atrial systole. The reduced LV filling also reduces LV preload and contractile function, further lowering the stroke volume. The drop in systemic blood pressure that creates the paradoxical pulse in pericardial tamponade results from the dramatic inspiratory reduction in LV filling in inspiration. The inspiratory blood pooled in the lung is subsequently returned to the LA and the LV during expiration, and the blood pressure rises as the stroke volume increases again. In the most extreme cases of tamponade, the aortic valve may open only during expiration. A paradoxical pulse from tamponade may not occur in the presence of extreme hypotension, in patients with severe aortic insufficiency, in the presence of an atrial septal defect or a single ventricle, or in some cases of acute LV infarction. Table 57.1 outlines the major hemodynamic differences between constrictive pericarditis and pericardial tamponade.

Clinical Examination, Chest X-Ray, and Electrocardiography

The physical examination may be deceptive when hypotension and shock predominate (see Fig. 57.3). Tachycardia is the rule (although the heart rate may be lower in myxedema or in some uremic patients). As described previously, the expected findings include marked elevation

Acute pericardial effusion

◀▪▪▪▶

hours/days

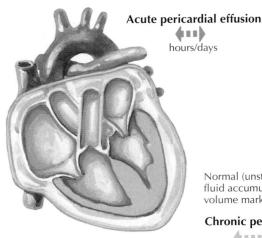

Acute effusion

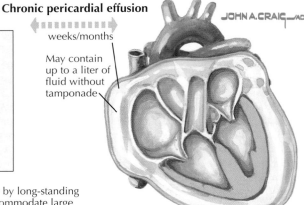

Pressure / Volume

Tamponade threshold (~250 cc)

Normal (unstretched) pericardium is able to accommodate acute fluid accumulation up to ~250 cc, beyond which additional volume markedly increases intrapericardial pressure.

Chronic pericardial effusion

◀▪▪▪▪▪▪▪▪▪▪▪▪▶

weeks/months

May contain up to a liter of fluid without tamponade

JOHN A. CRAIG—AD

Chronic effusion

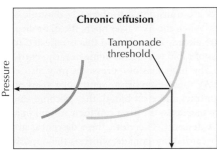

Pressure / Volume

Tamponade threshold

Pericardium that has been stretched over time by long-standing effusion is more distensible and is able to accommodate large fluid volume without critical increase in intrapericardial pressure.

Echocardiographic findings in cardiac tamponade

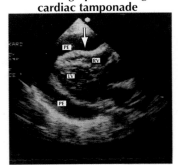

Long-axis view shows RV collapse due to large PE.

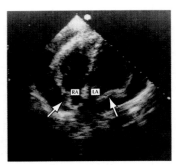

Four-chamber view demonstrates collapse of both RA and LA due to tamponade.

FIG 57.6 Pressure–Volume Relationship of Pericardium and Echocardiographic Examples of Pericardial Tamponade Physiology. *LA,* Left atrial; *LV,* left ventricular; *PE,* pulmonary embolism; *RA,* right atrial; *RV,* right ventricular. (With permission from Spodick DH. Pericardial diseases. In: Braunwald E, Zipes DP, Libby P, eds. *Heart Disease.* Philadelphia: WB Saunders; 2001:1842–1857.)

TABLE 57.1 Major Hemodynamic Differences Between Constrictive Pericarditis and Pericardial Tamponade

Constrictive Pericarditis	Pericardial Tamponade
Atrial pressures elevated with rapid *y* descent	Atrial pressures elevated with blunted *y* descent
y descent greater than *x* descent	*x* descent greater than *y* descent
Kussmaul sign often present	Kussmaul sign occasionally present
Square root sign in diastole	Blunted early filling in diastole
Nadir of early ventricular pressure near zero	Elevated early ventricular diastolic pressure
Paradoxical pulse uncommon	Paradoxical pulse common
Normal heart size on chest radiograph	Water-bottle cardiac enlargement
Calcification of the pericardium occasionally present	Calcification rarely seen
Atria normal in size and shape on echo	Right atrial, right ventricular, and occasional left atrial diastolic collapse
No or trivial pericardial effusion on echo, CT, or MRI	Pericardial effusion present
Often, thickened pericardium seen on CT or MRI	Normal or minimally thickened pericardium seen on CT or MRI

in the JVP (in the absence of hypovolemia), with loss of the decline in the *y* descent (which is occasionally detectable if the opposite carotid is palpated and a descent in the JVP with ventricular systole is noted). Kussmaul sign is usually not present. There may be signs for right heart failure, but often the patient is markedly dyspneic, with sinus tachycardia and either a paradoxical pulse or marked hypotension. Pericardial rubs are variable and may exist even in the presence of large effusions. At times, a large pericardial effusion produces dullness to percussion and bronchial breathing between the left scapula and spine (Bamberger-Pins-Ewart sign). The cardiac impulse may not be palpable.

The chest x-ray may reveal clear lung fields with a "water bottle" shape to the heart. Identification of the cardiac fat pad in the lateral view may reveal that the cardiac enlargement is from an increase in the extracardiac space. The SVC and the azygous veins may be dilated as well. Nonspecific findings such as PR depression, ST-segment elevation, and low voltage may be seen in pericardial tamponade related to active pericarditis. When the pericardial effusion is large, the heart may swing within the pericardium, producing an electrical alternans that primarily affects the QRS waves and not the T waves. Atrial arrhythmias are common.

Echo-Doppler Measurements

Two-dimensional echocardiography is critical in the diagnosis of a pericardial effusion and helpful in deciding whether tamponade is present. An echo-free space must be demonstrated and differentiated from epicardial fat. Normal separation of the pericardial layers is seen only in systole; separation in both systole and diastole is associated with >50 mL of pericardial fluid. For confusion to be avoided with a pleural effusion, which can be seen on echocardiography, pericardial effusions result in fluid being seen between the heart and descending aorta. Loculation of the pericardial fluid is not uncommon. Epicardial fat can usually be distinguished from fluid because it is brighter than the myocardium and moves with the heart. The amount of fluid is often quantitated by the size of the echo-free space (small: <10 mm; moderate: 10–20 mm; large: >20 mm). Some stranding or clots may also be observed.

In large effusions, the heart may swing within the pericardial fluid, correlating with electrical alternans on the surface ECG (beat-to-beat variation in direction or amplitude of the QRS complex). Systolic LV function is typically preserved. During inspiration, the aortic valve may demonstrate early closure, and the LV ejection time may decrease with the inspiratory reduction in the LV stroke volume. With tamponade, there is evidence of a smaller RV size and early diastolic RV collapse. The RV collapse is most marked in expiration, as the LV actively fills and expands, which results in increased pericardial pressure and reducing RV filling. The duration of RV diastolic collapse is directly related to the pericardial pressure. RV collapse is a more sensitive and specific marker of tamponade physiology than RA collapse. The RA free wall may show late diastolic collapse that lasts for at least one-third of the cardiac cycle (see Fig. 57.6). Occasionally, the LA free wall is also indented. The SVC and IVC diameters are usually enlarged (usually >2.2 cm), and these diameters collapse <50% with inspiration or during a brief sniff. The inspiratory increase in the RV size, the septal shift, the reduced LV size, the delayed mitral valve opening, and the decreased mitral valve E-F slope all reflect the hemodynamic changes that characterize pericardial tamponade.

Doppler studies reflect the flow variations that occur with respiration. Many of these changes in flow are like those seen in constrictive pericarditis, including a >25% variation in the mitral peak E wave with inspiration. Because of the loss of early ventricular diastolic filling due to the compression of the heart, much of the systemic and pulmonary venous flow to the heart must occur during ventricular systole (atrial diastole). These reciprocal changes with respiration are also present in the respective pulmonary venous flow or mitral annular movements (tissue Doppler) and in the hepatic venous flows. The hepatic venous flow may also demonstrate marked atrial reversal of diastolic flow with expiration. These Doppler changes are outlined in Fig. 57.5. The LV ejection time (related to stroke volume) decreases as the RV ejection time increases.

Computed Tomography

It is not uncommon that pericardial effusions are incidental findings on CT performed for other reasons. It can better define loculation of

the fluid compared with echo. Chest CT is important because it can often uncover disease of adjacent structures that may be responsible for the pericardial effusion. CT can also characterize the pericardial effusion using Hounsfield attenuation units; this may be useful in cases of potential chylous pericardial fluid, hemorrhage, and purulent or malignant effusions. Pericardial thickening of >4 mm can also be observed, and the association of both fluid and constrictive pericardial findings can be useful at times.

Cardiac Magnetic Resonance Imaging

CMR provides similar data as CT and echo, and can detect small effusions. Signal intensity can also provide some insight into the fluid characteristics. The use of CMR to detect associated constrictive or restrictive physiology or abnormal late enhanced gadolinium may be of benefit in some patients. CMR can demonstrate the swinging heart.

Cardiac Catheterization

Cardiac catheterization is generally done as a therapeutic measure with percutaneous pericardiocentesis; extensive hemodynamics are rarely investigated. Figs. 57.2 and 57.4 summarize the expected findings. When the issue of mixed disease (i.e., effusive–constrictive disease) is present, pericardiocentesis to remove the tamponade component reveals an underlying constrictive physiology. To help analyze effusive–constrictive disease, it is useful to remeasure the intracardiac pressures once the pericardial fluid has been removed. Classic tamponade physiology may change to constrictive physiology if both are contributory. The analysis of the fluid itself is rarely useful except to diagnosis bacterial infection and occasionally to confirm malignancy. Transudates, exudates, and bloody pericardial effusion can result from a variety of causes. At times, polymerase chain reaction of the fluid may be useful to diagnose tuberculosis or for viral identification, and centrifuged fluid may provide tumor cytology.

SUMMARY OF COMPARISONS BETWEEN CONSTRICTIVE PERICARDITIS AND CARDIAC TAMPONADE

A summary of the major hemodynamic differences between constrictive pericarditis and cardiac tamponade is provided in Table 57.1. Differences in the physical examination of patients with constrictive pericarditis and pericardial tamponade are summarized in Table 57.2. Comparison of the echo/Doppler observations is summarized in Table 57.3. From a hemodynamic standpoint, all of the studies document the fundamental problem of an inability to fill the heart in diastole with resultant elevated right heart pressures occurring in the presence of normal pulmonary arterial pressures.

TABLE 57.2 **Differences in the Physical Examination of Patients With Constrictive Pericarditis Versus Patients With Pericardial Tamponade**

Constrictive Pericarditis	Pericardial Tamponade
Clear lung fields	Clear lung fields, with occasional Ewart sign in large pericardial effusions
Ascites often present; peripheral edema occasionally present	Ascites and peripheral edema rare
Evidence of pleural effusions common	Pleural effusions uncommon
JVP markedly elevated; rapid x and y descents	JVP moderately elevated; loss of y descent evident
Pericardial rub rare	Pericardial rub common
Apical pulse localized and may retract with systole	Apical pulse large and diffuse
Loud filling sound ("knock") occasionally present with normal S_1 and S_2	Heart sounds often diminished

JVP, Jugular venous pressure.

TABLE 57.3   Comparison of the Echo-Doppler Findings in Constrictive Pericarditis Versus Pericardial Tamponade

Constrictive Pericarditis	Pericardial Tamponade
Pericardial effusion small or not present	Pericardial effusion evident and often large
Atria normal in size	Atria demonstrate free wall collapse
Right ventricle is normal in size. Septal shift is occasionally noted with inspiration.	Right ventricle (especially outflow) may demonstrate free wall collapse. Septal shift with inspiration common
Distinct interventricular septal bounce in early ventricular diastole	No interventricular septal bounce
Mitral valve motion usually normal	Delayed mitral valve opening and reduced E-F slope of mitral opening are evident. Aortic valve may close prematurely with inspiration.
With inspiration, LVET normal or slightly shortened and RVET prolonged	With inspiration, LVET shortened and RVET prolonged
Mitral valve E wave initially high with short deceleration and reduced "A" wave	Mitral valve E-wave height usually blunted
With inspiration or sniff, IVC does not decrease >50% in diameter.	Similarly, with inspiration or sniff, IVC does not decrease >50% in diameter.
With inspiration, >25% decline in mitral valve E-wave height	Similarly, with inspiration, >25% decline in mitral valve E-wave height
With inspiration, RV pressure may rise (as noted on tricuspid regurgitation jet, if present).	With inspiration, RV systolic pressure may fall normally or rise modestly.
With inspiration, tricuspid valve E wave increases >40%, and mitral valve E wave decreases.	Similarly, with inspiration, tricuspid valve E wave increases >40%, and mitral valve E wave decreases.
With inspiration, hepatic vein flow increases and pulmonary vein flow decreases.	Similarly, with inspiration, hepatic vein flow increases and pulmonary vein flow decreases.

IVC, Inferior vena cava; *LVET,* left ventricular ejection time; *RV,* right ventricular; *RVET,* right ventricular ejection time.

FUTURE DIRECTIONS

Despite improvements in the diagnosis and treatment of pericardial disease, opportunities for advances still exist. A better understanding of the inflammatory mechanisms involved is needed. The impact of associated myocardial involvement is still unclear. Prevention of chronic disease is the major goal and supersedes diagnostic and therapeutic advances. There is evidence that colchicine, among other antiinflammatory agents, appears to markedly reduce recurrences of pericarditis, and with it is the hope that the incidence of constrictive pericarditis will decline. Emerging therapies with human immunoglobulins and anakinra are being investigated. Better focused radiation beam control for the treatment of lymphoma and other chest tumors should also help greatly reduce the incidence of constrictive pericarditis compared with the wide radiation windows that were used previously. Positron-emission tomographic scanning may have a role in identifying active inflammation and helping to decide the duration of active therapy. Surgical pericardial windows via video-assisted thoracotomy has become important because it helps permanently drain many chronic pericardial effusions that have had a tendency to recur with percutaneous draining only. Newer percutaneous techniques that are less invasive than the current video-assisted thoracoscopic surgery procedure would be welcomed. Little has been done to improve the diagnostic yield from pericardial effusion analysis, and further use of polymerase chain reaction and genomic techniques may emerge to improve the assessment of pericardial fluid.

ADDITIONAL RESOURCES

Adler Y, et al. ESC Guidelines for the Diagnosis and Management of Pericardial Diseases of the European Society of Cardiology. Endorsed by the European Association of Cardio-Thoracic Surgery. *Eur Heart J.* 2015;36:2921–2964.

Comprehensive overview of the diagnosis and management of both acute and chronic pericardial disease. Discusses both cardiac tamponade and constrictive pericarditis in detail, including a discussion of transient constrictive pericarditis, effusive–constrictive pericarditis and chronic constrictive pericarditis. The diagnosis and treatment of individual causes for pericardial disease are broken down and specific recommendations with associated evidence are provided for reference.

Cremer PC, et al. Complicated pericarditis. Understanding risk factors and pathology to inform imaging and treatment. *J Am Coll Cardiol.* 2016;68:2311–2328.

Good discussion of causes of pericarditis, with comments on future investigations, especially regarding the use of CMR and steroid-sparing treatments. Analysis of autoinflammatory and autoimmune pericarditis, and a state-of-the-art review.

Garcia M. Constrictive pericarditis versus restrictive cardiomyopathy. *J Am Coll Cardiol.* 2016;67:2061–2076.

Comprehensive review of the hemodynamics of constriction and its role in heart failure with preserved ejection fraction compared with restrictive cardiomyopathy.

Klein AL, et al. American Society of Echocardiography Clinical Recommendations for Multimodality Cardiovascular Imaging of Patients with Pericardial Disease. Endorsed by the Society for Cardiovascular Magnetic Resonance and the Society of Cardiovascular Computed Tomography. ASE Expert Consensus Statement. *J Am Soc Echocardiogr.* 2013;26:965–1012.

Excellent summary of the literature and a review of the use of each of the noninvasive imaging modalities used in acute pericarditis, cardiac tamponade, and constrictive pericarditis. Includes many teaching graphics, and a review of hemodynamics and pathology. Good images of how the various imaging modalities add to the diagnosis of pericardial disease.

EVIDENCE

Schutzman JJ, Obarski TP, Pearce GL, Klein AL. Comparison of Doppler and two-dimensional echocardiography for assessment of pericardial effusion. *Am J Cardiol.* 1992;70:1353–1357.

A classic article on assessing the hemodynamic significance of pericardial effusions and noninvasive determination of the presence of pericardial tamponade.

Sengupta PP, Krishnamoorthy VK, Abhayavata WP, et al. Disparate patterns of left ventricular mechanics differentiate constrictive pericarditis from restrictive cardiomyopathy. *JACC Cardiovasc Imaging.* 2008;1:29–38.

Overall review of diagnostic intricacies of pericardial constriction and restrictive cardiomyopathy.

Talreja DR, Nishimura RA, Oh JK, Holmes DR. Constrictive pericarditis in the modern era: novel criteria for diagnosis in the cardiac catheterization laboratory. *J Am Coll Cardiol.* 2008;51:315–319.

Comprehensive discussion of invasive criteria for diagnosing constrictive pericarditis using the ratios of the RV and LV pressure-time areas.

Peripheral Vascular Disease

58

Renal Artery Stenosis and Renal Denervation

George A. Stouffer, Walter A. Tan

Obstructive disease in the renal arteries can decrease blood flow to the kidneys, which can result in activation of the renin-angiotensin system, hypertension, ischemic nephropathy, and other pathological changes. Technological advances, including intraarterial stenting, have generated enthusiasm for revascularization as a treatment for hypertension and progressive renal dysfunction caused by renal artery stenosis (RAS). However, there is no effect on mortality, and measurable beneficial outcomes (e.g., blood pressure [BP] improvement or stabilization of renal function) occur in only approximately 50% to 70% of patients who undergo successful revascularization, underlining the limited understanding of this disease and the importance of careful patient selection.

ETIOLOGY AND PATHOGENESIS

The predominant cause of obstructive RAS is atherosclerosis (Fig. 58.1). The atherosclerotic process can involve the renal artery or the aorta, with disease of the latter affecting the ostium of the renal artery.

Obstructive RAS can also be caused by fibromuscular dysplasia (FMD), although this is rare and occurs in <10% of cases of RAS. FMD is a collection of vascular diseases characterized by intimal or medial hyperplasia. It is commonly bilateral and affects women more often than men. The middle and distal portions of the vessel are the most commonly involved sites, with a typical angiographic appearance of "beads on a string" (see Fig. 58.1). FMD can cause hypertension but rarely leads to major loss of renal function, although progressive renal impairment has been described in smokers with FMD.

Regardless of its underlying pathological cause, decreased renal perfusion results in compensatory activation of the renin-angiotensin system (Fig. 58.2), which can cause systemic hypertension, salt retention, and activation of the neurohormonal system. RAS also causes ischemic changes within the kidney (ischemic nephropathy) and increased systemic markers of oxidative stress. Other pathological effects have been postulated but have not been proven to result from RAS.

Natural History

Hemodynamically significant RAS is associated with an increased incidence of major adverse cardiovascular events, including cardiac death, myocardial infarction, and stroke. In the Cardiovascular Health Study, a prospective, multicenter cohort study of Americans aged older than 65 years, the presence of renovascular disease, as determined by duplex ultrasonography, increased the risk of short-term adverse cardiovascular outcomes by approximately twofold. This risk persisted after controlling for coronary artery disease risk factors and existing cardiovascular disease, and was not dependent on the effects of increased BP. In other studies, 4-year survival was only 57% in patients with severe RAS discovered incidentally at the time of cardiac catheterization and 74% in a multicenter study of patients who underwent

percutaneous renal revascularization. In a single-center study of 748 patients with severe renal artery disease who required percutaneous revascularization, 10-year survival was only 41%.

RAS is a progressive disease in which the rate of progression is a function of the disease severity and BP. Studies of patients with documented RAS have shown that progression of atherosclerotic disease in renal arteries occurs in approximately 25% of patients at 1 year, 35% at 3 years, and 50% at 5 years. The rate of progression to total occlusion at 5 years has been reported to be approximately 10% in arteries with lesions of <60% stenosis. In another study, in which the average stenosis at the time of enrollment was 72%, 16% of the patients randomly assigned to receive medical treatment had total occlusion at 1 year.

Clinical Presentation

Most patients with hypertension have essential hypertension. Overall, renovascular disease is the etiology in 0.5% to 2% of patients with hypertension (Fig. 58.3), but it is more common in patients who present with new-onset severe hypertension. RAS is more common in white than in black individuals, and the prevalence increases with age. Clinical factors that increase the likelihood of RAS include age, recent onset or sudden worsening of hypertension, and the presence of an abdominal bruit. The prevalence of RAS is also higher in patients with atherosclerosis in other vascular beds. Hemodynamically significant RAS is found in 6% to 23% of patients with hypertension who are undergoing cardiac catheterization. Significant RAS was found in 10.4% of patients at autopsy after a cerebrovascular accident.

Atherosclerotic renovascular disease has been estimated to cause renal failure in 5% to 10% of Medicare patients who are starting dialysis for end-stage renal disease. The mortality in individuals with RAS and end-stage renal disease is staggering; survival rates reported at 2, 5, and 10 years are 56%, 18%, and 5%, respectively.

The American Heart Association Working Group for RAS has proposed that a grading classification for patients with RAS be used to facilitate trial design and reporting. Grade I is RAS plus no clinical manifestations (normal BP and renal function). Grade II is RAS plus medically controlled hypertension and normal renal function. Grade III is RAS plus uncontrolled BP, abnormal renal function, and/or evidence of volume overload.

DIFFERENTIAL DIAGNOSIS

The primary entity in the differential diagnosis is essential hypertension (see Chapter 15), although several other less common causes of hypertension must also be considered (see Fig. 58.3). The point at which renal artery atherosclerosis becomes physiologically significant and leads to increased BP and ischemic nephropathy is not completely understood. Recognition of lesions that compromise blood flow to the kidney is essential to identify patients whose conditions will improve with renal

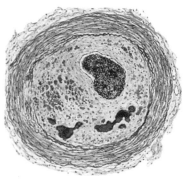

Severe concentric atherosclerosis with lipid deposition and calcification complicated by thrombosis (composite, ×12)

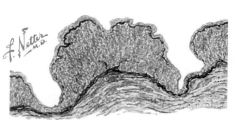

Medial fibroplasia (longitudinal section) with variation in mural thickness, chiefly of media, and aneurysmal evaginations (Verhoeff-Van Gieson stain, ×20)

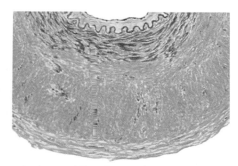

Subadventitial fibroplasia with concentric ring of dense collagen between media and adventitia (Masson trichrome stain, ×80)

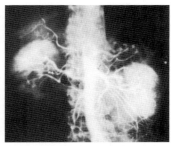

Aortorenogram showing atherosclerotic narrowing and poststenotic dilatation of both renal arteries

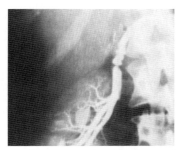

Renal arteriogram showing characteristic beaded appearance caused by alternate stenoses and aneurysmal dilatations

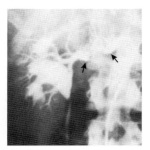

Arteriogram showing extensive, varied stenosis of right renal artery

FIG 58.1 Etiologies of Renal Artery Disease Likely to Cause Hypertension.

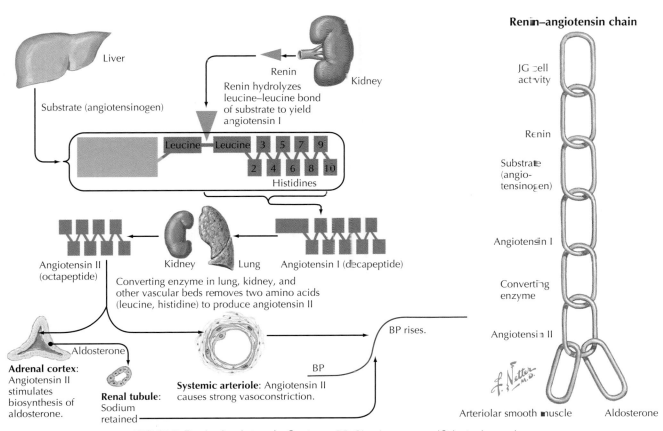

FIG 58.2 Renin-Angiotensin System. *BP*, Blood pressure; *JG*, juxtaglomerular.

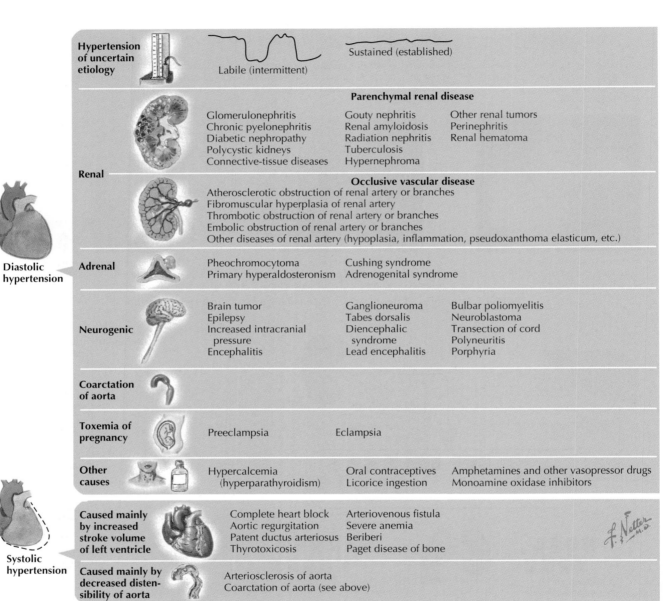

Hypertension of uncertain etiology

Labile (intermittent)   Sustained (established)

Diastolic hypertension

Renal

Parenchymal renal disease

Glomerulonephritis
Chronic pyelonephritis
Diabetic nephropathy
Polycystic kidneys
Connective-tissue diseases

Gouty nephritis
Renal amyloidosis
Radiation nephritis
Tuberculosis
Hypernephroma

Other renal tumors
Perinephritis
Renal hematoma

Occlusive vascular disease

Atherosclerotic obstruction of renal artery or branches
Fibromuscular hyperplasia of renal artery
Thrombotic obstruction of renal artery or branches
Embolic obstruction of renal artery or branches
Other diseases of renal artery (hypoplasia, inflammation, pseudoxanthoma elasticum, etc.)

Adrenal

Pheochromocytoma
Primary hyperaldosteronism

Cushing syndrome
Adrenogenital syndrome

Neurogenic

Brain tumor
Epilepsy
Increased intracranial
  pressure
Encephalitis

Ganglioneuroma
Tabes dorsalis
Diencephalic
  syndrome
Lead encephalitis

Bulbar poliomyelitis
Neuroblastoma
Transection of cord
Polyneuritis
Porphyria

Coarctation of aorta

Toxemia of pregnancy

Preeclampsia   Eclampsia

Other causes

Hypercalcemia
  (hyperparathyroidism)

Oral contraceptives
Licorice ingestion

Amphetamines and other vasopressor drugs
Monoamine oxidase inhibitors

Systolic hypertension

Caused mainly by increased stroke volume of left ventricle

Complete heart block
Aortic regurgitation
Patent ductus arteriosus
Thyrotoxicosis

Arteriovenous fistula
Severe anemia
Beriberi
Paget disease of bone

Caused mainly by decreased distensibility of aorta

Arteriosclerosis of aorta
Coarctation of aorta (see above)

FIG 58.3 Etiology of Hypertension.

some experts to advocate a measurement of translesional pressure gradients in these patients to determine hemodynamic significance. There are limited data that correlate translesional gradients to clinical outcomes, and there is no consensus on whether absolute systolic, peak systolic, or mean pressure should be used; whether the pressure should be measured during a resting or hyperemic state; and what level constitutes a lesion that would benefit from revascularization. Although not validated in large clinical studies or included in current guidelines, early work on renal fractional flow reserve (rFFR) has been promising in that it appears to have good predictive value relative to patient outcomes. rFFR is a proportional determinant of the severity of a stenosis by comparing the pressure distal to a stenosis with aortic pressure during hyperemia.

DIAGNOSTIC APPROACH

The renal arteries can be visualized with arteriography, magnetic resonance angiography (MRA), and spiral CT. Arteriography, with the direct injection of contrast dye into the renal artery, remains the gold standard for identifying and quantifying obstructive lesions (Fig. 58.5). MRA and spiral CT are noninvasive methods with excellent sensitivity and good, but not optimal, specificity for identifying RAS.

MANAGEMENT AND THERAPY

Optimum Treatment

Renal Artery Revascularization

Renal artery obstructive disease can be treated by either surgical or percutaneous approaches. Surgical renal artery revascularization generally involves aortorenal bypass (using a hypogastric artery, a saphenous vein, or polytetrafluoroethylene grafts), ileorenal, splenorenal (for left RAS), or hepatorenal (for right RAS) approaches (Fig. 58.6). Results of surgical renal artery revascularization show operative mortality rates of 2% to 6%, with improvement of hypertension observed in 79% to 95% of patients. With advances in percutaneous revascularization, surgical renal artery revascularization is rarely used and mainly reserved for patients with severe aortic disease that requires treatment.

Percutaneous balloon angioplasty for RAS, first reported by Gruentzig and colleagues in 1978, has resulted in varying rates of improvement in hypertension (36%–100% of patients in uncontrolled studies) (Fig. 58.7). Success rates with balloon angioplasty are better for nonostial stenoses as opposed to ostial stenoses. Restenosis has been reported in 10% to 47% of cases.

Stenting has been advocated as the preferred percutaneous treatment for RAS, especially when the lesion is ostial (Fig. 58.8). The use of stenting, as opposed to balloon angioplasty, is associated with higher rates of technical success and lower rates of restenosis. Procedural success rates are generally >95%, with long-term angiographic patency rates of 86% to 92%. Major complications occur in approximately 2% of patients and include parenchymal perforation, cholesterol emboli, embolized stents, and aortic dissection.

Percutaneous intervention is generally preferred over medical management in patients with FMD, because it reduces hypertension in approximately 75% of patients. Balloon angioplasty is successful in 82% to 100% of patients, with restenosis in 10% to 11%.

INDICATIONS FOR REVASCULARIZATION IN ATHEROSCLEROTIC RENAL ARTERY STENOSIS

Despite the poor prognosis associated with RAS, several large randomized trials have shown no benefit on mortality or cardiovascular outcomes with percutaneous renal artery stenting. The Cardiovascular Outcomes

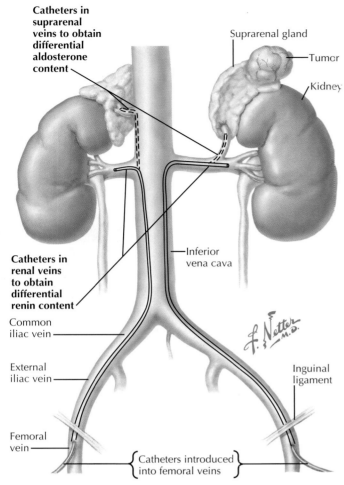

FIG 58.4 Differential Renin/Aldosterone Concentrations.

revascularization. This is especially important, because of the high rate of essential hypertension in patients with RAS.

There is as yet no consensus on how to identify significant RAS. In part this reflects that there is not a one-to-one correlation with stenosis severity and favorable outcomes after the stenosis has been reduced by percutaneous interventions. Although many surrogates have been proposed, one well-controlled study found that the only clinical factors that predicted a beneficial BP response to renal artery revascularization were a preprocedure mean arterial pressure >110 mm Hg and bilateral RAS. Other studies have indicated that measurement of split-vein renin levels may be a means to determine who will benefit from renal artery revascularization (Fig. 58.4). A renal vein renin ratio of 1.5:1 correlates with BP improvement in some studies. Likewise, using captopril as a provocative agent coupled with nuclear imaging (scintigraphy) may be of value in identifying patients who will benefit from renal artery revascularization, with a sensitivity of approximately 75% and a specificity of 90%.

Doppler ultrasonography, although technologically demanding, is a promising technique. The measurement of a resistance index by Doppler can be used as a predictive tool. Patients with resistance index values >80 show much poorer results (no improvement in BP, worsening renal function) after revascularization than do patients whose values are <80. There is general agreement that lesions ≥70% by angiography are hemodynamically significant, whereas lesions ≤50% have no hemodynamic effect. The significance of lesions between 50% and 70% varies, leading

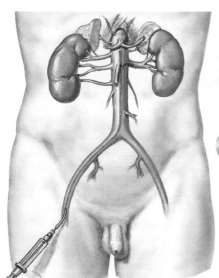

Catheter introduced via femoral artery to desired level of aorta and contrast medium injected, which then flows into normal and accessory renal arteries and possibly also into other aortic branches (aortorenal angiography), or catheter may be made to enter renal arteries for direct injection (selective renal angiography)

Seldinger technique for catheterization of femoral artery

1: Needle introduced into artery

2: Guide wire passed through needle

3: Needle withdrawn

4: Catheter introduced over wire

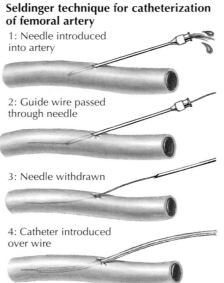

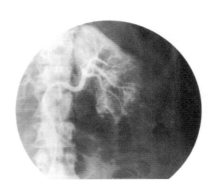

Selective left renal arteriogram. Multiple tumor vessels in lower pole of left kidney suggestive of highly vascular tumor (hypernephroma)

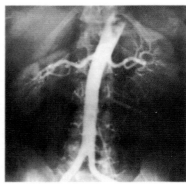

Aortorenal angiogram. Beaded appearance of left renal artery is evidence of fibromuscular hyperplasia; aneurysm at bifurcation of right renal artery

FIG 58.5 Aortorenal and Selective Renal Angiography (Transfemoral Approach).

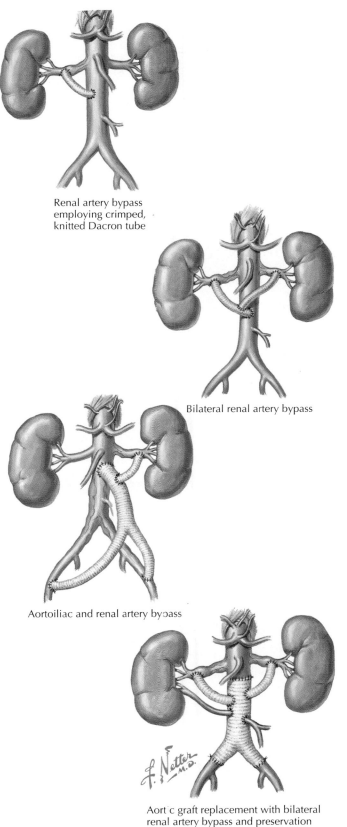

Renal artery bypass
employing crimped,
knitted Dacron tube

Bilateral renal artery bypass

Aortoiliac and renal artery bypass

Aortic graft replacement with bilateral
renal artery bypass and preservation
of an accessory renal artery

FIG 58.6 Surgical Renal Revascularization.

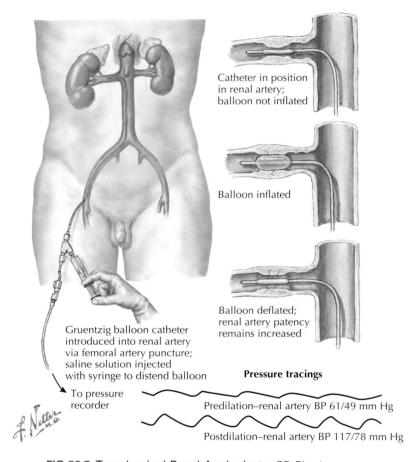

Catheter in position
in renal artery;
balloon not inflated

Balloon inflated

Balloon deflated;
renal artery patency
remains increased

Gruentzig balloon catheter
introduced into renal artery
via femoral artery puncture;
saline solution injected
with syringe to distend balloon

To pressure
recorder

Pressure tracings

Predilation–renal artery BP 61/49 mm Hg

Postdilation–renal artery BP 117/78 mm Hg

FIG 58.7 Transluminal Renal Angioplasty. *BP*, Blood pressure.

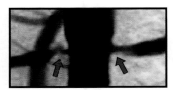

Pretreatment arteriogram–
stenotic lesions (*arrows*).

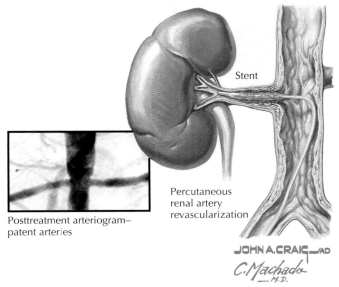

Stent

Percutaneous
renal artery
revascularization

Posttreatment arteriogram–
patent arteries

JOHN A. CRAIG _AD
C. Machado _M.D.

Patients with hypertension and atherosclerotic renal artery stenosis
most likely to respond to balloon angioplasty percutaneous renal artery
revascularization are those with onset of hypertension within the past
5 years, those without primary renal disease, and middle-aged men
with atherosclerotic renal artery stenosis and malignant hypertension
not caused by primary renal disease. A positive captopril renogram
predicts cure or improvement of hypertension after revascularization.

FIG 58.8 Percutaneous Revascularization of Stenotic Renal Arteries.

in Renal Atherosclerotic Lesions (CORAL) trial, the largest randomized study of patients with RAS ever performed, found that renal artery stent implantation did not provide any benefit beyond optimal medical therapy in the occurrence of death, cardiovascular events, or renal events in patients with moderately severe atherosclerotic RAS. There was a modest improvement in systolic BP that favored the stent group, but no difference in adverse clinical outcomes. The CORAL results were similar to findings from the Angioplasty and Stenting for Renal Artery Lesions (ASTRAL) Trial and the Stent Placement and Blood Pressure and Lipid-Lowering for the Prevention of Progression of Renal Dysfunction Caused by Atherosclerotic Ostial Stenosis of the Renal Artery (STAR) trial.

All of these studies have been criticized primarily for enrollment of patients with hemodynamically insignificant RAS and/or exclusion of patients who the treating physician thought would likely benefit from revascularization.

Hypertension

The most common indication for renal artery revascularization is to improve BP control. Improvement occurs in most patients, but complete resolution of hypertension is uncommon. Factors that predict improvement include pretreatment BP (mean arterial pressure >110 mm Hg) and the presence of bilateral RAS. Because renovascular and non-renovascular hypertension often coexist in an older adult population

with atherosclerotic disease, patient selection is critical in deciding whether to undertake renal artery revascularization.

Renal Preservation

Renal artery revascularization can stabilize and even reverse progressive decreases in renal function in selected patients. In a meta-analysis of six studies, revascularization in patients with ischemic nephropathy resulted in an improvement in renal function in 46%, stabilization of renal function in 31%, and worsening of renal function in 22%. Unfortunately, there are still limited data regarding appropriate identification of patients with ischemic nephropathy who will improve with revascularization.

Pulmonary Edema

Acute pulmonary edema with respiratory failure and death can occur in patients with RAS, especially in patients with bilateral (but usually not unilateral) RAS. Successful revascularization can virtually eliminate recurrent episodes.

Avoiding Treatment Errors

One of the major difficulties in treating RAS is identifying patients who will benefit from revascularization. Clinical trials have found that measurable beneficial outcomes occur in only approximately 50% to 70% of patients who undergo successful renal artery revascularization. The

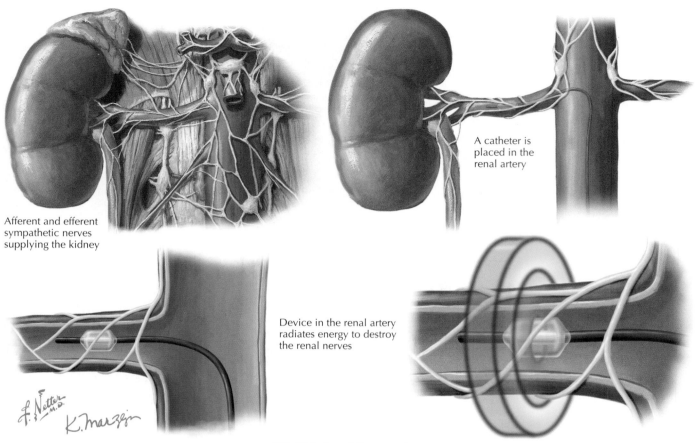

Afferent and efferent sympathetic nerves supplying the kidney

A catheter is placed in the renal artery

Device in the renal artery radiates energy to destroy the renal nerves

FIG 58.9 Renal Denervation.

possibility that clinical benefits independent of the traditional endpoints (primarily BP reduction and renal function preservation) occur with renal artery revascularization is being studied in the CORAL trial. In addition, many techniques are being evaluated to assess the hemodynamic significance of renal artery lesions with the goal of better identifying patients who will improve following treatment of RAS.

Renal Denervation

Interruption of afferent and efferent sympathetic nerves supplying the kidney (i.e., renal denervation [RD]) has the ability to reduce BP in patients with resistant hypertension. Originally done during an open surgical procedure, this technique fell out of favor with the advent of oral medications. The recent development of catheter-based methods to achieve RD has led to a revival of interest in this approach to reducing BP (Fig. 58.9).

The efferent renal sympathetic nerves innervate the renal arterial resistance vasculature, all tubular segments of the nephron, and the juxtaglomerular granular cells. Increases in efferent renal sympathetic nerve activity produce: (1) renal vasoconstriction that leads to reductions in renal blood flow and the glomerular filtration rate; (2) increases in renal tubular sodium and water reabsorption throughout the nephron; and (3) increases in the renin secretion rate. Increased renal sympathetic nerve stimulation results in a rightward shift of the pressure-natriuresis curve (meaning that a higher arterial pressure is required to achieve natriuresis). The kidneys influence central regulation of cardiovascular hemodynamics via afferent fibers that carry impulses centrally to structures that govern global sympathetic tone.

The first significant trial of catheter-based RD in humans was a multicenter proof-of-concept study that enrolled 50 patients with a mean office BP of 177/101 ± 20/15 mm Hg despite treatment with an average of 4.7 antihypertensive medications. The results were striking; office BP was reduced by −22/−11 mm Hg when measured 6 months after the procedure. Subsequently, the Symplicity Hypertension (HTN)-2 trial enrolled 106 patients with resistant hypertension at 24 centers in Europe, Australia, and New Zealand. The baseline office BP was 178/97 ± 18/16 mm Hg in the RD group (on an average of 5.2 medications) and 178/98 ± 16/17 mm Hg in control subjects (on an average of 5.3 medications). Six months after treatment, BP was reduced by 32/12 ± 23/11 mm Hg in the treatment group, whereas there was no change in BP in the control group.

Symplicity HTN-3 was performed in the United States and enrolled 535 patients who were randomized to RD (n = 364) or to a sham procedure (n = 171). Baseline characteristics were similar between the two arms, with a mean systolic BP of 180 mm Hg; the mean 24-hour ambulatory BP (ABP) was 159 mm Hg despite a mean of 5.1 antihypertensive medications. There were significant reductions in office systolic BP in both the RD (−14 mm Hg) and sham procedure (−11.7 mm Hg) arms at 6 months, with no significant difference between the groups. Similar results were observed on 24-hour ABP monitoring; mean systolic BP decreased to a significant degree in both groups. There was no difference in safety endpoints, including major adverse events (1.4% of patients in the denervation arm compared with 0.6% in the sham procedure arm; $P = 0.67$), mortality (0.6% in each arm), serum creatinine elevation >50% (1.4% vs. 0.6%), and new RAS >70% (0.3% vs. 0%).

The major criticism of Symplicity HTN-3 was that consistent and effective RD was not achieved with the Ardian catheter (Medtronic, Minneapolis, Minnesota). There were also questions about patient selection, and subsequently, the Renal Denervation for Hypertension (DENERHTN) trial showed a benefit of RD + optimal medical therapy over optimal medical therapy alone. Currently, there are several trials testing second-generation technology in patients with resistant hypertension who are on multiple medications and in patients with mild hypertension in the absence of medications.

FUTURE DIRECTIONS

Important areas of future study of RAS include identifying characteristics that predict which patients will benefit from renal artery intervention, determining whether RAS has deleterious effects independent of hypertension and ischemic nephropathy, and optimizing renal artery revascularization. For RD, the focus is on improving technology to enhance RD and in optimizing patient selection.

ADDITIONAL RESOURCES

Gulati R, Raphael CE, Negoita M, Pocock SJ, Gersh BJ. The rise, fall, and possible resurrection of renal denervation. *Nat Rev Cardiol.* 2016;13:238–244.
A review of renal denervation.
Hildreth CJ, Lynm C, Glass RM. JAMA patient page. Renal artery stenosis. *JAMA.* 2008;300:2084.
A description of RAS in language that a patient can understand.
Rooke TW, et al. Management of patients with peripheral artery disease (compilation of 2005 and 2011 ACCF/AHA Guideline

Recommendations): a report of the American College of Cardiology Foundation/American Heart Association Task Force on Practice Guidelines. *J Am Coll Cardiol.* 2013;61(14):1555–1570.
Guidelines summarizing current data regarding RAS and the benefits and risks of revascularization.
The Agency for Healthcare Research and Quality (AHRQ) guidelines on renal artery stenosis. Available at <https://effectivehealthcare.ahrq.gov/topics/renal-update/research>.
An evidence-based approach to treating patients with RAS.

EVIDENCE

Bhatt DL, Kandzari DE, O'Neill WW, D'agostino R, Flack JM, Katzen BT, Leon MB, et al. A controlled trial of renal denervation for resistant hypertension. *NEJM.* 2014;370(15):1393–1401.
Results of the Symplicity HTN 3 study.
Cooper CJ, Murphy TP, Cutlip DE, et al. Stenting and medical therapy for atherosclerotic renal-artery stenosis. *NEJM.* 2014;370(1):13–22.
Results of the CORAL study, the largest trial of renal artery revascularization.
Dworkin LD, Cooper CJ. Renal-artery stenosis. *NEJM.* 2009;361(20):1972–1978.
A good overview of RAS.
Slovut DP, Olin JW. Fibromuscular dysplasia. *N Engl J Med.* 2004;350:1862–1871.
A good overview of FMD.
Todd J, Stouffer GA. Hemodynamics of renal artery stenosis. *Catheter Cardiovasc Interv.* 2008;72:121–124.
An overview of the hemodynamic changes in renal perfusion associated with RAS and the ways these changes are used in various diagnostic modalities to determine hemodynamically significant disease.

59

Interventional Approaches for Peripheral Arterial Disease

Jason Crowner, Martyn Knowles, Mark A. Farber

Charles Dotter and Melvin Judkins first introduced catheter-based interventions for atherosclerotic disease in 1964. Major technological advances now make interventions possible for a vast array of conditions, benefiting millions of patients with coronary, cerebral, or peripheral arterial disease. Percutaneous interventions have greatly expanded therapeutic options, often complementing and occasionally replacing drugs or surgery. This chapter reviews the indications for endovascular therapy for relatively common extracardiac arterial diseases. Cerebrovascular and cardioembolic disease are discussed in Chapter 61.

UPPER EXTREMITY DISEASE

The innominate and subclavian arteries contribute the main blood supply to the upper extremities, but also provide flow to the brain via the carotid and vertebral arteries. In cases of coronary artery bypass grafting, they can also provide blood flow to the heart through a transposed internal thoracic (mammary) artery often referred to as a right or left internal mammary artery bypass. Symptoms of disease in the innominate or subclavian arteries generally present in the form of arm pain, coolness, or discoloration; alternatively, patients can also present with angina, cerebrovascular, and vertebrobasilar insufficiency, depending on the location of disease.

There are no randomized comparisons of surgical and percutaneous revascularization for occlusive diseases involving the aortic arch vessels. The use of percutaneous angioplasty and stenting continues to be a mainstay in the treatment for innominate and subclavian artery stenosis, unless contraindications of severe calcification exist, with patency rates and symptom relief being as high as 95%. Patency rates may be decreased when complete occlusion is encountered because these procedures are more technically difficult and require more manipulation, which can lead to increased complications such as stroke. Multiple surgical approaches for revascularization of arch vessels exist with variations in patency rates, some being as high as 98%. Percutaneous interventions are associated with vascular access and embolization complications, which can lead to further interventions, depending on location and severity. Dissection, thrombosis, and embolization involving the cerebrovascular arteries, internal thoracic artery, vertebral, and upper extremity territories are complications associated with both approaches and are uncommon.

Nonatherosclerotic pathologies can also affect the upper extremity vasculature and involve extrinsic compression of the subclavian or axillary artery or vein as it crosses the thoracic outlet. Thoracic outlet syndrome can involve the artery, vein, or nerve secondary to a cervical rib, fusion of the first and second rib, or repetitive motion trauma. The latter is most commonly seen in athletes and most commonly affects the vein (Paget-Schroetter syndrome). Surgical management is considered the definitive treatment, with decompression of the thoracic outlet by first rib resection. Catheter-directed thrombolysis can be used in the setting of venous thrombosis. Further endovascular intervention with stent placement is relatively contraindicated because it can lead to stent fracture or kinking secondary to continued extrinsic compression with resultant re-thrombosis. However, percutaneous intervention can be used after appropriate first rib resection.

DISEASES OF THE VISCERAL ARTERIES

Chronic mesenteric ischemia is classically described as postprandial abdominal pain presenting 30 to 60 minutes after a meal, with associated weight loss from food avoidance or "food fear." It can present acutely as the result of embolic disease. In this situation, patients typically present with severe abdominal pain that is characteristically out of proportion to the physical examination. In chronic conditions, formation of multiple collateral pathways develop between the three major intestinal branches of the abdominal aorta: the celiac artery, the superior mesenteric artery, and the inferior mesenteric artery. The differential diagnosis includes atherosclerosis, compression of the celiac artery from the median arcuate ligament, and nonocclusive etiologies, such as heart failure with low cardiac output and visceral artery vasospasm from cocaine, ergot, or vasopressors. Renal artery stenosis is discussed in Chapter 58.

Open revascularization for chronic mesenteric ischemia has short-term success rates of nearly 100% and primary patency rates of 89% at 6 years, with a perioperative mortality of 3% to 4%. Endovascular interventions can be performed with percutaneous transluminal angioplasty (PTA) alone or in conjunction with stenting. The patency rates for PTA range from 79% to 95%, with an improvement to 92% to 100% when a stent is used. Recently, there has been a trend for using covered stents to decrease recurrence rates. Major complications are rare, but procedural failures can happen in the form of thrombosis, distal embolic ischemia, or continued stenosis secondary to extrinsic compression from the median arcuate ligament.

Comparison of endovascular revascularization versus open revascularization for treatment of chronic mesenteric ischemia is difficult due to the selection criteria used for each approach. In a study by the Mayo clinic, a risk-stratified comparison demonstrated that open revascularization had similar mortality but higher morbidity with longer hospitalizations than endovascular therapy in both low- and high-risk patients. Symptom improvement was effective by both methods of revascularization, but endovascular revascularization demonstrated an increased incidence of restenosis, recurrent symptoms, and reinterventions. Both approaches have their advantages and disadvantages, with the decision of which intervention to perform being based on center preference and patient risk factors. However, this may change in the future to reflect more preferential use of endovascular revascularization as technological advances in the procedure are made.

Acute mesenteric ischemia is most often caused by either thrombosis from atherosclerotic disease or an embolus (generally from a cardiac source). The primary cause has shifted in recent years and now is thought to be secondary to thrombosis; although the nidus has changed, the primary treatment strategy remains exploratory laparotomy, with possible bowel resection and revascularization. The revascularization treatment depends largely on the etiology; embolus is treated most commonly with an embolectomy or mesenteric bypass, and thrombosis is most commonly treated by mesenteric bypass, mesenteric endarterectomy, or percutaneous stenting.

LOWER EXTREMITY DISEASE

Peripheral arterial disease affects approximately 12% of the adult population in the United States. This population has a higher risk of death (three to four times that of age-matched control subjects), which is mostly attributed to cardiac and cerebrovascular diseases. Claudication is the most common presenting symptom, which involves pain in the legs or buttocks with ambulation that subsides with rest. Intermittent claudication is present in approximately 2% of the population aged older than 65 years, with a rate of progression to amputation of 1% per year. Surgical revascularization is primarily reserved for advanced disease (lower extremity ulcers or rest pain); however, endovascular therapies have increased the therapeutic options for claudication.

The Trans-Atlantic Inter-Society Consensus (TASC) on the Management of Peripheral Artery Disease, first published in 2000 and revised in 2007 (TASC II), was created to provide a guideline for the treatment of peripheral arterial disease. The document received multidisciplinary input from 16 societies and leading physicians who stressed the medical management of the disease, but it also evaluated the evidence of therapies based on morphological classification. Revised recommendations support endovascular therapies for lesions in the superficial femoral artery (SFA) <10 cm in length (TASC II type A) and surgical revascularization for occlusive lesions of the SFA >20 cm in length (TASC II type D) (Fig. 59.1). For intermediate lesions (TASC II type B or C lesions), the comorbidities and fully informed preferences of the patient and the experience of the operator, as well as long-term outcomes, must be considered.

The initial treatment for intermittent claudication is centered on risk factor modification, smoking cessation, and a structured exercise program. Conservative management can help improve symptoms of intermittent claudication, walking distance, and quality of life. In conjunction with an exercise program, cilostazol has demonstrated benefit in improving walking distance in those patients with intermittent claudication due to peripheral arterial disease, as demonstrated by a recent Cochrane review.

Failure of conservative management or the presence of life-style limiting claudication warrants further intervention, with angiography

Lower extremity arterial disease (PTA or PTAS)

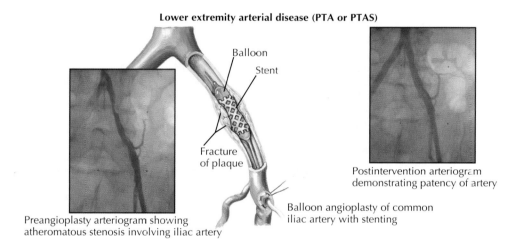

Preangioplasty arteriogram showing atheromatous stenosis involving iliac artery

Balloon
Stent
Fracture of plaque
Balloon angioplasty of common iliac artery with stenting

Postintervention arteriogram demonstrating patency of artery

Isolated iliac versus multilevel disease

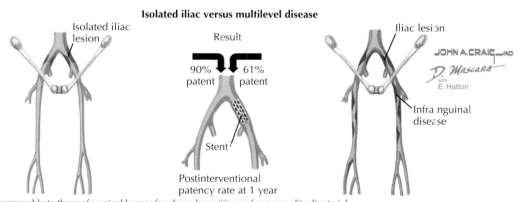

Isolated iliac lesion

Result
90% patent   61% patent
Stent
Postinterventional patency rate at 1 year

Iliac lesion

Infrainguinal disease

JOHN A. CRAIG—MD
D. Mascaro with E. Hatton

Clinical results of PTA are comparable to those of surgical bypass for above-knee (iliac or femoropopliteal) arterial disease that does not include multiple serial stenoses or long occlusions. The subset of patients with stenosis confined to iliac arteries benefits most from PTA or stenting.

FIG 59.1 Interventional Approaches to Peripheral Arterial Disease. *PTA,* Percutaneous transluminal angioplasty; *PTAS,* percutaneous transluminal angioplasty with stenting.

generally being the initial approach. Multiple studies have been done to distinguish the effect of PTA alone compared with PTA with bare metal stenting on vessel patency in patients with symptomatic peripheral vascular disease. A Cochrane review of "Angioplasty versus bare metal stenting for superficial femoral artery lesions" found only a short-term gain in primary patency for stenting of lesions of the SFA. There was no evidence of a sustained benefit in patients who underwent primary stenting. These results demonstrated that either intervention is a suitable initial choice and suggest that both interventions will have similar results in the long term, most likely from progression of disease. Continued risk factor modification and exercise therapy in conjunction with a peripheral vascular intervention should confer the overall best outcomes.

Advanced peripheral vascular disease generally presents with pain at rest or ulcerations; these constellation of symptoms are referred to as critical limb ischemia (CLI) and are associated with a significant risk of limb loss. At this point, most conservative and minimally invasive measures have been exhausted, and patients require high-risk endo-vascular interventions, bypass operations, or amputation. The Best Endovascular versus Best Surgical Therapy in Patients with CLI (BEST-CLI) trial is an on-going multicenter, open label, randomized trial comparing best endovascular therapy with best open surgical treatment in patients eligible for both. The trial hopes to establish primary end-points that include amputation rates, repeat interventions, and mortality, with a full evaluation of cost-effectiveness and quality-of-life outcomes between each modality.

The subset of patients with stenosis confined to the iliac arteries is one group that substantially benefits from PTA or stenting. In one study in which 37% of the randomized patients had iliac artery stenosis, the 1-year patency rate was 90% for the iliac subgroup, but this rate decreased to 61% when patients with infrainguinal disease were included. Although surgical revascularization seems to confer better long-term patency, complication rates are higher, especially in patients with significant comorbidities. The Covered versus Balloon Expandable Stent Trial (COBEST) demonstrated 5-year results with an enduring patency advantage of covered stents over bare metal stents in both the short and long term.

Many other modalities are being used in the lower extremities, including atherectomy devices, drug-eluting stents and/or balloons, absorbable metal stents, and a multitude of variations on the simple angioplasty balloon. Although data are lacking to support the routine use of any such device, unique situations exist wherein such devices may prove useful in experienced hands.

FUTURE DIRECTIONS

The systemic nature of atherosclerosis can result in disease throughout the arterial system. Patients with peripheral vascular disease are at an increased risk for death, most commonly from cardiac or cerebral events. These cohorts of patients are also at an increased risk of aortic aneurysms secondary to similar risk factors: hypertension, tobacco use, hyperlipidemia, and family history. As the population continues to live longer, the number of overall atherosclerotic patients continues to increase. A multidisciplinary collaboration among primary care providers, geriatricians, cardiologists, interventional radiologists, endocrinologists, neurologists, surgeons, and other healthcare team members is required to combat the rising prevalence of this disease. Multidisciplinary care maximizes prevention, health maintenance, and optimal selection of patients and procedures (diagnostic and therapeutic). As medications and technology improve, the treatment patterns and algorithms will continue to change and hopefully lead to enhanced quality of life.

ADDITIONAL RESOURCES

Mozaffarian D, Benjamin EJ, Go AS, Arnett DK, Blaha MJ, Cushman M, Howard VJ. Executive summary: Heart Disease and Stroke Statistics— 2016 update: a report from the American Heart Association. *Circulation.* 2016;133(4):447.

The American Heart Association guide to heart and stroke statistics.

Norgrena L, Hiattb WR, Dormandy JA, et al; on behalf of the TASC II Working Group. Inter-society consensus for the management of peripheral arterial disease. *J Vasc Surg.* 2007;45(1, Jan suppl):S5–S67.

The TASC document on management of peripheral arterial disease was published in January 2007 as a result of cooperation among 14 medical and surgical vascular, cardiovascular, vascular radiology, and cardiology societies in Europe and North America.

EVIDENCE

Bedenis R, Stewart M, Cleanthis M, Robless P, Mikhailidis D, Stansby G. Cilostazol for intermittent claudication. *Cochrane Database Syst Rev.* 2014;(10):Art. No.: CD003748, doi:10.1002/14651858.CD003748.pub4.

Review of 15 double-blind randomized controlled trials that compared cilostazol with placebo and demonstrated improved walking distance results in those taking cilostazol for intermittent claudication caused by peripheral arterial disease. There was no evidence of reduction in all-cause mortality or cardiovascular events.

Chowdhury M, McLain A, Twine C. Angioplasty versus bare metal stenting for superficial femoral artery lesions. *Cochrane Database Syst Rev.* 2014;(6):Art. No.: CD006767, doi:10.1002/14651858.CD006767.pub3.

Review of 11 trials with 1387 patients examined the outcome of angioplasty alone versus angioplasty with stenting in lesions of the SFA. Primary patency benefit was demonstrated in the stenting group, but was not sustained in the long term.

Farber A, Rosenfield K, Menard M. The BEST-CLI trial: a multidisciplinary effort to assess which therapy is best for patients with critical limb ischemia. *Tech Vasc Interv Radiol.* 2014;17:221–224.

The BEST-CLI trial is a pragmatic, multicenter, open label, randomized trial that compared best endovascular therapy with best open surgical treatment in patients eligible for both treatments. The trial aims to provide clinical guidance for CLI management.

Hadjipetrou P, Cox S, Piemonte T, Eisenhauer A. Percutaneous revascularization of atherosclerotic obstruction of aortic arch vessels. *J Am Coll Cardiol.* 1999;33:1238–1245.

Subclavian and brachiocephalic artery obstruction can be effectively treated by primary stenting or surgery. Comparison of stenting and the surgical experience demonstrated equal effectiveness but fewer complications, and suggested that stenting should be considered as first-line therapy for subclavian and brachiocephalic obstruction.

Lane R, Ellis B, Watson L, Leng GC. Exercise for intermittent claudication. *Cochrane Database Syst Rev.* 2014;(7):Art. No.: CD000990, doi:10.1002/14651858.CD000990.pub3.

Review of 30 trials involving 1816 participants with stable leg pain that demonstrated significant benefit of exercise programs compared with placebo in improving walking time and distance in those patients with leg pain from intermittent claudication.

Mwipatayi B, Sharma S, Daneshmand A, Thomas S, Vijayan V, Altaf N, Garbowski M, Jackson M, et al. Durability of the balloon-expandable covered versus bare-metal stents in the Covered versus Balloon Expandable Stent Trial (COBEST) for the treatment of aortoiliac occlusive disease. *J Vasc Surg.* 2016;64:83–94.

Demonstrated the 5-year results of the initial COBEST. Covered stents had a better and enduring patency advantage over bare metal stents in both the short and long term. This was more prevalent with treatment of the TASC C and D lesions.

Oderich G, Bower T, Sullivan T, Gloviczki P. Open versus endovascular revascularization for chronic mesenteric ischemia: risk-stratified outcomes. *J Vasc Surg.* 2009;49:1472–1479.

Comparison of endovascular versus surgical revascularization from a risk-stratified standpoint, with similar mortality and symptom relief in both groups, but increased incidence of symptom recurrence, restenosis, and reintervention in the endovascular group.

Schillinger M, Sabeti S, Loewe C, et al. Balloon angioplasty versus implantation of nitinol stents in the superficial femoral artery. *N Engl J Med.* 2006;354:1879–1888.

In the intermediate term, treatment of SFA disease by primary implantation of a self-expanding nitinol stent yielded results that were superior to those with the currently recommended approach of balloon angioplasty with optional secondary stenting.

Weijer M, Vonken E, Vries J, Moll F, Vos J, Borst G. Technical and clinical success and long-term durability of endovascular treatment for atherosclerotic aortic arch branch origin obstruction: evaluation of 144 procedures. *Eur J Vasc Endovasc Surg.* 2015;50:13–20.

Treatment of aortic arch branch origin obstruction using endovascular treatment is safe and efficacious, with good mid-term durability. Endovascular means can also be safely used to treat recurrent symptomatic lesions.

60

Surgery for Peripheral Vascular Diseases

Jason Crowner, Robert Mendes, Martyn Knowles, and Mark A. Farber

Peripheral vascular disease (PVD) encompasses the pathologies of both the arterial and the venous circulations. Advanced disease of either system can be debilitating and disabling. The clinical presentation and therapeutic choices for patients with PVD vary widely, depending on the vascular distribution involved and the severity of the disease. This chapter focuses on the common problems that require surgical intervention. Although PVD includes venous pathologies, these are less likely to result in serious morbidity and mortality; thus, this chapter focuses on arterial pathologies.

Atherosclerosis involving the infrarenal aorta and the iliac and infrainguinal arteries is the most common cause of arterial insufficiency of the lower extremities, and is typically multifactorial (Fig. 60.1). PVD can be subdivided into categories based on location: inflow (infrarenal aorta, iliac), outflow (femoral, popliteal), and runoff (tibial, peroneal) vessels. These categories help define the risks and benefits of intervention and treatment options.

A detailed history and physical examination can identify the anatomical distribution of vascular pathology. Invasive and noninvasive imaging augments clinical findings and aids decision-making. Several open surgical and endovascular interventions, discussed later, provide significant benefits to patients with PVD.

Other important areas of the vascular system affected by occlusive disease include the carotid arteries and the visceral vessels. Surgical and other interventional approaches to treating atherosclerosis of the carotid and visceral arteries are also discussed in this chapter.

ETIOLOGY AND PATHOGENESIS

Embolic disease, thrombosis, or trauma may also cause arterial occlusion (Fig. 60.1). However, the most common cause of lower extremity arterial occlusion is atherosclerosis. The etiology and pathogenesis of atherosclerosis are discussed in Chapter 14.

LOWER EXTREMITY ATHEROSCLEROSIS

Clinical Presentation

With the tendency for development of collateral circulation in the lower extremities, patients with lower extremity atherosclerosis may be asymptomatic despite significant arterial insufficiency. In addition, many of these patients have comorbid conditions (e.g., cardiac disease) that restrict their activity and preclude them from having symptoms until advanced disease is present. For individuals who can ambulate, claudication—muscle "cramping" or discomfort after walking a specific distance, with relief of the pain upon resting—is often the chief complaint. This pain is reproducible and consistent with pathophysiology that limits muscular blood supply during exertion, causing lactic acid accumulation.

Claudication of the proximal muscles of the leg, buttock, or hip usually indicates inflow disease, commonly referred to as aortoiliac occlusive disease. Leriche syndrome may develop in some patients with severe disease. Patients with Leriche syndrome exhibit the characteristic triad of sexual dysfunction, buttock claudication, and absent femoral pulses. The association between aortoiliac occlusive disease and proximal muscle complaints is variable, and some patients may complain of calf claudication despite the presence of significant occlusion more proximally. Atheromatous embolization from aortoiliac lesions can lodge in the distal vessels, creating localized ischemia of the digits with resulting cyanosis. Because this is an embolic process, patients with the "blue toe syndrome" often have palpable distal pulses, and may, depending on the degree of involvement, experience resolution of their clinical symptoms with time or medical therapy, or both.

Patients with atherosclerosis involving the femoropopliteal (outflow) vessels or with multilevel distribution of the disease can present with complaints ranging from claudication, the mildest presentation, to the most severe symptoms of pain at rest and tissue loss. Patients with mild complaints often never seek medical attention because they attribute symptoms to arthritis or old age. However, as the disease worsens and pain at rest ensues, a persistent burning or aching sensation over the dorsum of the foot often prompts individuals to seek help. Although usually of little benefit, patients may keep the ischemic limb in a dependent position, in an attempt to have gravity aid blood flow. Other signs characteristic of severe ischemia include dependent rubor, muscle atrophy, skin changes, lower extremity alopecia, ulcerations, and lack of palpable distal pulses. Although these signs and symptoms of severe ischemia occur in nondiabetic individuals, with the increasing prevalence of diabetes, a higher proportion of patients who present with femoropopliteal disease are diabetic (Fig. 60.2).

Isolated lesions at a single level rarely result in lower extremity pain at rest and nonhealing ulcerations. Patients who present with concomitant lower extremity infections and persistent ulcerations despite medical therapy should be thoroughly evaluated for significant arterial insufficiency. In many instances, these patients require lower extremity revascularization to salvage the limb.

Assessment by a noninvasive vascular laboratory can provide extensive critical information on the location and hemodynamic significance of lower extremity arterial obstruction. The ankle-brachial index provides an overall estimate of limb perfusion pressure, whereas analysis of velocity waveforms in the arteries at the groin, knee, and ankle helps to classify the obstruction location as inflow (aortoiliac), outflow (superficial femoral artery), or runoff (tibioperoneal vessels), as well as its hemodynamic impact of extremity perfusion. Photoplethysmography waveforms in the toes and toe pressures help diagnose even more distal disease. Transcutaneous oxygen measurements aid in the quantification of tissue ischemia, and may be used to analyze ischemia and predict wound healing.

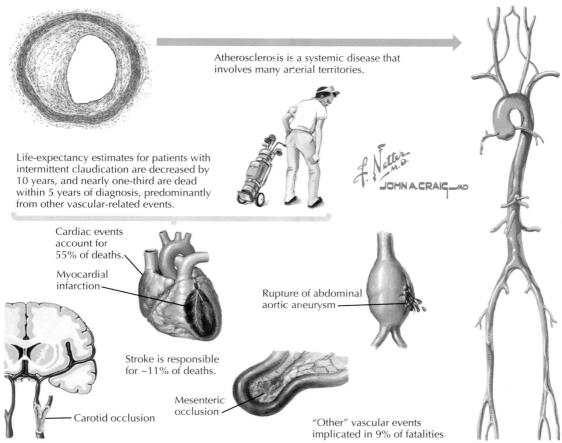

Atherosclerosis is a systemic disease that involves many arterial territories.

Life-expectancy estimates for patients with intermittent claudication are decreased by 10 years, and nearly one-third are dead within 5 years of diagnosis, predominantly from other vascular-related events.

Cardiac events account for 55% of deaths.

Myocardial infarction

Rupture of abdominal aortic aneurysm

Stroke is responsible for ~11% of deaths.

Mesenteric occlusion

Carotid occlusion

"Other" vascular events implicated in 9% of fatalities

FIG 60.1 Multiterritorial Atherosclerotic Disease.

Management and Therapy
Optimum Treatment

All patients should undergo aggressive evaluation and treatment for hyperlipidemia and other genetic disorders associated with progressive atherosclerosis. Reducing risk factors, most importantly, cessation of smoking, will slow disease progression. In addition, patients should integrate diet modification, exercise regimens that encourage collateral circulation, and prevention of lower extremity trauma and infection into their lifestyles. Drug therapy with an antiplatelet drug or cilostazol can provide symptomatic improvement in some patients.

Ischemic pain at rest, ulceration, and gangrene of the digits are indications for arterial reconstruction if anatomically feasible. Decisions about operations for lifestyle-impairing claudication must be based on patient comorbidities and the anatomical distribution of the disease. The decision as to which operative approach is best for an individual (and whether a surgical approach is indicated) should be based on the natural history of the disease, the overall condition of the patient, and the risks and benefits specific to the procedure and individual (Fig. 60.3). The goal of the procedure (e.g., limb salvage, wound healing, relief of pain at rest, exercise tolerance) must be determined before surgical intervention. The Best Surgical Therapy in Patients with Critical Limb Ischemia (BEST-CLI) trial is an on-going multicenter, open label, randomized trial that is comparing best endovascular therapy with best open surgical treatment in patients eligible for both. The trial hopes to establish primary endpoints that include amputation rates, repeat interventions, and mortality with a full evaluation of cost-effectiveness and quality-of-life outcomes between each modality. Endovascular procedures such as balloon angioplasty or stenting increase the options for therapy and are discussed in detail in Chapter 59.

If inflow disease is present, it should be addressed first, because surgical correction can relieve symptoms and obviate the need for the less successful infrainguinal bypass surgery. Patients with symptomatic inflow disease can be treated with endovascular therapies, in-line arterial reconstructions, or extra-anatomic bypass. In making the decision about surgical therapy, consideration of both the perioperative risk of the patient and the influence of anatomy and comorbidities of the patient on graft survival is important. For instance, comorbidities may exclude one approach or another. Other issues, such as cigarette smoking, may also influence therapeutic decisions. Many vascular surgeons will not perform reconstructive surgery on patients who are still smoking, because smoking lowers bypass patency rates dramatically.

Bilateral aortoiliac disease is best treated with aortobifemoral grafting, using a prosthetic graft. The patency of this graft is approximately 80% to 90% at 5 years and approximately 70% at 10 years. Mortality risks for this procedure are <5%. The descending thoracic aorta can be used as an alternative inflow source in patients with a history of abdominal infection, previous irradiation, abdominal stomas, or multiple abdominal operations (all of which increase operative morbidity rates). The thoracobifemoral bypass achieves patency rates of 75% to 85% at 5 years, with perioperative mortality rates of <5% when experienced vascular surgeons perform the bypasses. Extra-anatomic bypasses (grafts that course through an anatomic pathway that is significantly different from the native arteries) should be performed in patients who cannot tolerate major aortic reconstructive surgery because of comorbidities. The most common extra-anatomic procedures are axillobifemoral and femorofemoral bypass grafts. Axillobifemoral reconstruction, used for aortoiliac occlusive disease, has a 5-year patency rate of 50% to 60%.

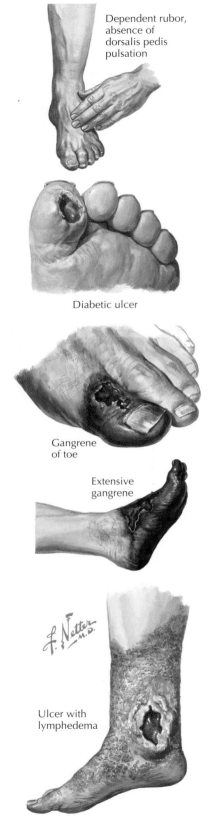

Dependent rubor, absence of dorsalis pedis pulsation

Diabetic ulcer

Gangrene of toe

Extensive gangrene

Ulcer with lymphedema

FIG 60.2 Complications of Diabetic Vasculopathy and Neuropathy.

For patients with unilateral iliac disease not amenable to angioplasty, femorofemoral bypass has a 5-year patency rate of 50% to 80%.

Critical ischemia or tissue loss from infrainguinal occlusive disease is best treated with arterial reconstruction. With respect to patency and resistance to infections, autologous vein grafts are superior to other conduits, especially when reconstruction below the knee is necessary. Availability, quality, and length requirements may necessitate a search for alternate sites for veins, such as the arms (basilic, cephalic) or the posterior leg (lesser saphenous vein). If possible, an autologous graft rather than synthetic material should be used for infrainguinal bypasses. Prosthetic material in lower extremity bypass procedures is reserved mainly for patients without other conduit options. In some cases, prosthetic material may be used for reconstructions above the knee.

Comparison of the use of an autologous saphenous vein with polytetrafluoroethylene grafts in above-the-knee (femoropopliteal) and below-the-knee (distal femoropopliteal and femorodistal) bypass procedures showed equivalent 2-year patency rates in grafts to the same level, but patency rates were significantly different at 4 years for infrapopliteal bypasses but not for above-the-knee procedures. Prosthetic graft material for distal bypasses is a better option than primary amputation in patients with suboptimal autologous vein options.

An excellent summary of the diagnosis and treatment of patients with lower extremity ischemia may be found in the American College of Cardiology/American Heart Association 2011 Practice Guidelines for the management of patients with peripheral arterial disease.

Avoiding Treatment Errors

Patients often attribute calf or thigh pain to orthopedic conditions. Individuals with lower extremity pain associated with exercise should have a complete vascular evaluation.

CAROTID DISEASE

Clinical Presentation

Most patients with carotid artery stenosis are asymptomatic (see also Chapter 61). For patients with symptoms, complaints range from short-lived symptoms consistent with a transient ischemic attack—which may include contralateral extremity weakness, ipsilateral facial weakness, slurred speech, or temporary monocular blindness (amaurosis fugax)—to fully developed stroke deficits.

Management and Therapy
Optimum Treatment

Carotid endarterectomy has been the mainstay of treatment of carotid artery disease for decades. Large multicenter trials, such as the Asymptomatic Carotid Atherosclerosis Study (ACAS) and the North American Symptomatic Carotid Endarterectomy Trial, validated the safety and efficacy of carotid endarterectomy in treating and preventing strokes in patients with carotid artery stenosis. Surgical therapy involves exposure of the carotid bifurcation under general or regional anesthesia. After arresting flow and removing the intima and the media of the diseased section, the artery is closed. The procedural stroke rate is approximately 1%. Adjacent nerve injuries and hematomas are the most common complications. By using routine carotid patch closure, long-term restenosis rates are significantly reduced and rarely seen. Patients recover quickly from this procedure (1 week), and hospitalizations are routinely <24 hours.

Carotid angioplasty with stenting is decreasing in frequency. Although early studies showed an increased risk of stroke after carotid angioplasty, the safety of carotid angioplasty stenting has improved by using distal protective devices. Most trials in this area are "noninferiority studies" to determine whether the outcomes of carotid artery angioplasty

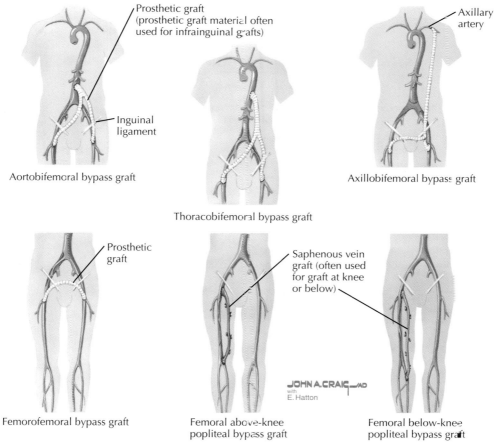

FIG 60.3 Surgical Management of Peripheral Arterial Disease of the Lower Extremities.

stenting equal those with carotid endarterectomy. The results of these trials have been equivocal. There is no consensus on whether any intervention (carotid endarterectomy or carotid artery stenting) is indicated with asymptomatic carotid stenosis. The results of the ACAS supported revascularization for asymptomatic individuals with significant carotid artery stenosis. However, it should be noted that the ACAS was conducted in an era when aspirin therapy was considered optimal medical management. No similar study has been done with a combination of aspirin and a P2Y12 inhibitor (e.g., clopidogrel) in asymptomatic patients.

Avoiding Treatment Errors

The optimum treatment for asymptomatic carotid stenosis remains somewhat controversial, as discussed previously. Careful consideration should be given to advocating an invasive procedure in asymptomatic patients. Risk reduction has improved with aggressive medical treatment, including hypercholesterolemia treatment, aspirin, and excellent blood pressure control. These same agents are being used in the surgically treated patients; thus, allowing us to reduce the procedural risks of cardiac and cerebrovascular complications. In general, there is a slow trend toward managing asymptomatic patients medically unless progression of disease is detected.

VISCERAL DISEASE

Clinical Presentation

Patients who have atherosclerotic lesions involving visceral arteries typically present with end-organ ischemia that manifests as chronic abdominal pain. Although abdominal bruits are often detected, the natural history of the disease indicates that patients rarely become symptomatic and that symptoms generally occur only when the disease is far advanced. There is considerable debate about whether (and how) asymptomatic stenoses of visceral arteries should be treated. Duplex scanning can be used to identify patients with significant visceral stenosis.

Management and Therapy
Optimum Treatment

In patients with mesenteric ischemia, collateral flow can come from several vascular distributions, including the iliac arteries, the supraceliac aorta, and the thoracic aorta. Because of the low prevalence of the disease, individual series are small, and results are difficult to compare. After surgical repair, long-term patency is difficult to assess without follow-up angiography. Based on relief of symptoms, surgical approaches are highly successful; symptom-free disease is experienced by 80% to 100% of patients. Because of the limited involvement of the thoracic aorta in atherosclerotic disease, some surgeons prefer that the bypass originate from the thoracic aorta. Graft failures are unusual with this approach in patients followed longitudinally by duplex ultrasonography. Surgical mortality and morbidity rates are also low. Bypass techniques for the renal arteries typically use a replacement aortic graft, or for in flow, the splenic or hepatic artery. However, with advances in endovascular therapies, fewer open surgical procedures are being performed on visceral arteries.

Avoiding Treatment Errors

The major symptoms associated with the superior mesenteric artery and celiac stenosis are postprandial pain and weight loss. If both these symptoms are present, strong consideration should be given to ultrasound or angiographic evaluation, or both.

FUTURE DIRECTIONS

As the development of endovascular devices continues, more and more traditional surgical vascular procedures will be replaced with minimally invasive procedures because of patient preference and outcomes. The minimally invasive techniques include branched devices for aneurysmal disease, and drug-eluting stents or other devices such as absorbable stents (analogous to those used in coronary artery disease; see Section IV) to inhibit intimal hyperplasia and arrest the aneurysmal disease process in adjacent arteries. Standard surgical management algorithms will center on endovascular therapies with combined open and endovascular treatments for patients with complex problems not amenable to endovascular approaches alone. Until treatment options involve only endovascular percutaneous therapies—with proven long-term success rates comparable to the success rates of surgical treatments—physicians trained to perform both endovascular and surgical treatments are best suited to provide care.

New drugs used in the treatment of cardiovascular disease are described elsewhere in this publication, and it is likely that further implementation of preventative strategies will be increasingly important for patients at risk for PVD. In the future, medical treatment may be used to treat smaller aneurysms, stabilize plaques, prevent atherosclerosis, and vascularize ischemic chronic lower extremity ulcers.

ADDITIONAL RESOURCES

Benjamin E, Blaha M, Chiuve S, et al. Heart disease and stroke statistics—2017 update: a report from the American Heart Association. *Circulation.* 2017;135:e146–e603.

The American Heart Association guide to heart and stroke statistics.

Norgrena L, Hiattb WR, Dormandy JA, et al. on behalf of the TASC II Working Group. Inter-society consensus for the management of peripheral arterial disease. *J Vasc Surg.* 2007;45(1, Jan suppl):S5–S67.

The Trans-Atlantic Inter-Society Consensus (TASC) Document on Management of Peripheral Arterial Disease was published in January 2007 as a result of cooperation among 14 medical and surgical vascular, cardiovascular, vascular radiology, and cardiology societies in Europe and North America.

EVIDENCE

Farber A, Rosenfield K, Menard M. The BEST-CLI trial: a multidisciplinary effort to assess which therapy is best for patients with critical limb ischemia. *Tech Vasc Interv Radiol.* 2014;17:221–224.

The BEST-CLI trial is a pragmatic, multicenter, open label, randomized trial that compares best endovascular therapy with best open surgical treatment in patients eligible for both treatments. The trial aims to provide clinical guidance for critical limb ischemia management.

Farber MA. Visceral vessel relocation techniques. *J Vasc Surg.* 2006;43(supplA): 81A–84A.

The main advantage of visceral relocation techniques is the decrease in visceral ischemia that may occur with long periods of aortic cross-clamping.

Gerhard-Herman MD, Gornik HL, Barrett C, et al. 2016 AHA/ACC guideline on the management of patients with lower extremity peripheral artery disease: executive summary: a report of the American College of Cardiology/American Heart Association Task Force on Clinical Practice Guidelines. *J Am Coll Cardiol.* 2017;69:1465–1508.

These are guidelines published by joint vascular societies for the treatment of patients with peripheral vascular pathology.

Khaodhiar L, Dinh T, Schomacker KT, et al. The use of medical hyperspectral technology to evaluate microcirculatory changes in diabetic foot ulcers and to predict clinical outcomes. *Diabetes Care.* 2007;30:903–910.

Hyperspectral imaging is a new technology that compares oxygenated and deoxygenated hemoglobin. It may prove useful is assessing lower extremity ischemia and in the prediction of wound healing potential.

Mwipatayi B, Sharma S, Daneshmand A, Thomas S, Vijayan V, Altaf N, Garbowski M, Jackson M, et al. Durability of the balloon-expandable covered versus bare-metal stents in the Covered versus Balloon Expandable Stent Trial (COBEST) for the treatment of aortoiliac occlusive disease. *J Vasc Surg.* 2016;64:83–94.

This demonstrated the 5-year results of the initial COBEST trial. Covered stents have a better and enduring patency advantage over bare metal stents in both the short and long term. This was more prevalent when TASC C and D lesions were treated.

Oderich G, Bower T, Sullivan T, Gloviczki P. Open versus endovascular revascularization for chronic mesenteric ischemia: risk-stratified outcomes. *J Vasc Surg.* 2009;49:1472–1479.

Comparison of endovascular versus surgical revascularization from a risk-stratified standpoint, with similar mortality and symptom relief in both groups, but increased incidence of symptom recurrence, restenosis, and reintervention in the endovascular group.

61

Carotid Artery Revascularization

Martyn Knowles, Jason Crowner, Mark A. Farber

Cerebrovascular accidents (CVAs) are a major cause of disability and death worldwide. There are two broad categories of stroke: hemorrhage and ischemia. Hemorrhage is characterized by bleeding within the closed cranial cavity, whereas ischemia is regarded as too little blood to supply the needed amount of oxygen and nutrients to a specific part of the brain. The morbidity caused by a CVA can be debilitating, causing permanent disability such as aphasia, paralysis, blindness, numbness, or weakness. Transient symptoms, which last <24 hours, are called a transient ischemic attack (TIA) and manifest with similar symptoms. The long-term sequelae of CVAs can have lasting financial and social burdens on the patient, family, and the healthcare system.

Of the two major etiologies of CVAs, ischemic causes account for approximately 70% to 80% of all cases. Ischemic CVAs occur usually from thrombosis, embolism, or systemic hypoperfusion. The sources of thrombosis or embolic disease can be from large vessels (e.g., the aorta or extracranial carotid system), the heart, or small vessels within the intracerebral arterial system. The extracranial carotid artery system is a common source of thrombotic and embolic CVAs.

Atherosclerotic plaque at the carotid artery bifurcation is a common cause of CVA, accounting for approximately 40% to 60% of all ischemic strokes (Figs. 61.1 and 61.2). Since the introduction of carotid artery endarterectomy (CEA) in 1954, operative treatment of carotid artery occlusive lesions has decreased the risk of subsequent ipsilateral ischemic strokes. Recently, new endovascular carotid artery stenting (CAS) techniques have been introduced; however, their role in the management of carotid artery disease remains controversial.

The origin of the carotid artery at the aortic arch is a common site of atherosclerotic disease and can be a cause of ischemic CVA. Diagnosis is often more difficult because of the location of disease in the chest. Treatment involves either extrathoracic or extra-anatomic surgical repair, or more recently, endovascular management with angioplasty and stenting.

This chapter provides a review of the epidemiology, pathophysiology, diagnosis, and treatment options for carotid artery disease.

EPIDEMIOLOGY

Worldwide, CVA is the second most common cause of mortality and the third most common cause of disability. Although incidence appears to be decreasing in the United States, it seems to be increasing in low-income countries. In the United States, the annual incidence of new or recurrent stroke is approximately 800,000; approximately 600,000 of these are first strokes. At younger ages, men have a higher risk of stroke than women, which reverses, with women having a higher risk at age 75 years or older. The risk of stroke appears to be affected by race, with whites having a lower incidence than blacks and Hispanics in the United States. Recently, stroke has decreased from the third leading cause of

death in the United States to the fourth, likely due to improvements in acute stroke care over the last few years. The risk factors for stroke include age older than 55 years, male sex, hypertension, family history, atrial fibrillation, smoking, hypercholesterolemia, diabetes, obesity, renal insufficiency, and alcohol use. Overall, five factors cause a significant number of strokes: hypertension, smoking, obesity, diet, and physical inactivity.

PATHOGENESIS OF STROKE

The incidence of stroke due to ischemia worldwide is approximately 70%; however, in the United States, the incidence is closer to 90%. Ischemia includes thrombosis, embolism, and hypoperfusion. Thrombosis refers to in situ obstruction of an artery, typically from atherosclerosis, dissection, or fibromuscular dysplasia. A stroke occurs from reduced flow distal to the thrombosis, and can be due to occlusion of either a large or a small vessel. Large vessels include the extracranial carotid and proximal intracranial arteries. Small vessel disease includes branch vessels from the intracranial vessels. Embolism refers to debris that arises from a source, such as the heart or arterial segment, that becomes free and flows downstream until lodging in a small vessel. Hypoperfusion refers to a more global circulatory problem, which typically requires a more extensive pattern of occlusive disease involving multiple vessels. There is often a combination of etiologies that leads to a stroke (e.g., a preexisting lesion) that becomes a source of emboli.

Atherosclerosis is the most common cause of occlusive disease in the extra- and/or intracranial carotid arteries, and remains a major preventative cause of ischemic stroke. Large-vessel cervical disease is believed to be a cause of stroke in approximately 15% of cases. Furthermore, CVA from carotid artery etiology has the highest rate of recurrence at 30 days.

The carotid artery bifurcation is the most likely area to have atherosclerosis, which is at least partially due to alterations in flow and shear stress at this location. There is a separation of flow between the high-resistance external carotid artery system and the low-resistance internal carotid artery (ICA) system. These alterations in flow can cause shearing stress, injuring the vessel and making it prone to plaque formation, which typically forms on the wall opposite from the flow divider. The inciting event is intimal injury, followed by platelet deposition, smooth muscle proliferation, fibroplasia, and loss of the luminal diameter. As the lumen diameter becomes smaller, the flow velocities and turbulence increase, which can lead to hypoperfusion or atheroembolization. With progressive atherosclerotic disease at the ICA, it is common to develop a necrotic core rich with lipids and cholesterol. A fibrous cap develops, which can easily rupture and causes plaque disruption that typically leads to a clinical event.

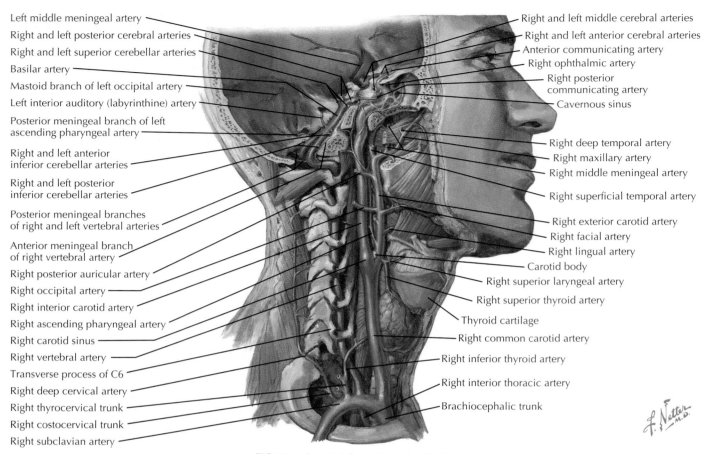

Left middle meningeal artery

Right and left posterior cerebral arteries

Right and left superior cerebellar arteries

Basilar artery

Mastoid branch of left occipital artery

Left interior auditory (labyrinthine) artery

Posterior meningeal branch of left ascending pharyngeal artery

Right and left anterior inferior cerebellar arteries

Right and left posterior inferior cerebellar arteries

Posterior meningeal branches of right and left vertebral arteries

Anterior meningeal branch of right vertebral artery

Right posterior auricular artery

Right occipital artery

Right interior carotid artery

Right ascending pharyngeal artery

Right carotid sinus

Right vertebral artery

Transverse process of C6

Right deep cervical artery

Right thyrocervical trunk

Right costocervical trunk

Right subclavian artery

Right and left middle cerebral arteries

Right and left anterior cerebral arteries

Anterior communicating artery

Right ophthalmic artery

Right posterior communicating artery

Cavernous sinus

Right deep temporal artery

Right maxillary artery

Right middle meningeal artery

Right superficial temporal artery

Right exterior carotid artery

Right facial artery

Right lingual artery

Carotid body

Right superior laryngeal artery

Right superior thyroid artery

Thyroid cartilage

Right common carotid artery

Right inferior thyroid artery

Right interior thoracic artery

Brachiocephalic trunk

FIG 61.1 Arterial Supply to the Brain.

CLINICAL MANIFESTATIONS OF STROKE

Symptoms related to carotid artery disease correspond with the location of symptoms. A left ICA symptomatic lesion should cause right-sided symptoms and vice versa. Symptomatic carotid artery disease is classically believed to be a TIA, CVA, or amaurosis fugax that corresponds to the territory of the diseased artery. A TIA is a neurological event similar to a stroke; however, symptoms last for <24 hours. These are considered a precursor of a more serious event, and a large number of those who experience a TIA will progress to a CVA. Motor symptoms can include hemiparesis contralateral to the affected hemisphere. Sensory deficits can also occur in a similar fashion, such as numbness or paresthesia. Aphasia, dysphagia, or dysarthria can also occur. Amaurosis fugax is the temporary monocular blindness from cholesterol embolization to the retinal artery via the ophthalmic artery. Dizziness, syncope, vertigo, seizures, bowel or bladder incontinence, or migraines are not typically related to carotid disease; therefore, other causes must be sought. Once the symptoms persist for <24 hours, the TIA becomes a full CVA. The full severity of a stroke can often take weeks to manifest as the penumbra either recovers or does not recover. Global ischemia is generally uncommon with carotid artery disease, with the exception of involvement of multiple carotid and vertebral arteries.

DIAGNOSTIC EVALUATION

Carotid artery duplex ultrasonography (DUS) is typically the first diagnostic modality performed for diagnosis of carotid artery disease. There

are limited data to suggest a value in screening for carotid artery disease; however, any patient with concerning symptoms should undergo DUS. DUS can accurately identify occlusive carotid artery disease, while avoiding radiation. Due to the sensitivity and specificity of DUS for carotid artery disease, no further imaging modality is required to identify the need for treatment. A complete examination includes evaluation of the common, external, and internal carotid arteries, as well as the vertebral arteries and often the subclavian arteries. The peak systolic velocity, end-diastolic velocity, and the ratio of velocities in the common carotid artery (CCA) to ICA (CCA/ICA) are used to determine the severity of stenosis. Although laboratories differ in their ranges, patients are typically classified as either normal—mild, 1% to 49%; moderate, 50% to 69%; severe, 70% to 99%—or occluded. DUS also detects troubling plaque morphology that identifies high-risk plaque, which can estimate the risk of neurological symptoms. Magnetic resonance angiography (MRA) and computerized tomographic angiography (CTA) are also frequently used for identification of carotid artery disease; both of these modalities have benefits and limitations. CTA provides excellent resolution and imaging but involves contrast and radiation. In contrast, MRA avoids radiation and contrast but has a lower resolution, cannot detect calcifications, and can overestimate blockages. Both modalities do provide useful information regarding intracranial collateral circulation, location of high carotid lesions, proximal brachiocephalic disease, vessel tortuosity, and high-risk features for endovascular management. Angiography remains the gold standard for diagnosis; however, the procedure itself carries approximately 1% risk of CVA.

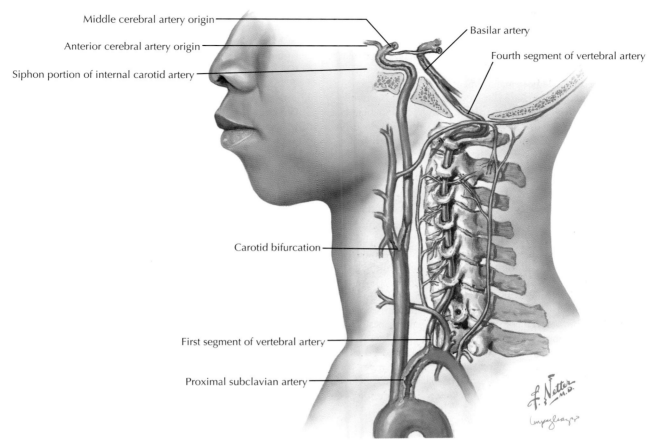

Middle cerebral artery origin

Anterior cerebral artery origin

Siphon portion of internal carotid artery

Basilar artery

Fourth segment of vertebral artery

Carotid bifurcation

First segment of vertebral artery

Proximal subclavian artery

FIG 61.2 Common Sites of Cerebrovascular Occlusive Disease.

TREATMENT OF CAROTID ARTERY OCCLUSIVE DISEASE

Symptomatic

Patients with carotid artery occlusive disease are placed into two main categories: asymptomatic or symptomatic disease. Patients with a recent (<6 months) TIA, CVA, or amaurosis fugax are considered symptomatic. In patients who have a TIA, 15% will go on to a CVA, 10% within 90 days. Due to the risk of recurrence or progression to severe ipsilateral CVA, surgical management is required for risk reduction of stroke. The degree of stenosis corresponds with the risk for ipsilateral CVA. The degree of stenosis was correlated with CVA risk and validated in multiple trials, most prominently in the North American Symptomatic Carotid Endarterectomy Trial (NASCET) study. A stenosis <50% was unlikely to cause neurological manifestations. In patients with stenosis >50%, patients treated medically were more likely than those who underwent surgical management with a CEA to experience ipsilateral stroke. Although this benefit was found in all patients with >50% stenosis, those in the 70% to 99% group benefited the most from surgery. After 2 years, there was a significant reduction in ipsilateral stroke in those who underwent a CEA. In patients with 50% to 69% stenosis, 22.2% of medically treated patients and 16.7% of surgically treated patients had an ipsilateral CVA in 5 years. In patients with 70% to 99% stenosis, 26% of medically treated patients and 9% of surgically treated patients had an ipsilateral CVA over a 2-year period. The European Carotid Surgery Trial (ECST) found similar results for severe stenosis, but no benefit for those with moderate stenosis. These trials included medical

therapy with only aspirin, and since then, there have been multiple improvements in medical therapy, including antiplatelet medications such as clopidogrel and hydroxy-3-methylglutaryl coenzyme A reductase inhibitors (statins). Aspirin is an important medication for secondary stroke prevention, and the addition of clopidogrel is recommended in symptomatic patients for the prevention of stroke. Statins lower stroke risk by 30% by stabilizing plaque and are important for the reduction of stroke.

Timing of intervention continues to be debated. Traditionally, surgeons would wait at least 6 weeks after a neurological event before intervention; however, patients have a high risk of recurrence within 30 days, and some patients have secondary events. The apprehension of performing surgery too soon is due to the concern of a hemorrhagic conversion of a new ischemic lesion, a risk that decreases with time. Currently, most surgeons recommend intervention between 2 days and 2 weeks after the event; however, if the patient has had a large dense deficit, it is best to wait a few weeks. Patients with crescendo TIAs or an evolving stroke have a much higher risk of stroke and require urgent intervention.

Asymptomatic

Treatment for patients with asymptomatic carotid artery disease is not as well defined as treatment in those with symptomatic disease. Asymptomatic patients with carotid artery stenosis can be identified during physical examination when a bruit is found or during DUS for screening. The major trial that evaluated asymptomatic patients with carotid artery disease was the Asymptomatic Carotid Atherosclerosis Study (ACAS) trial. Asymptomatic patients with >60% stenosis were randomly assigned to either medical management or CEA. After 5 years, the best medical therapy was found to be inferior to surgery with regard to ipsilateral CVA (11% for medical management vs. 5.1% for CEA over 5 years). Therefore, with endarterectomy, there was a risk reduction of stroke of 53%. In Europe, the Asymptomatic Carotid Surgery Trial (ACST) showed similar results. Medical management at that time included aspirin, and again did not include statins or clopidogrel. Currently, most accept that surgical intervention in the asymptomatic patient is indicated for a stenosis of ≥80%; however, for those with a 60% to 79% stenosis, surgery remains controversial. Currently, clinical trials are comparing carotid intervention versus best medical management in the treatment of asymptomatic carotid stenosis.

TREATMENT

There is widely accepted consensus that intervention is warranted in symptomatic (>50% stenosis) and asymptomatic (>80% stenosis) patients. The next decision is which treatment modality should be undertaken. CEA traces back to the 1950s and is considered the gold standard for treatment of occlusive carotid artery stenosis.

CEA is a surgical technique that involves direct carotid artery exposure, removal of plaque, and repair of the artery with a patch (Fig. 61.3). CEA can be done under local, regional, or general anesthesia. There are techniques to monitor for stroke during the procedure. Typically under general anesthesia, there is a choice of using electroencephalography, transcranial Doppler, stump pressure measurement, or somatosensory-evoked potentials for evaluation of collateral intracerebral flow during the procedure. If these techniques show a concern for low collateral flow, a shunt can be placed from the CCA to the ICA that maintains flow during the procedure. The evaluation of stump pressure can also be performed. Measuring stump pressure requires clamping the common and external carotid artery while maintaining patency of the ICA using a transducer to check the back pressure. A mean pressure of <40 mm Hg is the most widely accepted measurement for the threshold regarding shunting.

The patient is positioned to expose the neck, and an incision is made along the anterior border of the sternocleidomastoid muscle. The platysma muscle is divided, and the sternocleidomastoid is identified and retracted laterally. The facial vein is ligated from the internal jugular vein, which exposes the carotid artery. Dissection is carefully performed to avoid injury to the cranial nerves, with the vagus nerve being the most likely to be injured. The CCA is carefully dissected out, as well as the external artery and ICA. Once the vessels are clamped, and the evaluation of possible shunt performed, the patient is heparinized (typically 100 U/kg), and then the artery is opened from the CCA into the ICA, past the distal aspect of the stenosis, and the endarterectomy is performed. The endarterectomy removes the intima and the superficial media layer of the carotid artery plaque. All debris and small flaps are removed or tacked down with sutures. Special care is taken with the distal aspect of the endarterectomy, to ensure that no flap is left after the initiation of flow again. Careful irrigation is performed to remove any remaining clot or debris. Once the endarterectomy is completed, the artery is closed using a patch repair, usually bovine pericardium. All vessels are allowed to backbleed and are flushed, and then flow is restored. After all bleeding is controlled, the neck is closed in multiple layers and the patient is woken up and taken to the intensive care unit

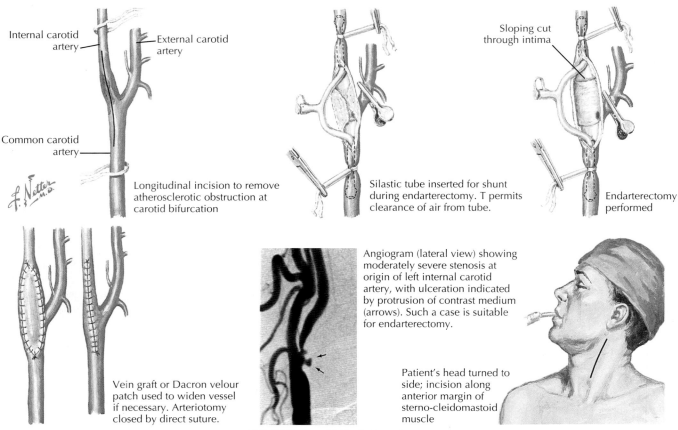

Internal carotid artery

External carotid artery

Common carotid artery

f. Netter M.D.

Longitudinal incision to remove atherosclerotic obstruction at carotid bifurcation

Silastic tube inserted for shunt during endarterectomy. T permits clearance of air from tube.

Sloping cut through intima

Endarterectomy performed

Vein graft or Dacron velour patch used to widen vessel if necessary. Arteriotomy closed by direct suture.

Angiogram (lateral view) showing moderately severe stenosis at origin of left internal carotid artery, with ulceration indicated by protrusion of contrast medium (arrows). Such a case is suitable for endarterectomy.

Patient's head turned to side; incision along anterior margin of sterno-cleidomastoid muscle

FIG 61.3 Carotid Endarterectomy.

for neurological and blood pressure monitoring. The patient is continued on aspirin indefinitely.

Since the Food and Drug Administration approved CAS in 2004, there has been a proliferation of technology development and use of this treatment for symptomatic and asymptomatic carotid disease. High-risk patients, for anatomical or medical reasons, as well as older adult patients, were thought to benefit from CAS over CEA. Initially, CAS was reserved for high-risk patients due to evidence that showed improvements in results over CEA. The Stenting and Angioplasty with Protection in Patients at High Risk for Endarterectomy (SAPPHIRE) trial examined CAS versus CEA for high-risk patients (medical comorbidities and anatomic features), and CAS was associated with a lower risk of major events at 1 year, with a greater advantage in asymptomatic patients. The Endarterectomy Versus Angioplasty in Patients with Symptomatic Severe Carotid Stenosis (EVA-3S) trial was a European trial for symptomatic patients with >60% stenosis that was stopped prematurely due to higher 30-day stroke risk with CAS. However, using an embolic protection device (Fig. 61.4) was optional, and its use was associated with similar results to CEA. The Stent-Supported Percutaneous Angioplasty of the Carotid Artery versus Endarterectomy trial (SPACE) trial examined patients with ≥70% symptomatic stenosis and failed to prove the noninferiority of CAS compared with CEA. Recently, the Carotid Revascularization Endarterectomy versus Stenting Trial (CREST) examined CAS versus CEA in standard risk symptomatic and asymptomatic patients. Overall, there appeared to be no difference between the two techniques in the long-term, but there appeared to be a higher rate of myocardial infarction with CEA and a higher rate of stroke with CAS. Currently, the Centers for Medicare and Medicaid Services limits

reimbursement for CAS to only high-risk symptomatic patients with carotid stenosis >70%.

However, there are some patients that do better with one technique over the other. Advanced age, initially believed to be a benefit for CAS, has actually been found to have a higher risk of stroke. Furthermore, symptomatic patients who have undergone CAS appear to have a higher risk of stroke or death if performed early (<7 days). Outside of anatomic factors—such as previous neck radiation, contralateral vocal cord paralysis, a high lesion, or severe medical comorbidities—there does not appear to be sufficient data to support CAS for treatment of asymptomatic patients. Currently, the CREST 2 trial is enrolling patients and is designed to answer further questions regarding the role of stenting in the management of carotid artery disease.

CAS requires careful patient identification and preoperative imaging to aid in a safe, successful procedure. Axial imaging is highly recommended before the procedure. Axial imaging can assist in the evaluation of the intracranial collateral circulation and anatomic factors related to the case, including the identification of disease within the aortic arch, arch type, tortuosity within the carotid artery, or morphology of the carotid artery lesion. Specific lesion characteristics could make stenting more risky, such as hypoechoic plaque, ulceration, long lesion length, circumferential calcification, or thrombus. A physical examination must be performed to help identify an appropriate access site to decrease the risk of complications. Commonly, patients with carotid artery disease also have peripheral arterial disease with aortoiliac occlusive disease that would make access difficult. Although the transfemoral approach is the most common approach, there are a variety of other approaches that are possible, including transcervical or transradial.

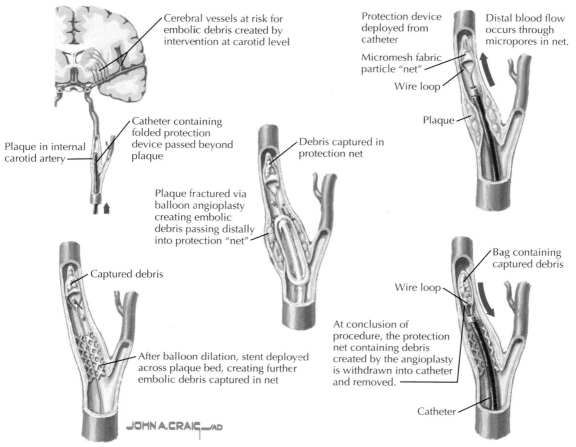

FIG 61.4 Cerebrovascular Emboli Protection Device.

COMPLICATIONS

The most serious complication after both CEA and CAS is a neurological event. An acute ipsilateral CVA is a dramatic complication after CEA or CAS, and can occur secondary to hypoperfusion or embolization during the procedure. Hypoperfusion is related to poor collateral flow, and embolization can occur from thrombus formed during the procedure, clamp site injury, or inadequate flushing at the end of the procedure. There are technical issues that can occur during CEA that include intimal flap, platelet adhesion to the patch, dissection, and stenosis from repair. CREST showed a periprocedural risk of death of 0.3%, CVA of 2.3%, and myocardial infarction of 2.3% after endarterectomy. For CAS, the periprocedural risk of death was 0.7%, CVA risk was 4.1%, and myocardial infarction risk was 1.1%. Cranial nerve injuries are a common complication after CEA; however, the incidence varies greatly, with a range between 1% and 30%.

CONCLUSIONS

Worldwide, CVA remains a significant cause of morbidity and mortality. Carotid artery atherosclerosis accounts for a large percentage of CVAs from embolism or thrombosis. Surgical management with CEA is the gold standard for treatment of symptomatic and asymptomatic carotid artery disease. Carotid stenting remains an excellent option for patients at high risk for endarterectomy, and further trials are evaluating its place in the management of carotid artery disease. Brachiocephalic occlusive disease can cause similar symptoms to carotid bifurcation disease, and requires intervention via endovascular or surgical means.

ADDITIONAL READING

Barnett HJ, Taylor DW, Eliasziw M, et al. Benefit of carotid endarterectomy in patients with symptomatic moderate or severe stenosis. North American Symptomatic Carotid Endarterectomy Trial Collaborators. *N Engl J Med.* 1998;339:1415–1425.
Large, multicenter trial that investigated the use of medical management versus surgery for symptomatic carotid artery disease and found a significant improvement in the avoidance of ipsilateral stroke with surgery.
Berguer R, Morasch MD, Kline RA. Transthoracic repair of innominate and common carotid artery disease: immediate and long-term outcome for 100 consecutive surgical reconstructions. *J Vasc Surg.* 1998;27:34–41, discussion 2.
Large single-center retrospective review of brachiocephalic disease treated with a transthoracic approach with excellent long-term results.
Brott TG, Hobson RW 2nd, Howard G, et al. Stenting versus endarterectomy for treatment of carotid-artery stenosis. *N Engl J Med.* 2010;363:11–23.
Large, multicenter trial (CREST study) that compared the use of stenting versus endarterectomy for symptomatic and severe asymptomatic carotid artery stenosis

in normal risk patients, which found no significant overall difference between the two groups.
Brott TG, Howard G, Roubtin GS, et al. Long-term results of stenting versus endarterectomy for carotid-artery stenosis. *N Engl J Med.* 2016;374: 1021–2031.
Ten-year follow-up of the CREST study that showed no significant difference between patients who underwent stenting and those who underwent endarterectomy with respect to the risk of periprocedural stroke, myocardial infarction, or death, and subsequent ipsilateral stroke.
Byrne J, Darling RC 3rd, Roddy SP, et al. Long term outcome for extra-anatomic arch reconstruction. An analysis of 143 procedures. *Eur J Vasc Endovasc Surg.* 2007;34:444–450.
Large single-center retrospective review of extrathoracic reconstruction for brachiocephalic disease with excellent long-term results.
Endarterectomy for asymptomatic carotid artery stenosis. Executive Committee for the Asymptomatic Carotid Atherosclerosis Study. *JAMA.* 1995;273:1421–1428.
The ACAS trial was a large multicenter trial that investigated the management of asymptomatic carotid artery disease for stenosis >60% using medical or surgical management, and found a significant improvement in 5-year outcomes with surgery.
Gurm HS, Yadav JS, Fayad P, et al. Long-term results of carotid stenting versus endarterectomy in high-risk patients. *N Engl J Med.* 2008;358:1572–1579.
Large multicenter trial that compared the use of stenting versus endarterectomy for symptomatic and severe asymptomatic carotid artery stenoses, which found no differences between the two treatment modalities at 3 years.
Mas JL, Chatellier G, Beyssen B, et al. Endarterectomy versus stenting in patients with symptomatic severe carotid stenosis. *N Engl J Med.* 2006;355:1660–1671.
Multicenter randomized trial that examined the treatment of symptomatic carotid artery stenosis with endarterectomy versus stenting, which was stopped short due to a higher risk of stroke in the stenting group.
Przewlocki T, Kablak-Ziembicka A, Pieniazek P, et al. Determinants of immediate and long-term results of subclavian and innominate artery angioplasty. *Catheter Cardiovasc Interv.* 2006;67:519–526.
Single-center review of endovascular management for occlusive brachiocephalic disease that showed good short- and mid-term results with angioplasty.
Rerkasem K, Rothwell PM. Systematic review of operative risks of carotid endarterectomy for recently symptomatic stenosis in relation to timing of surgery. *Stroke.* 2009;e564–e725.
Study that examined the appropriate timing for carotid endarterectomy for symptomatic carotid artery stenosis.
Warlow CP. Symptomatic patients: the European Carotid Surgery Trial (ECST). *J Mal Vasc.* 1993;18:198–201.
Large, multicenter trial that investigated the use of medical management versus surgery for symptomatic carotid artery disease, which found similar results in patients with severe stenosis to the NASCET trial.

62

Diseases of the Aorta

Martyn Knowles, Jason Crowner, Mark A. Farber

There is a wide spectrum of diseases that can affect the aorta. Aneurysmal disease is the second most frequent disease of the aorta after atherosclerosis. The most common location for aneurysmal disease is the infrarenal aorta, but it can also affect the thoracic, ascending, and arch portions of the aorta, as well as the iliac vessels. Typically, aneurysmal disease is a silent pathology that is found incidentally on imaging or physical examination. Although, in the past, the etiology for aneurysmal disease was believed to be secondary to atherosclerosis, recently, it has been found to be multifactorial. Most patients are asymptomatic and undergo treatment because the aneurysm is large or increasing in size, and thus puts them at risk for rupture. Symptoms of aneurysmal aortic disease include abdominal pain, back pain, and flank pain, and portend a risk of rupture. Endovascular aneurysm repair (EVAR) of the abdominal aorta has emerged as an effective and safe approach for repair of aortic aneurysms. Alternatively, thoracic aortic disease (aneurysms, dissections, transections) can be treated with thoracic endovascular aneurysm repair with excellent results. Recently, advancement of stent technology has allowed incorporation of more complex anatomy involving the visceral and renal vessels, as well as the hypogastric and supraaortic trunk vessels.

Acute aortic syndrome (AAS) is a collection of pathologies that includes acute aortic dissection, aortic rupture, intramural hematoma, and penetrating atherosclerotic ulcer. These entities have a high morbidity and mortality, and require immediate recognition and management to improve outcomes. Aortic transection from blunt aortic injury has seen an improvement in patient outcomes with the introduction of endovascular techniques for repair.

There are also a variety of less common aortic pathologies, such as vasculitis, inflammatory and/or mycotic aneurysms, and connective tissue diseases. Takayasu disease and giant cell arteritis are two large vessel vasculitides that involve the aorta and major branch vessels. Inflammatory and/or mycotic aneurysms are rare causes of aneurysms, but require recognition for proper treatment and correct surgical repair. Ultimately, care must be taken to identify genetic disorders such as connective tissue diseases as potential causes for aneurysms, because incorrect diagnosis can lead to an increase in morbidity and mortality.

This chapter provides a review of the various aortic pathologies, with an evaluation of the epidemiology, pathophysiology, diagnosis, and treatment options.

ANEURYSMAL DISEASE

Aneurysmal disease usually involves large arteries, most commonly, the infrarenal aorta and iliac arteries, and it less often involves other major arteries, including the thoracic aorta and the femoral and popliteal arteries (Figs. 62.1 and 62.2). Although small aneurysms have been reported to rupture, the risk of rupture is believed to rise exponentially with an increasing diameter, according to Laplace law—that the greater the radius of an artery, the greater the tension on the arterial wall. Atherosclerosis is an important contributor to aneurysmal dilatation as are hypertension and tobacco use, with up to one-third of patients having a genetic predisposition for aneurysmal disease.

Etiology and Pathogenesis

For many years, the etiology of aneurysmal disease was believed to be primarily related to atherosclerosis, largely because aneurysmal disease occurs predominantly in older adult hypertensive individuals and is associated with tobacco use. The etiology is now believed to be multifactorial. Genetic predisposition may be involved in up to one-third of patients with aneurysms. Microscopic analysis indicates that deficiencies in elastin, collagen, or both, may be crucial factors. Collagen-degrading matrix metalloproteinases are probable culprits in aneurysm formation, and current research focuses on their role in the pathogenesis of aneurysmal disease. Elastin and collagen breakdown, which may be accelerated based on a genetic predisposition to produce matrix metalloproteinases, may precipitate an inflammatory reaction. This inflammatory reaction can then contribute to weakening of the arterial wall and eventual dilatation. The presence of several cytokines and systemic biomarkers has been shown to correlate with the presence and size of abdominal aortic aneurysms (AAAs), and it is likely that a causative relationship exists.

Clinical Presentation

Each year, approximately 9000 deaths occur from ruptured abdominal aortic aneurysms (rAAAs), and this disease is the 13th leading cause of death in the United States, despite advances in diagnostic imaging, screening programs, and heightened awareness. Abdominal pain may indicate rapid enlargement or impending rupture of an AAA. Other symptoms of an AAA include nausea, early satiety, and back pain from compression of adjacent structures; however, approximately 75% of patients are asymptomatic at presentation, and the presence of an AAA is detected by physical examination or screening of high-risk individuals.

Management and Therapy
Optimum Treatment

Management guidelines center on evaluation of rupture risk. When the risk of rupture exceeds the risk of surgical repair, replacement of the aneurysmal segment of the artery is indicated. For an asymptomatic AAA, the risk of rupture varies with the diameter of the aneurysm; an AAA of 5 cm has a 5% rupture risk per year, and an AAA of 6 cm has an estimated 10% to 15% rupture risk per year. Patients with saccular aneurysms, chronic obstructive pulmonary disease, or hypertension are believed to have a higher than average risk of aneurysm rupture. Treatment is indicated for aneurysms that are greater than twice the

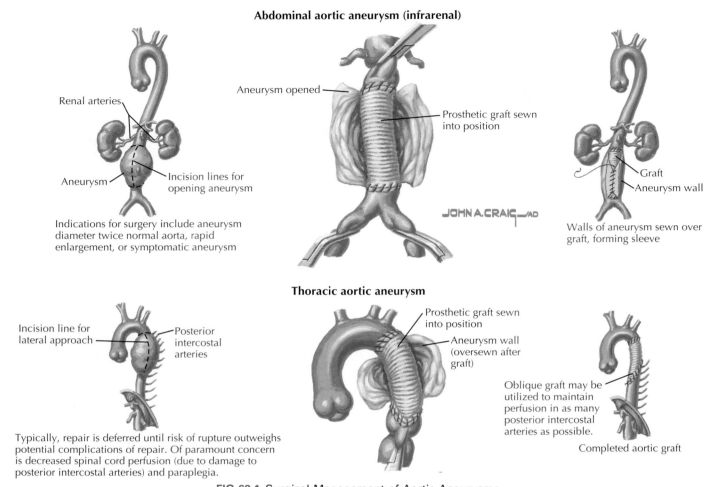

Abdominal aortic aneurysm (infrarenal)

Renal arteries

Aneurysm opened

Prosthetic graft sewn into position

Aneurysm

Incision lines for opening aneurysm

Indications for surgery include aneurysm diameter twice normal aorta, rapid enlargement, or symptomatic aneurysm

JOHN A.CRAIG_AD

Graft
Aneurysm wall

Walls of aneurysm sewn over graft, forming sleeve

Thoracic aortic aneurysm

Incision line for lateral approach

Posterior intercostal arteries

Prosthetic graft sewn into position

Aneurysm wall (oversewn after graft)

Oblique graft may be utilized to maintain perfusion in as many posterior intercostal arteries as possible.

Completed aortic graft

Typically, repair is deferred until risk of rupture outweighs potential complications of repair. Of paramount concern is decreased spinal cord perfusion (due to damage to posterior intercostal arteries) and paraplegia.

FIG 62.1 Surgical Management of Aortic Aneurysms.

normal artery diameter, that are enlarging rapidly (>0.5 cm in 6 months), or that are symptomatic; the major symptoms are pain or evidence of distal emboli potentially related to the aneurysm.

The number of patients in the United States with the diagnosis of a rAAA has declined in recent years from 23.2 to 12.8 per 100,000 Medicare beneficiaries, as did repairs of rAAAs (15.6–8.4 per 100,000). These data reflect increased surveillance for AAAs and the increased use of EVAR. With the increasing number of EVARs, the threshold for intervention based on size has become more controversial. Some evidence suggests that observation of AAAs of <5.5 cm is the proper course, whereas other observers believe that EVAR should be offered to patients earlier in the course of their disease. This question is being addressed in a large randomized study that, when complete, should provide much needed direction on when to intervene in patients with AAAs.

During the past 50 years, the surgical technique for AAA repair has remained essentially unchanged, with outcome improvements resulting from advances in preoperative screening and risk stratification, improved anesthetic practice, and intensive care management. Notably, however, the use of more durable synthetic grafts in recent years (rather than using homografts for AAA repair) has also contributed to the improved long-term outcome after AAA repair. Aneurysmorrhaphy involves mobilization and exposure of the aneurysm and the normal artery above and below the diseased section. Blood flow through the artery is arrested for inline replacement of the diseased artery with an artificial one, resulting in major cardiovascular stress during the procedure and for several days after. The combination of cardiovascular stress and the

advanced age and comorbid conditions of the patient increases the procedure-associated morbidity and mortality rates. Patients usually require 7 to 10 days of hospitalization and 6 to 8 weeks to recover. However, once patients fully recover from the procedure, long-term follow-up indicates that few patients need further intervention. When further intervention is needed, generally it is because progression of the disease has occurred in adjacent arteries. Ongoing research focuses on the identification of mechanisms to arrest the disease process to prevent spread and inhibit the inflammatory process.

As general medical care and nutrition have improved, the mean age in the United States and industrialized countries has increased, and accordingly, there have been an increasing number of individuals with AAAs. As the age and medical comorbidities of patients with an AAA have increased, so has the interest in less invasive procedures for treatment, which resulted in the development of minimally invasive techniques for the treatment of aneurysmal disease. AAA endovascular repair techniques involve the insertion of a new lining into the diseased artery using hooks or stents to secure the lining to the arterial wall. Four devices have been approved by the U.S. Food and Drug Administration for the treatment of infrarenal AAAs. The indications for treatment with endovascular devices are identical to those for open surgical repair. The procedure can be performed under local, regional, or general anesthesia, and typically involves exposure of the common femoral arteries for device insertion. Although insertion has been accomplished with percutaneous techniques, most devices are too large for insertion by routine percutaneous treatment methods. Once the aorta is accessed,

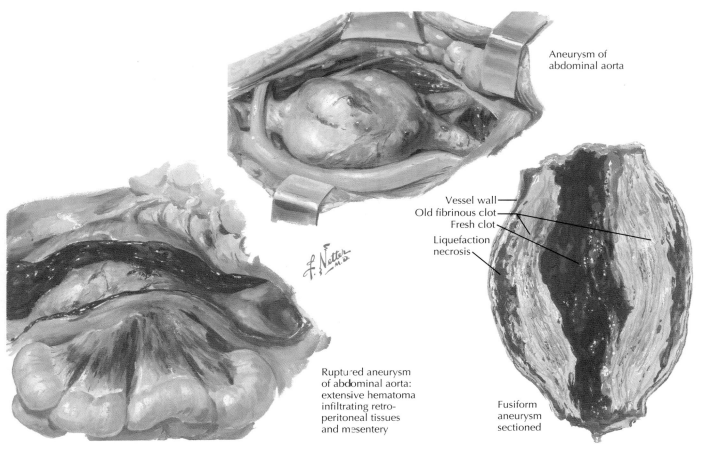

Aneurysm of
abdominal aorta

Vessel wall
Old fibrinous clot
Fresh clot
Liquefaction
necrosis

Ruptured aneurysm
of abdominal aorta:
extensive hematoma
infiltrating retro-
peritoneal tissues
and mesentery

Fusiform
aneurysm
sectioned

FIG 62.2 Surgical View of Aortic Aneurysms.

imaging methods guide device implantation just below the renal arteries, where the aorta and its endothelium are the healthiest. Most patients are hospitalized for 1 day and are fully recovered from the procedure within 1 week. Successful implantation has been accomplished in >98% of patients.

Patient selection is crucial to outcomes with EVAR. Seal failures (endoleak) are more likely to occur in patients with short, angled, or diseased proximal infrarenal arteries. During follow-up, complications associated with endoleaks or migration develop in 6% to 15% of patients. Many of these complications can be treated with secondary endovascular interventions and do not necessitate conversion to open repair and removal of the device. Iliac artery access issues (smaller or diseased arteries) may also create complications associated with implantation. Although new design techniques and lower profile devices have overcome many of these problems, complications occur in 1% to 2% of patients.

Prospective studies have shown a reduction in the mortality rates and major morbidities by 50% with EVAR procedures compared with open surgery. Blood loss and time required to return to an active lifestyle are also significantly reduced. Interim data also suggest that patient survival is greater after EVAR than after traditional open surgical treatment, and this has resulted in the increased use of this approach. Notably, a report from the Agency for Healthcare Research and Quality stated that EVAR did not improve longer term overall survival or health status and was associated with greater complications, need for reintervention, long-term monitoring, and costs.

In 2008, approximately 50% of AAAs were treated with endovascular therapy. As branched designs and other innovations are incorporated

and durability concerns are addressed, the use of EVAR technology will most likely increase.

Avoiding Treatment Errors

With both the endovascular and open approaches, the anatomy of the aneurysm must be determined. This includes proximity to the renal arteries as well as the angulation of the neck of the aneurysm and the status of the inferior mesenteric artery. Failure to revascularize the inferior mesenteric artery may result in postoperative visceral ischemia, whereas graft impingement on the renal arteries may result in renal failure. Placement of an endograft in a patient with a severely angulated neck can be associated with a type I endoleak.

THORACIC ANEURYSMS

Clinical Presentation

Thoracic aneurysms are less prevalent than AAAs. The clinical presentation of thoracic aneurysms is similar to that of AAAs, in that most patients are asymptomatic. The most common clinical presentation results from compression of adjacent structures, which can produce chest pain, hoarseness from recurrent laryngeal nerve injury, back pain, or pulmonary problems from compression of bronchial structures.

Management and Therapy
Optimum Treatment

As is the case for surgical repair of infrarenal disease, surgical repair of thoracic aneurysms usually requires replacement of the diseased artery

(Fig. 62.2). However, the risks associated with surgical repair of thoracic and thoracoabdominal aneurysms are significantly higher than those of AAA repair. One major risk associated with thoracoabdominal aneurysm repair is paraplegia, because perfusion to the spinal cord must be interrupted during the repair. Several approaches have been developed to limit the amount of ischemia, including the use of barbiturates, hypothermia, and spinal cord drainage to increase perfusion pressure via collaterals. Even with these protective approaches, for extensive aneurysms involving the area from the left subclavian artery to the aortic bifurcation, the risk of paraplegia is as high as 25%. For small aneurysms involving a short section of the aorta, the risk of paraplegia is not negligible (2%–8%). Because of the high risk, treatment is delayed until the risk of rupture is greater than the risk of repair, typically when an aneurysm is 6 cm in diameter. Individuals with Marfan disease or other collagen vascular diseases represent an important subset in whom the risk of dissection and/or rupture is increased even at smaller aneurysm diameters; thus, these patients require earlier surgical intervention.

Recent treatment of thoracic aneurysms with endografts has lowered the risk associated with treating this problem and increased the number of patients who are candidates for treatment. The results of endovascular therapy trials being conducted for the treatment of thoracic diseases are promising. Although an association between endovascular therapy and paraplegia exists in patients with a concomitant or previous infrarenal repair, the association between the length of the aneurysm and paraplegia as a complication of surgical repair is not present when the aorta is covered by the endograft. Other thoracic aortic pathologies being treated include aortic dissections, aortic transections, penetrating ulcers, and ruptured plaques, all with promising results.

In the past, repair of many extensive thoracoabdominal aneurysms involved using atriofemoral bypass. In patients with visceral ischemia, especially to the kidneys and liver, the potential for renal failure and serious coagulopathy was significant with conventional surgical repair. Fortunately, recent studies have demonstrated that visceral revascularization techniques performed in conjunction with placement of an endograft have decreased the morbidity associated with thoracic aortic cross-clamping.

Avoiding Treatment Errors

There are few clinical manifestations associated with thoracic aneurysms. The diagnosis is by chest x-ray or CT scan in patients at high risk for systemic aneurysms.

THORACOABDOMINAL AORTIC ANEURYSMS

Thoracoabdominal aortic aneurysms (TAAAs) are more extensive aneurysms that are classified according to the DeBakey classification (types I–IV) and involve the descending thoracic aorta, and to varying degrees, the abdominal aorta. Clinical presentation is similar to other aortic aneurysms; however, the surgical treatment is significantly more invasive. Until recently, open surgical repair was the mainstay of treatment, which often required reimplantation of the visceral vessel. This can be associated with significant morbidity and mortality because of the comorbid medical condition in many of these patients. The most concerning of these complications is paraplegia, and depending on the extent of repair, this can occur in up to 15% of patients. More recently, endovascular techniques with fenestrated and branched devices have shown a significant reduction in major complications. Although these devices are available throughout Europe, they are currently only available at a few investigational institutions within the United States. As with other minimally invasive techniques, major morbidity and mortality is reduced by >50%.

AORTIC DISSECTION

Aortic dissection is defined as disruption of the medial layer of the aorta and separation with formation of a true and false lumen, with or without communication (Fig. 62.3). In most cases, an intimal tear is seen as the initiating condition, exacerbated by severe hypertension. The process is either followed by aortic rupture in the case of adventitial disruption, or reentering into the aortic lumen through a distal secondary reentry tear. The dissections can either be anterograde or retrograde. An acute dissection occurs with a time course of <14 days, subacute occurs between 15 and 90 days, and chronic dissection occurs at >90 days. The classification for aortic dissection is via the DeBakey system (divided into types I, II, and III) or the Stanford classification (type A or B). In the DeBakey system, type I includes involvement of the ascending and descending thoracic aortas. Type II only involves the ascending aorta. Type III involves the descending thoracic aorta distal to the left subclavian artery. There are subtypes within type III, with IIIa aortic dissections being confined to the descending thoracic aorta, whereas type IIIb aortic dissections extend into the abdominal aorta. In the Stanford classification, a type A dissection is when the tear begins in the ascending aorta and progresses throughout the vessel, often extending as far as the arteries in the leg. Type B dissection includes cases in which the tear is located only in the descending aorta and may extend into the abdomen.

The most common risk factor for acute aortic dissection is hypertension, with a preponderance in men. Chest pain is the most frequent symptoms of acute aortic dissection. An abrupt onset of severe chest or back pain is classic; the pain may be sharp, ripping, tearing, or knife-like. In addition, with distal extension of the dissection, back, abdominal, and lower extremity pain may be observed. A pulse deficit is common in up to 30% of patients, with changes in the left upper extremity or bilateral lower extremity pulses. End-organ dysfunction can be related to aortic dissection if it involves the visceral vessels and renal vessels, causing kidney failure, and paraplegia can be present due to occlusion of the spinal arteries (1% of the time). Furthermore, patients can have a cerebral malperfusion due to extension of the dissection into the supraaortic branches. Development of cardiac complications is common, with aortic regurgitation from dilation of the aortic root, with possible tearing of the annulus or valve cusps, and pericardial tamponade or congestive heart failure. Approximately 10% to 15% of patients with aortic dissection can have obliteration of the coronary vessel origins and may present with ST-elevation myocardial infarction.

Axial imaging is imperative to rule out acute aortic dissection in patients with concerning clinical symptoms. CT angiography (CTA) and magnetic resonance angiography are particularly useful and are able to identify true and false lumens, location of entry tears, malperfusion, or ischemia. Transesophageal echocardiography or gated CT scan can be useful in identifying ascending dissections. CTA is the most commonly used imaging technique due to speed, sensitivity, and rapid availability.

Treatment of acute aortic dissection depends on the location. For a type A dissection, surgery is a treatment of choice. The mortality rate within the first 48 hours if not operated on is 50%; however, perioperative mortality is approximately 25%, with a risk of neurological complications of 20%. Open repair involves either replacement of the ascending aorta, and depending on aortic valve involvement, often requires aortic valve replacement and reimplantation of the coronary arteries as needed. Extension into the aortic arch is often needed, with a hemi-arch or full arch replacement with a classic "island" technique. If the descending thoracic aorta is involved, often a "frozen elephant trunk" repair is performed, which maintains a free-floating graft in the descending thoracic aorta that can be used to dock with a thoracic endograft procedure in the future.

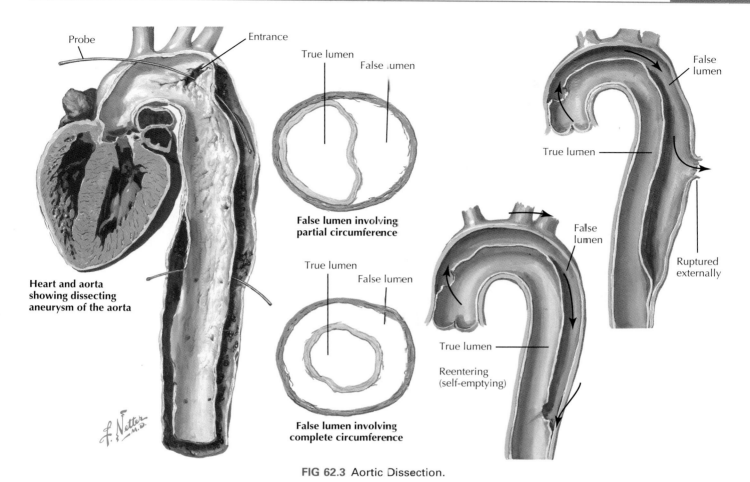

Probe

Entrance

True lumen

False lumen

False lumen involving
partial circumference

True lumen

False lumen

**Heart and aorta
showing dissecting
aneurysm of the aorta**

False lumen involving
complete circumference

False lumen

True lumen

False lumen

Ruptured
externally

False lumen

True lumen

Reentering
(self-emptying)

True lumen

FIG 62.3 Aortic Dissection.

Treatment of a type B aortic dissection depends on whether it is complicated or uncomplicated. The initial therapy for complicated aortic dissections is medical therapy with antiimpulse therapy, including intravenous β blockade. Rapid blood pressure control to maintain a systolic blood pressure of <120 mm Hg, and a heart rate of <70 beats/min is imperative. In the presence of malperfusion (spinal, visceral, lower extremity), rupture, uncontrolled hypertension, or continued symptoms, despite optimal medical therapy to decrease blood pressure, requires urgent repair. Thoracic endovascular aortic repair can be performed to cover the proximal tear, stabilize the dissected aorta, and prevent late complications by inducing aortic remodeling. Redirecting flow to the true lumen can assist in improving distal perfusion, thus ameliorating malperfusion.

CONCLUSIONS

Aortic disease can occur from a variety of vastly different pathologies that creates complexity in tailoring repair to these specific problems. Aneurysmal disease can involve the entirety of the aorta, and based on anatomic and morphological criteria, it can be repaired with simple endovascular stenting or require more invasive repairs with complex devices to incorporate branch vessels. Acute aortic syndromes are a significant cause of morbidity and mortality, and require rapid identification and management for improvement in results. Experience and

knowledge in a variety of surgical and endovascular techniques is required for best patient outcomes.

ADDITIONAL READING

Azizzadeh A, Keyhani K, Miller CC 3rd, Coogan SM, Safi HJ, Estrera AL. Blunt traumatic aortic injury: initial experience with endovascular repair. *J Vasc Surg.* 2009;49:1403–1408.
Single-center trial that examined the use of endovascular repair for blunt aortic injuries with results far superior to open repair.

Coselli JS Bozinovski J, LeMaire SA. Open surgical repair of 2286 thoracoabdominal aortic aneurysms. *Ann Thorac Surg.* 2007;83:S862–S864.
Large single-center retrospective study that showed excellent outcomes with open repair of thoracoabdominal aneurysms.

EVAR trial participants. Endovascular aneurysm repair versus open repair in patients with abdominal aortic aneurysm (EVAR trial 1): randomised controlled trial. *Lancet.* 2005;365:2179–2186.
Randomized multicenter study that evaluated the repair of infrarenal aortic aneurysms with either endovascular or open repair that showed no advantage to EVAR.

Greenberg RK, Lytle B. Endovascular repair of thoracoabdominal aneurysms. *Circulation.* 2008;117(17):2288–2296.
Review article that examined the use of fenestrated and branched endovascular devices for the repair of thoracoabdominal aneurysms

Lederle FA, Wilson SE, Johnson GR, Reinke DB, Littooy FN, Acher CW, et al. Immediate repair compared with surveillance of small abdominal aortic aneurysms. *N Engl J Med.* 2002;346:1437–1444.

Randomized multicenter trial that compared watchful waiting until 5.5 cm size versus early management of infrarenal aortic aneurysms, which found no benefit to early repair.

Pape LA, Awais M, Woznicki EM, Suzuki T, Trimarchi S, Evangelista A, et al. Presentation, diagnosis, and outcomes of acute aortic dissection:

17-year trends from the International Registry of Acute Aortic Dissection. *J Am Coll Cardiol.* 2015;66(4):350–358. doi:10.1016/j.jacc.2015.05.029.

Review of a multicenter database for the presentation, diagnosis, and outcomes of aortic dissection.

63

Deep Vein Thrombosis and Pulmonary Embolism

David W. Lee, Eric D. Pauley, Matthew A. Cavender

ETIOLOGY AND PATHOGENESIS

Venous thromboembolism (VTE) is common and has an annual incidence of approximately 0.1% in the general population. VTE is a broad term used to include patients with both deep venous thromboembolism (DVT) and pulmonary embolism (PE). These conditions warrant consideration together because up to 90% of PEs are secondary to DVT in the iliac, femoral, or popliteal venous systems. Less common sources of PE include calf vein thrombosis, pelvic vein thrombosis, thrombus formation from right heart abnormalities, upper extremity thrombosis, invasive tumors (renal cell carcinoma), and fat embolism secondary to trauma.

Venous thrombosis occurs when there is stasis of blood flow, endothelial injury, and hypercoagulability (commonly known as Virchow triad). Stasis of blood flow can occur when venous outflow is obstructed (e.g., May-Thurner Syndrome, which is left iliac venous obstruction secondary to an overlying right common iliac artery) or situations that lead to immobility (Fig. 63.1). Any travel resulting in immobility for >4 hours increases the risk of DVT by at least twofold, and this risk can persist for several weeks after travel. Although all hospitalized patients who are immobile are at increased risk of DVT, those in the postoperative setting have an additional risk. Surgery and trauma affect each element of the Virchow triad by decreasing venous flow in the setting of immobilization, allowing the exposure of tissue factor through endothelial damage, and increasing hypercoagulability via depletion of endogenous anticoagulants. Hypercoagulability can be inherited or acquired. Factor V Leiden mutation, prothrombin gene mutation, protein S deficiency, protein C deficiency, and antithrombin III deficiency are inherited conditions that account for approximately 10% of DVTs. Of these conditions, patients with protein S deficiency are most likely to have a DVT in their lifetime. Acquired hypercoagulable conditions include antiphospholipid syndrome, nephrotic syndrome, inflammatory bowel disease, heparin-induced thrombocytopenia, pregnancy, oral contraceptive pills, hormone replacement therapy, myeloproliferative disorders, and malignancy.

The pathogenesis of PE begins with the embolization of DVT (Fig. 63.2). PE results in a ventilation and/or perfusion (V/Q) mismatch by obstructing perfusion of pulmonary alveoli that have normal ventilation, leading to impaired gas exchange and/or hypoxemia, and possibly even infarction of the lung. An inflammatory process can contribute to atelectasis, which leads to intrapulmonary shunting and stimulation of the respiratory drive and respiratory alkalosis with hypocapnia. PE can also lead to acute pulmonary infarction if small emboli occlude the distal segmental and subsegmental vessels. The resulting parenchymal necrosis and pleural inflammation can cause pleuritic chest pain. Finally, PE can lead to obstructive shock and cardiovascular collapse if the thrombus burden is large enough to obstruct cardiac output from the right ventricle (Fig. 63.3). Large PEs can cause increased pulmonary vascular resistance, pulmonary hypertension, acute right ventricular (RV) failure, and RV dilatation. Due to the RV dilatation and reduced RV output, the left ventricular (LV) preload decreases and the cardiac output decreases, leading to systemic hypotension and obstructive shock.

CLINICAL PRESENTATION

When evaluating patients with possible DVT and/or PE, it is important for the clinician to be familiar with risk factors for VTE. The most important risk factors are immobilization or prolonged bedrest, recent surgery, tobacco use, obesity, previous VTE, lower extremity trauma, malignancy, hormone or oral contraceptive use, pregnancy or postpartum status, and stroke. A history of DVT and malignancy are the strongest predictors of VTE.

Deep Vein Thrombosis

The most common presenting symptoms of DVT are unilateral pain (46%), edema (40%), swelling (25%), and tenderness (27%) of the lower extremity. The location of symptoms does not always correlate with the location of the DVT. Patients with an isolated calf DVT can have pain throughout the leg, whereas patients with symptoms predominantly in the calf may have a proximal DVT. Physical examination findings consistent with DVT are calf erythema, calf warmth, and difference in calf diameter. Patients may have evidence of Homan sign, which is seen when there is resistance or pain with dorsiflexion of the foot. However, this sign is of little clinical usefulness because it is neither sensitive or specific for a DVT. The absence of calf swelling and/or difference in calf diameter are the most clinically useful findings when attempting to rule out DVT because each have a negative likelihood ratio greater than two.

Pulmonary Embolism

Patients with PE can have a variety of different presentations that range from no symptoms to shock and/or hemodynamic collapse. The most common presenting symptoms, in order of prevalence, are dyspnea, pleuritic chest pain, leg pain and/or swelling due to DVT, cough, orthopnea, wheezing, and hemoptysis. Less common presentations include arrhythmias, presyncope, syncope, and shock. Dyspnea, especially due to proximal infarction of a proximal vessel, is typically sudden in onset, with patients noticing worsening breathlessness over a matter of seconds. Distal vessel infarction can cause pleural inflammation and pleuritic chest pain. It is important to note that the preceding symptoms may be absent, even in the setting of significant amount of thrombus burden, and up to 25% of patients will not report the presence of dyspnea. Signs of PE, in order of prevalence, include hypoxemia, tachypnea, lower extremity pain and/or swelling, tachycardia, rales, decreased breath

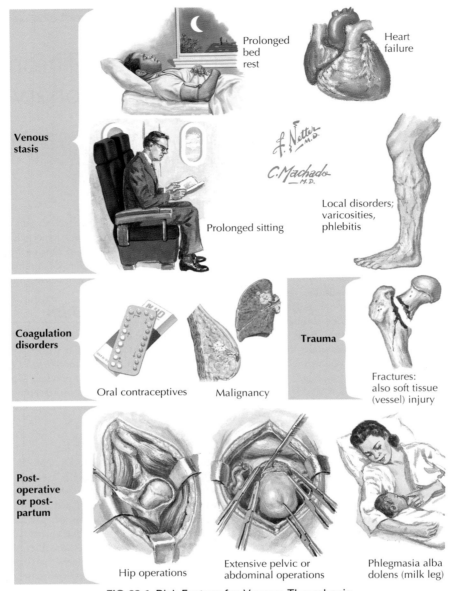

Prolonged bed rest

Heart failure

Venous stasis

Prolonged sitting

Local disorders; varicosities, phlebitis

Coagulation disorders

Oral contraceptives

Malignancy

Trauma

Fractures: also soft tissue (vessel) injury

Post-operative or post-partum

Hip operations

Extensive pelvic or abdominal operations

Phlegmasia alba dolens (milk leg)

FIG 63.1 Risk Factors for Venous Thrombosis.

sounds, loud pulmonic component of the second heart sound, jugular venous distention, and fever (Fig. 63.4).

DIFFERENTIAL DIAGNOSIS

Deep Vein Thrombosis

The differential diagnosis for DVT includes other disorders that cause redness, swelling, and/or pain of the lower extremities. Muscular injuries are a frequent cause of swelling and pain, and are typically apparent by history. Immobility that results from these musculoskeletal injuries can predispose patients to DVT. Baker cysts are the result of fluid collection that can result in swelling behind the knee. When these cysts rupture, they can cause calf pain and appear similar to a DVT. Large cysts can compress the popliteal vein, and cause concomitant DVT via venous stasis. Lymphangitis, inflammation of the lymphatic vessels, can be caused by both infectious and noninfectious causes. In patients with lymphangitis, it is important to evaluate the distal extremity for

evidence of skin abrasions or infection. Cellulitis is a common cause of acute unilateral edema, pain, redness, and swelling of the extremity, and can present with a fever. It is more common in patients with chronic venous insufficiency and lymphedema. Patients with lower extremity edema from either increased venous pressure (heart failure, constrictive pericarditis, venous outflow obstruction, stasis, or insufficiency) or loss of oncotic pressure (malnutrition, liver disease) can have presentations similar to that of a DVT.

Pulmonary Embolism

The differential diagnosis of PE includes processes that cause acute dyspnea, chest pain (especially pleuritic), hemoptysis, tachycardia, and/or hypoxia. Pneumothorax, a collection of air between the visceral and parietal pleura that results in collapse of the lung, can cause acute dyspnea and chest pain. Tension pneumothorax is a life-threatening condition that must be recognized and treated quickly. Acute coronary syndrome (ACS), which is also life-threatening, typically manifests with

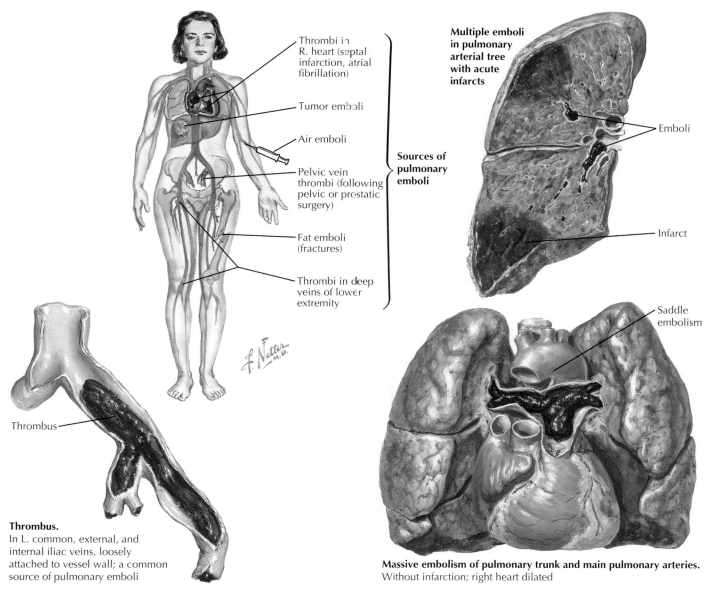

Thrombi in R. heart (septal infarction, atrial fibrillation)

Tumor emboli

Air emboli

Pelvic vein thrombi (following pelvic or prostatic surgery)

Fat emboli (fractures)

Thrombi in deep veins of lower extremity

Sources of pulmonary emboli

Multiple emboli in pulmonary arterial tree with acute infarcts

Emboli

Infarct

Saddle embolism

Thrombus.
In L. common, external, and internal iliac veins, loosely attached to vessel wall; a common source of pulmonary emboli

Thrombus

Massive embolism of pulmonary trunk and main pulmonary arteries.
Without infarction; right heart dilated

FIG 63.2 Pathogenesis of Acute Pulmonary Embolism.

angina rather than pleuritic chest pain. Dyspnea and hypoxia are not as profound in ACS as in patients with a PE, and hemoptysis is rare. Pneumonia manifests as fever, cough, and consolidation on imaging, which can help differentiate this condition from PE. Vasculitis, with or without diffuse alveolar hemorrhage, can lead to hypoxia and hemoptysis, but should have evidence of an interstitial infiltrate on imaging. Primary pulmonary malignancies or metastases can cause acute intrapulmonary complications leading to hemoptysis, hypoxia, chest pain, and pleural effusions. Likewise, the worsening of underlying lung disorders, such as chronic obstructive pulmonary disease (COPD), asthma, bronchiectasis, and congenital heart diseases, can also cause respiratory decompensation.

DIAGNOSTIC APPROACH

Laboratory Evaluation

Laboratory data can be helpful in the clinical assessment of patients, but these data do not have sufficient specificity to diagnose DVT or PE.

Patients with PE may have respiratory alkalosis, hypocapnia, hypoxemia, and an increased alveolar–arterial oxygen gradient on an arterial blood gas at room air. However, a normal arterial blood gas does not exclude the diagnosis of PE. Patients with VTE typically have an elevated plasma D-dimer. The D-dimer assay measures a degradation product released by the lysis of a cross-linked fibrin clot, and elevated levels have a 99.5% sensitivity for the diagnosis of DVT and PE. However, D-dimer has poor specificity, and can be elevated in a variety of clinical scenarios, including in patients with advanced age, sepsis, recent surgery, pregnancy, chronic inflammatory disease, and malignancy. Finally, patients with PE and RV dysfunction typically have elevated troponin and/or pro-brain natriuretic peptide (pro-BNP) levels as a result of myocardial injury and/or stretch. Although these cardiac biomarkers cannot be used to diagnose PE, they can be helpful in the risk stratification of patients with PE.

Electrocardiography

ECG is not useful in the diagnosis of PE due to poor sensitivity and specificity. The most common ECG findings in patients with PE include:

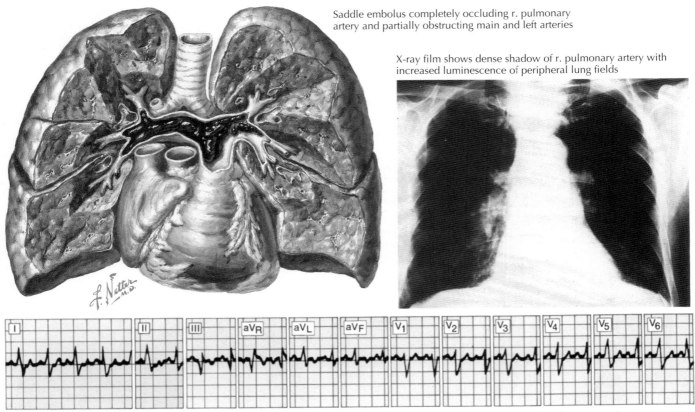

Saddle embolus completely occluding r. pulmonary artery and partially obstructing main and left arteries

X-ray film shows dense shadow of r. pulmonary artery with increased luminescence of peripheral lung fields

Characteristic electrocardiographic findings in acute pulmonary embolism. Deep S_1; prominent Q_3 with inversion of T_3; depression of S-T segment in lead II (often also in lead I) with staircase ascent of S-T_2; T_2 diphasic or inverted; r. axis deviation; tachycardia

FIG 63.3 Saddle Embolus.

sinus tachycardia; an incomplete or complete right bundle branch block; an S wave in lead I with a Q wave and an inverted T wave in lead III (S1, Q3, T3 pattern); and inverted T waves in leads V_1 through V_4. However, a normal ECG does not exclude the diagnosis of PE.

Echocardiography

Although limited in its ability to diagnose PE, transthoracic echocardiography can be used to risk stratify patients and identify those with submassive or massive PE. The common echocardiographic findings in patients with submassive or massive PE include RV dilatation (defined as a RV-to-LV dimension ratio of ≥0.9), RV systolic dysfunction (tricuspid annular plane systolic excursion <1.7 cm), and interventricular septal flattening. The presence of McConnell sign, which is defined as hypokinesis of the RV free wall with normal contraction of the RV apex, can help differentiate RV dysfunction due to a PE from causes of global RV dysfunction (e.g., pulmonary hypertension). Furthermore, a transthoracic echocardiogram can help narrow the differential diagnosis by ruling out pericardial effusion, LV systolic dysfunction, and focal wall motion abnormalities that may suggest myocardial infarction. At times, it may be possible to see a clot in transit either in the right atrium, the RV, or main pulmonary arteries.

Imaging

Lower extremity venous compression ultrasound has 100% sensitivity and 99% specificity for proximal DVT, and 93% sensitivity for calf DVT. CT venography, magnetic resonance venography, and invasive catheter-based contrast venography can also be used to diagnose DVT

with high sensitivity and high specificity. Although invasive venography was previously considered the gold standard, venous compression ultrasound is sufficient to diagnose DVT and has become the preferred diagnostic modality for DVT because it is accurate, safe, widely available, and cost-effective. Ultrasonic or venographic evidence of DVT in patients with PE symptoms confirms the diagnosis of PE. However, a normal venous compression ultrasound or venography does not exclude the diagnosis of PE, and chest imaging should be obtained in patients with suspected PE and normal lower extremity venous studies.

Chest radiography in patients with PE may demonstrate the Hampton hump (defined as a dome-shaped density in the lung periphery resulting from pulmonary infarction in the presence of vessel occlusion) or the Westermark sign (focal hypovolemia resulting from vessel collapse distal to the PE), but radiography may also be normal and is typically not useful in the diagnosis of PE. CT pulmonary angiography (CTPA) has at least 90% sensitivity and 96% specificity for PE (Fig. 63.5). Magnetic resonance pulmonary angiography and invasive catheter-based, contrast-enhanced pulmonary angiography can also be used to diagnose PE with high sensitivity and high specificity. Although invasive pulmonary angiography was previously considered the gold standard, CTPA is sufficient to diagnose PE and has become the preferred diagnostic modality for PE because it is accurate, safe, widely available, and cost-effective. In patients with any contraindications to CTPA or inconclusive results on CTPA, V/Q scans can be performed to assess for perfusion defects. The major limitations of V/Q scans include test results that are characterized as normal, low probability, intermediate probability, or high probability (rather than a diagnosis); the high

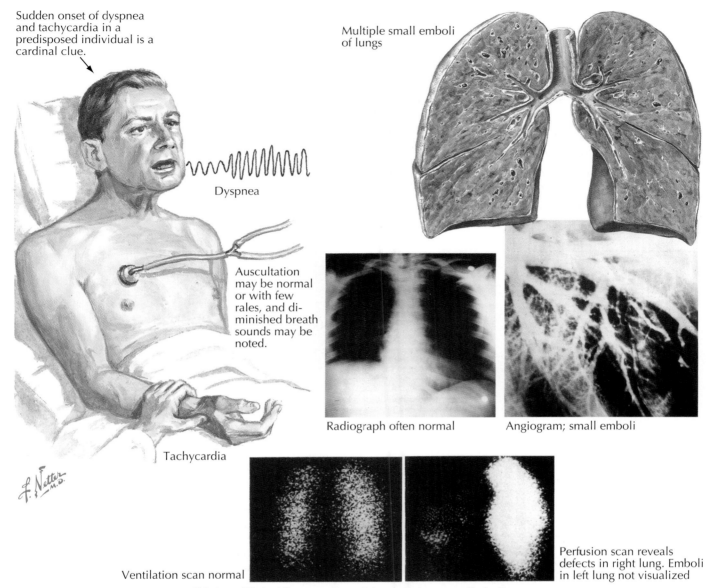

Sudden onset of dyspnea and tachycardia in a predisposed individual is a cardinal clue.

Dyspnea

Auscultation may be normal or with few rales, and diminished breath sounds may be noted.

Tachycardia

Multiple small emboli of lungs

Radiograph often normal

Angiogram; small emboli

Ventilation scan normal

Perfusion scan reveals defects in right lung. Emboli in left lung not visualized

FIG 63.4 Clinical Presentation of Acute Pulmonary Embolism.

false-positive rate; and indeterminate results in the setting of abnormal chest radiographs.

Strategy for Diagnostic Evaluation

Because the history, physical examination, and laboratory data of patients with suspected DVT and PE are fairly nonspecific, clinical prediction models can be used to determine the pretest likelihood of VTE and guide diagnostic evaluation. Wells and colleagues developed a risk score that has been validated to determine the pretest likelihood of VTE (Table 63.1). Based on the Wells score, patients can be identified as having a low, intermediate, or high pretest likelihood of VTE and can be referred for specific diagnostic studies. Patients with a low pretest likelihood of VTE can be initially evaluated with a plasma D-dimer level. The diagnosis of VTE can be excluded in patients with a low pretest likelihood and a normal D-dimer level. In patients with an intermediate or high pretest likelihood or those with an elevated D-dimer level, a venous compression ultrasound or a CTPA can be performed

in patients with suspected DVT or PE, respectively. In patients with suspected PE and a contraindication to CTPA or inconclusive results on CTPA, either a V/Q scan to evaluate for PE or a venous compression ultrasound to evaluate for DVT can be performed. Finally, in patients with suspected DVT or PE and inconclusive results on the preceding studies, invasive contrast venography or pulmonary angiography can be performed, respectively.

MANAGEMENT AND THERAPY

Early Risk Stratification

Patients with symptomatic acute PE have a 10% risk of early mortality, and should undergo rapid risk stratification to guide management upon diagnosis (Table 63.2). High-risk PE, or massive PE, constitutes acute PE associated with cardiac arrest, sustained hypotension and/or shock (defined as systolic blood pressure <90 mm Hg for at least 15 minutes or requiring inotropic support), or persistent bradycardia (defined as

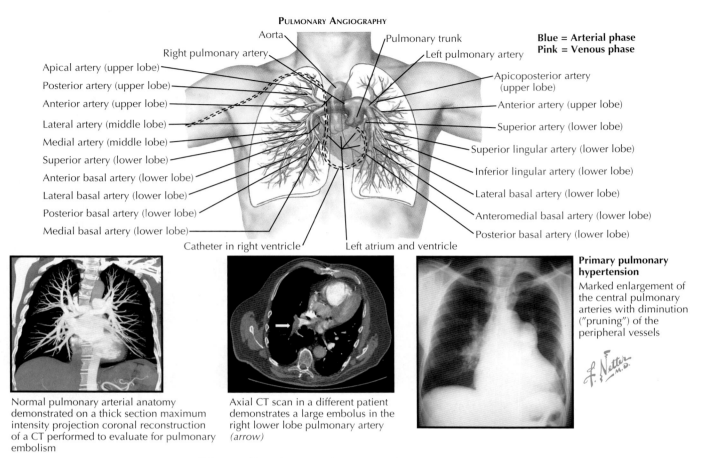

PULMONARY ANGIOGRAPHY

Blue = Arterial phase
Pink = Venous phase

Normal pulmonary arterial anatomy demonstrated on a thick section maximum intensity projection coronal reconstruction of a CT performed to evaluate for pulmonary embolism

Axial CT scan in a different patient demonstrates a large embolus in the right lower lobe pulmonary artery *(arrow)*

Primary pulmonary hypertension
Marked enlargement of the central pulmonary arteries with diminution ("pruning") of the peripheral vessels

FIG 63.5 Chest Imaging for Acute Pulmonary Embolism.

TABLE 63.1 Wells Model for the Pretest Likelihood of Deep Venous Thrombosis

Criteria	Points
Signs and Symptoms	
• Entire leg swelling	1
• Calf swelling at least 3 cm, compared with the asymptomatic leg	1
• Pitting edema confined to the symptomatic leg	1
• Collateralization of superficial veins	1
• Localized tenderness along the deep veins	1
Risk Factors	
• Previous diagnosis of VTE	1
• Active malignancy	1
• Paralysis, paresis, or recent immobilization of lower extremity	1
• Recently bedridden for at least 3 days, or major surgery within the previous 12 wks requiring regional or general anesthesia	1
Clinical Judgment	
• Alternative diagnosis at least as likely as DVT	−2

Total points for low likelihood <1, intermediate likelihood 1 to 2, high likelihood >2.
DVT, Deep venous thrombosis; *VTE,* venous thromboembolism.

heart rate <40 beats/min). Intermediate-risk PE, also known as submassive PE, includes acute PE associated with CT evidence of RV dilatation, echocardiographic evidence of RV dilatation or systolic dysfunction, or elevated cardiac biomarkers (i.e., troponin or pro-BNP). Patients with low-risk PE have evidence of PE but do not have any of these high-risk features.

Systemic Anticoagulation

Systemic anticoagulation is the standard therapy for all patients with acute DVT and PE. Because of the risk of early mortality associated with PE, patients in whom there is a high suspicion for PE should be treated immediately with systemic anticoagulation before further diagnostic evaluation is performed. Patients with suspected DVT who do not have signs consistent with PE can wait for anticoagulation until after a confirmatory test. Intravenous unfractionated heparin (UFH) or subcutaneous low-molecular-weight heparins (LMWHs; enoxaparin, dalteparin) have historically been the preferred therapies during the initial treatment phase. Intravenous UFH is typically administered as an 80 U/kg bolus followed by a continuous infusion initiated at 18 U/kg per hour, with periodic rate adjustments made based on the activated partial thromboplastin time or factor Xa level. Subcutaneous LMWH, or enoxaparin, is typically administered as a 1 mg/kg injection every 12 hours with dose adjustments made based on renal function. Direct oral anticoagulants (DOACs), which are increasingly being used as initial therapy in patients with confirmed DVT and/or PE, are appropriate, especially for low-risk patients in whom fibrinolytic therapy (either systemic or catheter directed) is not needed. Before starting treatment,

TABLE 63.2 Contemporary Risk Stratification and Management of Acute Pulmonary Embolism

Category	Criteria (Only Need 1)	Mortality Risk	Management

Massive	• Survived cardiac arrest
	• Sustained hypotension with:
	  • SBP <90 mm Hg for at least 15 min, or
	  • Obstructive shock requiring inotropic support
	• Persistent profound bradycardia (HR <40 beats/min)
		High	• Anticoagulation
			• Systemic thrombolysis
			• Surgical embolectomy
			• Catheter-based intervention[a]

Submassive	• RV dysfunction with:
	  • RV dilatation (RV/LV ratio >0.9) on CT, or echocardiogram, or
	  • RV systolic dysfunction on echocardiogram, or
	  • Elevated BNP or N-terminal pro-BNP
	• Myocardial necrosis, defined as elevated troponin
		Intermediate	• Anticoagulation
			• Systemic thrombolysis, surgical embolectomy, or catheter-based intervention, if poor prognosis
			• Ultrasound-assisted, catheter-directed thrombolysis

Low risk	None of the above	Low	• Anticoagulation

[a]In patients with contraindications to systemic fibrinolysis or in whom fibrinolytic therapy failed.
BNP, Brain natriuretic peptide; *HR*, heart rate; *LV*, left ventricular; *RV*, right ventricular; *SBP*, systolic blood pressure.

TABLE 63.3 Anticoagulation Therapies for Venous Thromboembolism

Drug	Mechanism of Action	Benefits	Risks
Warfarin	Vitamin K antagonist	• Reversal possible with vitamin K and FFP • Safe in all age groups • Largest evidence base • Widely available • Low cost	• Slow onset and offset • Long half-life • Numerous drug interactions • Need for frequent monitoring • Unpredictable pharmacokinetics • Diet restrictions
Dabigatran	Direct thrombin inhibitor	• Reversal possible with antidote (idarucizumab) • Quick onset and offset • Short half-life	• Inability to monitor drug • Less evidence base • High cost • Increased risk of GI bleed
Apixaban Rivaroxaban Edoxaban	Direct factor Xa inhibitor	• Rapid onset and offset • Short half-life • Few drug interactions • Predictable pharmacokinetics • No dietary restrictions	• Not reversible • Inability to monitor drug • Less evidence base • High cost

FFP, Fresh frozen plasma; *GI, gastrointestinal.*

the presence of absolute or relative contraindications to anticoagulation (i.e., active bleeding, bleeding diathesis) must be carefully assessed.

Patients with VTE require long-term therapy (Table 63.3). In patients with active malignancy, LMWH has been shown to provide a significant lower recurrence rate of VTE compared with warfarin. For all other patients, long-term therapy with an oral anticoagulant is appropriate. Warfarin, a vitamin K antagonist that inhibits factors II, VII, IX, X, and proteins C and S, has historically been the most common oral anticoagulant used in clinical practice for the treatment of VTE. It can be reversed with vitamin K and fresh frozen plasma in the setting of active bleeding. The major limitations of warfarin include slow onset with a long half-life, numerous drug–drug and drug–food interactions, and the need for frequent monitoring due to variability in pharmacodynamics. The DOACs have rapid onset with a short half-life, fewer drug–drug or drug–food interactions, and do not require frequent monitoring. As a result, these agents are being used at a high frequency in clinical practice. Currently available DOACs include a direct thrombin inhibitor (dabigatran) and direct factor Xa inhibitors (apixaban, rivaroxaban, edoxaban). Although dabigatran can be reversed with an antidote (idarucizumab), the direct factor Xa inhibitors do not have specific reversal agents at this time.

The optimal duration of therapeutic anticoagulation depends on the presence of any reversible risk factors for thrombosis (recent surgery, recent bedrest, recent limb immobilization, pregnancy, oral contraceptives, hormone replacement therapy) and the risk of bleeding while on anticoagulation. Acute VTE in the presence of major risk factors for thrombosis can be classified as provoked or secondary VTE, and is typically treated with anticoagulation therapy for at least 3 months (assuming the risk factor has resolved). Acute VTE in the absence of these major risk factors is classified as unprovoked or idiopathic VTE, and is typically treated with a longer duration of anticoagulation therapy. Randomized trials that have evaluated the duration of anticoagulation in patients with unprovoked VTE have found lower rates of recurrence in patients treated with extended duration of DOACs. Decisions regarding the duration of therapy must account for both the risk of future VTEs and the risk of bleeding with extended anticoagulation. VTE in the setting of malignancy and recurrent VTE are also treated with anticoagulation indefinitely.

Systemic Thrombolysis

In addition to systemic anticoagulation with UFH, systemic thrombolysis is standard therapy for patients with massive PE, including those patients with shock. Thrombolysis rapidly dissolves thromboembolism and relieves the obstructive shock that causes hemodynamic collapse in patients with massive PE. Alteplase is the only Food and Drug Administration–approved thrombolytic agent for the treatment of massive PE, and is administered intravenously as a continuous infusion of 100 mg over 2 hours. Systemic anticoagulation is typically discontinued during the infusion of thrombolytic therapy. The decision to administer systemic thrombolytic therapy in patients with massive or submassive PE must be made only after carefully considering the benefits, risks, indications, contraindications, and alternatives of thrombolysis. The most significant risks of systemic thrombolysis are major bleeding (up to 19% incidence) and intracranial hemorrhage (up to 3% incidence). Absolute contraindications to systemic thrombolysis include active bleeding, bleeding diathesis, previous intracranial hemorrhage or conditions that may increase the risk of bleeding (i.e., intracranial neoplasm, arteriovenous malformation, aneurysm), ischemic stroke in the past 3 months, head or facial trauma in the past 3 months, and suspected aortic dissection. Relative contraindications to systemic thrombolysis include any previous ischemic stroke >3 months ago, severe uncontrolled hypertension, recent internal bleeding, noncompressible vascular puncture, recent invasive procedure, anticoagulant use with an international normalized ratio >1.7 or prothrombin time >15 seconds, pregnancy, and age older than 75 years.

Surgical Embolectomy

Surgical embolectomy is indicated in patients with massive PE and those with contraindications to systemic thrombolysis or failure of systemic thrombolysis. In addition, patients who have evidence of VTE trapped within a patent foramen ovale or the RV can benefit from surgical embolectomy. Although it involves cardiopulmonary bypass with circulatory arrest, surgical embolectomy is associated with lower rates of recurrent PE, major bleeding complications, and mortality in patients who have failed systemic thrombolysis compared with repeat thrombolytic therapy.

Catheter-Based Intervention

Multiple percutaneous interventions have shown efficacy in reducing clot burden through fragmentation and/or embolectomy, and can be used in patients with massive PE who have contraindications to systemic thrombolysis or in whom systemic thrombolysis has failed. Suction embolectomy catheters allow for the manual aspiration of thrombus through the catheter; however, these devices have limited usefulness in PE because of the typical size of the thrombus. The AngioJet (Boston Scientific, Marlborough, Massachusetts) is a rheolytic embolectomy device, and involves the injection of a fibrinolytic agent through the distal tip of a catheter to thrombolyze and mechanically disrupt thrombus. After allowing the fibrinolytic agent to dwell within the affected area for 15 to 20 minutes, aspiration of the thrombus can be done through the same catheter. Rotational embolectomy catheters are also available that are designed to fragment thrombus while continuously aspirating clot fragments.

The EKOS device (BTG, Philadelphia, Pennsylvania) combines an infusion catheter for thrombolytic therapy with an ultrasound component designed to further reduce thrombus burden. Catheter-directed, ultrasound-assisted thrombolytic therapy using the EKOS device is increasingly being used for the treatment of submassive PE. The Ultrasound-Accelerated Thrombolysis of Pulmonary Embolism (ULTIMA) study randomized 59 patients with intermediate-risk PE to either UFH or EKOS. Patients treated with EKOS had greater improvement in the ratio of the RV-to-LV dimension. There were no differences in major bleeding compared with UFH alone. The SEATTLE II study showed that, in patients with submassive or massive PE, EKOS therapy followed by UFH significantly decreased RV dilation, reduced pulmonary hypertension, and decreased anatomic thrombus burden. The effects of EKOS on mortality and other clinical outcomes remain unknown.

FUTURE DIRECTIONS

Challenges in the evaluation and management of acute PE include: the nonspecific clinical presentation of patients; the potential for rapid clinical deterioration; the significant risk of early mortality; the need for quick and accurate diagnosis, as well as the need for risk stratification; and the need to consult with multiple specialties for the optimal treatment strategy. Multidisciplinary teams called PE response teams have formed at numerous medical centers across the nation to address these challenges. The purpose of these teams are to create a mechanism that prioritizes effective, safe, and rapid care in patients with suspected or known PE; to create a platform that unifies clinicians from different specialties to discuss patients and agree on the optimal treatment strategy; and to provide a platform for data collection that will establish better evidence-based practice.

ADDITIONAL RESOURCES

Dudzinski DM, Piazza G. Multidisciplinary pulmonary embolism response teams. *Circulation.* 2016;133(1):98–103.
Reference on the rationale and implementation of PE response teams.
Fesmire FM, Brown MD, Espinosa JA, Shih RD, et al. Critical issues in the evaluation and management of adult patients presenting to the emergency department with suspected pulmonary embolism. *Ann Emerg Med.* 2011;57(6):628–652.
Perspective on the evaluation and management of PE, published by the American College of Emergency Physicians.
Jaber WA, Fong PP, Weisz G, Lattouf O, et al. Acute pulmonary embolism: with an emphasis on an interventional approach. *J Am Coll Cardiol.* 2016;67(8):991–1002.
Council perspective on the management of acute PE, published by the American College of Cardiology.
Jaff MR, McMurtry MS, Archer SL, Cushman M, et al. Management of massive and submassive pulmonary embolism, iliofemoral deep vein thrombosis, and chronic thromboembolic pulmonary hypertension: a statement from the American Heart Association. *Circulation.* 2011;123(16):1788–1830.
Guidelines on the management of PE and DVT, published by the American Heart Association.
Kearon C, Akl EA, Ornelas J, Blaivas A, et al. Antithrombotic therapy for VTE disease: CHEST guideline and expert panel report. *Chest.* 2016;149(2):315–352.
Guidelines on antithrombotic therapy for VTE, published by the American College of Chest Physicians.
Raja AS, Greenberg JO, Qaseem A, Denberg TD, et al. Evaluation of patients with suspected acute pulmonary embolism: best practice advice from the Clinical Guidelines Committee of the American College of Physicians. *Ann Intern Med.* 2015;163(9):701–711.
Guidelines on the evaluation of suspected PE, published by the American College of Physicians.

EVIDENCE

Kearon C. Natural history of venous thromboembolism. *Circulation.* 2003;107:I-22–I-30.
Review of the natural history of VTE.
Konstantinides SV, Barco S, Lankeit M, Meyer G. Management of pulmonary embolism: an update. *J Am Coll Cardiol.* 2016;67:976–990.
Review of the management of PE.

Kucher N, Boekstegers P, Muller OJ, Kupatt C, et al. Randomized, controlled trial of ultrasound-assisted catheter-directed thrombolysis for acute intermediate-risk pulmonary embolism. *Circulation.* 2014;129(4):479–486.
Prospective multicenter randomized controlled trial that compared ultrasound-assisted, catheter-directed thrombolysis plus UFH versus UFH alone in acute intermediate-risk PE.

Piazza G, Hohlfelder B, Jaff MR, Ouriel K, et al. A prospective, single-arm, multicenter trial of ultrasound-facilitated, catheter-directed, low-dose fibrinolysis for acute massive and submassive pulmonary embolism: the SEATTLE II study. *JACC Cardiovasc Interv.* 2015;8(10):1382–1392.
Prospective multicenter registry of ultrasound-facilitated, catheter-directed thrombolysis, in acute massive and submassive PE.

Cardiac Considerations in Specific Populations and Systemic Diseases

64

Cardiovascular Disease in Pregnancy

Patricia P. Chang, Thomas S. Ivester

Cardiovascular conditions are among the most common causes of maternal mortality in the United States. As more women delay childbearing into their thirties and forties, the interaction among coronary disease, its risk factors, and pregnancy is becoming increasingly important in prenatal care. In addition, more women with congenital heart disease are reaching childbearing age. Thus, a multidisciplinary approach is needed to achieve optimal maternal and fetal outcomes. Understanding normal physiological adaptations to pregnancy and their potential effect on cardiovascular hemodynamics is central to the management of pregnant women with and without heart disease.

PHYSIOLOGICAL ADAPTATIONS TO PREGNANCY

Changes During Pregnancy

Two important hematologic parameters that affect hemodynamic changes during pregnancy are increases in red blood cell mass and plasma volume. Plasma blood volume generally increases by approximately 50%, and red blood cell mass concomitantly increases by 20% to 30% (Fig. 64.1). This rise in total blood volume creates a relative physiological anemia of pregnancy. The etiology of this blood volume increase is multifactorial and due mainly to activation of the renin-angiotensin-aldosterone system by estrogen. Other pathways responsible for water retention are stimulated by other pregnancy-related hormones. Another important hematologic change is that blood becomes hypercoagulable because of estrogen-induced increases in coagulation factors and vascular stasis.

Cardiac output (CO) increases by 45% to 50% during a normal pregnancy, starting as early as 5 weeks after the last menstrual period, predominantly from an increase in stroke volume (during the first and second trimesters) and an increase in heart rate (10–20 beats/min during the third trimester). Most of the increase in CO occurs by gestational week 16. This increase is followed by a further, slower increase in CO that peaks at week 24 until week 32. There is also a 34% decrease in the systemic vascular resistance (SVR) by 20 weeks due to decreased aortic compliance and arteriovenous shunting in the uterus. Subsequently, in the final weeks of pregnancy, there is a slight decrease in CO, which is primarily caused by decreased stroke volume and increased SVR (Fig. 64.1, middle panel).

Structural changes of the heart are related to these hemodynamic changes. The left ventricular (LV) mass increases because of increased LV end-diastolic volume, decreased LV end-systolic volume, and increased wall thickness. There is also an increase in the valvular cross-sectional area, which results in more physiological regurgitation and affects the tricuspid and pulmonary valves more commonly than the mitral valve, but which rarely results in audible murmurs. Because of hormone-mediated changes to the thoracic cavity, the heart is typically displaced slightly cephalad and laterally, and the lung apices rise higher into the thoracic inlet.

Positional changes also have hemodynamically significant effects on the pregnant woman. Of particular importance is the supine hypotension syndrome characterized by symptoms of near-syncope and/or syncope, which is caused by compression or occlusion of the inferior vena cava (IVC) by the gravid uterus when she lays supine. The symptoms can be relieved by assuming another position, particularly tilting to the left or lying in the left lateral decubitus position (Fig. 64.1, lower panel). Supine hypotension syndrome is one of the primary reasons to advise pregnant women against exercising in the supine position at approximately 20 to 23 weeks. IVC compression also reduces CO by 8% at 24 weeks and by 25% at 33 weeks. This positional effect is especially important if the pregnant woman, particularly in the second or third trimester, needs cardiopulmonary resuscitation, in which case, she should be placed in the left lateral decubitus position.

Changes During Labor and Delivery

Marked increases occur in stroke volume, heart rate, and, subsequently, CO during labor and delivery. Blood pressure (BP; both systolic and diastolic) and oxygen consumption also increase significantly. The degree of pain and anxiety during labor has a dramatic effect on these parameters, but modulation via analgesia, sedation, or both may help. With each contraction, SVR typically increases by 10% to 25% because of autotransfusion of 300 to 500 mL of blood. CO also increases as labor progresses, by 17% early on, and by 34% when cervical dilation is approximately 8 cm. Heavy Valsalva maneuvers may decrease preload during the second stage of labor (when the cervix is completely dilated through the birth of baby).

Significant hemodynamic changes occur with both vaginal delivery and cesarean section (C-section). The decision to pursue cesarean delivery should be individualized and based on the status of the fetus and the hemodynamic state of the mother. Although counterintuitive, vaginal delivery causes fewer hemodynamic alterations than C-section and is generally better tolerated even in women with heart disease. Therefore, vaginal delivery is the recommended mode of delivery unless there is an obstetric indication for C-section. Exceptions include those with a markedly dilated aortic root (>5.5 cm) as seen in Marfan syndrome (in whom a hypertensive episode might cause aortic dissection), women with severe aortic coarctation with poorly controlled hypertension, and in the setting of acute severe cardiovascular decompensation. Another alternative is to offer an assisted second-stage labor (forceps or vacuum), which avoids the maximal stresses incurred with maternal expulsive efforts. In addition, special precaution should be given regarding epidural or spinal anesthesia in women with certain conditions, including aortic stenosis (AS), complicated coarctation of the aorta, tetralogy of

Hematologic changes in pregnancy

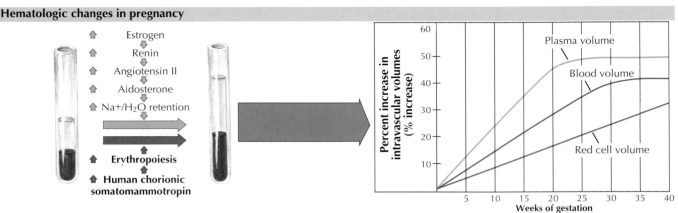

Multifactorial stimulation of fluid retention and erythropoiesis in pregnancy results in a 50% increase in plasma volume and a 30% increase in red cell mass, creating a relative "physiological" anemia and an increased blood volume.

Changes in cardiac output

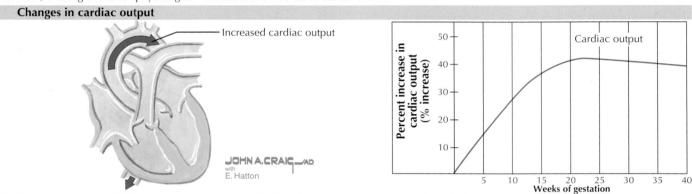

Cardiac output increases 50% in normal pregnancy, predominantly from increased stroke volume in first and second trimesters and increased pulse rate in third trimester.

Postural changes

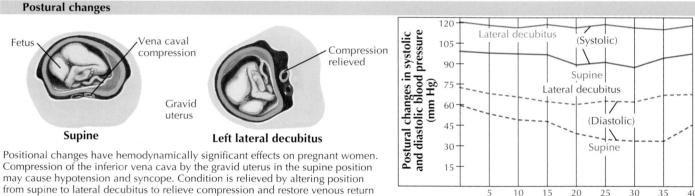

Positional changes have hemodynamically significant effects on pregnant women. Compression of the inferior vena cava by the gravid uterus in the supine position may cause hypotension and syncope. Condition is relieved by altering position from supine to lateral decubitus to relieve compression and restore venous return and cardiac output.

FIG 64.1 Cardiovascular Adaptations to Pregnancy. *Na+,* Sodium.

Fallot, hypertrophic obstructive cardiomyopathy, pulmonary hypertension, and Eisenmenger syndrome.

Changes in the Postpartum Period

After delivery, CO again increases because of increased venous return from relief of IVC compression, autotransfusion of uterine blood, and fluid mobilization. CO returns to prelabor values within 1 hour of delivery and through 2 to 6 weeks after vaginal delivery. Fluid shifts are greatest in the first 48 to 72 hours postpartum because typical blood loss at delivery is 300 to 1000 mL. Caution should be exercised in volume administration in postpartum patients with heart failure (HF).

CLINICAL PRESENTATION

Cardiac Examination During Normal Pregnancy

The symptoms of normal pregnancy, which often include fatigue, dyspnea, palpitations, and even near-syncope, in association with the normal signs of pregnancy, including augmentation of the jugular venous pulsations, normal heart sounds or murmurs, and a modest amount of lower extremity edema, may be misinterpreted as those of cardiac disease. Conversely, pathological signs and symptoms at times may be attributed to normal pregnancy. Thus, knowledge of the normal cardiac examination of pregnancy is crucial (Table 64.1).

TABLE 64.1 Normal Physical Findings for the Cardiac Examination During Pregnancy

Examination	Findings
Precordial palpation	Laterally displaced left ventricular impulse
	Palpable right ventricular impulse
Heart sounds	Increased intensity of S_1 and S_2
	Splitting of S_1
	Increased physiological splitting of S_2
Heart murmurs	Midsystolic murmurs (common; usually grade I and II/VI), heard best at left lower sternal border
	Diastolic murmurs (rare; soft, medium to high pitched), heard best over the pulmonic area and over the left sternal border
	Continuous murmurs:
	Cervical venous hum: heard best over the right supraclavicular fossa
	Mammary souffle (may also be heard as only a systolic murmur): heard best in the left 2nd to 4th intercostal space; decreased by pressing stethoscope firmly against the chest wall and the upright position

Although the presence of an S_3 had been previously believed to be a normal finding in pregnancy and in young adults, it is still relatively rare in the healthy pregnant state. An S_4 is unusual and usually pathological. Because of increased plasma volume and CO, new or more prominent systolic flow murmurs may be detected during pregnancy. Although diastolic murmurs have been reported in normal pregnancy, if a diastolic murmur is identified, echocardiography should be performed to exclude valvular pathology. With more plasma volume, the pregnant woman may show mild jugular venous distention and peripheral edema, and the pulse pressure becomes more widened with more of a decrease in the diastolic BP than in the systolic component.

DIFFERENTIAL DIAGNOSIS

Distinguishing between normal pregnancy and pathological symptoms during pregnancy is often difficult. Whether cardiac in origin or not, common cardiac symptoms include chest pains, palpitations, exertional dyspnea or fatigue, and peripheral edema. Chest pains are rarely cardiac in etiology, but should warrant an ECG if symptoms are worrisome for angina. During pregnancy, nonspecific ST- and T-wave changes and left-axis deviation may be present on ECG due to physiological changes (a laterally displaced and slightly enlarged LV). Palpitations are frequently premature atrial or ventricular beats, but a Holter monitor may be useful. Dysrhythmias may be related to the physiological hypokalemia of pregnancy and increased myocardial stretch. Previously quiescent or treated reentrant tachycardia syndromes may resurface. Differentiating normal pregnancy symptoms from HF symptoms may be difficult; however, certain physical examination signs are always pathological, such as crackles and precordial heaves.

DIAGNOSTIC APPROACH

Taking a comprehensive history of the pregnant patient is important in identifying preexisting cardiac conditions that will be best managed by a maternal-fetal medicine subspecialist together with a cardiologist. Peripartum cardiac complications are rare (<1%) and mostly related to hypertension and preexisting chronic cardiovascular disease. The most severe cardiac complications of peripartum onset are peripartum cardiomyopathy and acute myocardial infarction. The remainder of this chapter describes the evaluation and management of the common cardiovascular conditions in the pregnant woman.

PREEXISTING DISEASE STATES AND PREGNANCY

Maternal and fetal risks of cardiac disease generally depend on the underlying cardiovascular lesion and the functional class of the mother. Overall, women in New York Heart Association (NYHA) functional classes III and IV have a relatively high mortality rate (>7% during pregnancy) compared with those in NYHA functional classes I and II (<1%). A risk index to better risk-stratify pregnant women with heart disease includes four predictors of primary events: previous cardiac events or arrhythmias; baseline NYHA functional class more than II or cyanosis; significant left heart obstruction (mitral valve area of <2 cm^2, aortic valve area of <1.5 cm^2, or peak LV outflow tract gradient >30 mm Hg by echocardiography); and reduced systemic ventricular systolic function (ejection fraction [EF] <40%). Women can be categorized by a modified World Health Organization (WHO) classification into four pregnancy risk classes according to their cardiac condition (Table 64.2).

Ideally, pre-pregnancy counseling provides the patient with information about case-specific maternal and fetal risks to prepare for the safest pregnancy possible. This also allows the physician and patient to discuss risk factor modification and potential prenatal surgical correction of the underlying defect if pregnancy is desired.

Congenital Heart Disease

Congenital heart disease is believed to be multifactorial in origin, arising from a genetic predisposition combined with environmental factors. In general, the risk to offspring is 3% to 5%. However, reported rates vary between 1% and 18%, depending on the specific type of maternal lesion and the number of affected siblings. Maternal congenital heart disease confers different risks to both the mother and fetus, depending on the type of lesion (Table 64.2).

Uncomplicated acyanotic lesions, including atrial and ventricular septal defects, patent ductus arteriosus (with left-to-right shunting), and aortic coarctation, are usually well tolerated during pregnancy. Patients with coarctation who develop severe hypertension are at risk for HF, cerebral aneurysm rupture, and aortic dissection. Therefore, modest, but not aggressive, BP control is warranted for this population.

The maternal and fetal outcomes of pregnancy in acyanotic and cyanotic women with congenital heart disease depends significantly on the type of lesion, state of surgical repair (if any), ventricular function, degree of pulmonary hypertension, magnitude of hypoxemia, and NYHA functional class of the mother. Hence, it is important to address each case individually.

Pulmonary Vascular Disease and Eisenmenger Syndrome

The spectrum of pulmonary vascular disease includes primary pulmonary hypertension, secondary vascular pulmonary hypertension, and Eisenmenger syndrome. Although the morbidity and mortality of these disease states are high in general, these conditions, combined with pregnancy, produce an exceptionally high risk of poor maternal and fetal outcomes (WHO class IV). Maternal mortality rates vary based on the etiology of pulmonary vascular disease: 36% for Eisenmenger syndrome, 30% for primary pulmonary hypertension, and 56% for secondary vascular pulmonary hypertension. Risk is further increased if hematocrit is >65% or room air pulse oximetry is <85%. Typically, women with pulmonary vascular disease and Eisenmenger syndrome die shortly after delivery from sudden or progressive HF, arrhythmias, or thromboembolic events. It also appears that late hospitalization,

TABLE 64.2 Maternal Congenital and Valvular Heart Disease and Maternal and/or Fetal Risk During Pregnancy

Very High Risk WHO Class IV[a]	Moderate to High Risk WHO Class III[b]	Low to Moderate Risk WHO Class II[c]	Very Low Risk WHO Class I[d]
• Severe systemic ventricular dysfunction (EF <30%) with NYHA Class III or IV symptoms • Severe pulmonary hypertension with (e.g., Eisenmenger syndrome) or without septal defects • Cyanotic heart disease with pulmonary hypertension • Severe LV outflow tract obstruction (severe MS, severe symptomatic or asymptomatic AS) • Severe valvular disease (AS, AR, MS, MR) with LVEF <40% or with severe pulmonary hypertension (pulmonary pressure >75% of systemic pressures) • Aortic dilation >4.5 cm with Marfan syndrome, or >5.0 cm with bicuspid aortic valve • Severe native aortic coarctation • Previous peripartum cardiomyopathy with impaired LV contraction	• Systemic right ventricle (TGA after atrial switch procedure, congenitally corrected TGA) • Cyanotic lesions without pulmonary hypertension • Fontan-type circulation • Other complex congenital heart disease • Mechanical valve • Aortic dilation 4.0–4.5 cm with Marfan syndrome, or 4.5–5.0 cm with bicuspid aortic valve	• Unoperated septal defects (ASD, VSD) • Coarctation of the aorta (repaired)[e] • Tetralogy of Fallot • Mildly impaired LV contraction[e] • Hypertrophic cardiomyopathy[e] • Native or tissue valvular heart disease (not considered WHO I or IV, e.g., mild severity and NYHA class I or II)[e] • Marfan syndrome without aortic dilation[e] • Aortic dilation <4.5 cm with bicuspid aortic valve[e] • Most arrhythmias	• Small, mild or uncomplicated pulmonary stenosis, PDA, mitral valve prolapse • Repaired simple congenital lesions (ASD, VSD, PDA, anomalous pulmonary venous drainage) • Isolated atrial or ventricular ectopic beats

AR, Aortic regurgitation; *AS*, aortic stenosis; *ASD*, atrial septal defects; *EF*, ejection fraction; *LV*, left ventricular; *MR*, mitral regurgitation; *MS*, mitral stenosis; *NYHA*, New York Heart Association; *PDA*, patent ductus arteriosus; *TGA*, transposition of the great arteries; *WHO*, World Health Organization; *VSD*, ventricular septal defects.
[a]Extremely high risk of maternal mortality or severe morbidity such that pregnancy is not advised.
[b]Significant increase in maternal mortality or severe morbidity.
[c]Small increase in maternal mortality or a moderate increase in morbidity.
[d]No detectable increased risk of maternal mortality and either no or a mild increase in morbidity.
[e]Possible WHO Class III depending on the individual.
Adapted from the ACC/AHA guidelines for the management of patients with valvular heart disease (Bonow et al, 2008) and from a WHO classification of pregnancy risk for cardiac lesions (Thorne et al, 2006).

operative delivery, pulmonary vasculitis of a systemic disease, and illicit drug use are risk factors associated with maternal death in the secondary but not primary pulmonary hypertension group.

Because of the significant mortality rate, women with pulmonary vascular disease and Eisenmenger syndrome should be advised against pregnancy. If these states are diagnosed in gestation, early termination of the pregnancy is recommended. If the patient refuses termination or if the disease is diagnosed late in pregnancy, physical activity should be limited, bed rest should be advised for the third trimester, and the patient must be closely monitored. Early hospitalization has decreased mortality in pregnant women with secondary vascular pulmonary hypertension and Eisenmenger syndrome.

Standard drug therapies include calcium channel blockers, inhaled nitric oxide, and inhaled or intravenous (IV) prostaglandins. Anticoagulation prophylaxis is often recommended if clinically indicated (e.g., when hospitalized, but not during delivery), while the woman is considered hypercoagulable (especially during the third trimester and for at least 8 weeks postpartum). Spontaneous vaginal delivery is preferred, with attempts to shorten the second stage of labor using forceps or vacuum extraction. The use of pulmonary artery catheters during labor remains controversial.

Marfan Syndrome

Marfan syndrome is an autosomal dominant connective tissue disorder and can have significant cardiovascular involvement, most commonly, mitral valve prolapse and dilation of the aortic root at the level of the sinuses of Valsalva. Mitral regurgitation, aortic regurgitation, and aortic dissection can develop before or during pregnancy. Pregnant women with Marfan syndrome and only minor cardiovascular involvement, as well as an aortic root diameter of <40 mm usually tolerate pregnancy without difficulty and have little change in aortic root diameter. However, pregnant women with Marfan syndrome and an aortic root measuring >40 mm, aortic regurgitation, or a history of aortic dissection are at higher risk.

Because of the risks, women with Marfan syndrome and aortic root dilation are often advised against becoming pregnant. When pregnant, women with Marfan syndrome should be advised to avoid vigorous activity. Because β-blockers decrease the rate of aortic root dilation and aortic complications in the general population with Marfan syndrome, they are routinely administered to all pregnant women with Marfan syndrome. Serial echocardiograms are usually performed.

Valvular Heart Disease

Rheumatic heart disease is the most common cause of valvular disease in developing countries. Regurgitant valvular lesions, unless severe, are usually well tolerated in pregnancy because of a physiological afterload reduction (decreased SVR), increased plasma volume, and hyperdynamic and tachycardic states. Mitral valve prolapse is the most common valvular disease and most common cause of mitral regurgitation in young women, but it may resolve during pregnancy due to stretching of the mitral annulus and LV enlargement. Mitral valve prolapse is generally well tolerated, with no increased risk of complications unless there is significant mitral regurgitation. Both mitral and aortic regurgitation can usually be managed medically with diuretics for pulmonary congestion and vasodilator therapy only if the patient is hypertensive. Rarely, valve surgery is required because of severe NYHA functional class III to IV symptoms.

Pregnant women with stenotic valvular lesions require close monitoring throughout pregnancy, labor, and delivery, as well as prompt intervention on rare occasions. Mild AS, mild mitral stenosis, and mild to moderate pulmonic stenosis are fairly well tolerated. Ideally, women with more significant stenotic valvular lesions should either have their valves repaired or replaced before pregnancy or be counseled against becoming pregnant. Valvuloplasty of severe aortic, mitral, and pulmonic stenosis has also been successfully performed during pregnancy. Infrequently, aortic and mitral valves have been replaced during pregnancy for refractory symptoms or deterioration of functional class; however, because of the significant risk to the mother and the fetus, surgical valve replacement should be considered only as a last resort.

Mitral stenosis often becomes symptomatic and may be newly diagnosed during pregnancy. Symptoms usually develop in the later part of pregnancy from the increase in stroke volume and heart rate, leading to an increase in the transvalvular gradient. In addition, higher left atrial pressure can precipitate pulmonary edema; decreased diastolic filling occurs with tachycardia; and there is a higher risk of atrial arrhythmias. Therefore, institution of a modest diuretic (to relieve congestion) and β-blocker therapy (to avoid tachycardia), as well as salt, fluid, and activity restriction are effective. Digoxin may be useful if valvular atrial fibrillation develops. If the stenosis is moderate to severe with NYHA functional class III or IV symptoms, and medical therapy is unsuccessful, percutaneous balloon valvuloplasty should be considered before labor and delivery. These women are preload dependent and may benefit from invasive hemodynamic monitoring during labor and delivery.

Most AS in pregnant women is congenital. In the case of a bicuspid aortic valve, aortic root dilatation or aortopathy may be an associated finding, with a potential risk of spontaneous aortic dissection in the third trimester, especially if there is aortic coarctation. Ideally, moderate to severe AS should be corrected before conception. In the pregnant patient with severe AS who is asymptomatic or with mild symptoms during pregnancy, conservative management is often sufficient with bed rest, oxygen, and β-blockers. However, for the pregnant patient with symptomatic severe AS, percutaneous balloon valvuloplasty or surgery should be considered before labor and delivery; if surgery is pursued, the Ross procedure has historically been preferred.

For most valvular disease, routine antibiotic prophylaxis to prevent bacterial endocarditis is not recommended for uncomplicated vaginal delivery or C-section unless infection is suspected. Antibiotic prophylaxis is optional for high-risk patients, including those with a prosthetic valve, any degree of valvular stenosis, moderate or severe regurgitant valvular disease, history of endocarditis, complex congenital heart disease, or surgically constructed systemic–pulmonary conduits.

The pregnant patient with a prosthetic valve is challenging because pregnancy is both a hypercoagulable and hyperdynamic state. The thrombogenic mechanical prosthetic valves require long-term anticoagulation with warfarin, which is associated with a 15% to 25% risk of embryopathy in the first trimester, but the alternatives to warfarin (e.g., heparin) are less effective. Although the less thrombogenic bioprosthetic valves do not require anticoagulation, they are less durable and carry a higher risk of accelerated degeneration during pregnancy. Thus, the current recommendations for anticoagulation in the pregnant patient are the following: heparin (either low molecular weight subcutaneous or unfractionated IV) for gestational weeks 6 to 12; if desired, a change to warfarin until week 36, then a change back to heparin after week 36; and resume warfarin postpartum as soon as the obstetrician approves.

Heart Failure

Managing pregnant women with some form of preexisting cardiomyopathy (dilated, hypertrophic, or restrictive) is becoming more common.

Pre-pregnancy counseling is important and should be individualized based on risk-benefit analysis. When pregnant, medical management should be optimized and not significantly altered beyond substituting medications that are potentially teratogenic with nonteratogenic alternatives (e.g., replacing an angiotensin-converting enzyme [ACE] inhibitor with hydralazine). In addition, close monitoring of the EF with echocardiography is warranted in those with or at risk of a decreased EF, particularly during the third trimester when hemodynamic changes are greatest. Invasive hemodynamic monitoring might be helpful during labor, delivery, and early postpartum management.

CARDIOVASCULAR DISEASE UNIQUE TO PREGNANCY

Hypertension in Pregnancy

In 2009, the American Society of Hypertension updated the classification of hypertension in pregnancy and suggested guidelines for management. High BP during pregnancy (≥140 mm Hg systolic or ≥90 mm Hg diastolic) is classified into four categories: chronic hypertension, gestational hypertension, preeclampsia superimposed on chronic hypertension, and preeclampsia–eclampsia. These categories can help predict the course of hypertension and the necessity for treatment. Preeclampsia (pure or superimposed) is most often associated with severe maternal-fetal-neonatal complications (including fatalities). If pharmacological treatment is required in addition to lifestyle modifications, methyldopa has traditionally been used as a first-line agent due to its safety profile. However, tachyphylaxis and limited efficacy have limited its value. Other first-line agents include calcium channel blockers (e.g., nifedipine) and β-blockers (e.g., labetalol and others, but avoid atenolol, which has been associated with fetal growth effects). Certain diuretics, such as hydrochlorothiazide, are used as second-line agents.

Chronic hypertension is defined as hypertension diagnosed before pregnancy, before the 20th week of gestation, or during pregnancy that does not resolve postpartum. This is more common in African Americans, patients with diabetes, patients with chronic renal disease, and obese patients. Most of the increased risk in this population occurs with superimposed preeclampsia.

Gestational hypertension is high BP diagnosed for the first time after week 20 with no accompanying proteinuria. Preeclampsia does not develop, and BP returns to normal by 6 to 12 weeks postpartum. However, if postpartum BP remains high, the final diagnosis is chronic hypertension.

Preeclampsia superimposed on chronic hypertension is diagnosed when a patient with hypertension, but without proteinuria before the 20th week of gestation, develops proteinuria. This diagnosis is also made when a patient with hypertension and proteinuria before the 20th week has a sudden increase in proteinuria, sudden increase in BP, platelet count drop to <100,000, or acute elevation in serum transaminases (aspartate aminotransferase [AST] or alanine aminotransferase [ALT]) or other signs or symptoms of preeclampsia.

Finally, the classification of preeclampsia–eclampsia applies to women who develop increased BP associated with proteinuria after the 20th week of gestation (Fig. 64.2). Confirmatory signs of the diagnosis include systolic BP of ≥160 mm Hg and/or diastolic BP ≥110 mm Hg, proteinuria of >2.0 g/24 hours, increased serum creatinine concentration, platelet count <100,000, and/or evidence of microangiopathic hemolytic anemia and elevated AST or ALT concentrations. Additional symptoms that should raise concern include persistent epigastric discomfort, headaches, visual disturbances, and other central nervous system complaints.

The etiology of preeclampsia–eclampsia is unknown, although there are many risk factors (Table 64.3). Endothelial dysfunction is the hallmark of this disease. This systemic disease is associated with significant

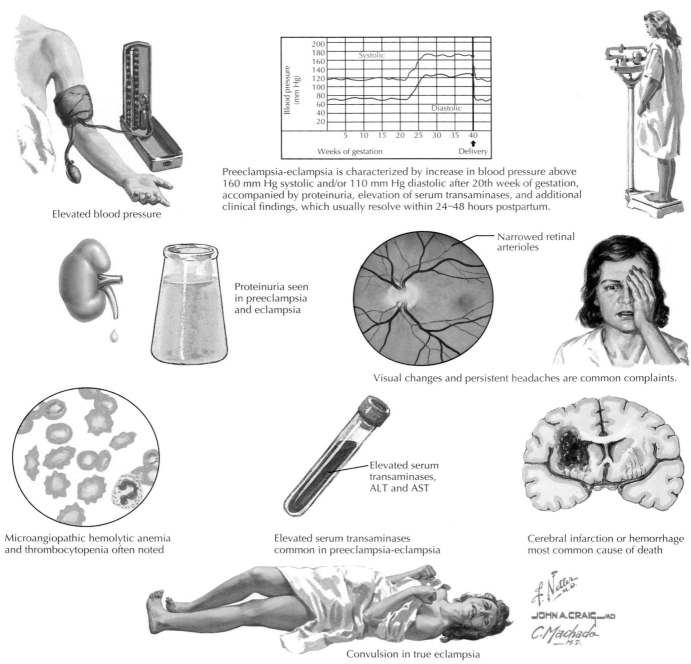

Preeclampsia-eclampsia is characterized by increase in blood pressure above 160 mm Hg systolic and/or 110 mm Hg diastolic after 20th week of gestation, accompanied by proteinuria, elevation of serum transaminases, and additional clinical findings, which usually resolve within 24–48 hours postpartum.

Elevated blood pressure

Proteinuria seen in preeclampsia and eclampsia

Narrowed retinal arterioles

Visual changes and persistent headaches are common complaints.

Microangiopathic hemolytic anemia and thrombocytopenia often noted

Elevated serum transaminases, ALT and AST

Elevated serum transaminases common in preeclampsia-eclampsia

Cerebral infarction or hemorrhage most common cause of death

Convulsion in true eclampsia

FIG 64.2 Preeclampsia–Eclampsia. *ALT,* Alanine aminotransferase; *AST,* aspartate aminotransferase.

increased morbidity and mortality for the mother and fetus. The severity of preeclampsia varies from mild to severe, and it may progress rapidly and unpredictably. In general, patients with mild preeclampsia may be closely supervised. Those with preeclampsia with severe characteristics should be admitted to a tertiary care center and monitored closely for signs of maternal or fetal distress. Preeclampsia can progress to eclampsia, a convulsive phase that may be fatal (Fig. 64.2). It can also lead to pulmonary edema, renal damage, and liver damage. Cerebral infarction and hemorrhage account for most deaths in preeclampsia–eclampsia. Hydralazine (IV), labetalol (IV or intramuscularly), and nifedipine (per os) are commonly used to treat severe hypertension; nitroprusside (IV) is considered an agent of last resort because of possible cyanide toxicity.

Magnesium sulfate is recommended to prevent seizures in preeclampsia and also to treat and prevent recurrent seizures in eclampsia. Delivery timing should be based on maternal and fetal conditions, including gestational age. Delivery is the cure for preeclampsia; signs and symptoms usually regress within 24 to 48 hours postpartum but can last longer. Therefore, it is important to monitor postpartum women with preeclampsia–eclampsia until BP and other abnormal parameters have normalized.

Peripartum Cardiomyopathy

Peripartum cardiomyopathy (PPCM) is a rare form of HF that affects otherwise healthy young women. It is defined as the onset of cardiac

TABLE 64.3 Risk Factors for Preeclampsia, Peripartum Cardiomyopathy, and Peripartum Acute Myocardial Infarction

	Risk Factors
Preeclampsia	Maternal age ≥30 yrs
	Multiple gestation
	Black race
	Hypertension
	Obesity
	Insulin resistance
	Diabetes
	Increased circulating testosterone
	Thrombophilias
	Sickle cell disease
	Collagen vascular disease
	Autoimmune diseases
	Renal disease
Peripartum cardiomyopathy	Maternal age ≥30 yrs
	Multiparity
	Multiple gestation
	African descent
	Preeclampsia or sustained hypertension
	Long-term tocolysis
Acute myocardial infarction	Maternal age ≥30 yrs
	Hypertension
	Thrombophilia
	Smoking
	Transfusion
	Diabetes mellitus
	Postpartum infection

failure, with a LVEF of <45% with or without LV dilation, without an identifiable cause, with onset in the last month of pregnancy or within 5 to 6 months after delivery in the absence of preexisting heart disease. Incidence is estimated at 1 in 2500 to 4000 live births in the United States, but rates have been higher in Africa (1 in 1000) and highest in Haiti (1 in 300). The etiology of this disorder remains unknown but is believed to be multifactorial, potentially related to inflammation, infection, nutrition, hormones, an autoimmune process, and genetic predisposition. There is an association with oxidative stress involving the prolactin-cleaving protease cathepsin D that produces a 16-kDa prolactin fragment, which promotes vasoconstriction and impairs cardiomyocyte function. Risk factors for developing PPCM are shown in Table 64.3. Women with pregnancy-associated cardiomyopathy diagnosed earlier than the last gestational month have similar characteristics.

The outcome of patients with PPCM is highly variable and dependent on whether the LV size and function normalizes. Most studies report mortality rates of 25% to 50%, with most deaths occurring in the first 3 months after diagnosis. In up to 50% of patients, EF returns to normal or near normal within 6 months postpartum. The remaining patients demonstrate persistent cardiac dysfunction or deteriorating function, and experience the symptoms and complications associated with chronic HF. PPCM accounts for approximately 5% of reported pregnancy-related deaths in the United States, with higher mortality among black women.

Management of PPCM is supportive and includes standard treatment for HF, including an intraaortic balloon pump or LV assist device or cardiac transplantation when necessary. The risks and benefits of evidence-based HF medications should be reviewed before administration, especially if the patient is still pregnant. If the cardiomyopathy is diagnosed before delivery, hydralazine is the afterload-reducing agent of choice (because ACE inhibitors are teratogenic); however, ACE inhibitors are favored postpartum and are safe for breastfeeding patients. Beta-blockers are generally safe during pregnancy. Aldosterone antagonists should be avoided during pregnancy because of antiandrogenic effects. PPCM patients who received bromocriptine therapy in addition to standard HF therapy have had favorable outcomes.

Advisability of future pregnancies is controversial because recurrence with subsequent pregnancies is common. In patients with persistent LV dysfunction, future pregnancies should be avoided because of risk of further decrease in LV function and clinical deterioration. However, in patients whose EF returned to normal after the initial incident, the recommendations are not as steadfast. Relapse of LV dysfunction can occur, albeit less frequently and perhaps less severely than in those with persistent systolic dysfunction. Mechanistically, impaired contractile reserve, which can be demonstrated by dobutamine stress echocardiography, may be contributory. Based on these observations, even for women with PPCM with normalized EF and normal contractile reserve, subsequent pregnancy should be considered with caution.

Pulmonary Edema Induced by Tocolytic Therapy

Tocolytic agents are sometimes used to prevent preterm labor, and some patients are exposed to more than one agent. Common agents include nifedipine, indomethacin, magnesium sulfate, and terbutaline. Although these agents can delay delivery, they have significant side effects: tachycardia (ventricular tachycardia has been reported), chest pain without ECG changes, electrolyte abnormalities, and noncardiogenic pulmonary edema. The rate of pulmonary edema induced by these agents is low. However, among pregnant women with pulmonary edema, tocolytics have been implicated in approximately 25% of cases. The increased incidence of pulmonary edema seen in women treated with tocolytic therapy is most often associated with short-term (<48 hours) IV infusions. There has been at least one report associating long-term (>4 weeks) oral tocolytic therapy with development of PPCM.

Acute Myocardial Infarction

As more older women get pregnant, the prevalence of coronary artery disease and risk of acute myocardial infarction (AMI) during pregnancy may rise. In addition to traditional coronary risk factors, pregnancy increases the risk of AMI three- to fourfold. The incidence of AMI in pregnancy ranges from 3 to 100 per 100,000 deliveries. The maternal case fatality is as high as 11%, with an associated fetal mortality of 9%. Risk factors for AMI are listed in Table 64.3. The most common etiology is atherosclerosis with or without intracoronary thrombus, but this has been seen in only 40% of cases; other causes include coronary thrombus without atherosclerotic disease, coronary dissection, and possible coronary vasospasm. Patients who develop AMI should be treated with revascularization as appropriate. Medical management may be difficult because of the risk of hemorrhage and teratogenesis with antiplatelets and anticoagulants. However, the risk of fetal death is usually associated with maternal death, emphasizing the importance of optimizing maternal health.

OPTIMUM TREATMENT

Because many cardiovascular diseases may affect the pregnant woman, treatment must be individualized yet follow the standards of care. Ideally, multidisciplinary antenatal discussions should be shared among obstetricians, cardiologists, and primary care providers. Outcomes are improved for both mother and child when there is a thoughtful care plan in place.

Avoiding Treatment Errors

Because drugs are rarely tested in pregnant women, safety information on most pharmaceuticals in this population is limited. Most cardiovascular drugs cross the placenta and are also secreted in breast milk. Therefore, when possible, it is advisable to avoid the use of prescription and over-the-counter drugs during pregnancy and during the postpartum period if the mother is breast-feeding. However, newly pregnant women receiving treatment for cardiovascular disorders should not discontinue important medications before consultation with a maternal-fetal medicine specialist. Ideally, prospective mothers should undergo preconceptional counseling.

When this is not possible, every effort should be made to use a medication that has been shown to be safe during pregnancy. The Food and Drug Administration (FDA) has previously categorized drugs according to their potential to cause birth defects, based on data from human and animal studies. The categories range from class A drugs (no documented fetal risks) to class X drugs (contraindicated in part or all of pregnancy due to proven teratogenicity). Few cardiovascular drugs are class B (animal studies suggest risk, but results are unconfirmed in controlled human studies); examples include methyldopa, lidocaine, and sotalol. Most cardiovascular drugs currently in use are class C (animal studies have demonstrated adverse fetal effects, but no controlled human studies are available); examples include most β-blockers (e.g., labetalol, metoprolol, propranolol), hydralazine, and calcium channel blockers. Finally, class D drugs demonstrate some evidence of human fetal risk, but the benefits from use during pregnancy may be acceptable if the drug is needed because safer drugs cannot be used or are ineffective. However, this system of categories is gradually being replaced with more descriptive information (Pregnancy and Lactation Labeling Rule, effective 2015). Drugs that are FDA-approved since 2015 do not have this rating. This FDA classification will be phased out for older medications by 2018. In general, if pharmacological therapy is needed, drugs that have been in use for longer periods prescribed at the lowest possible dosages are recommended.

FUTURE DIRECTIONS

The increased survival rate of women with congenital heart disease combined with the trend toward delaying childbearing until later years will continue to increase the likelihood that healthcare providers of pregnant women will manage complex cardiovascular disease. Ideally, a multidisciplinary approach to these patients at a tertiary care center is recommended to optimize outcomes for mother and child. Because pregnant women are frequently excluded from clinical trials, the evidence for the management of cardiovascular disease during pregnancy is modest and mostly based on case series and registries. As standard therapies are extrapolated from studies in more generalized populations, further investigation is needed in this specialized population.

ADDITIONAL RESOURCES

https://medlineplus.gov/pregnancyandmedicines.html and https://reprotox.org/.
Online resources for medication risks in pregnancy.

https://toxnet.nlm.nih.gov/newtoxnet/lactmed.htm (LactMed).
Online resource for medication risks in lactation (for breastfeeding mothers).

EVIDENCE

Bonow RO, Carabello BA, Chatterjee K, et al. 2008 Focused update incorporated into the ACC/AHA 2006 guidelines for the management of patients with valvular heart disease: a report of the American College of Cardiology/American Heart Association Task Force on Practice Guidelines (Writing Committee to revise the 1998 guidelines for the management of patients with valvular heart disease). Endorsed by the Society of Cardiovascular Anesthesiologists, Society for Cardiovascular Angiography and Interventions, and Society of Thoracic Surgeons. *J Am Coll Cardiol.* 2008;52(13):e1–e142.
These guidelines provide current recommendations for treatment of valvular heart disease based on available data and consensus opinion (classes I, IIa, IIb, III; levels A, B, C).

Canobbio MM, Warnes CA, Aboulhosn J, et al. Management of pregnancy in patients with complex congenital heart disease: a scientific statement for healthcare professionals from the American Heart Association. *Circulation.* 2017;135(8):e50–e87.
These guidelines provide current recommendations for the management of the pregnant patient with complex congenital heart disease based on available data and consensus opinion (classes I, IIa, IIb, III; levels A, B, C).

European Society of Gynecology (ESG); Association for European Paediatric Cardiology (AEPC); German Society for Gender Medicine (DGesGM), Regitz-Zagrosek V, Blomstrom Lundqvist C, et al. ESC guidelines on the management of cardiovascular diseases during pregnancy: the Task Force on the Management of Cardiovascular Diseases during Pregnancy of the European Society of Cardiology (ESC). *Eur Heart J.* 2011;32(24):3147–3197.
These guidelines provide current recommendations for the management of the pregnant patient with cardiovascular disease.

Ismail S, Wong C, Rajan P, Vidovich MI. ST-elevation acute myocardial infarction in pregnancy: 2016 update. *Clin Cardiol.* 2017 Feb 13 [Epub ahead of print, PMID: 28191905].
This review provides current overview of the management of the pregnant patient with ST-elevation myocardial infarction.

Jeejeebhoy FM, Zelop CM, Lipman S, et al. Cardiac arrest in pregnancy: a scientific statement from the American Heart Association. *Circulation.* 2015;132(18):1747–1773.
This report provides current recommendations regarding cardiopulmonary resuscitation during pregnancy, based on consensus opinion.

Lindheimer MD, Taler SJ, Cunningham FG. American Society of Hypertension. ASH position paper: hypertension in pregnancy. *J Clin Hypertens (Greenwich).* 2009;11(4):214–225.
This report from the American Society of Hypertension provides current classification of and recommendations for treatment of hypertension during pregnancy based on available data and consensus opinion.

Sliwa K, Hilfiker-Kleiner D, Petrie MC, et al. Current state of knowledge on aetiology, diagnosis, management, and therapy of peripartum cardiomyopathy: a position statement from the Heart Failure Association of the European Society of Cardiology Working Group on peripartum cardiomyopathy. *Eur J Heart Fail.* 2010;12(8):767–778.
This review provides current classification of and recommendations for treatment of PPCM based on consensus opinion.

Thorne S, MacGregor A, Nelson-Piercy C. Risks of contraception and pregnancy in heart disease. *Heart.* 2006;92(10):1520–1525.
This consensus document provides a WHO classification of maternal risk of pregnancy associated with specific cardiovascular conditions.

65

Neuromuscular Diseases and the Heart

Rebecca E. Traub

Neuromuscular disorders are a subset of neurology that affects the peripheral nervous system, including lower motor neuron projections from the spinal cord, spinal nerve root, peripheral nerve, neuromuscular junction, and muscle. A number of neuromuscular diseases have effects on the heart. Most often, diseases of muscles (myopathy), both acquired and hereditary, can affect cardiac muscle and therefore cause cardiomyopathy or conduction disease. Peripheral nerve disease can also affect the autonomic nervous system, causing arrhythmias or effects on blood pressure. Other genetic or acquired syndromes may have both neuromuscular and cardiac abnormalities. It is critical for the neurologist seeing neuromuscular patients to be aware of which conditions may be associated with cardiac complications, to ensure appropriate cardiac screening and monitoring. Cardiologists also need to be aware of when an underlying neurological disorder may be contributing to the cardiac condition of a patient. This chapter reviews many of the neuromuscular conditions associated with cardiac disease.

MYOPATHIES

Myopathies include all diseases of muscle, including hereditary and acquired. Genetic myopathies, including muscular dystrophies, congenital myopathies, and metabolic myopathies, depending on specific genetic cause, can affect cardiac muscle. Some acquired myopathies can also have cardiac effects.

Muscular Dystrophies

Traditionally categorized by mode of inheritance, age of onset, severity, and pattern of clinical presentation, the inherited muscular dystrophy disorders generally present with progressive muscle weakness in childhood or young adulthood.

Dystrophinopathies: Duchenne and Becker. Duchenne and Becker muscular dystrophies are X-linked recessive disorders that are caused by mutations in the dystrophin gene; therefore, they have reduced or absent expression of the dystrophin protein, which is an essential component of the cytoskeleton of skeletal and cardiac muscle. Progressive weakness and pseudohypertrophy of muscles, particularly the calves, are characteristic of both.

Clinical manifestations of Duchenne muscular dystrophy typically present in early childhood, with contractures and with proximal muscle weakness more than distal muscle weakness. The Gower maneuver, which is the use of the arms when trying to stand up from the floor, is a characteristic physical examination finding (Fig. 65.1). Nonprogressive cognitive impairment or global development delay is common. There is steady progression to wheelchair use within 10 years, and death usually occurs in the second or early third decade of life from respiratory or cardiac failure, although use of corticosteroids may slow this progression.

Duchenne muscular dystrophy causes a dilated cardiomyopathy with left ventricular fibrosis, as well as arrhythmias and conduction abnormalities. Fibrosis of the posterobasal left ventricular wall can demonstrate the characteristic ECG changes of tall right precordial R waves with an increased R/S ratio and deep Q waves in leads I, aVL, and V_5 to V_6. Mitral regurgitation may occur secondary to progression of the cardiomyopathy. The symptoms related to cardiomyopathy in Duchenne muscular dystrophy are often not appreciated until later in the disease course, but they can be detected by ultrasound before symptom onset.

Becker muscular dystrophy, in which there is altered or decreased dystrophin expression, but with some retained function, presents with a less severe phenotype, often at a later age. The severity of the Becker phenotype varies greatly. Cardiomyopathy also occurs with Becker muscular dystrophy and is sometimes more severe than the degree of generalized weakness might suggest. Right ventricular involvement occurs early in Becker patients, with later development of left ventricular dysfunction, which is related to a fibrotic process that results in heart failure. Conduction abnormalities may also be seen.

The diagnosis of Duchenne or Becker muscular dystrophy is often considered in a boy or young adult with the typical distribution of weakness, calf pseudohypertrophy, and high creatine kinase levels. Electrodiagnostic testing with electromyography confirms a myopathic process, and many patients now have diagnosis confirmed by genetic testing of the *DMD* gene, looking for deletions and/or duplications or point mutations. In atypical cases or when genetic testing is not readily available, muscle biopsy demonstrates a dystrophic process with reduced or absent dystrophin staining (Fig. 65.1).

Treatment of Duchenne muscular dystrophy includes glucocorticoids, which have been demonstrated to slow progression of muscle weakness and scoliosis, and to improve pulmonary function. Several nonrandomized studies have described benefit in delaying the onset and progression of cardiomyopathy in Duchenne muscular dystrophy with steroid use, but further research is needed.

Aside from steroid use, treatment for Duchenne and Becker muscular dystrophy is supportive, with surgical management of scoliosis, noninvasive and invasive methods of ventilator support, and management of cardiac complications. In Becker muscular dystrophy, some patients with disproportionate cardiac involvement have successfully undergone cardiac transplantation.

Emery-Dreifuss Muscular Dystrophy. Emery-Dreifuss muscular dystrophy (EDMD) is a genetically heterogeneous disorder characterized by early contractures of the elbows, ankles, and posterior cervical muscles, as well as slowly progressive muscle weakness in a scapulohumeroperoneal distribution, often accompanied by cardiac disease, including conduction defects, arrhythmias, and cardiomyopathy. Genes associated with EDMD phenotype include *EMD* (encoding emerin), *FHL1*, *LMNA*, *SYNE1*, *SYNE2*, and *TMEM43*. Dilated cardiomyopathy

Gower maneuver

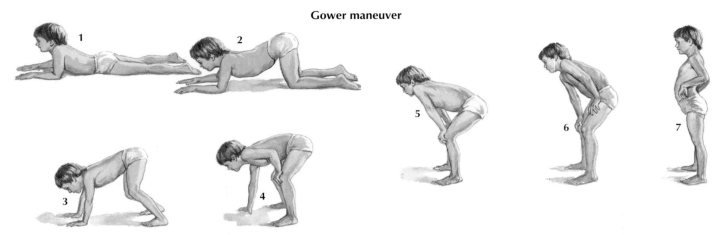

Characteristically, the child arises from prone position by pushing himself up with hands successively on floor, knees, and thighs because of weakness in gluteal and spine muscles. He stands in lordic posture.

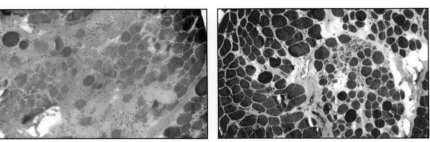

Muscle biopsy specimens showing necrotic muscle fibers being removed by groups of small, round phagocytic cells (**left**, trichrome stain) and replaced by fibrous and fatty tissue (**right**, H & E stain).

FIG 65.1 Duchenne Muscular Dystrophy. *H&E,* Hematoxylin and eosin.

is common in these disorders, often with associated conduction abnormalities. Sudden cardiac death has been described in patients without overt muscle weakness.

Diagnosis of EDMD is suspected in any patient with scapulohumeroperoneal weakness with contractures and cardiac involvement, as well as studies suggestive of a myopathic process. Diagnosis is confirmed by genetic testing for the previously described genes associated with the EDMD phenotype and may preclude muscle biopsy in some cases.

Treatment for the muscle weakness is symptomatic. Cardiac monitoring is critical, and a pacemaker or implantable defibrillator may be indicated for patients with conduction disease or arrhythmias.

Myotonic Dystrophy. Myotonic dystrophy includes two genetic muscular dystrophies that share the clinical phenotype of a dystrophic myopathy, with either the clinical or electromyographic finding of myotonia. The physical examination finding of myotonia is of delayed muscle relaxation after contraction or muscle percussion (Fig. 65.2). Electrographic myotonia describes the waxing and waning high-frequency discharges seen on needle electromyography.

There are two genetic subtypes of myotonic dystrophy, both autosomal dominant, including type 1 (DM1), which is related to an expansion of the CTG triplet repeat of the dystrophia myotonica protein kinase *(DMPK)* gene, and type 2 (DM2), which is related to expansion of a CCTG repeat in the zinc finger protein *(ZNF9)* gene (also known as the *CNBP* gene).

DM1 is more typical of a distal myopathy, and is accompanied by facial weakness, ptosis, bulbar weakness, temporal wasting, and frontal balding. DM2 shares many clinical features with DM1, but tends to be overall less severe, demonstrates more proximal rather than distal limb weakness, and shows less clinical myotonia. The diagnosis of myotonic dystrophy is often suspected based on clinical and electrodiagnostic features, and confirmed with genetic testing. In some cases, muscle biopsy is performed and typically shows myopathic changes with a notable increase of internalized nuclei.

Patients with DM1, and to a lesser degree, those with DM2, are at risk for cardiac conduction abnormalities, as well as atrial fibrillation and ventricular arrhythmias. Cardiomyopathy is less common in these disorders. Occasionally, sudden cardiac death is the presenting symptom of DM1. Therefore, patients with myotonic dystrophy are recommended for at least an annual cardiac screening with ECG, and in some cases, longer cardiac monitoring. Pacemakers or implantable defibrillators are occasionally warranted.

Limb Girdle Muscular Dystrophy. Limb girdle muscular dystrophy (LGMD) is a genetically heterogeneous group of autosomal-dominant (type 1) or autosomal-recessive (type 2) myopathies characterized by weakness and wasting of the shoulder and pelvic girdle muscles. The limb-girdle phenotype may overlap with other hereditary myopathies, and occasionally, acquired muscle diseases. There are currently 8 identified autosomal dominant LGMD subtypes (named LGMD1A-H) and 23 autosomal recessive subtypes (named LGMD2A-W).

Some genetic subtypes of LGMD are more likely to affect cardiac function, which is one primary rationale for establishing a genetic diagnosis in a patient suspected of having LGMD. The LGMD subtypes most commonly associated with cardiac involvement include LGMD1B, LGMD1E, LGMD2E, and LGMD2I. Others in which cardiac involvement

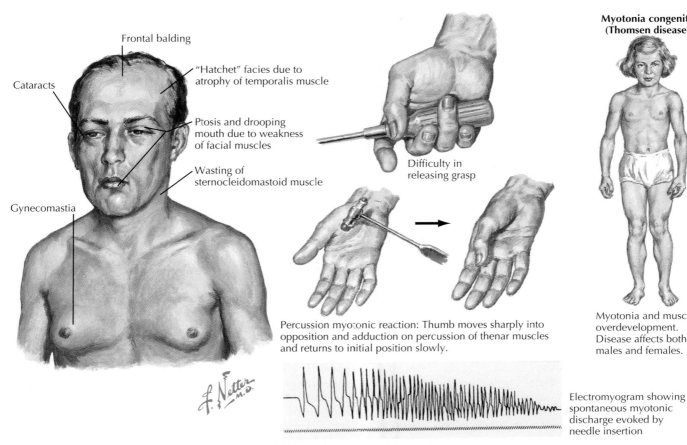

Myotonia congenita (Thomsen disease)

Frontal balding

"Hatchet" facies due to atrophy of temporalis muscle

Cataracts

Ptosis and drooping mouth due to weakness of facial muscles

Wasting of sternocleidomastoid muscle

Gynecomastia

Difficulty in releasing grasp

Percussion myotonic reaction: Thumb moves sharply into opposition and adduction on percussion of thenar muscles and returns to initial position slowly.

Myotonia and muscular overdevelopment. Disease affects both males and females.

Electromyogram showing spontaneous myotonic discharge evoked by needle insertion

FIG 65.2 Myotonic Dystrophy.

may also be seen are summarized in Table 65.1. Subtypes in which cardiac involvement is unusual include LGMD1C, LGMD2A, LGMD2B, and LGMD2L. Because cardiac involvement is generally common with LGMD, screening for associated cardiomyopathy is advised when exact genetic diagnosis cannot be established.

In a patient clinically suspected of having LGMD based on history and physical examination, with confirmatory creatine kinase testing and electrodiagnostics suggestive of a myopathic process, diagnosis is often made directly with genetic testing.

Distal Myopathies. Distal myopathies, or muscular dystrophies, are a genetically heterogeneous group of hereditary muscle diseases that clinically present with distal weakness greater and sooner than proximal weakness. The most common distal myopathy is Welander distal myopathy. Most of the genetic mutations categorized as distal myopathies do not have significant cardiac involvement, although conduction defects are occasionally noted. Myotonic dystrophy and myofibrillar myopathies may present with prominent distal weakness, but are more strongly associated with cardiomyopathy or cardiac conduction abnormalities.

Myofibrillar Myopathies. Myofibrillar myopathies are another genetically heterogeneous group of hereditary muscle diseases associated with mutations of the Z-disk–related proteins. Myofibrillar myopathies are often associated with cardiomyopathy, conduction abnormalities, and arrhythmias, and in some cases, the cardiac involvement may be the most prominent or exclusive manifestation of disease. Gene mutations described to cause myofibrillar myopathies include desmin, αB-crystallin, *ZASP*, myotilin (allelic with LGMD1A), filamin C, *BAG3*, *SEPN1*, and *FHL1*.

TABLE 65.1 Limb Girdle Muscular Dystrophy Subtypes Associated With Cardiac Involvement

Type	Locus	Gene	Protein
LGMD1A	5q31	*MYOT*	Myotilin
LGMD1B	1q11-q21	*LMNA*	Lamin A/C
LGMD1D(E)	7q	*DNAJB6*	DnaJ homolog subfamily B member 6
LGMD2C	13q12	*SGCG*	Gamma-sarcoglycan
LGMD2D	17q12-q21	*SGCA*	Alpha-sarcoglycan
LGMD2E	4q12	*SGCB*	Beta-sarcoglycan
LGMD2F	5q33-q34	*SGCD*	Delta-sarcoglycan
LGMD2G	17q11-q12	*TCAP*	Telethonin
LGMD2H	9q31-q34	*TRIM32*	Tripartite motif containing 32
LGMD2I	19q13.3	*FKRP*	Fukutin-related protein
LGMD2J	2q24.3	*TTN*	Titin
LGMD2K	9q34.1	*POMT1*	Protein-O-mannosyl transferase 1
LGMD2M	9q31	*FKTN*	Fukutin
LGMD2N	14q24	*POMT2*	Protein-O-mannosyl transferase 2
LGMD2O	1p34.1	*POMGnT1*	Protein O-linked mannose β1,2-N-acetylglucosaminyl transferase
LGMD2P	3p21	*DAG1*	Dystroglycan

Facioscapulohumeral Muscular Dystrophy. Facioscapulohumeral muscular dystrophy (FSHD), the third most common muscular dystrophy, consists of two genetic subtypes. Type 1 is related to contraction in the D4Z4 macrosatellite repeat at the 4q35 gene locus, and type 2 is caused by a mutation in the *SMCHD1* gene. Cardiac involvement is not common in FSHD, but some studies have reported an increased risk of cardiac arrhythmias in FSHD patients, so screening is advised.

Congenital Myopathies

Congenital myopathies are the group of muscle diseases that typically present at birth, although in some cases, presentation may be in later childhood and adulthood. The most common congenital myopathies are nemaline myopathy, central core disease, and centronuclear or myotubular myopathies. The clinical weakness of congenital myopathies typically affects distal or axial and respiratory muscles. Cardiomyopathy may occur in many of the congenital myopathies, particularly nemaline myopathy. Central core disease is associated with an increased risk of malignant hyperthermia.

Metabolic Myopathies

Metabolic myopathies include a group of muscle diseases associated with genetic defects in energy storage and metabolism. Subgroups of metabolic myopathies include disorders of glycogen metabolism, disorders of lipid metabolism, and mitochondrial disorders, all of which may have cardiac manifestations.

Disorders of Glycogen Metabolism. Glycogen storage diseases result from deficiency or partial loss of enzymes in the glycogen degradation pathway. Glycogen metabolism disorders present with episodes of rhabdomyolysis, liver dysfunction, episodes of hypoglycemia, gross motor delay, peripheral neuropathy, or cardiomyopathy. Many genetic defects that result in glycogen storage disease have been identified; the most important, from a cardiac standpoint, is acid maltase deficiency. Acid maltase deficiency (type 2 glycogenosis, Pompe disease, LGMD2V) is an autosomal recessive disease that causes deficiency of α-1,4-glucosidase, which may present in infancy, childhood, or adulthood depending on the degree of residual enzyme activity. Infantile onset is severe and multisystemic, and nearly always has cardiac involvement. Adult-onset forms are less likely to have cardiac involvement, but cardiomyopathy does sometimes occur. Enzyme replacement therapy with recombinant α-glucosidase benefits the infantile-onset disease and probably helps in later onset phenotypes. Cardiomyopathy particularly appears to improve with enzyme replacement therapy.

Other glycogen storage diseases commonly manifesting with cardiomyopathy include muscle glycogen synthase deficiency and lysosome-associated membrane protein 2 deficiency (Danon disease).

Disorders of Lipid Metabolism and Carnitine Deficiency. Metabolic myopathies related to abnormalities of lipid metabolism include carnitine deficiency, fatty acid transport defects, defects of β-oxidation, neutral lipid storage disease, and lipin-1 deficiency. Symptoms associated with these disorders typically are triggered by metabolic stressors. Primary carnitine deficiency is the lipid storage myopathy most often associated with cardiomyopathy. Clinical features of carnitine deficiency can range from severe metabolic decompensation in infancy, to myopathy with cardiomyopathy in childhood or adult presentations. Diagnosis can be established by screening with serum carnitine levels and confirmed with cultured skin fibroblasts, low carnitine levels in muscle biopsy, or genetic testing. Treatment is with oral supplementation of L-carnitine and measures to avoid hypoglycemia.

Mitochondrial Disorders. Mitochondrial disease includes genetic defects of either mitochondrial or nuclear DNA that affect proteins necessary for mitochondrial function of oxidative phosphorylation to produce adenosine triphosphate. Mitochondrial disease can present with a wide range of phenotypes, but organ systems most likely to be affected are those with high-energy requirements, including the brain, heart, and skeletal muscle. Kearns-Sayre syndrome typically presents with progressive external ophthalmoplegia, cardiac conduction block, and mitochondrial myopathy, and occasionally with central nervous system involvement. Leber hereditary optic neuropathy primarily presents with a progressive optic nerve degeneration but may have associated cardiac conduction abnormalities. Some mitochondrial myopathies may present with selective or prominent cardiomyopathy, either with hypertrophic or dilated forms. Treatment is generally symptomatic and supportive, although some respiratory chain cofactors are tried as oral supplementation. Because of the variability of phenotypic expression of mitochondrial disease based on the specific mutation and tissue expression, screening for cardiac conduction disease and cardiomyopathy in any patient diagnosed with a mitochondrial disorder is generally advised.

PERIODIC PARALYSIS SYNDROMES

Periodic paralysis syndromes are a rare group of neuromuscular disorders related to muscle channel ion defects that result in episodes of muscle weakness, which are often triggered by exercise, fasting, or high carbohydrate intake (Fig. 65.3).

Hypokalemic periodic paralysis, an autosomal dominant disorder related to either calcium channel or sodium channel mutations, presents with episodes of weakness associated with low serum potassium levels. Cardiac arrhythmias rarely occur during episodes of severe hypokalemia. Treatment includes potassium supplementation and acetazolamide.

Andersen syndrome, or Anderson-Tawil syndrome, is a rare subtype of periodic paralysis related to potassium channel mutation; it is characterized by periodic paralysis, ventricular arrhythmia, and dysmorphic features. Potassium levels vary with Andersen syndrome but are most often low. Diagnosis of periodic paralysis disorders is typically suspected based on clinical history, may show suggestive findings on electrodiagnostic testing, and can be confirmed with genetic testing. Any patient with a periodic paralysis disorder should be screened for an increased QT interval.

Acquired Myopathies

A number of muscle diseases acquired later in life, including inflammatory, toxic, and degenerative disorders, may manifest with cardiac involvement.

Inflammatory Myopathies. Myositis includes a group of immune-mediated muscle diseases that cause inflammation and damage in skeletal muscle, and in severe cases, may also affect cardiac muscle. Subtypes of myositis include polymyositis, dermatomyositis, necrotizing autoimmune myopathy (NAM), and inclusion body myositis.

Dermatomyositis is a vasculopathy of muscle and skin, typically presenting with rash, proximal muscle weakness, and high creatine kinase levels. Muscle pathology shows perimysial and perivascular inflammation. Polymyositis presents with similar clinical features as dermatomyositis, without the associated rash, but pathologically instead shows primarily endomysial inflammation and muscle fiber necrosis. Both dermatomyositis and polymyositis are inflammatory conditions, and are occasionally paraneoplastic or seen in association with other connective tissue disease. They are treated similarly, with high-dose steroids and steroid-sparing therapies. Although these disorders primarily affect skeletal muscle, in severe cases, cardiac muscle can be involved with associated cardiomyopathy or cardiac conduction defects that improve with immunotherapy (Fig. 65.4).

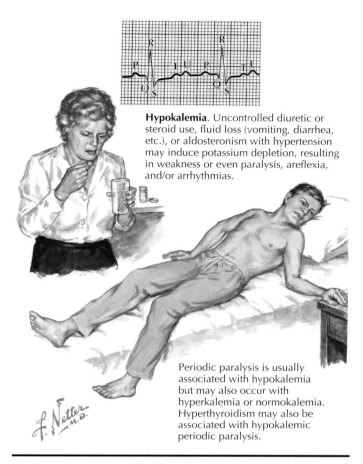

Hypokalemia. Uncontrolled diuretic or steroid use, fluid loss (vomiting, diarrhea, etc.), or aldosteronism with hypertension may induce potassium depletion, resulting in weakness or even paralysis, areflexia, and/or arrhythmias.

Periodic paralysis is usually associated with hypokalemia but may also occur with hyperkalemia or normokalemia. Hyperthyroidism may also be associated with hypokalemic periodic paralysis.

Hyperkalemia. Addison disease (primary adrenocortical insufficiency), characterized by bronzing of skin, weakness, weight loss, and hypotension, is associated with elevated serum potassium. Manifestations may be mild in early stages, with weakness predominating.

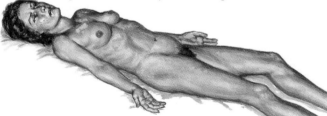

FIG 65.3 Myopathies Related to Disorders of Potassium Metabolism.

NAM is a distinct autoimmune myopathy presenting with similar symptoms as polymyositis, including proximal weakness with high creatine kinase levels, although often with a more severe phenotype. The pathology of NAM is distinct, with myofibril necrosis with little or no inflammatory response. It is often seen in association with anti-signal recognition particle antibodies or HMGCR antibodies, which are sometimes associated with statin exposure. Cardiac involvement, either conduction abnormalities or cardiomyopathy, appears to be common with NAM, but large series have not been well studied.

Inclusion body myositis is a distinct subset of acquired muscle disease that has both inflammatory and neurodegenerative features. Cardiac involvement is not common.

Sarcoidosis is a systemic autoimmune granulomatous disorder that typically affects the lungs, but can have manifestations in any system of the body. Cardiac involvement can occur with sarcoidosis, either in combination with systemic disease, a generalized myopathy, or as an isolated finding. Manifestations of cardiac sarcoidosis include conduction abnormalities, arrhythmias, or cardiomyopathy. Cardiac MRI typically suggests this diagnosis, but endomyocardial biopsy may be necessary in a patient in whom sarcoidosis has not been otherwise histologically confirmed. Treatments include corticosteroids and steroid-sparing immunotherapy.

Peripheral Neuropathy

Peripheral neuropathy, or polyneuropathy, refers to a broad spectrum of disease that affects the peripheral nerves extending from the nerve root to skin and neuromuscular junction. Shared symptoms of peripheral neuropathy generally include some combination of sensory loss, paresthesias, pain, weakness, and autonomic dysfunction, depending on the subset of peripheral nerve types affected. Most peripheral neuropathy does not affect cardiac function. However, when neuropathy is severe or associated with significant autonomic involvement, cardiovascular manifestations may be prominent.

Diabetic Neuropathy

Peripheral neuropathy is common in patients with diabetes. The most common manifestations are distal sensory loss in the feet, sometimes with associated pain. A generalized sensory or sensorimotor neuropathy in diabetes can be accompanied by autonomic neuropathy, often affecting both the sympathetic and parasympathetic systems. Cardiovascular manifestations of diabetic autonomic neuropathy include orthostatic hypotension, resting tachycardia, and an increased risk of silent myocardial infarction and mortality.

Immune-Mediated Neuropathies

Guillain-Barré syndrome. Guillain-Barré syndrome (GBS) describes monophasic acute immune-mediated neuropathies that are often postinfectious and typically demyelinating in pathophysiology. The typical clinical features are acute onset, progressing over hours to days, ascending sensory loss and weakness, and occasionally, with cranial and respiratory involvement. Treatment with intravenous immunoglobulin or plasma exchange speeds recovery, and supportive management, including respiratory support, is critical. Autonomic involvement with GBS is common, including hypotension or labile blood pressures, with episodes of severe hypertension, tachyarrhythmias, bradyarrhythmias, and vagal dysfunction. Close cardiac and blood pressure monitoring during hospitalization for GBS, even in patients with relatively mild disease at onset, is critical for preventing life-threatening complications.

Chronic Immune-Mediated Autonomic Neuropathy. Chronic autonomic neuropathy, which is sometimes associated with a more generalized sensory or sensorimotor polyneuropathy, may occur related to an underlying autoimmune cause. Autonomic neuropathy may also occur in association with certain cancers as a paraneoplastic phenomenon, most often small cell lung cancer with anti-Hu antibodies. When severe, cardiovascular involvement may manifest with orthostatic hypotension or tachyarrhythmia. Treatment is aimed at the underlying autoimmune or malignant process.

Amyloidosis

Amyloidosis includes a range of disorders that result in extracellular deposition of fibrils composed of low molecular weight subunits of a variety of proteins with typical pathological appearance. Neuromuscular involvement is common in both hereditary (TTR) and AL (plasma cell dyscrasia–associated) amyloidosis, typically with peripheral neuropathy and autonomic dysfunction. Cardiac involvement in the form of cardiomyopathy is also commonly seen with AL and hereditary amyloidosis (Fig. 65.5).

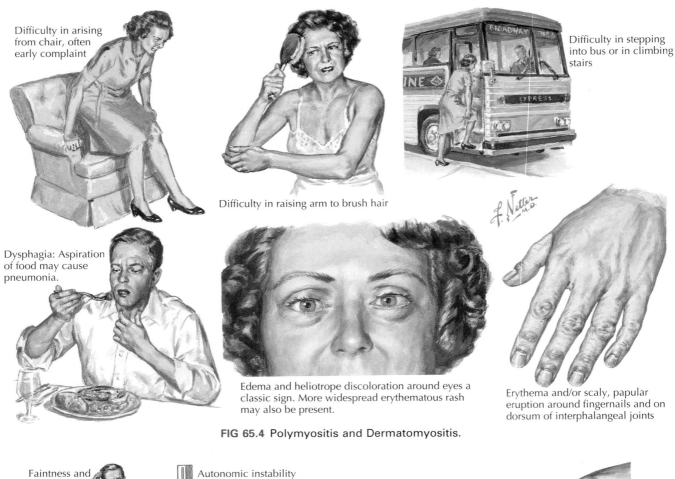

Difficulty in arising from chair, often early complaint

Difficulty in raising arm to brush hair

Difficulty in stepping into bus or in climbing stairs

Dysphagia: Aspiration of food may cause pneumonia.

Edema and heliotrope discoloration around eyes a classic sign. More widespread erythematous rash may also be present.

Erythema and/or scaly, papular eruption around fingernails and on dorsum of interphalangeal joints

FIG 65.4 Polymyositis and Dermatomyositis.

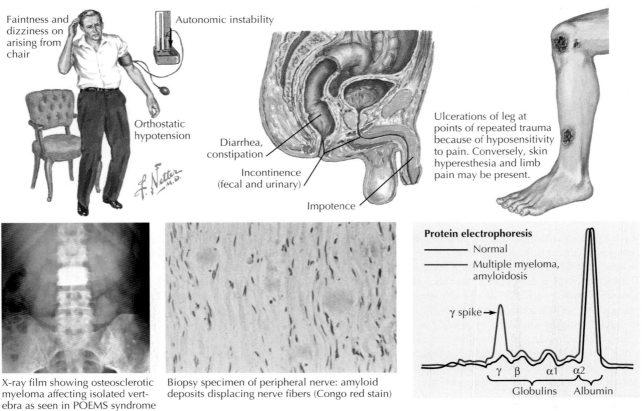

Faintness and dizziness on arising from chair

Autonomic instability

Orthostatic hypotension

Diarrhea, constipation

Incontinence (fecal and urinary)

Impotence

Ulcerations of leg at points of repeated trauma because of hyposensitivity to pain. Conversely, skin hyperesthesia and limb pain may be present.

X-ray film showing osteosclerotic myeloma affecting isolated vertebra as seen in POEMS syndrome

Biopsy specimen of peripheral nerve: amyloid deposits displacing nerve fibers (Congo red stain)

Protein electrophoresis
— Normal
— Multiple myeloma, amyloidosis

γ spike

γ   β   α1   α2

Globulins   Albumin

POEMS, polyneuropathy-organomegaly-endocrinopathy-monoclonal gammopathy, skin changes.

FIG 65.5 Amyloid Neuropathy.

Hereditary Neuropathies

A genetic subset of hereditary neuropathies affects small fiber and autonomic involvement; these are phenotypically grouped as the hereditary sensory and autonomic neuropathies. The degree of autonomic and cardiovascular effects of autonomic dysfunction in this group of disorders varies by genetic subtype.

There are also a number of genetic diseases that commonly manifest with a combination of peripheral neuropathy and cardiac disease, including Friedreich ataxia, abetalipoproteinemia, Refsum disease, and porphyrias.

ADDITIONAL RESOURCES

Claeys KG, Fardeau M. Myofibrillar myopathies. *Handb Clin Neurol.* 2013;113:1337–1342.
A review of the myofibrillar myopathies, including their cardiac manifestations.
Gorman GS, Chinnery PF, DiMauro S, et al. Mitochondrial diseases. *Nat Rev Dis Primers.* 2016;2:16080.
A comprehensive review of mitochondrial disorders, including cardiac manifestations.
Mckeon A, Benarroch EE. Autoimmune autonomic disorders. *Handb Clin Neurol.* 2016;133:405–416.
A review of autoimmune and paraneoplastic autonomic disorders.
Schwartz T, Diederichsen LP, Lundberg IE, Sjaastad I, Sanner H. Cardiac involvement in adult and juvenile idiopathic inflammatory myopathies. *RMD Open.* 2016;2(2):e000291.
A review of cardiac involvement in inflammatory myopathies.
Spurney CF. Cardiomyopathy of Duchenne muscular dystrophy: current understanding and future directions. *Muscle Nerve.* 2011;44(1):8–19.
A comprehensive review of clinical features and management of cardiomyopathy in Duchenne muscular dystrophy.
Washington University Neuromuscular Disease Center website. http://neuromuscular.wustl.edu/.
An excellent online reference with up-to-date clinical, genetic, and pathological information on all neuromuscular disorders.
Wicklund MP. The muscular dystrophies. *Continuum (Minneap Minn).* 2013;19(6 Muscle Disease):1535–1570.
An excellent clinical overview of the muscular dystrophies.

EVIDENCE

Barber BJ, Andrews JG, Lu Z, et al. Oral corticosteroids and onset of cardiomyopathy in Duchenne muscular dystrophy. *J Pediatr.* 2013;163(4):1080.
In this study of boys with Duchenne muscular dystrophy, oral corticosteroid treatment was associated with delayed cardiomyopathy onset.
Groh WJ, Groh MR, Saha C, et al. Electrocardiographic abnormalities and sudden death in myotonic dystrophy type 1. *N Engl J Med.* 2008;358(25):2688–2697.
In this study of patients with type 1 myotonic dystrophy, a severe abnormality on ECG or clinical history of atrial tachyarrhythmia predicted sudden cardiac death.
Narayanaswami P, Weiss M, Selcen D, et al. Evidence-based guideline summary: diagnosis and treatment of limb-girdle and distal dystrophies: report of the guideline development subcommittee of the American Academy of Neurology and the practice issues review panel of the American Association of Neuromuscular & Electrodiagnostic Medicine. *Neurology.* 2014;83(16):1453–1463.
An evidence-based review and guidelines with specific recommendations regarding cardiac care in patients with LGMDs.
Nicolino M, Byrne B, Wraith JE, et al. Clinical outcomes after long-term treatment with alglucosidase alfa in infants and children with advanced Pompe disease. *Genet Med.* 2009;11(3):210.
In this study of infants and children with Pompe disease, enzyme replacement therapy prolonged survival and improved measures of cardiomyopathy and motor skills.
Pop-Busui R, Evans GW, Gerstein HC, et al; Action to Control Cardiovascular Risk in Diabetes Study Group. Effects of cardiac autonomic dysfunction on mortality risk in the Action to Control Cardiovascular Risk in Diabetes (ACCORD) trial. *Diabetes Care.* 2010;33(7):1578.
In this trial of glucose management in type 2 diabetes, patients with cardiac autonomic neuropathy had increased risk of mortality.

66

Cardiovascular Manifestations of Endocrine Diseases

David R. Clemmons

Endocrine system diseases generally affect multiple organ systems, because hormones secreted into the general circulation act on multiple tissues that are distant from their sources of synthesis and secretion. Nearly all hormones and accompanying hormonal disorders may be associated with a pathophysiological disarrangement of some component of the cardiovascular system. This chapter focuses on the most common disorders and those with the most important deleterious consequences for cardiovascular function.

PITUITARY GLAND DISORDERS

The seven peptide hormones secreted by the anterior pituitary gland and the two hormones secreted by the posterior pituitary gland all affect the cardiovascular system. Most of these hormones cause changes in salt or water metabolism that indirectly alter the system, but some directly affect vascular tone. The anterior pituitary hormones and their direct and indirect effects on cardiovascular function are listed in Table 66.1. Three disorders can result in major changes in cardiovascular function: hypopituitarism, acromegaly, and antidiuretic hormone (ADH) secretion disorders.

Hypopituitarism

Hypopituitarism in adults often results from mass lesions that arise in the hypothalamus or the pituitary fossa. Growth hormone (GH) deficiency and gonadotropin deficiencies are often present. If the lesion causing the deficit is extensive, thyroid-stimulating hormone (TSH) (thyrotropin) and adrenocorticotrophic hormone (ACTH) secretion may also be impaired. GH deficiency per se does not lead to cardiomyopathy or loss of vascular tone; however, patients with GH deficiency most commonly present with a lack of energy and stamina. Therefore, cardiac output (CO) may not be adequate to sustain peak exercise activity, and endurance may be moderately impaired. Treatment with GH replacement therapy for as long as 3 years improves treadmill performance, which suggests that GH deficiency leads to a decrease in exercise tolerance. However, whether this improvement is due solely to GH stimulation of myocardial function is unclear, because GH also increases red cell mass, which could alter exercise tolerance. TSH and ACTH deficiencies lead to changes in cardiovascular function, as discussed in the sections on hypothyroidism and hypoadrenalism. Loss of gonadotropin secretion, particularly in men, can lead to low testosterone concentrations. This can lead to impaired exercise performance, loss of skeletal muscle mass, and decreased stamina. Replacement with testosterone improves muscle function and exercise performance.

Acromegaly

Sustained hypersecretion of GH by a pituitary tumor can lead to overgrowth of several tissues and to several cardiovascular changes (Fig. 66.1). Cardiovascular function is an important determinant of morbidity and mortality in untreated acromegaly. The most common comorbid cardiovascular condition accompanying acromegaly is hypertension, which is present in 60% of inadequately treated patients. Hypertension in acromegaly is usually mild but can be difficult to manage conventionally. Left ventricular (LV) mass can be significantly increased compared with that of normotensive patients. Curing the acromegalic condition is the most effective way to lower blood pressure (BP). Some patients can develop a concentric ventricular hypertrophic cardiomyopathy unassociated with hypertension but which is associated with long-standing acromegaly, which can result in both diastolic and systolic dysfunction. Cardiomegaly can be disproportionate to the changes in size that occur in other organs in severe acromegaly. The severity of cardiomyopathy correlates with the duration of exposure to high levels of GH. Diastolic dysfunction and hypertrophy develop first and are common in untreated patients. These changes are reversible with adequate treatment of excessive GH. If left untreated, there is progression to systolic dysfunction, and heart failure and severe ventricular arrhythmias can occur. Histological evaluation of the myocardium in patients with long-standing acromegaly can show interstitial fibrosis, lymphocytic infiltration, and occasionally, necrosis.

Other changes in acromegaly can lead to secondary effects on the cardiovascular system. Some patients have sleep apnea that causes chronic recurrent hypoxemia, approximately 25% of patients have diabetes mellitus, and up to 40% of patients have hypertriglyceridemia. Premature mortality is increased in acromegaly, and cardiovascular diseases are the cause of death in 38% to 62% of patients. Normalizing GH and insulin-like growth factor 1 concentrations with conventional treatment restores normal life expectancy, preventing the premature death that results from cardiovascular disease.

Disorders of Antidiuretic Hormone Secretion

Unlike diseases of the anterior pituitary gland, the etiology of ADH deficiency is often hypothalamic lesions (in ~60% of patients). Most cases of ADH deficiency are acquired, and many result from attempts to remove the pituitary tumor surgically, which can damage the pituitary stalk or the posterior pituitary. Severe ADH deficiency leads to polyuria, polydipsia, and, if untreated, vascular collapse. The most common hypothalamic causes are mass lesions, which are primarily tumors of the hypothalamus (e.g., craniopharyngioma and dysgerminoma).

ADH is a potent pressor agent that stimulates direct vasoconstriction of blood vessels. This action is conferred at the level of the regional arterioles, and physiological concentrations can induce this effect. Loss of ADH leads to a significant increase in serum osmolarity of >295 mOsm/L, with inappropriately dilute urine of <300 mOsm/L. The diagnosis is established by detecting abnormally high serum osmolarity with low plasma vasopressin and low urinary osmolarity.

Administering vasopressin quickly reverses the changes in these parameters. Vasopressin acts on the kidney to decrease free-water

TABLE 66.1 Pituitary Hormones and Their Actions on the Cardiovascular System

Hormone	Direct	Indirect
ACTH	Stimulates cortisol secretion Stimulates aldosterone	Cortisol increases arteriolar tone. Aldosterone stimulates Na⁺ retention and K⁺ excretion.
TSH	Stimulates thyroxine and triiodothyronine synthesis	Thyroxine stimulates HR, pulse pressure, and LV contractility.
LH	Stimulates estrogen and testosterone synthesis	Estrogen acts as a vasodilator.
ADH	Stimulates water retention, increases plasma volume; acts through a central mechanism to increase vasoconstriction	
GH	Stimulates vasomotor force and LV function	Through IGF-1, it stimulates HR.

ACTH, Adrenocorticotrophic hormone; *ADH*, antidiuretic hormone; *GH*, growth hormone; *HR*, heart rate; *IGF-1*, insulin-like growth factor I; *K⁺*, potassium; *LH*, luteinizing hormone; *LV*, left ventricular; *Na⁺*, sodium; *TSH*, thyroid-stimulating hormone.

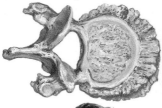

Thoracic vertebra in acromegaly: Hyperostosis, especially marked on anterior aspect

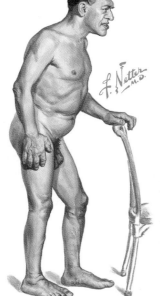

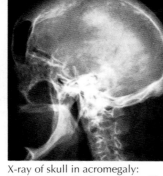

X-ray of skull in acromegaly: Enlargement of sella turcica, with occipital protuberance, thickening of cranial bones, enlargement of sinuses and of mandible

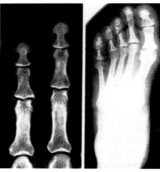

Tufting of phalanges in hands and narrowing of phalanges in feet

FIG 66.1 Acromegaly.

clearance. It also affects the brain to maintain central BP control; these brain actions are probably necessary for the maintenance of normal upright BP. The use of ADH antagonists illustrates the importance of endogenous arginine vasopressin for maintaining normal BP.

Syndrome of Inappropriate Antidiuretic Hormone Secretion

Several central nervous system and primary pulmonary diseases, as well as medications, can cause inappropriately high concentrations of ADH, leading to decreases in plasma osmolarity. In these syndromes, high levels of ADH secretion continue, despite low osmolarity. Arginine vasopressin concentrations can be increased up to 10 to 20 times greater than normal in this disorder. This does not lead to hypertension per se, but rather to water intoxication. Serum sodium continues to decrease because free-water clearance is consistently impaired, thus leading to severe hyponatremia, which sometimes manifest as seizures. Identification of the source of inappropriate ADH secretion or correction of the underlying lesion is needed for successful treatment. Empiric treatment severely restricts free-water intake. Recently, a new class of ADH receptor antagonists (vaptans) has been shown to improve hyponatremia associated with euvolemic inappropriate secretion of ADH. These drugs are approved for the in-hospital treatment of severe euvolemic hyponatremia.

THYROID DISORDERS

Hyperthyroidism

Hyperthyroidism causes some of the most impressive and sustained disarrangements of cardiovascular function related to endocrine abnormalities. Graves disease, the most common cause of hyperthyroidism, is triggered by an autoimmune process in which thyroid antigens that are recognized as foreign stimulate the production of an autoantibody that stimulates the TSH receptor. The autoantibody directly binds to the TSH receptor on thyroid tissue and stimulates thyroid function. The effect of this stimulating antibody is unremitting and necessitates specific therapy to block thyroid hormone synthesis. The second most common cause of hyperthyroidism is a toxic multinodular goiter. This condition can account for 40% of cases in patients older than 60 years of age.

The most common symptoms of cardiac dysfunction that occur in thyrotoxicosis include fatigue, palpitations, dyspnea, heat intolerance, increased sweating, and weight loss. Tachycardia and palpitations occur in 80% to 90% of untreated patients (Fig. 66.2). Older adult patients who develop Graves disease may also experience heart failure. In this circumstance, the failing heart cannot meet the metabolic requirements that are raised by the increased thyroid hormone, which results in overt congestive heart failure (CHF). Similarly, angina pectoris may be an important symptom in older adult patients with hyperthyroidism. Myocardial oxygen consumption can increase by as much as 70% in untreated hyperthyroidism. In the presence of fixed coronary lesions, blood flow may be inadequate to supply the increased metabolic need. In younger patients, thyrotoxicosis is associated with increased inotropic and chronotropic effects on the heart. Palpitations, and, occasionally, atrial arrhythmias, are the initial symptoms. Atrial fibrillation occurs in 33% to 47% of patients who are older than 60 years. Vascular resistance is decreased by peripheral vasodilation; the net effect is a marked increase in CO, which results in increased oxygen consumption. Peripheral edema is the most common symptom of overt heart failure in Graves disease, although dyspnea on exertion can also be prominent.

Physical findings typically include a hyperdynamic precordium, accentuated heart sounds, and a systolic murmur that can be heard over the precordium because of increased flow across the aortic valve.

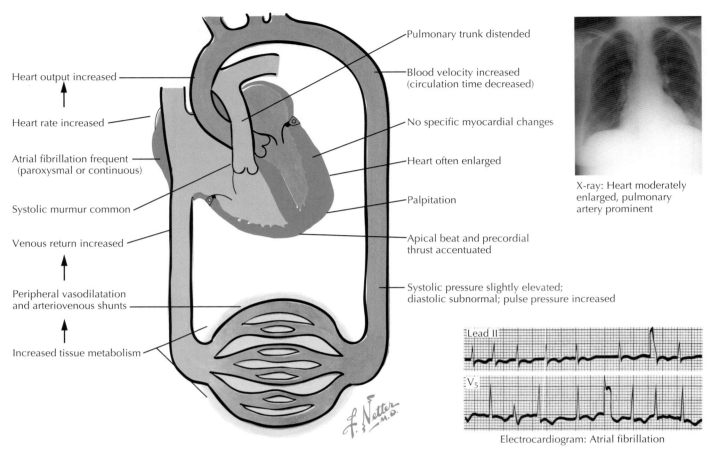

Heart output increased

Heart rate increased

Atrial fibrillation frequent (paroxysmal or continuous)

Systolic murmur common

Venous return increased

Peripheral vasodilatation and arteriovenous shunts

Increased tissue metabolism

Pulmonary trunk distended

Blood velocity increased (circulation time decreased)

No specific myocardial changes

Heart often enlarged

Palpitation

Apical beat and precordial thrust accentuated

Systolic pressure slightly elevated; diastolic subnormal; pulse pressure increased

X-ray: Heart moderately enlarged, pulmonary artery prominent

Lead II

V_5

Electrocardiogram: Atrial fibrillation

FIG 66.2 The Hyperthyroid Heart.

Arrhythmias can range from sporadic premature beats to overt atrial fibrillation. Thyrotoxicosis is present in approximately 11% of patients with atrial fibrillation who are older than 60 years of age. Atrial fibrillation due to either hyperthyroidism or hypothyroidism is common enough that thyroid disease must be excluded at an early stage in the evaluation of this arrhythmia. ECG findings are nonspecific. Heart failure in younger patients is generally reversible with adequate treatment. Whether a distinct thyrotoxic cardiomyopathy exists is debated; however, extensive cardiac remodeling occurs in some patients. This may also be aggravated by long-standing tachyarrhythmias. In older adult patients in whom underlying cardiac abnormalities exist, heart failure can be severe and may trigger atrial fibrillation. Acceleration of angina pectoris can be dramatic in older adults, and overt myocardial infarction can occur in these patients if left untreated.

The diagnosis is established by elevated serum thyroxine (T_4) in the presence of a suppressed TSH concentration. Early in the disease, triiodothyronine (T_3) is elevated, which is usually followed by an increase in T_4.

Initial treatment of Graves disease with antithyroid drugs blocks thyroid hormone synthesis. Treatment of the thyroid disease does not always restore normal sinus rhythm. If patients fail to undergo remission in a reasonable period on antithyroid drugs, or if they do not tolerate these medications, they are generally treated with radioactive iodine. In older adult patients with multiple cardiac complications, initial therapy with radioactive iodine may be indicated. Although reversal of the thyrotoxic state generally restores cardiac abnormalities due to thyrotoxicosis to normal in younger patients, this is not always the case in older adult patients. Both sets of patients may benefit initially from therapy with β-blockers, which limits most effects of catecholamines on the cardiovascular system—effects that are accentuated in Graves disease. If a toxic multinodular goiter is present, the usual treatment is radioactive iodine.

An increasingly recognized important cause of hyperthyroidism in cardiac patients is amiodarone-induced thyrotoxicosis (AIT). This usually occurs in patients during the first year of therapy. There are two different pathophysiological mechanisms that induce hyperthyroidism. In the first (AIT type I), the iodine in amiodarone induces hyperthyroidism. These patients have a low radioactive iodine uptake, and color flow Doppler shows increased vascularity. They respond to potassium perchlorate and antithyroid drugs. Type II AIT patients have a distinctive thyroiditis induced by an amiodarone metabolite. These patients have a low radioactive iodine uptake and absent vascularity. They respond to high-dose corticosteroid therapy.

Hypothyroidism

Like hyperthyroidism, hypothyroidism is usually caused by autoimmune thyroid disease. The most common cause of thyroid failure is Hashimoto thyroiditis, which occurs in 80% of women with hypothyroidism. In this disease, an autoantibody to the thyroid gland is produced that blocks thyroid function and thyroid hormone action. Eventually, this may result in destruction of the thyroid gland as a result of cytotoxic lymphocytic infiltration. However, this occurs over a period of several years, so the onset and progression are usually insidious and unrecognized by the patient. Hypothyroidism also develops in almost all patients who receive radioactive iodine treatment for hyperthyroidism. Hypothyroidism can result from a pituitary tumor or other causes of anterior pituitary gland destruction, but these are rare compared with Hashimoto thyroiditis. Patients who have thyroid damage due to antibodies or

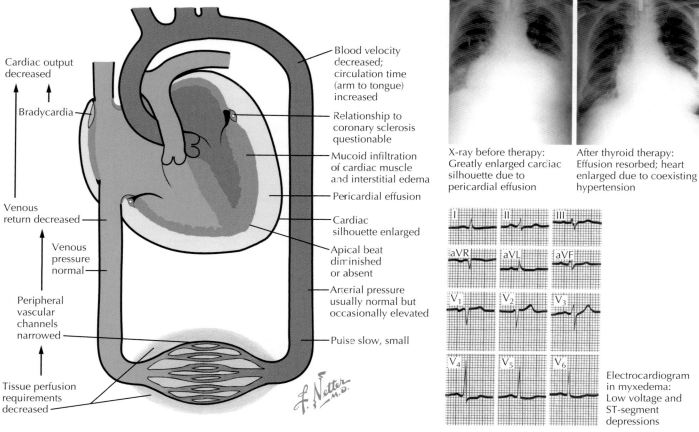

X-ray before therapy: Greatly enlarged cardiac silhouette due to pericardial effusion

After thyroid therapy: Effusion resorbed; heart enlarged due to coexisting hypertension

Electrocardiogram in myxedema: Low voltage and ST-segment depressions

FIG 66.3 Cardiovascular Effects of Hypothyroidism/Myxedema.

radiation are highly susceptible to suppression of thyroid function by exogenous iodine. Therefore, administration of contrast agents or ingestion of drugs that contain iodine (e.g., amiodarone) can induce severe hypothyroidism.

Changes in the cardiovascular system are also common in patients with severe long-standing hypothyroidism (Fig. 66.3). These patients have an increased peripheral vascular resistance, decreased stroke volume, and, as a result, decreased CO. Although systolic pressure may be decreased and diastolic pressure increased in these individuals, mean arterial pressure is often normal. The mechanism of increased vascular resistance is related to reduced compliance and impaired nitric oxide availability. The preejection and isovolumetric contraction times are prolonged, and the ventricular relaxation rate during diastole is slower. The mechanism of reduced cardiac contractility is multifactorial. T_3 stimulates the synthesis of calcium regulatory proteins that have been implicated in the cardiac manifestations of hypothyroidism. Blood volume is decreased, and pericardial and pleural effusions are common. Echocardiographic evidence of pericardial effusion is present in approximately 40% of patients.

Physical examination reveals a slow pulse, diastolic hypertension, and soft first and second heart sounds. Cardiac enlargement, when present, is generally caused by a pericardial effusion. Peripheral edema may be present, but it is generally nonpitting and not caused by heart failure. The ECG may show bradycardia and low voltage with nonspecific ST-segment or T-wave changes and a prolonged QT interval. First-degree heart block is also common. There is decreased myocardial contractility and slowing of the isovolumic relaxation phase of diastolic function. In hypothyroid patients with known coronary artery disease

(CAD), silent myocardial ischemia may occur. Although symptomatic angina is not common, it can occur during thyroid hormone replacement therapy, particularly in patients with severe long-standing hypothyroidism. This problem is accentuated by the anemia that is often present in hypothyroidism. Hypothyroidism secondarily results in severe lipoprotein abnormalities, including hypercholesterolemia and low concentrations of high-density lipoprotein cholesterol (HDL-C). Increased homocysteine levels may also occur in hypothyroidism.

The treatment of hypothyroidism is thyroid hormone replacement therapy. Young patients can tolerate full replacement doses; however, older adult patients with angina need extremely low-dose therapy with gradual incremental increases as tolerated.

PARATHYROID DISORDERS

Hyperparathyroidism is an unusual cause of vascular pathogenesis. In one study, 69% of patients with primary hyperparathyroidism were found to have systolic and diastolic hypertension. Generally, the degree of BP elevation is minimal. The cause of hyperparathyroidism in 85% of patients is a parathyroid hormone–producing tumor, which leads to hypercalcemia, the most common presenting sign. The hypercalcemic state can also cause LV hypertrophy, increased heart muscle contractility, and arrhythmias. Calcium deposition in the myocardium, the heart valves, or the coronary arteries occurs in up to 69% of patients with hyperparathyroidism compared with 17% of age-matched controls. Usually, these changes occur with severe long-standing hyperparathyroidism. However, in recent years, the presentation and treatment of hyperparathyroidism have changed markedly, and a much lower percentage of patients have these abnormalities at the time of diagnosis because they are diagnosed and treated much earlier in the course of their illness. Secondary hyperparathyroidism (not due to a parathyroid gland tumor) is common in patients with chronic renal failure. These patients have elevated serum phosphorus that leads to a secondary increase in parathyroid hormone. Vascular calcification and reduced arterial compliance are common. Although patients with primary hyperparathyroidism are usually treated by surgical removal of the tumor, until recently, there was no effective treatment for secondary hyperparathyroidism. The development of a calcium-sensing receptor antagonist (cinacalcet) has provided an effective means for treating secondary hyperparathyroidism. One study showed that treatment of patients with end-stage renal disease and secondary hyperparathyroidism had modest improvement (13%) in a composite index of vascular events.

ADRENAL DISORDERS

Both glucocorticoid and mineralocorticoid excesses can lead to marked cardiovascular abnormalities.

Cushing Disease and Syndrome

The most common cause of glucocorticoid excess is from pituitary tumors that overproduce ACTH, termed "pituitary Cushing disease." Less common but equally deleterious to cardiovascular function are primary adrenal adenomas that overproduce glucocorticoids or ectopic tumors (tumors outside the pituitary) that overproduce ACTH.

Cushing syndrome, or excess glucocorticoid production, often leads to severe skeletal muscle myopathy, because glucocorticoids inhibit protein synthesis in muscle (Fig. 66.4). Because of its rapid onset, dramatic presentation, and severe deleterious effects, Cushing syndrome is generally treated before severe atrophic cardiomyopathy develops. Therefore, it is rare for patients to present with cardiomyopathic symptoms. Hypertension is common in Cushing syndrome because of mineralocorticoid overproduction that leads to increased plasma volume and sodium retention. In addition, glucocorticoids enhance the vasopressive effects of endogenous catecholamines. Severe hypokalemia can cause characteristic ECG changes. Whether atherosclerosis occurs

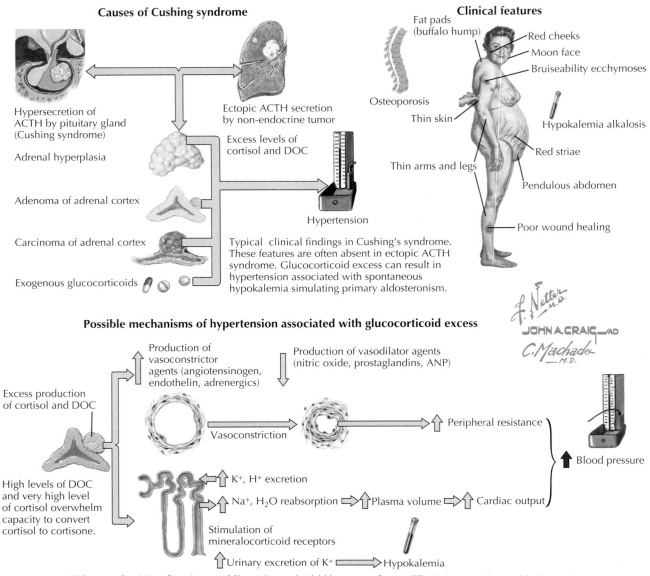

FIG 66.4 Cushing Syndrome–Mineralocorticoid Hypertension. *ACTH*, Adrenocorticotrophic hormone; *ANP*, atrial natriuretic peptide; *DOC*, deoxycorticosterone; *H⁺*, hydrogen; *K⁺*, potassium; *N⁺*, sodium.

independently of the changes in lipoprotein metabolism that result from excess glucocorticoid is not clear. However, marked increases in atherosclerosis in patients who receive long-term glucocorticoid therapy in pharmacological doses have been reported.

Treatment involves removing the cause of the excess cortisol or ACTH. Generally, the cardiovascular abnormalities are easily ameliorated. Patients who receive pharmacological doses of glucocorticoids for prolonged periods for underlying inflammatory disorders are just as susceptible to cardiovascular complications. Cushing syndrome may precipitate CHF in susceptible patients, because the resulting increase in mineralocorticoids causes salt retention.

Addison Disease

Hypoadrenalism is most often caused by a primary autoimmune disorder, Addison disease, in which the adrenal glands are progressively destroyed, leading to marked sodium loss with increased serum potassium. Orthostatic hypotension and decreased plasma volume are generally present. Decreased plasma volume can manifest as a reduction in the size of the cardiac silhouette on chest radiographs.

Occasionally, patients with undiagnosed chronic adrenal insufficiency develop acute adrenal insufficiency, usually in the setting of underlying physical stress, such as a car accident or bacterial infection. During stress, healthy individuals secrete up to 10 times more cortisol than under normal conditions. Because this requirement cannot be met in patients with adrenal failure, symptoms of acute adrenal insufficiency develop: nausea and vomiting, hypotension, dizziness, and eventually, vascular collapse and shock. The diagnosis should be suspected in patients with these findings and a low serum sodium concentration, a high potassium concentration, and evidence of low plasma volume. It is confirmed by administering 1 µg of cosyntropin (synthetic ACTH) intravenously and measuring the plasma cortisol level after 30 or 60 minutes. A normal response to the ACTH challenge is a peak cortisol level of 18 µg/dL. Treatment consists of fluid replacement and administration of hydrocortisone.

Several other hormones also have profound effects on salt and water balance, and therefore, on cardiovascular function. The most important of these are atrial natriuretic peptide (ANP), brain natriuretic peptide (BNP), and endothelin. ANP is a 28-amino acid peptide produced by the left atrium. A circulating precursor form, 1-126, is believed to be biologically inactive. Normally, ANP-28 is made solely in the left atrium; however, in pathological states such as LV hypertrophy or failure, ANP-28 can also be released from the left ventricle. Atrial wall tension is the primary factor that controls synthesis and secretion of ANP-28. Therefore, ANP-28 is increased in acute and chronic volume expansion, CHF, and other conditions associated with elevated intraatrial pressure. It functions to stimulate vasodilation in both small and large arteries. Negative feedback regulation of ANP-28 occurs, and volume contraction decreases its synthesis and secretion. ANP-28 binds to specific receptors in the kidney, where it increases capillary permeability, glomerular filtration rate, renal filtration fraction, urinary filtration, and excretion of sodium. This, in turn, lowers plasma volume and decreases BP. ANP is active in patients with acute renal failure, and its administration improves glomerular function.

A related peptide, BNP, is released by neural tissue. BNP is also stored in nerve endings in the atrium. This site of synthesis and release can be stimulated by many of the same stimuli that cause release of ANP-28. In general, BNP is released in response to more chronic changes in plasma volume. BNP acts on the same renal receptors that are activated by ANP and has similar effects on kidney function. Both peptides have direct effects on arterial smooth muscle cells and bring about vasodilatation. Administration of ANP or BNP to patients with heart failure results in beneficial effects on plasma volume and CO; however,

patients with severe heart failure become refractory to monotherapy. A recent trial using combined treatment with an inhibitor for ANP degradation and an angiotensin II receptor blocker showed a significant reduction in morbidity and mortality. Recent reports also suggested that plasma BNP levels provide useful information in monitoring the longitudinal treatment of patients with CHF (see Chapter 23).

Endothelin is a small peptide that is released by vascular endothelium and whose three isoforms are closely related. Endothelin receptors are present on vascular smooth muscle cells, cardiac myocytes, and renal glomerular endothelium. Endothelin is a potent vasoconstrictor, an action that can be opposed by the release of nitric oxide, and a potent vascular mitogen. In addition to its effects on blood vessels and kidney function, endothelin also has direct inotropic and chronotropic effects on the heart; however, endothelin also decreases coronary blood flow because of its vasoconstrictive effects. Endothelin may also act secondarily to decrease plasma volume by increasing the release of ANP and BNP.

Mineralocorticoid Disorders

In addition to glucocorticoids, the adrenal gland synthesizes a group of steroids with sodium-retaining activity. Aldosterone is the principal steroid among this group. Unlike cortisol, which is regulated primarily by ACTH secretion, the primary stimulus for aldosterone synthesis is the renin-angiotensin system. In hypovolemic states, the afferent arterioles of the kidney contain specialized juxtaglomerular cells that sense low-flow or low-pressure states in these vessels. These states trigger the release of the enzyme renin directly from the kidney into the blood. Renin acts on angiotensinogen, a peptide precursor that is synthesized in the liver, which enzymatically converts angiotensinogen into angiotensin I. Angiotensin I passes through the pulmonary circulation and is cleaved by a second enzyme, termed angiotensin-converting enzyme (ACE), to angiotensin II. Angiotensin II is the most biologically active component of the renin-angiotensin system. This peptide, although labile, has direct vasoconstrictive effects on blood vessels and serves as a stimulus to maintain arteriolar tone. This stimulus is particularly important in maintaining normal BP when a person is assuming an upright posture. In addition to its acute effects on arteriolar tone, angiotensin II stimulates the adrenal gland to synthesize aldosterone. This is the principal mechanism for regulating aldosterone production.

Aldosterone acts on the distal convoluted tubule and collecting duct to increase sodium absorption (Fig. 66.5). This effect occurs via a sodium-potassium transporter. For each molecule of sodium that is reabsorbed, the tubular cells secrete a molecule of potassium. Under normal circumstances, this maintains a normal sodium–potassium balance and a normal plasma volume. Expansion of the plasma volume results in increased flow through the renal afferent arterioles, and this signals the system to decrease renin, thus maintaining equilibrium.

Another important stimulus that controls the release of angiotensin II is potassium, which directly stimulates angiotensin II and aldosterone production. ACTH can also stimulate aldosterone secretion and is needed to maintain normal rates of aldosterone synthesis.

Primary disorders of this system are uncommon causes of hypertension and plasma volume expansion. Primary tumors in which aldosterone is the principal secretory product are the most common disorder. Of patients with hyperaldosteronism, approximately 60% have an aldosterone-producing adenoma. Another 34% have idiopathic bilateral enlargement of the zona glomerulosa in both adrenal glands and overproduce aldosterone, which leads to increased sodium retention and potassium excretion. These patients usually present with mild hypertension, evidence of volume overload, and hypokalemia. Other than direct effects on the vasculature, hyperaldosteronism also leads to increased salt retention, which can precipitate CHF in older adult patients.

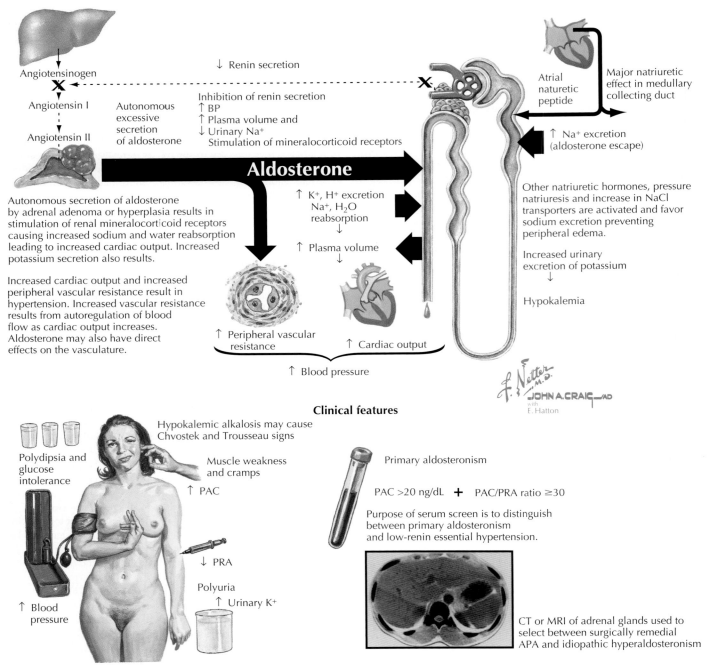

Angiotensinogen

↓ Renin secretion

Angiotensin I

Angiotensin II

Autonomous excessive secretion of aldosterone

Inhibition of renin secretion
↑ BP
↑ Plasma volume and
↓ Urinary Na⁺
Stimulation of mineralocorticoid receptors

Aldosterone

↑ K⁺, H⁺ excretion
Na⁺, H₂O reabsorption
↓

↑ Plasma volume
↓

Autonomous secretion of aldosterone by adrenal adenoma or hyperplasia results in stimulation of renal mineralocorticoid receptors causing increased sodium and water reabsorption leading to increased cardiac output. Increased potassium secretion also results.

Increased cardiac output and increased peripheral vascular resistance result in hypertension. Increased vascular resistance results from autoregulation of blood flow as cardiac output increases. Aldosterone may also have direct effects on the vasculature.

↑ Peripheral vascular resistance

↑ Cardiac output

↑ Blood pressure

Atrial naturetic peptide

Major natriuretic effect in medullary collecting duct

↑ Na⁺ excretion (aldosterone escape)

Other natriuretic hormones, pressure natriuresis and increase in NaCl transporters are activated and favor sodium excretion preventing peripheral edema.

Increased urinary excretion of potassium
↓

Hypokalemia

Clinical features

Polydipsia and glucose intolerance

Hypokalemic alkalosis may cause Chvostek and Trousseau signs

Muscle weakness and cramps
↑ PAC

↓ PRA

Polyuria
↑ Urinary K⁺

↑ Blood pressure

Primary aldosteronism

PAC >20 ng/dL **+** PAC/PRA ratio ≥30

Purpose of serum screen is to distinguish between primary aldosteronism and low-renin essential hypertension.

CT or MRI of adrenal glands used to select between surgically remedial APA and idiopathic hyperaldosteronism

FIG 66.5 Primary Hyperaldosteronism–Mineralocorticoid Hypertension. *APA,* Aldosterone-producing adenoma; *BP,* blood pressure; *H⁺,* hydrogen; *K⁺,* potassium; *Na⁺,* sodium; *NaCl,* sodium chloride; *PAC,* plasma aldosterone concentration; *PRA,* plasma renin activity.

The diagnosis is usually established by obtaining the ratio of plasma aldosterone to renin. Because renin is suppressed by the increased plasma volume, this ratio is usually >20:1, necessitating further investigation. Multiple drugs that are used to treat hypertension can alter renin and aldosterone, and they should be discontinued before diagnostic testing. Adrenal MRI often confirms the diagnosis of an aldosterone-producing tumor.

Treatment for an adrenal adenoma consists of surgical removal, which cures hypertension in approximately 60% of patients. Patients with bilateral hyperplasia and no tumor respond well to drugs that directly antagonize the effects of aldosterone, such as spironolactone. Eplerenone is a more selective aldosterone antagonist. It has little affinity for other steroid receptors, thus reducing the incidence of bothersome adverse effects, such as gynecomastia and menstrual irregularities that are experienced with spironolactone. These drugs are effective in inhibiting the sodium-retaining and vasoconstrictive properties of aldosterone. They can induce hyperkalemia; therefore, their usefulness is limited to patients with a glomerular filtration rate of >30 mL/min. ACE inhibitors are effective for the treatment of CHF in which secondary hyperaldosteronism is present.

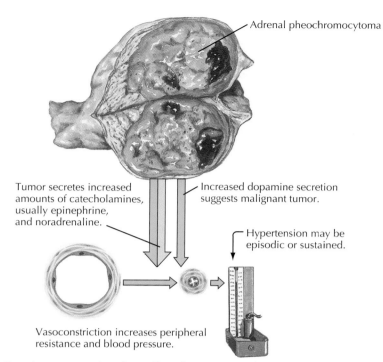

Adrenal pheochromocytoma

Tumor secretes increased amounts of catecholamines, usually epinephrine, and noradrenaline.

Increased dopamine secretion suggests malignant tumor.

Hypertension may be episodic or sustained.

Vasoconstriction increases peripheral resistance and blood pressure.

Pheochromocytoma is a chromaffin cell tumor secreting excessive catecholamines resulting in increased peripheral vascular resistance and hypertension.

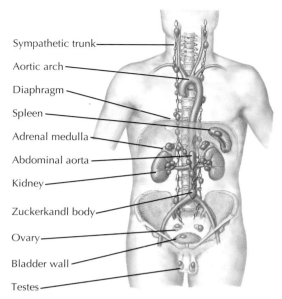

Potential sites of pheochromocytoma

Sympathetic trunk
Aortic arch
Diaphragm
Spleen
Adrenal medulla
Abdominal aorta
Kidney
Zuckerkandl body
Ovary
Bladder wall
Testes

Most pheochromocytomas are adrenal in origin, but can occur in various sites in sympathetic ganglia and may be associated with multiple endocrine neoplasia syndromes. Most are sporadic, but some are hereditary.

Clinical features of pheochromocytoma

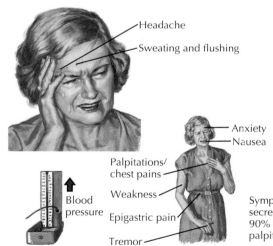

Headache
Sweating and flushing
Anxiety
Nausea
Palpitations/chest pains
Weakness
Blood pressure
Epigastric pain
Tremor

Random urine sample
24-hour urine sample

Abnormal random urine assay for creatine and metanephrine or 24-hour urine assay of metanephrine and free catecholamines used in diagnosis

Symptoms are secondary to excessive catecholamine secretion and are usually paroxysmal. More than 90% of patients with pheochromocytoma have headaches, palpitations, and sweating alone or in combination.

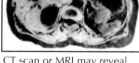

CT scan or MRI may reveal presence of tumor.

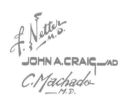

J. Netter M.D.
JOHN A. CRAIG—MD
C. Machado—M.D.

FIG 66.6 Pheochromocytoma.

Adrenal Medullary Tumors

Pheochromocytoma, although rare, is an important cause of acute changes in BP and cardiovascular function. These tumors are generally unilateral, but they can occur bilaterally and outside the adrenal medulla (e.g., anywhere in the sympathetic ganglia chain) (Fig. 66.6). The rapid release of norepinephrine or epinephrine from the tumor results in dramatic cardiovascular signs and symptoms.

Because catecholamines work directly on arterioles to cause severe vasoconstriction, the principal signs are rapid elevation of BP, palpitations, sweating, tremulousness, anxiety, and nervousness. Other symptoms can include headache, chest pain, extreme weakness, and fatigue. Acute symptoms occur in approximately 50% of patients and include severe

headache, dyspnea, palpitations, sweating, and tremor. Signs that are notable on physical examination are hypertension, postural hypotension, tachycardia, weight loss, increased respiratory rate, and tremor. A postural reduction in BP (e.g., >10 mm Hg) occurs in approximately 90% of patients as a result of contraction of intravascular volume. Patients with underlying angina pectoris or heart failure may severely decompensate in the presence of an untreated pheochromocytoma. The diagnosis is established by measuring plasma catecholamines, urinary catecholamines, and the principal metabolites of epinephrine and norepinephrine, which include metanephrine.

Administration of β-adrenergic blocking agents can precipitate a hypertensive crisis by leaving α-adrenergic activity unopposed. Other medications that can precipitate a crisis include monoamine oxidase inhibitors, tricyclic antidepressants, and catecholamine reuptake inhibitors. Hypertension responds well to α-adrenergic blocking agents, including phenoxybenzamine (dibenzyline). Management is usually surgical, unless the tumor is malignant, in which case long-term therapy with α-blockers is required.

DIABETES

Both types of diabetes (type 1 from severe insulin deficiency and type 2 primarily from insulin resistance combined with insulin deficiency in the later stages) accelerate the development of atherosclerosis. Hypertension is also common in patients with long-standing diabetes, which contributes to the high incidence of vascular disease in these patients. Patients, in whom even moderate degrees of azotemia develop, often become seriously hypertensive as a result of diabetic nephropathy.

Significant lipoprotein abnormalities also develop in most patients who have long-standing diabetes. Therefore, multiple risk factors all contribute to extensive vascular disease, which occurs in 80% of patients with long-standing diabetes. As a factor that increases the relative risk for CAD, diabetes ranks second, only behind smoking.

It is difficult to separate the degree of risk conferred by diabetes from that conferred by hyperlipidemia. However, both are independent risk factors. It should be noted that the dyslipidemic syndrome that occurs in diabetes involves a profile that confers high risk for CAD. The lipoprotein phenotype common to patients with diabetes is overproduction of triglycerides and apolipoprotein B. Low-density lipoprotein cholesterol (LDL-C) levels are normal in approximately 65% of patients, but the small dense LDL-C fraction is often elevated, particularly in patients with extreme hypertriglyceridemia and low HDL-C levels. This is due in part to the activity of hepatic lipase, which is increased in type 2 diabetes and results in processing of LDL-C to small dense particles. Likewise, overproduction of triglycerides can lead to suppression of HDL-C, particularly the most important subfraction, HDL_2. This combination of abnormalities constitutes the dyslipidemic syndrome that is common in patients with type 2 diabetes. The presence of nephropathy further aggravates the dyslipidemic syndrome in diabetes. Hypertriglyceridemia and a low HDL-C level are often accentuated, and dialysis can further worsen the profile.

A low HDL-C level is a strong predictor of coronary heart disease in patients with diabetes. Total triglycerides seem to have some predictive value, although the predictive value of total cholesterol in diabetic individuals is debated. The non–HDL-C fraction of cholesterol, which includes LDL-C plus very low-density lipoprotein cholesterol, is an excellent predictor of risk. Intimal medial thickness is increased in patients with diabetes, suggesting the presence of a diffuse atherosclerotic process, even in those who have not had a myocardial infarction. Fatality rates after an ischemic event are substantially higher among patients with diabetes. Treatment of hyperlipidemia is usually uses statins, which have been shown to reduce vascular events in diabetics. The recently developed PCSK9 inhibitors are potent drugs for lowering LDL-C, but whether they reduce vascular events in diabetics compared with other hypolipidemic agents has not been determined.

The low HDL-C levels in persons with diabetes are associated with poor glycemic control. Improving glycemic control often lowers triglycerides and raises HDL-C. Treatment with oral hypoglycemic agents or insulin improves both triglyceride and HDL-C levels. Weight loss also improves both of these parameters. Two recently developed classes of antidiabetic drugs have been associated with a decrease in cardiovascular events. These include glucagon-like peptide-1 (GLP-1) agonists and sodium glucose co-transporter 2 (SGLT2) inhibitors. GLP-1 agonists function primarily to enhance insulin secretion postprandially. SGLT2 inhibitors block renal reabsorption of glucose. Although both drugs reduce cardiovascular events in part by reducing blood glucose, the findings suggest that they may also function by other as yet unidentified mechanisms.

Not surprisingly, peripheral vascular disease is also widespread in patients with diabetes. Many patients with coronary disease also have disease in the large peripheral arteries. Leg and foot amputations are far more frequent in patients with diabetes. Bilateral occlusive disease in medium-sized arteries below the knee is common in patients with long-standing disease. Medical treatment of peripheral vascular disease generally has limited success. Vascular surgery is the only option for many patients. Indications for Doppler ultrasonography, followed by arteriography, are pain at rest, ulcerations that fail to heal, and gangrene.

Cardiomyopathy

The possibility of a distinct diabetic cardiomyopathy has been debated. Postmortem examinations reveal cardiomegaly and myocardial fibrosis. Unexplained CHF occurs in a substantial number of patients with diabetes. Echocardiography of patients with extensive microvascular disease shows compromised cardiac function. Impaired diastolic filling has been demonstrated in a substantial number of patients with type 1 diabetes with long-standing disease. A delayed increase in the ventricular ejection fraction during dynamic exercise is present in 29% of patients. The pathogenesis seems to be varied and multifactorial.

FUTURE DIRECTIONS

Several recently developed drugs have been tested for their ability to improve the cardiovascular manifestations of endocrine disorders. Major new findings have been reported for GLP-1 agonists and SGLT2 inhibitors. Both these classes of drugs have been shown to reduce vascular events. Future studies are likely to focus on defining the subgroups of patients who are most responsive to these agents and whether different classes of drugs will benefit different types of patients in terms of reducing cardiovascular events.

Major progress has also been made in improvement of hyperlipidemia and reducing vascular events associated with hyperlipidemia. Specifically, PCSK9 inhibitors and the maximum tolerated dose of statins have been shown to reduce vascular events. Future studies are likely to address the subpopulation within this group who have diabetes. Specifically, a trial needs to be conducted exclusively in diabetic patients to determine whether the addition of PSCK9 inhibitors will lower vascular events in this particular group. These drugs offer the potential to lower LDL-C to extremely low levels and therefore partially compensate for the deleterious effects of chronic hyperglycemia on vascular function. Additional studies are likely to continue studying the role of non–HDL-C versus LDL-C in precipitating vascular events in patients with diabetes.

Another important area of improvement in therapy has been heart failure. Specifically, the combined use of inhibitors of ANP and BNP degradation with angiotensin receptor blocking agents has been shown to be efficacious in terms of lowering morbidity and mortality in this patient population. These studies are likely to be expanded to determine the optimum time of intervention and the optimum dosing regimens that will obtain the maximum benefit. Studies of aldosterone receptor antagonists have clearly shown some benefit in patients with heart failure. In addition, there is an increase in reaction reactive oxygen species generation in patients with poorly controlled diabetes. Trials to assess the efficacy of these agents alone or in combination with ACE inhibitors in reducing vascular events in diabetics should be forthcoming. Studies to assess the safety and efficacy of calcium-lowering agents in patients with late stage diabetic nephropathy and vascular calcification are likely to continue. Because calcium receptor mimetics have shown some efficacy in this regard, there is hope that a further understanding of the pathophysiology of the process will lead to drugs that can be used successfully to reduce this complication.

Studies are continuing in the role of estrogen therapy alone in reducing vascular complications when administered in the first few years after menopause. Although studies to date have shown benefit, the exact benefit-to-risk ratio compared with the potential risk for ovarian and breast cancer has not been definitively determined.

EVIDENCE

Anabtawi A, Moriarty PM, Miles JM. Pharmacologic treatment of dyslipidemia in diabetes: a case for therapies in addition to statins. *Curr Cardiol Rep.* 2017;19(7):62–71.
A comprehensive review of the pathophysiology and treatment of diabetic dyslipemia.

Díez J. Chronic heart failure as a state of reduced effectiveness of the natriuretic peptide system: implications for therapy. *Eur J Heart Fail.* 2017;19(2):167–176.
A detailed analysis of the mechanism of action of each of the peptides and evidence for their reduced effectiveness in heart failure.

Jabbar A, Pingitore A, Pearce SH, et al. Thyroid hormones and cardiovascular disease. *Nat Rev Cardiol.* 2017;14(1):39–55.
A comprehensive review of the molecular changes that occur in the heart and blood vessels in response to thyroid hormones and the changes that occur in hyper- and hypothyroidism.

Lombardi G, Di Somma C, Grasso LF, et al. The cardiovascular system in growth hormone excess and growth hormone deficiency. *J Endocrinol Invest.* 2012;35(11):1021–1029.
A comprehensive review of the cardiovascular changes that occur in states of GH deficiency and excess.

Morselli E, Santos RS, Criollo A, et al. The effects of oestrogens and their receptors on cardiometabolic health. *Nat Rev Endocrinol.* 2017;13(6):352–364.
An in-depth analysis of the risks and benefits of estrogen on cardiovascular function.

Paneni F, Lüscher TF. Cardiovascular protection in the treatment of type 2 diabetes: a review of clinical trial results across drug classes. *Am J Cardiol.* 2017;120(1S):S17–S27.
An excellent review of the clinical trial results of the effects of these new drugs on cardiovascular outcomes in diabetics.

Pappachan JM, Raskauskiene D, Sriramar R, et al. Diagnosis and management of pheochromocytoma: a practical guide to clinicians. *Curr Hypertens Rep.* 2014;16(7):442–453.
A comprehensive review of the most recently discovered genetic causes of this disease, as well as a review of the most accurate and precise diagnostic tests, and information on how to interpret the results.

Pasqualetti G, Tognini S, Polini A, et al. Is subclinical hypothyroidism a cardiovascular risk factor in the elderly? *J Clin Endocrinol Metab.* 2013;98(6):2256–2266.
An excellent meta-analysis of a therapy trial of subclinical hypothyroidism and potential cardiovascular benefits.

Schumaecker MM, Larsen TR, Sane DC. Cardiac manifestations of adrenal insufficiency. *Rev Cardiovasc Med.* 2016;17(3–4):131–136.
A succinct summary of the cardiac manifestations of loss of adrenal function.

Toka HR, Pollak MR. The role of the calcium-sensing receptor in disorders of abnormal calcium handling and cardiovascular disease. *Curr Opin Nephrol Hypertens.* 2014;23(5):494–501.
A clearly written review of the efficacy of the calcium sensing receptor and pathophysiological alterations in primary and secondary hyperparathyroidism.

Valassi E, Crespo I, Santos A, et al. Clinical consequences of Cushing's syndrome. *Pituitary.* 2012;15(3):319–329.
A succinct summary of the changes that occur in metabolism in Cushing syndrome that increase cardiovascular risk as well as potential direct effects of steroids on the vascular tone.

Vinod P, Krishnappa V, Chauvin AM, et al. Cardiorenal syndrome: role of arginine vasopressin and vaptans in heart failure. *Cardiol Res.* 2017;8(3):87–95.
A detailed analysis of the mechanism of action of each of the peptides' effects on cardiovascular function and their involvement in pathophysiological changes.

67

Connective Tissue Diseases and the Heart

Rachel D. Romero, Beth L. Jonas

ETIOLOGY AND PATHOGENESIS

Autoimmune rheumatic diseases include a wide variety of illnesses, such as rheumatoid arthritis (RA) and systemic lupus erythematosus (SLE), in which changes to both the innate and adaptive immune system lead to tissue damage. The etiologies of these diseases are believed to be multifactorial. Genetic susceptibility is believed to play an important role, but is not sufficient for the development of disease. Environmental agents, infections, or drugs are possible inciting factors. For example, tobacco exposure has been identified as a strong risk factor for RA, and ultraviolet light exposure has been associated with the development of SLE. Infection may also play a role through molecular mimicry: studies have shown that Epstein-Barr virus may precede the development of SLE autoantibodies, which are amplified through epitope spreading. Certain major histocompatibility complex haplotypes have been found to be associated with increased risk of particular rheumatological diseases. Classic examples include the link between human leukocyte antigen HLA-B27 in spondyloarthropathy and HLA DRB1*044 in RA.

Autoimmune rheumatic diseases commonly affect the cardiovascular system. The endocardium, myocardium, pericardium, and conducting system may all be injured through different mechanisms by any rheumatological disease. Tissue damage may be due to direct immunologic injury (via direct antibody attack, immune complex formation, or cell-mediated destruction) to the myocardium, endocardium, or pericardium, or to the blood vessels supplying these tissues. Direct inflammatory infiltration or fibrosis frequently causes conduction system damage and various electrophysiological abnormalities. In utero conduction damage may be due to specific autoantibodies, including anti-Ro/SSA and anti-La/SSB passively transferred from maternal circulation through placental blood flow. In addition to the effects of the underlying disease process on the heart, many of the rheumatological diseases confer a higher risk of coronary artery disease (CAD), which is believed to be related to high levels of systemic inflammation.

CLINICAL PRESENTATION

Systemic Lupus Erythematosus

SLE is a multisystem autoimmune disorder characterized by the production of autoantibodies, with a striking female predominance in the reproductive years (10:1 female-to-male) (Fig. 67.1). The diagnosis of SLE requires both characteristic clinical features (e.g., malar rash, alopecia, arthritis, oral ulcers, or nephritis) in addition to supportive serologies. Diagnosis may be difficult due to the heterogeneity of the disease. Classification criteria have been developed by both the Systemic Lupus International Collaborating Clinics and the American College of Rheumatology (ACR) for research purposes, but may be useful as a reference when evaluating a patient with possible SLE. Cardiovascular diseases are one of the most important causes of morbidity and

mortality in SLE patients. Autoantibodies and the development of immune complexes with complement activation are believed to be the major mechanisms in cardiovascular injury in SLE. The cardiac manifestations of lupus may affect the pericardium, myocardium, valves, conduction system, and coronary arteries.

Serositis in SLE is often associated with disease flares. Pericarditis is the most common cardiac manifestation of lupus, with approximately 25% of all patients with SLE developing symptomatic pericarditis during the course of their disease. The prevalence by echocardiography and in autopsy studies is as high as 60% in individuals with SLE. Cardiac tamponade is rare and occurs in 1% to 2% of patients; however, some retrospective studies found 13% to 22% of patients with symptomatic pericarditis had tamponade. Constrictive pericarditis is even less common. Analysis of pericardial fluid has revealed decreased pH and neutrophil predominant inflammatory exudate. Pericardial biopsy has revealed mononuclear cells, fibrinous material, and immune complex deposition; however, biopsy is not necessary for diagnosis.

Myocarditis is clinically evident in <10% of patients but can cause severe systolic dysfunction. Cardiac MRI shows delayed gadolinium enhancement in lupus myocarditis, although this may be seen in myocarditis from other causes. Biopsy has a low yield and is not required for diagnosis; however, it may be of benefit in some patients. Myocarditis often develops with other organ involvement and may occur early in the course of disease. Treatment with steroids or cytotoxic agents can be lifesaving. Cardiomyopathy may be directly caused by SLE, but the most common cause is coexisting hypertension or CAD. Hydroxychloroquine, which is frequently prescribed for patients with SLE, is a rare cause of cardiomyopathy in SLE patients.

Asymptomatic valvular involvement, which is usually mitral and/or aortic, has been found in up to 70% of patients by transesophageal echocardiography. In a meta-analysis from 20 case–control studies that included 1117 SLE patients and 901 healthy control subjects from January 1, 1992 to July 31, 2013, patients with SLE who were evaluated with echocardiography had 11 times the increased risk of combined valvular alterations compared with healthy control subjects. There was a tenfold increase in mitral valve thickening, aortic valve thickening, mitral valve regurgitation, and mitral valve vegetation. Libman and Sacks first described sterile endocarditis-like lesions in SLE in 1924. These lesions most commonly involve the mitral valve, but may occur in any valve. These lesions consist of thrombotic-fibrinous clusters with proliferating endothelial cells, edema, and areas of necrosis, and have only rarely been reported to embolize. Antiphospholipid syndrome, which may accompany SLE, may be associated with valvular pathology. Acute valvular insufficiency in SLE can lead to hemodynamic instability and require surgical correction.

Conduction abnormalities, including atrioventricular (AV) block, bundle branch block, and dysautonomia, have been found in up to 10% of patients with SLE. However, most of these are not clinically

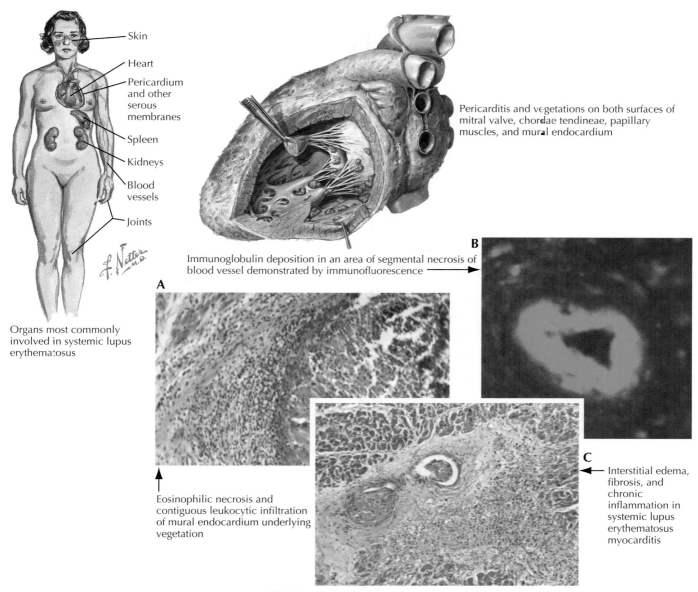

Skin

Heart

Pericardium and other serous membranes

Spleen

Kidneys

Blood vessels

Joints

Organs most commonly involved in systemic lupus erythematosus

Pericarditis and vegetations on both surfaces of mitral valve, chordae tendineae, papillary muscles, and mural endocardium

Immunoglobulin deposition in an area of segmental necrosis of blood vessel demonstrated by immunofluorescence

B

A

Eosinophilic necrosis and contiguous leukocytic infiltration of mural endocardium underlying vegetation

C

Interstitial edema, fibrosis, and chronic inflammation in systemic lupus erythematosus myocarditis

FIG 67.1 Lupus Erythematosus.

significant. In pregnant patients with SLE, screening for anti-Ro/SSA and anti-La/SSB antibodies is important to identify those at risk for having an offspring with neonatal lupus. In neonatal lupus, maternal autoantibodies cross the placenta, which affects the conduction system of the developing fetus. Complete heart block may occur, which is associated with fetal myocarditis. Two percent of fetuses develop heart block in the presence of anti-Ro/SSa antibodies, which rises to 18% in subsequent pregnancies if the first child is affected. Weekly fetal echocardiography between 17 and 24 weeks of gestation is recommended. Hydroxychloroquine use may reduce the risk of recurrent neonatal lupus in subsequent pregnancies. Although there is increased risk of having a child with neonatal lupus, adults with anti-Ro/SSA and anti-La/SSB are not prone to heart block. However, one study showed statistically significant prolongation of the QTc interval to 445 ms compared with 419 ms in control subjects.

Atherosclerosis remains the most prevalent and significant mortality risk in patients with SLE. The development of premature CAD in SLE patients is believed to be related to systemic inflammation. Some studies have shown a 2- to 10-fold increased risk of myocardial infarction. Long-term steroid use also increases the risk of subclinical cardiovascular disease and independently predicts the risk of cardiovascular events. Hydroxychloroquine modulates cardiovascular risk by improving both the lipid profile and glycemic control. Two prospective lupus cohort studies have shown a 50% to 60% decreased risk for cardiovascular disease with hydroxychloroquine use.

Rheumatoid Arthritis

RA is a systemic illness characterized by a symmetric, destructive polyarthritis, and occurs in 1% of most populations. The diagnosis of RA is based upon the presence of a chronic symmetric inflammatory arthritis, elevated inflammatory markers, and supportive serologies (rheumatoid factor and/or anti-CCP antibody). The 2010 ACR/European League Against Rheumatism classification criteria, developed for research purposes, uses a scoring system based on these domains. The presence of extra-articular manifestations in RA is associated with increased severity of disease and may involve the skin, eyes, lungs, hematologic system,

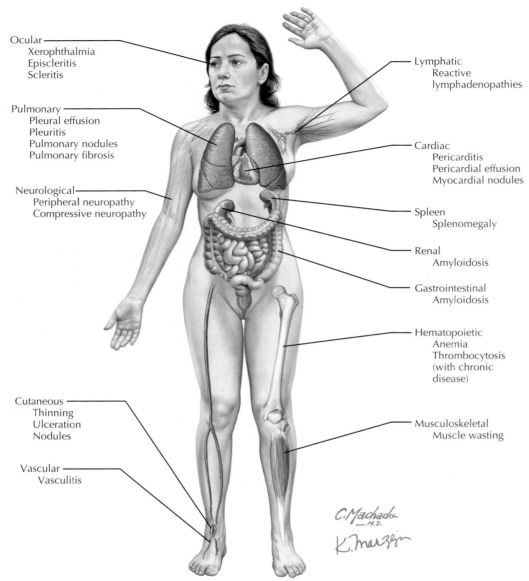

Ocular
Xerophthalmia
Episcleritis
Scleritis

Pulmonary
Pleural effusion
Pleuritis
Pulmonary nodules
Pulmonary fibrosis

Neurological
Peripheral neuropathy
Compressive neuropathy

Cutaneous
Thinning
Ulceration
Nodules

Vascular
Vasculitis

Lymphatic
Reactive
lymphadenopathies

Cardiac
Pericarditis
Pericardial effusion
Myocardial nodules

Spleen
Splenomegaly

Renal
Amyloidosis

Gastrointestinal
Amyloidosis

Hematopoietic
Anemia
Thrombocytosis
(with chronic
disease)

Musculoskeletal
Muscle wasting

FIG 67.2 Systemic Manifestations of Rheumatoid Arthritis.

nervous system, and the heart (Fig. 67.2). Cardiovascular disease causes almost one-half of all deaths in patients with RA. Manifestations include pericarditis, cardiomyopathy and/or myocarditis, cardiac amyloidosis, coronary vasculitis, arrhythmia, valvular disease, congestive heart failure (CHF), and CAD. The most frequent cardiac manifestations in RA patients are pericarditis and valvular heart disease. Pericarditis is seen in between 30% and 50% of autopsy cases and up to 30% by echocardiography; however, the clinical prevalence is lower. Pericarditis is more common in male, seropositive patients with nodular RA. Most patients develop pericarditis after the onset of arthritis, but rarely, it may be the initial manifestation of RA. Pericardial fluid is exudative, serosanguinous, or hemorrhagic with low glucose, neutrophilic predominance, and low pH. Cholesterol crystals may be seen in persistent effusions. Adhesions and loculations are common, often making pericardiocentesis difficult. A significant proportion of patients with clinical pericarditis have constriction or tamponade with a grave prognosis. These patients, under some circumstances, may benefit from surgical pericardiectomy.

Valvular lesions occur frequently (up to 70%); however, they are rarely symptomatic in RA. Pathologically, endocardial lesions can be caused by fibrosis, nonspecific inflammation, or less frequently, rheumatoid granulomas. Mitral or aortic valve insufficiency are the most common, with 30% to 80% and 9% to 33% frequency in a small case series, respectively. Myocarditis is rarely clinically evident but can be associated with arrhythmias. Cardiomyopathy secondary to RA may be from focal, nonspecific diffuse necrotizing or granulomatous myocarditis. In a small case series of 30 RA patients, cardiomyopathy was found in 37% by echocardiography. Restrictive cardiomyopathy from cardiac amyloidosis may rarely occur in RA. It should be noted that tumor necrosis factor (TNF)-α blockers, which are often used for treatment of RA and other rheumatic diseases should be used with caution in patients with known New York Heart Association functional class III or IV heart failure due to the risk of worsening CHF.

Vasculitis of coronary vessels has been described, although the clinical significance is unknown. It has been seen in up to 20% in postmortem studies. Increased cardiovascular risk occurs in RA independent of traditional risk factors and has been attributed to ongoing inflammation. The prevalence of cardiovascular disease in RA is increased to an extent that is comparable to that of the prevalence in the diabetic population. Arrhythmias may occur due to ischemia, as well as conduction abnormalities due to nodules, amyloidosis, and CHF. It has been hypothesized that increased sympathetic activity plays a role in development of ventricular tachyarrhythmias.

Idiopathic Inflammatory Myopathies

Idiopathic inflammatory myopathies (IIMs), including dermatomyositis, polymyositis, and inclusion body myositis, are chronic inflammatory muscle diseases characterized by muscle weakness, and histopathologically by inflammatory cell infiltration of skeletal muscle. The diagnosis is established based on clinical features, results of electromyography, and muscle biopsy. Clinically manifest cardiac involvement is rare, with CHF, conduction abnormalities, and CAD being the most frequently reported. The pathophysiological mechanisms are believed to include myocarditis, CAD, and involvement of the small vessels of the myocardium.

Congestive heart disease has been observed in between 3% and 45% of myositis patients. In a systematic review that observed frequencies of various clinical cardiac afflictions in IIM, CHF was the most common cause of death. Cardiomyopathy may be caused by myocarditis and has been identified on cardiac MRI in several case series. Myocarditis has been reported to be the most common cardiac manifestation in IIM, with 38% in cumulative prospective cohorts. Histologically, myocarditis appears similar to inflammation of skeletal muscle, with mononuclear inflammatory cells localized to the endomysium and perivascular areas with degeneration of the myocytes. Patients may also have myocardial fibrosis, which can lead to heart failure symptoms (both systolic and diastolic) and dysrhythmias. Pericarditis is unusual in IIM, with a reported frequency of approximately 10%. Pulmonary hypertension may occur if patients have associated interstitial lung disease or antisynthetase syndrome, which is characterized by antibodies to tRNA, with a constellation of clinical findings, including Raynaud syndrome, mechanic's hands, arthritis, and interstitial lung disease.

The risk of developing atherosclerotic CAD is increased twofold to fourfold in polymyositis and dermatomyositis. It is unclear how much of this risk is driven by traditional cardiovascular risk factors versus systemic inflammation. However, there have been recent studies that have shown increased prevalence of traditional cardiovascular risk factors in these patients. Small vessel disease may also cause angina pectoris. A rare form of myositis, immune-mediated necrotizing myopathy, has been associated with the use of statins and may have hydroxy-3-methylglutaryl coenzyme A reductase antibody positivity. Therefore, close monitoring and care must be taken with the use of statins in patients with IIMs.

Subclinical cardiac disease also occurs and is evidenced by ECG changes, including atrial and ventricular arrhythmias, bundle branch block, AV block, high grade heart bock, prolonged PR intervals, and nonspecific ST-T wave changes. In a systematic review, dysrhythmias were seen on 31.8% of ECGs in a cumulative prospective cohort.

Mixed Connective Tissue Disease

Mixed connective tissue disease (MCTD) is a connective tissue disorder characterized by high titers of anti-U1 ribonucleoprotein with clinical features that overlap with SLE, systemic sclerosis (SS), and polymyositis. Cardiac manifestations account for approximately 20% of mortality in MCTD. In a recent systematic review, the prevalence of cardiac disease in MCTD varied between 13% and 65%.

The most frequently reported manifestation is pericarditis, with two prospective studies showing prevalences of 30% and 43%. Myocarditis

may also occur. Cardiac noninvasive testing with ECG and echocardiography have revealed subclinical abnormalities, including conduction defects, pericardial effusions, and mitral valve prolapse. Similar to other chronic inflammatory diseases, MCTD patients also have a higher prevalence of accelerated atherosclerosis. The pathophysiological causes of cardiac disease in MCTD are believed to be similar to those seen in IIMs. Pulmonary hypertension may also occur due to small vessel disease, with autopsy studies showing intimal proliferation of small pulmonary arteries and arterioles with smooth muscle hypertrophy. The presence of pulmonary hypertension in MCTD patients is associated with an unfavorable prognosis and is usually refractory to immunosuppressive treatment.

Systemic Sclerosis

SS, or scleroderma, is a chronic connective tissue disorder characterized by autoimmunity, vascular damage, and fibrosis that affects the skin, blood vessels, joints, skeletal muscle and internal organs, such as the gastrointestinal tract, kidney, and lungs (Fig. 67.3). SS is classified as diffuse or limited cutaneous on the basis of the extent and distribution of skin involvement. The estimated clinical prevalence of cardiac disease in SS is 15% to 35%. It may affect both limited and diffuse disease, with a retrospective study of 254 patients over 4 years showing 7% prevalence in limited disease and 21% in diffuse disease.

Cardiac manifestations in SS may be classified as primary, which may manifest as myocardial damage, fibrosis, pericardial, and rarely, valvular disease, or secondary to indirect effects from damage to the kidneys and lungs. Primary myocardial disease is believed to be due to microvascular ischemia. Myocardial Raynaud phenomenon has been proposed as a mechanism for myocardial injury; however, in contrast to peripheral Raynaud syndrome, it demonstrates only infrequent luminal narrowing of the vessels of the heart. Early in SS, vasospasm of small coronary arteries and arterioles is an important manifestation. In late disease, there is reduced coronary flow reserve from fixed abnormalities. Because cardiac manifestations of SS may be indolent, they may progress silently, with clinical disease being a harbinger of poor prognosis. In one study, clinical cardiac disease in SS was associated with 70% mortality at 5 years. Myocardial fibrosis may arise, causing systolic and diastolic dysfunction and arrhythmias. Endomyocardial biopsy shows patchy fibrosis, which is a pathognomonic finding, in addition to contraction band necrosis, and involvement of the subendocardial layer (which is often spared in atherosclerotic disease). The prevalence of atherosclerosis of large epicardial coronary arteries has been shown to be similar to the general population. Symptomatic pericardial disease may occur in 5% to 16% of patients including pericarditis, pericardial effusions, and pericardial adhesions. In addition, conduction system defects, valvular disease, myocardial hypertrophy, and ischemia may also occur.

Scleroderma renal crisis and pulmonary hypertension, both manifestations of severe disease, may lead to cardiac dysfunction as a result of damage in the kidneys and lungs, respectively. Scleroderma renal crisis may cause severe systemic hypertension, which may lead to systolic dysfunction and CHF. The prevalence of pulmonary hypertension in SS is approximately 10% to 12%. It is often a poor prognostic indicator. Pulmonary hypertension may be isolated and secondary to vascular narrowing or associated with pulmonary fibrosis. Isolated pulmonary hypertension tends to be more severe and is more frequent in limited cutaneous (45%) than in diffuse cutaneous (26%) disease.

Seronegative Spondyloarthropathies

Seronegative spondyloarthropathies include ankylosing spondylitis, psoriatic arthritis, reactive arthritis, and arthritis associated with inflammatory bowel disease. All of these conditions are associated with HLA

Progressive Systemic Sclerosis (Scleroderma)

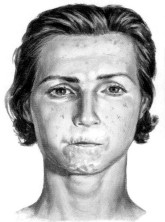

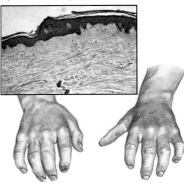

Typical skin changes in scleroderma. Extensive collagen deposition and some epidermal atrophy

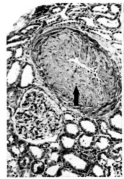

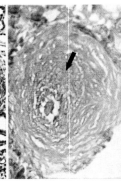

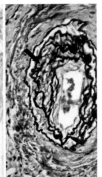

Characteristics. Thickening, tightening, and rigidity of facial skin, with small, constricted mouth and narrow lips, in atrophic phase of scleroderma

Sclerodactyly. Fingers partially fixed in semiflexed position; terminal phalanges atrophied; fingertips pointed and ulcerated

Arcuate artery in acute scleroderma. Mucoid swelling of intima in medium-sized artery of kidney, most often seen in acute cases

Arcuate artery in acute scleroderma. Colloidal iron stain, demonstrating that intimal swelling is composed largely of mucopolysaccharides

Arcuate artery in chronic scleroderma. Marked intimal thickening, consisting of dense, laminated matrix, rich in elastic fibers, and small amount of collagen

Scleroderma

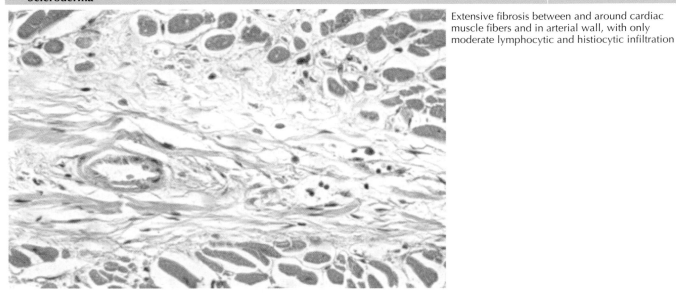

Extensive fibrosis between and around cardiac muscle fibers and in arterial wall, with only moderate lymphocytic and histiocytic infiltration

FIG 67.3 Systemic Sclerosis (Scleroderma).

B27, although the association is strongest in ankylosing spondylitis, which is considered the prototype seronegative spondyloarthropathy. Seronegative spondyloarthropathies share clinical manifestations, including enthesitis, uveitis, and others (Fig. 67.4). The aortic valve has been described as similar to an enthesis, and in ankylosing spondylitis, inflammation at its insertion points may lead to fibrosis of the aortic wall and shortened AV cusps. This may cause a dilated aortic root with secondary aortic regurgitation. Aortic regurgitation is often associated with long-standing disease of at least 10 to 15 years and older age. Aortic dissection or aortitis may also occur. In a recent retrospective cohort of >8000 patients with ankylosing spondylitis, the age- and sex-standardized prevalence ratio of aortic valvular heart disease compared with the general population was 1.58 (95% confidence interval: 1.31–1.91). There has been anecdotal evidence that progressive aortic

dilation in ankylosing spondylitis may respond to corticosteroids and cytotoxic therapies. In some cases, surgery may be necessary.

Mitral valve pathology is less common than aortic pathology and is characterized by leaflet fibrosis or regurgitation. Other mechanisms of mitral regurgitation include mitral valve prolapse and left ventricle dilation secondary to aortic regurgitation. Echocardiography may also show hyperechoic thickening of the aortic–mitral junction, which is a classic feature known as a subaortic bump. Heart failure due to myocarditis may also occur. Diastolic heart failure is more common than systolic heart failure, especially during the first 15 years of disease. In contrast to SLE and RA, symptomatic pericarditis is rare, only occurring in <1% of patients. AV conduction disturbances are usually caused by inflammation of the membranous septum. Electrophysiology studies show that AV block is often located in or below the node. It has been postulated

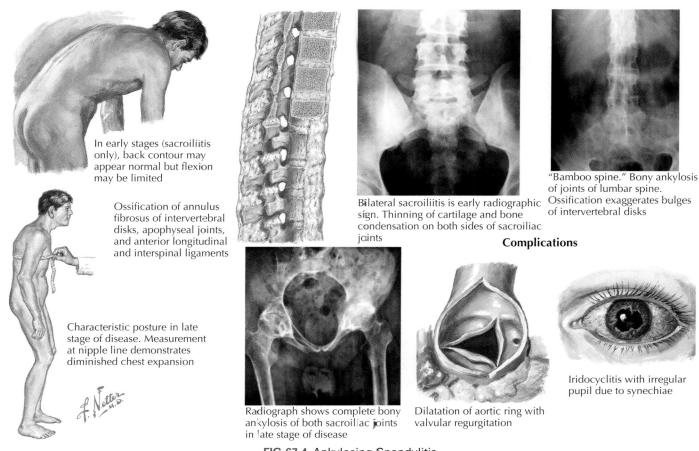

In early stages (sacroiliitis only), back contour may appear normal but flexion may be limited

Ossification of annulus fibrosus of intervertebral disks, apophyseal joints, and anterior longitudinal and interspinal ligaments

Characteristic posture in late stage of disease. Measurement at nipple line demonstrates diminished chest expansion

Bilateral sacroiliitis is early radiographic sign. Thinning of cartilage and bone condensation on both sides of sacroiliac joints

"Bamboo spine." Bony ankylosis of joints of lumbar spine. Ossification exaggerates bulges of intervertebral disks

Complications

Radiograph shows complete bony ankylosis of both sacroiliac joints in late stage of disease

Dilatation of aortic ring with valvular regurgitation

Iridocyclitis with irregular pupil due to synechiae

FIG 67.4 Ankylosing Spondylitis.

that HLA B27 plays a key role in the pathogenesis of severe AV block. Sinus node dysfunction, although rare, may lead to bradyarrhythmias in patients with HLA B27 seronegative spondyloarthropathies.

Vasculitis

The vasculitides are a group of disorders characterized by destruction of blood vessel walls secondary to inflammatory events such as direct antibody attack, immune complex formation, and cell-mediated destruction. Vasculitis may occur as a primary process or may be secondary to another underlying disease such as RA or SLE (Fig. 67.5). Generally, the vasculitides are classified according to the predominant size of the involved vessels: small vessel, medium vessel, large vessel, or variable vessel.

Among the small-vessel vasculitides, the three antineutrophil cytoplasmic antibody (ANCA)–associated vasculitides are granulomatosis with polyangiitis (GPA), eosinophilic granulomatosis with polyangiitis (EGPA), and microscopic polyangiitis (MPA). Among these, cardiac involvement is most commonly seen in EGPA, affecting up to two-thirds of adult patients (including both clinical and subclinical disease). EGPA, formerly known as Churg-Strauss syndrome, is characterized by chronic rhinosinusitis, asthma, and peripheral blood eosinophilia. Cardiac involvement is an important indicator of poor prognosis among EGPA patients. It is important to recognize the two subtypes of EGPA: ANCA-positive and ANCA-negative. ANCA-negative EGPA may be more difficult to diagnose and is more commonly associated with cardiac manifestations such as cardiomyopathy, myocarditis, and pericardial effusions than its counterpart. It has also been shown that EGPA patients

have a higher propensity to develop ventricular arrhythmias because of higher rates of QTc dispersion. Cardiac transplantation may be necessary for those patients with severe cardiac involvement. In GPA, cardiac involvement is rarer, with a North American cohort study of 517 patients showing a prevalence of only 3.3%. Pericarditis, myocarditis, valvular disease, cardiomyopathy, and conduction abnormalities may occur. Cardiac involvement in MPA has not been largely studied, but has also been described to rarely occur.

The medium-vessel vasculitides include polyarteritis nodosa (PAN) and the childhood vasculitis Kawasaki disease (KD) (Fig. 67.6). PAN rarely affects the heart; however, if present, it confers a twofold to threefold increased risk of mortality. PAN has been reported to cause coronary arteritis, pericarditis, myocardial involvement, and endocardial involvement. In KD, children may develop coronary artery dilatation that can regress with early therapy (standard therapy is intravenous immunoglobulin and aspirin), but 5% to 8% of patients may progress to coronary artery aneurysms. Coronary artery aneurysms may be seen in up to 25% of untreated children and pericardial effusions in 30%, along with myocarditis and valvular regurgitation. These patients have an increased risk of cardiovascular mortality, particularly those with coronary artery lesions; such patients may require long-term statin therapy.

Large-vessel vasculitides include Takayasu arteritis (TA) and giant cell arteritis (GCA). These primarily affect the aorta and main branches but may also involve medium-sized arteries, including the coronary arteries. TA is the most common large-vessel vasculitis, with cardiac

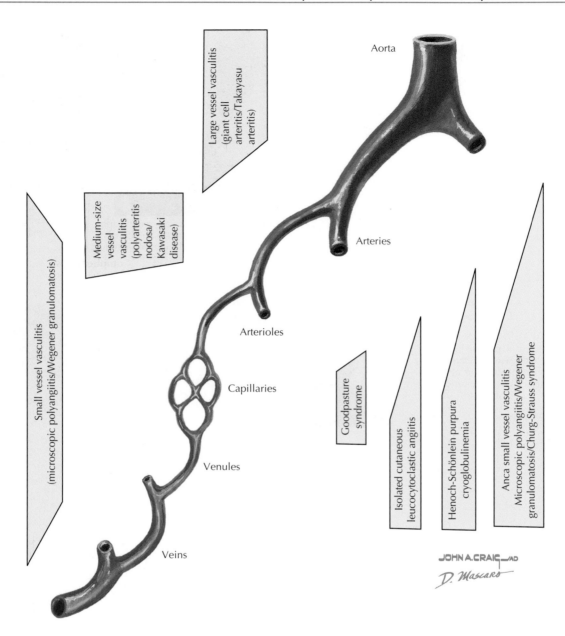

FIG 67.5 Distribution of Specific Vasculitis Syndromes.

manifestations including aortic regurgitation, pulmonary hypertension, myocarditis, and coronary disease. The presence of antiphospholipid antibodies in TA has been associated with increased risk of vascular complications (e.g., aortic regurgitation). There is an increased risk of thrombosis in TA that should respond to immunosuppressive treatment; however, there may be indications for anticoagulation in certain clinical settings (e.g., intracardiac thrombi, which have higher risk for embolization). GCA rarely affects the heart; however, there is an increased risk of CAD, particularly early in the disease course. Patients with GCA may develop inflammation of the aorta, aortic dilatation, or aneurysms, with thoracic aneurysms being three times more common than abdominal aneurysms.

Behcet disease (BD) is a variable-vessel disease because it can affect any size vessel, including both arterial and venous circulation. The disease is characterized by recurrent oral and genital ulcers, inflammatory ocular disease, skin involvement, and arthritis. Up to 6% of BD patients may have clinically apparent cardiac manifestations, which are more commonly seen in male patients. The spectrum of cardiac lesions that have been described in the literature include pericarditis, myocardial aneurysms, endocardial fibroelastosis, intracardiac thrombosis, and endocarditis with aortic valve involvement. Again, some patients with intracardiac thrombi require judicious use of anticoagulation. Anticoagulation should be used with caution because of the risk of fatal hemoptysis if pulmonary artery aneurysms are present. BD patients

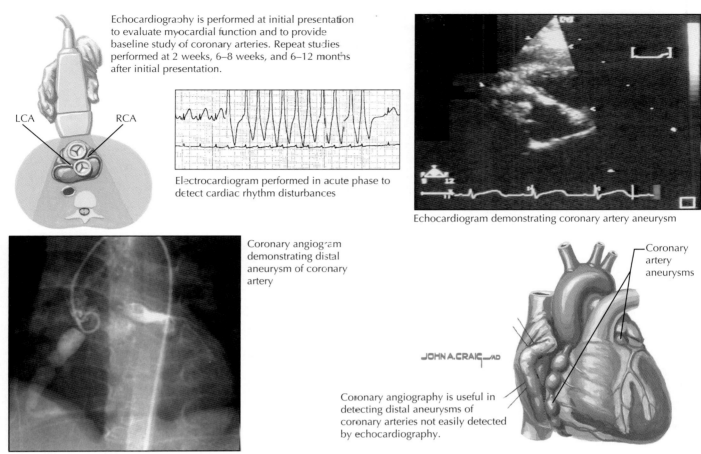

Echocardiography is performed at initial presentation to evaluate myocardial function and to provide baseline study of coronary arteries. Repeat studies performed at 2 weeks, 6–8 weeks, and 6–12 months after initial presentation.

LCA   RCA

Electrocardiogram performed in acute phase to detect cardiac rhythm disturbances

Echocardiogram demonstrating coronary artery aneurysm

Coronary angiogram demonstrating distal aneurysm of coronary artery

Coronary artery aneurysms

JOHN A. CRAIG—AD

Coronary angiography is useful in detecting distal aneurysms of coronary arteries not easily detected by echocardiography.

FIG 67.6 Cardiac Evaluation in Kawasaki Disease. *LCA,* Left coronary artery; *RCA,* right coronary artery.

may also have conduction abnormalities, including intraatrial and interatrial delay, prolonged QT, and other arrhythmias; they are likely to develop premature CAD.

DIAGNOSTIC APPROACH

The diagnostic approach for cardiovascular pathology in the presence of rheumatic diseases is similar to the approach in the general population. However, it is helpful to have an understanding of the more common cardiac manifestations in specific rheumatic diseases (Table 67.1). In addition to history and physical examination, noninvasive testing such as an ECG, echocardiography, and other imaging modalities are helpful. In vasculitides, CT angiography and magnetic resonance angiography are used. Invasive testing with cardiac catheterization may be necessary to evaluate for coronary ischemia or pulmonary hypertension. Recent studies have shown that cardiovascular MRI may detect occult lesions, such as edema, myocarditis, diffuse subendocardial fibrosis, and myocardial infarction at initial diagnosis of rheumatic diseases in treatment naïve patients. Interestingly, after 6 and 12 months of appropriate treatment, these imaging findings may be reversed.

MANAGEMENT AND THERAPY

Once a diagnosis is made, management of active autoimmune diseases is directed at controlling the systemic inflammation and preventing tissue damage. In most cases, the initial therapy may include corticosteroids due to their rapid and effective control of inflammatory symptoms. However, additional therapies are usually indicated both to spare the patient from long-term steroids and act as disease-modifying therapies.

Treatment of RA is aimed at early initiation of disease-modifying antirheumatic drugs (e.g., methotrexate or leflunomide), with the addition of biologics if necessary (e.g., TNF inhibitors), abatacept (costimulatory blocker CTLA4-Ig), tocilizumab (anti–interleukin-6), or rituximab (anti-CD20 monoclonal antibody). The efficacy of antimalarials (hydroxychloroquine) in preventing SLE flares has been well demonstrated and should be used in the treatment of all patients with SLE, unless contraindicated. In cases of organ involvement secondary to SLE, the use of other steroid-sparing agents, such as mycophenolate mofetil, azathioprine, or cyclophosphamide, may be necessary. Belimumab (which prevents stimulation of B cells) has now been approved by the Food and Drug Administration for the treatment of lupus. Treatment of scleroderma is often difficult and is targeted to organ-specific manifestations. For example, calcium-channel blockers for Raynaud phenomenon, proton-pump inhibitors for gastrointestinal reflux disease, and mycophenolate mofetil can be used in cases of interstitial lung disease (which may also help with skin thickening). As opposed to other rheumatic diseases, corticosteroids must be used with extreme caution in scleroderma due to the association with scleroderma renal crisis. The vasculitides are treated with high-dose corticosteroids, which also often require the use of other medications such as cyclophosphamide or rituximab. Tocilizumab is now being used in the treatment of large-vessel vasculitides as well.

TABLE 67.1   Overview of Cardiac Involvement in Specific Rheumatic Diseases

	Pericarditis	Myocarditis	Valvular Disease	Conduction Abnormalities	CAD	Pulmonary HTN
SLE	(++) Most common cardiac manifestation in SLE. Pericardial fluid is exudative.	(+) May cause severe systolic dysfunction.	(++) Mitral and aortic valve most commonly involved (ex. Libman-Sacks).	Rare. AV block, BBB. Anti-Ro/ anti-La associated with neonatal lupus and CHB.	(++) Increased risk	(+)
RA	(++) More common in seropositive males than females.	(+) Rare, but may lead to cardiomyopathy.	(++) Frequent in RA, but rarely symptomatic. Typically MV and AV.	(+) May be secondary to ischemia, nodules, amyloid, CHF.	(++) RA is considered an independent risk factor for CAD.	(+) May be isolated PAH or secondary to ILD.
Inflammatory myopathies	(+) Uncommon	(++) Most common cardiac manifestation in IIM. May cause CHF.	(+) Uncommon	(+) May be secondary to fibrosis.	(++) Close monitoring with initiation of statins which may cause myopathy.	(+) May be seen in anti-synthetase syndrome or ILD.
MCTD	(++) Most common cardiac manifestation in MCTD.	(+)	(+) MV prolapse has been reported.	(+) Typically subclinical.	(+)	(++) Poor prognostic indicator.
Scleroderma	(+) Less common	(+) Myocardial patchy fibrosis may lead to cardiomyopathy.	(+) Less common	(+) Secondary to fibrosis	(+)	(++) Isolated PAH or secondary to ILD. Poor prognostic indicator.
Seronegative spondyloarthropathies	Uncommon	Uncommon	(+) Aortitis, aortic valve regurgitation, mitral regurgitation.	(+)	(+)	
Small-vessel vasculitis (EGPA, GPA)	(+) Pericardial effusions	(+)	(+)	(+)	(+)	(+)
Medium-vessel vasculitis (polyarteritis nodosa, KD)	(+)	(+)	(+)	(+) KD: higher risk for ventricular arrhythmia	(+) KD: coronary aneurysms	(+)
Large-vessel vasculitis (Takayasu, GCA)	(+) in GCA	(+)	(+) Aortic regurgitation and mitral regurgitation most common.		(+)	(+)
Variable-vessel vasculitis (Behcet disease)	(+)	(+) Myocardial aneurysms and endocardial fibroelastosis.	(+) Aortic valve most commonly.	(+)	(+)	(+)

+, May occur; ++, occurs more frequently; *AV*, atrioventricular; *BBB*, bundle branch block; *CAD*, coronary artery disease; *CHB*, congenital heart block; *CHF*, congestive heart failure; *EGPA*, eosinophilic granulomatosis with polyangiitis; *GCA*, giant cell arteritis; *GPA*, granulomatosis with polyangiitis; *HTN*, hypertension; *IIM*, idiopathic inflammatory myopathy; *ILD*, interstitial lung disease; *KD*, Kawasaki disease; *MTCD*, mixed tissue connective disease; *MV*, mitral valve; *PAH*, pulmonary hypertension; *RA*, rheumatoid arthritis; *SLE*, systemic lupus erythematosus.

ADDITIONAL RESOURCES

American College of Rheumatology [home page on the Internet]. Available at: http://www.rheumatology.org/.
The ACR website is continually updated with information for patients and practitioners as well as physicians. It offers many patient resources in Spanish as well as English, and is easily searchable

European League against Rheumatism. Available at: http://www.eular.org/.
This website offers a variety of resources, including practice guidelines, meetings, and online courses on rheumatic diseases. Specialized reviews of specific diseases are also offered.

Firestein GS, Budd RC, Harris ED, et al, eds. *Kelley and Firestein's Textbook of Rheumatology.* 10th ed. Philadelphia: Elsevier; 2017.
An excellent text resource that also may be loaded onto the computer as a searchable database.

Koopman WJ, Moreland LW, eds. *Arthritis and Allied Conditions.* 15th ed. Philadelphia: Lippincott Williams & Wilkins; 2004.
This excellent text is also available for computer access and searching. It focuses on specific clinical dilemmas with expert opinion on management in challenging areas.

EVIDENCE

Chen J, Tang U, Zhu M, Xu A. Heart involvement in systemic lupus erythematosus: a systematic review and meta-analysis. *Clin Rheumatol.* 2016;35:2437–2448.
A recent systematic review that assessed cardiac abnormalities in SLE by echocardiography.

Gupta R, Wayangankar SA, Targoff IN, Hennebry TA. Clinical cardiac involvement in idiopathic inflammatory myopathies: a systematic review. *Int J Cardiol.* 2011;148(3):261–270
A systematic review of cardiac involvement in IIM that stresses the importance of early and comprehensive cardiac evaluation in these patients.

Lambova S. Cardiac manifestations in systemic sclerosis. *World J Cardiol.* 2014;6(9):993–1005.
Excellent review article of cardiac manifestations in SS, including the usefulness of different imaging modalities.

McMahon M, Skaggs B. Pathogenesis and treatment of atherosclerosis in lupus. *Rheum Dis Clin North Am.* 2014;40(3):475–495.
Review of cardiovascular disease in SLE and potential SLE-specific biomarkers and screening tests for cardiovascular disease.

Misra DP, Shenoy SN. Cardiac involvement in primary systemic vasculitis and potential drug therapies to reduce cardiovascular risk. *Rheumatol Int.* 2017;37(1):151–167.
Excellent concise review article of the cardiac manifestations in the primary systemic vasculitides, including frequencies and treatment strategies.

Voskuyl AE. The heart and cardiovascular manifestations in rheumatoid arthritis. *Rheumatology (Oxford).* 2006;45(suppl 4):iv4–iv7.
Overview of the epidemiological aspects of cardiovascular disease and their relevance in the diagnosis and treatment of RA.

68

Cardiac Tumors and Cardio-Oncology

Anna Griffith, Mark A. Socinski, Brian C. Jensen

CARDIAC TUMORS

Before the second half of the twentieth century, cardiac tumors were diagnosed almost exclusively at autopsy, and no treatment options existed for those rare instances of antemortem discovery. Despite advances in cardiac imaging that improve detection, cardiac tumors remain rare, although the advent of cardiopulmonary bypass has facilitated curative surgical therapy in selected cases.

Clinical Presentation

The clinical presentation of a cardiac tumor depends on its location. Endocardial tumors, such as myxomas, usually present with sequelae of embolism or symptoms of valvular obstruction. Emboli result from dislodgment of adherent thrombus or tumor fragments, causing various pathologies, ranging from small vessel vasculitis to stroke, infarction, or peripheral ischemia. Valvular obstruction presents similarly to valvular heart disease, most often mimicking mitral or tricuspid stenosis. Tumors that arise within the myocardium are more likely to produce arrhythmias and disruption of the conduction system, including atrioventricular block, and rarely, sudden cardiac death. Diffuse myocardial infiltration can result in heart failure from systolic or diastolic dysfunction. Epicardial and pericardial involvement may manifest as pain, pericardial effusion, or heart failure due to pericardial constriction or tamponade. Malignancy should be considered as a potential etiology for any pericardial effusion.

Differential Diagnosis

The differential diagnosis for an intracardiac mass should include thrombus, infectious endocarditis, and primary or secondary neoplasm.

Primary Benign Cardiac Tumors
Myxoma

Data from autopsy series place the prevalence of primary heart tumors at approximately 0.02%, of which 75% are benign (Table 68.1). Myxomas are the most common primary cardiac neoplasm, accounting for 50% of all benign cardiac tumors (Fig. 68.1). Myxomas are two to three times more common in women, and the median age of presentation is 50 years. Roughly 75% of myxomas are found in the left atrium, usually on the interatrial septum near the fossa ovalis. More than 90% of myxomas are solitary. Myxomas arise from multipotent mesenchymal cells. Histology reveals spindle-shaped or stellate cells within abundant myxoid stroma. Grossly, myxomas are gelatinous, pedunculated tumors with an average diameter of 4 to 8 cm.

Myxomas typically present with embolization or symptoms of valvular obstruction, although they may also cause systemic signs and symptoms similar to those of collagen vascular disease, endocarditis, vasculitis, and malignant neoplasms. In the setting of left atrial tumors, auscultation may reveal a tumor "plop" that occurs in early diastole and can be confused with an S_3 gallop. A mitral diastolic rumble or holosystolic murmur may be present.

Lipoma

Lipomas are the second most common benign primary cardiac tumor. Lipomas can occur at any age and have no predilection for either sex. They are encapsulated tumors, usually small, and located in the epicardium or the myocardium. Symptoms, when present, are usually referable to infiltration of the myocardium, with resultant arrhythmias or conduction defects. Bulky or symptomatic lipomas should be resected.

Rhabdomyoma

Rhabdomyoma is the most common benign cardiac tumor of infancy and childhood. Multiple tumors usually occur within the ventricular myocardium, although some project into the ventricular cavity. One third of rhabdomyomas are associated with tuberous sclerosis. It is not uncommon for tumors to regress spontaneously; therefore, conservative management is recommended.

Fibroma

Fibromas are childhood tumors that occur in the ventricular myocardium, often in the interventricular septum. Symptoms and signs result from involvement of the conduction system and can include sudden death. Due to the location of the tumor, resection is usually not feasible, and cardiac transplantation may be the only treatment option.

Papillary Fibroelastoma

Papillary fibroelastomas are the most common tumors of the cardiac valves. These are not true neoplasms, but avascular growths with unclear pathogenesis. Formerly diagnosed only at autopsy, they frequently are seen during echocardiography and may be confused with valvular vegetations. Fibroelastomas do not cause valvular dysfunction and rarely are associated with thromboembolism.

Primary Malignant Cardiac Tumors
Sarcoma

Approximately 25% of primary cardiac neoplasms are malignant, and 95% of these are sarcomas (Table 68.2). Sarcomas are aggressive tumors that present most commonly in the third to fifth decade of life, with signs and symptoms of heart failure due to valvular obstruction or myocardial infiltration. Sarcomas derive from mesenchymal cells and therefore may present as distinct pathological subtypes, most commonly angiosarcoma and rhabdomyosarcoma. Angiosarcoma, including Kaposi sarcoma, is the more common subtype and exhibits a 2:1 male predominance. Angiosarcomas typically arise in the right atrium, whereas rhabdomyosarcomas have no chamber predilection and often are multifocal.

TABLE 68.1 Primary Benign Cardiac Neoplasms

| Benign Tumor | PERCENTAGE OF TUMORS | |
	Adults	Children
Myxoma	45	15
Lipoma	21	0
Papillary fibroelastoma	16	0
Rhabdomyoma	2	45
Fibroma	3	15
Hemangioma	5	5
Teratoma	1	13
Other	6	6

Reused with permission from Allard MF, Taylor GP, Wilson JE, et al. Primary cardiac tumors. In: Goldhaber S, Braunwald E, eds. *Atlas of Heart Diseases*. Philadelphia: Current Medicine; 1995:15.1–15.22.

TABLE 68.2 Primary Malignant Cardiac Tumors

| Malignant Tumor | PERCENTAGE OF ALL TUMORS | |
	Adults	Children
Angiosarcoma	33	0
Rhabdomyosarcoma	21	33
Mesothelioma	16	0
Fibrosarcoma	11	11
Lymphoma	6	0
Osteosarcoma	4	0
Thymoma	3	0
Neurogenic sarcoma	3	11
Leiomyosarcoma	1	0
Liposarcoma	1	0
Synovial sarcoma	1	0
Malignant teratoma	0	44

Reused with permission from Allard MF, Taylor GP, Wilson JE, et al. Primary cardiac tumors. In: Goldhaber S, Braunwald E, eds. *Atlas of Heart Diseases*. Philadelphia: Current Medicine; 1995:15.1–15.22.

Myxoma. Characteristically originating from interatrial septum and almost filling LA; RV hypertrophy

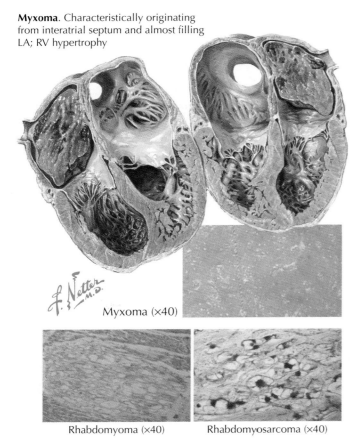

Myxoma (×40)

Rhabdomyoma (×40)   Rhabdomyosarcoma (×40)

FIG 68.1 Heart Tumors. *LA,* Left atrium; *RV,* right ventricular.

The prognosis for all pathological subtypes of cardiac sarcoma is poor. Optimal treatment requires complete resection, although the extent of myocardial infiltration often precludes surgery. Sarcomas grow quickly, and death due to heart failure or arrhythmia within a few weeks or months after diagnosis is typical.

Lymphoma

Primary cardiac lymphomas are almost exclusively non-Hodgkin and typically are diffuse B-cell lymphomas. Lymphoma constitutes approximately 1% of all cardiac tumors and 0.5% of extranodal non-Hodgkin

lymphoma, although it may be somewhat more common in immunosuppressed patients. Cardiac lymphomas can present with pericardial effusion, heart failure, or arrhythmia. Many patients die before initiation of chemotherapy due to rapid tumor progression.

Pericardial Mesothelioma

Pericardial mesothelioma is a rare tumor that occurs in young people, presenting as constriction or pericardial effusion, with or without tamponade. Myocardial invasion is uncommon. Chemotherapy and radiation therapy (RT) may give temporary improvement in a palliative setting, but the disease is uniformly and rapidly fatal.

Secondary Malignant Cardiac Tumors

Metastatic disease involving the heart is much more common than primary cardiac neoplasms. Only 10% of secondary tumors are symptomatic, although 1% of unselected individuals have secondary tumors of the heart at autopsy. Most symptomatic individuals have pericardial metastases, and pericardial effusion may be the primary presentation of metastatic malignancy. A diagnosis of cardiac metastasis should be considered when patients with known malignancy develop new-onset cardiac dysfunction (heart failure, arrhythmia, cardiomegaly, among others).

Lung and breast cancers involve the heart via local spread and subsequent infiltration of the pericardium, causing effusion and constriction. In myeloid leukemias, leukemic cells are seen on light microscopy infiltrating between myocytes. Non-Hodgkin lymphomas have a high rate of cardiac involvement—up to 25% of patients may have grossly visible epicardial or myocardial disease. Melanomas constitute a small portion of secondary cardiac tumors, but for unknown reasons, melanoma has the highest rate (~50%) of cardiac metastasis of any malignancy.

Diagnostic Approach

Transthoracic echocardiography is the most commonly used modality to diagnose cardiac tumors (Fig. 68.2). Cardiac MRI or CT scan can further assess pericardial disease and the extent of myocardial tumor infiltration. Biopsy of cardiac tumors typically is not warranted if

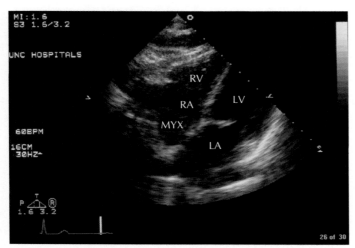

Image courtesy of Dr. Alan Hinderliter.

FIG 68.2 Echocardiographic Image of a Right Atrial Tumor. At the time of resection, the tumor was found to be a myxoma. *LA,* Left atrium; *LV,* left ventricle; *MYX,* myxoma; *RA,* right atrium; *RV,* right ventricle.

operative intervention is planned, because the risk of complication—particularly embolization—often outweighs the need for a preoperative diagnosis.

Management and Therapy

Advances in imaging and surgical technique have allowed for prompt diagnosis and safe, curative resection of most benign tumors. Because of the propensity of myxomas to cause life-threatening complications, surgical resection should be performed without delay. After resection, patients with sporadic myxomas have a recurrence rate of 1%, whereas patients with familial myxoma syndrome have a 7% to 22% rate of recurrence. In persons with a short life expectancy and serious comorbid conditions, the morbidity of operative resection may outweigh the benefits. In these instances, it is prudent to initiate lifelong anticoagulation to decrease risk of thromboembolism.

Unfortunately, malignant disease of the heart is largely a fatal disease, because resection for cure is typically not feasible. In addition, with the exception of lymphoma, most primary cardiac tumors are not sensitive to chemotherapy or RT. Cardiac transplantation is not an option for malignant cardiac tumors because of concerns for micrometastatic disease and the requirement for posttransplantation suppression of cell-mediated immunity.

THE FIELD OF CARDIO-ONCOLOGY

Cardiovascular disease is three to five times more common in survivors of cancer than age-matched control subjects and is the most common cause of death in women with stage 1 to 3 breast cancer, which suggests that either cancer or its treatment enhances cardiovascular risk. The developing field of cardio-oncology recognizes the fascinating interplay among cancer, cancer therapies, and cardiovascular disease, and seeks to optimize cardiovascular health in patients currently or formerly treated for cancer.

Anthracyclines

Anthracyclines, including doxorubicin, were introduced in the 1960s and remain a cornerstone of chemotherapeutic regimens for many malignancies, including lymphoma, leukemia, breast cancer, and small cell lung cancer. Anthracycline-induced cardiotoxicity has been described for decades; it is predominantly dose-dependent, but also can occur idiosyncratically at any time during the treatment course. Acute toxicities are less frequent than chronic toxicities and occur in the first weeks after initiating anthracycline treatment. There are numerous forms of acute toxicity, including arrhythmias, pericarditis, myocarditis, and ventricular dysfunction. Long-term anthracycline toxicity primarily manifests as dilated cardiomyopathy. Unfortunately, data from adult survivors of childhood cancers demonstrate that the risk of cardiomyopathy extends for decades beyond the final dose of anthracycline.

Etiology and Pathogenesis

Anthracycline cardiotoxicity likely arises from multiple underlying mechanisms. Oxidative stress and double-stranded DNA breaks, induced by anthracycline binding to topoisomerase-2, contribute to mitochondrial dysfunction and cell death. Collectively, these insults lead to diastolic dysfunction, then systolic dysfunction, and in some cases, heart failure.

The strongest risk factor for anthracycline-induced cardiotoxicity is the cumulative dose. Other risk factors include age, chest radiation, existing heart disease, hypertension, and diabetes. Monitoring guidelines have been established and include a pretreatment assessment of the left ventricular ejection fraction (LVEF) via transthoracic echocardiography, ECG, and serial LVEF assessment during therapy.

Management and Therapy

Prevention of anthracycline cardiotoxicity largely requires limitation of exposure. Current recommendations suggest limiting the cumulative dose of anthracyclines to 450 to 500 mg/m^2, although more recent studies have suggested that risk begins to rise after a cumulative dose of 300 mg/m^2.

Treatment of anthracycline-induced cardiotoxicity largely relies on standard heart failure therapies, β-blockers, and angiotensin-converting enzyme (ACE) inhibitors. The OVERCOME (preventiOn of left Ventricular dysfunction with Enalapril and caRvedilol in patients submitted to intensive ChemOtherapy for the treatment of Malignant hEmopathies) trial demonstrated that treatment with enalapril and carvedilol preserved LVEF after anthracycline compared with the placebo control. The PRADA (PRevention of cArdiac Dysfunction during Adjuvant breast cancer therapy) trial, one of the largest prospective studies in the cardio-oncology field, concluded that ACE inhibition protected against an early decline in LVEF. Dexrazoxane, an ethylene diamine tetraacetic acid derivative, has been shown to reduce cardiotoxicity, but concerns for decreased antitumor effects and increased risk of secondary malignancy limit its use.

Human Epidermal Growth Factor Receptor-2 Targeted Agents

Trastuzumab is a humanized monoclonal antibody that targets human epidermal growth factor receptor 2 (HER2). HER2 (ErbB2) is overexpressed in a subset of breast cancers, and targeting HER2 has dramatically improved the prognosis for patients with tumors harboring this oncogene.

Trastuzumab is used as adjuvant therapy in patients who are also being treated with conventional chemotherapy, including doxorubicin. Trastuzumab has clearly been associated with cardiotoxicity, although its actual incidence and clinical significance are debated. Clinical trials have reported a 3% to 19% rate of asymptomatic cardiac dysfunction and a 2% to 4% rate of symptomatic heart failure, although these trials likely underestimated the incidence of cardiomyopathy because they selected only low-risk patients. This notion was supported by a real-world registry that showed a 27% incidence of cardiotoxicity in unselected trastuzumab recipients.

Etiology and Pathogenesis

The cardiotoxicity of trastuzumab likely arises from direct effects on cardiomyocyte ErbB2 receptors, in part through antagonizing ErbB2 binding of neuregulin, which is released by myocardial endothelial cells. ErbB2 sends signals through recognized cardioprotective molecules (e.g., Akt) to promote cardiomyocyte survival and metabolic function. Trastuzumab-induced cardiomyopathy typically is reversible within weeks to months of withholding trastuzumab. However, experimental and clinical evidence has suggested that trastuzumab can induce irreversible cardiomyocyte damage, particularly in combination with anthracyclines. The cardiotoxicity of trastuzumab does not appear to be a class effect, because the HER2 targeted agent, lapatinib, appears to have limited effects on cardiac function.

Management and Therapy

Patients receiving trastuzumab or other HER2 targeted agents should have a baseline echocardiogram to establish LVEF before initiation of treatment, followed by serial assessment of LVEF every 3 months for the duration of treatment, typically for 1 year. Consensus recommendations suggest discontinuation of trastuzumab and initiation of ACE inhibition and β-blockade if the LVEF drops >10% or to <45%. Many patients tolerate rechallenge after a hiatus from HER2 antagonist therapy against a background of neurohormonal antagonism.

Kinase Inhibitors and Vascular Endothelial Growth Factor Inhibitors

Kinase inhibitors (KIs) have revolutionized treatment of hematologic malignancies like chronic myeloid leukemia, and solid tumors such as gastrointestinal stromal tumors and renal cell cancer. Chronic myeloid leukemia, which was once a fatal disease, has largely become a chronic condition with the advent of tyrosine kinase inhibitors (TKIs), such as imatinib, the first BCR-ABL-targeted TKI. However, this class of targeted therapies has been associated with a broad spectrum of cardiovascular toxicities, including hypertension, thrombosis, cardiomyopathy, and arrhythmia. Imatinib has been replaced by more effective second-generation TKIs, such as nilotinib, dasatinib, bosutinib, and ponatinib, although many of these agents also increase risk for cardiovascular events (Table 68.3). Specifically, dasatinib can cause pulmonary artery

TABLE 68.3 Cardiovascular Toxicity by Chemotherapeutic Class

Therapeutic Class	Examples of Therapies	Cardiovascular Toxicity
Anthracyclines	Doxorubicin, daunorubicin, epirubicin, idarubicin	Acute: arrhythmia, myocarditis; Acute or chronic: LV dysfunction
HER2 targeted therapies	Trastuzumab, pertuzumab, lapatinib	LV dysfunction
Tyrosine kinase inhibitors	Dasatinib, nilotinib, sorafenib, sunitinib, lapatinib	Hypertension, LV dysfunction, pulmonary hypertension
Angiogenesis inhibitors	Bevacizumab	Hypertension, LV dysfunction
Immune checkpoint inhibitors	Ipilimumab, nivolumab	Myocarditis
Thalidomides	Lenalidomide, thalidomide	Thromboembolism

HER2, Human epidermal growth factor receptor 2; LV, left ventricular.

hypertension, and nilotinib is associated with peripheral or cardiac ischemic events.

The cardiovascular toxicity of several other KIs deserves specific mention. The multitargeted KI sunitinib, used to treat GIST and renal cell carcinoma (RCC), has been associated with hypertension in 27% to 34% of patients, as well as decreased LVEF, and rare cases of deep vein thrombosis and pulmonary embolism. Sorafenib, which is used to treat hepatocellular carcinoma, RCC, and thyroid carcinoma, has also been associated with hypertension and decreased LVEF. Long-term KI therapy is indicated for many patients, so careful monitoring of blood pressure and other cardiac risk factors to minimize the risk of cardiovascular toxicity is increasingly important.

Vascular endothelial growth factor (VEGF) inhibitors are another important class of antitumor medications with significant cardiovascular effects. VEGF inhibitors block angiogenesis, a central determinant of the growth of most solid tumors. The most widely studied VEGF inhibitor is bevacizumab, which is used in the treatment of numerous malignancies, including colorectal, lung, renal, and ovarian cancers. Bevacizumab has been associated with a number of cardiovascular toxicities, including hypertension, cardiomyopathy, venous thromboembolism, and arterial thrombosis. Nearly all patients treated with VEGF inhibitors experience a dose-dependent increase in both diastolic and systolic blood pressure, and more than one-half of patients develop hypertension as a result. These toxicities are largely representative of an on-target class effect, because almost all VEGF inhibitors also increase the risk of vascular events and cardiomyopathy.

Immune Checkpoint Inhibitors

Two immune checkpoint inhibitors, ipilimumab and nivolumab, have transformed the treatment of melanoma. These therapies activate autoreactive T cells and have been associated with dermatitis, colitis, hepatitis, and pneumonitis. One high profile case report outlined two cases of fatal myocarditis, which both occurred approximately 15 days after initiation of treatment with both immune checkpoint inhibitors. A subsequent retrospective study of 20,500 patients treated with one or both immune checkpoint inhibitors demonstrated that the incidence and severity of myocarditis is significantly greater when both nivolumab and ipilimumab are given together.

Other immunomodulatory agents, such as lenalidomide and thalidomide, often used in the treatment of multiple myeloma and amyloidosis, have been associated with a high risk of thromboembolic disease. As a consequence, thromboprophylaxis is now a mandatory component of protocols that include these medications. Lenalidomide, when used in combination with dexamethasone, has been associated with increased risk of myocardial infarction.

Radiation Therapy

RT is used effectively in the treatment of numerous malignancies, including lymphoma and breast cancer. Mediastinal RT significantly increases the risk of subsequent coronary artery disease, valvular heart disease, pericardial disease, and restrictive cardiomyopathy. The pathogenesis of injury likely differs for each complication, although all involve microvascular damage and enhanced fibrosis. Technical advances such as conformal imaging and breath holding have decreased the incidence of RT-induced heart injury. Nevertheless, clinicians should maintain an increased index of suspicion for cardiovascular disease in cancer survivors who were treated with RT.

FUTURE DIRECTIONS

The underlying mechanisms and the incidence of cardiovascular toxicity related to targeted cancer therapies both remain unclear. Ongoing basic research will seek to clarify the biology of KI-induced toxicities, which may help inform both prevention of manifest cardiotoxicity and the future development of drugs that do not adversely affect the heart. Forthcoming clinical trials of new cancer therapies should enhance efforts at detection and systematize the reporting of adverse cardiovascular events, perhaps through revision of the National Cancer Institute Common Terminology Criteria for Adverse Events, which outlines specific guidelines for reporting adverse events in all oncological trials. Understanding the true incidence of cardiotoxicity associated with antineoplastic agents will be essential for effective prevention and treatment.

Cardiovascular disease and cancer remain the two leading causes of death in industrialized regions of the world. Cancer survivors are at increased risk of subsequently developing cardiovascular disease, and the number of cancer survivors will increase significantly in coming years due to advances in cancer therapy. It is likely that the field of cardio-oncology will continue to expand accordingly, with the ongoing goal of providing optimal comprehensive care to cancer patients.

ADDITIONAL RESOURCES

Roberts WC. Primary and secondary neoplasms of the heart. *Am J Cardiol.* 1997;80:671–682.
In-depth review of cardiac neoplasms.
Shapiro LM. Cardiac tumors: diagnosis and management. *Heart.* 2001;85:218–222.
Thorough, yet concise review of benign and malignant cardiac tumors and their management.

EVIDENCE

Burke A, Virmani R. *Atlas of Tumor Pathology. Tumors of the Heart and Great Vessels.* Washington, DC: Armed Forces Institute of Pathology; 1996:231.
An overview of the incidence and pathology of cardiac tumors.
Lenneman CG, Sawyer DB. Cardio-oncology: an update on cardiotoxicity of cancer-related treatment. *Circ Res.* 2016;188:1008–1020.
An overview of cardiovascular disease in cancer survivors treated with both chemotherapeutic agents and RT. This article also provides guidelines for treating and preventing cardiovascular effects of cancer therapy.
Lipshultz SE, Adams MJ, Colan SD, et al. Long-term cardiovascular toxicity in children, adolescents, and young adults who receive cancer therapy: pathophysiology, course, monitoring, management, prevention, and research directions: a scientific statement from the American Heart Association. *Circulation.* 2013;128(17):1927–1995.
An overview of current data on the lifelong cardiovascular effects of chemotherapy on pediatric patients.
Moslehi J. Cardiovascular toxic effects of targeted cancer therapies. *N Engl J Med.* 2016;375:1457–1467.
A review article outlining the cardiovascular effects of newer chemotherapeutic agents, including targeted therapies, and a broad overview of the emerging field of cardio-oncology.
Singal PK, Iliskovic N. Doxorubicin-induced cardiomyopathy. *N Engl J Med.* 1998;339:900–905.
A review of available literature on the history and research regarding doxorubicin-induced cardiomyopathy.

69

Pulmonary Hypertension

Lisa J. Rose-Jones, H. James Ford

ETIOLOGY AND PATHOGENESIS

Pulmonary hypertension (PH) is elevated pressure in the pulmonary arteries, which is hemodynamically defined as a mean pulmonary artery pressure (MPAP) of ≥25 mm Hg. It may occur in response to many different mechanisms. Regardless of how PH is uncovered, whether as part of a differential diagnosis or incidentally on an echocardiogram or right heart catheterization, a search for the etiology, and thus, the pathophysiology is worthwhile. PH creates increased afterload that the right ventricle (RV) was not designed to work against. The RV attempts to counterbalance this pressure with adaptive remodeling mechanisms, often initially through hypertrophy. However, over time it will reach a point where it can no longer compensate, and begins to dilate and fail. It is crucial that patients be appropriately diagnosed with the correct etiology of PH, because management varies widely, and specific treatments could be harmful if used in the wrong clinical scenario.

Hemodynamic profiles and concomitant diagnostic testing can help to determine the etiology of PH. Increased pulmonary blood flow from excess cardiac output may be the sole cause for some cases of PH. Conditions such as a febrile state, anemia, pregnancy, presence of an arteriovenous fistula, or thyrotoxicosis could contribute to this. The hallmark of this increased flow phenomena is that when pulmonary pressures are elevated, there is no true resistance elevation in the pulmonary circulation on right heart catheterization. However, left-sided heart disease is the most common reason for PH. Left atrial hypertension results in a passive retrograde transmission of pressure, which is believed to be a postcapillary issue and leads to increased hydrostatic pressure and resulting constriction, and thus, elevation in pulmonary artery pressures. Pulmonary arterial hypertension (PAH), another reason for increased pulmonary pressures, results from loss of the vascular cross-sectional area as a consequence of vasculopathy. In this condition, the vascular resistance is abnormal in the pulmonary bed. The World Health Organization (WHO) updated Fifth World Symposium classifies these diverse groups by their different histopathologic features (Fig. 69.1).

World Health Organization Group 1: Pulmonary Arterial Hypertension

PAH is a panvasculopathy of primarily the distal pulmonary arteries, arterioles, and capillaries. Medial hypertrophy, intimal proliferation and fibrosis, and ultimately, plexiform lesion formation, distinguishes this disease (Fig. 69.2). It is believed to be triggered by an imbalance in hormones that promote cellular proliferation, thrombosis, and vasoconstriction. There are numerous systemic conditions and heritable genetic mutations that are associated with the development of PAH. With the loss of the vascular lumen, there is restricted blood flow through the pulmonary arterial circulation, and thus, an increase in the resistance. This is hemodynamically defined as a MPAP of ≥25 mm Hg in the setting of a normal pulmonary artery wedge pressure (PAWP) or left ventricular end-diastolic pressure (LVEDP) of ≤15 mm Hg with a pulmonary vascular resistance (PVR) of >3 Wood units. Although it is the least common form of PH, with an estimated 50,000 to 100,000 cases in the United States, it is the most extensively studied to date. PAH has the bulk of the evidence base for pulmonary vasodilator use as treatment.

World Health Organization Group 2: Pulmonary Hypertension Due to Left Heart Disease

Often referred to as pulmonary venous hypertension (PVH), group 2 PH results from chronically elevated left atrial pressures as a consequence of left heart disease. Systolic or diastolic dysfunction of the left ventricle, as well as mitral or aortic valvular disease, can trigger this "backup" of venous pressure. This was previously referred to as a postcapillary process. It is hemodynamically differentiated by the presence of an elevated MPAP of ≥25 mm Hg in the setting of an elevated PAWP or LVEDP ≥15 mm Hg. There are an estimated 2 to 3 million Americans that fall into this category, thus making it the most common form of PH that clinicians encounter.

World Health Organization Group 3: Pulmonary Hypertension Due to Lung Diseases and/or Hypoxia

Chronic obstructive pulmonary disease, interstitial lung disease, and sleep-disordered breathing are the most common culprits of WHO group 3 PH. The exact prevalence of PH in chronic lung disease is unknown. Some of the proposed mechanisms for elevation of pulmonary pressures in chronic obstructive pulmonary disease include physical obliteration of the pulmonary vasculature, hyperinflation that causes compression of the alveolar vessels, and hypoxia-induced vasoconstriction and vascular remodeling.

World Health Organization Group 4: Pulmonary Hypertension Due to Chronic Thromboembolic Disease

This is the result of chronic thromboembolic disease and occurs in approximately 3% to 4% of patients with acute pulmonary emboli. Pulmonary arterial hypertensive arteriopathy is believed to be the causative mechanism of the pathological changes distal to the clot. Thus, it is hemodynamically similar to PAH but with the documented presence of chronic thromboembolic material. This etiology is crucial to identify, because it is the only form of PH that is potentially curable with pulmonary thromboendarterectomy (PTE).

World Health Organization Group 5: Pulmonary Hypertension Due to Unclear or Multifactorial Mechanisms

Lastly, WHO group 5 consists of several different disorders that have unclear pathogenesis and/or multifactorial mechanisms as to the

491

1. Pulmonary arterial hypertension (PAH)

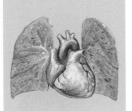

- Idiopathic pulmonary arterial hypertension
- Heritable
- Drug- and toxin-induced
- Persistent PH of newborn
- Associated with:
  - connective tissue disease
  - HIV infection
  - portal hypertension
  - coronary heart disease
  - schistosomiasis
  - chronic hemolytic anemia

1A. Pulmonary venoocclusive disease and pulmonary capillary hemangiomatosis

2. Pulmonary hypertension due to left heart disease

- Systolic dysfunction
- Diastolic dysfunction
- Valvular disease

3. Pulmonary hypertension due to lung diseases and/or hypoxia

- Chronic obstructive pulmonary disease
- Interstitial lung disease
- Other pulmonary diseases with mixed restrictive and obstructive pattern
- Sleep-disordered breathing
- Alveolar hypoventilation disorders
- Developmental abnormalities

4. Pulmonary hypertension due to chronic thrombotic and/or embolic disease

- Chronic thromboembolic pulmonary hypertension

5. Pulmonary hypertension with unclear multifactorial mechanisms

- Hematologic disorders
- Systemic disorders
- Metabolic disorders
- Others

Simonneau G et al. *J Am Coll Cardiol* 2009;54:S43–S54.

FIG 69.1 World Health Organization Classification System of Pulmonary Hypertension (PH).

causation of PH. Sarcoid lung disease, sickle cell disease, myeloproliferative disorders, and chronic renal failure are just a few relevant examples included in this category.

CLINICAL PRESENTATION

Dyspnea is the predominant complaint among almost all patients presenting with PH. Unfortunately, because of the broad differential diagnosis of breathlessness, >75% of patients do not end up with the correct diagnosis of PH until they have more advanced disease and evidence of right heart failure, such as lower extremity edema. Symptom severity is classified according to WHO functional classes I through IV, a modified form of the New York Heart Association classification of heart failure. Syncope is encountered with end-stage disease, and thus automatically classifies that patient into functional class IV. The mechanism

for syncope remains ill-defined, but it is prognostically associated with worse outcomes. Chest pain is often overlooked as a consequence of PH. Angina results from increased RV myocardial oxygen demand due to high wall stress, as well as a drop in systolic blood flow in coronary branches to the RV, and occasionally, compression of the left main coronary artery by a dilated main pulmonary artery.

Physical examination can also suggest the possibility of PH. In advanced PH, signs of right-sided heart failure may be present. The jugular venous pressure is typically elevated. With sustained pulmonary pressure elevations, the RV negatively remodels and can become increasingly dilated. This causes stretch of the tricuspid annulus and often significant tricuspid regurgitation. Tricuspid regurgitation creates a prominent *v* wave in the jugular venous pulsation. Because of elevated RV pressure and volume overload, there is a backup into the systemic veins. This can be evidenced by hepatomegaly, the presence of

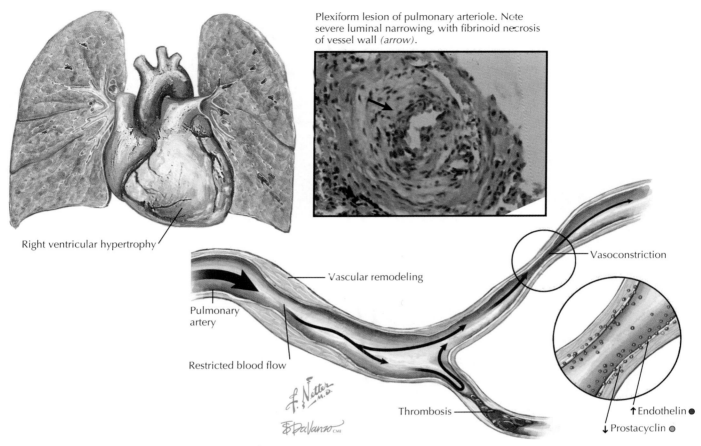

Plexiform lesion of pulmonary arteriole. Note severe luminal narrowing, with fibrinoid necrosis of vessel wall (arrow).

Right ventricular hypertrophy

Vascular remodeling

Pulmonary artery

Restricted blood flow

Vasoconstriction

Thrombosis

↑Endothelin ●
↓Prostacyclin ◉

FIG 69.2 Pathology of Pulmonary Hypertension.

hepatojugular reflux, and eventually ascites. The cardiac auscultatory examination will often reveal the tricuspid regurgitation murmur and an increased pulmonic component of the second heart sound (P2). With more advanced disease, a RV gallop may be heard, and the precordium may reveal an RV lift on palpation.

DIFFERENTIAL DIAGNOSIS

Most cases of breathlessness are secondary to heart and lung disease; for example, asthma, chronic obstructive lung disease, acute heart failure, or myocardial ischemia may be involved. Breathlessness may also be psychogenic in nature. The key to the correct diagnosis is to have PH on the differential diagnosis for dyspnea and exertional intolerance. A careful history to elicit any familial component, exposure to insults known to be related to the development of PH (anorexigen use, methamphetamine consumption, and so on), or presence of diseases associated with its development is crucial. During the physical examination, it is also prudent to note any signs and/or sequela of PH as listed previously. If a clinical suspicion of PH remains, a transthoracic echocardiogram is the next best step to conclude whether further diagnostic evaluation is warranted (Fig. 69.3).

DIAGNOSTIC APPROACH

The echocardiogram is vital to the diagnosis of PH. It provides an estimation of pulmonary artery systolic pressure (PASP) from the Doppler-derived velocity of tricuspid regurgitation jet. If estimated

PASP is ≥40 mm Hg, a closer look is warranted. It also provides a critical assessment of right atrial and RV size and function. The use of agitated saline contrast can exclude the presence of an intracardiac shunt. Most importantly, it can alert the clinician to the prevalent PVH secondary to left-heart disease.

Invasive hemodynamic testing is the gold standard in the diagnosis of PH. Right heart catheterization will reveal if there is true vascular obstruction, and thus, PAH. The key feature is a MPAP ≥25 mm Hg in the setting of an elevated PVR of >3 Wood units. The right heart catheterization will expose PVH if the PAWP is >15 mm Hg. If PAWP measurement is at all uncertain, LVEDP should be measured. The right heart catheterization not only provides a definitive diagnosis, but aids in determination of prognosis and allows for an assessment of pulmonary vasoreactivity. Vasodilator challenges can be an essential component of the invasive hemodynamics for individuals with group 1 PAH and preserved cardiac output. In particular, a positive test predicts safety of response to calcium channel blockers, which are more commonly observed in the idiopathic, heritable, and drug- and toxin-induced PAH groups.

A 6-minute walk test is an easy way to evaluate for hypoxemia and is strongly predictive of survival in the PAH population. Laboratory evaluation with antinuclear antibody, HIV, and liver function tests should also be obtained when looking for associated WHO group 1 diagnoses in suspect patients. Pulmonary function tests and overnight oximetry can help expose any underlying parenchymal lung disease or sleep-disordered breathing that could be the root of the PH. In addition, every patient with hemodynamics consistent with PAH needs a

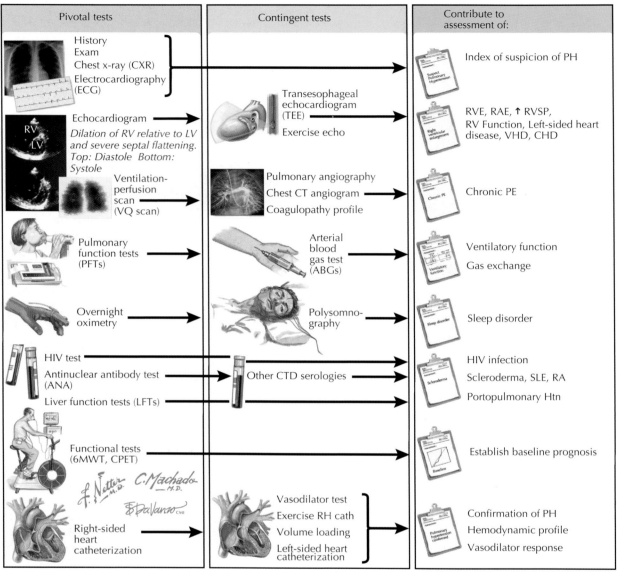

McLaughlin, V. V. et al. J Am Coll Cardiol 2009;53:1573-1619.

FIG 69.3 Important Investigations in the Workup of Pulmonary Hypertension. *6MWT,* Six-minute walking test; *CHD,* congenital heart disease; *CTD,* connective tissue disorder; *CPET,* cardiovascular pulmonary exercise test; *Htn,* hypertension; *PE,* pulmonary embolism; *RA,* rheumatoid arthritis; *RAE,* right atrial embolism; *RH,* right heart; *RV,* right ventricular; *RVE,* right ventricular embolism; *RVSP,* right ventricular systolic pressure; *SLE,* systemic lupus erythematosus; *VHD,* valvular heart disease.

ventilation and/or perfusion scan to rule out chronic thromboembolic PH (CTEPH). Spiral CT is not recommended in lieu of this because it can miss lower order, more distal vessel thromboembolic disease.

MANAGEMENT AND THERAPY

There have been tremendous advances in drug development and the number of approved therapies for PAH in the past two decades. All of the current PAH therapies work via one of three known major pathways involved in the pathogenesis of PAH: the prostacyclin pathway, the nitric oxide (NO) pathway, and the endothelin-1 pathway. Patients with PAH are known to have local imbalance in thromboxane and prostaglandin I2 (PGI2) production, such that there is a relative excess of thromboxane and a relative deficiency of PGI2. PGI2 promotes cardiac

inotropy, has antiproliferative effects on the vasculature, and inhibits platelet aggregation—all processes that are key in the development of PAH. As such, therapies that provide exogenous prostanoid (or agonize the prostacyclin receptor) are used to treat PAH. Furthermore, there is a relative excess of endothelin-1 in PAH patients. This molecule is a potent vasoconstrictor and also contributes to vascular proliferation and vascular smooth muscle hypertrophy. Antagonists of either one or both of the endothelin-1 receptors have been developed and approved to treat PAH. Finally, patients with PAH are deficient in bioavailable NO compared with normal healthy individuals. NO is a vasodilator that also deters vascular proliferation and smooth muscle hypertrophy. It is for this reason that drugs that inhibit the phosphodiesterase-5 (PDE-5) enzyme or directly stimulate soluble guanylate cyclase (SGC) (ultimately augmenting the downstream beneficial cellular effects of

NO) were studied and approved to treat PAH. Before an in-depth review of these three classes of PAH specific therapies is undertaken, attention should be given to more general therapeutic measures that have an important impact on the clinical course of PAH.

General Measures in the Treatment of Pulmonary Arterial Hypertension
Supplemental Oxygen Therapy
Assessment should be carried out for the presence of hypoxia in the resting state, with exertion, and during sleep. Any decrement in oxygenation saturation (generally, <90%) in any of these contexts should be corrected with administration of supplemental oxygen to achieve normal saturation. This prevents hypoxic pulmonary vasoconstriction from further elevating pulmonary artery pressures (on top of existing arteriopathy) and contributing to increased RV afterload and strain.

Assessment for and Correction of Hypoventilation and/or Sleep-Disordered Breathing
Comorbid untreated hypoventilation and/or sleep apnea also contribute to elevations in pulmonary artery pressure through hypercapnia and potential for associated hypoxia. Other neurohormonal mechanisms associated with obstructive sleep apnea also contribute to PH. As such, formal polysomnography should be performed in suspect patients, and appropriate application of positive airway pressure therapy based on the results should be used.

Diuretic Therapy
As RV dilatation and failure develop in the course of PAH, it is important to titrate diuretic therapy to levels required to minimize RV volume and pressure overload so that LV cavity size and function are not compromised, underscoring the importance of ventricular interdependence. This will aid in preventing systemic hypotension and compromised end-organ perfusion, particularly to the cerebral and renal vascular beds.

Anticoagulation
It had long been held belief, based largely on retrospective registry studies, that use of anticoagulation in idiopathic PAH (IPAH) and heritable PAH (HPAH) was associated with improved survival (believed to be associated with a reduction of in situ microthrombosis that is part of the arteriopathy seen in PAH). The international normalized ratio targets used were in the lower range (1.5–2.5) compared with anticoagulation for other indications. However, two recent registry analyses call into question the benefit of anticoagulation in IPAH, with one suggesting survival benefit and the other suggesting no benefit (COMPERA and REVEAL). For other forms of PAH, particularly PAH associated with connective tissue disorder, there was no survival benefit seen in COMPERA, and increased mortality was seen in REVEAL with use of warfarin. Although the recommendation to anticoagulate patients with IPAH persists in most PAH treatment guidelines, there remains much clinical equipoise for this practice. Novel anticoagulant agents such as direct thrombin and factor Xa inhibitors have not been studied in PAH.

Immunizations Against Respiratory Infections
Annual vaccination for influenza and appropriate interval comprehensive vaccination for pneumococcal infection are recommended for patients with all forms of PAH.

Avoidance of Valsalva Maneuvers
As much as possible, cough, excessive weight bearing, constipation, and other Valsalva-like maneuvers should be avoided and/or treated, particularly in the context of advanced RV failure. These maneuvers

transiently decrease venous return to the right heart, which can impair right-to-left filling and systemic cardiac output in the context of diseased pulmonary vasculature.

A Center-Based Treatment Approach
Because the proper diagnosis and treatment of PAH is quite complex, referral to a PH center with experienced clinicians, a multidisciplinary team approach, and availability of requisite resources is recommended by the guidelines.

Calcium Channel Blocker Therapy
As stated previously, the performance of acute vasodilator testing during right heart catheterization in patients with IPAH, HPAH, or drug- and toxin-induced PAH and preserved cardiac output can predict clinical response to calcium channel blocker therapy for PAH. This constitutes a small minority of PAH patients overall (~7%). However, it is important to determine because calcium channel blocker therapy is relatively much less expensive and less complex than PAH-specific therapies. A small number of patients can have a robust and long-term response to calcium channel blocker therapy. However, due diligence to close follow-up of these patients is required because up to 50% of patients may lose responsiveness to calcium channel blocker therapy with time and require initiation of PAH-specific therapy.

PULMONARY ARTERIAL HYPERTENSION–SPECIFIC THERAPIES
Parenteral Prostacyclins
The first PAH therapy to be approved was epoprostenol, a prostanoid molecule administered by continuous intravenous (IV) infusion via a tunneled central venous catheter and ambulatory infusion pump. The half-life of epoprostenol is 2 to 4 minutes, and the drug is not stable at room temperature, which requires drug cassettes to be packed in ice. Epoprostenol was shown, in a small, double-blind, randomized, placebo controlled trial versus conventional therapies alone (digoxin, diuretics, warfarin, and/or calcium channel blockers) to clearly improve mortality over 16 weeks in patients with IPAH. The drug was subsequently approved for use. Although it is complex in its administration, it remains a mainstay of PAH therapy in the current era. Epoprostenol is also currently available in a more thermostable form, minimizing the need for ice packs in most moderate temperature environments.

Treprostinil is the other continuous infusion prostanoid therapy that is approved for the treatment of PAH. It is a room temperature stable drug, with a half-life of approximately 4 hours. Treprostinil can be infused either IV or subcutaneously (SC), and generally requires doses approximately 1.5 to 2 times those used for epoprostenol to achieve the same therapeutic effect. Both epoprostenol IV and treprostinil SC/IV are titrated to effect (treatment goals in PAH—discussed in the following in further detail), and dosing is individualized to the patient. Both can cause significant side effects, particularly in the uptitration phase. Common side effects include headache, facial flushing, jaw pain, nausea, diarrhea, and pain and/or paresthesias of the upper and/or lower extremities. SC administration of treprostinil can also cause infusion site pain and inflammation. Patient reporting and treatment of side effects is important so they can be addressed, and uptitration of therapy can continue uninterrupted. Other pertinent information regarding these parenteral prostacyclin therapies is summarized in Table 69.1.

Endothelin-Receptor Antagonists
The first class of oral PAH therapy to be approved by the U.S. Food and Drug Administration (FDA) were the endothelin-receptor antagonists (ERAs), with the first being bosentan in 2001. Bosentan is dosed

TABLE 69.1	**Current Approved Therapies for Pulmonary Arterial Hypertension**			
Drug (Class) and Date of FDA Approval	**Route (Dosing)**	**Key Clinical Trial Data (Group 1 PAH Patients Unless Noted Otherwise)**	**Pertinent Adverse Effects**	**Special Considerations**
Bosentan (Tracleer) (ERA) Approved 2001	Oral (62.5 mg and 125 mg tabs, dosed twice daily; 62.5 mg bid for the first month)	BREATHE-1 trial: 213 patients. Randomized, double-blind. Significant change in 6MWD at 16 wks relative to placebo.	Potential for hepatotoxicity Teratogenicity Flushing, headache, nasopharyngitis, peripheral edema, anemia	Monthly liver transaminase monitoring required and pregnancy testing for women of childbearing potential. Potential for drug interactions (sildenafil, glyburide, cyclosporine, oral contraceptives)
Ambrisentan (Letairis) (ERA) Approved 2007	Oral (5 mg and 10 mg tabs, dosed once daily)	ARIES 1 (202 patients)/ARIES 2 (192 patients): functional class II–IV patients. Randomized, double-blind. Significant change in 6MWD compared to placebo at 12 wks.	Teratogenicity Headache, nasal congestion, peripheral edema, sinusitis, anemia	Monthly pregnancy testing required. Minimal drug interactions.
Macitentan (Opsumit) (ERA) Approved 2013	Oral (10 mg tabs, dosed once daily)	SERAPHIN trial: 742 patients, functional class II–IV; 45% reduction in morbidity and mortality composite endpoint in the 10 mg daily treatment group vs. placebo.	Teratogenicity Nasopharyngitis, headache, anemia	Monthly pregnancy testing required.
Tadalafil (Adcirca) (PDE-5i) Approved 2009	Oral (20 mg tabs, dosed 1 or 2 tabs once daily)	PHIRST trial: 405 patients, functional class predominantly II-III. Randomized, double-blind. Significant increase in 6MWD at 16 wks compared with placebo.	Headache, epistaxis, diarrhea	Contraindicated with use of nitrates.
Sildenafil (Revatio) (PDE-5i) Approved 2005	Oral (20 mg tabs, dosed up to 100 mg tid)[a]	SUPER-1 trial: 278 patients, functional class predominantly II-III. Randomized, double-blind. Significant increase in 6MWD at 12 wks compared with placebo.	Headache, epistaxis, diarrhea	Contraindicated with use of nitrates.
Riociguat (Adempas) (SGC-s) Approved 2013	Oral (0.5, 1.0, 1.5, 2.0, 2.5 mg tabs available, dosed up to 2.5 mg tid)	CHEST-1 trial: 261 patients with CTEPH (inoperable or persistent PH after PTE). Randomized, double-blind. Significant increase in 6MWD at 16 wks compared with placebo. PATENT-1 trial: 443 patients, functional class predominantly II-III. Randomized, double-blind. Significant increase in 6MWD at 12 wks compared with placebo	Teratogenicity Potential for systemic hypotension	Monthly pregnancy testing for women of childbearing potential. Drug is titrated up slowly over a few weeks with blood pressure monitoring before dose increases. Contraindicated with use of nitrates and PDE-5i.
Inhaled treprostinil (Tyvaso) (prostacyclin) Approved 2009	Inhalation (9 breaths, 4 times daily, via TD-100 system)	TRIUMPH-1 trial: 235 patients, functional class II–III. Randomized, double-blind. Significant change in 6MWD at wk 12 vs. placebo.	Cough, sore throat, flushing, nausea, vomiting, diarrhea, headache, muscle cramps	Proprietary nebulizer system required. Treatment 4 times daily.
Inhaled iloprost (Ventavis) (prostacyclin) Approved 2004	Inhalation (5 and 20 μg strengths, 6–9 treatments daily, via I-neb device)	AIR trials: 203 patients. Randomized, double-blind. Significant change in 6MWD at wk 12 vs. placebo.	Flushing, cough, nausea, vomiting, diarrhea, headache, muscle cramps	Proprietary nebulizer system required. Treatment 6–9 times daily.
Treprostinil injection (Remodulin) (prostacyclin) Approved 2002 (SC), 2004 (IV)	SC or IV, continuous (varies by patient, generally 50–120 ng/kg/min infusion)	470 patients, functional class II–IV. Randomized, double-blind. Significant change in 6MWD at wk 12 vs. placebo.	Flushing, jaw pain, nausea/vomiting, diarrhea, extremity pain/cramps Infusion site pain for SC route	Continuous infusion via tunneled catheter (for IV route)—associated risks of blood stream infection and thrombosis. Half-life 4–6 h. Stable at room temperature

TABLE 69.1	Current Approved Therapies for Pulmonary ArterialHypertension—cont'd			
Drug (Class) and Date of FDA Approval	Route (Dosing)	Key Clinical Trial Data (Group 1 PAH Patients Unless Noted Otherwise)	Pertinent Adverse Effects	Special Considerations
Epoprostenol injection (Flolan) (prostacyclin) Approved 1995	IV, continuous (varies by patient, generally 30–45 ng/kg/min infusion)	81 patients, functional class III–IV. Randomized, double blind. Significant improvement in mortality over 12 wks in epoprostenol + conventional therapy vs. conventional therapy alone.	Flushing, jaw pain, nausea/vomiting, diarrhea, extremity pain/cramps.	Continuous infusion via tunneled catheter—associated risks of blood stream infection and thrombosis Half-life 2–4 min. Not stable at room temperature.
Epoprostenol injection, room temp stable (Veletri) (prostacyclin) Approved 2010	IV, continuous (varies by patient, generally 30–45 ng/kg/min infusion)	Same as original epoprostenol data.	Flushing, jaw pain, nausea/vomiting, diarrhea, extremity pain/cramps.	Continuous infusion via tunneled catheter—associated risks of blood stream infection and thrombosis Half-life 2–4 min. Stable at room temperature.
Oral treprostinil (Orenitram) (prostacyclin) Approved 2013	Oral (0.125, 0.25, 1 and 2.5 mg tabs. Dosed every 8–12 hours, titration depending on patient tolerance)	FREEDOM-M: 349 patients, functional class II–III. Randomized, double-blind. Significant change in 6MWD at wk 12 compared with placebo.	Headache, diarrhea, nausea, flushing, jaw pain, pain in hands or feet, systemic hypotension.	Tablets must be taken with food. TID dosing may provide more consistent drug exposure
Selexipag (Uptravi) (prostaglandin receptor agonist) Approved 2015	Oral (200, 400, 600, 800, 1000, 1200, 1400, and 1600 μg tabs. Dosed bid, titrated to maximum tolerated dose or 1600 μg bid)	GRIPHON trial: 1156 patients, functional class predominantly II–III; 40% reduction in clinical worsening events compared with placebo group.	Headache, diarrhea, nausea, flushing, jaw pain, pain in hands or feet, systemic hypotension.	Drug interactions (strong inhibitors of CYP2C8, e.g., gemfibrozil). Avoid in severe hepatic impairment (Child-Pugh C). Dose adjustment required in Child-Pugh B.

6MWD, Six-minute walk distance; *bid*, twice daily; *CTEPH*, chronic thromboembolic pulmonary hypertension; *ERA*, endothelin receptor antagonist; *FDA*, Food and Drug Administration; *IV*, intravenous; *PAH*, pulmonary arteria hypertension; *PDE-5i*, phosphodiesterase type 5 inhibitor; *PH*, pulmonary hypertension; *PTE*, pulmonary thromboendarterectomy; *SC*, subcutaneous; *SGC*, soluble guanylate cyclase stimulator; *tid* three times daily.
[a]The use of doses of sildenafil >20 mg tid is off label and not approved by the FDA, although it was studied in the SUPER-1 trial at these dosing levels and often used clinically.

twice daily and carries a small potential for hepatotoxicity, which requires monthly liver transaminase monitoring. Newer generation ERA drugs were subsequently approved that are dosed once daily and do not have the risk for hepatotoxicity (ambrisentan and macitentan). All ERA drugs are possibly teratogenic, and monthly pregnancy testing is required in women of childbearing potential. A synopsis of pertinent clinical trial data and special considerations in the dosing and administration of ERA therapies is presented in Table 69.1.

Phosphodiesterase-5 Inhibitors and Soluble Guanylate Cyclase Stimulators

The second oral PAH therapy approved by the FDA was sildenafil, a PDE-5 inhibitor that had been previously approved to treat erectile dysfunction. Sildenafil was shown to improve 6-minute walking distance over 12 weeks relative to placebo at a dose of 20 mg three times daily. Subsequently, another PDE-5 inhibitor, tadalafil, was also studied in PAH and approved at a dose of 40 mg/day based on the findings of the Pulmonary Arterial Hypertension and Response to Tadalafil (PHIRST) trial, which also showed superior improvements in 6-minute walking distance compared with placebo over 16 weeks in patients with PAH.

Riociguat is a first-in-class SGC stimulator that was studied in patients with group 1 PAH and in patients with CTEPH who were either inoperable or had persistent PH after PTE surgery. This agent was studied in the Chronic Thromboembolic Pulmonary Hypertension Soluble Guanylate Cyclase-Stimulator Trial-1 (CHEST-1) and the Pulmonary Arterial Hypertension Soluble Guanylate Cyclase-Stimulator Trial-1 (PATENT-1) (PAH population), both of which showed significant improvements in 6-minute walking distance relative to placebo in both populations. These studies led to the approval of riociguat for both indications. Riociguat is typically titrated up over a period of a few weeks to a maximum dose of 2.5 mg three times daily, with attention paid to systemic blood pressure, because hypotension is a potential adverse effect. Additional pertinent trial data, adverse effect information, and dosing considerations for both PDE-5 inhibitors and riociguat are presented in Table 69.1.

Inhaled Prostacyclins

Prostanoid therapies are also available via the inhalation route. The first drug approved in this class was iloprost in 2004. Iloprost has been used as a parenteral prostacyclin in Europe for many years as well. It has a relatively short half-life and requires inhalation six to nine times daily during waking hours to minimize the amount of time that patients experience trough drug levels. Administration of inhaled iloprost is accomplished through a proprietary aerosol device that is designed to deliver iloprost only. Treprostinil is also available as an inhaled formulation. With a longer half-life, trough exposure can be minimized with only four times daily dosing. This must also be administered through a proprietary nebulizer system via a series of subsequent breaths inhaled during each treatment. The current approved dose is nine breaths, four times daily. Many patients are titrated up to doses higher than this to achieve additional therapeutic effect, although this strategy remains off-label currently. Treatment times for each dose for both of these inhaled therapies are approximately 5 to 10 minutes.

Oral Prostacyclins and Prostacyclin Receptor Agonists

Treprostinil is the only PAH therapy that is available in parenteral (IV and SC), inhaled, and oral formulations. The oral formulation is the first oral prostacyclin drug approved in the United States, although globally it was preceded by the availability of oral beraprost for the treatment of PAH in Japan. Oral treprostinil is dosed either twice or three times daily, and is approved for patients with functional class II to III limitations to improve exercise capacity.

More recently, the prostacyclin receptor agonist selexipag has been studied in a large event-driven trial that examined clinical worsening as the primary endpoint. This placebo-controlled, randomized, double-blind trial allowed for patients with an existing background PAH therapy and showed a significant treatment affect even with 80% of the enrolled patients being on an existing background PAH treatment. The duration of this trial, much like the SERAPHIN (Study with an Endothelin Receptor Antagonist in Pulmonary arterial Hypertension to Improve cliNical outcome) trial in which macitentan was studied, was much longer and enrolled many more patients than earlier PAH drug clinical trials.

Combination Therapy

The use of combinations of different classes of PAH therapy has essentially become the standard of care. Traditionally, this approach has involved sequential addition of different classes of PAH therapy in patients who were not meeting treatment goals or who were progressively worsening, despite existing therapy. The benefit of this approach has been deduced from a number of PAH drug trials that enrolled patients on existing background PAH therapy and showed benefit in the primary endpoint (usually 6-minute walking distance over 12 to 24 weeks). One recent area of interest has asked the question as to whether initial, upfront combination PAH therapy is more beneficial than PAH monotherapy alone, or if the relatively slower sequential, add-on approach is more beneficial. This strategy was studied in the Ambrisentan and Tadalafil in Patients with Pulmonary Arterial Hypertension (AMBITION) trial, in which initial combination therapy with ambrisentan and tadalafil was shown to be superior to the pooled monotherapy group of either tadalafil or ambrisentan alone. This was an event-driven trial (time to first clinical failure event) that enrolled 600 patients who were in the study for an average of <1.5 years. Although the usefulness of combination therapy seems to be clearer, the question remains as to which particular combinations are most efficacious and in which subsets of PAH patients the strategy is best used.

Treatment of Chronic Thromboembolic Pulmonary Hypertension

Once strong evidence for CTEPH has been obtained with a positive ventilation perfusion scan, performance of pulmonary angiography is needed (often in conjunction with right heart catheterization and pulmonary hemodynamic measurements) to fully assess the extent and location of chronic thromboemboli and determine if PTE surgery is feasible. The lesions present in CTEPH are fibrotic material that is deeply incorporated into the vessel wall (Fig. 69.4). PTE is a long and complex surgery, involving sternotomy, creation of a bloodless surgical field, and cardioplegia, such that appropriate visualization and adequate dissection of thromboembolic material can be achieved. This is accomplished by full cardiopulmonary bypass and deep hypothermic circulatory arrest. Significant improvements in pulmonary hemodynamics are usually observed, because PVR is reduced by the removal of chronic clot. This procedure was pioneered at the University of California, San Diego by Dr. Stuart Jameison and colleagues. It is best performed in a center with sufficient surgical volume and experience to optimize patient outcomes, particularly with respect to morbidity and mortality.

In patients with disease that is too distal to perform PTE effectively, riociguat is an option for medical therapy; it has been approved for this indication, as noted previously, based on the results of the CHEST trial. Likewise, patients that have residual PH after PTE can also be treated medically with riociguat.

Treatment Goals in Pulmonary Arterial Hypertension

The main goals of treatment in PAH, apart from the utmost goal of prolonging survival, are to restore right heart size and function to normal or near normal, and to improve functional capacity. Serial interval imaging of the right heart, usually achieved through transthoracic echocardiography, is the cornerstone of assessing RV size and contractility. Cardiac MRI can also be performed (and generally is considered superior to transthoracic echocardiography for this purpose), although cost and logistical challenges preclude its routine use for this purpose. Interval measurement of pro–brain natriuretic peptide levels is often used as an adjunct tool with cardiac imaging to further assess RV strain. Functional capacity is usually assessed both objectively (6-minute walking distance or formal cardiopulmonary exercise testing) and subjectively (WHO and/or New York Heart Association functional class assessment by the clinician via patient symptom and physical activity history). In some instances, definitive repeat assessment of pulmonary arterial hemodynamics by right heart catheterization is needed to better understand treatment effects and to determine need for additional or alternative PAH therapies. The specific treatment goals for PAH as defined at the 2013 Fifth World Symposium on Pulmonary Hypertension are outlined in Table 69.2.

Atrial Septostomy

For patients in whom multimodality PAH therapy is failing and who have advanced right heart failure with severe right heart volume and pressure overload, the creation of an atrial septostomy is an option to serve as a pressure release mechanism. This is rarely done and usually reserved for situations where it would serve as a bridge to a more definitive therapy (e.g., lung transplantation). In countries with limited access to PAH therapies, atrial septostomy can also be performed for symptom relief or palliation. Care must be taken that the procedure is carried out in a graded fashion, to minimize the amount of hypoxemia that accompanies the creation of this right-to-left shunt.

Lung Transplantation

The definitive therapy for PAH is bilateral lung transplantation. Patients who are maximized on all three classes of PAH therapy, usually including a parenteral prostacyclin therapy, and who have persistent right heart failure, are candidates for lung transplantation evaluation. Most patients do not require cardiac transplantation as well, because restoration of a normal pulmonary circulation and the associated sharp decrease in RV afterload usually allows for recovery of normal RV size and function. Of note, patients who undergo lung transplantation for PAH

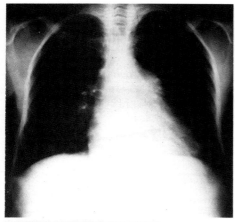

CXR is often largely unremarkable except for evidence of an enlarged main pulmonary artery.

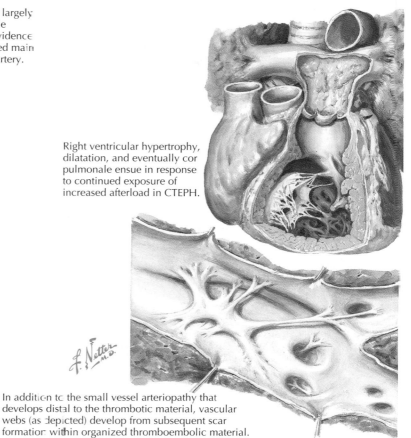

Right ventricular hypertrophy, dilatation, and eventually cor pulmonale ensue in response to continued exposure of increased afterload in CTEPH.

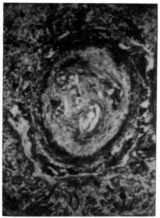

Organized thromboembolic material with accompanying intimal thickening of the pulmonary arterial wall.

In addition to the small vessel arteriopathy that develops distal to the thrombotic material, vascular webs (as depicted) develop from subsequent scar formation within organized thromboembolic material.

FIG 69.4 Chronic Effects of Pulmonary Embolism (Cor Pulmonale). *CTEPH*, Chronic thromboembolic pulmonary hypertension; *CXR*, chest x-ray.

TABLE 69.2 Treatment Goals for Pulmonary Arterial Hypertension

Hemodynamics	Right atrial pressure <8 mm Hg
	Cardiac index ≥3 L/min/m²)
WHO/NYHA Functional Class	I or II
6-min walk distance	≥380–440 m
Right heart appearance on cardiac imaging (echocardiography or cardiac MRI)	Normal/near normal right ventricular size and function
Natriuretic peptide levels (BNP, pro-BNP)	Normal
Cardiopulmonary exercise testing	Peak VO₂ >15 mL/kg/min
	VE/VCO₂ at anaerobic threshold <36

BNP, Brain natriuretic peptide; *NYHA*, New York Heart Association; *VCO₂*, carbon dioxide output; *VE*, minute ventilation; *WHO*, World Health Organization.

have a higher immediate-term (30 day) postoperative mortality compared with patients undergoing lung transplantation for other pulmonary diseases. This is usually due to acute rejection. Beyond this 30-day window, the intermediate and longer term survival is on par with that for other pretransplantation lung diseases.

FUTURE DIRECTIONS

New, potentially first-in-class therapies are currently under clinical investigation for the treatment of PAH. These include therapies that target the production of proinflammatory leukotriene B4 (ubenimex) and cellular metabolic modifiers (bardoxalone methyl) that promote mitochondrial respiration and reduce the formation of reactive oxygen species and associated inflammation. Other potential new classes of therapy for PAH include FK506 (tacrolimus) to promote BMPR2 signaling, and rituximab to suppress endothelial cell apoptosis that may be driven by autoimmunity in systemic sclerosis patients and drive the development of pulmonary arteriopathy.

Apart from the potential for new classes of therapy, innovations in the delivery of existing therapies are also being studied, the most notable of which is a wholly implantable pump and catheter system to deliver treprostinil infusion. This is accomplished through an implantable pump that can be refilled percutaneously at intervals and also controlled through an external transducer device (i.e., setting flow rate).

As the genetic underpinnings of PAH become better understood, the potential for gene therapy to augment expression of pertinent enzymes (such as NO synthase) or ligands known to interact with BMPR2 (such as BMP9) becomes of increasing interest. There is much work underway in this regard currently, although none are ready for clinical application yet.

The ability to provide targeted individualized therapies for PAH patients is of great interest. Variability in treatment response within the same class of drug from one individual to another remains apparent. The reasons for this variability are not well understood currently (in the way they are in the field of oncology and cancer chemotherapeutics). Efforts are underway to better understand the phenomics of PH of various forms through the multicenter National Institutes of Health Pulmonary Vascular Disease Phenomics (PVDOMICS) initiative.

ADDITIONAL RESOURCES

Galiè N, Corris PA, Frost A, et al. Updated treatment algorithm of pulmonary arterial hypertension. *J Am Coll Cardiol.* 2013;62(25 suppl):D60–D72.

Update from the Fifth World Health Symposium on the management of PAH patients as it relates to general health measures, supportive therapies, and pulmonary vasodilators, with discussion of approaches to patients with advanced disease and an inadequate response.

Humbert M, Lau E, Montani D, et al. Advances in therapeutic interventions for patients with pulmonary hypertension. *Circulation.* 2014;130:2189–2208.

Excellent review of targets of pharmacotherapy and pulmonary vasodilators that were approved by late 2014.

McLaughlin VV, Gaine SP, Howard LS, et al. Treatment goals of pulmonary hypertension. *J Am Coll Cardiol.* 2013;62(25 suppl):D73–D81.

Reviews currently accepted goals that correlate with improved long-term outcomes for patients on active treatment.

Simonneau G, Gatzoulis M, Adatia I, et al. Updated clinical classification of pulmonary hypertension. *J Am Coll Cardiol.* 2013;62(25 suppl):D34–D41.

Fifth World Symposium revision to the PH classification scheme that attempts to categorize the underlying pathology more precisely.

Vachiéry JL, Adir Y, Barberà JA, et al. Pulmonary hypertension due to left heart diseases. *J Am Coll Cardiol.* 2013;62:D100.

An excellent comprehensive review of the most common form of PH that is due to left heart disease.

EVIDENCE

Barst RJ, Rubin LJ, Long WA, et al. A comparison of continuous intravenous epoprostenol (prostacyclin) with conventional therapy for primary pulmonary hypertension. *N Engl J Med.* 1996;334:296–301.

The landmark clinical trial that paved the way for the use of pulmonary vasodilators in PAH.

Benza RL, Miller DP, Barst RJ, et al. An evaluation of long-term survival from time of diagnosis in pulmonary arterial hypertension from the REVEAL registry. *Chest.* 2012;142(2):448–456.

A look at the contemporary US PAH registry from the mid-2000s and trends in survival caused by many new pulmonary vasodilator therapies compared with the older National Institutes of Health PAH registry.

Christie JD, Edwards LB, Kucheryavaya AY, et al. The registry of the International Society for Heart and Lung Transplantation: twenty-seventh official adult lung and heart-lung transplant report—2010. *J Heart Lung Transplant.* 2010;29:1104–1118.

Despite advancements of disease-specific medical therapies for PH, transplantation remains the gold standard for patients in whom medical therapy fails. These data review referral trends, outcome analyses, and survival comparisons with other lung disease states.

Delcroix M, Lang I, Pepke-Zaba J, et al. Long-term outcome of patients with chronic thromboembolic pulmonary hypertension: results from an international prospective registry. *Circulation.* 2016;133:859–871.

European registry documenting improved long-term outcomes in patients with underlying CTEPH who underwent surgical treatment with PTE.

Pengo V, Lensing AW, Prins MH, et al. Incidence of chronic thromboembolic pulmonary hypertension after pulmonary embolism. *N Engl J Med.* 2004;350:2257–2264.

The prospective trial that demonstrated the risk at 2 years of developing CTEPH was 3.8% in patients with acute pulmonary embolism.

70

HIV and the Heart

Michelle A. Floris-Moore, Kristine B. Patterson, Joseph J. Eron

HIV and AIDS affect >36 million people worldwide. Increased survival among HIV-infected persons who have access to effective combination antiretroviral therapy (ART) and rising rates of new diagnoses among older adults have resulted in growing numbers of older people living with HIV.

Some cardiac manifestations more commonly seen before availability of effective ART, such as dilated cardiomyopathy (DCM), myocarditis, and pericarditis, are now relatively rare in individuals treated for HIV. Instead, traditionally age-related illnesses, like atherosclerotic cardiovascular disease (ASCVD), have become increasingly important in HIV care. This chapter explores common cardiac diseases in HIV-infected individuals and the ways in which etiologies differ compared with the general population (Fig. 70.1). Optimal care of cardiac disease in the HIV-infected patient should be integrated among the cardiologist, the HIV care provider, and the primary care provider.

ETIOLOGY AND PATHOGENESIS

The etiology underlying cardiac diseases in HIV infection is multifactorial and may include one or more of the following categories: (1) direct viral effect of HIV and associated chronic inflammation; (2) HIV-associated infections and/or opportunistic diseases; (3) antiretroviral medications; and (4) risk factors common to the general population that are highly prevalent in populations affected by HIV (e.g., hyperlipidemia, smoking, and hypertension). Treatment of cardiac disease in HIV-infected patients should address pathways underlying the disease process and modifiable risk factors.

CLINICAL PRESENTATION

Dilated Cardiomyopathy

In the pre-ART era, DCM was found in 20% to 40% of patients with long-standing HIV infection, even in the absence of an AIDS-defining diagnosis. Currently, HIV-associated DCM is rare and may be related to impaired immune function, direct cardiotoxic effects of HIV or HIV proteins, drug-related toxicity, and/or nutritional deficiencies.

Specific opportunistic infections implicated include viral (cytomegalovirus, herpes simplex), protozoal (*Toxoplasma gondii*), bacterial (*Mycobacterium tuberculosis, Mycobacterium avium-intracellulare*), and fungal (*Cryptococcus neoformans, Aspergillus fumigatus, Histoplasma capsulatum, Coccidioides immitis,* and *Candida* spp.) infections and should be considered in evaluation of the HIV-infected patient with DCM. Ability to identify the causative agent of DCM is often limited, and clinical management focuses on treatment of heart failure and supportive measures. In patients who have uncontrolled HIV, effective ART is also indicated, and virological control can lead to a significant improvement in cardiac function.

Pulmonary Hypertension

Although uncommon, pulmonary arterial hypertension (PAH) independently predicts mortality among people living with HIV. The prevalence of PAH is estimated to be 1 in 200 in HIV-infected individuals compared with 1 in 200,000 in the general population, and rates remain essentially unchanged despite use of effective ART. The pathogenesis underlying PAH in HIV infection remains unclear but may be related to duration of infection, effects of HIV on endothelial function, or sequelae of opportunistic pulmonary infections. Early recognition and treatment of PAH is recommended because clinical management of more advanced disease and cardiopulmonary complications is challenging. Treatment of PAH in HIV-infected patients is the same as for other nonidiopathic PAH. Initiation of ART, although important for control of HIV, has not been shown to improve PAH.

Pericardial Effusions and Pericarditis

Pericardial effusions are commonly seen in HIV-infected individuals. Clinical manifestations include asymptomatic effusions detected on echocardiography, pericarditis with and/or without constriction, and tamponade. The clinical presentation of pericarditis alone is not different in HIV-infected and uninfected individuals, and etiology is most often not determined. Specific considerations in this population include infections (viral, fungal, and mycobacterial, with tuberculosis as a particular concern in patients at high risk for this coinfection), malignancies (e.g., Kaposi sarcoma [KS] and non-Hodgkin lymphoma [NHL]), and other HIV-associated diseases (e.g., nephropathy).

Infective Endocarditis

Infective endocarditis in HIV-infected individuals has similar prevalence to that in individuals with the same risk behaviors and similar clinical presentation. *Staphylococcus aureus* and *Streptococcus viridans* are the major responsible organisms. As in all cases of endocarditis, exposure history can help guide assessment of likely pathogens (e.g., intravenous drug use increases risk for *S. aureus*). However, certain organisms are seen more frequently in HIV-infected individuals who are at higher risk of *Salmonella* bacteremia, which results in endocarditis, than are seen in immunocompetent patients. Other than *Candida* species, fungal endocarditis (*Aspergillus fumigatus, Histoplasma capsulatum,* and *Cryptococcus neoformans*) is also more common in HIV-infected individuals; however, this remains relatively rare. Individuals with late-stage HIV infection and advanced immunosuppression have a worse prognosis and higher mortality than those who are earlier in the disease course.

Cardiac Neoplasms

Both KS and NHL, the two most common malignancies associated with HIV/AIDS, may involve the heart. Cardiac KS is always associated with disseminated KS, and physical examination findings (e.g., skin

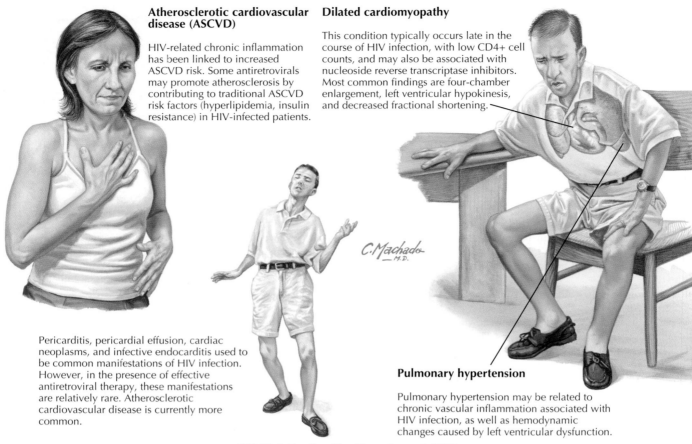

Atherosclerotic cardiovascular disease (ASCVD)

HIV-related chronic inflammation has been linked to increased ASCVD risk. Some antiretrovirals may promote atherosclerosis by contributing to traditional ASCVD risk factors (hyperlipidemia, insulin resistance) in HIV-infected patients.

Dilated cardiomyopathy

This condition typically occurs late in the course of HIV infection, with low CD4+ cell counts, and may also be associated with nucleoside reverse transcriptase inhibitors. Most common findings are four-chamber enlargement, left ventricular hypokinesis, and decreased fractional shortening.

Pericarditis, pericardial effusion, cardiac neoplasms, and infective endocarditis used to be common manifestations of HIV infection. However, in the presence of effective antiretroviral therapy, these manifestations are relatively rare. Atherosclerotic cardiovascular disease is currently more common.

Pulmonary hypertension

Pulmonary hypertension may be related to chronic vascular inflammation associated with HIV infection, as well as hemodynamic changes caused by left ventricular dysfunction.

FIG 70.1 Cardiac Manifestations of AIDS.

lesions) may provide evidence to suggest the diagnosis. Cardiac findings are usually subclinical; however, fatal cardiac tamponade and pericardial constriction may occur. Pericardiocentesis is considered a high-risk procedure because of the vascular nature of KS lesions. In suspected cases, a pericardial window is preferred for providing decompression in addition to establishing the diagnosis.

NHL is usually high grade, of B-cell origin, and disseminates early. Cardiac involvement of NHL may present with intractable heart failure, pericardial effusion, cardiac tamponade, or arrhythmias. Patients with mechanical obstruction may benefit from surgical resection.

Cardiac toxicity from chemotherapy for either malignancy is also possible depending on the agents used.

ATHEROSCLEROTIC CARDIOVASCULAR DISEASE

HIV-infected individuals appear to have greater risk for ASCVD and may develop clinical ASCVD at younger ages than the general population. Observational studies suggest that, compared with seronegative individuals, HIV-infected adults have twice the risk of myocardial infarction (MI) and a fourfold increase in risk of sudden cardiac death. Although this may be partly attributable to a high prevalence of traditional risk factors (e.g., smoking and hypertension), studies also show increased MI rates among HIV-infected individuals with no traditional ASCVD risk factors. Other factors implicated include direct and indirect impacts of HIV and ART. HIV or ART may (1) alter traditional risk factors (e.g., dyslipidemia), or (2) affect underlying ASCVD pathogenesis

(e.g., viral effects, proinflammatory processes, and endothelial dysfunction). Thus far, there is no clear evidence that any one of these factors supersedes the others.

Impact of Immunosuppression

The severity of pretreatment immunosuppression may contribute to ASCVD risk in HIV-infected patients. In the San Francisco General Hospital Observational Cohort Evaluating Long-Term Consequences of Virologic Failure (SCOPE) cohort and the Multicenter AIDS Cohort Study (MACS), lower nadir CD4+ cell counts were independently associated with more rapid progression of carotid intima media thickness and higher CVD event rates, respectively. In contrast, the HIV Outpatient Study found associations of CVD events with the CD4+ cell count at baseline but not with nadir CD4. Although the impact of the CD4+ cell count on ASCVD remains unclear, low nadir CD4 (<200 cells/mm^3) could be considered a potential risk factor in cardiac assessment.

HIV-Related Inflammation

Despite causing profound immunodeficiency, HIV induces chronic immune activation and increased expression of proinflammatory mediators by activated T cells and macrophages, promoting leukocyte recruitment and extracellular remodeling of the arterial endothelium. Increased inflammatory and monocyte activation marker levels are associated with subclinical and clinical CVD among HIV-infected adults. In addition, HIV viral proteins may contribute to endothelial activation. Although ART may ameliorate this process, it does not completely suppress the cascade.

Antiretroviral Medications

Although ART has radically improved survival and health status of HIV-infected people, some studies have linked ART medications to increased ASCVD risk. The Strategies for Management of Antiretroviral Therapy (SMART) study demonstrated increased ASCVD among patients who episodically discontinued ART on the basis of CD4 count—presumably due to the proinflammatory state seen with uncontrolled viral replication. The risk decreased on reinstitution of ART but did not return to baseline. Additional data suggested improvement in endothelial function after ART initiation, but another recent study showed persistent arterial inflammation despite restoration of immune function after starting ART.

Other data indicate that specific antiretroviral medications may increase CVD risk. One large cohort, the Data Collection on Adverse Events of Anti-HIV Drugs (D:A:D Study), detected a relative risk of 16% for MI associated with protease inhibitor (PI) use for every year of ART exposure. However, PI-associated risk was lower than the annual risk associated with age, male sex, or tobacco usage.

In the D:A:D study, current and/or recent use of abacavir was associated with a twofold increase in the risk of a cardiovascular event, after adjusting for confounders. Findings of the SMART study and North American AIDS Cohort Collaboration on Research and Design (NA-ACCORD) showed similar associations of abacavir with higher CVD risk. A criticism of earlier nonrandomized studies was that individuals with risk factors for renal insufficiency, some of which also increased ASCVD risk, might have received abacavir instead of tenofovir disoproxil fumarate because of the concern for renal toxicity of tenofovir disoproxil fumarate, which increased rates of ASCVD in the abacavir group. Some of those analyses have been updated, and findings of increased ASCVD risk persist. However, there was no increased CVD risk seen in a longitudinal observational study for individuals enrolled in clinical trials with randomization to abacavir and/or non-abacavir arms. These studies and others evaluated changes in inflammatory markers associated with abacavir use, and showed that platelet hyperreactivity and worsening endothelial function were seen with abacavir. The impact of abacavir on CVD risk has yet to be definitely determined. However, because of this uncertainty, abacavir should be avoided in individuals with and/or at high risk for ASCVD.

Traditional Modifiable Risk Factors

As in the general population, cigarette smoking, hypertension, diabetes, and obesity are all strong predictors of CVD among people with HIV infection. Smoking rates are consistently higher among HIV-infected adults than age-matched control subjects. HIV infection is also associated with low high-density lipoprotein cholesterol (HDL-C) levels, which persists even after immunologic recovery. Some patients on ART gain weight as their health improves, and develop obesity and associated metabolic complications, like insulin resistance (IR) and dyslipidemia. Use of specific ART medications is also independently associated with metabolic complications.

Dyslipidemia

ART is linked to lipid perturbations, but the pathogenesis is not well understood. Differences exist between and within ART classes, and effects cannot be generalized. Of the PIs, lopinavir-ritonavir is associated with a greater increase in triglycerides (TGs) and low-density lipoprotein cholesterol (LDL-C) levels than other medications in that class, whereas atazanavir appears to have the least deleterious impact on lipid levels.

The non-nucleoside reverse transcriptase inhibitors (NNRTIs) are variably associated with increases in total cholesterol, LDL-C, and TGs, but in some studies, they have also been linked to favorable increases

in HDL-C. Dolutegravir and raltegravir, both integrase strand transfer inhibitors (INSTIs), appear to be more lipid-neutral than PIs and/or efavirenz. Thus, for some HIV-infected patients with hyperlipidemia, switching to an INSTI-based ART regimen may be beneficial. Of note, elvitegravir, another INSTI, is given in conjunction with cobicistat, a pharmacokinetic booster that is associated with increases in lipids, which is similar to that seen with low doses of ritonavir.

Insulin Resistance

IR in HIV infection is multifactorial. Important contributors include traditional diabetes risk factors (genetics, physical inactivity, obesity) and HIV-related factors, such as the effects of specific antiretrovirals (indinavir, thymidine analogs), and consequences of the lipodystrophy syndrome. Screening for diabetes and/or impaired glucose tolerance with measurement of fasting glucose and/or glycosylated hemoglobin A_{1C} (HgbA$_{1C}$) is recommended as part of routine care for HIV-infected adults. Treatment of IR should include exercise, dietary modifications, and consideration of a more metabolically friendly ART regimen.

Management of Cardiovascular Disease Risk in HIV-Infected Patients

A fasting lipid profile and fasting glucose or HgbA$_{1C}$ should be obtained before initiation of ART and at 3 to 6 months later. Data on the best risk assessment tool for estimation of ASCVD risk in HIV-infected patients vary. Some studies suggest that risk assessment tools used in the general population underestimate CVD risk in HIV-infected adults and favor the use of specific risk scores that incorporate HIV-related information. A CVD risk prediction model, developed in the D:A:D study and recently updated in 2015, includes the CD4+ cell count, and cumulative exposure to PIs, NRTIs, and abacavir (a restricted version omits the antiretroviral medication history, which is not always readily available). Although some studies report improved accuracy of prediction with the D:A:D risk score, others suggest that the previously used Framingham Risk Score and the current Pooled Cohort Equation (PCE) recommended by the 2013 American Heart Association (AHA) Guidelines, performs well in HIV-infected populations. Because there is no clear guidance regarding superiority of a particular tool for this population, the PCE should be used to assess ASCVD risk among HIV-infected adults aged 40 to 75 years (age limits per AHA guidelines). For younger HIV-infected patients, or those in whom HIV-related factors are believed to play a major role in CVD risk, the D:A:D CVD risk score may be used.

Statin use should be implemented based on PCE ASCVD risk score, with intensity of statin based on AHA guidelines; however, potential drug interactions must be considered because many ART medications affect statin levels. In general, PIs and cobicistat increase statin levels, and initial statin doses for patients on these drugs should therefore be relatively low and gradually increased as tolerated to reach goal. Lovastatin and simvastatin are contraindicated in such patients. The statins most frequently used in HIV-infected patients on ART include pravastatin, atorvastatin, and rosuvastatin. Monitoring for muscle toxicity and hepatotoxicity should be performed on a regular basis. With refractory hypertriglyceridemia and hypercholesterolemia, both a fibrate and a statin may be necessary, although the risk of toxicity may be compounded. Niacin lowers LDL-C but potentially worsens IR, and should be avoided in patients taking PIs.

As with the general population, lifestyle modifications (diet and moderate exercise) should be incorporated into treatment of dyslipidemia or hyperglycemia. In individuals with established CVD, medical intervention should be initiated concurrently. CVD risk management of HIV-infected individuals should be in conjunction with the primary care and HIV providers. In some instances, ART may be altered to assist in the management of dyslipidemia.

Avoiding Drug Interactions

Several drugs used to treat cardiac disease interact with ART. Some of the more commonly encountered drug interactions are presented here, but this is not an exhaustive list. Consultation with an HIV specialist is recommended when starting any new medications for a patient who is also taking ART.

Most statins are metabolized by cytochrome P450 3A4 (CYP3A4), which may be inhibited or induced by HIV therapeutics. There is increased risk of skeletal muscle toxicity (myalgias, rhabdomyolysis) and hepatotoxicity from increased statin levels when coadministered with PIs or cobicistat (which inhibit CYP3A4). Lovastatin and simvastatin are extensively metabolized by CYP3A4 and are contraindicated in patients receiving PIs or cobicistat. Atorvastatin is partially metabolized by CYP3A4, and can be administered with PIs, but should be started at low dose. Pravastatin and rosuvastatin are not metabolized by CYP3A4, but levels are significantly increased when administered with darunavir, and the statin dose should be decreased. Nevirapine, efavirenz, and etravirine induce CYP3A4, thus lowering statin concentrations and decreasing efficacy of most statins. Pitavastatin, however, is metabolized primarily by glucoronidation and not by CYP3A4, and therefore, has minimal drug interactions with ART medications.

Dolutegravir, an INSTI, has no interaction with statins, but interacts with metformin, leading to increased metformin levels if coadministered. It is therefore recommended that metformin doses be decreased by half when given to a patient who also takes dolutegravir.

Antiplatelet agents often have clinically significant drug interactions with ART. Levels of prasugrel, tirofiban, ticagrelor, and clopidogrel may be elevated when co-administered with PIs and decreased when given with some NNRTIs, potentially leading to increased risk of bleeding or decreased efficacy, respectively. Similarly, anticoagulants (e.g., warfarin, rivaroxaban) and thrombolytics (e.g., altepase) have variable drug interactions with PIs and NNRTIs. The impact of drug interactions between ART and the medications in drug-eluting stents is unclear and is not currently believed to be clinically significant.

Many antiarrhythmic drugs interact with ART, and some are contraindicated in patients on specific antiretrovirals. Amiodarone and flecainide interact with many antiretrovirals, and consultation with a pharmacist is advised when using these medications in patients on ART. Amiodarone levels are increased in the presence of all PIs and cobicistat, which requires careful monitoring of levels, and is contraindicated in patients on ritonavir, nelfinavir, indinavir, or saquinavir. Efavirenz, nevirapine, and rilpivirine also interact with amiodarone, potentially decreasing levels and prolonging the QT interval; co-administration should be avoided. Close monitoring of drug levels and ECG should be used if use of these therapies cannot be avoided. Flecainide is subject to similar drug interactions with ART. Dronedarone is contraindicated for use with PIs because of increased levels and risk for cardiac (QT prolongation, arrhythmia) and other adverse effects, and should also be avoided in patients on efavirenz or nevirapine. Digoxin levels are increased when coadministered with PIs, and the dose should be decreased by 15% to 30%, with close monitoring of levels.

Expert consultation with an HIV specialist and pharmacist is recommended to assess risk of clinically significant drug interactions and to determine if ART medications need to be modified in patients who also require treatment for cardiac disease.

FUTURE DIRECTIONS

Since the introduction of ART, the overall incidence of nonatherosclerotic cardiac disease (e.g., pericarditis and DCM), in HIV-infected individuals has significantly decreased. This likely reflects increased control of HIV replication, improved immune function, and consequent decrease in opportunistic infections. However, non-AIDS defining conditions, such as ASCVD, have become major contributors to morbidity and mortality. Accumulating evidence indicates that HIV-infected patients are at excess risk for ASCVD; however, the mechanisms underlying this risk remain poorly understood. Future investigation to clarify those mechanisms could facilitate development of novel interventions targeting immune modulation to augment ASCVD risk reduction strategies and decrease cardiovascular morbidity and mortality.

At the same time, existing data show that traditional modifiable ASCVD risk factors remain important predictors of ASCVD in HIV-infected patients, and control of these risk factors is essential. Routine CVD risk factor screening and strategies to control risk should be implemented into the standard treatment of HIV-infected individuals. These should include lifestyle modifications, smoking cessation, and initiation of statins when indicated. Treatment of cardiac disease in the HIV-infected patient is complex, and should include a team approach of the cardiologist, HIV specialist, and primary care provider.

ADDITIONAL RESOURCES

Aberg JA, Gallant JE, Ghanem KG, et al. Primary care guidelines for the management of persons infected with HIV. *Clin Infect Dis.* 2014;58:1–10.
Updated guidelines for primary care of HIV-infected adults, including recommendations for screening and/or management of metabolic comorbidities (diabetes, dyslipidemia) and other ASCVD risk factors.
Friis-Møller N, Ryom L, Smith C, et al. Updated prediction model of the global risk of cardiovascular disease in HIV-positive persons: the D:A:D study. *Eur J Prev Cardiol.* 2016;23:214–223.
A global CVD risk equation for estimating risk among HIV-infected adults, developed in the multicenter D:A:D cohort, includes CD4+ cell count and antiretroviral history, as well as traditional ASCVD risk factors. The D:A:D model predicted risk more accurately than a Framingham study model.
Janda S, Quon BS, Swiston J. HIV and pulmonary arterial hypertension: a systematic review. *HIV Med.* 2010;11:620–634.
Systematic review synthesizes available data on PAH in HIV. Provides important information on clinical presentation, radiographic and pathological findings, treatment, and clinical outcomes of an uncommon disease.
Lumsden RH, Bloomfield GS. The causes of HIV-associated cardiomyopathy: a tale of two worlds. *Biomed Res Int.* 2016;2016:8196560.
Discusses pathogenesis of cardiomyopathy in HIV infection, role of inflammation, immunologic changes, opportunistic infections, and drug toxicity. Addresses differences in cardiomyopathy rates and etiologies in resource-poor compared with high-income countries.
Stein JH, Currier JS, Hsue PY. Arterial disease in patients with human immunodeficiency virus infection: what has imaging taught us? *JACC Cardiovasc Imaging.* 2014;7:515–525.
Discussion of mechanisms underlying associations between HIV infection and ASCVD risk and results of different arterial imaging modalities (carotid ultrasound, cardiac CT, brachial artery ultrasound, and FDG-PET).

EVIDENCE

El-Sadr WM, Lundgren JD, Neaton JD, et al. CD4+ count-guided interruption of antiretroviral treatment. The Strategies for Management of Antiretroviral Therapy (SMART) Study Group. *N Engl J Med.* 2006;355:2283–2296.
Pivotal clinical trial that randomly assigned participants to continue or interrupt ART based on CD4 cell counts and demonstrated that interruption of therapy was associated with greater mortality and increased CVD events.
Freiberg MS, Chang CH, Kuller LH, et al. HIV infection and the risk of acute myocardial infarction. *JAMA Intern Med.* 2013;173:614–622.
Data from the Veterans Affairs Cohort Study, demonstrating increased MI risk among HIV-infected veterans, compared with demographically similar uninfected controls, adjusted for Framingham risk factors, comorbidities, cigarette smoking, and alcohol and/or cocaine use.

Llibre JM, Hill A. Abacavir and cardiovascular disease: a critical look at the data. *Antiviral Res.* 2016;132:116–121.

Compiled data on associations between abacavir and CVD, and provides a concise assessment of conflicting findings regarding impact of recent and/or cumulative abacavir exposure with MI in several HIV cohorts.

Subramanian S, Tawakol A, Burdo TH, et al. Arterial inflammation in patients with HIV. *JAMA.* 2012;308:379–386.

Cross-sectional study providing evidence of greater arterial inflammation in treated and virologically-controlled HIV-infected adults compared with uninfected control subjects with a similar low Framingham risk score. Arterial inflammation in HIV-infected participants was similar to that seen in a second uninfected comparison group with known ASCVD, and associated with markers of monocyte and/or macrophage activation.

Zanni MA, Toribio M, Robbins GK, et al. Effects of antiretroviral therapy on immune function and arterial inflammation in treatment-naive patients with HIV infection. *JAMA Cardiol.* 2016;1:474–480.

Longitudinal study of treatment-naïve HIV-infected adults without history of coronary artery disease that assessed impact of ART initiation on arterial inflammation and coronary plaque, showing persistent arterial inflammation despite improvement in immunologic parameters and a decrease in lymph node inflammation.

71

Sleep Disorders and the Cardiovascular System

Bradley V. Vaughn, Elizabeth Boger Foreman

NORMAL SLEEP PHYSIOLOGY

The state of sleep is determined by an array of coordinated neuronal processes. Sleep is typically divided into stages based on electroencephalographic (EEG) features, eye movements (electrooculography), and muscle tone (electromyography). Stages N1 through N3 are collectively called nonrapid eye movement sleep. Stage N1 sleep is frequently associated with the perception of drowsiness and is characterized by EEG features of mild slowing and vertex sharp waves. Stage N2 (light sleep) is characterized by the presence of K complexes or sleep spindles. In stage N3 (deep sleep), high-amplitude slow waves predominate in EEG activity. Rapid eye movement (REM) sleep (or stage R) is characterized by a low-amplitude, mixed-frequency pattern on the EEG, absence of muscle tone in voluntary muscles, and intermittent REMs. Dreams can occur in all stages of sleep but are more vividly recalled from REM sleep. Healthy adults display a reproducible pattern of sleep organization. They enter sleep through stage N1, progress to stage N2, and after 15 to 25 minutes progress to stage N3, followed by reemergence of stage N2 sleep. The first REM sleep period occurs after approximately 90 minutes. This pattern repeats approximately every 90 minutes throughout the sleep period, with progressively less slow-wave sleep and longer periods of REM sleep in each cycle.

All of these stages have other physiological correlates. As individuals progress normally through the stages of sleep, there are variations in heart rate, blood pressure, peripheral vascular tone, oxygen delivery, coronary blood flow, and respiration. In a healthy individual, transitional periods between quiet wakefulness and light sleep are characterized by mild instability in breathing, making these periods particularly subject to periodic breathing. As the individual becomes drowsy, the heart rate may decrease, with a subtle drop in blood pressure. In sustained nonrapid eye movement sleep, parasympathetic regulation of cardiovascular activity predominates, characterized by decreased blood pressure, greater high-frequency heart rate variability, and more regular breathing compared with quiet wakefulness. In REM sleep, skeletal muscles are paralyzed, except for a select few, including the diaphragm. This muscle atonia results in a decrease in peripheral vascular tone. Surges in sympathetic and parasympathetic output cause increased variability of heart rate, blood pressure, and respiratory rate. This fluctuation in autonomic output leads to accelerations and slowing of the heart rate and breathing, as well as increased afterload. This, combined with the decreased respiratory response to hypercapnia and hypoxia, makes individuals with underlying cardiac disease (e.g., heart failure, conduction disturbances, coronary artery disease) or pulmonary disease vulnerable during REM sleep and may increase the risk of arrhythmias and reduced coronary blood flow.

SLEEP LENGTH AND HEALTH

Our society has progressively shortened the amount of time dedicated to sleep. At the beginning of the 20th century, it was estimated that

individuals spent approximately 9 to 10 hours per night in bed. As of 2008, the average working American sleeps <7 hours per night. Sleep deprivation in the short term is associated with autonomic instability, higher blood pressure, increased appetite, higher cortisol levels, and increased inflammatory markers. Epidemiological studies suggest that chronic sleep deprivation is associated with weight gain and obesity. In addition, individuals who sleep <5 hours per night are at higher risk for vascular disease, development of diabetes, and a shorter life span. Similarly, individuals who sleep >9 hours also appear to have a shorter life span. The underlying mechanism for the link of sleep deprivation and disease is unclear. Yet, some believe that dysregulation of the endocrine and autonomic nervous systems, as well as increases in inflammation contribute to the development of hypertension, vascular disease, and weight gain. Regardless of the mechanism, sleep duration may affect cardiovascular health.

SLEEP-RELATED BREATHING DISORDERS

Sleep can be disrupted by several disorders (Box 71.1), many of which have not been extensively studied for their relationships to cardiovascular health. Patients presenting to a sleep specialist are typically those with sleep-related breathing disorders. Common sleep problems, including obstructive sleep apnea (OSA), central sleep apnea (CSA), and obesity hypoventilation, can adversely affect cardiovascular health. Sleep-related breathing patterns, such as Cheyne-Stokes respiration (CSR), may reflect underlying cardiovascular issues. These disorders offer an opportunity to identify predisposing and exacerbating factors of cardiovascular disease and improve long-term risks.

Obstructive Sleep Apnea

In OSA, apneas are defined in adults as the absence of airflow for ≥10 seconds as a result of collapse of upper airway structures, in the setting of continued respiratory effort (Fig. 71.1). Hypopneas are defined in adults as impairment of airflow by >30% and are associated with oxygen desaturation of at least 3% or an EEG arousal. Some insurance programs only allow counting those events associated with a 4% desaturation. Significant pathophysiology is also seen with apnea and hypopnea events, including swings in blood pressure, heart rate, and vascular resistance. The number of apnea and hypopnea events per hour, termed the apnea–hypopnea index (AHI), is used to determine disease severity (Table 71.1). Population studies estimate that more than one in five middle-aged individuals have at least mild disease, with incidence being more prevalent in males. The mechanisms for this airway obstruction are linked to airway compromise, typically at multiple levels: the nose, retropalatal and retroglossal regions, and the pharynx (Box 71.2, Fig. 71.2). Common factors associated with an increased risk of OSA include male sex, older age, obesity, anatomically small airway, and others (Box 71.3).

BOX 71.1 Categories of Sleep Disorders

Insomnias
Sleep-related breathing disorders
Hypersomnias
Circadian rhythm disorders

Parasomnias
Sleep-related movement disorders
Other disorders

BOX 71.2 Symptoms of Obstructive Sleep Apnea

Snoring
Daytime sleepiness
Witnessed apneas or gasping events
   during sleep
Insomnia

Hypertension
Decreased cognition
Morning headaches
Sexual dysfunction

BOX 71.3 Mechanisms of Obstructive Sleep Apnea

Neural
- Pharyngeal muscular relaxation (neural control, medication or drug effect)
- Diminished response to upper airway load
- Upper airway neural impairment (vibration injury of sensory nerves, neuropathy, neuromuscular junction disease)

Structural
- Infiltration of pharyngeal tissues (adiposity, tumor, mucopolysaccharidoses)
- Tonsillar or adenoid hypertrophy
- Retrognathia or micrognathia
- Macroglossia
- Nasal obstruction
- Chronic mucosal edema (vibration injury allergies, sinusitis, gastroesophageal reflux)

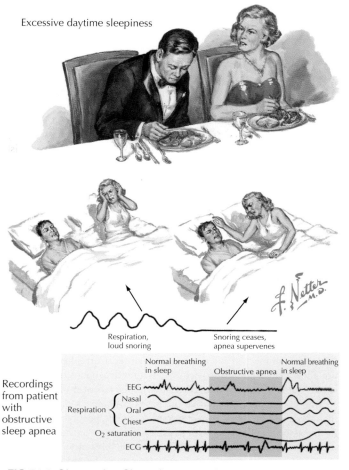

Excessive daytime sleepiness

Respiration, loud snoring

Snoring ceases, apnea supervenes

Recordings from patient with obstructive sleep apnea

Respiration { Nasal, Oral, Chest }

Normal breathing in sleep

Obstructive apnea

Normal breathing in sleep

EEG
O₂ saturation
ECG

FIG 71.1 Obstructive Sleep Apnea. *EEG,* Electroencephalogram.

TABLE 71.1 Apnea Severity

AHI	Apnea Severity (Events/Hour)
0–4.9	Normal
5–14.9	Mild
15–29.9	Moderate
≥30	Severe

AHI, Apnea-hypopnea index.

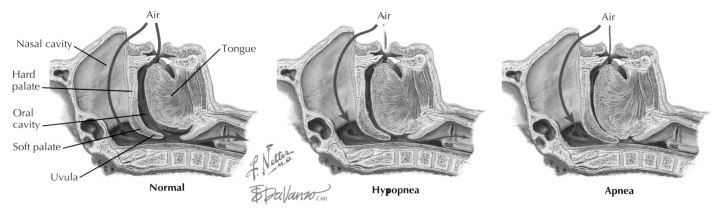

Air   Air   Air

Nasal cavity   Tongue
Hard palate
Oral cavity
Soft palate
Uvula

Normal   **Hypopnea**   **Apnea**

FIG 71.2 Anatomic Representation of Obstructive Sleep Apnea.

OBSTRUCTIVE SLEEP APNEA LINK TO HYPERTENSION

OSA is associated with a series of vascular changes. During each respiratory event, a gradual increase in peripheral vascular tone and decrease in cardiac output occurs. This is followed by a sudden opening of the airway, and the cardiac output increases against high peripheral vasoconstriction and results in a dramatic increase in blood pressure. Beyond the repetitive respiratory events, other influences may increase systemic blood pressure. Possible mechanisms of causation include intermittent, repeated hypoxia episodes that cause chemoreceptor stimulation, increased sympathetic activation, decreased baroreceptor responsiveness, cardiovascular remodeling, decreased mechanisms of vascular relaxation, and activation of the renin-angiotensin system. Epidemiological studies suggest a moderate link between OSA and hypertension. Analysis of data from the Wisconsin Sleep Cohort shows a linear relationship between severity of the AHI and elevations in 24-hour blood pressure monitoring. Similar relationships were seen in the Sleep Heart Health Study.

OSA can also precede the appearance of hypertension, as evident in the prospective analysis of this group. Clinicians should suspect OSA in patients who have failed to respond to two or more antihypertensive medications and especially in patients lacking a physiological nocturnal dip in blood pressure. This relationship of sleep apnea to hypertension provides therapeutic opportunities. Although nocturnal oxygen therapy does not appear to decrease the elevated blood pressure in patients with OSA, short-term studies have shown that treatment with continuous positive airway pressure (CPAP) decreased sympathetic activity during sleep and modestly improved both nocturnal and daytime blood pressure. These studies are encouraging, and more studies are needed to determine longer term outcomes.

OBSTRUCTIVE SLEEP APNEA AND CARDIAC DISEASE

Evidence from the Sleep Heart Health Study, a cross-sectional study of >6000 adults, indicates that blood oxygen desaturations correlate with a higher prevalence of cardiovascular disease, independent of other risk factors. The study showed a greater effect for events associated with at least 4% desaturation, but events associated with 3% desaturation also appeared significant. Untreated OSA is associated with an increased incidence of hypertension, myocardial ischemia, infarction, early cardiac death, heart failure, pulmonary hypertension, and arrhythmias (particularly, atrial fibrillation). Although several studies showed the benefits of CPAP, a recent study in the *New England Journal of Medicine* found that CPAP did not prevent cardiovascular events more than usual care alone. This study was criticized because of the high inclusion of patients who were noncompliant with the therapy, with a cohort average of only 3.3 hours per night of CPAP use. OSA is frequently found in patients with congestive heart failure (~11%–50% have OSA) and is more common in men of any age and in women older than 60 years. OSA can lead to and exacerbate heart failure by repeated oxygen desaturations, increased sympathetic activation, and increased afterload. In addition, increased swings in intrathoracic pressure caused by untreated OSA can also lead to increased myocardial oxygen demand. The greater negative intrathoracic pressure also results in atrial stretch, causing the release of atrial natriuretic peptide, which can result in nocturia. Compounding the effect is an inflammatory response that appears to advance coronary artery disease and elevate C-reactive protein levels, and release of vasoactive substances (e.g., endothelin and nitric oxide synthetase), which leads to endothelial dysfunction.

Cardiovascular diseases can also have a significant impact on sleep. Heart failure can disrupt normal sleep architecture, selectively decreasing REM sleep and leading to REM sleep deprivation. Untreated OSA results in more fragmented, less restorative sleep, due to frequent arousals.

TREATMENT OF HEART FAILURE AND OBSTRUCTIVE SLEEP APNEA

The dynamic feedback loop of heart to brain that influences regulation of the respiratory cycle can play an important role in sleep continuity. Respiratory dysfunction leads to frequent arousals and sleep fragmentation. Optimal management of fluid status in heart failure can improve cardiac cycle times and the time of blood flow from the heart to the brain, reducing respiratory events and AHI.

The effect of the treatment of OSA on heart failure is better established. Usage of CPAP improves left ventricular ejection fraction, subjective dyspnea, and daytime sleepiness. In addition, in a randomized controlled study of 55 patients with heart failure, CPAP used for 3 months improved left ventricular function, reduced left ventricular end-systolic diameter, reduced urinary norepinephrine, lowered blood pressure, and lowered heart rate. Other studies have shown improvement with CPAP use in right heart function, pulmonary artery pressures, reduced hospitalizations, and mortality rates.

OBSTRUCTIVE SLEEP APNEA AND ATRIAL FIBRILLATION

There are data to support that treatment of OSA with CPAP reduces recurrence of atrial fibrillation after electrical cardioversion or pharmacological therapy. The mechanisms behind this have not been clearly identified, but the repeated adrenergic surges that accompany untreated OSA are likely a contributor. Identification and treatment of individuals with OSA is important to the success of treatment for arrhythmias, and clinicians should have a low threshold for screening or referral.

OBSTRUCTIVE SLEEP APNEA AND STROKE

OSA also is implicated as a risk factor for stroke. Current evidence does not allow clear establishment of OSA as an independent risk factor for stroke, but OSA severity does correlate with the risk of stroke. Individuals who have experienced stroke and have OSA have a higher mortality than those without OSA. Similar to cardiac disease, possible mechanisms for the association of OSA with stroke include hypertension, reduction in cerebral blood flow, release of vasoactive substances that lead to endothelial damage, and proinflammatory states. In addition, snoring and apnea may cause intimal thickening of carotid arteries. Observational studies show individuals who are compliant with therapy for OSA have lower rates of recurrent events and better functional recovery from acute stroke.

CLINICAL PRESENTATION AND DIAGNOSTIC APPROACH

Common symptoms of OSA include snoring and daytime sleepiness, but nearly half of individuals with OSA do not express somnolence (Box 71.4). The Epworth Sleepiness Scale is a validated measure of sleepiness, and other tools such as the STOPBANG (Snoring, Tiredness, Observed apnea, high blood Pressure, Body mass index, Age, Neck circumference, and Gender) questionnaire identify patients with potential OSA (Box 71.5). Although obesity is a risk factor, patients with OSA do not have to be obese or have narrow upper airways. Overnight pulse oximetry has limited usefulness in OSA screening due to lack of sensitivity. Many individuals with normal lung function will not exhibit repetitive oxygen desaturations on overnight pulse oximetry and yet

BOX 71.4 Risk Factors Associated With Increased Risk of Obstructive Sleep Apnea

Male	High-arched palate
Age older than 50 years	Large adenoids and/or tonsils
Obesity (body mass index of ≥30 kg/m²)	Snoring
Micrognathia or retrognathia	Neck size >17 inches

BOX 71.5 Individuals Who Need Further Evaluation for Obstructive Sleep Apnea

Snoring With
- Excessive daytime sleepiness
- Insomnia

Excessive Daytime Sleepiness, Insomnia, or Snoring in
- Coronary artery disease
- Heart failure
- Hypertension
- Stroke
- Malignant arrhythmias
- Recurrent atrial fibrillation
- Chronic obstructive pulmonary disease
- Asthma
- Neuromuscular disease
- Metabolic syndrome
- Diabetes type 2
- Pulmonary hypertension

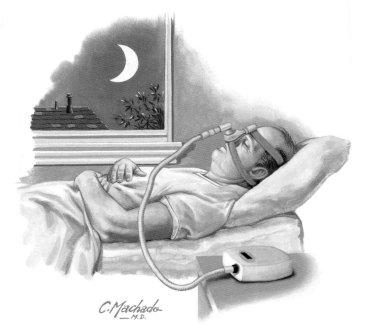

FIG 71.3 Continuous Positive Airway Pressure Therapy for Obstructive Sleep Apnea.

still have mild to moderate disease. The gold standard for diagnosis of OSA is attended polysomnography in which EEG, electrooculography, electromyography, ECG, two parameters of respiratory flow (nasal temperature and nasal pressure), and chest and abdominal movements and pulse oximetry are monitored continuously. Unattended respiratory monitoring has been approved by the Center for Medicare Service for use in patients without cardiovascular or respiratory comorbidities with a high pretest probability for OSA, under the supervision of an experienced sleep specialist. These studies are not sensitive nor accurate for distinguishing individuals with mild disease from normal, nor do they identify other types of sleep-related breathing disorders, such as hypoventilation or CSR.

DIFFERENTIAL DIAGNOSIS

The constellation of snoring, excessive sleepiness, and witnessed apnea is highly associated with OSA. Other disorders that may present with similar features include primary snoring, CSR with obstructive features, and obesity hypoventilation. Adding to the dilemma is that individuals may vary from night to night in the degree of upper airway obstruction. Although at baseline, patients may have some mild variation in severity, factors that influence upper airway patency such as alcohol, nasal congestion, and position may contribute significantly to changes in severity.

MANAGEMENT AND THERAPY

Optimum Treatment

In addition to maximizing treatment of comorbid conditions, treatment options for OSA include CPAP therapy, surgery, custom-fit oral appliances, weight loss, and, in specific cases, positional therapy (Fig. 71.3).

CPAP is the first-line therapy indicated for all patients with an AHI >10 and those with an AHI between 5 and 10 with symptoms. Key points to successful compliance relate to the inclusion of the patient in the decision-making, education of the patient, comfortable mask or interface, quick response to therapeutic hurdles, and frequent patient follow-up. Oral appliances advancing the mandible are best targeted for patients with mild to moderate sleep apnea with appropriate dentition.

If a surgical approach is chosen, all three areas of concern in OSA (nose, retroglossal and retropalatal regions, and posterior oropharynx) should be evaluated and treated to achieve best success. This may require several surgeries, possibly including septoplasty, radiofrequency ablation of turbinates, genioglossus advancement, tongue reduction, bimaxillary advancement, uvulopalatopharyngoplasty, tonsillectomy, and adenoidectomy. Although not commonly performed since the introduction of CPAP, tracheostomy is curative, ensures compliance, and may be the best choice in morbidly obese patients. Alternatively, neural stimulation therapy of the hypoglossal nerve is approved by the Food and Drug Administration and has been shown to improve the AHI in carefully selected patients.

Often a combination of treatment approaches is used in severe cases. The key element is partnering with the patient as they develop acceptance of the therapy. All patients with sleep-disordered breathing should avoid excessive alcohol intake and medications that suppress the respiratory drive.

Avoiding Treatment Errors

Treatment errors typically occur in three realms: CPAP titration, device setup, and patient usage. CPAP titrations, to meet the gold standard of optimum therapy, must be performed in an accredited sleep center and result in complete resolution of breathing disturbance in the supine position in REM sleep. Treatment errors can arise if the titration does not demonstrate resolution of events in all sleep states or positions. Another pitfall may occur if the titration is not performed with the same physiological challenges the patient incurs at home (e.g., allergies, alcohol, medication effect). Setup errors may occur from the assumption that the ordered therapy is the one delivered, or that the patient is using the device correctly. This can be avoided by physicians requiring patients to bring the device to the clinic and demonstrate its usage. Physicians can quickly determine the proficiency of the patient with the equipment by watching patients don the mask and headgear, and turn on the machine. Patients who have difficulty putting on the mask or are unfamiliar with the buttons on the machine are unlikely to be using the device. Compliance and pressure settings may be verified by examining the machine's pressure setting, blower, and therapeutic hours (standard on all newer machines). Finding that a patient is not adequately using the machine offers an opportunity to delve into barriers to patient success with therapy.

Central Sleep Apnea

CSA results from a loss of ventilatory effort and airflow for ≥10 seconds. Brief respiratory pauses are commonly seen even in healthy individuals during transitions from wakefulness to light sleep. However, when these events become lengthy, frequent (more than five per hour), persist into deeper stages of sleep, and/or are accompanied by oxygen desaturations or arousals, daytime consequences may ensue. Central apneas typically indicate a dysfunction of the regulatory process controlling breathing. CSR, one common form of central apnea, is described in the next section. CSA, excluding CSR, may occur from endogenous brain dysfunction inducing a high carbon dioxide (CO_2) apnea threshold, increased CO_2 sensitivity, or abnormal primary respiratory cycling. Central apneas also occur with narcotic and/or muscle relaxant use, excessive alcohol, increasing age (older than 65 years), and acute brain injury or stroke. Individuals with CSA may complain of insomnia or disrupted sleep, or have bed partners noting apneas, but snoring is absent. Clinicians should evaluate for underlying heart failure, thyroid, or neurological disease, or narcotic use that suppresses respiratory drive. For some individuals, a high CO_2 apnea threshold is an underlying driver and can be identified by the presence of apnea with a concurrent decrease in end-tidal CO_2 level. For other patients, brain imaging may be helpful in identifying possible central neurological structural issues.

Maximal medical therapy for the underlying condition and removal of respiratory suppressants are the primary treatments. Other treatment options include respiratory stimulants, supplemental oxygen, and bilevel positive airway pressure with a backup respiratory rate. The role of CPAP in these individuals is unclear at present but may be helpful in some patients.

Due to the complexity of etiology in central apneas, treatment errors may arise by not recognizing the underlying drivers of the respiratory disturbance. Patients who use narcotics or respiratory suppressants should have medication minimized. Heart failure patients should have cardiac output maximized, and individuals who are CO_2 or oxygen responsive should have therapies directed toward these drivers. In addition, some individuals will need further pulmonary or neurological evaluation to assess primary organ issues.

Cheyne-Stokes Respiration

CSR, a form of central apnea, is characterized by a repetitive crescendo–decrescendo pattern (Fig. 71.4). This breathing pattern is typically related to heart failure or central nervous system deficits. CSR is an example of an underdamped oscillator, swinging from hyperventilation to hypoventilation. Classic CSR becomes more apparent during light sleep, and improves in REM sleep and slow-wave sleep due to the diminished response to CO_2. Underlying mechanisms of CSR include a high-sensitivity response to CO_2 and hypoxemia, a high apnea CO_2 threshold, and prolonged cardiac cycle time (present in heart failure). In heart failure patients with CSR, sympathetic nervous system activity is higher

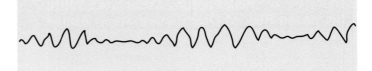

FIG 71.4 Cheyne-Stokes Respiration.

during day and night compared with healthy individuals, and the presence of daytime CSR indicates a poorer prognosis.

Patients may present with symptoms of snoring at night, witnessed apneas, paroxysmal nocturnal dyspnea, frequent awakenings, and unrefreshing sleep, or they may make no sound with sleep. Clinicians should have a high index of suspicion. All patients with heart failure should be queried regarding the presence of symptoms of sleep-disordered breathing and if the patient finds their sleep refreshing. In-laboratory diagnostic polysomnography is the best study to detect this breathing disorder. Therapy for patients with CSR focuses on two key elements: maximization of cardiac output and improving ventilation. In some patients, supplemental oxygen and increasing end-tidal CO_2 improve the ventilator pattern, whereas other patients may need noninvasive ventilator support. CSR is sensitive to positive airway pressure and changes in overall health. Patients with heart failure should have the positive airway pressure titration performed once cardiac output is maximized. Patients with strokes should be retitrated after brain function has stabilized, typically after 3 months. In both cases, a common error occurs by increasing the positive airway pressure settings, which often increases the central apnea component. Recent studies have shown that the use of adaptive servoventilation (ASV), may be associated with a higher mortality rate in patients with congestive heart failure. This noninvasive ventilator therapy appears to improve the breathing pattern but may place patients at additional cardiovascular risk. Currently, individuals who have an ejection fraction <45% are not candidates for this device.

Obesity Hypoventilation

The true Pickwickian syndrome describes an obese individual who is excessively sleepy and probably experiencing obesity hypoventilation syndrome. This disorder is defined as a body mass index >30 kg/m² and a resting arterial partial pressure of CO_2 >45 mm Hg. These individuals may present with daytime sleepiness, fatigue, unrefreshing sleep, insomnia, or morning headache, but may lack a history of snoring. Because of their large thoracic and abdominal girth, these patients have lower pulmonary functional reserve capacity and breathe at lower overall lung volumes in wakefulness. During sleep, the loss of muscle tone translates into further reduction of lung volume, especially the functional reserve capacity, which results in events of prolonged oxygen desaturation. These events are more pronounced during REM sleep because of the associated skeletal muscle atonia. Thus, the diaphragm must push unaided against a large abdomen. The diagnosis of sleep-related hypoventilation is attained on overnight polysomnography with calibrated continuous end-tidal CO_2 measurements and correlated with morning arterial blood gas sampling. A surrogate measure predicting obesity hypoventilation is venous bicarbonate levels >27 mmol/L. Untreated obesity hypoventilation is associated with higher posthospitalization mortality rates. Observational studies suggest individuals with obesity hypoventilation experience higher rates of other vascular events, even when controlled for obesity. This syndrome can be readily treated with positive airway pressure, but patients may require ventilation beyond pressure support.

OTHER SLEEP DISORDERS

Restless Legs Syndrome

Restless legs syndrome (RLS) is defined by four criteria: an uncomfortable urge to move, the symptoms are improved by movement, the symptoms are made worse by rest, and there is a circadian pattern of increased symptoms in the evening (Box 71.6). This disorder is associated with periodic limb movements in sleep, but these are not necessary for the diagnosis. In observational studies, individuals with RLS have higher risks of hypertension and potentially cardiovascular events. The mechanistic link is unclear, but suggestions that RLS may be related to increased sympathetic activity, sleep fragmentation, and low iron all need further investigation. Similar studies that show the effect of treatment on vascular consequences are lacking. RLS is a complex disorder that requires investigation into potential etiologies such as renal failure, spinal cord disease, inherited neuropathy, anemia, and medications. However, the most common form is idiopathic, and this appears to have familial features. Treatment focuses on improving underlying identifiable causes and symptom management, but therapy does not appear to alter the progression of the disorder.

Cardiovascular Medications and Sleep

The commonly used cardiovascular medications have not been well studied in sleep, although some effects are known. Angiotensin-converting enzyme inhibitors commonly cause cough and low-grade nasal and pharyngeal edema, which may worsen OSA. In patients with OSA, angiotensin-converting enzyme inhibitors, when not producing airway edema, are more effective in lowering nocturnal blood pressures than are other choices of therapy. Alpha 2-adrenergic agonists such as clonidine cause a decrease in REM sleep and consequently the opportunity for REM-related apnea events; however, these agents may exacerbate daytime somnolence. Beta-adrenergic antagonists (β-blockers) seem to have varying effects on lowering nocturnal versus daytime blood pressures but as a class do not provide significant reduction of nocturnal blood pressures related to sleep apnea. This class of medicines also blocks the release of melatonin, thus reducing the ability of the brain to synchronize the body circadian clock. Beta-blockers are associated with fatigue, nightmares, insomnia, depression, and mental cloudiness. Diuretics dosed in the evening can result in significant nocturia and disruption of sleep.

Conversely, some patients with hypersomnia are treated with stimulant medications that may increase daytime blood pressure and increase risk of cardiovascular events.

FUTURE DIRECTIONS

The complex interaction of sleep and cardiovascular diseases challenges astute clinicians to be aware of the diagnostic and therapeutic opportunities in sleep and heart health. Treatment of sleep-related breathing disorders offers great hope in providing risk reduction of further events and mortality. CSR in sleep may serve as a marker of cardiac function. Current knowledge highlights the importance of diagnosing and adequately treating sleep-disordered breathing to improve overall health and maximize daytime function. However, research is needed to clarify these interactions and the impact of treatment of both cardiovascular disease and sleep. Our understanding of the mechanisms involved in the effects of sleep disorders have on the cardiovascular system is rapidly expanding. Further work is needed in understanding the mechanisms by which sleep balances the immune, autonomic, and endocrine systems, and how these pathways may be beneficial to the heart. Through these opportunities, we can offer novel therapies that incorporate the circadian and neural systems in improving function and quality of life.

ADDITIONAL RESOURCES

American Academy of Sleep Medicine. *The International Classification of Sleep Disorders.* 3rd ed. Westchester, Ill: American Academy of Sleep Medicine; 2014.
Reviews the characteristic features, requirement for diagnosis, and associated findings for all recognized sleep disorders.
Gottlieb DJ, Somers VK, Punjabi NM, Winkelman JW. Restless legs syndrome and cardiovascular disease: a research roadmap. *Sleep Med.* 2016. pii: S1389-9457(16)30147-2. doi:10.1016/j. [Epub ahead of print.]
This article reviews the evidence of the interaction of RLS and cardiovascular events, and draws correlations from the evidence of sleep-disordered breathing.
Kryger M, Roth T, Dement W. *Principles and Practice of Sleep Medicine.* 6th ed. Philadelphia: Elsevier Saunders; 2017.
Comprehensive review of all sleep physiology, sleep disorder pathophysiology, and treatment, including technical features of sleep studies. An excellent reference with insightful chapters and sections highlighting current knowledge in sleep medicine.
Pearse SG, Cowie MR. Sleep-disordered breathing in heart failure. *Eur J Heart Fail.* 2016;18:353–361.
This review examines the data of sleep-disordered breathing in heart failure and the role of central and obstructive apnea play in the application of therapy.
Somers VK, White DP, Amin R, et al. Sleep apnea and cardiovascular disease: an American Heart Association/American College of Cardiology Foundation Scientific Statement from the American Heart Association Council for High Blood Pressure Research Professional Education Committee, Council on Clinical Cardiology, Stroke Council, and Council on Cardiovascular Nursing. *Circulation.* 2008;118:1080–1111.
American Heart Association/American College of Cardiology scientific statement for association of OSA and cardiovascular disease; an excellent review of evidence.

EVIDENCE

Cowie MR, Woehrle H, Wegscheider K, et al. Adaptive servo-ventilation for central sleep apnea in systolic heart failure. *N Engl J Med.* 2015;373: 1095–1105.
This study showed an increased mortality in those patients with an ejection fraction <45% who used ASV therapy for CSR.
Dediu GN, Dumitrache-Rujinski S, Lungu R, et al. Positive pressure therapy in patients with cardiac arrhythmias and obstructive sleep apnea. *Pneumologia.* 2015;64:18–22.
This trial shows that adding CPAP has favorable effects on preventing recurrences, heart rate control in patients with atrial fibrillation, and in reducing frequency and/or severity of ventricular extrasystoles.
Huang Z, Liu Z, Luo Q, et al. Long-term effects of continuous positive airway pressure on blood pressure and prognosis in hypertensive patients with coronary heart disease and obstructive sleep apnea: a randomized controlled trial. *Am J Hypertens.* 2015;28:300–306.
This small but significant study showed that treatment of OSA with CPAP improves uncontrolled hypertension in individuals with coronary disease.
McEvoy RD, Antic NA, Heeley E, et al. CPAP for Prevention of Cardiovascular events in obstructive sleep apnea. *N Engl J Med.* 2016;375:919–931.
This study randomized 2700 patients with OSA and compared those on usual care with CPAP or usual care alone. The study particularly shows no clear difference, but inadequate compliance was a major flaw in the study.
Punjabi NM, Newman A, Young T, et al. Sleep disordered breathing and cardiovascular disease: an outcome based definition of hypopneas. *Am J Respir Crit Care Med.* 2008;177:1150–1155.
Examines data from the Sleep Heart Health Study to demonstrate what features of hypopnea are associated with cardiovascular events, particularly showing that desaturation plays an important role.

72

Cardiovascular Disease in Women and Vulnerable Populations

Paula Miller

The US population continues to become more diverse, and because of this diversity there are challenges in providing good cardiovascular care. The emerging diversity necessitates a broader understanding of cardiovascular disease (CVD) in special and underserved populations. These populations include women, older adult patients, various ethnic groups, and an often forgotten population, the intellectually disabled. Looking at sex alone, in 2014, there were 125.9 million women compared with 119.4 million men in the United States. In the age group older than 85 years (older adults), there were twice as many women than men alive. The Latino, African American, and Asian populations are also growing, and there are challenges specific to their ethnicity. We need to understand the individual risks and challenges, and learn how to address primary and secondary prevention in all these populations.

Age-adjusted events from CVD in the general population are decreasing, but in these special populations, the number of cardiovascular events are staying the same or increasing. Women in general (including women in ethnic and special subgroups) have seen no significant changes in CVD morbidity or mortality. This chapter reviews some of these special populations and makes suggestions on identifying, managing, and modifying risk factors, with the goal of decreasing the overall burden of CVD.

GERIATRIC POPULATION

CVD can occur at any age, but the absolute risk increases incrementally as the population ages and is greatest in the population of patients older than the age of 65 years. This portion of the population is increasing because the baby boomers are entering the older than 65 years population. According to the Population Reference Bureau, in early 2016, the number of Americans aged 65 years and older is projected to more than double from 46 million today to >98 million by 2060, and those in the population who are aged 65 years and older will rise to nearly 24% from 15%. In addition, the older population is becoming more racially and ethnically diverse. Between 2014 and 2060, the share of the older population that is non-Hispanic white is projected to drop by 24%, from 78.3% to 54.6%. This group, which has a higher prevalence of CVD, will further increase the demand on the healthcare system, which underscores the importance of treatment strategies for older adults (Fig. 72.1, top).

Clinically, coronary heart disease (CHD) in older adults and/or geriatric patients often presents in an atypical manner. The initial presentation may be dyspnea on exertion, decreased exercise tolerance, fatigue, or heart failure. The patient may also have no symptoms. Because the symptoms are atypical or there are no symptoms, this often delays diagnosis and treatment. This delay, combined with an increase in comorbidities and the underuse of proven beneficial therapies (pharmacological and interventional), contributes to increased rates of morbidity and mortality among older adult patients with post–myocardial infarction (MI). The increased incidence of comorbid conditions contributes to polypharmacy in older adult patients—with the attendant risk of adverse effects—and prevents the addition of medications that would probably lower cardiac risk.

Despite the need for multiple medical therapies, risk factor modification in older adult patients translates into decreased cardiovascular events. Elevated low-density lipoprotein cholesterol (LDL-C) has an important role in the pathogenesis and lifelong risk of CHD, and demonstration that reduction of LDL-C levels decreases risk of cardiovascular events has been found in the older adult/geriatric population. Studies that are more recent have included patients aged older than 65 years and even those aged older than 80 years, and thus recommendations are changing. The decision whether to treat high or high-normal lipids in an older adult individual needs to be individualized and based upon both chronological and physiological age. A patient with a limited life span due to severe comorbid illness is probably not a candidate for drug therapy, whereas an otherwise healthy older adult individual should not be denied drug therapy simply based on age. Preventive therapies (pharmacological and nonpharmacological) in older adult individuals may decrease cardiovascular events even more dramatically than in younger patients, probably because of the increased risk and incidence of CVD in older adult individuals. Age should not exclude patients from treatment for lowering of LDL-C, especially as a therapeutic strategy for secondary prevention, but there is not a large amount of data in patients aged older than 80 years. In primary prevention, the treatment of elevated LDL-C is more controversial. There are benefits of preventive treatment in this population that are substantiated by several smaller trials and by the Heart Protection Study, which included patients up to the age of 80 years. The recommendations from the Adult Treatment Panel III (ATP III) emphasize therapeutic lifestyle changes as an important component of therapy to reduce LDL-C and do not rule out statin therapy.

Hypertension is a common problem in older adults (age older than 60–65 years with a prevalence as high as 60%–80%). In the participants in the National Health and Nutrition Examination Survey, hypertension was observed in 67% of adults aged 60 years or older. Newer guidelines from the Joint National Commission on Blood Pressure suggests target blood pressures based on underlying disease and age. For an older adult with hypertension only, a goal of <150/90 mm Hg is reasonable. Hypertension is a major risk factor for stroke, heart failure, and CHD. Although hypertension was once considered part of normal aging, the benefit of treating older adult patients with elevated systolic and/or diastolic blood pressure is clear. Treatment of isolated systolic hypertension can provide a 30% reduction in the combined fatal and nonfatal stroke rate, a 26% reduction in the rates of fatal and nonfatal cardiovascular events, and a 13% reduction in the total mortality rate.

Diabetes mellitus

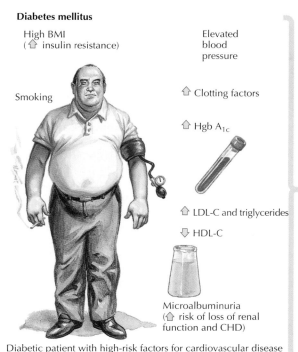

High BMI (⬆ insulin resistance)

Smoking

Elevated blood pressure

⬆ Clotting factors

⬆ Hgb A₁c

⬆ LDL-C and triglycerides

⬇ HDL-C

Microalbuminuria (⬆ risk of loss of renal function and CHD)

Diabetic patient with high-risk factors for cardiovascular disease

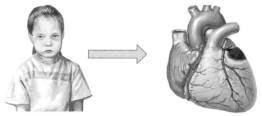

Acute MI

Acute MI is often first symptom of cardiovascular disease.

Stroke

Atherosclerotic peripheral vascular disease frequently involves distal vessels in diabetes.

Morbidity and mortality from cardiovascular and other atherosclerotic diseases involving cerebral and peripheral vessels are 2 to 3 times higher among persons with diabetes.

Increased incidence of type II diabetes in children and adolescents raises the likelihood premature CHD will develop.

Management goals

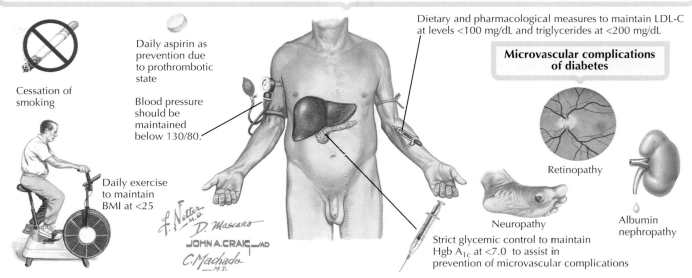

Cessation of smoking

Daily aspirin as prevention due to prothrombotic state

Blood pressure should be maintained below 130/80.

Daily exercise to maintain BMI at <25

Dietary and pharmacological measures to maintain LDL-C at levels <100 mg/dL and triglycerides at <200 mg/dL

Microvascular complications of diabetes

Retinopathy

Neuropathy

Albumin nephropathy

Strict glycemic control to maintain Hgb A₁c at <7.0 to assist in prevention of microvascular complications

FIG 72.1 Cardiovascular Disease in Diabetes. *BMI,* Body mass index; *CHD,* coronary heart disease; *HDL-C,* high-density lipoprotein cholesterol; *HgbA₁c,* glycosylated hemoglobin A₁c; *LDL-C,* low-density lipoprotein cholesterol; *MI,* myocardial infarction.

WOMEN

CVD is the leading cause of death in men and women. In women, CVD and stroke cause one in three deaths in women each year, killing approximately one woman every 80 seconds. In 1984, the number of deaths for women exceeded that for men, but most recent numbers show the incidence is about the same, but more women die from their disease. In 2013, CHD was responsible for the deaths of 289,758 women in the United States, which is approximately one in every four female deaths, with an estimated 44 million women in the United States affected by CVD.

Ethnicity also plays a part in the chance of women developing heart disease. Heart disease is the leading cause of death for African American and white women in the United States, and among Hispanic women, heart disease and cancer cause roughly the same number of deaths each year. In Native American, Alaska Native, Asian, or Pacific Islander women, heart disease is second only to cancer as a cause of death. In the most recent Centers for Disease Control and Prevention data (CDC), approximately 5.8% of all white women, 7.6% of black women, and 5.6% of Mexican American women have CHD (a form of CVD). In this CDC data, it is noted that almost two-thirds (64%) of women who die suddenly from CHD events have no previous symptoms.

Despite increases in awareness over the past decade, only 54% of women recognize that heart disease is their number one killer. Women will still answer "cancer" as the response to the question "what do you think you will die from?" Educating women on their risks, signs, and symptoms of heart disease and available treatments is the number one tool in reducing deaths from heart disease. In addition to receiving information on disease prevalence, women must be taught that CHD and/or CVD symptoms can differ from symptoms that men commonly report. Women often have dyspnea on exertion, heartburn, fatigue, decreased exercise tolerance, or back pain as their presenting symptom, or the anginal equivalent. When questioning women further, they may also describe some subtle typical symptoms with these atypical symptoms. However, the presence of somewhat vague or confusing symptoms often contributes to the delayed or missed diagnoses of CHD (Fig. 72.1, bottom).

Most CHD risk factors and strategies for preventing disease applicable to men also apply to women. Risk factors beyond the typical risk factors that frequently occur in women include an isolation postmenopausal state, depression, and lower socioeconomic status. The magnitude of the effects of these typical and atypical risk factors and prevention strategies may be different. For example, diabetes is an even more powerful risk factor for CHD in women (Fig. 72.2). It is associated with a three- to sevenfold increase in the frequency of CHD development, and a diabetic woman is twice as likely to have a recurrent MI compared with a man with equal risk factors.

Smoking is also a stronger risk factor for MI in women than in men. The incidence of MI is increased sixfold in women and threefold in men who smoke at least 1 pack per day (20 cigarettes) compared with individuals who never smoked. In the worldwide INTERHEART study of patients from 52 countries, smoking accounted for 36% of the population-attributable risk of a first MI. In another systematic review and meta-analysis of 75 cohorts that evaluated the risks of smoking on CHD and adjusted for the effects of other known CHD risk factors (>2.4 million persons with >44,000 CHD events), female smokers were 25% more likely than male smokers to develop CHD.

Smoking in women is a concern because smoking rates are declining at a slower rate among women than among men.

Hypertension is more prevalent in men up until the age of 45 years. From age 45 to 54 years, the incidence of hypertension for men and women is similar. After the age of 54 years, a significantly higher percentage of women have high blood pressure. Because this is a modifiable risk factor, education of women about the dangers of hypertension and intensive screening becomes important.

Dyslipidemias, especially elevated triglycerides and low high-density lipoprotein cholesterol (HDL-C), are more commonly seen with CHD in women and are most commonly seen in postmenopausal women. Low HDL-C in postmenopausal women is a potent risk factor for CHD events. Strategies to reduce LDL-C with statins provide at least an equivalent reduction in risk in women compared with men. In some studies, the risk of primary or secondary cardiovascular events was more favorably influenced by statin therapy in women than in men. Menopause, with its associated estrogen loss and effect on the lipid profile, presents a challenge. Hormone replacement therapy (HRT) and estrogen replacement therapy recommendations have evolved over the past 30 to 40 years. Historically, a cardioprotective effect of HRT in women was inferred, based largely on observational data and regardless of the CVD status of the woman. However, no benefit in the rates of nonfatal MI or death from CHD in women with known heart disease receiving combined HRT was found in the largest randomized clinical trial conducted. An increase in CHD events was observed during the first year of HRT use in that trial. A large-scale trial that investigated the primary prevention benefits of combined HRT was stopped early, principally because of the

risk of associated invasive breast cancer. However, a significant increase in cardiovascular events was also observed. Taken together, clinical trials do not support the use of combined HRT in primary or secondary prevention of cardiovascular events. The American Heart Association released a statement for healthcare professionals recommending that HRT not be initiated for prevention of heart attack or stroke in women with CVD, which was reemphasized in their 2011 guidelines for treatment of women. Prediction of 10-year mortality by the ATP III guidelines has been advanced by the Reynolds Risk Score. This model includes variables such as diabetes mellitus, family history, and high-sensitivity C-reactive protein, an inflammatory marker. The Reynolds risk predictor can be adjusted for age with predictions for CVD at current age as well as 10, 20, or 30 years into the future, providing a projection of how treatment of certain risk factors might improve risk.

The updated 2011 American Heart Association/American College of Cardiology guidelines for prevention of CVD in women continue to recommend a heart healthy diet (increased fresh fruits and vegetables), increased activity (30 minutes a day to maintain weight and 60–90 minutes to lose weight), eating oily fish in their diet at least twice a week or using fish oil supplements, and the use of aspirin routinely in women aged older than 65 years and earlier in those at high risk.

RACIAL AND ETHNIC CONSIDERATIONS

The US population has become increasingly diverse, with an increase in Hispanics, African Americans, Native Americans, and Asian/Pacific Islanders. Ethnicity refers to a group of people who share a geographic area, religion, culture, or language. The prevalence and incidence of CVD varies among these ethnic and racial groups in the United States. Race refers to common characteristics passed down through the genes. Non-Hispanic whites (63%) have roots in Europe, the Middle East, or North Africa. Blacks (13%) have origins in any of the black racial groups of Africa or Afro-Caribbean countries. Asians (5%) may have ancestors anywhere from India to Japan. This geographic diversity within racial groups means that there are often greater genetic differences within groups than between certain groups. These variations are important in developing strategies for prevention and treatment as these minority populations increase in number.

CVD mortality rate varies significantly by US region, with a greater than twofold difference between states with the lowest and the highest rates. From 2008 to 2010 in the United States, the highest death rates from CVD were in the south, and the lowest rates were in the west. Factors influencing these differences are complex. As an example, in the southern United States, >25% of individuals are obese. This, in turn, puts the population at a higher risk for diabetes mellitus and CVD. The key to reducing CVD in these populations lies in education and intervention on dietary choices and treatment of diabetes. However, many do not have health insurance and do not see a doctor regularly despite the availability for most with the Affordable Care Act. Improved access to health care coupled with education and modification of risk factors can reduce cardiovascular events. The highest mortality rates from CVD are seen in the Mississippi Delta, Appalachia, and the Ohio River Valley, where the numbers of people in the lower socioeconomic category are highest. The areas with the highest CVD mortality in the United States are frequently poor and rural.

African Americans have the highest mortality rates in the United States for CHD and stroke. In 2014, the overall death rate from CHD in the United States in African American men was 232 deaths per 100,000 population compared with 167 per 100,000 in white men. In white women, the rate was 205 per 100,000, and in African American women, it was 277 per 100,000. The mortality rate from CHD is lower among the Hispanic, Asian, and Native American populations. Among Asians,

Cardiovascular disease in the elderly

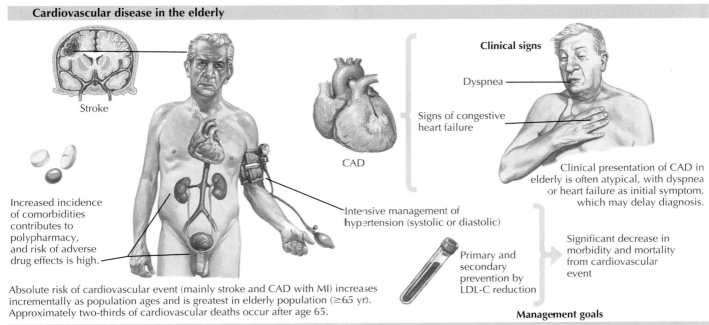

Stroke

Increased incidence of comorbidities contributes to polypharmacy, and risk of adverse drug effects is high.

CAD

Clinical signs

Dyspnea

Signs of congestive heart failure

Clinical presentation of CAD in elderly is often atypical, with dyspnea or heart failure as initial symptom, which may delay diagnosis.

Intensive management of hypertension (systolic or diastolic)

Primary and secondary prevention by LDL-C reduction

Significant decrease in morbidity and mortality from cardiovascular event

Management goals

Absolute risk of cardiovascular event (mainly stroke and CAD with MI) increases incrementally as population ages and is greatest in elderly population (≥65 yr). Approximately two-thirds of cardiovascular deaths occur after age 65.

Cardiovascular disease in women

Risk factors

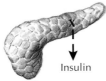

Insulin

Diabetes in women is a more powerful risk factor than in men, associated with 3 to 7 times increase in CHD development.

Smoking is a stronger risk factor for MI in middle-aged women than men.

Hormone replacement is contraindicated as cardio-protection in postmenopausal women.

Treatment of dyslipidemias (⬆LDL-C, ⬇HDL-C, ⬆triglycerides) offers reduction in cardiovascular event risk

Clinical presentation

Women may present with "heartburn"-type symptoms due to CHD.

Back pain is a common "anginal equivalent" in women.

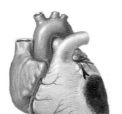

Cardiovascular disease is leading cause of death in both men and women. More women die from cardiovascular disease than from breast cancer.

Fatigue and dyspnea on exertion with decreased exercise tolerance are common complaints.

CHD symptoms reported by women often differ from those reported by men. These vague or confusing symptoms may contribute to a delayed or missed diagnosis.

FIG 72.2 Cardiovascular Disease in Women and Older Adults. *CAD,* Coronary artery disease; *CHD,* coronary heart disease; *HDL-C,* high-density lipoprotein cholesterol; *LDL-C,* low-density lipoprotein cholesterol; *MI,* myocardial infarction.

probably because of the high prevalence of hypertension, the mortality rate from stroke is higher.

Racial differences in healthcare outcomes are well documented in the United States. Members of minority populations, especially African American individuals, are less likely to receive invasive cardiovascular procedures, which are shown to improve outcomes; are less likely to see doctors and other healthcare providers; and tend to smoke more than nonminority populations. As the ethnic populations increase, more attention must be directed toward identifying those at risk and intervening with recommended therapies.

LOWER SOCIOECONOMIC GROUPS

Socioeconomic differences in CVD mortality rates are reported for many countries, including the United States. In most reports, a clear gradient in mortality rates exists; the CVD mortality rate is higher in individuals with lower education levels and in those in lower occupational classes. Socioeconomic status is a more potent risk factor in women. Unfortunately, reports suggest that the gap in the CVD mortality rates between the poor and undereducated and the wealthy and well educated has not narrowed and may even be widening.

INTELLECTUALLY DISABLED

The intellectually disabled have seen their incidence of cardiovascular events increase as people have been moved from institutional living to more home care and/or group home arrangements. The change may be related to a more diverse food selection and lack of arranged exercise. Further investigation is needed, but in the interim, these individuals should be identified and advised similarly to any patient of similar race or ethnicity.

FUTURE DIRECTIONS

Future directions for prevention of CHD in special populations must target the special needs of each population. Clinical trials testing new strategies must establish appropriate guidelines for the individual patient taking their race and ethnicity into the equation.

CVD in older adults, the most rapidly expanding US subgroup, is an important public health issue. Prevention efforts in this group must be aggressive. Older adults must be included in clinical trials, and comprehensive risk factor identification and modification pursued. Because of the potentially debilitating nature of cardiovascular events, primary and secondary prevention therapies in older adults are especially beneficial.

Major federal initiatives have been launched to eliminate the racial and ethnic differences in cardiovascular outcomes, and these need to continue. The challenges of changing behavior and CVD risk are magnified among those of lesser educational background and lower economic income; the needs of those who may be lacking the resources to understand and afford necessary measures should be addressed. Developing effective interventions for risk factor reduction among lower socioeconomic groups must be a priority.

ADDITIONAL RESOURCE

Ridker PM, Buring JE, Rifai N, et al. Development and validation of improved algorithms for the assessment of global cardiovascular risk in women. The Reynolds Risk Score. *JAMA*. 2007;297:611–619.

The Reynolds Risk Score provides a way to further risk-stratify women using the traditional ATP III risk factors while incorporating family history and high-sensitivity C-reactive protein. The tool can be accessed on the internet at: http://www.reynoldsriskscore.org; Accessed March 22, 2010.

EVIDENCE

Centers for Disease Control and Prevention (CDC). Million hearts: strategies to reduce the prevalence of leading cardiovascular disease risk factors—United States, 2011. *MMWR Morb Mortal Wkly Rep*. 2011;60:1248–1251.

The authors summarized data including that from NHANES (National Health and Nutrition Examination Survey), and this includes analysis of the main risk factors for cardiovascular disease.

Foody JM, Cole CR, Blackstone EH, Lauer MS. A propensity analysis of cigarette smoking and mortality with consideration of the effects of alcohol. *Am J Cardiol*. 2001;87:706–711.

Examination of mortality from smoking, as well as smoking and the association with alcohol consumption.

Garcia M, Mulvagh SL, Merz CN, Buring JE, Manson JE. Cardiovascular disease in women, clinical perspectives. *Circ Res*. 2016;118:1273–1293.

This is a comprehensive review focusing on unique aspects of cardiovascular health in women and sex differences as they relate to clinical practice in the prevention, diagnosis, and treatment of cardiovascular disease.

Mosca L, Benjamin EJ, Berra K, et al. Effectiveness-based guidelines for the prevention of cardiovascular disease in women—2011 update: a guideline from the American Heart Association. *Circulation*. 2011;123:1243–1262.

Recommendations for prevention in women with respect to primary and secondary prevention, including disease processes, lifestyle, and medications/supplements.

Njølstad I, Arneson E, Lund-Larsen PG. Smoking, serum lipids, blood pressure, and sex differences in myocardial infarction. A 12-year follow up of the Finnmark Study. *Circulation*. 1996;93:450.

The authors demonstrate a correlation with the selected risk factors noted in the title and the impact of sex differences.

73

Cardiovascular Disease in the Elderly

Xuming Dai, Walter A. Tan

Aging is a normal physiological process associated with a decline in organ system function. Changes of cardiovascular physiology intertwine with pathophysiology of cardiovascular disease (CVD). Although disease should not be misconstrued as an inevitable consequence of aging, distinctions are often arbitrarily defined, and the difference between diminished biological reserve and overt dysfunction can be thought of as quantitative rather than qualitative. Although the role of genetics in aging in the broadest spectrum remains poorly understood, examples of hereditary syndromes of premature aging, such as Hutchinson-Gilford syndrome (progeria) and Werner syndrome (wherein affected individuals typically die between the second and fourth decades of life), support the notion that aging is at least partly genetically programmed (see Chapter 3).

Age is a strong independent risk factor for CVD, and a powerful predictor of cardiovascular disability, morbidity, and mortality. Our society is aging, and the healthcare system is therefore facing a challenge to care for the growing older adult population with CVD. Unfortunately, patients older than 75 years of age are underrepresented in clinical studies that assess safety and efficacies of diagnostic and therapeutic approaches. Therefore, the clinical evidence obtained from younger populations may not be readily applicable to older populations. Understanding key aspects of cardiovascular physiology in older adults, their unique clinical characteristics, and responses to therapy can serve a foundation to guide clinical practice. Frailty, depression, and other confounding comorbidities in older adults add yet another layer of complexity in discerning which changes are attributable to aging and which ones to disease or environment (Table 73.1). This chapter summarizes the cardiovascular physiology of older adults, describes clinical features of common CVD, and considers strategies that may decrease the risk of death and disability from these diseases in older adults.

CARDIOVASCULAR PHYSIOLOGY IN OLDER ADULTS

As a result of decades of complex molecular and cellular aging, which are processes that are under the influence of both genetics and environmental factors, cardiovascular physiology in older adults is characterized by (1) increased arterial stiffness; (2) increased ventricular stiffness, and reduced ventricular compliance and cardiac reserve; (3) impaired β-adrenergic, parasympathetic function, and autonomic reflexes; and (4) degenerative changes of the conduction system.

Increased Vascular Stiffness

Age-related changes occur throughout the arterial wall (Fig. 73.1). Decreased distensibility or increased stiffness of the large central arteries is a hallmark of vascular aging. Processes include complex molecular mechanisms such as oxidative stress, endothelial dysfunction (decreased production of nitric oxide), inflammation, matrix production and/or

degradation, vascular cell migration and proliferation, and vascular calcification. Senile cardiac transthyretin-related amyloidosis and other β-sheet protein accumulations are also associated with arterial aging. Blood flow in the aging arterial system becomes less laminar as vessels become more tortuous and endothelial cells show greater heterogeneity in size, shape, and axial orientation. These changes together result in large artery stiffening, decreased compliance and recoil, and a diminished capacity to absorb the pulsatile wavefront produced by the ejecting heart. Hemodynamic consequences of these changes include: (1) increased systolic pressure and pulse pressure; (2) increased left ventricular (LV) afterload, contraction, and oxygen requirements; and (3) decreased coronary filling pressure.

The peripheral arterial tree also shows morphological and physiological decline. The average aortic root size is approximately 14 mm/m² for both sexes in the early twenties and increases to 17 mm/m² in healthy octogenarians. With increases in the aortic diameter, individuals have an increased risk of aneurysm formation and aortic dissection. Large-caliber vessels thicken progressively. The intima-medial wall thickness of carotid arteries is 0.03 mm in the young and doubles by the age of 80 years. After the fourth decade of life, renal blood flow per gram of kidney weight decreases progressively, probably because of increased renal arterial resistance.

Peak oxygen use ($VO_{2\,max}$), a measure of work capacity and physical conditioning, declines by approximately 50% by 80 years of age compared with the $VO_{2\,max}$ of a 20-year-old individual (~10% loss per decade of life). Aside from age-associated decline in cardiac function, up to one-half of the $VO_{2\,max}$ impairment is attributable to poor peripheral oxygen extraction and use, largely from inefficient redistribution of blood flow to skeletal muscles.

Reduced Ventricular Compliance and Cardiac Reserve

Primary changes in cardiomyocytes during aging include: an increase in size; a decrease in numbers, with an alteration in the myocyte-to-fibroblast ratio; and an increase in the abundance of lipids and their peroxidation products, including amyloid, collagen, fat, fibrotic foci, and advanced glycation products. These processes result in gross hypertrophy. Aging also diminishes the capacity for regeneration and repair of injured cardiomyocytes. The intrinsic myocardial contractility is diminished with age, in large part as a result of higher vascular afterload and compensatory effects of sympathetic overactivity. Although at rest, the normal sitting and submaximal end-systolic volume index is similar in adults between the ages of 20 and 85 years, the response to maximal exercise (seated cycle exercise to >100-W workload) is significantly attenuated in older adults. A young person can increase the LV ejection fraction by almost 50% to accommodate the demands of intense exercise, from a baseline LV ejection fraction of approximately 62% to 87%. In the older adult heart, only one-fifth of this contractile reserve is seen (increasing LV ejection fraction from ~63% to only ~70%), despite the

TABLE 73.1 Cardiovascular Changes in Older Adults Without Overt Disease

Measured Change	Functional Consequence
Myocardium	
Increased interventricular septal thickness; increased cardiac mass per body mass index in women	Increased propensity for diastolic dysfunction
Prolonged action potential, calcium, transient, and contraction velocity (in animal models); desensitization of myocardial β-adrenergic receptors	Decreased intrinsic contractile reserve and function
Reduced early and peak left ventricular filling rate and increased pulmonary capillary wedge pressure	Greater dependence on atrial kick, and physiological S_4 heart sound
Cardiac Valves	
Fibrosis and calcification of the aortic valve and the mitral annulus	Valvular stiffening
Vasculature	
Thickening of the media and subendothelial layers; increased vessel tortuosity	Decreased vessel compliance; increased hemodynamic shear stress and lipid deposition in the arterial walls
Large elastic arteries (e.g., aorta, carotid artery) become thicker, tortuous, and more dilated.	Increased peripheral vascular resistance and earlier reflected pulse waves, and consequent late augmentation of systolic pressure
Impulse Formation and Propagation	
Substantial decrease in sinoatrial pacemaker cell population, with separation from atrial musculature due to surrounding fatty tissue accumulation	Diminished intrinsic sinus and resting heart rates
	Slight PR interval prolongation; increased incidence of ventricular ectopy
Increase in collagenous and elastic tissue in all parts of the conduction system	Propensity toward bundle branch blocks and abnormal conduction
Decreased density of bundle fascicles and distal conduction fibers	Lower threshold for atrial and ventricular arrhythmias; increased fibrosis and myocyte death
Reduced threshold for calcium overload and for diastolic after-depolarizations and ventricular fibrillation	
Autonomic System	
Diminished autonomic tone, especially parasympathetic; increased sympathetic nerve activity and circulating catecholamine levels	Decreased spontaneous and respiratory-related heart rate variability

Frank-Starling mechanism and increased LV diastolic pressures. In older adults, the isovolumic relaxation time may also be prolonged (i.e., the interval increases between the closure of the aortic valve and the opening of the mitral valve) because of slowed ventricular relaxation. The peak rate of LV diastolic filling is also reduced approximately 50% with aging. Together, these changes lead to the increased propensity toward diastolic dysfunction in older adults and the increased dependence on atrial contraction ("kick") for augmentation and completion of diastolic LV filling. This diminished diastolic capacity makes older adults more vulnerable to the hemodynamic and symptomatic consequences of atrial fibrillation (AF). With aging, cardiac output may no longer be able to meet increased demands of exertion, illness, or severe physical or emotional stresses.

In addition, the left atrium tends to enlarge with advancing age, increasing the likelihood that AF will develop. Fibrosis and calcification of the aortic valve and the mitral annulus may lead to valvular dysfunction.

Impaired Beta-Adrenergic and Parasympathetic Function

Decreased responses to β-adrenergic and parasympathetic stimulation and reflex are other hallmarks of aging. Age-related postsynaptic signaling deficits attenuate β-adrenergic modulation of heart rate variability and vascular tone, muting compensatory increases in heart rate and exercise reserve capacity. The maximum heart rate achieved in 20-year-old individuals is approximately 180 beats/min, but it is only approximately 120 beats/min in octogenarians. The maximal cardiac index therefore decreases approximately 30% over six decades. Older cardiomyocytes secrete more stress-related products, such as atrial natriuretic

factor and opioid peptides. Moreover, ambient plasma catecholamine levels are elevated, and the production of nitric oxide is reduced, which all contribute to increased afterload and a lowered cardiac output. These age-related changes often diminish the normal response to stressors, such as standing up rapidly, volume loss, or exercise, which results in orthostatic hypotension and syncope.

Degenerative Changes of Conduction System

Significant changes in the cardiac conduction system occur during the normal aging process of the heart as a result of structural remodeling of the extracellular matrix, modifications of cell-to-cell coupling between neighboring cardiomyocytes, and changes in active membrane properties. Older adults have an increased risk of arrhythmias. The sinoatrial node may separate physically from the atrial tissue as fat accumulates around it, and the absolute number of pacemaker cells in the sinus node declines substantially after 60 years of age. The number of pacemaker cells in a 75 year old may be only 10% compared with that in young adulthood. These changes are major contributors to the increased prevalence of sick sinus syndrome with aging. Sinoatrial function slows with age, but healthy octogenarians and nonagenarians with resting heart rates <40 to 45 beats/min or sinus pauses >2 seconds should be followed carefully. This group of patients carries an increased risk of syncope and other heart rate–related problems. Other age-related abnormalities in the conduction system include an increase in fibrous tissue in the internodal tracts and a diminished density of left bundle fascicles and distal conducting fibers. These conduction abnormalities are exacerbated by the increase in polyunsaturated fatty acids in cardiac cellular membranes that occurs with aging, resulting in changes in ion thresholds and exchange, as well as in myocardial changes that are proarrhythmic.

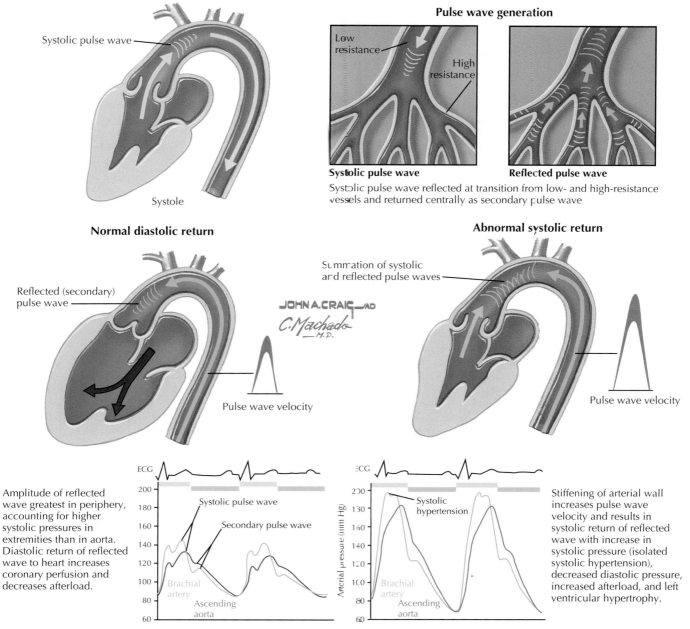

Pulse wave generation

Systolic pulse wave

Systole

Low resistance

High resistance

Systolic pulse wave

Reflected pulse wave

Systolic pulse wave reflected at transition from low- and high-resistance vessels and returned centrally as secondary pulse wave

Normal diastolic return

Reflected (secondary) pulse wave

Pulse wave velocity

Abnormal systolic return

Summation of systolic and reflected pulse waves

Pulse wave velocity

JOHN A. CRAIG _MD
C. Machado _M.D.

Amplitude of reflected wave greatest in periphery, accounting for higher systolic pressures in extremities than in aorta. Diastolic return of reflected wave to heart increases coronary perfusion and decreases afterload.

Systolic pulse wave

Secondary pulse wave

Brachial artery

Ascending aorta

Systolic hypertension

Brachial artery

Ascending aorta

Stiffening of arterial wall increases pulse wave velocity and results in systolic return of reflected wave with increase in systolic pressure (isolated systolic hypertension), decreased diastolic pressure, increased afterload, and left ventricular hypertrophy.

FIG 73.1 Wave Reflection and Isolated Systolic Hypertension.

Atrial ectopic beats were found in 6% of adults older than 60 years of age by resting electrocardiography, in 39% with maximal treadmill exercise, and in 88% on 24-hour ambulatory monitoring. Short runs of paroxysmal supraventricular tachycardia are nearly twice as prevalent in octogenarians as in septuagenarians, and are observed in approximately one-half of those 65 years of age or older. The prevalence of ventricular ectopic beats rises from 0.5% in those younger than 40 years of age to 11.5% in those 80 years of age and older, and increases further in those with associated cardiac disease. The PR interval is slightly prolonged with age, primarily from delayed conduction proximal to the His bundle, and the prevalence of first-degree atrioventricular block is 6% to 8% in octogenarians. There is an increased incidence of progression from first-degree atrioventricular block to second- and third-degree block in older adults as well.

CARDIOVASCULAR PATHOLOGY IN OLDER ADULTS

CVD is both the leading cause of death and the most frequent diagnosis in men and women older than 65 years. Approximately one in four individuals in the United States and one in five worldwide will be aged 65 years or older by 2030, and it is projected that 80% of all cardiovascular deaths will occur in this cohort.

Coronary Artery Disease

Age is the strongest independent risk factor for the development of atherosclerotic CVD. From asymptomatic coronary artery atherosclerosis, stable and unstable angina, to acute myocardial infarction (MI), coronary artery disease (CAD) in older adults has unique clinical characteristics and challenges in diagnosis and treatment. Recognition of angina or acute coronary syndromes can be difficult in older adults, because up to 90% of patients present with symptoms other than classic chest pain. Between the ages of 65 and 85 years, the prevalence of silent or misclassified ischemia increases by 50% in men and by nearly 300% in women. Higher prevalence of baseline abnormalities on ECG reduces the specificity in diagnosing acute coronary syndrome in older adults. Lower exercise capacity associated with aging limits the sensitivity of stress ECG diagnosis of ischemia. Increased prevalence of coronary calcification and difficulties with satisfactory breath-hold reduce the accuracy of coronary CT angiography evaluation of CAD in older adults. Coronary angiography remains the gold standard for diagnosis of epicardial CAD. It is generally safe in older adults, but as expected, there is a slightly increased risk of bleeding, stroke, contrast-induced kidney injury, as well as adverse reactions to even routine procedural sedation.

Older adults have a higher prevalence of multivessel or left main CAD, with significant calcification and tortuosity, and reduced cardiac function. The 30-day mortality rate for acute MI in older adults can exceed 20%. Even non–Q-wave MI has a significant age gradient of 1-year cardiac mortality rate: 29% in those 70 years of age or older compared with 14% in younger patients. Corresponding all-cause 1-year mortality rates were recently reported to be 36% and 16%, respectively, highlighting the hazard from competing comorbidities in geriatric patients.

For stable ischemic heart disease (SIHD), guideline-directed medical therapy (GDMT) is as effective in the older adult population as in the younger population, with a favorable benefit-to-risk ratio. GDMT should be the initial approach in treating older adults with SIHD. Revascularization should be considered in patients with refractory symptoms (despite GDMT), who have evidence of moderate to severe ischemia and obstructive CAD. In the Trial of Invasive versus Medical Therapy in Elderly Patients (TIME) study, faster symptom relief and improved exercise capacity were achieved by revascularization in comparison to GDMT alone in older adult SIHD patients. Revascularization also reduces the risk of repeat hospitalization and non-fatal MI and improves survival in older adult patients. In the setting of ST-elevation MI, although age is not a contraindication for thrombolytic therapy, its benefit diminishes in older adults, and bleeding risk increases. In the current era, emergent primary percutaneous coronary intervention is preferred over thrombolytic therapy in older adult patients with ST-elevation MI. Over the last decade, the advancement of equipment and technique has made percutaneous coronary intervention safer for even very elderly patients (≥90 years of age), with high success rates and a declining risk of major complications. One study of elective angioplasty showed similar rates of cardiac death or recurrent angina in patients 75 years of age or older compared with those of their younger counterparts (mean age 55 years) when complete revascularization was achieved. Although coronary artery bypass grafting (CABG) offers a greater survival advantage in patients with highly complex CAD (high SYNTAX [Synergy Between Percutaneous Coronary Intervention With Taxus and Cardiac Surgery] score) and diabetes, the operative mortality and risk of complications such as stroke and cognitive impairment in older adults after CABG are substantial. A special consideration for older adult patients undergoing invasive procedures or open heart surgery is the risk of stroke or multiorgan atheroemboli, which are commonly attributed to severe atherosclerosis and calcification of the aortic arch and peripheral vessels. Foreknowledge of the concomitant vascular disease distribution and consequent adaptation of surgical technique may minimize these perioperative complications. Prolonged hospitalization and postsurgery recovery in older adults is also significant. Therefore, revascularization and alternatives should be carefully discussed and planned after considering the whole patient with their family. Shared decision-making is influenced not only by coronary anatomy, technical feasibility, and

risks, but takes into consideration comorbidities and functional reserve, patient values, as well as realistic goals of care and life-expectancy.

Valvular Heart Disease

The most common valvular diseases requiring treatment in older adults are calcific aortic stenosis and mitral regurgitation from myxomatous degeneration or annular dilatation. Aortic stenosis prevalence in adults older than 62 years of age is reported to be approximately 10% for mild stenosis, 6% for moderate stenosis, and 2% for severe stenosis.

Physical examination and screening for significant valvular disease in older adults are less reliable than in younger individuals for several reasons. First, many older adults may be asymptomatic, either because they are sedentary by nature or because they have adapted their lifestyles to the constraints of severe valvular and coronary disease. Second, up to half of older adults have systolic murmurs that are of little clinical consequence. Third, many comorbidities in older adults, including kyphosis, chronic obstructive pulmonary disease, and decreased blood flow velocity across the valves (related to decreased cardiac output), may obscure the classic signs of aortic stenosis or mitral regurgitation. Fourth, peripheral pulsus parvus et tardus (diminished and slow carotid artery pulses, an excellent indicator of aortic stenosis in young individuals) can be confounded by aortic and carotid arterial stiffening, heart failure (HF), or β-blocker use. Therefore, especially for patients who are in declining health, clinicians should have a lower threshold for suspecting reparable valvular disease.

The relief of aortic stenosis is associated with substantial improvements in quality of life even in very old individuals, with long-term survival rates similar to age-matched individuals who do not require treatment. Of the septuagenarians and older patients who had operations for aortic stenosis in three studies, more than two-thirds were in New York Heart Association functional classes III to IV at baseline. Most (80%–90%) improved to functional class I status and independent living after surgery. Although the risk-to-benefit ratio is acceptable for individuals who are otherwise healthy, the surgical mortality rate doubles with age older than 75 years (12.4% for patients older than 75 years of age, compared with 6.6% for younger patients). The mortality risk increases more when concomitant CABG or other procedures are required. Other predictors of complications after aortic valve replacement in older adults are impaired LV function, diabetes mellitus, nonsinus rhythm, urgency of surgery, and severe renal or lung disease. Operative mortality with mitral valve surgery in the older adult population is even higher, mostly because of complex underlying etiologies and the likelihood that LV dysfunction resulting from mitral regurgitation will not improve after surgery. In recent years, percutaneous transcatheter aortic valve replacement has been proven advantageous over surgical valve replacement in high-risk or nonoperable patients, especially older adults, as well as moderate-risk individuals (see details in Chapter 54). Percutaneous mitral valvuloplasty is a proven therapeutic method for mitral stenosis with good long-term results. The favorable long-term outcomes reported for mitral valvuloplasty are based predominantly on young cohorts who had rheumatic mitral stenosis, and this approach has not been extensively studied in older adults with more calcific valvular disease. The procedural complication-free success rate is lower for older cohorts with degenerative and calcific mitral valve disease (see details in Chapter 46).

Heart Failure

Cardiovascular aging predisposes to the development of clinical HF, particularly HF with preserved ejection fraction (HFpEF). HF is relatively uncommon before 45 years of age. Its incidence grows linearly thereafter, and geometrically after 85 years of age, with the mean age of the first episode being at 80 years old. More than 500,000 hospital admissions per year are for HF in patients older than 65 years of age. The diagnosis of HF in older adults can be difficult due to atypical presentations: a higher prevalence of comorbidities such as aortic stenosis, undiagnosed CAD, AF, hypertension, lung or kidney disease, cerebrovascular accident, anemia, and malignancy; a sedentary baseline lifestyle; a high prevalence of HFpEF; and communication barriers. Peripheral edema may result from benign causes such as venous stasis, or it may result from other organ failure (liver or renal). Unfortunately, older adult HF patients are less likely to be referred to specialist care, less likely to receive effective diagnostic procedures, and less likely to adhere to evidence-based medical therapy. Furthermore, clinical trials of HF tend to exclude an older adult population, resulting in unvalidated extrapolations of current guidelines to the care of older adults.

One additional therapeutic issue of particular importance in older adults is polypharmacy. The clinician must be vigilant against agents considered benign by the patient that may actually exacerbate HF, such as nonsteroidal antiinflammatory drugs. The potential for drug interactions (e.g., with warfarin or digitalis) or intolerance from altered renal or hepatic metabolism is magnified, particularly with the standard multidrug therapy for HF.

Finally, it is noteworthy that the prognosis of HF in older adults is worse than the prognosis of most cancers (<20% 5-year survival rate). It may thus be appropriate for physicians to help patients ponder and prepare for "end-of-life" concerns for their own and their families' welfare.

Arrhythmias

Myocardial fibrosis, atrial dilation, valvular heart disease, and degenerative changes of the sinus node and conduction system in the aging heart predispose older adult patients to AF. AF is the most common arrhythmia in older adult patients. In the general population, the prevalence of AF is increasing in parallel to the aging of the population. Of patients with AF, approximately 70% are 65 to 85 years of age. CAD also doubles the risk of AF for men, whereas HF increases the risk of AF by 8-fold in men and by 14-fold in women. The treatment goal for AF in older adults is to prevent thromboembolic episodes and to improve quality of life, by reducing symptoms and hospitalizations related to AF. Both the CHADS2 and CHA2DS2-VASc scores emphasize the significant increase of risk of stroke with age. Although the incidence of stroke is only approximately 6% to 7% in patients with AF in their sixties, stroke afflicts 26% of nonagenarians with AF. Therefore, older adult patients with AF should be treated with anticoagulation, taking into consideration their increased propensity to falls and bleeding.

Both vitamin K antagonists and novel oral anticoagulants are effective in older adults, with the latter showing significant reductions in stroke, intracranial hemorrhage, and mortality with comparable major bleeding events when dosed appropriately and with preserved renal function. A growing number of older adult patients have concomitant AF and CAD that require stent placement, and the duration and type of dual antiplatelet therapy with anticoagulation ("triple therapy") need to be balanced with the increased risk of bleeding.

With regard to rhythm versus rate control for AF in older adults, the general consensus is that rate control should be the firstline therapy, especially for older adults with asymptomatic AF. Beta-blockers are the most effective agents as shown in the substudy of the Atrial Fibrillation Follow-up Investigation of Rhythm Management (AFFIRM) trial. Nondihydropyridine calcium channel blockers (verapamil and diltiazem) are alternatives for patients with preserved ejection function. Rhythm control in older adult symptomatic patients with AF is reasonable. Compared with other antiarrhythmic agents, amiodarone is relatively safe, keeping in mind the considerable extracardiac side effects. The efficacy and safety of catheter ablation of AF in older adults has not been well established. As a last resort, atrioventricular node ablation and permanent pacemaker implantation has been done for highly symptomatic older adult patients with AF.

Cerebrovascular Disease

Age is the most important nonmodifiable risk factor for all strokes and associated outcomes. After the age of 55 years, for each successive decade the stroke rate doubles in both men and women. Seventy-five percent to 89% of strokes occur in individuals aged older than 65 years, and of these, 50% occur in people aged 70 years or older, and approximately 25% occur in individuals aged 85 years or older. Isolated systolic hypertension increases with age, most likely because of increased vascular impedance, with a recalibration in baroreceptor reflex thresholds (Fig. 73.1). Fortunately, the absolute and relative risk reductions in stroke from antihypertensive therapy increase with age as well, with a 50% relative risk reduction in the 5-year stroke rate in those older than 80 years of age, compared with a 30% relative risk reduction with treatment in sexagenarians. AF and HF gain increasing importance as risk factors for stroke with age. The attributable risk of stroke from AF is 1.5% in the fifth decade of life, rising exponentially to 23.5% by the eighth decade of life. For HF, the corresponding attributable risks are 2.3% and 6%.

Aging-related changes in cerebral vessels reduce cerebrovascular reserves and increase the susceptibility of the brain to vascular insufficiency and ischemic injury, thereby increasing the morbidity and mortality rates after an ischemic stroke in older adults. The consequences of stroke are more severe in the very old; for those aged 85 years or older, the in-hospital mortality rate from an acute stroke is >25% compared with 13.5% for those younger than 85 years of age. Among those who survive to be discharged, only one-fifth have minimal or no neurological deficit compared to one-third of a younger cohort. One third of older adult stroke survivors had dementia (based on a Mini-Mental Status Exam score <24), which is a threefold higher prevalence than stroke-free subjects in the same age group. Because dementia is the largest contributor to disability in basic activities of daily living (e.g., dressing, bathing, and transfers), the estimated 18.4% population-attributable risk of dementia from stroke should be recognized as an important target for prevention.

For acute ischemic stroke, the fundamental approaches for treatment are reperfusion and neuroprotection. Thrombolytic therapy for acute ischemic stroke in patients older than 80 years is controversial because these patients have been significantly underrepresented in clinical trials. As with other therapies, the risk of treatment is higher in older adults. Even given the increased risk, therapeutic interventions may reduce mortality and morbidity compared with conservative therapy. For instance, older adults with severe carotid stenosis are at high risk if treated with medications alone, but, when patients are carefully selected, carotid endarterectomy reduces the risk of stroke and stroke-related death (Fig. 73.2).

Peripheral Arterial Occlusive and Aneurysmal Disease

Peripheral arterial occlusive disease can be considered a late-stage manifestation of atherosclerosis. Although the mean age in clinical trials of European patients who require coronary interventions is 55 years of age, the average ages for those with extracoronary occlusive disease who require revascularization are 59, 65, 67, and 72 years, respectively, for those with iliac, renal, carotid, and infrainguinal artery stenoses (Fig. 73.3; see also Chapters 58 to 62). The incidence of abdominal aortic aneurysms increases fourfold in individuals older than 65 years of age compared with those 55 years of age or younger. These data should heighten awareness and diagnosis of peripheral arterial disease.

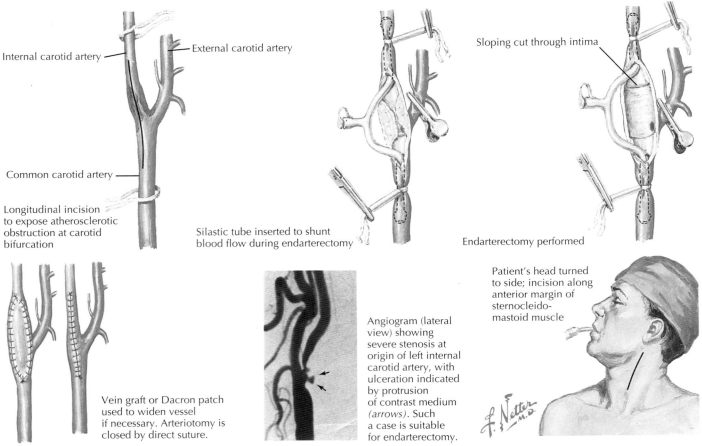

Internal carotid artery

External carotid artery

Common carotid artery

Longitudinal incision to expose atherosclerotic obstruction at carotid bifurcation

Silastic tube inserted to shunt blood flow during endarterectomy

Sloping cut through intima

Endarterectomy performed

Vein graft or Dacron patch used to widen vessel if necessary. Arteriotomy is closed by direct suture.

Angiogram (lateral view) showing severe stenosis at origin of left internal carotid artery, with ulceration indicated by protrusion of contrast medium (arrows). Such a case is suitable for endarterectomy.

Patient's head turned to side; incision along anterior margin of sternocleido-mastoid muscle

FIG 73.2 Endarterectomy for Atherosclerosis of the Extracranial Carotid Artery.

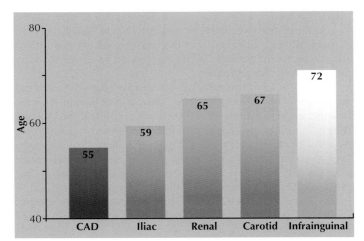

FIG 73.3 Average Age at Which Different Arteries Require Revascularization. *CAD,* Coronary artery disease. With permission from Tan WA, Yadav JS, Wholey MH. Endovascular options for peripheral arterial occlusive and aneurysmal disease. In: Topol EJ, ed. *Textbook of Interventional Cardiology.* 4th ed. Philadelphia: WB Saunders; 2002:481–522.

FUTURE DIRECTIONS

The narrower physiological reserve that accompanies advancing age elevates cardiovascular risk and narrows the therapeutic benefit. However, outcomes have improved markedly with advances in medical and interventional therapies, particularly in more vulnerable populations such as older adult patients. A progressive decrease in 30-day acute MI mortality rate has been documented in octogenarians from 55% in the 1970s to 31% in the 1980s to 22% by 1991. This represents a 72% decrease after statistical adjustment for comorbidities and MI severity. Better and safer monitoring and anesthetic techniques permit necessary surgery even for high-risk patients. Endovascular therapies are less invasive, offering very old patients short- and medium-term outcomes that formerly could be obtained only with major surgery (e.g., transcatheter aortic valve replacement for aortic stenosis and stent grafting for abdominal aortic aneurysms).

The benefits of prevention and therapy should be extended more aggressively to all age groups, with careful consideration of individual risk profiles and preferences. More importantly, simply extending life span no longer suffices. The key challenge for health care in the 21st century is the extension of the "health span" or quality of later life for our older patients.

ADDITIONAL RESOURCES

Dai X, Hummel SL, Salazar JB, Taffet GE, Zieman S, Schwartz JB. Cardiovascular physiology in the older adults. *J Geriatric Cardiology.* 2015;12:196–201.

Contemporary review of the cardiovascular physiology in the older adult population with illustration of their mechanisms and clinical impacts.

National Institutes of Health, National Institute on Aging. The Baltimore Longitudinal Study of Aging (BLAS). Available at: http://www.blsa.nih.gov. Accessed March 14, 2017.

For >5 decades, >1400 men and women have been followed in America's longest-running scientific study of human aging, sponsored by the National Institute on Aging.

Schwartz JB, Zipes DP. Chapter 80 Cardiovascular Disease in the Elderly. In: Bonow RO, Mann DL, Zipes DP, Libby P, eds. *Braunwald's Heart Disease: a Textbook of Cardiovascular Medicine.* 9th ed. Philadelphia, PA: Elsevier Saunders Ltd.; 2012.

Comprehensive overview of cardiovascular physiology, epidemiology, clinical manifestations, and treatment approaches of CVD in the older adult population.

EVIDENCE

de Boer J, Andressoo JO, de Wit J, et al. Premature aging in mice deficient in DNA repair and transcription. *Science.* 2002;296:1276–1279.

The consequence of XPD mutation in this mouse model was increased vulnerability to oxidative DNA damage. The phenotype for humans with the same mutation, however, is not osteoporosis and early graying as observed in mice, but more typically growth retardation, neurological abnormalities, and brittle hair and nails, attributed to the depressed RNA synthesis.

Julien DJ, Elbaz A, Ducimetière P, et al. Slow walking speed and cardiovascular death in well functioning older adults: prospective cohort study. *BMJ.* 2009;339:b4460.

Slow gait speed predicted approximately a threefold increase in cardiovascular deaths but not cancer deaths. This illustrates complex interactions among aging, disease, mind-body interactions, and environment.

Lakatta EG. So! What's aging? Is cardiovascular aging a disease? *J Mol Cell Cardiol.* 2015;83:1–13.

In this special issue on cardiovascular aging, one of the principal investigators for the Baltimore Longitudinal Study of Aging provides a candid and broad perspective of this complicated area.

Mackey RH, Sutton-Tyrrell K, Vaitkevicius PV, et al. Correlates of aortic stiffness in elderly individuals: a subgroup of the Cardiovascular Health Study. *Am J Hypertens.* 2002;15:16–23.

In these 356 subjects aged 70 to 96 years, baseline insulin resistance, increased common carotid intima-media thickness, elevated heart rate, and decreased physical activity correlated with higher aortic pulse wave velocity years later.

Schoenhofen EA, Wyszynski DF, Andersen S, et al. Characteristics of 32 supercentenarians. *J Am Geriatric Soc.* 2006;54:1237–1240.

Fascinating cohort and well-validated database of people who have lived 110 years and beyond.

The TIME Investigators. Trial of Invasive versus Medical therapy in Elderly patients with chronic symptomatic coronary-artery disease (TIME): a randomised trial. *Lancet.* 2001;358:951–957.

Prospective randomized clinical trial to compare medical therapy versus invasive treatment for older adult patients (mean age 80 years; range 75–91 years) with symptomatic SIHD. The TIME trial suggested that invasive treatment provides greater benefit than optimized medical therapy in symptom relief, improvement of quality of life, and early mortality.

Page numbers followed by *f* indicate figures; *t*, tables; *b*, boxes.

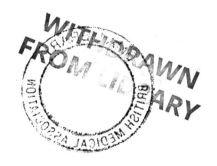

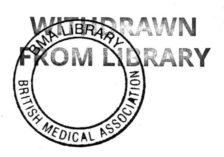